Basic Surgery

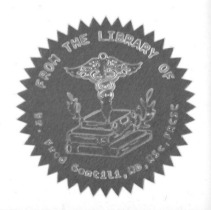

CONTRIBUTORS

Harold W. Bales, M.D.

Arthur E. Baue, M.D.

John R. Border, M.D.

David R. Boyd, M.D., C.M.

Gerard P. Burns, M.Ch.(Belf.), F.R.C.S.(Eng. & Edin.)

Richard G. Caldwell, M.D.

Frederic A. de Peyster, M.D.

Alexander Doolas, M.D.

Alexander S. Geha, M.D.

Gordon D. Glennie, M.B., F.R.C.P.(Can.)

Robert N. Green, M.D., F.R.C.P.(Can.)

Loren J. Humphrey, M.D., Ph.D.

W. Rodger Inch, Ph.D.

William R. Jewell, M.D.

James Kyle, D.Sc., M.Ch., F.R.C.S.(Eng.), F.R.C.S.(Ire.)

Bernard Langer, M.D., F.R.C.S.(Can.), F.A.C.S.

John A. McCredie, M.B., B.Ch., B.A.O., M.Ch.(Belf.),
F.R.C.S.(Eng. & Edin.), F.R.C.S.(Can.), F.A.C.S.

Robert E. Madden, M.D.

Stanley Mercer, F.R.C.S.(Can.)

Eugene R. Mindell, M.D.

John F. Mullan, M.B., F.R.C.S.(Eng.)

G. William Odling-Smee, F.R.C.S.(Eng.)

Donald H. Pearson, M.D.

Fred R. Plecha, M.D.

Walter J. Pories, M.D., F.A.C.S.

George P. Reading, M.D.

David L. Roseman, M.D.

Worthington G. Schenk, Jr., M.D.

John H. Schneewind, M.D.

R. Roderick Shepherd, F.R.C.S.(Can.)

Nicholas R. St. C. Sinclair, B.Sc., M.D., Ph.D.

Robert M. Stone, F.R.C.S.(Can.)

Alvin L. Watne, M.D.

Thomas A. Watson, F.A.C.R., D.M.R.(Eng.), F.R.C.P.(Can.)

Richard B. Welbourn, M.D., F.R.C.S.(Eng.)

Richard W. Williams, M.D.

Basic Surgery

EDITED BY

John A. McCredie
M.B., B.Ch., B.A.O., M.Ch.(Belf.),
F.R.C.S.(Eng. & Edin.), F.R.C.S.(Can.), F.A.C.S.

Associate Professor of Surgery and Therapeutic Radiology,
University of Western Ontario

ILLUSTRATED BY

Carol Donner
B.F.A., A.M.I.

Member, Society of Illustrators

MACMILLAN PUBLISHING CO., INC.
New York

COLLIER MACMILLAN CANADA, LTD.
Toronto

BAILLIÈRE TINDALL
London

MACMILLAN PUBLISHING CO., INC.
866 Third Avenue, New York, New York 10022

COLLIER MACMILLAN CANADA, LTD.
BAILLIÈRE TINDALL · London

Library of Congress Cataloging in Publication Data

Main entry under title:

Basic surgery.

Includes bibliographies and index.
1. Surgery. I. McCredie, John A. II. Donner, Carol.
[DNLM: 1. Surgery. W0100 B311]
RD31.B37   617   76-1929
ISBN 0-02-378740-6

Baillière Tindall SBN 0 7020 0628 9

Printing: 1 2 3 4 5 6 7 8   Year: 7 8 9 0 1 2 3

PREFACE

Basic Surgery has been prepared as a textbook and text supplement for the medical student, intern, and surgical resident. The book should also be of value to the practicing physician and surgeon as well as the surgical nurse—as a guide to understanding pathophysiologic processes and explaining clinical phenomena.

The 35 chapters are grouped into four units. Unit I, "Basic Considerations," stresses the basic medical sciences because of their importance in surgery. Many patients who previously would have died now survive because of the application of scientific principles. For example, an understanding of the regulation of homeostasis is essential in the care of the critically ill, as is knowledge about wound healing and surgical infections. The immune response and the principles of cancer therapy have practical clinical application and, therefore, are included in this unit. Controlled clinical trials, which are discussed in a separate chapter, are often needed to determine the best treatment when several options are available.

Unit II, "Total Care of the Surgical Patient," describes the general principles common to the care of all surgical patients. Emphasis is placed on consideration of all body systems and the psychological approach to surgical patients. Pain is described in detail because of the recent advances in understanding pain mechanisms and the development of new procedures for its relief. Improvements in preoperative and postoperative care, anesthesia, and operating room management, which have resulted in decreased morbidity and mortality, are the subjects of four chapters. Burns are also included in this unit, to stress their widespread effects on all body systems.

In Unit III, "Principles of General Surgery," the important surgical diseases of individual organs are presented. The clinical features are explained in terms of altered pathophysiology. Principles of therapy, rather than details of surgical technique, are emphasized throughout.

The selection of subjects for Unit IV, "Principles of Specialty Surgery," was particularly difficult. Presented therein are the fundamentals of orthopedic surgery and fractures, cardiopulmonary surgery, peripheral vascular surgery, urology, reconstructive and plastic surgery, neurosurgery, and pediatric surgery that are essential for all students and practitioners. Obstetrics and gynecology, ophthalmology, and otolaryngology are not discussed.

Hundreds of illustrations, including a four-color atlas of surgical anatomy, appear throughout the text. They are designed to reinforce the written word, stress important points, and simplify difficult concepts. An effort has been made to make these line drawings and halftones as simple and clear as possible without extraneous detail. The legends (captions) of the illustrations are sufficiently detailed to enable the reader to quickly review the chapter and to stress important points.

Wherever possible, references are cited that constitute a review of a particular subject. The suggested bibliography for additional reading, which appears at the end of most chapters, includes books and articles that describe the subject in greater depth.

A number of people have assisted the editor and illustrator by reviewing manuscripts and preliminary artwork for many of the chapters. We are indebted for comments, criticisms, and suggestions by Drs. E. W. R. Campsall, J. H. Duff, D. P. Girvan, R. L. Holliday, I. Ramzy, and A. C. Webster, of London, Ontario; Dr. G. P. Burns, of Buffalo, New York; Dr. N. Delarue, of Toronto, Ontario; and Dr. W. Cole, of Asheville, North Carolina. In addition, great help was given by two surgical residents, Drs. Marg Paul and Tony Viidik, and a fourth-year medical student, Mr. Paul Walker. We also wish to pay tribute to the cooperation of the 36 contributors to the book, and to Miss Lynda Springer for typing and/or retyping many of the manuscripts. Special thanks are due Miss Joan Carolyn Zulch, medical editor of Macmillan Publishing Co., Inc., for acting as the catalyst for creation and production of this book.

JOHN A. McCREDIE
CAROL DONNER

CONTRIBUTORS

Bales, Harold W., M.D.   Late Associate Professor of Plastic Surgery, University of Rochester School of Medicine and Dentistry; Attending Surgeon, Highland Hospital, Rochester, New York

Baue, Arthur E., M.D.   Professor and Chairman, Department of Surgery, Yale University School of Medicine, New Haven, Connecticut

Border, John R., M.D.   Professor of Surgery, School of Medicine, State University of New York at Buffalo; Director, Trauma Research Center, Buffalo, New York

Boyd, David R., M.D., C.M.   Director, Division of Emergency Medical Services, U.S. Department of Health, Education, and Welfare, Hyattsville, Maryland

Burns, Gerard P., M.Ch.(Belf.), F.R.C.S.(Eng. & Edin.)   Associate Professor of Surgery, School of Medicine, State University of New York at Buffalo; Attending Surgeon, E. J. Meyer Memorial Hospital and V. A. Hospital, Buffalo, New York

Caldwell, Richard G., M.D.   Assistant Professor of Surgery, Rush Medical College; Associate Attending Surgeon, Rush–Presbyterian–St. Luke's Medical Center, Chicago, Illinois, and Lutheran General Hospital, Park Ridge, Illinois

de Peyster, Frederic A., M.D.   Professor of Surgery, Rush Medical College; Attending Surgeon, Rush–Presbyterian–St. Luke's Medical Center and Cook County Hospital, Chicago, Illinois

Doolas, Alexander, M.D.   Associate Professor of Surgery, Rush Medical College; Associate Attending Surgeon, Rush–Presbyterian–St. Luke's Medical Center, Chicago, Illinois

Geha, Alexander S., M.D.   Associate Professor of Surgery, Washington University School of Medicine; Assistant Director of Surgery and Director of Thoracic and Cardiovascular Surgery and Research, Jewish Hospital of St. Louis, St. Louis, Missouri

Glennie, Gordon D., M.B., F.R.C.P.(Can.) Director of Dental Anesthesia, Dental School, University of Western Ontario; Consultant in Anesthesia, St. Joseph's Hospital, London, Ontario, Canada

Green, Robert N., M.D., F.R.C.P.(Can.) Associate Professor and Coordinator, Section of Endocrinology, University of Western Ontario, London, Ontario, Canada

Humphrey, Loren J., M.D., Ph.D.   Professor and Chairman, Department of Surgery, University of Kansas School of Medicine, Kansas City, Kansas

Inch, W. Rodger, Ph.D.   Professor of Therapeutic Radiology, University of Western Ontario; Radiobiologist, Ontario Cancer Treatment and Research Foundation, London, Ontario, Canada

Jewell, William R., M.D.   Associate Professor of Surgery, University of Kansas School of Medicine; Attending Surgeon, V.A. Hospital, Kansas City, Kansas

Kyle, James, D.Sc., M.Ch., F.R.C.S.(Eng.), F.R.C.S.(Ire.)   Senior Clinical Lecturer in Surgery, University of Aberdeen; Consultant Surgeon, Aberdeen Royal Infirmary, Aberdeen, Scotland

Langer, Bernard, M.D., F.R.C.S.(Can.), F.A.C.S.   Associate Professor of Surgery, University of Toronto Faculty of Medicine; Head, Division of General Surgery, Toronto General Hospital, Toronto, Ontario, Canada

McCredie, John A., M.B., B.Ch., B.A.O., M.Ch.(Belf.), F.R.C.S.(Eng. & Edin.), F.R.C.S.(Can.), F.A.C.S.   Associate Professor of Surgery, University of Western Ontario; Member, Surgical Staff, Victoria Hospital, London, Ontario, Canada

Madden, Robert E., M.D.   Professor of Surgery, New York Medical College; Attending Surgeon, Flower and Fifth Avenue Hospitals, New York, New York

Mercer, Stanley, F.R.C.S.(Can.)   Associate Professor of Surgery (Pædiatric), University of Ottawa Faculty of Medicine; Chief of Surgery, Children's Hospital of Eastern Ontario, Ottawa, Ontario, Canada

Mindell, Eugene R., M.D. Professor and Chairman, Department of Orthopedic Surgery, School of Medicine, State University of New York at Buffalo; Chief of Orthopedic Surgery, E. J. Meyer Memorial Hospital, Buffalo, New York

Mullan, John F., M.B., F.R.C.S.(Eng.) Professor and Chairman, Division of Neurosurgery, Pritzker School of Medicine, University of Chicago; Attending Surgeon, University of Chicago Hospitals and Clinics, Chicago, Illinois

Odling-Smee, G. William, F.R.C.S.(Eng.) Senior Lecturer in Surgery, The Queen's University of Belfast; Consultant Surgeon, The Mater Infirmorum and Royal Victoria Hospital, Belfast, Northern Ireland

Pearson, Donald H., M.D. Associate Professor of Neurosurgery, Southern Illinois University School of Medicine, Springfield, Illinois

Plecha, Fred R., M.D. Associate Professor of Surgery, Case Western Reserve University School of Medicine; Associate Surgeon, Cleveland Metropolitan General Hospital, Cleveland, Ohio

Pories, Walter J., M.D., F.A.C.S. Professor and Associate Director, Department of Surgery, Case Western Reserve University School of Medicine; Chief of Surgery, Cleveland Metropolitan General Hospital and Cuyahoga County Hospital, Cleveland, Ohio

Reading, George P., M.D. Associate Professor of Plastic Surgery, University of Rochester School of Medicine and Dentistry; Senior Associate Surgeon, Strong Memorial Hospital, Rochester, New York

Roseman, David L., M.D. Associate Professor of Surgery, Rush Medical College; Assistant Attending Surgeon, Rush–Presbyterian–St. Luke's Medical Center, Chicago, Illinois

Schenk, Worthington G., Jr., M.D. Professor and Chairman, Department of Surgery, School of Medicine, State University of New York at Buffalo; Director of Surgery, E. J. Meyer Memorial Hospital and Director of Surgical Research Laboratories, Buffalo, New York

Schneewind, John H., M.D. Late Associate Professor of Surgery, University of Illinois College of Medicine; Chief of Emergency Services, University of Illinois Research and Educational Hospitals, Chicago, Illinois

Shepherd, R. Roderick, F.R.C.S.(Can.) Instructor in Surgery, University of Western Ontario; Member, Surgical Staff, Victoria, St. Joseph's, and University Hospitals, London, Ontario, Canada

Sinclair, Nicholas R. St. C., B.Sc., M.D., Ph.D. Professor of Bacteriology and Immunology, University of Western Ontario, London, Ontario, Canada

Stone, Robert M., F.R.C.S.(Can.) Assistant Professor of Surgery, University of Toronto Faculty of Medicine; Member, Surgical Staff, Toronto General Hospital, Toronto, Ontario, Canada

Watne, Alvin L., M.D. Professor and Chairman, Department of Surgery, West Virginia University School of Medicine, Morgantown, West Virginia; Consultant, V.A. Hospital, Clarksburg, West Virginia

Watson, Thomas A., F.A.C.R., D.M.R.(Eng.), F.R.C.P.(Can.) Professor and Head, Department of Therapeutic Radiology, University of Western Ontario; Director, Ontario Cancer Foundation, London Clinic, London, Ontario, Canada

Welbourn, Richard B., M.D., F.R.C.S.(Eng.) Professor of Surgery, University of London; Director, Department of Surgery, Royal Postgraduate Medical School and Hammersmith Hospital, London, England

Williams, Richard W., M.D. Assistant Professor of Surgery, School of Medicine, State University of New York at Buffalo; Attending Surgeon, V.A. Hospital, Buffalo, New York

CONTENTS

INTRODUCTION   *John A. McCredie*   1

Unit I
Basic Considerations

1. METABOLIC RESPONSE TO STARVATION, SEPSIS, AND TRAUMA
   John R. Border   7
2. PULMONARY AND CARDIOVASCULAR FAILURE   *John R. Border*   41
3. FLUID, ELECTROLYTE, AND ACID-BASE BALANCE   *John A. McCredie*   92
4. IMMUNE RESPONSE IN TISSUE TRANSPLANTATION AND CANCER
   Nicholas R. St. C. Sinclair and *John A. McCredie*   103
5. TISSUE HEALING   *Walter J. Pories* and *Fred R. Plecha*   117
6. SURGICAL INFECTIONS   *G. William Odling-Smee*   125
7. CANCER: SPREAD AND PRINCIPLES OF TREATMENT
   John A. McCredie and *W. Rodger Inch*   141
8. CONTROLLED TRIALS IN SURGERY   *Richard B. Welbourn*   158

Unit II
Total Care of the Surgical Patient

9. MODERN CONCEPTS IN THE CARE OF THE CRITICALLY INJURED
   David R. Boyd   167
10. MANAGEMENT OF PAIN   *Donald H. Pearson* and *John F. Mullan*   181
11. PREOPERATIVE ASSESSMENT AND CARE   *Robert E. Madden*   199
12. OPERATIVE ANESTHESIA   *Gordon D. Glennie*   222
13. OPERATING ROOM MANAGEMENT   *John A. McCredie* and *Gerard P. Burns*   233
14. POSTOPERATIVE CARE AND COMPLICATIONS
    Arthur E. Baue and *Alexander S. Geha*   241
15. BURNS   *George P. Reading*   261

Surgical Anatomy
(following page 268)

   I.   Skin
  II.   Anterior view of the head and neck showing relation of deep structures to surface anatomy
 III.   Lateral view of the head and neck
 IV.   Contents of the thoracic and abdominal cavities
  V.   Transverse sections of the pleural and peritoneal cavities
 VI.   Stomach, duodenum, pancreas, liver, gallbladder, spleen, and small bowel
VII.   Blood supply of the colon
VIII.   Pelvis, rectum, and anus

Unit III
Principles of General Surgery

16.	HEAD AND NECK	*Harold W. Bales*	273
17.	ESOPHAGUS	*John A. McCredie* and *Gerard P. Burns*	285
18.	STOMACH AND DUODENUM	*John A. McCredie*	296
19.	LIVER AND BILIARY TRACT	*Bernard Langer* and *Robert M. Stone*	314
20.	PANCREAS	*James Kyle*	340
21.	JEJUNUM AND ILEUM	*Alvin L. Watne*	354
22.	COLON, APPENDIX, RECTUM, AND ANUS		
	Alexander Doolas, Richard G. Caldwell, David L. Roseman, and		
		Frederic A. de Peyster	371
23.	INTESTINAL OBSTRUCTION AND HERNIA	*Richard W. Williams*	411
24.	LYMPHORETICULAR SYSTEM	*William R. Jewell* and *Loren J. Humphrey*	425
25.	SKIN AND SOFT TISSUES	*John A. McCredie* and *Thomas A. Watson*	435
26.	BREAST	*John A. McCredie*	445
27.	THYROID, PARATHYROID, AND ADRENAL GLANDS	*Robert N. Green*	474
28.	HAND	*George P. Reading* and *John H. Schneewind*	494

Unit IV
Principles of Specialty Surgery

29.	ORTHOPEDIC SURGERY AND FRACTURES	*Eugene R. Mindell*	507
30.	CARDIOPULMONARY SURGERY	*Robert E. Madden*	526
31.	PERIPHERAL VASCULAR SURGERY	*Worthington G. Schenk, Jr.*	549
32.	UROLOGY	*R. Roderick Shepherd*	563
33.	RECONSTRUCTIVE AND PLASTIC SURGERY	*George P. Reading*	586
34.	NEUROSURGERY	*Donald H. Pearson* and *John F. Mullan*	599
35.	PEDIATRIC SURGERY	*Stanley Mercer*	629
	INDEX		643

INTRODUCTION

John A. McCredie

ROLE OF SURGERY

The place of surgery in society is continually changing. Initially the surgeon drained pus and cared for the injured patient, who always had a deformity or an established disease. The surgeon's scope then extended to prevention. Patients were immunized against infections, and those with hernias were operated on before strangulation. Now the surgeon deals with auto safety, organization of trauma centers, public education for prevention and early detection of cancer, and organization of health care. In the face of this extended scope a number of ethical problems have arisen. For example, it has been necessary to redefine death because of progress in tissue transplantation; the use of special procedures to prolong life has had to be questioned under certain circumstances; and the justification for allowing patients to participate in controlled clinical trials has become increasingly important. Naturally the education of the surgeon has changed over the years. He/she is no longer simply a skilled technician but is concerned equally with preoperative and postoperative care. Indeed the competent surgeon must understand thoroughly the many contributions of the basic sciences to clinical medicine.

Major advances in surgery have tended to occur sporadically and have often been the result of progress in other disciplines. In the second half of the nineteenth century advances in anesthesiology and bacteriology led to the introduction of antiseptic and aseptic techniques and in turn to the present era in the art of surgery. In the mid-nineteenth century it was believed that death would inevitably follow the opening of the peritoneal cavity, and more recently it was thought that it would never be possible to operate on the heart. Quite possibly the 1970s and 1980s will produce great steps forward that will exceed those of the last 100 years.

DEVELOPMENT OF SURGERY

Surgery was initially an art rather than a science. The university-trained philosophic physicians and the drug-dispensing apothecaries were on a level superior to that of the technical mechanics, the barbers and surgeons. The surgeon's knowledge of anatomy and physiology was remarkably poor. In civilian practice his role was to drain abscesses, perform amputations, treat deformities and cut for stone; during war he dressed wounds and amputated limbs. The scientific approach to surgery was not introduced until the latter half of the eighteenth century, chiefly by John Hunter who emphasized human and comparative anatomy, questioned old dogmas, and encouraged careful patient observation and detailed documentation of histories. The amalgamation of the schools of surgery with the universities in the early 1800s broadened the surgeon's education and encouraged a multidisciplinary scientific approach that fostered the great advances of the latter half of the nineteenth century. The science of anesthesia developed from the nitrous oxide–sniffing "frolicks" of the 1820s. It is now difficult to understand the controversy that raged after Simpson gave chloroform to Queen Victoria for the birth of one of her children. The development of antiseptic and then aseptic surgery was interdisciplinary. The obstetrician Semmelweiss observed that puerperal sepsis was the result of infection carried from patient to patient on the hands of doctors and that infections were less frequent when women were delivered at home than in the hospital. The chemist Pasteur recognized that certain diseases were caused by bacteria. Lister applied this knowledge to surgery. He recommended the use of phenol to kill microorganisms in the air, on the surgeon's hands, on instruments, and on the patient's skin, and later he introduced aseptic technique. The surgeon's hands were cleaned by scrubbing, the skin was sterilized with an antiseptic, and instruments were sterilized by boiling.

It is not surprising that major advances in surgery have frequently resulted from wartime experience. During World War I immunization against tetanus, delayed closure of wounds, and blood transfusion were introduced. The clinical use of a sulfonamide in 1935 and penicillin in 1941 marked the beginning of drugs that effectively combated the important staphylococcal and streptococcal infections. The improved organization of surgical services during World War II decreased morbidity and mortality. Patients were rapidly evacuated to efficient surgical units and emphasis was placed on their rehabilitation. Knowledge gained from the Korean and Vietnam wars resulted in emphasis on rapid resuscitation and on a multidisciplinary approach to care of the critically injured patient. Intravenous fluid replacement was often commenced within minutes of injury and continued during rapid transit by helicoptor to a well-equipped and well-staffed surgical unit.

During the last 50 years growth in knowledge has been so great that specialization has become necessary. The surgeon in the nineteenth century looked after all surgical diseases. The obstetricians and gynecologists were the first to establish their own independent discipline and were soon followed by the otolaryngologists. Only during the present century have the surgical specialties —urology, orthopedics, pediatric surgery, neurosurgery, cardiovascular surgery, and plastic and reconstructive surgery—become established. The surgeon must now work as a member of a team and must frequently consult with an anesthesiologist, an internist, a radiologist, a bacteriologist, and a clinical chemist. The development of closely integrated multidisciplinary groups, such as nephrourology, neurologic science, and gastroenterology, has resulted in improved patient care and better timing of surgical treatment. More recently cooperation with a number of nonmedical people, such as the electronic engineer, computer scientist, and physicist, has led to the development of new techniques.

The establishment of the principles of tissue transplantation dates mainly from the work of Medawar in the 1940s. Understanding the cell-mediated immune response against foreign tissues led to attempts to inhibit allograft rejection. Total-body or local radiotherapy, prednisone, azathioprine, then antilymphocytic serum and globulin were used to suppress the immune response. The histocompatibility genes have been partially mapped out in humans, as was done in detail more than 20 years earlier in the mouse. This has resulted in better matching of the donor and recipient and generally a weaker attempt at rejection by the host.

The increase in trauma cases has shifted emphasis in the care of surgical patients. The most common cause of death in people below

40 years is trauma, and about one third of the active treatment beds in North America are now occupied by injured patients. The immensity of the problem has prompted efforts to reduce death and morbidity. These have included analyzing the nature of injuries at home and on the road and suggesting safety measures. Improved safety belts, better roads, and safer cars have resulted. Intensive-care units and trauma centers have upgraded care and lessened mortality and morbidity. Emphasis is now on rapid transport to adequately staffed and equipped hospitals where the critically injured patient receives immediate care of his airway, control of bleeding, and rapid fluid replacement.

Manual dexterity in the operating room has not changed significantly since the end of the nineteenth century. The present-day surgeon, however, can proceed more slowly because of improvements in anesthesia and better treatment of fluid loss and can perform major operations with a lower morbidity and mortality. Surgical instruments also have not been altered to any important extent. Automatic suturing devices have increased slowly in popularity but not with the enthusiasm that might have been anticipated. The surgeon and the engineer have worked together, mainly in Russia, to improve automatic instrumentation. Microsurgery has produced great advances in eye and ear surgery, but its application to suture of small blood vessels has been slow.

The role of plastic surgery was initially confined to the correction of deformities and defects. Recently it has been used increasingly to correct cosmetic defects such as wrinkles, minor nasal deformities, and racial characteristics, to enlarge or decrease the size of breasts, and to remove fat pads.

SURGERY TODAY

At present there is considerable interest in the surgeon's role in the education of doctors and in total health care. The position of surgery as a major subject in the undergraduate medical curriculum has been challenged. It has been suggested that the management of patients with surgical diseases be taught by physicians and that the only contact the student have with a surgeon occur when he/she is taking a surgical elective. Certainly this would be a backward step. The surgeon's knowledge of the pathophysiology of surgical diseases is greater than that of any other specialist in medicine. It is therefore essential that the surgeon continue to play the major role in teaching surgical diseases. In recent years the surgeon's role has been broadened to include organization of trauma centers, advice on rapid transport of the injured patient, prophylaxis of industrial, road, and domestic accidents, and prevention and early diagnosis of cancer. The growth in knowledge and the change in importance of major surgical diseases have necessitated modifications in the surgical curriculum. Since most medical students do not intend to pursue a surgical career, an effort has been made to present the principles of surgery that all students should understand. Emphasis now rests on integrating the basic sciences with clinical surgery, on understanding principles, and on evaluating the total care of the surgical patient.

The surgeon must also consider new ethical problems. The increasing incidence of tissue transplantation has made it necessary to define death with greater precision. Discussions about euthanasia and special measures to prolong life have become frequent. The growth in knowledge has made it essential for consideration of relicensing surgeons, possibly every five years. The ethics of performing clinical trials is under strict scrutiny; therefore it has been necessary to establish committees to examine carefully every controlled clinical trial.

FUTURE OF SURGERY

It is difficult to predict the future of a particular branch of medicine. For example, the dermatologist played a dominant role a century ago, but the chest physician, who looked after patients with tuberculosis, and the fever doctor have virtually disappeared. The decrease in the number of patients with serious infections and the increase in those suffering from the effects of trauma have changed the pattern of surgery. Growth in specialization and development of rapid transport systems may markedly decrease the number of "general surgeons." There will almost certainly be a further increase in transplantation of tissues, development of artificial organs, and traumatic and cosmetic surgery. Changes in surgery for cancer and atherosclerosis will depend upon advances in the basic sciences.

The surgeon's role will undoubtedly increase outside the hospital. He/she will lead in developing statewide trauma services and in training paramedical personnel to help staff health centers. The surgeon will be called on more frequently to participate in public education, especially in preventive medicine, and will become increasingly involved in the politics of health-care administration.

In addition he may be called upon to use different tools. A number of pilot studies have focused on the use of computers in hospitals, in statistical surveys, and in the diagnosis and treatment of patients, and they will almost certainly come to play a major role in surgery.

UNIT I
BASIC CONSIDERATIONS

Chapter 1

METABOLIC RESPONSE TO STARVATION, SEPSIS, AND TRAUMA

John R. Border

CHAPTER OUTLINE

Normal Hepatic Functions
Interrelations of Hepatic and Systemic Body
    Functions
Neuroendocrine Regulation
Normal State
Starvation
Hypercatabolic State
    Modifications of the Basal Hypercatabolic
        Response
    Shock
    Muscle Mass
    Gastrointestinal Tract
    Circulation
    Stress Catabolic State

Insulin Resistance
Metabolic Rate, Temperature, and the
    Stress Catabolic State
The Depleted Patient
    Acute Depletion
    Chronic Depletion
    Summary
Alterations in the Basic Response
    Hepatic
    The Systemic Body—Reflections of Hepatic
        Dysfunction
        Summary of Systemic Body Responses
Manipulation of the Metabolic Response
Summary

The acute survival of the patient with severe sepsis or trauma largely depends on managing his circulatory and pulmonary failure and preventing renal failure that follows this management. The long-term survival is related principally to prevention of sepsis and metabolic management. Successful metabolic management is aimed at preserving or restoring function to the liver and skeletal muscle, with the management of the other organ failures largely flowing from this. Organ function is related chiefly to protein content in the long-term situation. Patients with severe sepsis or trauma clearly have a total body protein catabolic state of considerable magnitude relative to that associated with starvation. This is characterized by increased urea in the urine with urea excretion at the peak on the fifth to seventh day commonly reaching four to five times the amount encountered for starvation.[15,27,64,70] Ureagenesis occurs only in the liver. Protein catabolism, because of hydration, generally produces about one calorie per gram of weight loss; therefore large weight losses are associated with these protein catabolic states. It is clear that the larger and more acute the weight loss is in the septic or traumatized patient, the more likely the patient is to die. Weight losses are very difficult to measure in these patients because of their rapidly changing water balance. However, protein loss and weight losses of 30 to 40 percent or more clearly enhance the possibility of death.[60,62] Weight losses of 10 to 20 percent are common in the severely ill patient who survives.

The weight loss indicates largely total body protein loss. It is, however, clear that protein loss confined largely to the muscles of ambulation in a bed-resting man is a very different problem acutely from an equal protein loss from the liver, heart, kidneys, or muscles of respiration. It is this interorgan distribution of protein loss and its controls that is of the utmost importance in successful management of the critically ill patient. Thus it is probably true that the route and nature of the nutritional support may alter the interorgan distribution of total body protein loss in a deleterious or beneficial way in a sick man and thus affect the outcome.

The acute response to life-threatening trauma and sepsis shows an elevation in the plasma growth hormone, aldosterone, antidiuretic hormone, adrenocorticotropic hormone, glucocorticoids, epinephrine, glucagon, and a diminished insulin.[15] There are in addition many observations that suggest generally enhanced sympathetic nervous system activity and diminished parasympathetic nervous system activity. These changes are associated with hyperglycemia together with a relatively increased plasma fatty acid for the plasma glucose and, if no mechanisms of circulatory failure are active, an increased cardiac output together with an increased temperature, leukocytosis, increased sedimentation rate, decreased clotting time, and sodium and water retention. The net result of these changes is an increased concentration of energetic substrate (glucose and fatty acids) plus the circulation required for delivery at a time when teleologically the body cells would need these changes for survival. Work in small animals shows that along with these changes there is gross loss of skeletal muscle protein with enhanced synthesis of all visceral protein, especially hepatic.[15]

Investigation of the components of the acute response to severe stress has a long history. The stress has varied from that of accidental trauma, deliberate trauma, surgical trauma, cold exposure, heat exposure, and severe exercise to pain and anxiety. Bernard spoke of the milieu interior and its control.[12] Cannon investigated the role of the sympathetic nervous system in the response to stress.[21] Moore,[71] Cuthbertson,[27] Johnston,[58] and many others looked into the total body protein catabolic state that results from trauma. Fleck,[42] Levenson,[63] and others investigated the relationships between organ protein synthesis and organ protein loss in response to sepsis or burns.

Kinney has explored the total body metabolic rate changes that occur with various kinds of trauma and sepsis.[61] Howard and others have studied glucose tolerance and insulin resistance following trauma.[55] Goodall[46] and Harrison[52] probed the relationship of the plasma fatty acids to urinary catecholamine end product excretion in burns. Wilmore has investigated the plasma glucose, fatty acid, glucagon, and insulin relationships to urinary catecholamine end product excretion.[101] Caldwell,[20] Cuthbertson and Tilstone,[38] and Wilmore[100] have studied the relationship of altered environmental temperature to the protein catabolic state and metabolic rate in the burn patient and animal and the multiple fracture patient. Allison and others have investigated the response of glucose and insulin to a glucose tolerance test following burns, surgery, and myocardial infarction.[3] Allison has explored the effect of glucose,

potassium, and insulin on the protein catabolic state secondary to burns.[4] Blackburn has investigated the effect of amino acids without glucose on the protein catabolic state following surgical trauma.[40] Dudrick has investigated the uses of intravenous hyperalimentation in similar patients.[34] Hartroft has studied the role of the calorie-nitrogen ratio in hepatic fat accumulation with per os feeding,[53] while Frederickson and Levy have described the normal physiology of hepatic lipoprotein synthesis as a transport form for hepatic lipids.[43] Cahill and various associates have described the biochemical-endocrine adaptation to starvation.[19] Unger and associates have investigated the role of glucagon in response to a variety of states.[95] Exton and Park and various associates have investigated the role of the glucagon and insulin on control of hepatic metabolism in the perfused liver.[34] Elwyn has explored the role of the liver in vivo in response to a meat meal in the dog.[33] Gump has investigated hepatic glucose output and blood flow in severely stressed man,[31] while Long investigated via radioisotopic tracers glucose turnover and oxidation.[65] In addition, Ban,[9] Frohman,[44] Bernardis,[44] Hume and Egdahl,[56] and many others have addressed the role of the central nervous system and especially the hypothalamus in neuroendocrine metabolic control.

Typically all of these investigations over many years have been presented in a textbook of surgery basically as parallel threads of a very complicated story with the admonition that too much nitrogen loss was associated with death. It has now become apparent that all of the responses described are parts of an integrated controlled system that has a major effect upon survival. The integration for this system occurs in the hypothalamus, liver, pancreas, and in the periphery. The result is controlled mobilization of energetic and synthetic substrate from the liver to the periphery in the anabolic state and from the periphery to the liver in the catabolic state. The central organ in either state is the liver. Intelligent therapeutic manipulation of the metabolic response to sepsis and trauma must begin with a detailed knowledge of hepatic function and its control.

NORMAL HEPATIC FUNCTIONS

The normal functions of the liver are:

1. Modulation of plasma amino acids except leucine, isoleucine, and valine which are controlled principally by skeletal muscle.

2. Modulation of plasma proteins.

3. Control of the rate of glucose entry into the systemic body.

4. Control of plasma alanine and ammonia via ureagenesis.

5. Modulation of the plasma pyruvate-lactate ratio and therefore the redox potential of the blood.

6. Clearance of gut bacterial toxins.

7. Clearance of amino acids in excess of a complete mixture except for leucine, isoleucine, and valine so that amino acid imbalances are corrected for the systemic body.

8. Temporary storage as glycogen, triglycerides, and proteins of nutrients ingested in excess of immediate needs with release between meals under neuroendocrine control to the systemic body.

9. Interconversion of excess nutrients ingested so that a balanced nutrient mixture is presented to the liver and the systemic body. Excess glucose, whether ingested per se or synthesized from glucose precursors such as amino acids, is converted to fat.

10. Modulation of portal venous pressure. Portal venous blood flow is primarily controlled by the regulation of intestinal blood flow.

11. Transport of the essential fat-soluble vitamins via synthesis of transport proteins such as retenone-binding protein which transports vitamin A from storage in the liver to the body, particularly the gastrointestinal mucosa and skin.

12. Modulation of the systemic blood levels of glucagon, insulin, serotonin, and other hormones generated in the portal venous bed.

13. Catabolism of several hormones not generated in the portal venous bed such as glucocorticoids, catecholamines, estrogens, androgens, thyroid hormone, and aldosterone.

14. Synthesis of somatomedin from growth hormone, probably the active principle.

15. Clearance of bacteria and particulate matter via the reticuloendothelial system.

16. Synthesis of acute phase glycoproteins whose metabolism is largely unknown. One alpha-2HS-glycoprotein is important in opsonizing bacteria for leukocyte phagocytosis.

17. Ketogenesis, a water-soluble fat product for systemic oxidation where long-chain fatty acids cannot be oxidized. Hepatic ketogenesis indicates hepatic fat oxidation.

18. Synthesis of carnitine, a water-soluble quaternary ammonium compound, required for long-chain fatty acid oxidation by most organ mitochondria.

19. Synthesis of plasma lipoproteins for transport of excess hepatic triglycerides from the liver to the body.

20. Clearance of many body-generated or infused materials such as bilirubin, Cardio-Green, drugs, amino acids, fatty acids, glucose, glycerol, lactate, and many others.

INTERRELATIONS OF HEPATIC AND SYSTEMIC BODY FUNCTIONS

The liver functions primarily in relationship to the other organs of the body whether as an organ of temporary storage and interconversion, as occurs with food ingestion, or as the organ that receives materials released by the systemic body and interconverts them to the desired materials, as occurs with the lack of oral intake.[92] In the first case the liver is passively presented with widely varying nutrients in nature and quantity depending upon the vagaries of intake, and in the second neuroendocrine controls of the peripheral organs determine what materials the liver is to receive.

The liver at all times clears plasma amino acids and releases plasma proteins.[30] It appears probable that plasma proteins are a transport form for amino acids from the liver to the periphery and that albumin is the specifically controlled form. Thus the normally carefully controlled plasma albumin level not only strongly modulates blood volume but simultaneously provides a constant supply of amino acids to the periphery.

Hepatic glucose output is carefully controlled via the neuroendocrine system.[44] The neuroendocrine system is controlled by glucose sensors in the ventromedial nucleus of the hypothalamus and in the pancreatic islets (Figure 1–1). These sensors control via the autonomic nervous system and the release of glucagon and/or insulin into the portal venous system the rate of hepatic gluconeogenesis, glycogen synthesis or breakdown, and hepatic glucose output. Simultaneously the sympathetic nervous system and the pancreas-hepatic-controlled systemic plasma insulin modulate adipose tissue fat mobilization or deposition and peripheral protein synthesis.[76] Fat is the preferred fuel of all organs except the brain and those areas that derive energy from the glycolytic cycle.[94] Glucose is largely burned in the absence of fat.[75] The result is that the rate of fat oxidation is directly related to the plasma fatty acid and that, as this rises, less and less glucose is oxidized except for the brain. The plasma glucose and fatty acids normally bear within certain limits a reciprocal relationship that results in a constant blood-borne fuel supply to the body but allows progressive diversion of glucose to the brain from the systemic body as hypoglycemia occurs and progressive utilization of glucose by the systemic body as

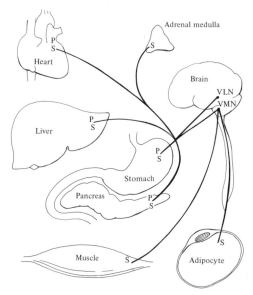

Figure 1–1. Neural organ modulation. Essentially, all organs have their functions modulated through neural connections by changes produced in their blood flow, or by direct cellular innervation. The most widespread control is by the sympathetic nervous system (*s*) that supplies most organs and, in general, modulates blood flow and cellular metabolism. Function of the sympathetic nervous system is under the control of the ventromedial nucleus of the hypothalamus which, in turn, is modulated by other hypothalamic nuclei and tracts which pass through the hypothalamus to other regions in the brain. Thus the central nervous system can respond through the ventromedial nucleus to essentially any stressful stimulus, either physiologic or psychologic. The ventromedial nucleus is also a glucose sensor and, through the sympathetic nervous system, modulates the plasma glucose by increasing glucose production and by mobilizing fatty acids so that less glucose is consumed. The sympathetic nervous system, in addition to its effects on cardiac output and blood flow, mobilizes energetic substrate from the body, directly and through its effect on the secretion of other hormones.

The parasympathetic nervous system (*p*) has a more restricted distribution to the heart, liver, gut, and pancreas and, in general, operates in opposition to the sympathetic nervous system to enhance energy intake by the gut and energy storage in the liver, both directly and through its effect on hormone secretion and energy storage. Stimulation of the parasympathetic innervation of the liver reduces glucose output and stimulates glycogen synthesis, while sympathetic stimulation increases breakdown of glycogen and output of glucose.

The parasympathetic and sympathetic nervous systems interact in the control of the pancreatic islets. In normal man the predominant control is the level of plasma glucose and cer-

hyperglycemia occurs.[76] The result is that glucose concentration is maintained relatively constant for the brain and has very little relationship to the rate of hepatic glucose output but that the plasma fatty acid concentration has a very good relationship to its rate of release from adipose tissue and its oxidation.

The neuroendocrine regulation of the plasma concentrations of glucose and fatty acids is superimposed on intracellular enzyme adaptations. Thus a state of fat oxidation by virtue of intracellular enzyme adaptations not only shuts off glucose oxidation but also most intracellular synthetic uses of glucose, such as glucose liponeogenesis.[75,94] In contrast, a state of glucose oxidation is also associated with increased cellular utilization of glucose for all synthetic processes including protein synthesis, reesterification of fatty acids, glycogen synthesis, and liponeogenesis. Thus a state of glucose oxidation stimulates many different uses of glucose and inhibits fat mobilization via intracelluar enzyme adaptations. The state of glucose oxidation actually involves increased intracellular consumption of pyruvate derived from glucose. Intracellular pyruvate may also come from plasma pyruvate or alanine. The plasma glucose, pyruvate, and alanine are in equilibrium so that they rise and fall together. Thus, in general, states of glucose oxidation are also states of enhanced plasma pyruvate and alanine direct oxidation and enhanced synthetic utilization.[96]

The plasma glucose, probably because of its relationship to cerebral function, is very carefully controlled, particularly in terms of preventing hypoglycemia. This control is exercised by control of the rate of glucose input to the body and the rate of fat mobilization.[8,44,76] Under normal conditions this may be translated as control of hepatic glucose output[44] and under conditions of prolonged fasting both hepatic and renal glucose output.[19,76] The liver is an organ not only of interconversion but also of temporary storage. Therefore glucose input to the liver must be under different controls from hepatic glucose output. Glucose input to the liver via oral ingestion is controlled by the vagaries of oral intake. Under conditions of more than enough oral glucose intake relative to protein, essentially all amino acids are

---

tain amino acids. In sick man, the sympathetic nervous system has dominant control by increasing the output of glucagon. The parasympathetic and sympathetic nervous systems interact in control of pancreatic exocrine secretion, motility of the stomach and colon, and to a lesser extent the small intestine.

utilized for protein synthesis except those present in imbalance. In inadequate glucose intake relative to protein, increasing amounts of amino acids are diverted to glucose so that the proper ratio of glucose to amino acids exists for the liver. The changes from the first condition to the second depend upon the hepatic pass-through of glucose and the amino acids, leucine, isoleucine, and valine and their effect upon the systemic blood and therefore the pancreatic islets. Thus intake of a mixed meal with excess glucose stimulates insulin release and impedes glucagon release, while intake of a meal rich in protein relative to glucose stimulates both insulin and glucagon release. In the first case insulin stimulates both glycogen and protein synthesis, but in the second case the effect of insulin coexists with the effect of glucagon.[95] The result is stimulation of glycogen and protein synthesis plus hepatic amino acid gluconeogenesis so that the desired glucose to protein ratio is achieved for the liver.

Glucose input to the liver under conditions of no oral intake is largely regulated by the neuroendocrine controls of release of gluconeogenic substrate from the periphery.[19,76] Thus the control of lipolysis also controls the release of glycerol, which is converted by the liver to glucose. The controls of glycolytic metabolism control release of the gluconeogenic substrate lactate. Finally the controls of skeletal muscle metabolism control the release of the gluconeogenic substrates alanine and glutamine.[17] Glutamine is utilized for renal ammoniagenesis with secondary renal gluconeogenesis.[47] The result of this arrangement is that the bulk of gluconeogenesis is controlled by processes not directly related to the plasma glucose, and only one small portion of the gluconeogenic substrate, alanine, appears to be directly controlled by the need for glucose.[36] This appears to be a common biologic control mechanism: bulk delivery not directly controlled with a finely tuned control mechanism superimposed on the bulk process.

The balance between glucose input and output occurs by virtue of glycogen storage and glucose liponeogenesis. In fact, hepatic glucose output appears to be most directly and immediately modulated by the autonomic nervous system control of the rate of glycogen synthesis or breakdown.[22,44] Thus stimulation of the sympathetic innervation of the liver activates the enzymes of glycogen breakdown, while stimulation of the parasympathetic innervation activates the enzymes of glycogen synthesis.[44] Stimulation of the ventromedial nucleus of the hypothalamus, which directly modulates the sympathetic nervous system, also enhances hepatic glucose output, while stimulation of the ventrolateral nucleus, which modulates the parasympathetic nervous system, reduces hepatic glucose output.[8,9,44]

Thus the acute minute-to-minute modulation of hepatic glucose output appears to be a function of the ventromedial nucleus of the hypothalamus which is exercised via direct autonomic innervation of the liver. Longer term modulation is achieved by the humoral controls related to glucagon and insulin[44] (Figure 1–2). These humoral hormones are present in locally high concentrations in portal venous blood. Their clearance by the liver and the dilution of hepatic venous blood flow into cardiac output before formation of systemic blood ensures that their portal venous concentration will always be higher than their systemic concentration. Insulin has been best studied and is cleared by the liver to the extent of 40 to 90 percent of the rate of presentation in portal venous blood.[37] The hepatic clearance of glucagon and insulin is probably very carefully modulated. Almost nothing is known of this element of metabolic control. A general property of the liver revealed in perfusion studies where neuroendocrine control is not active is that of increased clearance rate with increased concentrations in the portal venous blood. This appears to be true of glucose, fatty acids, and triglycerides (lipoproteins) and is also true of insulin in vivo. The result is that all factors that enhance portal venous concentrations stimulate hepatic clearance and therefore storage via synthetic process.[92] Consequently the concentrations of substrate in hepatic venous blood are normalized. This basic biochemical characteristic is further modulated by the humoral hormones. Thus, in general, insulin stimulates all hepatic anabolic synthetic processes, while glucagon stimulates all hepatic catabolic breakdown energy mobilization processes and particularly gluconeogenesis, glycogenolysis, protein breakdown, ureagenesis, and ketogenesis.[34]

Another basic biochemical characteristic of the liver appears to be that glucose in excess of storage capacity and hepatic glucose output is converted to fat.[53] This occurs whether the glucose is presented per se or in the form of gluconeogenic substrate such as amino acids. The amino acids utilized for gluconeogenesis are those presented in excess of hepatic protein synthetic capacity.[33] These may be in excess because of a delivery rate of a complete mixture of amino acids exceeding the rate at which they are consumed by protein synthesis.[33,45] or because of amino acid imbalances in which the amino acids in isolated excess are consumed for

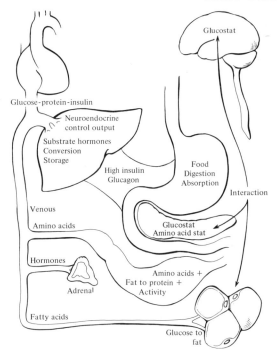

gluconeogenesis and ureagenesis.[45,103] Amino acid imbalances induce synthesis of destructive enzymes for the amino acids in excess.[103] The possible rate of hepatic ureagenesis as judged by infusion of single amino acids and therefore a state of amino acid imbalance always grossly exceeds that utilized physiologically. It therefore appears probable that the rate of ureagenesis is normally controlled by the balance between the rate of amino acid presentation in the portal vein and consumption by hepatic protein synthesis.[33] The rate of presentation of portal vein amino acids in vivo is normally delayed by their digestion in the gut, mucosal transport, and temporary utilization for protein synthesis in the gastrointestinal mucosa. This delay factor allows more efficient hepatic utilization of the amino acids ingested with lower ureagenesis as well as quick presentation to the liver of those amino acids exceeding the requirements for synthesis.[74]

The result of this system in terms of hepatic venous blood amino acids is that their concentrations are largely controlled by hepatic protein synthesis and not by portal venous concentration.[33] There are three exceptions to this. Leucine, isoleucine, and valine may be utilized by the liver for protein synthesis or produced by proteolysis but are not catabolized by the liver. These amino acids, when in excess, must pass through the systemic circulation to skeletal muscle for catabolism and disposal. The nitrogen balance of the liver is therefore that of the plasma amino acids arriving, variations in hepatic protein content, and of ureagenesis, plasma proteins leaving the liver; and a constant level of plasma amino acids leaving the liver.[33] The plasma amino acids have a daily fluctuation in concentration called a circadian

Figure 1–2. Humoral organ modulation. Blood flow and metabolism of organs are modulated by the autonomic nervous system and hormones. Anatomic relations are important. Thus the release of insulin and glucagon into the portal system presents the liver with locally high concentrations. Their removal by the liver insures a low concentration in the systemic circulation. The local interaction of hormones within their organ of origin is important. Glucagon and insulin influence each other's secretion in the pancreatic islets, and glucocorticoids within the adrenal cortex influence the metabolism and release of epinephrine within the adrenal medulla.

The anatomic relation with the liver is also important with gastrin and other gastrointestinal hormones. Most hormones, such as aldosterone, glucocorticoid, antidiuretic hormone, the catecholamines, estrogen, growth hormone, and many others, are presented to the liver in the same concentrations as in the systemic body circulation.

The lung also has a role in limiting the distribution of hormonal effects. Thus the lung clears prostaglandins E and F, serotonin, bradykinin, and epinephrine. Therefore, in general, the levels of hormones in arterial blood are different from those in mixed venous blood.

The systemic plasma hormones also interact upon given organs. Fat mobilization is stimulated by low insulin, high glucocorticoids, epinephrine, glucagon, and growth hormone. Muscle release of amino acids is stimulated by high glucocorticoids and low insulin. Epinephrine impedes insulin release and probably stimulates glucagon release so that the adrenal

medulla interacts not only with adrenal cortex but also with the pancreatic islets. In addition, there is further interaction with the hypothalamus. Thus electrical stimulation of the ventromedial nucleus of the hypothalamus stimulates not only the sympathetic nervous system with its humoral ramifications but also the release of ACTH, growth hormone, prolactin, and antidiuretic hormone. The hypothalamus has no blood-brain barrier so that all hormones and substrates have the potential to interact with the hypothalamus. In addition, the blood flow to the hypothalamus, unlike the rest of the brain, is modulated by the sympathetic nervous system. Central nervous system function is also linked to systemic body function through the competitive transport of the six neutral amino acids across the blood brain barrier. The amino acids are leucine, isoleucine, valine, tryptophan, phenylalanine, and tyrosine.

rhythm. This rhythm must be taken into account when defining constant.

Hepatic protein synthesis appears to be generally stimulated by increased amino acid supply plus caloric substrate and insulin.[73,74] Glucose is probably a better caloric substrate than fat both because of the enhanced insulin release it induces to the liver and because of the intracellular enzyme adaptations that occur.[74] The hepatic sinusoidal endothelium has large fenestrations, no basement membrane, and is a single cell thick.[66] This endothelial characteristic probably allows direct access of the plasma proteins to the hepatocyte and of hepatocyte-synthesized proteins to the plasma via the space of Disse and hepatocyte cilia. This local endothelial characteristic grossly reduces the sinusoidal colloid osmotic pressure and allows a very special hepatocyte microenvironment that is much closer to plasma than the interstitial fluid in other organs. As a result plasma proteins and the materials bound to them are able to directly influence hepatocyte metabolism. Thus plasma colloid osmotic pressure as evaluated against an impermeable membrane modulates hepatocyte albumin synthesis and secretion,[87] and protein-bound substrate, such as fat-soluble vitamins, fatty acids, tryptophan, bilirubin, and venous drugs and dyes, also modulates hepatocyte metabolism.

Hepatocyte protein metabolism is thus modulated by a number of factors that affect hepatic synthesis and storage and a number of factors that modulate protein release into the plasma. Under normal conditions the factors modulating protein synthesis appear to affect synthesis of all proteins. However, there appears to be a hierarchy in this. Structural protein probably has first priority, clotting protein second, and the other plasma proteins third priority. Transferrin, cerulloplasmin, albumin, vitamin A transport protein, and lipoproteins all appear to be in the third priority group. This has some advantages in that the plasma concentrations of these substances may be used within certain limits as an index of hepatic protein synthesis. The limitations relate to alterations in the sinusoidal endothelium and alterations in peripheral consumption. Thus cirrhosis commonly is associated with the conversion of the fenestrated, single cell, no basement membrane endothelium to a multicellular layer without fenestration, and with a basement membrane. This has been called capillarization,[88] and it must necessarily limit free access of proteins from hepatocyte to plasma and its reverse and thus alter the microenvironment of the hepatocyte. Under this condition access of hepatocyte-synthesized proteins to the general circulation can only be via the space of Disse to the lymphatic to the thoracic duct and then into venous blood. This appears to be one of the mechanisms of the increased thoracic duct flow and pressure in cirrhosis.[102] Capillarization has the distinct disadvantage of altering hepatocyte protein microenvironment but does increase sinusoidal colloid osmotic pressure and therefore reduces hepatic edema and hypoxia-limited metabolism.

The liver lobule extends from the portal vein to the central vein. Oxygen is consumed in this transit. The central venous end of the liver lobule appears normally to have hypoxia-limited metabolism. The portal venous end of the liver lobule appears to be the major site of cellular regeneration and probably protein synthesis. The enzyme patterns revealed on histochemistry also vary from aerobic patterns at the portal venous end to much more anaerobic patterns at the central venous end. The number of mitochondria per cell similarly vary. The essential effect is a large alteration in cell functions with anatomic distance from portal vein to central vein and abnormal sensitivity of hepatic function to hypoxia whether generated by arterial hypoxia, reduced hepatic blood flow, or increased central venous pressure hepatic edema.[84]

Evaluation of hepatic protein synthesis and release by plasma protein concentration is made hazardous by virtue of altered rates of peripheral consumption. Thus hypoalbuminemia in the severe stress states occurs probably both on the basis of reduced hepatic albumin output and increased peripheral consumption.[31,57] Certainly it is possible in severely stressed man to give far more albumin than the liver normally puts out per day under conditions where third-space sequestration simply cannot be active and still not be able to return the plasma albumin to normal. It is therefore probably better to use transferrin or vitamin A-binding prealbumin as plasma indexes of hepatic protein synthesis than albumin.

Fat enters the hepatocyte from plasma fatty acids, plasma triglycerides, and glucose lipogenesis. Fat leaves the hepatocyte via partial oxidation with ketogenesis and via lipoproteins (triglycerides, cholesterol, and phospholipids).[67] The liver appears normally with per os ingestion to be the major site of glucose liponeogenesis with adipose tissue glucose liponeogenesis as a backup mechanism in man.[76] The normal caloric balance, therefore, appears to be that glucose is utilized for oxidation energy, as required for glycogen synthesis and hepatic glucose output. Excess glucose is converted to lipids.[7,53] The glucose may be derived from portal venous glucose or hepatic gluconeo-genesis.

These lipids are then added to those cleared from the blood as fatty acids and as gut-generated chylomicrons (lipoproteins). Hepatic fat balance is then maintained by mobilization of lipids from the liver to the systemic body as very low-density lipoproteins containing choles-terol, triglycerides, and phospholipids.[67] These lipoproteins are then cleared from the blood by lipoprotein lipase which appears to be largely bound to capillary endothelium.[7] This system of hepatic glucose liponeogenesis with hepatic lipoprotein release operates most intensively in the presence of hyperglycemia and insulin but will probably operate with hyperglycemia alone without much insulin response.[13] Hyperglycemia with insulin response is associated with low plasma fatty acids. The insulin response, however, activates lipoprotein lipase.[7] The result is that in the presence of hyperglycemia with an insulin response and low plasma fatty acids those organs of the body with a restricted ability to oxidize glucose, such as red skeletal muscle, are supplied fatty acids for oxidation via lipoproteins and activation of lipoprotein lipase. A second result is that, in the presence of hyperglycemia and insulin, excessive glucose may be converted to lipids in the liver and then mobilized to the systemic body for storage in adipose tissue. The diabetic has milky plasma related in part to hyperglycemia-enhanced hepatic glucose liponeogenesis with enhanced hepatic output of lipoproteins but restricted peripheral clearance of lipoprotein because of inadequate insulin for lipoprotein lipase activation.[13]

Any factor that restricts hepatic protein synthesis restricts lipoprotein synthesis and therefore limits hepatic fat mobilization.[67] This may occur experimentally or clinically because of protein synthetic poisons, defi-ciencies such as choline, or inadequate amino acid supply relative to calories (an increased calorie to nitrogen ratio with per os ingestion).[53] This last condition may be readily produced in the protein-depleted patient or animal with intravenous infusion or per os glucose and depends upon the hyperglycemia induction of an insulin response that limits the normal skeletal muscle release of a complete mixture of amino acids for hepatic protein synthesis.[82] This condition simultaneously limits fat mobilization from the liver by limiting hepatic fat oxidation and therefore hepatic ketogenesis. Hepatic ketogenesis appears to be the major mechanism of hepatic fat mobilization under conditions of starvation.[19,76] Under these conditions the major source of hepatic fat appears to be plasma

fatty acids, and enhanced hepatic ketogenesis is associated with hypoglycemia, hypoinsulinemia, and hyperglucagonemia relative to the glucose and increased plasma fatty acids.[19]

In the stressed, depleted patient or animal the hyperglycemic insulin-induced, enhanced glu-cose, liponeogenetic fatty liver is associated not only with reduced release of lipoprotein but also with reduced hepatic structural protein, hypo-albuminemia, reduced transferrin, and reduced plasma vitamin A-binding prealbumin. Thus all hepatic protein synthetic activity appears to be reduced, probably by a reduction in supply of a complete mixture of amino acids from skeletal muscle.[91,97] In association with the reduced plasma albumin and vitamin A there is also reduced wound healing strength. In fact wound healing strength, plasma albumin, and hepatic protein mass correlate well under these con-ditions.[28] In contrast with starvation and hypo-glycemia, hepatic protein mass is reduced acutely relative to the fed state and then becomes stable in association with stable plasma proteins, suggesting reduced levels of hepatic protein synthesis relative to the fed state but a stable rate adequate to meet systemic plasma protein demands.[74]

Variations in the skeletal muscle delivery rate of a complete mixture of amino acids for hepatic protein synthesis have no necessary relationship to the rate of hepatic amino acid gluconeo-genesis. Thus in the stressed, severely depleted patient the hyperglycemic fatty liver is asso-ciated with several evidences of reduced hepatic protein synthesis in general but an enhanced rate of hepatic ureagenesis relative to the starved hypoglycemic patient. There are probably several reasons for this, all of which add up to endogenous generation of an amino acid im-balance by interconversion of amino acid, probably largely in skeletal muscle, so that one or more amino acids are present in excess of a balanced mixture. Thus in starvation the rate of hepatic amino acid gluconeogenesis and urea-genesis appears to be largely controlled by the plasma alanine, which is, in turn, controlled by the balance between skeletal muscle generation from other amino acids and hepatic consump-tion.[36] In induced hyperglycemia in the septic animal without oral intake, the plasma alanine rises and, although hepatic alanine gluconeo-genesis shuts off as it should, direct alanine oxidation is enhanced because of the rise in concentration.[96] Alanine may be converted to the pyruvate directly used for oxidation as well as glucose and enter the cell under different controls than glucose. Alanine, pyruvate, and glucose are in equilibrium. The rise in alanine in association with hyperglycemia is also associated with a rise in pyruvate and probably enhanced direct oxidation of plasma pyruvate.

Thus the induced hyperglycemia state described in the septic animal, although associated with evidence of reduced hepatic protein synthesis, is also associated with enhanced hepatic ureagenesis but reduced hepatic amino acid gluconeogenesis.[96] These relationships almost undoubtedly require enhanced skeletal muscle release of alanine at the same time that a reduced skeletal muscle release of a complete mixture of amino acids occurs. This is indicated by the gross imbalance in plasma amino acid concentrations with high tryptophan and very low concentrations of leucine, isoleucine, and valine.[96]

There is another possible component to this problem. Skeletal muscle has a very limited ability to oxidize glucose and a strong requirement for fatty acids or ketone bodies as a fuel.[86] The hyperglycemic, protein-depleted patient without oral intake has low plasma fatty acids and ketone bodies plus low lipoproteins. Therefore plasma delivery of all acceptable fuel to skeletal muscle has been compromised by the hyperglycemia and insulin response. The only other sources of fuel are endogenous fats and proteins, both of which are limited. In skeletal muscle the amino acids leucine, isoleucine, and valine may be utilized as an endogenous source of ketone bodies for oxidation.[86] The remaining amino acids are gluconeogenic and subject to all the limitations of oxidation as glucose, unless they can be converted within skeletal muscle to lipids. If this mechanism is operative and there is no skeletal muscle lipogenesis, then all amino acids except leucine, isoleucine, and valine will become in excess and will be released either per se or as alanine for hepatic gluconeogenesis with subsequent disposal either as glucose or lipids. Thus hyperglycemia will be associated with hypergluconeogenesis and restricted hepatic protein synthesis.

NEUROENDOCRINE REGULATION

The acute neuroendocrine regulatory systems may be divided into those that mobilize energetic and synthetic substrate (catabolic) and those that deposit energetic and synthetic substrate (anabolic).[15,40,74,89] The catabolic neuroendocrine system is composed of the ventromedial nucleus of the hypothalamus, growth hormone, adrenocorticotropic hormone and glucocorticoids, the sympathetic nervous system, epinephrine, and glucagon.[9] The anabolic neuroendocrine system is composed of the ventrolateral nucleus of the hypothalamus, the parasympathetic nervous system and insulin.[9] Growth hormone is listed on the catabolic side because of its acute direct activity in mobilizing fat and because its more chronic active anabolic component appears to be either a product of hepatic metabolism of growth hormone called somatomedin, enhanced insulin secretion, or some as yet undefined activity of growth hormone per se.

Energy mobilization or deposition is a product of the balance between the catabolic and anabolic neuroendocrine systems in individual organs. The catabolic and anabolic neuroendocrine systems have many cross and longitudinal interrelations. Under normal conditions the balance between these systems and their interrelations are largely controlled by the plasma glucose and perhaps plasma amino acids. Under abnormal conditions the catabolic neuroendocrine system, and therefore indirectly the anabolic neuroendocrine system, may be modulated by many factors in addition to the plasma glucose. It is clear that a total body protein catabolic state may be brought about by cold exposure, severe exercise, physically induced hyperthemia, experimental hypotension, atrial hypertension, arterial hypoxia, and hypoosmolality.[15] All of these stimuli have hypothalamic representation adjacent to the ventromedial nucleus and anatomic fiber tracts that interconnect the nuclei.[9] The ventromedial nucleus in addition acts as a glucose sensor and has blood vessels responsive to sympathetic control in contrast to the rest of the brain.[6,44] It therefore appears probable that ventromedial nucleus function is modulated by glucoceptors, baroceptors, chemoceptors, thermoceptors, osmoceptors, and by the cortical perception of anxiety and pain via connection with the limbic system. The hypothalamus is a very special area of the brain not only because of its unusual modulation of blood flow by the sympathetic nervous system but also because of the absence of a blood-brain barrier. It is connected to the systemic body not only by neural connections but also by all substrates carried in the blood. Thus in general all significant organ failures or severe stress will elicit enhanced ventromedial nucleus activity and a catabolic state.

The magnitude of the catabolic state will depend upon the cumulative strength of the stimuli. They may, however, be categorized in four major classes of a continuous process with many intermediate states: the hypercatabolic state, the stress catabolic state, the starvation catabolic state, and the depleted state. These categories are to be contrasted with the anabolic state induced by intravenous support which does

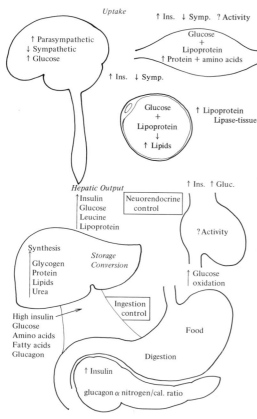

Figure 1–3. Hyperanabolic fed state. There is a response to insulin greater than that expected for the increase in plasma glucose compared with the same increase produced by intravenous glucose. Reasons are the parasympathetic stimulation during the cephalic phase of gastric secretion and the release of secretin, cholecystokinin, and gastrin. The glucagon response is just sufficient to convert relative excesses of amino acids to glucose so that the liver is presented with the proper ratio of glucose to amino acids. The hepatic parasympathetic-sympathetic response is one that insures maximum conversion of glucose to glycogen while admitting sufficient glucose to the systemic circulation to maintain the hyperglycemic state.

The neuroendocrine setting is such that there is maximal hepatic storage of ingested food as protein and glycogen. Excess amino acids are converted to glucose and urea while excess glucose is converted to fatty acids and then triglycerides. The triglycerides combine with phospholipids to form lipoproteins. Peripheral clearance of lipoproteins is increased as a result of an increase in activity of lipase. At the same time, the hyperinsulinemic response stimulates hepatic glycogen storage; it also stimulates the systemic utilization of glucose by decreasing fat mobilization and by enhancing cellular entry and consumption of glucose. It appears highly

not alter the basal glucose and the hyperanabolic state associated with food ingestion.

NORMAL STATE

This state vacillates between the fed energy storage state and the between-meal state with energy mobilization principally from the liver to the systemic body. In the fed state the gastrointestinal mucosa is first presented with regional hypernutrition that enhances local synthetic activity (Figure 1–3). The balance between the digestion and release of substrate, its local consumption, and absorption then presents the liver with locally high concentrations of substrate in the portal vein with the actual concentration dependent upon the balance between the rate of blood flow and the rate of delivery from the gut. The gut processes produce a longer period of lower concentration and allow a longer period of time for the hepatic processes.

The hypothalamic ventrolateral nucleus activation associated with the cephalic phase of digestion enhances insulin release[44] as does the local release of the gastrointestinal hormones such as secretin, pancreozymin, and cholecystokinin.[35] In addition the initial ventrolateral nucleus–parasympathetic activation stimulates hepatic glycogen synthesis. The hepatic pass-through of glucose by producing systemic hyperglycemia inhibits the ventromedial nucleus–sympathetic activation of fat mobilization[48] and inhibits the hepatic glycogenolytic enzymes while simultaneously further stimulating pancreatic islet insulin release and

probable that the regulators of hepatic protein synthesis largely control the hepatic venous blood levels of amino acids. It is clear that leucine, isoleucine, and valine are either utilized by the liver for protein synthesis or released during hepatic proteolysis but are not catabolized by the liver.

The hyperanabolic fed state is therefore one of maximal hepatic storage of ingested material and maximal dispersal of materials in excess to the systemic body with minimal concentration changes. The supply of substrate to the liver under these conditions is under ingestion-digestion control, while hepatic storage and dispersal to the systemic body is under neuroendocrine control, particularly insulin.

Between meals, the material stored in the liver is mobilized to the systemic body under neuroendocrine control based largely upon the plasma glucose and its effects upon the pancreatic islets (insulin-glucagon) and upon the ventromedial nucleus–sympathetic nervous system to the liver (increased glucose output) and adipose tissue (fat mobilization).

inhibiting glucagon release. The hepatic pass-through of amino acids then activates glucagon release as needed, while the reduced sympathetic activity also decreases glucagon release.[95] As a result the liver is presented simultaneously with locally high concentration of substrate and insulin plus the concentration of glucagon required for sufficient glucose to produce the desired ratio of glucose to protein. Thus all hepatic synthetic activities are stimulated, and substrate is maximally deposited in the liver while the plasma glucose is maintained at hyperglycemic levels relative to basal. This process lasts as long as systemic hyperglycemia is maintained by hepatic pass-through glucose.[76] Simultaneously with these hepatic events the decreased sympathetic nervous system activity plus the systemic hyperinsulinemia secondary to hepatic pass-through inhibits fat mobilization and stimulates systemic body consumption of glucose and amino acids, so that the increased hepatic output is consumed systemically with minimal increased glucose concentration changes to mark the increased hepatic output. During this same period hepatic glucose beyond that required for glycogen and hepatic glucose output is being converted to lipids and being mobilized from the liver to the systemic body as lipoproteins.[53] Since the systemic hyperinsulinemia also activated the lipoprotein lipase which clears the lipoproteins from the blood to the systemic tissues, once again a considerable increase in hepatic output of substrate is attended by minimal plasma concentration change.[7]

All of these processes result therefore not only in maximal hepatic storage and constant composition but also maximal dispersion of excess nutrient from the liver to the systemic body for storage largely under control of the plasma glucose.

After this period the liver has increased in mass and glycogen content but is otherwise constant in composition. At this point the plasma glucose falls to a basal level, the ventro-medial nucleus sympathetic system is activated,[48] the ventrolateral nucleus–parasympathetic system deactivated,[44] pancreatic insulin output falls, and pancreatic glucagon output rises.[95] The result is increased fat mobilization and oxidation with attendant decreased glucose consumption. Simultaneously hepatic glycogen is mobilized to maintain hepatic glucose output at the level that prevents hypoglycemia, and if the glycogen stores are significantly decreased, hepatic gluconeogenesis is enhanced by glucagon so that they are maintained. Considerable decrease in hepatic glucose output results with minimal change in the plasma glucose and the

hepatic glycogen but consumption of hepatic protein and the gluconeogenic substrates of glycerol, plasma amino acids, and lactate. Thus between meals the material contained in the liver is mobilized under glucose neuroendocrine control to the body in the form it needs.

In normal man the catabolic and anabolic neuroendocrine system plus the intracellular enzyme adaptations to fat or glucose oxidation are carefully poised so that rapid shifts may be made in either direction. As a result glucose tolerance tests show rapid disappearance.

STARVATION

The transient period between feeding and the onset of a stable starvation state is characterized by continued mobilization of substrate from the gut and liver with reduction in mass of both organs[74] (Figure 1–4). This mobilization is based on reduction in nutritional support from one of regional hypernutrition to one of equivascular nutrition plus neuroendocrine mobilization. Under these conditions the plasma glucose falls from the basal value for overnight fasted man to a lower value of 50 to 60 mg percent. The exact glucose level achieved is lower in women than men.[68] Simultaneously the plasma insulin falls,[18] and the ventromedial nucleus–sympathetic system is further activated with enhanced fat mobilization and oxidation.[48] As the insulin and glucose fall, the glucagon response increases until about the third day when there is a slight but detectable peak both in ureagenesis[18] and the systemic plasma glucagon.[95] As fat oxidation is enhanced, the plasma insulin falls below that expected for the plasma glucose presumably because of enhanced sympathetic activity and pancreatic islet oxidation of fat, while the plasma glucagon rises above the level expected for the plasma glucose presumably for the same reasons.[95,100] As these changes occur, hepatic ketogenesis is increased because of the reduced hepatic glycogen, hypoglycemia, enhanced plasma fatty acids, and the increase in glucagon relative to insulin.[18] Simultaneously the reduced insulin enhances skeletal muscle release of amino acids, both as a complete mixture of amino acids and as an excess of alanine and glutamine.[17] Thus in time the factors that mobilize amino acids from the liver as glucose or protein come into balance with the factors that increase the supply of amino acids to the liver. This balance appears to be based upon the effect of insulin on skeletal muscle and the effects of insulin and the sympathetic nervous system on adipose tissue.

The result is that in stable starvation hepatic output of substrate is controlled by the factors controlling peripheral release of substrate from

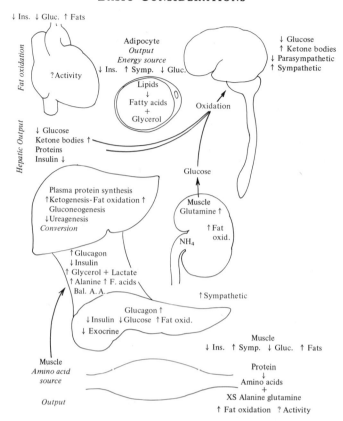

Figure 1–4. Starvation catabolic state. Increased neuroendocrine activity results in maximum gluconeogenesis and ketogenesis in the liver. In the skeletal muscles there are release of amino acids and mobilization of fat in adipose tissues. There are a decrease in secretion of insulin and an increase in glucagon. Hepatic gluconeogenesis is equivalent to hepatic output of glucose. The gluconeogenic substrates are glycerol, lactate, and alanine. Of these, both glycerol and alanine are directly controlled by insulin. Skeletal muscle also releases glutamine which is utilized by the kidney for gluconeogenesis and ammoniagenesis.

The starvation catabolic state is characterized by intracellular enzyme adaptations that stop the use of glucose except in the brain. The hepatic ketogenesis allows the brain, by bypassing the blood-brain barrier's impermeable characteristics to long-chain fatty acids, to oxidize fat in the form of ketone bodies for about 50 percent of its needs and further conserves glucose and therefore protein.

Starvation is initially characterized by mobilization of hepatic protein and protein from the gut and pancreas. The gut has decreased motility, decreased digestive capacity, and decreased absorptive capacity, except for amino acids. Thus, refeeding is, in general, associated with emesis, diarrhea, and restricted ability to eat until the gastointestinal tract has once again adapted by synthesis of more protein as muscle, mucosa, and pancreatic exocrine secretions.

the various organs, with the liver largely passively processing what is delivered. Under these conditions hepatic protein mass appears to be about one half that seen in the fed animal, and glycogen is essentially absent.

Systemic body glucose input under conditions of prolonged fasting occurs from both the liver and the kidney.[19] In the liver gluconeogenesis occurs on the basis of fat mobilization, glycerol release, glycolytic cycle lactate release, and a carefully controlled skeletal muscle alanine release.[18] In the kidney gluconeogenesis occurs

on the basis of renal ammoniagenesis from skeletal muscle glutamine release for urinary cation conservation and not on the basis of glucose need.[47] A largely uncontrolled bulk gluconeogenesis results with a finely tuned skeletal muscle alanine release gluconeogenesis superimposed. The passive nature of the hepatic response may be tested by infusing alanine and observing a sudden spurt of hyperglycemia.[36]

In stable starvation ketonemia occurs. This in effect converts the water-insoluble, long-chain fatty acids to short-chain, water-soluble fatty acids. The restriction on brain long-chain, fatty acid oxidation appears to be based upon the impermeability of the blood-brain barrier since all necessary enzymes are present for fat oxidation. Prolonged starvation is associated with the brain's consuming approximately one half of its caloric needs as ketone bodies and thus a further reduction in the consumption of glucose derived from protein consumption.[19]

As a result of all of these changes in starvation all of the body consumes fat for oxidation either directly or indirectly as ketone bodies except for about one half of the brain's needs, protein is conserved while fat is consumed, and most of these changes depend upon hypoglycemia.

Under these conditions both neuroendocrine regulation and intracellular adaptation are shifted grossly toward fat oxidation. Because of this, glucose tolerance tests, after a stable starvation state is achieved, show gross glucose intolerance.[18]

HYPERCATABOLIC STATE

The hypercatabolic state is characterized by enhanced activity of all catabolic neuroendocrine components and reduced activity of all anabolic components[15] (Figure 1–5). The hypercatabolic state has a generalized increase in sympathetic nervous system activity[101] together with its humoral endocrine extensions, epinephrine[98] and glucagon,[95] and a generalized reduction in the parasympathetic nervous system activity together with its humoral endocrine extension insulin.[3] Because of the venous drainage of the pancreatic islets and its autonomic nervous system innervation under these conditions, the liver is exposed to enhanced concentrations of glucagon, sympathetic nervous system activity, minimal concentrations of insulin, and parasympathetic nervous system activity. As this occurs, the plasma glucocorticoids rise,[56] and in general the patient goes from an active life to one of bed rest. The muscles are therefore exposed to a humoral environment of low insulin and high glucocorticoids. The result is a gross increase in skeletal muscle release of all amino acids.[17] Simultaneously the liver is exposed to a low insulin,[34] high glucagon,[34] high glucocorticoid activity plus large amounts of amino acids from muscle,[72] resulting in enhanced hepatic protein synthesis and of all gluconeogenesis including amino acids. Glucocorticoids not only stimulate hepatic protein synthesis generally both directly and by amino acid supply but also specifically stimulate synthesis of the enzymes of gluconeogenesis so that increased gluconeogenesis is encouraged to continue beyond the acute

hypercatabolic neuroendocrine state.[72] Simultaneously with the preceding changes, because of the enhanced glucagon and sympathetic nervous system activity plus the reduced insulin and parasympathetic nervous system activity, hepatic glucose output as well as hepatic gluconeogenesis, ureagenesis, and proteolysis are enhanced and hyperglycemia occurs. The magnitude of the hyperglycemia should depend largely upon the magnitude of the hepatic glycogen stores and the fatty acid response, and its duration upon the rate at which those stores are repleted by gluconeogenesis, assuming a constant hypercatabolic state.

As these changes occur in skeletal muscle and liver, the adipose tissue is exposed to an environment of enhanced sympathetic nervous system activity plus enhanced plasma glucagon, glucocorticoids, epinephrine, growth hormone, and reduced insulin. These are all stimuli that enhance adipose tissue fat mobilization.[7] However, hyperglycemia directly enhances reesterification of fatty acids in adipose tissue and therefore limits fat mobilization.[7] The plasma-fatty acid response depends upon the balance between these factors but, in general, should be higher than expected for a given glucose in basal man.

Finally the pancreatic islets are exposed to directly enhanced sympathetic nervous system activity plus enhanced plasma levels of glucose and epinephrine. The enhanced sympathetic nervous system activity and epinephrine causes enhanced glucagon output,[95,101] relative to the plasma glucose, while the enhanced epinephrine limits insulin output relative to glucose.[22]

Modifications of the Basal Hypercatabolic Response

Shock. The patterns of the response even in the hypercatabolic state may be grossly changed by organ failures or preceding disease or depletion. With acute shock the adipose tissue blood supply in general is grossly reduced so that fatty acid mobilization is reduced even though the neuroendocrine set calls for lipolysis. Simultaneously muscle blood flow is also reduced, reducing amino acid mobilization. However, the same event also reduces hepatic blood flow and therefore hepatic amino acid consumption, as well as reducing tissue oxidative consumption of both glucose and fatty acids. Under these conditions the liver may release amino acids rather than consume them. The lactic acidosis implies not only increased generation in the tissues but also decreased hepatic consumption of lactate. Thus many contradictory factors are at work, and the plasma fatty acids may be almost any value. But in general hyperglycemia and increased

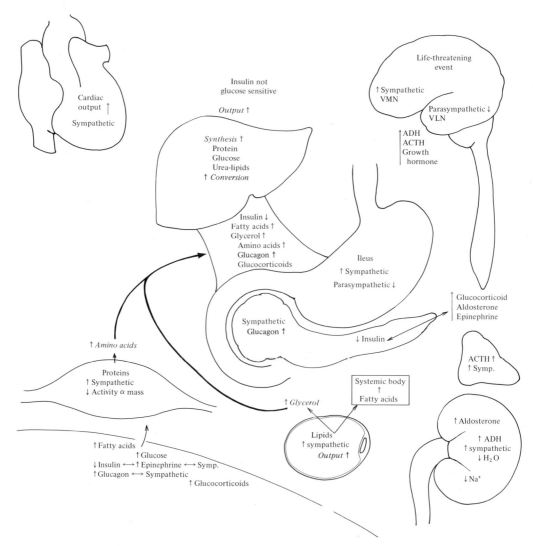

Figure 1–5. Hypercatabolic state. The hypercatabolic state occurs secondary to life-threatening stress and has as its major characteristic a lack of response of insulin to glucose, secondary to enhanced epinephrine release. In general, it lasts only until resuscitation has occurred from life-threatening organ failure and is then superseded by the stress catabolic state. There are an increase in the activity of the catabolic neuroendocrine system and suppression of the anabolic neuroendocrine system. All the characteristics of this state can be produced by generalized electrical stimulation of the ventromedial nucleus of the hypothalamus. Increased sympathetic activity results in changes in blood flow, direct changes in metabolism, and release of epinephrine and glucagon. In addition, there are an increase in antidiuretic hormone, increased adrenocorticotropic hormone, and increased growth hormone and, secondary to these, an increase in glucocorticoids and aldosterone. There is maximal mobilization of amino acids, fatty acids, and glycerol from the periphery with maximal hepatic protein synthesis and maximal hepatic gluconeogenesis and hepatic glucose output. Secondary to these changes, both the plasma glucose and fatty acids are simultaneously elevated, while there is increased hepatic output of plasma proteins and urea. In addition, if there is no circulatory failure mechanism there is maximal cardiac output. Thus, in general, energetic and synthetic substrates are maximally mobilized at the same time that the circulation is maximally mobilized to deliver substrate from organ to organ. The increase in antidiuretic hormone and aldosterone conserves body water and salt so that minimal exogenous supplies are required. At the same time the blood becomes hypercoaguable so that areas of bleeding are controlled more quickly.

plasma amino acids are present. Clearly the exogenous fuel of choice at this time is glucose, but this alone will do no good unless the basic shock mechanisms are diagnosed and treated.

Muscle Mass. The magnitude of the total body catabolic state as judged by the magnitude of peak urine urea excretion on the fifth to seventh day varies considerably. If the initial trauma is graded in terms of the statistical possibility of death, it is clear that within certain limits the greater the magnitude of trauma the greater the protein catabolic state.[15,27,70] This is probably related to the magnitude of the neuroendocrine response going from starvation through stress catabolic through hypercatabolic. Superimposed on this is another variable probably related to muscle mass. Young, healthy, vigorous, muscular males exposed to a given level of trauma have a greater total body protein catabolic response than malnourished thin males of similar age for this same sort of trauma.[15,27,70] Females in general have a smaller protein catabolic response than males, and aged malnourished individuals, especially female, have the smallest protein catabolic response. Finally, an individual exposed to a sequential, apparently identical challenge such as recurrent malarial fever has a progressively smaller total body protein catabolic response for each challenge as he has a greater cumulative nitrogen loss presumably from skeletal muscle.[54] In general, as the muscle mass decreases, the total body protein catabolic state decreases, but the probabilities of death from the insult increase.

The hypercatabolic response provides amino acids from skeletal muscle to the liver both for protein synthesis and amino acid gluconeogenesis. The magnitude of the response is clearly related to the magnitude of the neuroendocrine response and the magnitude of the skeletal muscle mass. This would be expected in principle since a given change of humoral hormones per unit muscle mass would then involve more units of muscle mass.

Skeletal muscle protein synthesis is clearly modulated by the humoral hormones with insulin stimulating synthesis and the glucocorticoids stimulating breakdown.[17] Glucagon in physiologic systemic doses probably has no skeletal muscle effect.[16] However, in spite of the effect of humoral hormones mechanical activity is a far more important stimulus to protein synthesis. It is therefore probably true that most of the amino acids mobilized come from the muscles put at rest. This in bed-resting man would particularly include the muscles of ambulation and would not generally include the myocardium or muscles of respiration in spontaneously breathing man. In fact, if the myocardium or muscles of respiration must work harder at this time, they might well receive amino acids for protein synthesis from the muscles of ambulation, probably via albumin and plasma proteins synthesized by the liver. Extremities immobilized by traction or casts would be expected to be particular contributors to the systemic body amino acid economy. The muscles and bone collagen are known to disappear rapidly under these conditions, although attention is usually directed more at the loss of bone calcium (osteoporosis). The patient placed on the ventilator might also be expected to lose respiratory muscle to the extent that the muscles are put at rest. Thus in the patient on the ventilator with positive end expiratory pressure, the inspiratory muscles would be more affected than the expiratory muscles.

In summary, the skeletal muscle portion of the acute catabolic response is extremely important in acute survival but has as a necessary side effect increased hepatic ureagenesis and a total body protein catabolic response. The magnitude of this response and its localization may be varied by muscular management. This response, although important to acute survival, delays rehabilitation by loss of the ambulatory muscles. It is probably true that immediate internal fixation of shaft fractures of the femur could diminish the total body protein catabolic response and accelerate rehabilitation in a way that would not damage the desired response for acute survival.

Gastrointestinal Tract. These patients all have an ileus and no oral intake. The ileus reflects enhanced sympathetic tone relative to parasympathetic tone to the stomach and colon and, to a lesser extent, the small intestine. The lack of oral intake limits luminal gastrointestinal mucosal nutritional support. This problem is accelerated, particularly in the stomach, by vasoconstriction, which also limits vascular nutritional support. The result is stress ulceration of the gastric mucosa.[83] As the vasoconstriction recedes and circulation is restored, these ulcerations commonly bleed. This bleeding is generally self-limited if the blood is replaced and circulation maintained.

The enhanced mobilization of energetic and synthetic substrate provides vascular hypernutrition to the intestine and its ancillary endocrine organs. However, the lack of the normal luminal hypernutrition of the mucosa may be expected to be associated with loss of mucosal mass.

Circulation. The same neuroendocrine factors that enhance substrate mobilization also enhance cardiac output if no specific circulatory

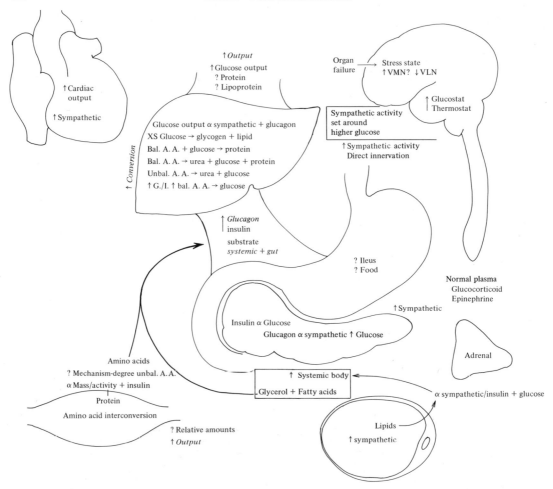

Figure 1–6. Stress catabolic state. The stress catabolic state is characterized by more restricted enhancement of the catabolic neuroendocrine system than during the hypercatabolic state. Three substates depend upon the insulin response to glucose. In substate I the insulin is hyperresponsive to glucose and the body is insulin resistant. The mechanism varies in different organs. In substate II insulin is normally responsive to glucose, and in substate III insulin has decreased responsiveness to glucose. The stress catabolic state merges at one end into the hypercatabolic state and at the other into the starvation catabolic state.

The plasma glucose in the stress catabolic state is modulated at a higher level than for the starvation catabolic state. Glucagon is modulated by the sympathetic nervous system and less by the plasma glucose and alanine. The plasma fatty acids are high relative to the plasma glucose compared with the starvation and hyperanabolic states, but the plasma fatty acids still bear a reciprocal relationship to the glucose. In the stress catabolic state, hepatic glucose output does not fall on infusing 5 percent glucose as in normal man. The plasma fatty acids and insulin, however, do respond so that there is no change in the concentration of plasma glucose. The urine output of urea is grossly increased during the transition from the hypercatabolic to stress catabolic state. However, when the stress catabolic state becomes stabilized, the urine output of urea with infusion of 5 percent glucose is only slightly increased. In spite of this characteristic the attainment of total body nitrogen balance requires nitrogen intakes greater than those required for normal man and calories in excess of measured expenditure. This state has a characteristic increased cardiac output and an increase in the thermoneutral zone so that cold exposure occurs at higher temperatures.

In the stress catabolic state, hepatic protein synthesis is highly dependent upon the nature, magnitude, and route of nutritional support because of the responsiveness of neuroendocrine controls and the setting of the liver toward gluconeogenesis by the increase in glucagon. Reduced hepatic protein synthesis is manifested by hypoalbuminemia, decreased transferrin, transcortin, vitamin A–binding protein, and by a fatty liver. These changes are secondary to decreased periph-

failure mechanism is active, such as hypovolemia. In general these patients may be expected to have high cardiac outputs, increased cardiac rates, and some degree of hypertension.[9] The hypercatabolic state is characterized by hypoinsulinemia. Insulin stimulates the entry of both glucose and potassium into all cells.[104] A portion of the potassium loss exceeding that produced by cellular destruction is probably related to the hypoinsulinemia. This potassium loss represents loss of intracellular potassium and therefore a change in transmembrane potential. If severe enough, this may be expected to have particular effects on contractility and rhythm in the heart. The use of glucose, potassium, and insulin in a way that does not produce hypoglycemia therefore appears rational, even though hyperglycemia is already present for the treatment of acute myocardial failure unresponsive to the normal positive inotropic agents. This has been reported with beneficial results on cardiac output in the low cardiac output shock state associated with sepsis and the hypercatabolic state.[25] Prolonged use of glucose, potassium, and insulin will interfere with skeletal muscle amino acid release and should therefore be accompanied by administration of intravenous amino acids for hepatic support.

Stress Catabolic State

The hypercatabolic state may be expected, with treatment of the more severe organ failures and alleviation of pain and anxiety, to be converted to the stress catabolic state[101] (Figure 1–6). This is a state of much more restricted enhanced sympathetic activity and much less ventromedial nucleus excitation. It is in general characterized by normal glucocorticoids and no epinephrine response but is associated with specific organ failures that enhance ventromedial nucleus activation relative to the starvation catabolic state. Thus it is characterized by enhanced urinary excretion of catecholamine end products[101] and plasma catecholamines in the high normal range[49] and, in addition, a high systemic plasma glucagon relative to the glucose,[101] but a normal or high insulin relative to the glucose.[101] Basal growth hormone levels are somewhat high relative to glucose.[100] The plasma glucose is somewhat high, and a diabetic glucose tolerance curve is present after intravenous glucose tolerance tests are done.[101] There is insulin resistance as judged by

the hypoglycemia induced by intravenous insulin.[55] The plasma fatty acids are high relative to the plasma glucose.[3] The cardiac output is high relative to starvation.[25] Hepatic glucose output does not decrease with intravenous glucose infusions that produce minimal hyperglycemia as it does in normal man,[50] but does with significant hyperglycemia.[96] An ileus may or may not be present. Fever is common, as is a leukocytosis and increased sedimentation rate. Urinary nitrogen output is somewhat high relative to a comparable state of starvation but not outstandingly high, as it is in the hypercatabolic state.[30]

The stress catabolic state is produced by specific organ failures and is best managed by treating those organ failures. One of these, cold exposure, will be discussed later. In the absence of effective immediate therapy the stress catabolic state is associated with very large nitrogen losses on a cumulative basis because it may last so long and not because of large daily losses.[15,62,64,70]

This state is characterized by evidence of enhanced sympathetic nervous system activity to the liver (glucose output not normally responsive to intravenous glucose without hyperglycemia),[50] to the pancreatic islets (enhanced glucagon relative to glucose),[101] to the adipose tissue (enhanced fat mobilization in the presence of normal insulin),[3] to the circulation (enhanced cardiac output),[25] and commonly to the stomach (ileus). It is, however, also one of a normal insulin response to glucose[101] (lack of enhanced epinephrine activity) and is therefore a glucose-responsive state.

The stress catabolic state for the liver is characterized by enhanced glucagon but relatively normal insulin and enhanced sympathetic activity relative to parasympathetic activity. In the absence of oral intake it is characterized by lack of the specific gastrointestinal hypernutrition the liver normally receives and by complete dependence of the liver upon release of energetic and synthetic substrate from the periphery. This is controlled in adipose tissue by the balance between sympathetic nervous system activity, insulin, and probably growth hormone and for skeletal muscle largely by variations in insulin levels.

The stress catabolic state is one of both enhanced fat and glucose oxidation and therefore enhanced hepatic glucose output.[50,96]

---

eral release of amino acids and increased hepatic conversion of amino acids to glucose and may be overcome by systemic infusion of amino acids or by absorption of nutrients from the small intestine. Since the effect of glucagon on the liver increases the calorie to nitrogen ratio, exogenous infusions or gastrointestinal tract nutritional support should be given with a low ratio of calories to nitrogen.

These functions are glucose-sensitive via pancreatic insulin and glucagon output. The pancreatic glucagon output is elevated relative to the glucose in starvation. This does not mean that it is not sensitive to glucose, but granted the function of other central mechanisms, more probably means that pancreatic glucagon output is modulated around a higher plasma glucose level. Pancreatic insulin output appears to be modulated around the normal glucose level or perhaps even a lower glucose level (relative hyperinsulinemia). However, both are normally released into the portal venous system, and the liver has its normal high concentrations relative to the systemic body.

The total body characteristics of this state are that, for nitrogen balance to be achieved, more carbohydrate calories must be given than measured energy and more protein (or amino acids) than normally required. In general, calories are required by 50 to 100 percent over measured expenditure and protein of 2 to 4 gm per kilogram per day in contrast to the normal 1 gm or for starved man 0.6 gm per kilogram per day. These observations have been repeated many times over many years for several different types of stress.[1,26,59] Any significant caloric requirement in excess of expenditure over other than a short time can only mean liponeogenesis. Granted a glucose caloric source and the fact that amino acids are cleared principally by the liver in the presence of a higher hepatic glucagon relative to insulin, these observations probably mean enhanced hepatic glucose liponeogenesis with the glucose coming both from amino acids and exogenous glucose. The glucose may also be utilized for adipose tissue liponeogenesis. This is shown in Long's measurements of radioactive glucose turnover as enhanced utilization of glucose for processes other than CO_2 production.[65]

There is an important feedback mechanism here that has been neglected. The supply of gluconeogenic substrate may be exogenously manipulated by intravenous amino acids, while their hepatic utilization is varied by the hepatic insulin-glucagon ratio of which both components are probably sensitive to plasma glucose. Thus if amino acids are infused at increasing rates, hepatic glucose output will increase as will plasma glucose, pancreatic insulin response, hepatic ureagenesis, and eventually pancreatic glucagon output will decrease. Finally as the hepatic insulin-glucagon ratio increases, more amino acids will be diverted into hepatic protein synthesis.[79] This will occur at higher rates of hepatic gluconeogenesis, ureagenesis, glucose liponeogenesis, and amino acid infusions than in the starved catabolic state but will

eventually occur with all of the expected beneficial effects of hepatic protein synthesis. The hepatic insulin-glucagon ratio may also be changed in cold exposure by increasing the temperature. In this circumstance the plasma proteins are also increased as well as ureagenesis being decreased.[41] The hepatic insulin-glucagon ratio may also be changed with the same results by administering insulin. However, since it is given systemically, the peripheral effects must be overcome by administration of glucose, potassium, and amino acids. This particularly includes hepatic mobilization of triglycerides as lipoproteins and of protein as plasma proteins.

This rationale probably accounts for the need of calories over measured expenditure and protein over predicted normal and accounts for the fact that nitrogen balance can be achieved if these are administered properly. Further, it predicts that the calorie-nitrogen ratio should be decreased as the stress catabolic state becomes more severe and that the calorie-nitrogen ratio may be increased as one goes from the stress catabolic state to the starvation catabolic state. Finally it also predicts that even in normal subjects a further increase in calorie-nitrogen ratio will be associated with the development of hepatic fatty infiltration as described by Hartroft because of inadequate amino acids for the lipoprotein mobilization of the hepatic triglycerides generated from the caloric support.[53]

To put the problem more practically, calorie-nitrogen ratios of 400 to 600 calories per gram of nitrogen may be utilized in starved man. In the stressed man the calorie-nitrogen ratio should not exceed 150 and the more severely stressed the patient, the lower the calorie-nitrogen ratio should be. With caloric support this may be as low as 75 to 100 and without caloric support (amino acids without glucose) about 25. In other words, so long as normal renal function exists and balanced amino acid mixtures are given, the body has a tremendous hepatic capacity to dispose of amino acids in excess but has very little capacity to defend itself against amino acid deficiencies, and the consequences are largely hepatic. When in doubt use lower calorie-nitrogen ratios.

Finally hepatic fat mobilization is best stimulated by the use of amino acids without glucose. In the starvation catabolic state this may be accomplished with 3 liters of isotonic amino acids with a ketonemia as an index of the starvation catabolic state. In the stress catabolic state two to three times as much amino acids may be required and because of the underlying neuroendocrine set, ketonemia is much less likely to occur. Intravenous hyperalimentation in the normal form (calorie-nitrogen ratio 200) is set up for the patient basically in the starvation catabolic state. The stress catabolic state requires a lower calorie-nitrogen ratio, which may be achieved by an additional peripheral venous infusion of amino acids without glucose or by increasing the amino acids relative to the glucose in the mixture.

The best hepatic nutritional support is achieved by use of the gastrointestinal tract. In normally starved man or animals the route of nutritional support probably makes little difference. This does not imply that information gained under these conditions may be extrapolated to stressed man, and in fact as discussed, the more severely stressed the individual is the more probable that the gastrointestinal route will show considerable benefits over the intravenous route.[2]

Insulin Resistance

Insulin resistance exists in terms of production of hypoglycemia by infused insulin.[55] The dosage of insulin utilized was large relative to physiologic release rates and given intravenously so that its systemic effects would occur before hepatic effects. The prime place that glucose insulin resistance would be expected under these conditions would be the liver because of its specific high glucagon level and adipose tissue because of the enhanced sympathetic activity that limits insulin's effect on fat mobilization and therefore the hypoglycemic effect. Insulin resistance in terms of fat mobilization and hepatic glucose output does not necessarily imply insulin resistance in terms of skeletal muscle amino acid mobilization or protein synthesis unless these are affected in some as yet unknown way. There are some indications that insulin resistance may also be present in skeletal muscle amino acid exchange and protein synthesis following trauma.[32] Allison has demonstrated that nitrogen balance can be achieved in the burn patient with the use of insulin, potassium, and glucose.[22] The insulin dosages required were 200 to 600 units per day, and 50 percent glucose had to be given to prevent hypoglycemia. These patients were simultaneously on per os feeding of mixed meals (protein) or intravenous hyperalimentation with amino acids. These observations are undoubtedly related to the need for protein in excess of normal and calories in excess of measured expenditure. The measured end point here is urine urea and therefore hepatic ureagenesis. The insulin is administered via systemic vein and produces the systemic effects before its hepatic effects. The administration of exogenous calories and amino acids is therefore very

important to success, since the administered insulin will block systemic mobilization of fats, gluconeogenic substrate, and amino acids. The dosage of insulin required is that which will produce a high enough portal vein insulin level to overcome the hepatic glucagon effect on ureagenesis. This is simply another way of achieving the same effect that can be achieved by administering amino acids in excess of normal requirements with endogenous pancreatic insulin release.

Finally insulin resistance does not imply lack of an effect, and the discussion would suggest that the degree of insulin resistance would vary for each organ and for each component of its function within an organ. This problem largely remains to be evaluated. However, it is clear that the insulin response to pure intravenous glucose which occurs under these conditions will, in principle, impede peripheral substrate mobilization and that a systemic hyperglycemic response relative to basal is more likely to occur with glucose infusion because of the more limited autonomic nervous system control of hepatic glucose output. The basal glucose can only be defined under these abnormal conditions as that plasma glucose that exists after several hours of infusion of only water and electrolytes and not by the statistical normal values of 75 to 125 mg percent.[18,40,68] Small changes in the plasma glucose relative to basal are very important in normal neuroendocrine regulation. All the alterations in neuroendocrine function observed in the stress catabolic state relative to starvation would suggest that the system is regulating around a higher plasma glucose level.

Intravenous glucose bypasses the normal controls of hepatic glucose output and must produce a neuroendocrine response. If this response is an autonomic nervous system–mediated decrease in hepatic glucose output, as apparently occurs in normal overnight fasted man,[22,36] so that systemic hyperglycemia does not occur and does not involve fat mobilization, then no great consequence may be expected because the factors controlling hepatic nutrition will not have been altered. On the other hand if fat mobilization is reduced without a change in plasma glucose or if hyperglycemia occurs with an insulin response, then the supply of substrate from the periphery to the liver will have been diminished and the balance between the organs changed in favor of hepatic malnutrition relative to starvation.[40]

The effects of hepatic malnutrition will depend upon its magnitude, duration, and exact components. A large glucose infusion with a considerable increase in plasma glucose and insulin response may be expected to severely limit peripheral amino acid mobilization while simultaneously stimulating hepatic glucose lipo-neogenesis under conditions in which hepatic fat mobilization is limited by no ketogenesis and very limited supplies of amino acids for lipoprotein synthesis.[28] This may produce considerable physiologic effects in terms of all the hepatic functions that depend on protein synthesis.

Metabolic Rate, Temperature, and the Stress Catabolic State

A stable body temperature indicates that the body's rate of heat production is equal to the rate of heat dissipation. Heat dissipation occurs via the skin of the face, neck and shoulders, arms and hands, and via the feet and lower legs. These areas have direct arteriovenous anastomoses to the subpapillary venous plexus which are modulated via the sympathetic nervous systems both by local sensors and by a hypothalamic thermoceptor sensor. This arrangement allows increased blood flow to warm a cold hand as a local phenomenon together with a generalized increase in blood flow to enhance total body heat dissipation. Heat dissipation that cannot be achieved by the increase in direct radiant and convective heat losses associated with the enhanced skin temperature produced by perfusion of the subpapillary venous plexus is then associated with sweating in the same areas, so that a component of water evaporation heat loss is added to those of radiant and convective heat loss.

The maintenance of body temperature requires that heat loss and production be balanced. Nonshivering thermogenesis appears to be predominantly modulated by the ventromedial nucleus–sympathetic nervous system with the various humoral hormone ramifications, such as glucagon, previously discussed under the stress catabolic state. Shivering thermogenesis is the mode of heat production of last resort and usually occurs with a drop in core temperature.

Both the dissipation of excess heat and the production of more heat require energy. Minimal total body energy expenditure occurs in the thermoneutral zone where the least energy is required for heat dissipation and for heat production to maintain the desired body temperature.[29,38,100] The thermoneutral zone for nude man is about 27° to 28°C and is probably somewhat less for nude females because of their increased adipose tissue insulation. Clothing and bed clothes in effect create a microenvironment which, when comfortably adjusted, approximates the thermoneutral zone for the skin.

The normal body temperature is about 37°C (98.6°F) for a thermoneutral skin temperature of 27°C. The body temperature of importance is not that in the rectum, esophagus, or mouth but rather that in the hypothalamus which may be approximated by ear tympanic membrane temperature. All the hepatic synthetic processes previously described generate heat which produces a local abdominal rise in temperature and therefore may dissociate to some degree the important hypothalamic temperature from the rectal temperature.

The body regulates heat dissipation and production to maintain a given hypothalamic temperature. The temperature selected depends upon the interplay of the hypothalamic thermoceptor center with the other hypothalamic nuclei and the factors that alter their activity. Essentially all factors either directly life-threatening or perceived by the cortex as life-threatening have effects that can only be interpreted as enhancing ventromedial nucleus activity and thus resetting the glucostat of the body to a higher level. The evidence also suggests that the thermostat of the body is reset to a higher level by the same factors.[100] Granted the fiber tract connections and the physiologic evidence for interaction between these centers, this is not unreasonable. Clearly both cold exposure (nude man below 27° to 28°C) and physically induced hyperpyrexia can produce a total body protein stress catabolic state which essentially duplicates that produced by clinical sepsis and trauma.[15]

It is not therefore unreasonable, granted the feedback system available, that the clinical response to severe sepsis and trauma should be attended both by an increase in the regulated temperature of the thermostat and an increase in the temperature of the thermoneutral zone of the skin.[20,38,100] To put it differently, the minimal total body metabolic rate occurs both at an increased body temperature in nude sick man and at an increased room temperature (i.e., above 27°C). Thus some degree of fever appears to be a normal component of the metabolic response to clinical trauma and sepsis. This does not mean that temperatures of 40 to 41°C (104 to 106°F) are to be condoned. It does mean that fever is much more difficult to interpret as good or bad and as evidence of sepsis alone since it may be caused by most life-threatening stresses.

A second aspect of the problem is that the metabolic rate and, as one component of this, the protein catabolic response will be enhanced by cold exposure at higher environmental temperatures. This is a stress catabolic state. The normal thermoneutral zone for nude man is 27°C (80°F). Most hospital room temperatures are a few degrees lower than this. Thus normal nude man is cold exposed in a hospital room. Injured septic nude man appears to have a thermoneutral zone of about 30.4°C (87°F) and may have one as high as 34°C (94°F) according to Wilmore.[100] The extra energy expenditure required to preserve body core temperature in going from a room temperature of 30°C to 20°C may account for as much as 2000 calories per day of nutritional support in addition to producing a nitrogen-wasting state.[101] For this reason a number of authors have recommended that burn patients, where the stress catabolic state is apt to last particularly long and where bedclothing covering is particularly difficult, be cared for in rooms heated to 30°C (86°F).[38,100] The same principle applies to other critically ill patients except that it is easier to achieve by bedclothes, and if the patient is conscious and alert, the bedclothes will be so arranged for comfort.

This, however, is not the case for the patient in traction or for the lethargic comatose patient. The patient in traction has an important heat dissipation area exposed that is particularly difficult to cover. He therefore has not only the local skeletal muscle metabolic and phlebothrombotic problem of immobilization but also the systemic neuroendocrine stress catabolic consequences and the pulmonary consequences, all of which contribute to his total body protein catabolic state.

The lethargic comatose patient with sepsis or trauma is particularly difficult to keep covered because of the uncovering that occurs with multiple treatments and examinations and because when covered, he is not covered to comfort.

In addition nutritional support is also not administered under the normal neuroendocrine control as it would be with spontaneous eating. This patient is particularly apt to suffer the neuroendocrine metabolic nutritional protein depletion consequences of cold exposure. The best defense against these changes is the alert conscious patient who controls his own caloric intake. The next best is to maintain environmental temperatures of about 30°C together with a caloric intake greater than needed by 50 to 100 percent with a high nitrogen content given via the gastrointestinal tract.

THE DEPLETED PATIENT

The depleted patient may be defined as one who is unable to mobilize or utilize effectively the energetic substrate required for the metabolic response to stress. This may be on the basis of metabolic demands exceeding the capacity for response, inadequate functional organ protein, limited circulation regionally or generally, inadequate mobilizable protein or fat for use in other organs, an inadequate neuroendocrine response to mobilize energetic substrate, or inadequate hepatic function to interconvert the substrate mobilized to the form desired by the body. One striking feature of this state may be best described as sympathetic nervous system exhaustion. This is characterized by reduced norepinephrine content of the sympathetic ganglia[47] and heart and reduced urinary excretion of catecholamine end products.[100]

Acute Depletion

Prolonged shock produces an acute depletion state based upon inadequate blood flow for mobilization in adipose tissue and muscle, inadequate blood flow for hepatic interconversion with secondary intracellular hepatocyte energy depletion, and inadequate blood flow for substrate delivery. Since the blood flow to the lung, heart, and brain is preferentially preserved, exogenous infusion of glucose may be expected to provide adequate energetic substrate to these organs so that their blood flow is preserved. Adipose tissue and skeletal muscle may withstand rather prolonged periods of limited blood flow. The kidney may be expected to fail, but this will not cause death if the electrolytes, especially potassium, can be adequately managed.

The problems in this sort of acute depletion revolve around the gut,[39] liver,[10,93] and neuroendocrine system.[39] The gut with its reduced blood flow may ulcerate and provide a portal for bacteria and toxins to enter the body. The liver may develop disorders of hepatocyte intracellular energy metabolism as well as depletion of essential protein systems or disorders of the reticuloendothelial clearance of toxins and bacteria. The brain's blood flow in major part is endogenously autoregulated independent of the sympathetic nervous system, as is the blood flow to the heart. The brain, however, has an important exception to its blood flow autoregulation and the protection given by the blood-brain barrier from systemic body events. Thus the hypothalamus has both a sympathetic nervous system–modulated blood flow and no functional blood-brain barrier. The hypothalamus is therefore susceptible to the same factors that limit systemic body blood flow and to the same toxin and compositional alterations as the systemic body. In addition to these hypothalamic alterations the systemic body portion of the neuroendocrine system is affected by low flow to the endocrine glands just as the rest of the body is.

Long-term survival from an episode of shock

therefore depends largely upon whether hepatic and neuroendocrine system function as a whole has been adequately preserved during shock so that adequate integrated functions can be resumed when the shock mechanism has been corrected. This system may go awry in many ways. Thus prolonged hemorrhagic shock is associated with inadequate hepatic glucose output, hypoglycemia, and brain death. This may be overcome with exogenous glucose.[70] Much has been made of the alteration of gastrointestinal mucosal permeability, the entry of endotoxin into the portal system, the limited hepatic clearance of endotoxin, and the altered hypothalamic neuroendocrine regulation with severe peripheral arteriolar vasoconstriction. Some authors believe that there is a common endotoxin mechanism between hemorrhagic shock and sepsis-associated shock.[39] This has led to attempts to preferentially increase gut and hepatic blood flow by blockade of the abdominal sympathetic nervous system or using systemic vasodilators to overcome the peripheral blood flow effects of the hypothalamic-increased sympathetic arteriolar constriction. It should be noted that such systemic vasodilators should also increase hypothalamic blood flow. Another approach has been the lytic cocktail which contains, in addition to sympathetic blockers, chlorpromazine to reduce hypothalamic noradrenergic activity and an analgesic to limit peripheral pain activation of the hypothalamus. Finally massive doses of glucocorticoids have also been used with various rationales but usually for peripheral vasodilation. These, however, should also have hypothalamic, skeletal muscle, and hepatic effects as previously discussed. The hepatic effects would also include stabilization of hepatic lyzosomes and limitation of hepatic damage by stabilization of the lyzosomal membrane and therefore limited release of the destructive lyzosomal enzymes.[90] It should be noted that the liver lyzosomes are normally much more active than those in the other organs.

Survival from shock has also been discussed in terms of the activity of the reticuloendothelial system, a large portion of which is contained in the liver. It is clear that shock is associated with reduced reticuloendothelial activity, and that factors enhancing reticuloendothelial activity are associated with enhanced survival from a variety of stressful situations including different kinds of shock.[5]

The essential point is that shock produces a state of acute depletion associated with altered gastrointestinal mucosal, hepatic, and neuroendocrine function. The exact alterations depend upon the exact circumstances of the shock. Thus shock in the animal anesthetized with Nembutal is very different from shock in the conscious animal. Shock in the malnourished animal is different from shock in the previously well-nourished animal. Shock in the dog is different from shock in the baboon or man. The shock state in previously healthy man is different from that in sick man and the differences depend upon how exactly the sick man is sick. However, in spite of these numerous qualifications, the common elements in long-term survival after resuscitation must involve largely the gut, liver, and neuroendocrine system. Acute survival depends largely upon intracellular energy metabolism in the various organs and the capacity to utilize blood energetic substrates to repair the damages of the low-flow state. Baue and others have directly infused high-energy phosphate in one form or another to provide the cell with exogenous high-energy phosphate at a time when its inherent capacity to generate it appears restricted.[24] This appears rational for acute survival but will make no difference if the pump priming produced does not stimulate the cell and the neuroendocrine system to sustained activity.

Chronic Depletion

The depleted patient is depleted in total body protein but has highly variable fat stores and may even be obese. The exact ratio of protein to fat depends upon the nature of the previous diet, and its duration, in addition to pathologic processes that convert protein to fat usually via hepatic amino acid gluconeogenesis.

The best studied prototypes of depletion are the infantile diseases known as marasmus and kwashiorkor.[97] These are complicated by the consumption of protein for growth. The child with marasmus has a very restricted intake of both calories and protein and is probably most comparable to adult man with pure starvation. The child with kwashiorkor has a nutritional intake in which calories (usually carbohydrate) grossly exceed nitrogen and therefore has a high calorie-nitrogen ratio (probably about 1000). The natural response of animals or children to nutritional intake with a high calorie-nitrogen ratio is to restrict total intake and thus convert from kwashiorkor to marasmus.[82] This may be overcome by forced feeding, either by the anxious mother or experimentally to produce kwashiorkor in the marasmic child or a similar picture in the animal. The child with kwashiorkor has also been called the "sugar baby," while the child with marasmus has been known as the forgotten one.

The child with marasmus is alert but apathetic, has a relatively normal body composition but of grossly restricted mass in both fat and protein, a very low metabolic rate per kilogram, relatively normal serum proteins, increased susceptibility to normally nonpathogenic organisms, and grossly reduced protein mass in the gut, exocrine pancreas, and liver.[97]

The child with kwashiorkor has a very fatty liver with increased glycogen and reduced protein. In addition he has reduced plasma levels of albumin, transferrin, transcortin, ceruloplasmin, prebeta-lipoprotein (triglycerides), vitamin A–binding protein, and, relative to the marasmic child, very reduced levels of several essential plasma amino acids, including especially the ones largely modulated by skeletal muscle (leucine, isoleucine, and valine).[97] The child with kwashiorkor typically has ascites in association with his fatty liver and generalized edema both intracellular and extracellular in association with hypoalbuminemia and disordered renal metabolism of water and electrolytes.[97] These observations are very similar to those in the depleted animal or septic man.[82]

The child with kwashiorkor therefore has, relative to the marasmic child, several signs of increased hepatic glucose liponeogenesis in the presence of inadequate amino acids for hepatic protein synthesis. The inadequate amino acids appear to be both due to inadequate oral intake and inadequate skeletal muscle release of a complete mixture of amino acids to the liver. Neither child has hypoglycemia relative to statistical normals.[77] However, the blood glucoses are at the lower limit of normal, and the blood glucose is slightly higher for the child with kwashiorkor as is the plasma insulin.[77] The child with marasmus has a higher excretion of epinephrine than the child with kwashiorkor, which may also be related to the lower plasma insulin. Refeeding and recovery produce a higher basal plasma glucose and plasma insulin in both diseases.[77]

The low metabolic rate is associated with reduced urinary excretion of dopamine and norepinephrine but not of vanillmandelic acid and epinephrine.[78] With refeeding and increased metabolic rate per kilogram, the urinary excretion of norepinephrine and dopamine rises per kilogram with the greatest statistical change in dopamine.[78] Dopamine is a precursor of both norepinephrine and epinephrine. These children appear to be able to respond in terms of epinephrine but not in terms of sympathetic nervous system direct innervation. The reduced metabolic rate secondary to this helps to preserve the duration of life while simultaneously limiting their capacity to respond to any stress. The same observations have been made in the severely depleted burn patient.[46,52,100]

In addition to these changes the response to oral glucose tolerance or standardized test meals is limited relative to intravenous tolerance tests in a way that suggests a deficiency of the gut insulinotropic factors.[81] The response to intravenous tests initially is also limited but not to the same degree. The result is that a test meal is followed by a smaller plasma glucose, plasma insulin, and smaller increment in metabolic rate.[85]

Animals with kwashiorkor-type syndromes may be readily prepared by feeding similar diets (calorie/nitrogen = 1000).[82] The hepatic increase in fat is regularly associated with an increase in glycogen, suggesting that a key hepatic change is increased hepatic glucose.[82] Increased hepatic glucose relative to amino acids may be produced by dietary means or by any stress that produces an increased hepatic glucagon response. The opinion of many authorities is that the marasmic child may be converted to the child with kwashiorkor either by carbohydrate feeding or by sepsis.[91,97] As previously discussed sepsis by virtue of the glucagon response produces both a protein-wasting state and presents the liver endogenously with a fuel of a higher calorie-nitrogen ratio just as carbohydrate feeding does. The difference would be largely one of fat mass in the body, with carbohydrate feeding producing a larger fat mass while the stress glucagon response would convert protein to fat and therefore be associated with a reciprocal change in mass and redistribution of mass from muscle to liver.

These syndromes exist in growing children where growth processes consume protein. Linear growth is severely restricted in both types of children in spite of high plasma growth hormones. However, it has now become apparent in children with kwashiorkor that a high plasma growth hormone is associated with a reduced plasma somatomedin.[80] Somatomedin is an hepatic product either of growth hormone or an hepatic substance produced under control of growth hormone. This dissociation between growth hormone and somatomedin probably is another reflection of hepatic dysfunction. With refeeding, growth hormone falls and somatomedin rises.[80]

The essential point is that the protein-depleted patient may respond to a stress glucagon response with hepatic fatty infiltration and reduced plasma levels of several very important proteins plus essential amino acids. These changes may be associated with signs of sympathetic nervous system exhaustion in response to stress so that the patient has a restricted ability to respond to stress in many ways and multiorgan failure. Acute resuscitation is possible, but the patient develops multiorgan system failure over several days and goes on to die. One of the causes of failure is infection with normally noninvasive organisms. Others are hypoalbuminemia, hypovolemia with oliguria, water retention, and hyponatremic hypochloridemic edema. Another is stress ulceration with massive bleeding secondary to decreased plasma vitamin A, increased portal venous pressure secondary to severe fatty infiltration of the liver, hypovolemia, and absent oral intake. Another organ failure is cerebral. In addition the patient is potassium- and magnesium-deficient and has not only skeletal muscle atrophy but also myocardial atrophy with secondary myocardial failure both on the basis of protein and potassium-magnesium depletion.

The therapeutic key of the chronically depleted patient is hepatic support. This involves initially nutritional support of a low calorie-nitrogen ratio. The lowest calorie-nitrogen ratio available is that of protein or equivalent amino acids. The first objective is circulatory support. By raising the plasma albumin so that the circulation is improved and tissue edema hypoxia limited, metabolism is relieved. The second objective is mobilization of hepatic fat to improve the hepatic circulation per se. This may be achieved by a few days of amino acids without glucose. The third objective is repletion of intracellular deficits of potassium, phosphate, and magnesium, especially of the heart. The fourth objective is total calorie-nitrogen electrolyte support with cellular synthesis via hyperalimentation. During this period a major objective is gut-pancreas protein synthesis so that the gastrointestinal tract may be utilized for nutritional support. This allows both the gastrointestinal mucosa and the liver to receive their normal regional hypernutrition while simultaneously allowing the normal controls of hepatic substate to the systemic body. The best hepatic nutritional support is obtained via the gastrointestinal tract.

Summary

The preceding discussion points out in depth the stress sympathetic nervous system response of Cannon, the stress glucocorticoid response of Selye, the protein catabolic states described by Moore, the increase in the thermoneutral zone described by Caldwell and Tilstone, the reversal of the protein catabolic state by an increase in room temperature as described by Cuthbertson, the altered insulin response to glucose described by Allison, the altered controls

of hepatic glucose output described by Gump *et al*. Several other characteristics of the metabolic response to trauma and sepsis are simply different facets of the neuroendocrine response to severe stress. All of these may be elicited by electrical stimulation of the ventromedial nucleus of the hypothalamus as described by Ban, while stimulation 2 mm away in the ventrolateral nucleus produces directly opposite changes that can only be described as hyperanabolic in contrast to the hypercatabolic state elicited in the ventromedial nucleus.[9] The response to trauma and sepsis is thus an integrated response that alters the balance between the catabolic and anabolic neuroendocrine systems to a more catabolic status. The magnitude may be great as in the hypercatabolic response with an epinephrine-limited insulin response or much less as in the stress catabolic response where insulin is normal or hypernormal relative to glucose, but the sympathetic glucagon response produces an elevated glucagon level for the glucose level. Glucose intolerance, as determined by glucose tolerance tests, implies only an altered transient neuroendocrine and tissue enzyme response and does not imply limited glucose metabolism. Thus, in general, the stress response is attended by both enhanced glucose oxidation and synthetic utilization (liponeogenesis) even though glucose intolerance is present. Simultaneously with enhanced glucose utilization enhanced fat oxidation also occurs. This is possible because of the enhanced metabolic rate. The enhanced metabolic rate is directly related to the sympathetic nervous system response and its ramifications, particularly the hepatic ramifications. This is probably the only organ in the body whose heat production may be widely varied by nutritional support and neuroendocrine controls. The hepatic response is therefore particularly important not only because of heat production but also because of its other functions.

ALTERATIONS IN THE BASIC RESPONSE

Hepatic

The role of the liver has been described in some detail. In addition to neuroendocrine-imposed changes the liver is subject to a large number of other challenges (Figure 1–7). Thus the absence of oral nutrition imposes a challenge in terms of loss of the liver's normal regional hypernutrition. Intravenous glucose sufficient to produce a neuroendocrine response may limit the peripheral release of amino acids and

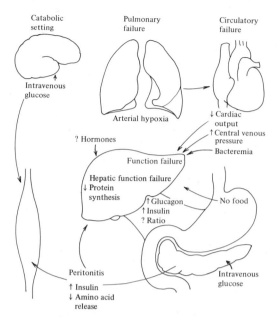

Figure 1–7. Stress catabolic hepatic insults. The sick patient has impaired hepatic function. Stimulation of the catabolic neuroendocrine apparatus results in a decrease in glucose, proteins, and lipoproteins in the liver. The liver is particularly susceptible because of its portal circulation. Circulatory failure results in decreased portal blood flow and arterial hypoxia. Both reduce the tissue oxygen tension in an organ that already has a marginal oxygen supply. The liver is adjacent to the heart and receives the full brunt of any increase in central venous pressure. An increase in central venous pressure produces hepatic edema and decreases the supply of oxygen to the hepatocyte.

The absence of food in the gastrointestinal tract results in hepatic malnutrition and loss of hepatic protein. The infusion of glucose results in release of insulin with a decrease in mobilization of fat and of amino acids from skeletal muscle. This further impairs nutrition. In the plasma there is a decrease in albumin, transferrin, vitamin A–binding protein, transcortin, and the opsonizing protein alpha 2HS glycoprotein. In peritonitis, bacteria and their toxins directly damage the liver. Their removal is impaired by the poorly functioning lymphoreticular system of the liver.

fatty acids to the liver. Pulmonary failure by increasing central venous pressure may add the challenge of hepatocyte edema hypoxia because of the lowered colloid osmotic pressure produced by the normally fenestrated sinusoidal endothelium. In addition to these problems hepatocyte metabolism may be further limited by arterial hypoxia or circulatory failure because of the normal architecture of the liver's

portal venous system. Finally peritonitis poses not only the systemic neuroendocrine response problems but also the problems with direct portal venous release of bacteria and bacterial toxins. The liver is therefore much like the lung in critically ill man in that it is susceptible to multiple insults.

The Systemic Body—Reflections of Hepatic Dysfunction

Hepatic function influences the function of essentially all other organs in the body (Figure 1–8). Cerebral function is influenced by the plasma levels of tryptophan, ammonia, and gut bacterial-generated false neurotransmitters such as octopamine. These factors alter cerebral neurotransmitters and therefore function. It is, therefore, not unexpected that hepatic dysfunction should be attended by cerebral dysfunction. One manifestation is the lethargic to comatose patient. Another factor may be altered neuroendocrine control from both altered hepatic control of systemic plasma glucagon and insulin and an altered setting of the hypothalamic nuclei because of altered neurotransmitters. Such alterations might have profound effects on the circulation and on all organs under neuroendocrine control.

The liver influences the circulation via the colloid osmotic pressure generated by albumin. This effect is progressively more important as higher and higher central venous pressures are required for adequate circulation because of increased pulmonary vascular resistance. High central venous pressures cannot be achieved chronically without a normal serum albumin. Hypoalbuminemia with increased pulmonary vascular resistance is commonly associated with moderately elevated central venous pressures (12–15 cm H_2O), restricted circulation, water retention with oliguria, hyponatremia, hypocholeridemia, and generalized edema. Normal blood volume under these conditions on a statistical basis is hypovolemia because of the increased blood volume required for venous distention.

The liver influences the peripheral metabolism of all organs by its control of the plasma amino acids and by the plasma albumin. Thus hypoalbuminemia is associated with limited wound healing and wound dehiscences. The limited wound healing is probably also related to the decreased plasma vitamin A which simultaneously occurs. This, however, must be only one small part of the general problem. Other facets may be related to the amino acids. Alanine is normally controlled by the liver and may be utilized as pyruvate for oxidation in place of glucose. An increase in plasma alanine secondary

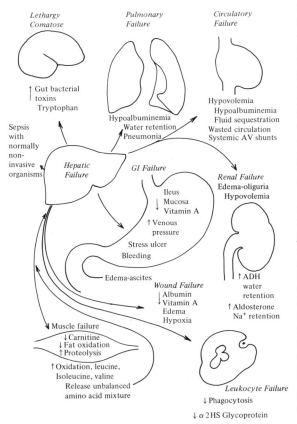

Figure 1–8. Hepatic failure corollaries. Impairment of hepatic function causes changes in distant organs and tissues similar to those that could be predicted from observation in chronically ill patients. False neurotransmitter amines, such as octopamine, derived from the action of bacteria in the gut, accumulate and impair cerebral function producing lethargy to coma. In addition, there are high concentrations of tryptophan and phenylalanine, and low concentrations of tyrosine, leucine, isoleucine, and valine. These changes are seen in hepatic encephalopathy and severe sepsis in the dog. Decreased plasma albumin is associated with decreased cardiac output, pulmonary edema, generalized edema, oliguria, hyponatremia and hypochloridemia. Contributory factors are an increase in antidiuretic hormone and aldosterone.

These patients also have sepsis with normally noninvasive organisms probably secondary to a decrease in hepatic macrophage activity. Hypoalbuminemia and a decrease in vitamin A lead to impairment of wound healing. Transferrin is decreased in the severely ill patient with sepsis and leads to anemia. It is also decreased, as a result of restricted hepatic protein synthesis, in the patient with impaired liver function.

Stress ulcer may occur, similar to that seen in the burn patient, as a result of decrease in

to inadequate hepatic clearance will be associated with a total body protein catabolic state on the basis of enhanced direct alanine oxidation generally throughout the body. The liver, together with skeletal muscle, normally ensures a balanced mixture of amino acids in the systemic plasma. This may go awry because of inadequate hepatic control of systemic plasma insulin with deposition of leucine, isoleucine, and valine in skeletal muscle and therefore a plasma amino acid mixture that cannot support hepatic protein synthesis. The system may also go awry because of unphysiologic concentrations of any other amino acid.

The liver influences skeletal muscle, long-chain fatty acid oxidation by supplying the required carnitine. Inadequate carnitine in skeletal muscle and heart must either restrict mechanical activity, or the energy requirements must be met by glucose, pyruvate, alanine, or the ketone bodies.[14] All of these alternatives in the absence of hepatic ketogenesis add up to enhanced protein catabolism or restricted muscle activity both mechanically and for sodium transport. The latter restriction will produce intracelluar edema. The liver also influences skeletal muscle function by its clearance of several hormones including the glucocorticoids. Thus the high plasma glucocorticoids associated with severe sepsis are in part related to decreased hepatic clearance.[11] The liver in-

plasma vitamin A and its binding protein synthesized in the liver. Contributory factors are that the absence of gastrointestinal food limits mucosal synthetic activity, decreases albumin, and predisposes to stress ulceration. Fatty infiltration of the liver increases the portal venous pressure and may increase bleeding from an ulcer.

A decrease in the essential amino acids leucine, isoleucine, and valine implies altered muscle metabolism and may limit protein synthesis generally. This altered muscle metabolism may occur because the liver does not properly clear insulin, resulting in hyperinsulinemia, or because the liver does not synthesize and release adequate carnitine. Carnitine is required for oxidation of long-chain fatty acid in muscle. The muscle can still burn ketone bodies.

The multiple organ failures which precede death in the chronically ill patient who does not die of circulatory or pulmonary failure occur at the same time as hepatic failure. They are therefore corollaries. An understanding of normal hepatic function plus the numerous observations made on such patients suggests that they are probably consequences of hepatic failure and of the mechanisms that produce it.

fluences antibacterial resistance both by direct clearance of bacteria and bacterial toxins via the reticuloendothelial system and by synthesis of acute phase glycoproteins. One of these, alpha 2-HS glycoprotein, is important as a bacterial opsonizing agent of leukocyte phagocytosis.[99]

The liver influences gastrointestinal function by clearing catecholamines, by delivering vitamin A via an hepatic-synthesized vitamin A–binding protein from hepatic vitamin A stores, and by modifying portal venous pressure. Vitamin A is an essential nutrient of the gastrointestinal mucosa for cell replication.[24] Limited hepatic protein synthesis with enhanced glucose liponeogenesis might therefore be expected to produce a fat-filled liver with high portal venous pressure and simultaneous gastric ulceration with maximal bleeding through minimal ulcerations. This problem would not be similar to the stress ulcer bleeding that occurs in the first few days based on limited microvascular flow, but would persist until death or reversal of the key hepatic lesions.

Summary of Systemic Body Responses. The hepatic insults discussed should lead with time to increasing hepatic dysfunction characterized predominantly in the liver as one that is fat-filled with moderate glycogen but protein poor. In addition cirrhotic changes would be expected so that clinically it would be a fatty cirrhotic liver. These changes would not be directly observable in vivo; rather one would see the systemic signs of the lethargic to comatose patient who is hypoalbuminemic with pulmonary failure and circulatory failure in association with oliguria, water retention, and generalized edema. In addition, such a patient would have poor wound healing and would be susceptible to infection from normally noninvasive organisms. This would particularly apply to gut bacteria and fungi, granted the changes in the gastrointestinal mucosa to be expected.

These findings are particularly common in the critically ill patient who has been ill for some time in the intensive care unit and supported on pure glucose.

MANIPULATION OF THE METABOLIC RESPONSE

The whole point to the detailed description of the neuroendocrine organ responses is to set up the concepts required for intelligently manipulating these processes in critically ill man.

Clearly the first priority is to treat those organ failures which produced enhanced ventromedial nucleus activity and thus convert the hypercata-bolic to the stress catabolic or starvation catabolic state. Then one must take advantage of the neuroendocrine state produced by exogenous infusion of substrate in such a way as to give maximal hepatic and therefore systemic support and, via this means, to alter the neuroendocrine response to that of starvation or the fed state. Once this is achieved, eating may be resumed unless there are organic bowel lesions.

All organ failures may produce a state of enhanced ventromedial nucleus activity. Hypovolemic shock in previously well man, quickly recognized and treated, produces a short-term hypercatabolic state followed by a relatively short stress catabolic state. This metabolic response clearly enhances survival and is so short that it has no significant lasting metabolic consequences. The same problem, if prolonged or if occurring in previously depleted man, may have considerable long-term consequences and may be much more difficult to reverse acutely. These are the conditions under which the use of glucose-potassium-insulin infusion may be of help after more conventional therapies have failed in circulation resuscitation. The rationale is that of the potassium-depleted myocardium and the use of insulin potassium to increase the transmembrane potential. Glucose must simultaneously be used because of the systemic body and hepatic effects of insulin in blocking energy mobilization. In principle the use of glucose, potassium, and insulin should also be associated with the use of amino acids to provide hepatic nutrition and hepatic protein synthesis.

The depleted patient in hypovolemic shock is prone to both hypoalbuminemia and the requirement for a high central venous pressure. For these reasons hypovolemic shock in these patients should be treated with much more plasma and albumin and much less in the way of crystalloids than hypovolemic shock in previously well-nourished man. Concentrated albumin may be used to the extent that there is generalized edema, particularly in the presence of oliguric renal failure. Plasma should be used in the absence of edema whether or not there is renal failure. Because the hypoalbuminemia also involves the interstitial fluid space and because these states are accompanied by enhanced albumin catabolism and reduced hepatic protein synthesis because of hypoxia, large quantities are required to achieve and maintain circulation resuscitation. Hypovolemic shock in the depleted patient is far different from hypovolemic shock in the previously well-nourished patient where much greater quantities of crystalloid and lesser quantities of colloid and blood may be utilized.

Acute and prolonged circulatory resuscitation

cannot be achieved in the presence of acute or progressive pulmonary failure. Therefore, it is of the utmost importance that pulmonary failure be diagnosed accurately, followed closely, and properly treated. Acute pulmonary resuscitation and prevention of progressive pulmonary failure is far easier to achieve than restoration of pulmonary function after pulmonary failure has been present for days.

The major problems that produce a prolonged stress catabolic response are sepsis, resistant pulmonary failure, burns, cold exposure, and head injuries. No progress with metabolic management can be achieved if these organ failures are not rigorously treated per se. The diagnosis of sepsis is particularly difficult in these patients since they have other reasons for fever, leukocytosis, pulmonary infiltrates, and bacteria in their tracheal aspirate. Intra-abdominal abscesses are commonly related to abdominal injury or surgery and are usually not present if these are absent or if the intestines are working. The presence of pus in the tracheal aspirate is required for the diagnosis of pneumonia but may be present with pulmonary injuries without pneumonia. Repeated cultures of all biologic fluids and repeated searches for physical evidence of sepsis are required in these patients to diagnose sepsis as early as possible. These patients are commonly blindly placed on antibiotics because one cannot be sure there is no sepsis and because of the signs of fever and leukocytosis. It must be remembered that antibiotics can mask the presence of infection and allow a large abscess to develop without localizing clinical signs. Abscesses are particularly apt to develop under normal-looking skin with crush injuries and hematoma contaminated by a previous bacteremia.

The whole problem of diagnosing sepsis in these patients is particularly difficult; however, no progress can be expected until abscesses are drained and the correct antibiotics utilized. For that reason it is best not to use antibiotics blindly but to repeatedly examine and evalutate the patient until localizing evidence of infection can be found. This approach is particularly difficult with intra-abdominal infections and infections deep to skeletal muscle.

Persistent pulmonary failure is most commonly associated with persistent sepsis, retained secretions, fat emboli, the supine position, the comatose lethargic state, and pulmonary contusions. If the pulmonary failure is persistent, the patient is very apt to require high central venous pressures and to develop, with time, several signs of hepatic dysfunction. If this combination of pulmonary failure, right ventricle failure, and hepatic dysfunction persists, then the lethargic comatose state together with irreversible stress ulcer bleeding will eventually cause death.

Progressive pulmonary failure on proper ventilator support with positive end expiratory pressure almost inevitably means retained secretions. These must be vigorously treated with suctioning with a Caude catheter and fiberoptic bronchoscopy. The supine position cannot be tolerated in the multiple trauma patient. Therefore, internal fixation of proximal shaft fractures is required to treat the pulmonary failure. This should be done a short time after admission before the patients develop pneumonia. It commonly needs to be done in the presence of fever and leukocytosis secondary to the supine position with pulmonary failure. Internal fixation is also important in the metabolic management of the leg and the prevention of cold exposure.

Burns are a particular problem because of their long-term requirements for healing and the attendant persistent skin failure with necrotic tissue infection, large insensible water losses, and accentuated cold exposure. The burn patient, however, has the peculiar advantage that, with proper wound management, oral intake is soon achieved and specific hepatic-gastrointestinal mucosa nutritional support provided. Basic principles of metabolic management require burn wound excision and skin grafting or, in the absence of this, maximum attempts to minimize cold exposure and burn wound sepsis together with maximum caloric support of high nitrogen content. The local environmental temperature of these patients should be maintained about 30°C either by covers or, when this is impossible, by increasing the room temperature. The conscious alert patient may be deliberately maintained so that he feels somewhat warm. For the lethargic comatose patient, temperatures somewhat higher than 30°C, but probably not above 34°C, should be employed. This has the double advantage of decreasing energy demands while increasing skin blood flow and therefore accelerating burn wound healing.

Burn wound therapy with local antibacterial agents is primarily utilized to prevent infection, but Sulfamylon may be used to treat existing infection, as may silver sulfadiazine, because of its penetration of the burn wound. The improper use of 0.5 percent aqueous silver nitrate by allowing the patient to lie in uncovered wet dressings in a pool of water is particularly apt to increase heat expenditure from evaporation of silver nitrate water. This treatment must be accompanied by a heated room, blankets, and a membrane impermeable to water so that evaporative water losses are minimized and a hot microenvironment is created.

Proper acute management of the life-threatening organ failures and the pain and anxiety associated with them converts the hypercatabolic state to the stress catabolic state. The stress catabolic state has as its essential characteristic a ventromedial nucleus sympathetic glucagon response and an insulin responsive or hyperresponsive to glucose. The liver is therefore set for increased glucose output and enhanced gluconeogenesis in the basal state via glucagon but is still insulin-responsive but at a higher level. Infusion of glucose under these conditions is particularly apt to interfere with peripheral amino acid release and, if the glucose infusion is great enough, to enhance glucose liponeogenesis. This does not represent a complete shutoff of peripheral amino acid release but rather a reset in the balance which takes time to produce hepatic damage.

In these patients pure intravenous glucose should not be used in high concentrations or for prolonged periods. The definition of a prolonged period clearly depends upon the preexisting state of nutrition. In previously healthy patients a week of 5 percent glucose will probably have no significant physiologic effect. In the previously depleted patient intravenous glucose should be used only for the period of resuscitation.

The next step in the metabolic management of these patients is the use of amino acids without glucose to provide maximum hepatic support in a way that minimally interferes with interorgan exchange of amino acids and allows normal neuroendocrine regulation of hepatic glucose output. Success with amino acids is largely measured by the development of ketonemia on the second to third day, secondary to hepatic fat oxidation and ketogenesis, and consistent with systemic fat oxidation. The greater the stress catabolic state the less likely this is to occur because of the glucagon-enhanced amino acid gluconeogenesis and hepatic glucose output together with a hyperglycemia-induced, hepatic insulin response-limiting ketogenesis. This, however, because of the other factors enhancing fat mobilization, does not necessarily imply limited systemic oxidation of long-chain fatty acids. This problem can only be evaluated by measuring urinary nitrogen and plasma glucose and fatty acids. If the urinary nitrogen ongoing from electrolyte or glucose support to amino acid support increases in an amount equal to the added amino acids, or if the plasma glucose does not fall with a rise in plasma fatty acids, then the added amino acids are not doing their selected job of enhancing fat oxidation because of their enhanced use for amino acid gluconeogenesis. This does not necessarily imply that they are not being utilized for hepatic protein synthesis, since skeletal muscle may be responsible for an endogenous amino acid imbalance for which it is consuming plasma proteins. Finally, if this response is present, then greater quantities of infused amino acids may produce hepatic protein synthesis by stimulating hepatic glucose output to the point where sufficient glucose insulin response exists for the hepatic insulin to overcome the hepatic glucagon responses.

Amino acids without glucose may also be utilized to mobilize hepatic fat by stimulating release of lipoproteins at the same time it minimizes glucose liponeogenesis. However, this is basically a holding action to prevent further organ failure from protein destruction and depends largely for calories on mobilization of endogenous fat. The severely cachectic patient, if he has been on pure glucose, commonly has hepatic fat infiltration and requires a period of pure amino acid support to mobilize this fat. However, this should be changed in a day or two to a regime designed to produce cellular protein synthesis.

Such a regime requires total caloric support. However, because this is administered on the stress catabolic background of a high glucagon and a normal or hyperresponsive insulin, together with systemic hyperglycemia, one may expect both enhanced amino acid gluconeogenesis and enhanced lipogenesis both in the liver and the adipose tissue. In part the route of administration may determine the site of liponeogenesis, since a greater systemic hyperglycemia would be expected with intravenous administration and a greater portal vein hyperglycemia with gastrointestinal tract administration. The enhanced amino acid gluconeogenesis plus the hepatic liponeogenesis requires that greater nitrogen be delivered per calorie of support than in normal man, and the gastrointestinal route probably requires greater nitrogen per calorie than the intravenous route with its adipose tissue liponeogenesis. The liponeogenesis requires that calories be administered in excess of measured expenditure to achieve nitrogen balance. Finally, it should be remembered that the primary goal is hepatic protein synthesis and that the liver has a very large capacity to handle excess nitrogen. Thus there are few dangers in reasonable excesses of nitrogen but considerable dangers in deficient nitrogen with respect to the development of a fatty liver. The situation is much like that of water and electrolyte balance in the patient with normal kidneys: There are no dangers in reasonable excesses but great dangers in cumulative small deficits.

It is therefore necessary in the stress catabolic state to give calories in excess of measured expenditure by at least 50 percent and protein in excess of the normal 1 gm per kilogram per day by 50 to 100 percent or more. These needs disappear as the patient enters the starvation catabolic state but even there, if protein synthesis is desired, the caloric supply and nitrogen supply must exceed maintenance. It is therefore the practice after a period of slowly rising intake of two to three days to allow cellular and neuroendocrine adaptation to maintain a patient on the higher levels required for nitrogen balance in the stress catabolic state so that as he goes into the starvation catabolic state with treatment of his primary disease energy and nitrogen will be supplied for cellular protein synthesis and repletion of body fat.

Normal bed-resting man expends about 1600 calories per day. With disease and stress this may commonly be increased 15 to 40 percent and with burns up to 100 percent. Thus 3000 calories per day will provide an excess of energy intake to all patients except the burn patient who will require 4000 to 5000 calories per day. Starved man will do well with a calorie-nitrogen ratio of 400 to 600. Critically ill man should probably have a calorie-nitrogen ratio no greater than 150, and a smaller ratio down to 100 (about 180 gm of protein for 3000 calories) would not overload his nitrogen disposal mechanisms, although it might waste some protein. This amount of protein is commonly catabolized at the peak of the acute protein catabolic response. Daily blood urea nitrogens should be obtained to be certain of this. Three thousand ml of the synthetic amino acid hyperalimentation fluid provides 18.75 gm of nitrogen per day and with 25 percent glucose provides 2550 calories of glucose plus 170 calories from the amino acids. This provides a calorie-nitrogen ratio somewhat over 150. If primary treatment successfully converts from the stress to the starvation catabolic state, this solution is more than adequate for support. However, if the patient remains septic or for any reason is thought to be remaining in the stress catabolic state, there should be no hesitation in increasing the amino acids administered by 100 to 200 percent. An increasing stress catabolic state in the stable patient on hyperalimentation is commonly signaled by increasing hyperglycemia and the hypercatabolic state by severe hyperglycemia. It is therefore of great value to follow the urinary glucose and expect to associate the onset of fever with increased hyperglycemia. Increased hyperglycemia also occurs for the same reason in the patient on amino acids without glucose.

Because of its hypertonic nature intravenous hyperalimentation should be administered via central venous catheter slowly throughout the 24 hours to simulate as much as possible the normal skeletal muscle release of amino acids and the normal hepatic output of glucose to the systemic body.

These desirable goals plus the normal specific gastrointestinal mucosa and liver hypernutrition may be better achieved by use of the gastrointestinal tract. This provides the additional benefit of absence of the septic complications of the intravenous route plus the use of many nutritional support materials that cannot be used intravenously. This route is commonly not used because of the existence of an ileus. An ileus involves predominantly the stomach and colon and the small intestine secondary to gas passing through the stomach. Clearly the gas- or fluid-distended intestine or obstructed intestine cannot be utilized. However, the patient with emesis and anorexia can commonly be supported via the gastrointestinal tract if the stomach is kept decompressed. This may be achieved by delivery of nutrient slowly throughout the 24 hours with the stomach on suction one-half hour out of each four. If this does not work, a long Cantor tube may be passed into the small intestine and a nasogastric tube passed. It is then possible to feed into the small intestine while decompressing the stomach. The same objectives may be achieved with multilumen tubes and with a gastrostomy and jejunostomy tubes. The objective is well worth the effort and risk involved.

Because the ileus involves the colon, this route of nutritional support should utilize one of the various elemental diets. These have the additional advantages of requiring minimal enzymatic digestion for absorption at a time when endocrine enzyme secretion may be restricted and of producing greater insulin release than the intravenous route so that hepatic synthetic activities are maximized. The hyperosmotic nature of the materials used plus the limitations of bowel mobility require 24-hour-a-day continuous slow delivery by pump much as with intravenous nutrition.

SUMMARY

Acute stress produces a catabolic state, one characteristic of which is a total body protein catabolic state. If this stress is perceived as acutely life-threatening, the hypercatabolic stress state is produced where insulin is either unresponsive or only slightly responsive to glucose. Resuscitation from the acute organ failures converts the hypercatabolic state to the stress catabolic state. The stress catabolic state is characterized by enhanced glucagon relative to glucose and an insulin that is normally or hyperresponsive to glucose. The stress catabolic state is secondary to a continuing organ failure or failures not immediately life-threatening and is best managed by treating the organ failure involved to convert the stress catabolic state to the starvation catabolic state. In the absence of effective immediate therapy such as of sepsis or continuing pulmonary failure, proper nutritional support is just as important as continued correct treatment of the primary organ failure. The stress catabolic state is a glucose-responsive state in such a way that intravenous glucose perpetuates total body protein catabolism and interference with the mobilization of a complete mixture of amino acids to the liver for hepatic protein synthesis. The prolonged use of pure intravenous glucose in this state is to be condemned, and the use of amino acids without glucose has much to commend in terms of supplying via the peripheral venous route specific hepatic nutrition and stimulating the oxidation of endogenous fat stores for energy. This, however, is basically a holding action with maximum effect on hepatic fat mobilization. Much preferred to the use of amino acids without glucose is the use of the elemental diet via the gastrointestinal tract because of its specific effects on gastrointestinal mucosa and liver hypernutrition and its restoration of the normal hepatic controls on input to the systemic body. This then allows normal neuroendocrine control of metabolism. The gastrointestinal tract may be utilized with appropriate precautions in the presence of an ileus but may not be utilized in small intestine distention or organic lesions. Under these conditions intravenous hyperalimentation is required. This should be administered continuously throughout the 24 hours to simulate as much as possible the normal skeletal release of amino acids and hepatic output of glucose.

CITED REFERENCES

1. Abbott, W. E.; Levey, S.; and Krieger, H.: Metabolic changes in surgical patients in relation to water, electrolytes, nitrogen and caloric intake. *Metabolism*, **8**:847–61, 1959.
2. Allardyce, D. B., and Groves, A. C.: A comparison of nutritional gains resulting from intravenous and enteral feeding. *Surg. Gynecol. Obstet.*, **139**:179–84, 1974.
3. Allison, S. P.: Carbohydrate and fat metabolism response to injury. In Lee, H. A. (ed.): *Parenteral Nutrition in Acute Metabolic Illness*. Academic Press, New York, pp. 197–211, 1974.
4. Allison, S. P.: High metabolic requirements states—

burns, severe multiple trauma. In Lee, H. A. (ed.): *Parenteral Nutrition in Acute Metabolic Illness*. Academic Press, New York, pp. 197–211, 1974.
5. Altura, B. M., and Hershey, S. G.: Reticulo-endothelial function in experimental injury and tolerance to shock. In Kovach, A. G.; Stoner, H. B.; and Spitzer, J. J. (ed.): *Neurohumoral and Metabolic Aspects of Injury*. Plenum Press, New York, pp. 545–71, 1973.
6. Angelakos, E. T.; King, M. P.; and Carballo, L.: Hypothalamic catecholamines and adrenergic innervation of hypothalamic blood vessels. In Kovach, A. G.; Stoner, H. B: and Spitzer, J. J. (eds.): *Neurohumoral and Metabolic Aspects of Injury*. Plenum Press, New York, pp. 509–19, 1973.
7. Avruch, J.; Carter, J. R.; and Martin, D. B.: The effect of insulin on the metabolism of adipose tissue. In Greep, R. O., and Astwood, E. B. (eds.): *Handbook of Physiology*. Vol. 1, Section 7. Williams & Wilkins, Baltimore, pp. 563–79, 1972.
8. Ban, T.: The hypothalamus and liver metabolism. *Med. J. Osaka Univ.*, **15**:275–91, 1965.
9. Ban, T.: The septo-preoptico-hypothalamic system and its autonomic function. *Prog. Brain Res.*, **21**:1–43, 1966.
10. Bane, A. E.; Sayeed, M. M.; and Wurth, M. A.: Potential relationships of changes in cell transport and metabolism in shock. In Kovach, A. G.; Stoner, H. B.; and Spitzer, J. J. (eds.): *Neurohumoral and Metabolic Aspects of Injury*. Plenum Press, New York, pp. 253–62, 1973.
11. Beisel, W. R., and Rapoport, M. I.: Inter-relations between adrenocortical functions and infectious illness. *N. Engl. J. Med.*, **280**:541–46, 596–604, 1969.
12. Bernard, C.: Leçons sur les phenomènes de la vie communs aux animaux et aux vegetaux. J. B. Bailliere, Paris, 1878.
13. Bierman, E. L.: Insulin and hypertriglyceridemia. In Shaffrin, E. (ed.): *Impact of Insulin on Metabolic Pathways*. Academic Press, New York, pp. 111–21, 1972.
14. Border, J. R.; Burns, G. P.; Rumph, C.; and Schenk, W. G.: Carnitine levels in severe infection and starvation: A possible key to the catabolic state. *Surgery*. (In press)
15. Border, J. R.: Metabolic response to short term starvation, sepsis and trauma. In Cooper, P., and Nyhus, L. M. (eds.): *Surgery Annual*. Appleton-Century-Crofts, New York, pp. 11–33, 1970.
16. Brennan, M. F.; Aoki, T. T.; Mueller, W. A.; and Cahill, G. F.: The role of glucagon as a catabolic hormone. *Surg. Forum*, **25**:72, 1974.
17. Cahill, G. F.; Aoki, T. T.; and Marliss, E. B.: Insulin and muscle protein. In Greep, R. O., and Astwood, E. B. (eds.): *Handbook of Physiology*. Vol. 1, Section 7. Williams & Wilkins, Baltimore, pp. 563–79, 1972.
18. Cahill, G. F.; Herrera, M. G.; Morgan, A. P.: Hormone fuel interrelationships during fasting. *J. Clin. Invest.*, **45**:1751–65, 1966.
19. Cahill, G. F.; Owen, O. E.; and Morgan, A. P.: The consumption of fuels during prolonged fasting starvation. *Adv. Enzyme Regul.*, **6**:143–50, 1968.
20. Caldwell, F. T.: Metabolic response to thermal trauma: II. Nutritional studies with rats at two environmental temperatures. *Ann. Surg.*, **155**:119–26, 1962.
21. Cannon, W. B.: *The Wisdom of the Body*. Morton, New York, 1932.
22. Cerasi, E., and Luft, R.: Pathogenesis of diabetes in man. In Shaffrin, E. (ed.): *Impact of Insulin on Metabolic Pathways*. Academic Press, New York, pp. 111–21, 1972.
23. Chaudry, I. H.; Planer, G. J.; Sayeed, M. M.; and

Baue, A. E.: ATP depletion and replenishment in hemorrhagic shock. *Surg. Forum*, **24**:77–79, 1973.

24. Chernov, M. S.; Cook, F. B.; Wood, Mac D.; and Hale, H. W.: Stress ulcer: A preventable disease. *J. Trauma*, **12**:831–33, 1972.

25. Clowes, G. H. A.; O'Donnell, T. F.; Ryan, N. T.; and Blackburn, G. L.: Energy metabolism in sepsis: Treatment based on different patterns in shock and high output stage. *Ann. Surg.*, **179**:684–96, 1974.

26. Coleman, W., and DuBois, E. F.: The influence of the high calory diet on the respiratory exchanges in typhoid fever. *Arch. Intern. Med.*, **14**:168–209, 1914.

27. Cuthbertson, D. P.: Physical injury and its effects on protein metabolism. In Munro, H. N., and Allison, J. B. (eds.): *Mammalian Protein Metabolism*. Vol. 2. Academic Press, New York, pp. 373–409, 1964.

28. Daly, J. M.; Steiger, E.; and Dudrick, S. J.: Postoperative nutrition and colonic wound healing, serum protein metabolism, and body weight. *Surg. Forum*, **23**:38–40, 1972.

29. Dudrick, S. J., and Copeland, E. M.: Parenteral hyperalimentation. In Nyhus, N. M. (ed.): *Surgery Annual*. Appleton-Century-Crofts, New York, pp. 69–97, 1973.

30. Duke, J. H.; Jorgenson, S. B.; Broell, J. R.; Long, C. L.; and Kinney, J. M.: Contribution of protein to caloric expenditure following injury. *Surgery*, **68**:168–74, 1970.

31. Eckhart, J.; Tempel, G.; Schreiber, U.; Schaaf, H.; Oeff, K.; and Schurnbrand, P.: The turnover of I^{125} labeled albumin after surgery and injury. In Wilkinson, A. W. (ed.): *Parenteral Nutrition*. Williams & Wilkins, Baltimore, pp. 93–99, 1972.

32. Egdahl, R. H.; Ryan, N. T.; George, B. C.; and Egdahl, D. H.: Chronic tissue insulin resistance following hemorrhagic shock. *Ann. Surg.*, **180**:402–408, 1974.

33. Elwyn, D.: The role of the liver in regulation of amino acid and protein metabolism. In Munro, H. N. (ed.): *Mammalian Protein Metabolism*. Vol. 4. Academic Press, New York, pp. 523–57, 1970.

34. Exton, J. A., and Park, C. R.: Interaction of insulin and glucagon in the control of liver metabolism. In Greep, R. O., and Astwood, E. B. (eds.): *Handbook of Physiology*. Vol. 1, Section, 7. Williams & Wilkins, Baltimore, pp. 437–56, 1972.

35. Fajans, S. S., and Floyd, T. C.: Stimulation of islet cell secretion by nutrients and by gastrointestinal hormones released during digestion. In Greep, R. O., and Astwood, E. B. (eds.): *Handbook of Physiology*. Vol. 1, Section 7. Williams & Wilkins, Baltimore, pp. 473–95, 1972.

36. Felig, P.: Interaction of insulin and amino acid metabolism in the regulation of gluconeogenesis. In Shaffrin, E. (ed.): *Impact of Insulin on Metabolic Pathways*. Academic Press, New York, pp. 111–21, 1972.

37. Field, J. B.: Insulin extraction by the liver. In Greep, R. O., and Astwood, E. B. (eds.): *Handbook of Physiology*. Vol. 1, Section 7. Williams & Wilkins, Baltimore, pp. 563–79, 1972.

38. Filstone, W. J.: The effects of environmental conditions on the metabolic requirements after injury. In Lee, H. A. (ed.): *Parenteral Nutrition in Acute Metabolic Illness*. Academic Press, New York, pp. 197–211, 1974.

39. Fine, J.: Shock and peripheral circulatory insufficiency. In Hamilton, W. F. (ed.): *Handbook of Physiology*. Vol. 3, Section 2. Williams & Wilkins, Baltimore, pp. 2037–71, 1965.

40. Flatt, J. P., and Blackburn, G. L.: The metabolic fuel regulatory system: Implications for protein-sparing therapies during caloric deprivation and disease. *Am. J. Clin. Nutr.*, **27**:175–87, 1974.

41. Fleck, A.; Ballantyne, F. C.; Filstone, W. J.; and Cuthbertson, D. P.: Environmental temperature and the metabolic response to injury-plasma proteins. In Kovach, A. G.; Stoner, H. B.; and Spitzer, T. T. (eds.): *Neurohumoral and Metabolic Aspects of Injury*. Plenum Press, New York, pp. 417–23, 1973.

42. Fleck, A., and Munro, H. N.: Protein metabolism after injury. *Metabolism*, **12**:783–89, 1963.

43. Frederickson, D. S.; Levy, R. I.; and Lees, R. S.: Fat transport in lipoproteins—an integrated approach to mechanisms and disorders. *N. Engl. J. Med.*, **276**:34–44, 94–103, 148–56, 215–25, 273–81, 1967.

44. Frohman, L. A.: The hypothalamus and metabolic control. *Pathobiol. Annu.*, **1**:353–72, 1971.

45. Furst, P.; Josephson, B.; and Vinnars, E.: The effect on the nitrogen balance of the ratio essential/nonessential amino acids in intravenously infused solutions. *Scand. J. Clin. Lab. Invest.*, **26**:319–26, 1970.

46. Goodall, Mc. C.; Stone, C.; and Haynes, B. W.: Urinary output of adrenaline and noradrenaline in severe thermal burns. *Ann. Surg.*, **145**:479–87, 1957.

47. Goodman, A. D.: Relationship of gluconeogenesis to ammonia production in the kidney. In Shaffrin, E. (ed.): *Impact of Insulin on Metabolic Pathways*. Academic Press, New York, pp. 111–21, 1972.

48. Goodner, C. J.; Tustison, W. A.; Davidson, N. B.; Chu, P. C.; and Conway, M. J.: Studies of substrate regulation in fasting. I. Evidence for central regulation of lipolysis by plasma glucose mediated by the sympathetic nervous system. *Diabetes*, **16**:576–89, 1967.

49. Groves, A. L.; Griffiths, J.; Leung, F.; and Meek, R. N.: Plasma catecholamines in patients with serious postoperative infection. *Ann. Surg.*, **178**:102–107, 1973.

50. Gump, F. E.; Long, C.; Killian, P.; and Kinney, J. M.: Studies of glucose intolerance in septic injured patients. *J. Trauma*, **14**:378–88, 1974.

51. Gump, F. E.; Long, C. L.; Geiger, J. W.; and Kinney, J. M.: The significance of altered gluconeogenesis in surgical catabolism. Submitted for publication to *J. Trauma*.

52. Harrison, T. S.; Seaton, J. F.; and Feller, I.: Relationship of increased oxygen consumption to catecholamine excretion in thermal burns. *Ann. Surg.*, **165**:169–72, 1967.

53. Hartroft, W. S.: The liver: Nutritional guardian of the body. In Gall, E. A., and Mostofi, F. K. (eds.): *The Liver*. Williams & Wilkins, Baltimore, pp. 131–50, 1973.

54. Howard, J. E.; Bigham, R. S.; and Mason, R. E.: Studies on convalescence. V. Observations on the altered protein metabolism during induced malarial infections. *Trans. Assoc. Am. Physicians*, **59**:242–47, 1946.

55. Howard, J. M.: Studies of the absorption and metabolism of glucose following injury. *Ann. Surg.*, **141**:321–26, 1955.

56. Hume, D. M.: Endocrine and metabolic response to injury. In Schwartz, S. I. (ed.): *Principles of Surgery*. McGraw-Hill, New York, pp. 1–65, 1969.

57. Jarnum, S.: Albumin synthesis after the administration of amino acid mixtures. In Wilkinson, A. W. (ed.): *Parenteral Nutrition*. Williams & Wilkins, Baltimore, pp. 93–99, 1972.

58. Johnstone, I. D. A.: Metabolic requirements after injury. In Lee, H. A. (ed.): *Parenteral Nutrition in Acute Metabolic Illness*. Academic Press, New York, pp. 273–78, 1974.

59. Johnston, I. D. A.; Tweedle, D.; and Spivey, J.: Intravenous feeding after surgical operations. In Wilkinson, A. W. (ed.): *Parenteral Nutrition*. Williams & Wilkins, Baltimore, pp. 189–98, 1972.

60. Keyo, A.: Caloric undernutrition and starvation with notes on protein deficiency. *JAMA*, **138**:500–511, 1948.

61. Kinney, J. M.; Duke, J. H.; Long, C. L.; and Gump, F. E.: Tissue fuel and weight loss after injury. *J. Clin. Pathol.*, **23**:(Suppl. 4) 65–72, 1970.

62. Kinney, J. M.: Energy significance of weight loss. In Cowan, G., and Schaetz, W. (eds.): *Intravenous Hyperalimentation*. Lea & Febiger, Philadelphia, pp. 84–96, 1972.

63. Levenson, S. M.; Braasch, J. W.; Mueller, H.; and Crowley, L.: Nitrogen metabolism following thermal injury. Cited by Levenson, S. M.; Pulaski, E. J.; and Del Guercio, L. R. M. Metabolic changes associated with injury. In Zimmerman, L. M., and Levine, R. (eds.): *Physiologic Principles of Surgery*. W. B. Saunders, Philadelphia, 1964.

64. Levenson, S. M.; Pulaski, E. J.; and Del Guercio, L. R. M.: Metabolic changes associated with injury. In Zimmerman, B. R., and Levine, R. (eds.): *Physiologic Principles of Surgery*. W. B. Saunders, Philadelphia, pp. 1–43, 1964.

65. Long, C. L.; Spencer, J. L.; Kinney, J. M.; and Geiger, J. W.: Carbohydrate metabolism in man: Effect of elective operations and major injury. *J. Appl. Physiol.*, **31**:110–16, 1971.

66. Majno, G.: Ultrastructure of the vascular membrane. In Hamilton, W. F. (ed.): *Handbook of Physiology*. Vol. 3, Section 2. Williams & Wilkins, Baltimore, pp. 2293–2377, 1965.

67. Masoro, E. J.: *Physiological Chemistry of Lipids in Mammals*. W. B. Saunders, Philadelphia, 1968.

68. Merimee, T. J., and Tyson, J. E.: Stabilization of plasma glucose during fasting. *N. Engl. J. Med.*, **291**:1275–78, 1974.

69. Moffat, J. G.; King, J. A. C.; and Drucker, W. R.: Tolerance to prolonged hypovolemic shock: Effect of infusion of an energy substrate. *Surg. Forum*, **19**:5–8, 1968.

70. Moore, F. D., and Ball, M. R.: *The Metabolic Response to Surgery*. Charles C Thomas, Springfield, Ill., 1952.

71. Moore, F. D.: *Metabolic Care of the Surgical Patient*. W. B. Saunders, Philadelphia, 1959.

72. Munro, H. N.: A general survey of pathological changes in protein metabolism. In Munro, H. N., and Allison, J. B. (eds.): *Mammalian Protein Metabolism*. Vol. 2. Academic Press, New York, pp. 267–321, 1964.

73. Munro, H. N.: Amino acids and metabolism and their relevance to parenteral nutrition. In Wilkinson, A. W. (ed.): *Parenteral Nutrition*. Williams & Wilkins, Baltimore, pp. 34–68, 1972.

74. Munro, H. N.: General aspects of the regulation of protein metabolism by diet and hormones. In Munro, H. N., and Allison, J. B. (eds.): *Mammalian Protein Metabolism*. Vol. 1. Academic Press, New York, pp. 382–483, 1964.

75. Neely, J. R., and Morgan, H. E.: Relationship between carbohydrate and lipid metabolism and the energy balance of heart muscle. *Annu. Rev. Physiol.*, **36**:413–59, 1974.

76. Owen, O. E., and Reichard, G. A.: Fuels consumed by man: The interplay between carbohydrates and fatty acids. *Prog. Biochem. Pharmacol.*, **6**:177–214, 1971.

77. Parra, A.; Garza, C.; Klish, W.; Garcia, G.; Argote, R.; Causeco, L.; Cuellar, A.; and Nichols, B. L.: Insulin-growth hormone adaptations in marasmus and kwashiorkor as seen in Mexico. In Gardner, L. I., and Amacher, P. (ed.): *Endocrine Aspects of Malnutrition*. Kroc Foundation, Santa Ynez, Ca., pp. 31–43, 1973.

78. Parra, A.; Serrano, P.; Chavez, B.; Garcia, G.; Argote, R.; Klish, W.; Cuellar, A.; and Nichols, B. L.: Studies of daily urinary catecholamines excretion in kwashiorkor and observed in Mexico. In Gardner, L. I., and Amacher, P. (eds.): *Endocrine Aspects of Malnutrition*. Kroc Foundation, Santa Ynez, Ca., pp. 31–43, 1973.

79. Parrilla, R.; Goodman, M. N.; and Toews, C. J.: Effect of glucagon: Insulin ratios on hepatic metabolism. *Diabetes*, **23**:725–31, 1974.

80. Pimstone, B.; Becker, D. T.; Hausen, J. D. L.: Human growth hormone and sulfation factor in protein calorie malnutrition. In Gardner, L. I., and Amacher, P. (eds.): *Endocrine Aspects of Malnutrition*. Kroc Foundation, Santa Ynez, Ca., pp. 31–45, 1973.

81. Pimstone, B.; Becker; Wenkove, C.; and Mann, M.: Insulin secretion in protein calorie manutrition. In Gardner, L. I., and Amacher, P. (eds.): *Endocrine Aspects of Malnutrition*. Kroc Foundation, Santa Ynez, Ca., pp. 31–43, 1973.

82. Platt, B. S.; Heard, C. R. C.; and Stewart, R. J. C.: Experimental protein-calorie deficiency. In Munro, H. N., and Allison, J. B. (eds.): *Mammalian Protein Metabolism*. Vol. 1. Academic Press, New York, pp. 382–483, 1964.

83. Pruitt, B. A.; Czaja, A. J.; and McAlhany, J. C.: Acute gastroduodenal disease after thermal injury: an endoscopic evaluation of incidence and natural history. *N. Engl. J. Med.*, **291**:925–29, 1974.

84. Rappoport, A. M.: Acinar units and the pathophysiology of the liver. In Rouiller, C. (ed.): *The Liver*. Academic Press, New York, pp. 266–330, 1963.

85. Robinson, H.; Cocks, T.; Kerr, D.; and Picou, D.: Fasting and postprandial levels of plasma insulin and growth hormone in malnourished Jamaican children during catch up growth and after recovery. In Gardner, L. I., and Amacher, P. (eds.): *Endocrine Aspects of Malnutrition*. Kroc Foundation, Santa Ynez, Ca., pp. 31–43, 1973.

86. Rosell, S., and Saltin, B.: Energy need, delivery and utilization in muscular exercise. In Bourne, G. (ed.): *The Structure and Function of Muscle*. Vol. 3. Academic Press, New York, pp. 186–223, 1973.

87. Rothschild, M. A.; Oratz, M.; and Schreiber, S. S.: Short-term measurements of serum protein synthesis. In Birke, G.; Norberg, R.; and Plantir, W. D. (eds.): *Physiology and Pathophysiology of Plasma Protein Metabolism*. Pergamon Press, New York, pp. 53–61, 1969.

88. Schaffner, F., and Popper, H.: Capillarization of hepatic sinusoids in man. *Gastroenterology*, **44**:239–42, 1963.

89. Schultz, K., and Beisbarth, H.: Post-traumatic energy metabolism. In Wilkinson, A. W. (ed.): *Parenteral Nutrition*. Williams & Wilkins, Baltimore, pp. 255–66, 1972.

90. Schumer, W., and Nyhus, L. M. (eds.): *Corticosteroids in the Treatment of Shock*. Illinois Press, Chicago, 1970.

91. Scrimshow, N.: Protein deficiency and infective disease. In Munro, H. N., and Allison, J. B. (eds.): *Mammalian Protein Metabolism*. Vol. 2. Academic Press, New York, pp. 569–93, 1964.

92. Shoemaker, W. C., and Elwyn, D. H.: Liver: Functional interactions within the intact animal. *Annu. Rev. Physiol.*, **31**:227–68, 1969.

93. Shoemaker, W. C.: *Shock*. Charles C Thomas, Springfield, Ill. 1967.

94. Spector, A.: Metabolism of free fatty acids. *Prog. Biochem. Pharmacol.*, **6**:130–76, 1971.

95. Unger, R. H., and Lefebvre, R. T.: *Glucagon: Molecular Physiology, Clinical and Therapeutic Implications*. Pergamon Press, New York, 1972.

96. Vaidynath, N.; Birkhahn, R.; Trietley, G.; Yuan, T. F.; Moritz, E.; Weissenhoffer, W.; McMenamy, R.; and Border, J. R.: Turnover of amino acids in sepsis and starvation: Effects of glucose infusion. Submitted to *J. Trauma*.

97. Viteri, F.; Behar, M.; Arroyave, G.; and Scrimshaw, N.: Clinical aspects of protein malnutrition. In Munro, H. N., and Allison, J. B. (eds.): *Mammalian Protein Metabolism*. Vol. 2. Academic Press, New York, pp. 523–69, 1964.

98. VonEuler, U. S.: Adrenal medullary secretion and its neural control. In Martini, L., and Ganong, W. F. (eds.): *Neuroendocrinology*. Vol. 2. Academic Press, New York, 1967.

99. VanOss, C. T.; Bronson, P. N.; and Border, J. R.: Changes in the serum alpha glycoprotein distribution in trauma patients. *J. Trauma* (in press).

100. Wilmore, B. W.; Orcutt, T. W.; Mason, A. D.; and Pruitt, B. A.: Alterations in hypothalamic function following thermal injury. Submitted for publication to *J. Trauma*.

101. Wilmore, D. W.; Moylan, J. A.; Lindsey, C. A.; Unger, R. H.; and Pruitt, B. A.: Hyperglucagonemia following thermal injury: Insulin and glucagon in the post traumatic catabolic state. *Surg. Forum*, **24**:99, 1973.

102. Witte, C. L.; Witte, M. H.; Dumont, A. E.; Frist, J.; and Cole, W. R.: Lymph protein in hepatic cirrhosis and experimental hepatic and portal venous hypertension. *Ann. Surg.*, **168**:567–77, 1968.

103. Wretland, A.: Amino acids. In Lee, H. A. (ed.): *Parenteral Nutrition in Acute Metabolic Illness*. Academic Press, New York, pp. 273–79, 1974.

104. Zierler, K. L.: Insulin, ions, and membrane potentials. In Greep, R. O., and Astwood, E. B. (eds.): *Handbook of Physiology*. Vol. 1, Section 7. Williams & Wilkins, Baltimore, pp. 347–69, 1972.

Chapter 2

PULMONARY AND CARDIOVASCULAR FAILURE

John R. Border

CHAPTER OUTLINE

Introduction
Acute Resuscitation
V—Stands for Ventilation
I—Stands for Infuse
P—Stands for Perfusion in Weil's Usage
P—Stands for Pulmonary Failure
R—Stands for Renal Resuscitation
Resuscitation Measurements
Ventilation
Acid-Base Balance
Bicarbonate
Summary: Acid-Base Balance
Blood Oxygen
  Oxygen Tension, Percent Oxyhemoglobin, Oxygen Content
  Arterial Oxygen Content, Arterial Hypoxia
  Mixed Venous Oxygen Tension, Cardiac Output, Oxygen Consumption
  Summary: Arterial Hypoxia in the Presence of Normal or Increased Ventilation
  Circulatory Failure, Shock
  Normal Physiology
  Venous Return to the Heart
    Summary
    Comment
  Blood Volume Regulation
  Interstitial Fluid Pressure
  Lymphatic Removal of Fluid from Interstitial Fluid
    Comment
  Cellular Fluid Volume Regulation
    Comment: Cellular Swelling, Interstitial Edema
    Comment: Blood Volume Regulation
  Shock Mechanisms
  Disorders of Peripheral Blood Flow
  Low Cardiac Output Shock
  Ventricular Outflow Obstruction
  Ventricular Failure
  Extracardiac Disorders of Diastolic Cardiac Filling

Valvular-Intracardiac Disorders
Disorders of Venous Return
Pulmonary Failure
Introduction
Normal Pulmonary Function
Relative Rate Consideration
Alveolar Barometric Pressure
  Summary
Carbon Dioxide Exchange
  Summary
The Lung as a Whole
Capillary Pressure
Pressure Flow Relationships
Effect of Lung Weight on Ventilation
Total Pulmonary Blood Volume Relative to Systemic Blood Volume
Summary: Control of Blood Flow Through Lung
Expiratory Ventilation
Physiology of Pulmonary Failure
Regional Hypoventilation
Blood Perfusion of Nonventilated Areas
Summary: Mechanisms of Arterial Hypoxia
Definition of Arterial Hypoxia
Mechanisms of Regional Hypoventilation
Extrapulmonic Causes of Regional Hypoventilation
Intrapulmonic Causes of Regional Hypoventilation
Perfusion of Nonventilated Alveoli (Atelectasis, Fluid-Filled Alveoli)
Summary: Regional Hypoventilation, Perfused Nonventilated Alveoli
Functional Residual Capacity
Regional Hyperventilation
Physiologic Dead Space
Interaction of Pulmonary Failure with the Rest of the Body
Management of Pulmonary Failure
Summary: Pulmonary Failure

Introduction

Cardiopulmonary failure is commonly acute, and there is nothing worse for the physician than the ordeal of watching a patient die and not knowing what to do. This is especially true for the young patient who has been in an accident or for the patient the surgeon has just operated upon. Every surgeon who has had any significant experience with patient care has, at some time or another, stood beside such a patient doing everything he could while watching a life slowly ebb away.

Lack of response of acute cardiopulmonary failure to therapy in general means inadequate therapy either in quantity, nature, or timing, and seldom means a disease process so advanced that it cannot be alleviated. The term cardiopulmonary failure has been carefully chosen here to be as specific as possible yet to include the spectrum of problems that can acutely cause death. It includes circulatory failure and pulmonary failure. The advanced circulatory failure which immediately precedes death is more popularly known as shock. Clinically, hypovolemic shock may be recognized as a state of diminished cerebration (apathy), diminished to absent urine output, arterial hypotension, tachycardia with tachypnea, pale cold skin, and absent peripheral veins. The exact shock mechanisms actively modify the clinical picture. Thus the patient with myocardial infarction and left ventricle failure may present with a primary picture not only of arterial hypotension but also of pulmonary edema and peripheral venous distention. The patient with severe sepsis early may have fever and arterial hypotension plus beet-red skin in the heat dispersal areas on the head, shoulders, forearms, and legs. Terminally when this patient develops the low cardiac output shock associated with sepsis, his temperature falls and the skin becomes cold and pale, but at much higher cardiac outputs than observed for the cold pale skin with hemorrhagic shock or myocardial infarction.

The experienced clinician can learn much from examination of the patient which, if combined with knowledge of the physiologic shock mechanisms to be elucidated subsequently, allows a much earlier start on the proper therapy. Shock is part of the act of dying, and early proper therapy is of the utmost importance.

Circulatory failure occurs separately from pulmonary failure essentially only in pure hypovolemic shock in the young healthy patient. Even under these conditions in the trauma patient severe pulmonary failure may and commonly does coexist with hypovolemic shock. In general, circulatory failure and pulmonary failure coexist, although one or the other may be dominant. The consequences of circulatory failure and pulmonary failure in terms of diminished oxygen delivery to the tissues are roughly the same. Also circulatory resuscitation cannot be achieved in the presence of severe arterial hypoxia nor can pulmonary resuscitation be achieved in the presence of severe circulatory failure. Therefore the objective is cardiopulmonary resuscitation with its two components of circulatory and pulmonary resuscitation. Such resuscitation can only be achieved by treatment aimed at reversing each and every one of the failure mechanisms active in both organ systems. Only acutely is it likely that circulatory or pulmonary failure will be due to one mechanism. Increased time in cardiopulmonary failure is associated with an increased number of active failure mechanisms until the situation becomes so complex that resuscitation cannot be achieved. The initial therapeutic decisions are therefore of the utmost importance.

In subsequent pages the physiologic mechanisms involved in normal circulation and pulmonary function will be presented and then analyzed in terms of cardiopulmonary failure. This is done because all rational therapy must aim to reverse all the physiologic mechanisms of failure. This subject has been very confused in the past because the clinician has tended to start therapy with clinical diagnoses which in one term may encompass several failure mechanisms. Thus the term "septic shock" encompasses a large number of circulatory failure mechanisms plus mechanisms of pulmonary and hepatic failure. This sort of clinical diagnosis has one major advantage in that it implies the septic process must be treated but major disadvantages in that no one therapy is apt to suffice for cardiopulmonary-hepatic resuscitation. The analysis of the problem into the physiologic mechanism of failure corrects this deficit and allows proper treatment.

Cardiopulmonary failure has a large number of metabolic consequences, and long-term survival demands that they be properly managed. This problem is considered in detail in the previous chapter on the metabolic response to sepsis, starvation, and trauma.

Acute Resuscitation

A patient who enters the emergency room or is found in the ward in acute life-threatening difficulties immediately becomes the focus of great activity. Uncontrolled, this may lead more to chaos than purposeful manipulation of physiologic parameters. A short concise guide, well-understood by all the members of the team, is required to guide therapeutic endeavors under these conditions. Weil has introduced, for cardiac patients, the VIP pneumonic.[1] *VIP* stands for "Very Important Person." We have converted it to *VIP—PROF* for general use. Very Important Person-Professor seemed sufficiently sarcastic that it was likely to be remembered.

V = Ventilation.

I = Infuse—the most common cause of shock is hypovolemia.

P = Perfuse in Weil's usage and pump failure in our usage, where the pump includes the ventricular outflow tracts, the pericardium, myocardium, and valves.

P = Pulmonary failure.

R = Renal failure.

ROF = Review organ failure—resuscitate all organs in failure, review antibacterial problems and take measures to prevent sepsis, review metabolic problems and consider especially hepatic problems. Review cerebral function and relationship to organ failures. Review and coordinate all problems.

V—Stands for Ventilation

Patients die most quickly of lack of ventilation. Difficulty in spontaneous ventilation may occur because of cerebral problems, upper airway problems, or thoracic-intrathoracic problems. The most common upper airway obstruction is the retracted tongue. This may be quickly corrected with an oropharyngeal airway or by turning the patient on his side or stomach. The patient with limited spontaneous ventilation who ventilates with ease passively, in general, has a cerebral limitation of ventilation. The patient with difficult passive ventilation has either upper airway or intrathoracic limitations of ventilation. The patient with upper airway disease, in general, has some degree of stridor with ventilation. All patients who are difficult to ventilate require immediate direct laryngoscopy and tracheal intubation. If these measures are not quickly successful, emergency tracheostomy is required. Repeated blind attempts at nasotracheal intubation should not be tolerated. If nasotracheal intubation does not succeed quickly, the patient should have direct laryngoscopy for diagnosis and intubation. This, again, should be done quickly or a tracheostomy performed. Tracheostomies are done most quickly by cutting down on the lower larynx and then passing a finger down the anterior tracheal wall, allowing all structures anterior to the trachea to be divided between the fingers so that any bleeders may be controlled by digital pressure until clamped. The trachea may then be entered via a simple stab wound for ventilation.

All patients with questionable ventilation of the slightest degree should be assisted with an oropharyngeal airway and face mask while being observed. Those difficult to ventilate should be intubated and placed on the ventilator in the emergency room while being observed. Those difficult to ventilate but without upper airway obstruction have intrathoracic-thoracic pathology that must be analyzed. The most common, and easily recognized, thoracic problem is a voluntary contraction of the expiratory muscles with bucking of ventilation. The other thoracic wall disorders, although they interfere with active ventilation, do not interfere with passive ventilation. Therefore, difficult ventilation unrelated to upper airway obstruction and voluntary bucking in general indicates intrathoracic pathology whose significance must be evaluated as discussed under pulmonary failure.

I—Stands for Infuse

Hypovolemia is statistically the most common cause of shock. Hypovolemic shock indicates a blood volume deficit of at least 1 liter and commonly more. Therefore, in general, one starts out to increase blood volume at least 1 liter. The rate of infusion and the fluids used will depend upon the blood pressure and the central venous pressure. Thus, if no blood pressure is present, two large-bore intravenous lines will be placed and the fluids pumped in as fast as they will go until a blood pressure is obtained. Ringer's lactate may be used acutely if the clinical characteristics suggest a low central venous pressure. If a high central venous pressure is present, secondary to right ventricle failure and not left ventricle failure, plasma should be used, because blood volume maintenance under these conditions is very dependent on colloid osmotic pressure. Ringer's lactate rapidly comes into equilibrium between the vascular and interstitial fluid volumes. Even under conditions of low central venous pressure only about one fourth of the volume administered stays in the vascular tree. Therefore, in general, to produce a prolonged increase in blood volume of 1 liter requires infusion of 4 to 5 liters of Ringer's lactate. Plasma and Ringer's lactate for blood volume resuscitation should be utilized only until blood is available. The patient who receives 2 to 3 liters of blood after external bleeding has stopped and then goes back into shock has either internal bleeding or pump failure.

P—Stands for Perfusion in Weil's Usage

It is better for rapid understanding to have P stand for pump failure. As used here, pump means all components of the heart including the pericardium and outflow arterial track. Failure of this combined mechanism is the second most common cause of circulatory failure. It is easiest to remember these mechanisms anatomically and by going in a direction opposite to blood flow. The mechanisms are:

Pump failure shock: Low cardiac output
A. Ventricular outflow obstruction
   Right versus left—most common on the right
B. Ventricular failure—pump failure
   1. Extracardiac disorders of cardiac filling
      The tamponades
      a. Pericardial
      b. Mediastinal
      c. Pleural
   2. Myocardial disorders
      a. Myocardial infarction
      b. Ventricular aneurysm
      c. Cardiac arrhythmias
      d. Myocardial failure
   3. Intracavitary disorders
      a. Acute valvular failure
      b. Acute septal defects

P—Stands for Pulmonary Failure

This is placed here so that the mechanisms of arterial hypoxia will be systematically explored. The results of arterial hypoxia without circulatory failure are largely the same as with circulatory failure since both produce tissue hypoxia. However, pulmonary failure with arterial hypoxia is much more dangerous since it is clinically not as obvious. We have seen arterial oxygen tensions of 27 in patients without cyanosis, cerebration disorders, or obvious clinical respiratory distress. These patients are the ones who seem to be doing well and then suddenly expire. They can only be detected when treatment is still possible by arterial blood gases. However, as detailed later, the analysis of arterial hypoxia requires simultaneous central venous blood gases and a known inspired oxygen so that the arterial hypoxia of circulatory failure may be differentiated from that due to pulmonary failure.

The mechanisms of arterial hypoxia are:
I. Circulatory failure
   Decreased mixed venous blood oxygen content. The arterial hypoxia will not respond to increased F_{IO_2}.
II. Pulmonary failure
   A. Regional hypoventilation–arterial oxygen responds to increased F_{IO_2}.
   B. Perfused nonventilated alveoli in the lung. The arterial oxygen does not respond to increased F_{IO_2}.

R—Stands for Renal Resuscitation.

The urine must be kept flowing at least 40 to 50 ml per hour or renal failure will occur. Oliguric renal failure is an extremely difficult situation in the patient who has had a recent laparotomy, a nasogastric tube, bleeding tendencies, and who is on the respirator with 100 percent humidity in the inspired gas and thus has essentially no insensible water loss.

If the electrolyte abnormalities, particularly of potassium, are controlled, patients do not die of renal failure. The high mortality rate associated with renal failure is largely secondary to the organ failures that produced the renal failure and not to the renal failure. The dominant organ system failure in this situation is circulatory failure. Oliguria must be analyzed first in terms of the mechanisms of circulatory failure. This does not necessarily imply arterial hypotension since this does not occur until cardiac output is reduced one third to one half. The most common cause of oliguria is hypovolemia. Our first maneuver is to increase the blood volume 1 liter under careful observation while getting central venous and arterial blood gases and considering the problem of systemic arteriovenous shunting in our interpretation of the central venous oxygen tension. The first hour the urine volume is less than 40 ml the patient will receive 80 mg of furosemide. If the urine volume does not improve the next one-half hour, he will receive 160 mg of furosemide and 25 gm of mannitol. If urine flow does not improve, the furosemide dose will be doubled half hourly until appropriate urine flows are obtained or 2000 mg of furosemide are given. We have seen urine flow begin at 2000 mg when it did not occur at 1000 mg and then continue.

Occasionally with this regime one will need to adjust the fluids for too much urine output. However, in these patients that is a rather easily manageable problem while oliguria or anuria can be very difficult to manage.

ROF stands for stop periodically, review organ function, and decide if the resuscitation is proceeding properly. If it is not, search promptly for errors in diagnosis or additional diagnoses. Someone in the resuscitation team must be the director and keep himself sufficiently free of the chaos to direct each individual into an harmonious whole, review the progress periodically, and consider possible additional measures.

Resuscitation Measurements

The most informative measures that can be made during resuscitation are the blood gases, blood pressure, central venous pressure, urine output, and urine specific gravity, Of these, the blood gases provide the single most informative measure of cardiopulmonary function, if both arterial and central venous blood are analyzed and the inspired oxygen is accurately known. Further, their analysis provides a detailed understanding of cardiopulmonary physiology. The blood gas measurements are oxygen tension, carbon dioxide tension, and pH. The carbon dioxide tension and pH allow calculation of the serum bicarbonate. These measurements in an emergency may be obtained in 10 to 20 minutes.

Ventilation

Arterial carbon dioxide tension provides the most direct measure of effective alveolar ventilation. The term "effective alveolar ventilation" is used here because of the calculated increase in physiologic dead space that occurs in critically injured man. Under these conditions normal mouth ventilation is consistent with alveolar hypoventilation. The normal minute mouth ventilation is about 5 liters. In these patients values of 10 to 20 liters are commonly required to maintain a normal arterial carbon dioxide tension. Normal arterial carbon dioxide tension ranges from 35 to 45 mm Hg. For reasons related to pulmonary failure to be discussed later, the patient on the ventilator commonly has a minute ventilation of 10 to 20 liters independent of his need for carbon dioxide control, and carbon dioxide tension is controlled by varying the external dead space between the head of the ventilator and the endotracheal tube. As little as zero and as much as 300 cc of dead space have been used. Arterial carbon dioxide tensions above 44 clearly indicate generalized hypoventilation. With one exception, this is in general only seen terminally or after medications which in one way or another interfere with ventilation. The exception involves the patient in severe pulmonary failure who has retained secretions. Here the tidal volume, although entering the major airways, is not evenly distributed to the alveoli. These patients typically have severe arterial hypoxia for their inspired oxygen (e.g., 50 mm Hg P_{O_2} on 100 percent oxygen), a rising arterial carbon dioxide tension, or, if on the ventilator, a decreasing dead space to maintain the same carbon dioxide tension, yet have been suctioned repeatedly with a straight catheter. They thus have a very high physiologic dead space with severe pulmonary failure. We have seen such patients respond dramatically to suctioning with a curved catheter (Caude) which truly suctions both bronchi. (e.g., 50 mm Hg P_{O_2} to 271 mm Hg P_{O_2} on 100 percent oxygen). This observation and several like it provide the primary reason why the measurement of tidal volume is not of great value by

itself in evaluating pulmonary function. In fact, we prefer to consider ventilatory failure as judged by mouth movement of air as an entirely different function from pulmonary failure although ventilatory failure eventually leads to pulmonary failure.

Acid-Base Balance

The calculated bicarbonate gives a measure of circulatory function in terms of the severe, rather prolonged failure compatible with shock if the serum sodium and chloride are simultaneously known. A metabolic alkalosis signifies *only* that the bicarbonate is increased and has no necessary relationship to pH without further assumptions. Similarly a metabolic acidosis signifies *only* that the bicarbonate is decreased and has no necessary relationship to pH without further assumptions. A respiratory acidosis signifies *only* that the carbon dioxide tension is increased and also carries no necessary implications about pH without further assumptions, although it does imply alveolar hypoventilation. Obviously a respiratory alkalosis implies *only* a decreased arterial carbon dioxide tension. Acid-base balance is so generally misunderstood that it is necessary to develop it somewhat in order to interpret blood gases.

The fundamental mass action equation which governs acid-base balance is:

1. $K = \dfrac{(H^+)\,(HCO_3{}^-)}{(H_2CO_3)}$

2. $(H_2CO_3) = k_1\,P_{CO_2}$

3. Statement 1 again

   $K = \dfrac{(H^+)\,(HCO_3{}^-)}{k_1\,P_{CO_2}}$

   The Henderson-Hesselbalch Equation

4. $(H^+) = \dfrac{K\,k_1\,P_{CO_2}}{(HCO_3{}^-)}$

Statement 4 makes it necessary to say something about both the respiratory state (P_{CO_2}) and metabolic state ($HCO_3{}^-$) in order to elucidate the hydrogen ion concentration. Since P_{CO_2} is generally measured these days and not calculated as it was when the fundamental relationship was explored in blood, it is far better simply to state the measured values and the calculated bicarbonate than to use any of the terms developed for early times.

Bicarbonate

The bicarbonate may be best understood as a filler anion. The law of electroneutrality requires that the sum of the positive cations equal the sum of the negative anions. The major cation in blood is sodium and the major anion is chloride. A chloride too high for the serum sodium produces a decrease in bicarbonate independent of the acidic products of anaerobic metabolism. The same thing occurs if the sodium is low and the chloride normal. Thus it is necessary to know the serum sodium and chloride in order to interpret the serum bicarbonate. The normal sodium is 140 to 145 and the normal chloride 100 to 105 with the difference in concentration about 40 mEq/L. This must be compared with a normal bicarbonate of 22 to 28 mEq/L. The burn patient who has been resuscitated with saline typically has a metabolic acidosis (decreased bicarbonate) on the basis of a normal serum sodium and a high serum chloride. Conversely the patient with voluminous acidic nasogastric suction has a metabolic alkalosis (high serum bicarbonate) on the basis of a low serum chloride relative to the serum sodium. These causes of metabolic acidosis or alkalosis may be readily discerned by measuring the serum sodium and chloride.

Hyperventilation may be secondary to a metabolic acidosis. We have seen a serum sodium of 135, serum chloride of 115, and serum bicarbonate of 9 without discernible circulatory difficulties in a patient who required large quantities of sodium and potassium and unfortunately received both as the chloride salt. This patient was severely hyperventilating and this was controlled by administering sodium bicarbonate.

In contrast to the changes that occur in the bicarbonate secondary to sodium and chloride are the changes that occur with circulatory failure sufficient to produce shock. Under these conditions the difference in concentration between the serum sodium and chloride is essentially normal, but the serum bicarbonate is grossly reduced. This reduction independent of sodium and chloride changes suggests the presence of an unmeasured anion. For shock this includes many anions; however, the predominant ones for anaerobic metabolism are lactate and pyruvate.

Summary: Acid-Base Balance

1. P_{CO_2} is a measure of alveolar ventilation. It decreases with hyperventilation and increases with hypoventilation.

2. Because of increases in the physiologic dead space, mouth hyperventilation is required to maintain a normal alveolar ventilation and normal P_{CO_2} in the critically ill patient.

3. The serum bicarbonate varies with the difference between the serum sodium and chloride.

4. A decreased bicarbonate in the presence of a normal serum sodium and chloride suggests the presence of unmeasured anions. When evidence for circulatory failure exists, this is generally lactate. A metabolic acidosis on this basis suggests severe circulatory failure with shock and responds to treatment of the circulatory failure.

5. The pH depends upon both the P_{CO_2} (respiratory state) and bicarbonate (metabolic state).

6. It is much better to give the measured values than to use the terms acidosis or alkalosis.

BLOOD OXYGEN
Oxygen Tension, Percent Oxyhemoglobin, Oxygen Content

The blood gas gives a value for oxygen tension (Figure 2–1). This is not the same as oxygen content or oxyhemoglobin but is related to these values by virtue of an equilibrium between oxygen in solution (oxygen tension) and hemoglobin to produce oxyhemoglobin. The amount of oxyhemoglobin present for a given oxygen tension depends upon the pH (Bohr effect), the temperature, and the concentration of 2-3 diphosphoglycerate in the red cell. Increases in pH, decreases in temperature, and decreases in 2-3 diphosphoglycerate increase the amount of oxyhemoglobin present for a given oxygen tension. This is a left shift curve (i.e., the percent oxyhemoglobin is greater for a given oxygen tension and the point is thus to the left of the normal curve).

The oxygen tension of arterial blood is normally 90 to 100 mm Hg with an oxygen content of about 20 cc (STPD) per 100 ml of blood (Figure 2–2). The oxygen tension of mixed venous blood is normally 40 mm Hg with an oxygen content of about 15 cc (STPD) per 100 ml of blood. Thus the arteriovenous oxygen content difference is about 5 cc per 100 ml of blood.

The oxygen tension–oxygen content relationship in blood is dependent upon the quantity of hemoglobin present per 100 ml of blood. This is normally about 14 gm per 100 ml.

Comments on Figure 2–1:

1. At the normal alveolar gas oxygen tension, the hemoglobin is essentially 100 percent oxyhemoglobin.

2. At the normal arterial oxygen tension hemoglobin is about 95 to 98 percent oxyhemoglobin.

3. Large increases in oxygen tension (inspired oxygen) above that required for 100 percent oxyhemoglobin produce only a small increase in oxygen content because the oxygen is free in solution.

4. Mixed venous blood has an oxygen tension of about 40 mm Hg and content of about 15 cc per 100 ml. However, because of the steep slope

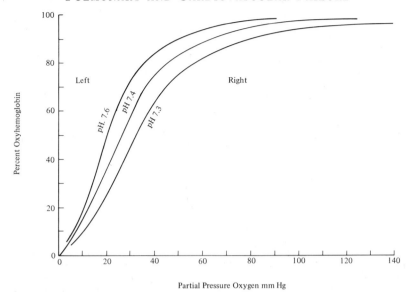

Figure 2–1. Percent oxyhemoglobin—P_{O_2}. This graph, incorporating the data of Hill, illustrates the effect of oxygen tension and pH on the reaction of oxygen with hemoglobin to form oxyhemoglobin. A shift of the curve to the left means that, for a given oxygen tension, oxygen is more firmly bound to hemoglobin, and the right shifted curve means that it is less firmly bound. A shift to the left occurs with an increase in pH, decrease in temperature, and decrease in 2-3 diphosphoglycerate in the red cells.

The effect of pH is important in normal oxygen transport since it aids oxygen pickup in the lungs and oxygen release in the tissues. It also shows how oxygen and carbon dioxide are related. About 80 percent of the carbon dioxide is transported from the tissues to the lungs without an increase in carbon dioxide tension.

As oxygen is picked up by hemoglobin in the alveolar capillary, carbon dioxide is evolved from plasma bicarbonate, and oxygen and carbon dioxide transport are linked. Therefore in regionally hypoventilated alveoli carbon dioxide is evolved only to the extent that oxygen is picked up. The opposite changes occur in the capillary so that oxygen release is linked to carbon dioxide pickup with minimal changes in carbon dioxide tension and therefore pH. However, to the extent that carbon dioxide tension and pH changes occur, they also act in the direction required to facilitate oxygen pickup in the lungs and release in the tissue.

2-3 diphosphoglycerate (2-3 DPG) is a normal product of the glycolytic energy cycle in the red cell which normally supplies the red cell with adenosine triphosphate for energy. It influences oxygen transport on a much longer term basis than the pH effect. An increase in 2-3 DPG decreases the affinity of hemoglobin for oxygen. A decrease in 2-3 DPG occurs in certain genetic enzymatic deficiency states characterized by a decrease in exercise tolerance and in bank blood stored in acid citrate dextrose. This problem may be alleviated by using fresh blood or glycerinated frozen red cells.

of the curve small changes in oxygen tension in the mixed venous blood are associated with large changes in oxygen content. Mixed venous oxygen tension is therefore a good index of oxygen content if the hemoglobin is known. We have seen mixed venous oxygen tensions as low as 13 mm Hg and as high as 62.

Arterial Oxygen Content, Arterial Hypoxia

The lung may be considered in the simplest analysis as having two sorts of blood which pass through it. One kind is exposed to alveolar gas and has the same oxygen tension. This normally constitutes 95 to 98 percent of cardiac output.

The second kind of blood has passed through the lungs without being exposed to alveolar gas and has the oxygen tension and content of mixed venous blood. This is normally 2 to 5 percent of cardiac output. This verbal statement may be rewritten mathematically where a = arterial, A = alveolar capillary blood, v = mixed venous blood, and c = oxygen content (solution plus that bound to hemoglobin).

1. $CaO_2 = XCAO_2 + YCvO_2$
   Normally $X = 0.98$ to 0.95 and $Y = 0.02$ to 0.05

One volume of arterial blood is therefore made up of X volumes of alveolar capillary

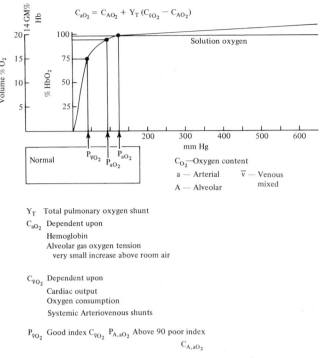

Figure 2–2. Arterial oxygen content. This presents the basic arterial oxygen content equation which is utilized in analyzing arterial hypoxia. The arterial oxygen content (C_{aO_2}) is dependent upon alveolar capillary blood oxygen content (C_{AO_2}), the relative volume of the total pulmonary shunt (Y_t), and the mixed venous oxygen content ($C_{\bar{v}O_2}$). The alveolar capillary blood oxygen content (C_{AO_2}) cannot be significantly increased by inspired oxygen once 100 percent oxyhemoglobin is reached (oxygen tension about 120 mm Hg at normal pH and 2-3 DPG) because the only increase is that of oxygen in solution. This increase in going from an oxygen tension of 120 to 600 mm Hg is less than 10 percent of the oxygen bound to hemoglobin. Thus large increases in oxygen tension above 120 mm Hg have very little effect on alveolar capillary blood oxygen content.

In contrast, because the mixed venous oxygen tension of 40 mm Hg is on the steep portion of the oxyhemoglobin dissociation curve small changes in mixed venous oxygen tensions are associated with large changes in mixed venous oxygen content. Mixed venous oxygen content is controlled by the rate of total body oxygen consumption, cardiac output, and systemic arteriovenous shunting.

In the presence of a perfect lung ($Y_t = O$) mixed venous oxygen content has no effect on arterial oxygen content. However, the greater the pulmonary shunt (increasing Y_t), the greater the effect of changes in mixed venous oxygen content. Under these conditions increasing mixed venous oxygen content increases arterial oxygen content and vice versa. The question must therefore always be asked as to how much of the arterial hypoxia is due to pulmonary failure and how much due to circulatory failure or, conversely, how much of an improved arterial oxygen tension is due to decreasing pulmonary failure and how much due to increasing cardiac output.

The point may be made differently; the difference between alveolar and arterial oxygen tensions may not be used to evaluate pulmonary failure alone because increasing pulmonary failure commonly coexists with increasing cardiac output so that increasing pulmonary failure may coexist with an unchanged difference between alveolar and arterial oxygen tension because of the increasing cardiac output.

Thus, in general, evaluation of the degree of pulmonary failure requires exact knowledge of the inspired oxygen, arterial oxygen content, and mixed venous oxygen content. Therefore, no method of oxygen delivery can be utilized which does not deliver a precisely known oxygen concentration. This means that in general nasal oxygen and masks should not be utilized unless the masks have a tight fit and that arterial oxygens cannot be evaluated without mixed venous oxygens. Practically, it is commonly necessary to utilize central venous oxygens in place of mixed venous oxygens.

blood plus Y volumes of mixed venous blood. Therefore

2. $1 = X + Y$ and $X = 1 - Y$

The initial equation may be rewritten substituting $(1 - Y)$ for X:

3. $CaO_2 = (1 - Y)CAO_2 + YCvO_2 = CAO_2 + Y(CvO_2 - CAO_2)$

Equation 3 is of the utmost importance in interpreting arterial hypoxia. In the second term $[Y(CvO_2 - CAO_2)]$ CAO_2 is always greater than CvO_2, and therefore this whole term is always subtracted from CAO_2 (first term) to decrease the alveolar capillary blood oxygen content to obtain arterial oxygen content. CAO_2 in the presence of normal alveolar ventilation cannot be significantly increased by increasing the inspired oxygen content above room air because the oxyhemoglobin is already saturated and the additional oxygen tension is expended in increasing the oxygen in solution. Therefore, the magnitude of the term to be subtracted to obtain the arterial oxygen content from the alveolar capillary blood oxygen content in normal ventilation on room air depends only upon the relative volume of mixed venous blood passing through the lungs without picking up oxygen (Y) and the oxygen content of mixed venous blood. The volume of blood passing through the lungs without picking up oxygen (Y) may be considered in terms of normal pulmonary function to pass through a pulmonary arteriovenous shunt. The exact nature of this shunt will be discussed later under pulmonary failure. The calculated value Y therefore constitutes a quantitative but inverse measure of the effectiveness of pulmonary oxygen transport from alveolar gas to alveolar capillary blood. We have seen calculated pulmonary arteriovenous shunts as high as 80 percent of cardiac output. However, the values in the severely ill patient are more commonly in the range of 20 to 60 percent.[8] An increasing calculated Y indicates increasing pulmonary failure.

Mixed Venous Oxygen Tension, Cardiac Output, Oxygen Consumption

The mixed venous oxygen tension is normally carefully controlled at about 40 mm Hg, and therefore oxygen content depends largely upon the quantity of hemoglobin and whether or not the oxyhemoglobin curve is in normal position for oxygen tension. The mixed venous oxygen tension depends upon the rate of oxygen consumption, the cardiac output, and the presence or absence of peripheral systemic arteriovenous

shunting. In the absence of systemic arteriovenous shunting, reduced mixed venous oxygen tensions indicate an inadequate cardiac output for the patient's metabolic needs. We have seen such values as low as 13 mm Hg in the presence of systemic arteriovenous shunting. A normal or high mixed venous oxygen tension may still not be compatible with a cardiac output great enough to maintain a normal arterial blood pressure. Under these conditions (usually in association with severe sepsis) we have seen arterial hypotension with mixed venous oxygen tensions as great as 62 mm Hg and have seen the arterial pressure rise with further increases in cardiac output and mixed venous oxygen tension. A reduced mixed venous oxygen tension has always been associated with a reduced cardiac output. However, a normal or high mixed venous oxygen tension, although compatible with normal or high cardiac output (relative to a statistical normal), does not necessarily mean that the cardiac output is as high as the patient needs. This can only be judged by arterial pressure, skin color, urine output, cerebration, and clinical condition.

The equation developed shows that arterial hypoxia may occur because of a reduction in mixed venous oxygen content and therefore a reduction in mixed venous oxygen tension. This only occurs with a reduction in cardiac output and therefore low cardiac output circulatory failure. In fact, the reduction in mixed venous oxygen tension occurs almost instantaneously, and therefore this measurement reflects circulatory failure considerably before a metabolic acidosis occurs and often before arterial hypotension ensues (see discussion of the relationship of arterial pressure to cardiac output under Circulatory Failure, Shock). This is of great value since the objective in managing the critically ill is not managing the clinical shock state but avoiding it.

In the equation developed for arterial oxygen content, the alveolar capillary blood oxygen content is reduced by the term Y $(CvO_2 - CAO_2)$. It is apparent that if both Y and CvO_2 increase this term may remain unchanged. Therefore increasing pulmonary failure associated with increased cardiac output may not result in arterial hypoxia. The arterial hypoxia produced by pulmonary failure may be alleviated or prevented by increased cardiac work in the form of increased cardiac output. For this reason a single arterial blood gas or the differences between alveolar gas and arterial oxygen tensions cannot by themselves be used as a measure of pulmonary failure because they do not take into account the variation that occurs in the mixed venous oxygen content.

Summary: Arterial Hypoxia in the Presence of Normal or Increased Ventilation

1. Arterial hypoxia may occur because of circulatory failure or pulmonary failure or both.

2. Pulmonary failure is characterized by an increased volume of mixed venous blood passing through the lungs without picking up oxygen [increased volume of shunt blood (Y)].

3. Low cardiac output circulatory failure is characterized by a low mixed venous oxygen tension and content.

4. A high cardiac output may prevent or alleviate the arterial hypoxia secondary to pulmonary failure by increasing the oxygen content of the mixed venous blood (Y) which passes through the lung without picking up oxygen.

5. Circulatory failure may occur with normal or high cardiac output (increased mixed venous oxygen content) as judged by excess serum lactate, arterial hypotension, decreased urine output, and a clinical shock state. These patients require control of their peripheral shunt and a higher cardiac output.

Circulatory Failure, Shock

Circulatory failure may be defined as a cardiac output less than the body's need. The extreme circulatory failure that, if not reversed, precedes death is known as shock. Shock may be defined as a generalized decrease in capillary blood flow to the extent that irreversible degenerative tissue changes occur in a relatively short time. Circulatory failure may in general occur because of factors that limit cardiac output (low cardiac output failure) or because of factors that alter the peripheral distribution of blood flow (e.g., systemic arteriovenous shunts, normal or high cardiac output shock).[6] To understand circulatory failure requires an understanding of the normal controls of cardiac output and arterial pressure.

Normal Physiology*

The blood flow to each organ is controlled by the metabolic activity of the organ with three exceptions. The exceptions are skin (heat

---

* This discussion is based largely on the work of Guyton and various associates.[25] The rational treatment of shock demands a complete understanding of normal cardiovascular physiology such as presented by Guyton. A simpler discussion is presented in his textbook of physiology.[26] There are a great number of small books available on the shock state. These include Thal,[49] Shoemaker,[45] and Weil and Shubin,[51] as particularly good personal views of the problem. Fine has summarized his views in the *Handbook of Physiology*.[17] Both Lillihei[30] and McLean[32] have summarized their views in textbooks.

dissipation), kidney (waste excretion), and the lung (must accept all cardiac output independent of metabolic needs). The controls of blood flow to each organ are placed at the arterioles since this is the region of greatest pressure drops. However, the controls of blood flow within the organ rest largely at the precapillary area with only a fraction of the capillaries being open at any one time. The arterioles are controlled largely by their sympathetic nervous system

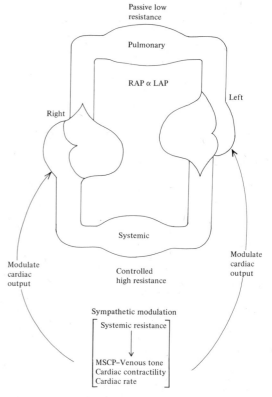

Figure 2–3. Normal circulation. Abbreviations: *RAP*, right atrial pressure; *LAP*, left atrial pressure; *MSCP*, mean systemic circulatory pressure.

The controls of cardiac output normally are those that regulate venous blood volume, cardiac contractility, and rate. They are modulated by the sympathetic nervous system. Normally the pulmonary circulation has a low resistance and does not influence cardiac output. The factors that control right ventricular output therefore also control left ventricle cardiac output (RAP is proportional to LAP). Any factor that increases cardiac output translocates blood from the systemic veins to the lungs and thus recruits capillaries so that, as cardiac output increases, increased oxygen transport occurs in the lungs not only because of increased flow rate, but also because of an increase in the number of capillaries.

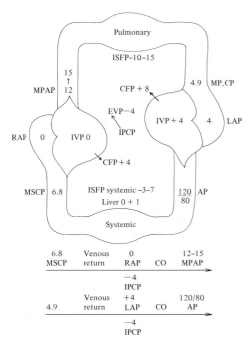

Figure 2–4. Normal circulation pressures. Abbreviations: *ISFP*, interstitial fluid pressure; *MSCP*, mean systemic circulatory pressure; *RAP*, right atrial pressure; *IVP*, intraventricular pressure; *MPAP*, mean pulmonary artery pressure; *MP,CP*, mean pulmonary circulatory pressure; *LAP*, left atrial pressure; *EVP*, extraventricular pressure; *CFP*, cardiac filling pressure; *AP*, arterial pressure; *IPCP*, intrapericardial pressure—synonymous with EVP. MSCP and MPCP are those pressures that exist if the heart is suddenly stopped and all pressures equalized before secondary hypoxic changes occur.

These values are those recorded by Guyton in the dog. There is constant flow with superimposed pulsations. Factors affecting the pressure are the osmotic pressure, blood volume, interstitial fluid volume, and transport of substrate from the circulation. The pressure available to cause blood to flow to the heart is MSCP-RAP and on the left MPCP-LAP. This difference must always be positive or blood will not flow from the periphery to the heart. Thus MSCP must always be greater than RAP and MPCP greater than LAP. The pressure available to fill the heart during diastole is the CFP, which is equal to IVP-EVP. Normally IVP is equal to the atrial pressure. Filling of the heart during diastole depends upon CFP, diastolic ventricular compliance, and the time available. Normally increased systolic contractility is associated with increased cardiac rate and diastolic compliance. Thus, the same factors that increase systolic ejection also increase diastolic cardiac filling, venous return, energetic substrate mobilization, and pulmonary oxygen and

innervation and secondarily by humoral substances.[24] There are two major exceptions. Both the brain and heart have a very careful autoregulated flow independent of the sympathetic nervous system. Thus sympathetic arteriolar vasoconstriction diverts blood flow to the heart and brain to meet their metabolic needs. This is not true of the hypothalamus in the brain where sympathetic modulation of blood flow occurs. In contrast the controls at the precapillary sphincter are largely based on metabolism in the immediate area. This allows minute-to-minute redistribution of blood flow from capillary to capillary as local metabolic needs change.

The control of organ blood flow at the arteriole is a changing resistance to flow mechanism. In order for such a mechanism to work, a reasonably constant pressure head is required in the larger arteries. This is provided by an elaborate system of pressure sensors which then feed back through the brain to control total peripheral resistance, myocardial contractility, and cardiac output by controlling the venous vasomotor tone and therefore mean circulatory pressure and ultimately venous return (Figure 2–3). The cardiac output is normally equal to the sum of the blood flow needs of the organs plus the blood flow required for heat dissipation and filtration of the blood for urine formation. The heart thus acts as a controlled pump set to pump whatever volume is required to maintain the inflow venous pressure and the outflow arterial pressure constant. Thus cardiac output

carbon dioxide transport. Cardiac rates above 180 interfere with diastolic filling and to a lesser extent at 140.

Interstitial fluid pressure is normally negative. Interstitial fluid volume is at a minimum, therefore the distance between circulation and tissue cells is minimal. The interstitial fluid pressure varies from organ to organ; it depends upon the capillary protein permeability, the capillary hydrostatic pressure, and lymphatic flow. An increase in capillary protein permeability lowers the colloid osmotic pressure. An increase in capillary hydrostatic pressure above the colloid osmotic pressure causes movement of fluid from the capillaries to the tissues. Edema occurs if this fluid is not removed equally rapidly by the lymphatic system. Edema fluid produces cellular malnutrition by increasing the distance of diffusion; the most critical nutrient is probably oxygen.

Normally the lung has the lowest interstitial fluid pressure and is the organ best protected against edema, while the liver, with its sinusoidal wall completely permeable to protein, is the least well protected and, because of its anatomic position, is the organ most exposed to high capillary hydrostatic pressures.

in the end is controlled by the controls of venous return.[25]

Venous Return to the Heart

In supine man without exercise there are no pumps on the venous side to aid return flow to the heart (Figure 2–4). The situation here is different from exercising man in whom muscular and tissue massage of the veins together with one-way valves produces a venous return pump. In supine nonexercising man the venous blood must be returned against the diastolic pressure within the ventricle. For blood to flow back to the heart there must be a pressure greater in the periphery than intraventricular diastolic pressure. Guyton and associates have established that this pressure is the mean circulatory pressure largely controlled by venous vasomotor tone and blood volume and largely independent of arterial pressure and arterial vasomotor tone. The mean circulatory pressure is that pressure which exists in the circulation if all flow is suddenly stopped and all pressures equalized before secondary hypoxic changes occur. In the dog it is 6.8 ± 1.2 mm Hg which together with a mean right atrial pressure of zero gives a pressure head for venous return to the heart of 6.8 ± 1.2 mm Hg. The mean circulatory pressure depends upon both blood volume and the sympathetic nervous system that controls venous vasomotor tone. In the dog mean circulatory pressure may be increased at constant blood volume to 20 mm Hg by infusion of epinephrine and at constant venous vasomotor tone is a function of blood volume. In order for blood to flow to the heart, the mean circulatory pressure must exceed the right atrial pressure. Since central venous pressures of 25 to 30 cm H_2O occur in man, it is apparent that the mean circulatory pressure must be capable of achieving values higher than 25 to 30 cm H_2O. Because it is the lowest pressure in the circulation independent of cardiac pumping activity the mean circulatory pressure is an important pressure in the controls of blood volume. Increases in mean circulatory pressure beyond the normal mean capillary hydrostatic pressure of 12 to 15 mm Hg must be counterbalanced by increases in capillary hydrostatic pressure. The increased capillary hydrostatic pressure must be expended against the plasma colloid osmotic pressure and tissue pressure. Increased central venous and therefore mean circulatory pressure of this magnitude can cause transudation of fluid from the vascular volume to the interstitial fluid space. If this is so severe that lymphatic activity cannot return it to the blood rapidly enough, edematous hypovolemia will occur and the mean circulatory pressure, central venous pressure, and venous return will be reduced. It is particularly important to maintain the colloid osmotic pressure by maintaining the serum albumin in patients whose central venous pressure cannot be lowered because of right ventricle diastolic cardiac filling considerations.

Summary. Venous return can be summarized as follows:

1. Cardiac output is normally controlled by the venous return so that central venous pressure remains relatively constant.

2. Venous return in supine nonexercising man is controlled by the difference in pressure between the mean circulatory pressure and the central venous pressure.

3. The mean circulatory pressure depends upon both venous vasomotor tone and blood volume.

4. Venous vasomotor tone is largely controlled by the sympathetic nervous system.

Comment. Hypovolemia produces a low cardiac output by a decreased mean circulatory pressure which in turn decreases central venous pressure, right ventricle diastolic cardiac filling pressure, and finally cardiac output. In the presence of normal lungs and a normal left ventricle, right atrial pressure accurately reflects left atrial pressure and left ventricle diastolic filling pressure. Therefore the mechanisms of venous return by controlling right ventricle cardiac output also control left ventricle cardiac output. This relationship is based upon the very low pulmonary vascular resistance. Any factor that increases pulmonary vascular resistance in principle requires a higher right atrial pressure to achieve the same left atrial pressure. Many such factors will be discussed later that increase pulmonary vascular resistance or decrease left ventricle contractility and thus distort the relationship between right atrial pressure and left atrial pressure. Endotoxemia in all species produces as one of several effects a decreased venous return in the presence of an unchanged blood volume. This is compatible with a decreased venous vasomotor tone. The same phenomenon occurs with spinal anesthesia and spinal cord transection shock. Blood losses exceeding 500 to 1000 ml occur in man with no great change in cardiac output or central venous pressure. This observation is compatible with changes in venous vasomotor tone sufficient to maintain the same mean circulatory pressure. It suggests strongly that measured blood volumes will not be of nearly as much value in the clinical management of bleeding as central venous pressure and more direct measurement of cardiac output versus the body's metabolic needs (e.g., central venous oxygen tensions).

Patients in severe cardiac failure have an increased norepinephrine output and serum level.[15] This is needed to support their high mean circulatory pressure. However, it also fixes their venous vasomotor tone. These patients have relatively rigid veins and therefore go into shock with much smaller blood losses and into pulmonary edema with much smaller increases in blood volume.

Blood Volume Regulation

Blood volume regulation results from a series of many independent processes. It is regulated acutely at the capillary level and by lymphatic activity which returns fluid from the interstitial fluid to the circulation via the thoracic duct and lymph node lymphatico-venous connections.[35] The lymphatico-venous connection returns crystalloid fluid devoid of protein, while the thoracic ducts return a protein-rich fluid.

Starling's law remains the basic law of the capillaries. However, it is now recognized that the pressures are different than those previously used. The colloid osmotic pressure depends upon the permeability of the membrane to which the colloid is exposed. The usual value given is about 25 mm Hg. However, this is the value obtained with a membrane in vitro completely impermeable to protein. The capillary endothelial membrane varies in permeability to protein from organ to organ and probably with disease states.[23,33] Thus the lung capillary membrane is normally very impermeable not only to protein but also to salts.[18,20] Therefore in the lung the plasma colloid osmotic pressure is close to that recorded in vitro. In contrast, the hepatic sinusoids are permeable to albumin and by electron microscopy have large pores.[33] Thus in the liver there should be no, or a very low, plasma colloid osmotic pressure in spite of the same serum concentration of protein. Other capillaries in the body vary between these extremes.[33] Effective plasma colloid osmotic pressure is thus not a constant function throughout the body.

The capillary hydrostatic pressure as measured directly by Landis was found to be about 25 mm Hg.[29] However, there are several difficulties with interpretation of this as the usual capillary hydrostatic pressure. First is that most of the time capillaries have no flow and thus the mean capillary hydrostatic pressure at any one time must be less than that in the capillaries with flow. Second, the mechanical act of cannulating a capillary obstructs flow so that the pressure measured will be the mean pressure in the flowing capillary plus the pressure drop that usually occurs due to flow. Thus the directly measured pressure must be greater than that

existing in the capillary with flow. The problem is further complicated by known organ variations. Thus the lung capillary hydrostatic pressure, granted the pressure which exists on both sides, cannot be much greater than about 10 mm Hg. The same sort of problem exists in the liver where most of the blood passes through under the very low gradient of pressure produced between the portal vein and the hepatic vein. It is obvious that in the liver, because of the very low effective colloid osmotic pressure, a very low sinusoidal pressure is required in order not to flood the liver with edema fluid. In the liver this is aided by fibrous tissues that allow increased interstitial fluid pressure. The systemic vessels in general have an arteriole that limits the pressure presented to the capillary. In contrast, the lung has no such arteriolar structure per se to protect it from increased pressures.

Capillary hydrostatic pressure is generally less than the 25 mm Hg measured directly by Landis. The exact value depends upon the organ and the physiologic condition at the time.[23]

Interstitial Fluid Pressure

Interstitial fluid pressure has in general been assigned a value close to zero. It is apparent now from the work of Guyton that the interstitial fluid pressure is negative with systemic values commonly in the range of -3 to -7 mm Hg.[23] A negative interstitial fluid pressure means that all excess fluid has been sucked out of the tissue so that its solid components are brought into apposition to maintain the shape of the organ. Interstitial edema is accompanied by a rise in interstitial fluid pressure to roughly zero or slightly positive. At this pressure large volumes of fluid may be added between the solid components without appreciably changing interstitial fluid pressure. In contrast, when the interstitial fluid volume and pressures are normal, removing small volumes of fluid produces a great increase in the negative pressure. Thus the compliance of the interstitial fluid system $(\Delta V/\Delta P)$ is biphasic with, at normal values, a very small compliance for further fluid removal but at edema levels and at normal levels a very large complicance for fluid addition. The negative interstitial fluid pressure therefore signifies that the interstitial fluid volume has been reduced to a minimum. It now seems clear that only a small percentage of the interstitial fluid is free and that most is bound to ground substance. The ground substance together with collagen and cells contitutes the solid elements of the tissue. The lymphatic system is basically a set of sewers with pumps produced by one-way valves, with tissue massage of the lymphatic vessel producing one-way movement. This system responds to uncleared free water in the tissues much as our sewers respond to liquid free water but not to water bound to dirt. In organs where the lymphatics do not reach the parenchyma, provision is made for movement of liquid water to the lymphatics. Thus it appears quite clear in the lung that free water can traverse the surface of the alveolus to reach the terminal lymphatics. Since the free water contains the transuded protein and salts, the lymphatics also control the interstitial fluid colloid osmotic pressure.

Lymphatic Removal of Fluid from Interstitial Fluid

The lymphatics empty into the veins either via the thoracic duct or via lymphatico-venous communications at the lymph nodes. The flow of lymph is thus delivered against venous pressure by rather weak pumps, and as might be expected, increased venous pressure decreases lymphatic flow. This has been most clearly demonstrated for thoracic duct flow. Thus the edema secondary to congestive cardiac failure is not only secondary to increased capillary hydrostatic pressure (increased mean circulatory pressure) but also to decreased lymphatic removal of fluid with increased interstitial colloid osmotic pressure. Inflammation is associated, at least in the rabbit ear, with obstruction of the lymphatics, probably on the basis of release of clotting elements through the now permeable capillary with clotting in the lymphatics. Inflammatory edema is therefore in part due to lymphatic obstruction.

Comment. In view of the preceding discussion it is possible to classify organs in terms of their resistance to edema. The lung has a negative interstitial fluid pressure of -10 to -15 mm Hg and is thus maximally protected against edema if the serum albumin is maintained and left ventricular failure does not occur. In contrast, as all clinicians know, the liver quickly enlarges with an increase in central venous pressure and is thus poorly protected against edema. Further the liver just as promptly diminishes in size as the cardiac failure and the central venous pressure are reduced.

Cellular Fluid Volume Regulation

Cellular volume is regulated independently of interstitial fluid volume by virtue of active ion transport across the cellular wall.[50,53] However, active ion transport requires energy usually contributed by consumption of adenosine triphosphate. Adenosine triphosphate may be synthesized by either aerobic metabolism or anaerobic glycolysis. The source of the ATP varies from organ to organ. Thus the red cell has no mitochondria, and transport energy is chiefly provided by anaerobic glycolysis. The renal medulla, although it has mitochondria, subsists in an area of regional tissue hypoxia and procures most of its energy from anaerobic glycolysis. Any factor that interferes with the supply of adenosine triphosphate, if severe enough, may lead to cellular swelling by the entrance of isotonic extracellular fluid into the cell.

Cellular swelling may also occur on an osmotic basis independent of active ion transport. The cell normally contains large protein molecules which are continually being broken down and resynthesized. Any factor that increases protein breakdown or decreases protein synthesis leads to the conversion of a few large osmotically active particles to many small osmotically active particles and thus an increase in osmolality which will then draw water into the cell. The forces involved in cellular swelling are based on osmosis and are capable of developing enormous pressures. This is in distinct contrast to the forces involved in interstitial edema which are at most those of capillary hydrostatic pressure.

Comment: Cellular Swelling, Interstitial Edema. Cellular swelling cannot be detected with the usual tracer compartment techniques. Shock has been shown to be associated with a reduced transcellular membrane potential compatible with decreased active ion transport. Further it is associated with an interstitial fluid pressure that remains more negative than usual when all the blood removed is returned and only reverts to normal with additional Ringer's lactate.[28] It is thus probable that cellular edema occurs generally with shock of sufficient intensity and duration to limit ATP synthesis.

The compartment syndromes provide a good clinical example of localized cellular swelling. These occur after prolonged interruption of the arterial blood supply and are characterized by very tense muscle compartments with total aseptic necrotic gangrene of the muscle if not relieved. Recognized early enough, they may be effectively treated by incising the fascial envelope of the muscle compartment. The pressures they generate are high enough to prevent arterial inflow and thus far above the pressures generated by interstitial edema. Cellular swelling does not become significant during the period of no flow but occurs after flow is restored. It is thus apparent that restoration of blood flow to an extremity after a prolonged interruption should be associated with a fasciotomy.

Burns provide an example of edema with multiple mechanisms. The charred area has been deprived of blood supply and the protein denatured. Little swelling occurs here. Underneath is an area of damaged cells with protein breakdown osmotic swelling. Deeper yet are cells damaged sufficiently to produce cellular swelling due to decreased active sodium transport. Associated with this area is also vascular damage with interstitial edema. Several years ago attempts were made to control extremity burn edema by placing the extremity in casts. Interstitial edema should be easily controlled this way; however, the observations were that the edema was under sufficient pressure to interfere with arterial blood flow, strongly suggesting a significant component of cellular swelling in burn edema.

Comment: Blood Volume Regulation. Blood volume regulation depends upon colloid osmotic pressure, external and internal fluid loss, and upon the rate of supply of exogenous extracellular fluid. With hypoalbuminemia, hypovolemia may coexist with generalized edema. Since interstitial fluid volume is normally at a minimum, little fluid can be mobilized from this area. In the absence of external supplies of Ringer's lactate, hemodilution secondary to blood loss occurs slowly in man, and the hematocrit is an unreliable indicator of changes in blood volume. With adequate external supplies of Ringer's lactate the hematocrit changes much more rapidly by virtue of the fluid administered, making the washout of albumin from tissue spaces and changes in hematocrit a much more reliable indicator of changes in blood volume. Cellular and interstitial edema constitute obligatory losses of vascular fluid and are associated with a rising hematocrit and hypovolemia in the absence of adequate external fluid supplies. Unreplaced external fluid losses (NG suction, fistula, insensible water loss) also produce hypovolemia, which in the pure state is associated with a rising hematocrit. Trauma and severe sepsis are associated with a rapidly falling serum albumin and edematous hypovolemia, which in the pure state is associated with a rising hematocrit. We have seen values as low as 1.25 gm percent in 24 hours in the previously depleted patient. To maintain an acceptable serum albumin we have had to give as much as 250 ml of plasma every two hours. When this is done, blood volume is well maintained, pulmonary edema is not a problem, and the peripheral edema is reduced even though the central venous pressure may measure 20 to 25 cm H_2O for weeks.

Blood volume is best maintained by giving more fluid in the form of Ringer's lactate and free water than the patient needs and by maintaining the serum albumin. Small excesses of Ringer's lactate are well tolerated. Continued small deficits lead to death.

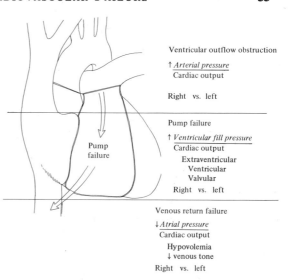

Figure 2–5. Low cardiac output shock mechanisms. Low cardiac output shock mechanisms are best thought of as ventricular outflow obstruction, pump failure, and failure of venous return. Factors affecting the right side must be differentiated from those affecting the left side. Ventricular outflow obstruction on the left side is uncommon, while right-sided obstruction, because of the filtering action of the lungs and the lesser myocardial mass, is common.

The pump failures are extraventricular, ventricular, and valvular. Extraventricular disorders affect both ventricles, while the most common ventricular and valvular disorders affect the left heart. The greater the pulmonary resistance to blood flow, the more important right ventricular pumping activity becomes.

Venous return failure in the presence of normal lungs primarily affects the right side of the heart and secondarily the left side of the heart. Causes are hypovolemia, spinal anesthesia, spinal cord transection, and sepsis.

Shock Mechanisms

The shock mechanisms physiologically may be divided into the following (Figure 2–5):

I. Disorder of peripheral blood flow
Physiologically equivalent to systemic arteriovenous shunting
High cardiac output shock

II. Pump failure
A. Ventricular outflow obstruction
B. Extracardiac disorders
The tamponades—pleural, mediastinal, pericardial
C. Ventricular failure
1. Disorders of contraction
a. Myocardial failure
b. Aneurysms—asynergy

2. Arrhythmias
3. Septal defects
D. Valvular disorders
1. Stenoses
2. Regurgitation
III. Disorders of venous return
A. Hypovolemia
B. Inadequate venous vasomotor tone

Disorders of Peripheral Blood Flow

This shock mechanism has the physiologic characteristics of systemic arteriovenous shunting.[10,46] These are a low total peripheral resistance, a low arteriovenous oxygen content difference with a high mixed venous oxygen content, and a high excess lactate indicating tissue hypoxia. Systemic arteriovenous shunting clearly occurs in the dermal subpapillary venous plexus and in the areas of inflammation. The subpapillary venous plexus is a heat dispersal mechanism of the body to which arterioles are connected via direct arteriovenous anastomoses. This mechanism is present in the extremities, head, neck, and shoulders. Patients with systemic arteriovenous shunting in these areas have very warm skin which may, in the presence of an adequate cardiac output, become beet red. Clearly these patients have large heat losses from these areas. If the cardiac output falls, these heat dispersal areas severely vasoconstrict. Blood flow through these areas therefore can be controlled, and the skin temperature in the heat dispersal areas is one guide as to whether or not cardiac output is adequate for all metabolic needs. The increased skin temperature is one reflection of the increase in the temperature of the thermoneutral zone of the sick patient which is also reflected by an increase in core temperature to febrile levels. This subject is discussed in depth in the chapter on the metabolic response. Systemic arteriovenous shunting behavior also exists in other areas of the body. This is most clearly seen in areas of inflammation and is not well understood.

Simultaneous with increased cardiac output due to a peripheral maldistribution of flow, the septic patient also has increased blood flow to the liver.[22] Thus the requirement for increased cardiac output with sepsis occurs on the basis of multiple mechanisms. There is no satisfactory universally accepted therapy for this peripheral maldistribution of blood flow. The major therapy available at present is to further increase cardiac output so that blood flow is adequate to meet the needs of the effective shunts plus the metabolic needs of the body.[46] This commonly means cardiac outputs two to three times the expected statistical normal. An adequate cardiac output under these conditions is one that maintains good urine output, warm pink skin, and good arterial pressure. This is achieved predominantly by high central venous pressures and the positive inotropic agents digitalis, isoproterenol, and glucagon. The height of the central venous pressure required depends largely on the degree of pulmonary failure present and the magnitude of the increase in pulmonary artery pressure required secondary to the pulmonary failure. The greater the central venous pressure required, the more it is dependent upon the colloid osmotic pressure and therefore maintenance of plasma albumin. As discussed under metabolism, there are many reasons for the plasma albumin to fall rapidly under these conditions. The plasma albumin must be carefully monitored and maintained if high central venous pressures are required.

Systemic arteriovenous shunting is seen most clearly in severely septic patients whose blood volume is well maintained and whose ventricular failure is properly treated. Systemic shunting also occurs in cirrhotic patients and probably in association with a variety of other shock mechanisms.[10,46] It is clear that there is a range of cardiac outputs in myocardial infarction patients where the degree of shock, as judged by plasma lactate, does not correlate well with the cardiac output. These patients probably have both a limitation of cardiac output and a peripheral maldistribution of blood flow. Hepatic dysfunction is commonly associated with this peripheral maldistribution of blood flow.[22] It is unknown whether or not this is cause and effect or whether both are effects of some as yet unknown cause. However, since the two coexist, it is wise to provide vigorous hepatic support while simultaneously treating the circulatory and pulmonary disorders of sepsis.

Patients with peripheral systemic arteriovenous shunting who do not respond quickly to measures designed to increase cardiac output should probably be treated with massive doses of steroids.[31] Clearly this should not be postponed until the steroids are given routinely to the dying patient as a sort of intravenous holy water. Methylprednisolone sodium succinate may be given in a dose of 30 mg per kilogram intravenously. An effect should occur in one to two hours, if all measures designed to increase cardiac output are maintained. The dose may then be repeated every four hours if there are signs of the effect wearing off.

The exact effect of massive doses of steroids has been very difficult to define. Clearly steroids should enhance the hepatic amino acid supply by enhancing skeletal muscle amino acid release. There is evidence that they may act as vasodilators. The steroids given do have access to the hypothalamus since this area has no blood-brain barrier and may have important effects there.

Berke has discussed the terminal syndrome of peripheral arteriovenous shunting when cardiac output falls with sepsis as a syndrome of increased beta adrenergic activity and has used beta adrenergic blockers to treat it with some success.[5] However, these simultaneously blockade an important positive inotropic effect and therefore must be accompanied by positive inotropic agents which do not act via beta receptors. Further the beta blockade was utilized in the presence of high central venous pressures and massive doses of steroids. This in effect means digitalis or glucagon.

Low Cardiac Output Shock

This occurs either because of pump failure or venous return failure. Pump failure may occur because of ventricular outflow obstruction, the cardiac tamponades, ventricular failure, or valvular failure.

Ventricular Outflow Obstruction

Ventricular outflow obstruction is common on the right side of the heart and uncommon on the left side (Figure 2–6). It may be central or peripheral. On the left side of the heart central ventricular outflow obstruction may occur because of dissecting aortic aneurysms or crossclamping of the aorta during vascular repairs. Peripheral left ventricular outflow obstruction is secondary to severe arteriolar vasoconstriction. This may occur secondary to exogenous infusion of vasoconstrictors in late shock of any cause, or secondary to increased intracranial pressure with endogenous severe sympathetic arteriolar vasoconstriction.[17] Left ventricle outflow obstruction leads to left ventricle failure because of the increased arterial pressure. The degree of increase in pressure required depends upon myocardial contractility. Thus the normal left ventricle can support very high arterial pressures, while the left ventricle in failure may have increased failure with rather moderate arterial pressure increases. Systemic vasodilating agents are used to treat left ventricle failure that does not respond adequately to positive inotropic agents.[31] This includes phenoxybenzamine, Regitine, and massive doses of steroids. Of these, massive doses of steroids are the safest to use. Isoproterenol has a vasodilating effect in addition to its positive inotropic effect. However, the vasodilation occurs principally in skeletal muscle and is therefore not in a desired area.

More important than the use of vasodilators in treating severe left ventricle failure unrespon-

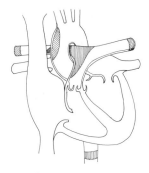

Central obstruction
    Right: Thromboemboli
    Left: Aneurysm

Peripheral obstruction
    Right: Pulmonary failure
        Emboli
        Fat
        Microthrombus

        Sepsis
        Local
        Distant
    Trauma
    Left: Vasoconstrictors
        Endogenous
        Exogenous

Figure 2–6. Ventricular outflow obstruction. Ventricular outflow obstruction may be central or peripheral. The central ventricular outflow obstructions are generally diagnosed by angiography, but peripheral obstructions must be inferred from an increase in vascular resistance. Ventricular outflow obstruction may result in acute myocardial failure. Ventricular outflow obstruction, because of the filtering action of the lungs, is much more common on the right side of the heart. It often occurs acutely, as in pulmonary embolism. Left ventricular obstruction is more often associated with chronic failure. An increase in intracranial pressure can cause vasoconstriction, left ventricular failure, and pulmonary edema, even in a previously healthy patient.

The many factors that contribute to pulmonary failure also contribute to right ventricular failure. However, if pulmonary function can be improved and there is adequate time, survival can occur.

sive to positive inotropic agents is the avoidance of vasoconstrictors so that peripheral circulation is normally controlled. There is one exception to this. The patient with left ventricle failure from coronary artery stenosis requires vasoconstrictors to produce a high enough pressure to provide blood flow to the uninfarcted but compromised left ventricle and thus treat its failure.[51] This is best given as norepinephrine so that a positive inotropic effect is simultaneously obtained. Thus the use of norepinephrine in the treatment of the left ventricle failure associated with myocardial infarction appears rational. However, it must be remembered that if given in too great a dose, it can induce left ventricle failure as well as several other undesirable changes. It is therefore generally given in a dose that produces an arterial systolic pressure about 20 mm Hg below normal and never in a dose that produces hypertension.

Right ventricle outflow obstruction is far more common than left ventricle outflow obstruction.

Central obstruction on this side is most commonly due to large pulmonary thromboemboli while peripheral obstruction may be due to fat emboli, microthromboemboli, pulmonary failure, or chronic obstructive lung disease. The right ventricle outflow obstructions are therefore largely due to structural changes in the lung which are unresponsive to chemotherapeutic agents. There is one significant exception related to pulmonary thromboemboli where the use of heparin may relieve associated vasoconstriction.[44] Right ventricle outflow obstruction is best handled by treatment of its associated right ventricle and pulmonary failure and prevention of further embolic phenomena while endogenous processes clear the emboli already present.

Right ventricle outflow obstruction alters the normal relationship between right venticle diastolic filling pressure and left ventricle diastolic filling pressure so that progressively higher right atrial pressures are required to achieve a given left atrial pressure. These patients may require central venous pressures of 25 to 30 cm H_2O in order to have an adequate cardiac output and are therefore in distinct contrast to patients with left ventricle failure where central venous pressure of 15 cm H_2O may be dangerous.

Ventricular Failure

Ventricular failure may occur on the right or left sides of the heart or on both sides and may be defined as a decreased cardiac output for a given diastolic cardiac filling pressure. The cardiac filling pressure is the difference between diastolic intraventricular and extraventricular pressures.[25] Intraventricular pressure is normally equal to the atrial pressure in the absence of atrioventricular valve disorders. The extraventricular pressure is equal to the intrapericardial pressure. Diastolic cardiac filling depends upon filling pressure and compliance. Normally any factor that increases systolic contractility also increases diastolic compliance, so that in a state of increased cardiac output a greater diastolic filling occurs for a given cardiac filling pressure. In general, increased sympathetic activity increases venous return, cardiac rate, diastolic cardiac filling, and systolic contractility so that all factors involved in increased cardiac output are simultaneously enhanced.[25]

Ventricular failure may occur on the basis of disordered contraction, myocardial failure, or both.[11] The contraction of the ventricle is a carefully coordinated process (Figure 2–7) that may become disordered from infarction or contusion so that one segment of the wall does

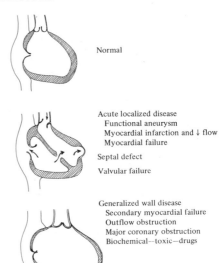

Normal

Acute localized disease
   Functional aneurysm
   Myocardial infarction and ↓ flow
   Myocardial failure
Septal defect
Valvular failure

Generalized wall disease
   Secondary myocardial failure
   Outflow obstruction
   Major coronary obstruction
   Biochemical—toxic—drugs

Electrical disorders
   Tachycardia
   Bradycardia
   Fibrillation

Figure 2–7. Acute ventricular failure. This may occur because of localized or generalized disease or because of electrical disorders. The patient with a myocardial infarction has a surrounding zone of hypoxia which has considerable potential for generating arrhythmias. This region, by virtue of its asynergy, may act as a functional aneurysm. Expansion of the infarction may be produced by anything that decreases blood flow or increases oxygen consumption in the region. Blood pressure must be maintained or expansion of the infarction will occur, and drugs that increase cardiac rate or myocardial oxygen consumption, such as isoproterenol, should not be utilized.

The infarcted area may also produce acute ventricular failure by production of septal defects or rupturing the chordae tendineae, producing acute mitral regurgitation. Trauma may also cause acute ventricular failure.

Factors that produce generalized wall disease are, in general, those that respond to positive inotropic agents. These agents alleviate the problem but do not reverse it until the primary cause is corrected.

not contract to the proper degree at the proper time. This is known as asynergy.[11] The area of asynergy is one of reduced blood flow and relative ischemia to infarction. It is therefore a focus of arrhythmias and an area of limited blood flow myocardial failure. The infarcted area and the area of blood flow myocardial failure may be extended by any factor that increases local oxygen consumption or reduces blood flow further. Local oxygen consumption may be increased by tachycardia, while reduction in blood flow may occur on the basis of hypotension. Recent advances in therapy have been

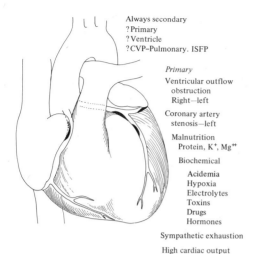

Always secondary
? Primary
? Ventricle
? CVP–Pulmonary. ISFP

Primary
Ventricular outflow
obstruction
Right—left

Coronary artery
stenosis—left

Malnutrition
Protein, K⁺, Mg⁺⁺

Biochemical

Acidemia
Hypoxia
Electrolytes
Toxins
Drugs
Hormones

Sympathetic exhaustion

High cardiac output
Failure

Figure 2–8. Myocardial failure. Myocardial failure is always a secondary process which may be alleviated by positive inotropic agents. However, complete reversal demands diagnosis of the primary cause and its treatment, as in septic shock, barbiturate intoxication, addisonian crisis, severe malnutrition, and severe acidemia.

predicated on increasing blood flow to this area with drugs and by increasing appropriately arterial pressure.[16] The most obvious example of asynergy is a ventricular aneurysm in which the contracting segments expel blood not only into the aorta but also into the aneurysm. The result is ventricular failure that may not be associated with myocardial failure and therefore not responsive to positive inotropic agents. Ventricular failure without myocardial failure may also occur because of acute septal defects.

Myocardial failure is by far the most common cause of ventricular failure and is essentially always a secondary process (Figure 2–8). The treatment of myocardial failure with positive inotropic agents should therefore always be associated with attempts to define the primary cause. Thus the myocardial failure secondary to ventricular outflow obstruction can be alleviated by positive inotropic agents but cannot be effectively treated unless the ventricular outflow obstruction is relieved. The myocardial failure secondary to coronary artery stenosis cannot be treated effectively without increasing coronary blood flow, although again it may be alleviated. The high cardiac output failure that occurs with sepsis is best handled by treatment of the septic process, although time may be purchased by positive inotropic agents and steroids. The circulatory failure that occurs secondary to acidosis, arterial hypoxia, or

electrolyte imbalances is best dealt with by treating these entities. The major exception to this lies in the disorders that occur secondary to shock where treatment of the shock mechanism is most important in reversing the arterial hypoxia and metabolic acidosis. The myocardial failure that occurs secondary to severe malnutrition is secondary to myocardial losses of protein, potassium, and magnesium and is best treated by management of these systemic body deficiencies. Insulin is important in the cellular transport of sodium and potassium and particularly important in the heart because of the link between potassium concentrations and myocardial contractility and arrhythmias. Low insulin concentrations with cellular potassium losses may occur with diabetic ketoacidosis and with the hypercatabolic state secondary to trauma or sepsis. If these are superimposed on a previous depleted state, restricted myocardial contractility may occur which responds to intravenous potassium, glucose, and insulin as described by Blackburn.[13]

The essential problem in ventricular failure is to differentiate the structural components from the biochemical components and then to differentiate the various biochemical components. The biochemical component left after correction of all blood electrolyte, hypoxia, and acid-base disorders is that responsive to positive inotropic agents. In practice this is done in a different way in the sense that blood volume is replaced until the patient is deliberately somewhat hypervolemic. Simultaneously electrolyte and acid-base disorders are corrected and then positive inotropic agents are given. The ventricular failure unresponsive to these measures is then investigated in terms of structural disorders and potassium depletion. This allows treatment of the statistically more common problems and limits the number of patients who must be screened for the more uncommon problems.

Extracardiac Disorders of Diastolic Cardiac Filling

Any factor that increases the extracardiac pressure requires a corresponding increase in the intraventricular pressure in order for adequate diastolic cardiac filling to occur (Figure 2–9). If the intraventricular pressure cannot be increased enough, diastolic cardiac filling will be limited and cardiac output will fall. Increases in extracardiac pressure may be produced by pericardial tamponade, mediastinal tamponade, and pleural tamponade. In general, an increase in the extracardiac pressure limits diastolic cardiac filling in both the right and left ventricles but is reflected only by an increase in the right atrial pressure. The major diagnostic problem is

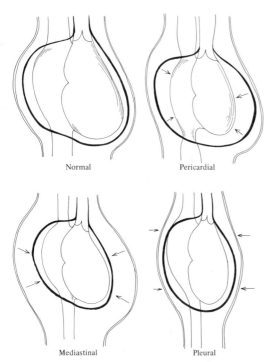

Normal   Pericardial

Mediastinal   Pleural

Figure 2–9. Extraventricular pump failure; tamponades—both ventricles. This form of pump failure occurs as a result of increase in the pressure outside of the heart and generally involves both ventricles. If the intraventricular pressures can be raised sufficiently, normal cardiac output may be achieved but at a higher atrial pressure. When the pressure outside of the heart rises high enough that increased atrial pressures can no longer compensate, cardiac output falls. In penetrating wounds of the heart, extraventricular pump failure may be associated with hypovolemia. Thus, with penetrating wounds, the patient commonly enters with hypovolemia and a low central venous pressure which then rises rapidly as blood volume is repleted.

differentiating the extracardiac tamponades from isolated right ventricle failure, usually secondary to right ventricle outflow obstruction.

Pericardial tamponade from penetrating injuries is usually easily differentiated as the blood loss is replaced and the central venous pressure rapidly rises from that of the initial hypovolemia to the high pressures of pericardial tamponade. Pericardial tamponade from blunt trauma or uremic pericarditis is far more difficult to differentiate, and the diagnosis can only be made for certain by pericardiocentesis with withdrawal of fluid and relief of the pericardial tamponade.[41]

Mediastinal tamponade typically occurs in the patient with ruptured mediastinal vessels,

usually the aorta. These are characterized, because of the common fibrous sheath of the superior mediastinal veins and arteries, by signs of superior vena cava obstruction, together with signs of blood loss both systemically and in the mediastinum. The typical picture is that of distended neck and hand veins together with a widened mediastinum by x-ray and arterial hypotension with a low central venous pressure. As blood volume is replaced, the central venous pressure rapidly rises just as it does with penetrating pericardial tamponade with blood loss.

Pleural tamponade may occur in the anxious gasping patient in the emergency room who by gasping is performing repeated Valsalva maneuvers. This problem is easily recognized if considered and quickly treated by reassurance. Sometimes, however, the patient cannot be reassured and also has arterial hypoxia secondary to his abnormal ventilatory patterns. These patients are recognized when they are intubated, their circulation improves, and their arterial hypoxia disappears. Pleural tamponade also occurs in the patient with compliant lungs who is placed on the ventilator with positive end expiratory pressure. In general this occurs with the patient who has relatively minimal pulmonary failure and who has arterial hypoxia largely on the basis of hypovolemic circulatory failure. This misuse of positive end expiratory pressure may be avoided if central venous blood gases and pressure are obtained simultaneously with the arterial blood gases. Positive end expiratory pressure is very poor therapy for hypovolemia.

Pleural tamponade secondary to positive end expiratory pressure may also occur in the patient who has had severe pulmonary failure and whose lungs have improved to the point that their compliance allows transmission of the pressure to the heart. In general if the patient is not hypovolemic, he can easily generate the additional 5 to 10 cm H_2O of pressure utilized in positive end expiratory pressure. Thus hypotension in response to the application of the usual positive end expiratory pressure is indicative of hypovolemia and is best treated both by removal of the positive end expiratory pressure and by transfusion of 500 to 1000 ml of blood. The patient is then placed back on positive end expiratory pressure.

Valvular-Intracardiac Disorders

Both myocardial infarction and cardiac trauma may produce not only areas of contusion or infarction but also rupture of chordae tendineae with valvular regurgitation and septal defects (Figure 2–7). These additional components of the circulatory failure will never be recognized unless they are kept in mind and searched for. In the presence of normal lungs both right ventricle valves may be excised and circulation well maintained because the central venous pressure can be increased enough to perfuse the lungs. The same considerations probably apply to right ventricle contusions and infarctions as long as the lungs are normal. Thus in the presence of right ventricle valvular damage every effort must be made to prevent pulmonary failure, pulmonary thromboemboli, and fat emboli in order to achieve survival.

The problems in the left ventricle are considerably different. Mitral regurgitation sufficient to raise the pulmonary capillary hydrostatic pressure equal to the colloid osmotic is regularly followed by immediate severe pulmonary edema. This may be treated, if not too great, by the use of the ventilator with positive end expiratory pressure in order to buy time for a more detailed consideration of the possibility of valve replacement surgery. Aortic regurgitation, by providing an additional source of filling during diastole, can raise the diastolic pressure and both limit diastolic filling and raise left atrial pressure. If left atrial pressure is sufficiently increased, pulmonary edema will also occur. If this does not happen, cardiac output will be reduced with the degree of reduction dependent upon the degree of regurgitation.

The effect of septal defects depends on their exact anatomy and the volume of flow. No further discussion will be undertaken since the point is that the diagnosis be considered with ventricular failure unresponsive to the usual therapy following trauma or myocardial infarction.

Disorders of Venous Return

Venous return may be limited because of hypovolemia or disorder of venous vasomotor tone.[25] Decreases in venous return produce a fall in central venous pressure and are easily recognized if they are isolated entities. However, when decreased venous return occurs concomitantly with any of the several shock mechanisms normally requiring an increased central venous pressure or an increase in central venous oxygen tension, the decision as to what central venous pressure indicates hypovolemia is very difficult.[7] Again if the problem is in the right ventricle a low central venous oxygen tension clearly indicates that the central venous pressure is not high enough. However, if the central venous oxygen tension is normal, this does not necessarily indicate that the central venous pressure is high enough unless arterial pressure, urine output, and skin temperature are normal.

Normovolemia in the severely ill patient is difficult to define. Statistical predictions as to normovolemia generally have an error of plus or minus a liter of blood unless corrections are made for fat masses. These corrections are difficult to make except on a statistical basis and may therefore be quite incorrect for the individual patient.[37] Any factor that increases central venous pressure produces some degree of venous distention and thus requires a blood volume in excess of the blood volume required at a normal central venous pressure. The large veins are the most compliant segments of the vasculature, and the distention produced by increased pressure may involve large volumes of blood unless there is a corresponding considerable increase in venous vasomotor tone. Because of the preceding problems measured blood volumes are of very little use, whereas the physiologic parameters of effective blood volume (i.e., central venous pressure, pulmonary artery wedge pressure, mixed venous oxygen tension) are of great use.

Edema and increased total body water have no necessary relationship to blood volume or to venous return. Venous return and cardiac output are related by the cardiac filling pressure, and under conditions of no increase in extracardiac pressure, changes in cardiac filling pressure may be equated to changes in atrial pressure. Capillary hydrostatic pressure must always be greater than atrial pressure in order for blood to flow to the heart. Any factor that increases capillary hydrostatic pressure so that it exceeds colloid osmotic pressure causes transudation of fluid from the vasculature to the tissues. Edema occurs if the transuded fluid is not removed equally rapidly by the lymphatics.[23,25]

Pulmonary edema regularly occurs in the unsupported dog if pulmonary capillary hydrostatic pressure is made to exceed colloid osmotic pressure[21] (Figure 2–10). That component of pulmonary edema which is intraalveolar and which produces a terminal airway cuffing (i.e., that portion which produces arterial hypoxia) may be treated by increased airway pressures as produced by the ventilator and positive end expiratory pressure.[43] It is much less clear whether or not this will treat interstitial pulmonary edema. Because lymphatics work largely with one-way valves and tissue massage, the increased pulsating airway pressures produced by the ventilator should also enhance pulmonary lymphatic flow as well as reduce transudation of fluid. This remains to be explored.

The systemic circulation is subject to the same considerations. However, a good part of the pressure drop in going from the capillaries to the

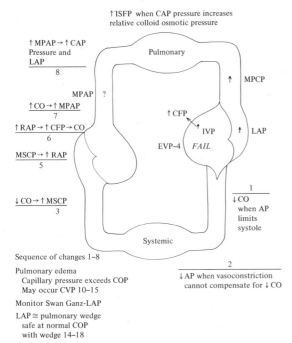

↑ISFP when CAP pressure increases
relative colloid osmotic pressure

↑ MPAP → ↑ CAP
Pressure and
LAP
8

↑ CO → ↑ MPAP
7

↑ RAP → ↑ CFP → CO
6

MSCP → ↑ RAP
5

↓ CO → ↑ MSCP
3

MPAP   ?

Pulmonary

↑   MPCP

↑ CFP
    IVP   ↑ LAP
EVP–4 *FAIL*

1
↓CO
when AP
limits
systole

Systemic

2
↓ AP when vasoconstriction
cannot compensate for ↓ CO

Sequence of changes 1–8

Pulmonary edema
  Capillary pressure exceeds COP
  May occur CVP 10–15

Monitor Swan Ganz-LAP

LAP ≅ pulmonary wedge
  safe at normal COP
  with wedge 14–18

Figure 2–10. Left ventricle failure. Abbreviations: *ISFP*, interstitial fluid pressure; *MPCP*, mean pulmonary circulatory pressure; *LAP*, left atrial pressure; *IVP*, intraventricular pressure; *EVP* extraventricular pressure; *CFP*, cardiac filling pressure; *CO*, cardiac output; *AP*, arterial pressure; *MSCP*, mean systemic circulatory pressure; *RAP*, right atrial pressure; *MPAP*, mean pulmonary artery pressure; *CAP*, capillary hydrostatic pressure; *COP*, colloid osmotic pressure.

Left ventricle failure is characterized by an increase in left cardiac filling pressure for a given cardiac output reflected by an increase in left atrial pressure that increases the mean pulmonary circulatory pressure. The difference between mean pulmonary capillary hydrostatic pressure and mean pulmonary circulatory pressure is much smaller than it is in the systemic circulation. Therefore, mean pulmonary capillary hydrostatic pressure begins to rise for a much smaller rise in left atrial pressure than the same phenomenon on the right side of the heart. In contrast, the pulmonary capillaries are relatively impermeable to protein so that, for edema to occur, the mean pulmonary capillary hydrostatic pressure must exceed the colloid osmotic pressure.

In left ventricular failure, the capillary hydrostatic pressure is influenced not only by the degree of left ventricular failure but also by right ventricular activity. Left ventricular failure, when it is sufficiently severe that the desired cardiac output cannot be generated against arterial pressure, is associated with a fall in cardiac output (*1*). There is compensatory arteriolar vasoconstriction (*2*), venous vaso-

right atrium is normally expended on the resistance to flow. As the veins are distended, the resistance to flow drops so that there is a period of increasing central venous pressure during which venous distention and decreased resistance to flow occur where capillary hydrostatic pressure does not rise significantly. However, when this is exhausted, a given increase in central venous pressure must be associated with the same increase in capillary hydrostatic pressure in order for blood to flow to the heart. In contrast, in the pulmonary circuit the resistance to flow from capillaries to left atrium is very low, and a given increase in left atrial pressure is almost immediately reflected in capillary hydrostatic pressure and, because of vascular recruitment, increased pulmonary blood volume.

The pulmonary and systemic circulations are also in contrast in terms of the relatively lower capillary hydrostatic pressure and increased impermeability of the pulmonary capillaries relative to the systemic capillaries.[23] The systemic capillaries differ between the organs as to protein impermeability and capillary hydrostatic pressure with the liver probably having the most permeable endothelium at the lowest hydrostatic pressure.

Because of all these considerations plus disease processes that affect in large part either the left ventricle or the right ventricle, no necessary inference can be drawn from systemic edema as to pulmonary edema or from pulmonary edema as to systemic edema apart from the fact that lowered colloid osmotic pressure lowers the capillary hydrostatic pressure at which both vascular beds have transudation of fluid. Left ventricle failure lowers the central venous pressure at which pulmonary edema will occur (Figure 2–10), while right ventricle failure or outflow obstruction raises the central venous pressure at which pulmonary edema will occur (Figure 2–11). Left ventricle failure can be satisfactorily managed by the use of

constriction, and an increased mean systemic circulatory pressure (*3*).

Pulmonary edema occurs when the pulmonary capillary hydrostatic pressure exceeds the pulmonary colloid osmotic pressure. The pulmonary capillary hydrostatic pressure is affected by both left and right ventricular function. A central venous pressure of 10 to 15 cm H_2O may be dangerous and should not be extrapolated to pulmonary capillary hydrostatic pressure. The best monitor is then the left atrial pressure. The pulmonary wedge pressure measured with a Swan Ganz catheter gives an accurate measurement provided that the patient is not on high positive end expiratory pressure.

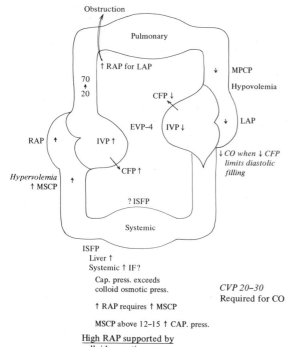

Figure 2–11. Right ventricle outflow obstruction. Abbreviations: *RAP*, right atrial pressure; *LAP*, left atrial pressure; *MPCP*, mean pulmonary circulatory pressure; *CFP*, cardiac filling pressure; *EVP*, extraventricular pressure; *IVP*, intraventricular pressure; *CO*, cardiac output; *CVP*, central venous pressure; *ISFP*, interstitial fluid pressure; *MSCP*, mean systemic circulatory pressure.

Pulmonary emboli, fat emboli, microthromb-emboli, and pulmonary failure cause a rise in pulmonary artery pressure and a fall in left atrial pressure. If the right ventricle can generate sufficient flow at a high enough pulmonary arterial pressure, the left atrial pressure and cardiac output are restored to normal. If the right ventricle cannot respond adequately, the right atrial pressure rises, the left atrial pressure drops, and the cardiac output decreases (RAP for LAP). The increased right atrial pressure requires an increase in mean systemic circulatory pressure (MSCP). This is provided by an increase in venous vasomotor tone and systemic venous blood volume. This condition may be aptly called right hypervolemia–left hypovolemia.

To restore cardiac output it is necessary to raise blood volume above normal and thus increase left atrial pressure and left ventricular cardiac output. The right ventricular outflow obstruction is, in general, at a precapillary level so that very high central venous pressures have little relationship to pulmonary edema. In general, the worse the right ventricle outflow obstruction, the higher the central venous pres-

pulmonary artery wedge pressures as a reflection of left atrial pressure.[48] These may be maintained between 14 and 18 cm H_2O if the colloid osmotic pressure is maintained at normal levels.[47] Positive end expiratory pressures of 10 cm H_2O or greater cause the pulmonary artery wedge pressure to be disassociated from left atrial pressure so that higher wedge pressures are produced by the same left atrial pressure.

Central venous pressures in the presence of normal lungs and absence of right ventricle failure accurately reflect left atrial pressure and are very useful (Figure 2–3). This is so essentially only in normal man with pure hypovolemia. In critically ill man with his usual pulmonary failure, central venous pressure seldom reflects left atrial pressure.

In right ventricle outflow obstruction and failure in general an increased central venous pressure is required to achieve a given left atrial pressure (Figure 2–11). The degree of increase required depends largely upon the increase in pulmonary artery pressure and the magnitude of the right ventricle failure. Systemic edema under these conditions depends upon the balance between fluid intake and output and the balance between capillary hydrostatic pressure and colloid osmotic pressure. Fluid intake exceeding output produces systemic edema independent of the balance between

sure required to achieve a given left atrial pressure. These are the patients who may require a further increase in blood volume when the central venous pressure is already 20 to 30 cm H_2O and who respond with an acute short-term increase in central venous pressure to yet higher levels but in whom cardiac output increases and remains increased, presumably as the blood is redistributed so that more remains in the left atrium and left ventricle.

The mean systemic capillary pressure must always be greater than the mean systemic circulatory pressure (MSCP) which in turn must be greater than the right atrial pressure (RAP) if blood is to flow from the periphery to the heart. Thus central venous pressures above 12 to 15 mm Hg are usually associated with increased capillary hydrostatic pressures.

The transudation of fluid from the capillary to the tissues as edema fluid depends upon the balance between capillary hydrostatic pressure and colloid osmotic pressure. Thus, with low colloid osmotic pressures high right atrial pressures cannot be generated because any increase in pressure causes a decrease in blood volume and an increase in edema. Sufficient albumin is given to maintain the albumin above 3 gm percent. A chronic central venous pressure above 25 to 30 cm H_2O may then be maintained without producing overt peripheral tissue edema.

capillary hydrostatic pressure and colloid osmotic pressure. Central venous pressures that produce an increase in capillary hydrostatic pressure in excess of colloid osmotic pressure produce hypovolemic edema with water retention and thereby lower urine output. The effect is to lower both central venous and capillary hydrostatic pressure to the point where they can be supported by the colloid osmotic pressure. Thus with hypoalbuminemia high central venous pressures cannot be generated, right ventricle cardiac filling pressure is reduced, and cardiac output is reduced to the level that can be supported by the colloid osmotic pressure. These patients are therefore edematous, oliguric, hyponatremic, hypochloridemic, hypoalbuminemic, and do not generate central venous pressures in excess of 12 to 15 cm H_2O chronically, although they may for a short while acutely. In general they are also in pulmonary failure, have arterial hypoxia relative to the inspired oxygen, and have several signs of hepatic dysfunction.

Under these conditions increasing the plasma albumin to the normal range is associated with a chronically higher central venous pressure (commonly 20 to 30 cm H_2O), an increase in cardiac output, mobilization of edema fluid with enhanced urine output, an increase in skin temperature, a return of the serum sodium and chloride to normal, increase in arterial oxygen tension, and a clearing of the usual metabolic acidosis.

Limited venous return may be defined as one which cannot generate the diastolic cardiac filling pressure required by the ventricle. Sufficiently severe right ventricle outflow obstruction limits the left ventricle filling pressure and thus limits cardiac output. Because of the associated increased right atrial pressure and decreased left atrial pressure this may be best described as right ventricle hypervolemia–left ventricle hypovolemia. This contrasts with left ventricle failure where the primary problem is left ventricle hypervolemia with a severe tendency toward pulmonary edema.

Right ventricle limitations of venous return may occur on a basis of hypovolemia or loss of systemic venous vasomotor tone. Pure hypovolemia with normal lungs produces both right and left ventricle hypovolemia. Hypovolemia may occur because of external fluid loss (electrolyte or blood) or a redistribution of fluid volume from the blood to the extravascular space. Redistribution may result from external forces sequestering fluid such as areas of sepsis, burns, venous obstruction, or from intravascular pressures (high central venous pressure) producing transudation of fluid from the blood to the extravascular space.

Limited venous return may also occur from loss of appropriate vasomotor tone. Spinal anesthesia, by sympathetically blockading the anesthetized area with loss of venous vasomotor tone, reduces venous return if the unparalyzed venous areas cannot vasoconstrict enough to compensate. The same phenomenon occurs with spinal cord transection. Both of these may be treated by increasing blood volume, and under normal central venous pressure this may be largely accomplished by Ringer's lactate. When a high central venous pressure is needed, spinal anesthesia in general should not be used or, if used, blood should be administered to maintain the mean circulatory pressure.

PULMONARY FAILURE

Introduction

Not more than 5 to 10 years ago there was a group of patients, apparently doing well initially, who were later recognized to have ventilatory arrest or who were found dead in bed. They had nurses' and doctors' notes indicating they were doing well or, if not, at least were not considered very sick. At postmortem these patients were found to have heavy edematous lungs, commonly with blood-filled capillaries and alveolae, hyaline membranes, bronchopneumonia, and atelectasis. This phenomenon has been called congestive atelectasis pathologically and by many terms clinically, including shock lung, the wet lung syndrome, Da Nang lung, and the adult acute respiratory distress syndrome.

Originally this condition was commonly recognized clinically at the time of a ventilatory arrest. The treatment was ventilatory support without any significant appreciation of the subtle nuances required for proper ventilatory support. Most of these patients died, either suddenly without ventilatory support or after several days of the most sophisticated support then available. Many were young people who on admission had a clear chest x-ray and one or more fractures. Then respiratory distress would be recognized on the third to seventh day, and the patients would then go on to die despite ventilatory support. Each such death was a great tragedy that the physician remembered well. Alfano and Hale have discussed our early experience under the title "Pulmonary Contusion."[1]

At that time ventilator therapy began with the clinical recognition of acute respiratory distress and was associated with a high mortality rate blamed by many physicians on the ventilator as much as the original disease. Consequently ventilators were used as a last resort, and there was great pressure to remove the patient from the ventilator as soon as possible. The result was that the patients would improve somewhat, be removed from the ventilator, and die of another episode of acute respiratory distress. The picture was not much better for patients left on the ventilator, but they did take longer to die.

Several such deaths excited my interest in this subject in 1964. Out of that experience came the recognition that the problem was not only ventilatory failure but also pulmonary failure and that, after this had persisted awhile, the patient died of both pulmonary and circulatory failure.[7] The pulmonary failure studied at that time had arterial oxygen tensions that hardly responded to increased inspired oxygen. When the calculated pulmonary shunts were analyzed as a function of inspired oxygen, there was no change over a rather wide range of inspired oxygens.[8] This was correctly interpreted as shunting through perfused nonventilated alveoli. However, no patient showed evidence of shunting through areas of regional hypoventilation. Sixteen out of 17 patients died. In the light of present knowledge it would be clear that we were studying a group of patients with severe advanced terminal pulmonary failure because we waited for clinical recognition of the acute respiratory distress syndrome. At that time this was not recognized so that although pulmonary and circulatory failures were now added to the obvious ventilatory failure, no significant advance in therapy occurred—with one exception. One patient received by hand several hyperinflations per hour. Although she eventually died of sepsis, this patient never developed as large a pulmonary shunt as the other patients, and the deduction was properly drawn that atelectasis contributed to perfused nonventilated alveolar shunt and that the patients should be hyperinflated.[8] This deduction seemed to be confirmed when experimental studies of the crushed chest in dogs showed severe compressive atelectasis with a minimal component of pulmonary contusion.[9] This, again, did not advance treatment significantly because regional hypoventilation was still not recognized.

Recognition was delayed until the studies of the group in Denver revealed the value of positive end expiratory pressure in experimental pulmonary failure.[2,3] These were subsequently extended to man. Positive end expiratory pressure had previously been studied rather extensively in normal man and animals where it did not significantly improve pulmonary function and did very significantly impair the circulation. Thus, based upon extrapolation from the normal, there was no reason to expect any significant benefit from positive end expiratory pressure and good reason to expect bad effects. The extrapolations, as so commonly happens when going from normal man to sick man, were all wrong because they ignored the changes in pulmonary compliance that occurred in pulmonary failure and the effect this would have on transmitting increased airway pressure to the heart and thus limiting diastolic cardiac filling. At almost the same time Moore and others published a very valuable book on *Post-Traumatic Pulmonary Insufficiency.*[36]

Pontoppidan later organized much of the knowledge available in a very valuable chapter,[38] using, however, the original terminology. This terminology is confusing to all except the person with the most dedicated interest in pulmonary failure. Rahn and Farhi, several years before, had discussed the mechanisms of increased difference between the alveolar and arterial oxygen tension in a chapter based upon basic physical principles that was intellectually clean with a few basic concepts.[40] This chapter is also somewhat confusing in that disorders of the ventilation perfusion distribution ratio are discussed as a single entity as opposed to diffusion limitations and perfused nonventilated alveoli. The concepts are quite correct, but much can be obtained for intelligent clinical management by considering disorders of the ventilation perfusion distribution ratio in terms of its components of regional hypoventilation and regional hyperventilation.

These basic concepts, although valuable, are still not of significant help until they can be analyzed so that effective specific therapy can be utilized. One should not treat the pulmonary failure secondary to elevated diaphragm in the patient in traction or with abdominal distention with the ventilator if the fractures can be internally fixed or the intestines decompressed and the pulmonary failure grossly improved by the sitting or standing position. This problem has been long recognized in the patient with the fractured hip. It seems astonishing that it has taken us so long to recognize it in other patients. A very important paper in this light was that of Burke *et al.* on high output respiratory failure in patients with abdominal distention.[12] The analysis of pulmonary failure to allow specific therapy depends upon a detailed understanding of normal pulmonary function, and the textbook of Bates has a particularly valuable section on this subject.[4] The analysis of regional hypoventilation and its relationship to decreased functional residual capacity rests particularly on the work of Powers and associates.[39] This chapter will attempt to synthesize the preceding material in a way that allows specific clinical therapy.

Normal Pulmonary Function*

The alveolus is essentially a membrane separating gas and fluid spaces with very efficient stirring mechanisms for moving the gas and fluid past the membrane. In addition the fluid phase moves in only one direction, and although the gases enter in simple solution, the membrane contains a binding mechanism with nonlinear characteristics for one gas (oxygen). Because of its chemical structure the membrane simultaneously converts the ionized form of a second gas (HCO_3^-) to the neutral form (H_2CO_3); thus as oxygen is bound and the oxygen tension increased, bicarbonate is converted to H_2CO_3, then to CO_2 via carbonic anhydrase and the carbon dioxide tension rises. Because of the unidirectional flow of blood this is not an equilibrium situation but rather a steady state. Therefore one must consider the relative rates of supply and removal of the various gases.

Relative Rate Consideration

The diffusion rate of any substance depends upon the concentration difference, the distance across which this occurs, and a diffusion constant characteristic of the medium through which diffusion occurs. The maximal diffusion rate for oxygen out of the alveolus will determine the difference in oxygen tensions between the alveolar gas and the mixed venous blood. The rate at which oxygen is supplied to the alveolus will be the volume of inspiratory ventilation multiplied by the concentration of oxygen in the inspired air.

The rate at which oxygen is removed by the blood will depend upon the concentration of hemoglobin, the velocity of the hemoglobin in the capillary, and the rates at which oxygen reacts for a given increase in oxygen tension in the fluid surrounding the hemoglobin. The oxygen tension in the fluid surrounding the hemoglobin will depend upon diffusion of oxygen in the plasma, through the red cell membrane, and through the intracellular fluid to a single hemoglobin molecule. In a steady state the rate of the process before and the rate of the next process determine the concentration at any single stage of the process. Thus the concentration of oxygen in the alveolus is determined by the rate at which oxygen is supplied by ventilation and the rate at which it is removed by diffusion through the alveolar membrane. The same considerations determine the concentration of oxygen in the plasma

---

* This discussion is based largely on the book by Bates, Macklem, and Christie and articles by Fishman, and Rahn and Farhi.

between the alveolar membrane and the red cell. Key to these considerations therefore are the rates of oxygen reaction with hemoglobin, the velocity at which hemoglobin passes through the capillary, and the length of the capillary. It would appear that the hemoglobin molecule spends some time between 0.1 and 1.0 second in the capillary, with the figure commonly quoted under normal conditions of 0.5 second. The calculations suggest that on room air the hemoglobin is in equilibrium with the alveolar gas in about 0.2 second. Since the rate of oxygen delivery to the hemoglobin depends upon the oxygen tension difference between alveolar gas and the red cell, water lowering the inspired oxygen, thus the alveolar gas oxygen tension increases the time to equilibrium. At an alveolar gas oxygen tension of 55 mm Hg, the rate of diffusion is slowed relative to the rate the hemoglobin moves so that equilibrium is reached only at the end of the capillary (i.e., 0.5 second). Obviously as the alveolar gas oxygen tension rises, equilibrium is approached earlier than 0.2 second, or as the velocity of blood flow increases the equilibrium is approached at a greater distance along the capillary. The timing is such that if the velocity of alveolar capillary blood flow more than triples, equilibrium will not be reached unless high concentrations of oxygen are inspired. Under these conditions increasing cardiac output further may, instead of alleviating it, increase arterial hypoxia unless the mixed venous oxygen increases sufficiently to overcome the relative limitations between diffusion, hemoglobin oxygen reaction, and the blood flow velocity. This situation is unlikely to occur in normal man because as cardiac output increases, additional capillaries are perfused, but it may occur if significant portions of the pulmonary vascular bed are occluded and the total cardiac output is directed to a limited portion of the lung.

Alveolar Barometric Pressure

The total gas pressure in the ventilated alveolus must equal the sum of the partial pressures of the various gases (i.e., H_2O, CO_2, O_2, N_2). This is the alveolar barometric pressure that equals atmospheric barometric pressure minus the pressure required to produce flow. This pressure is generally minimal relative to the barometric pressure with quiet breathing. This apparent trivial consideration, when properly expanded and applied to the physiology of the lung, led to major new insights into the function of the lung. Oxygen hypoventilation may be defined as a rate of delivery of oxygen to the alveolus by inspiratory ventilations lower than the blood is capable of removing it. As a result the alveolar gas oxygen tension falls. Since the alveolus is still ventilated, the constant barometric consideration demands, under these conditions, that some other gas rise in tension to maintain the sum constant. The water vapor pressure is fixed by temperature and osmotic pressure. The carbon dioxide tension cannot rise above the mixed venous tension to any significant degree (Bohr effect only). The body can store large quantities of carbon dioxide so that even with a complete lack of ventilation the carbon dioxide tension rises slowly. As a result, for each mm Hg drop in oxygen tension secondary to oxygen hypoventilation, there must be a rise to 1 mm Hg in nitrogen. In other words, oxygen is removed by the blood at a greater rate than it is supplied by ventilation, and because of this nitrogen accumulates in the hypoventilated area so that there is a mm Hg rise in nitrogen tension for each mm Hg fall in oxygen tension.

The rate at which oxygen is delivered to the alveolus depends upon the rate of inspiratory ventilation times the concentration of oxygen. Obviously under conditions of hypoventilation, increasing the inspired oxygen tension will alleviate arterial hypoxia by increasing the rate at which oxygen is supplied to the alveolus by ventilation. The worse the hypoventilation, the greater the oxygen concentration required. Thus in order to clearly reveal the mechanisms of arterial hypoxia secondary to hypoventilation, it is necessary to shift from a given inspired gas oxygen tension with an inert gas (normobaric) to the same inspired gas oxygen tension without the inert gas (hypobaric). Under conditions of oxygen hypoventilation with an inert gas at atmospheric pressure, the rate of oxygen removal from the alveolus by the blood is matched to the rate of supply because as the inert gas accumulates the alveolar gas oxygen tension falls and thus limits the rate of oxygen removal by the blood. When the inspired gas is 100 percent oxygen at a reduced barometric pressure so that the inspired oxygen tensions are equal, the alveolar gas oxygen tension does not drop with hypoventilation because there is no inert gas to accumulate. As a result the rate of removal by the blood is not limited, the alveolar volume rapidly drops, and atelectasis occurs within minutes. The inert gas, in addition to providing the mechanism of arterial hypoxia with hypoventilation, also supplies an important mechanism to keep the alveoli expanded. Because the blood perfusing the hypoventilated alveolus is in equilibrium with its nitrogen tension as well as all the other gases, it would be predicted and has been observed that under these conditions the nitrogen tension of the blood rises. The magnitude of the rise is of course directly related to the volume of blood that passes through the hypoventilated area and the degree of hypoventilation. The rise in nitrogen tension depends upon hypoventilation and does not occur with the perfused nonventilated alveolus. Therefore the rise in nitrogen tension can be used to quantitate regional hypoventilation arterial hypoxia independent of perfused nonventilated alveolus arterial hypoxia.[44,48]

Summary. Arterial hypoxia secondary to alveolar hypoventilation will respond to an increase in the inspired oxygen. The magnitude of the increase required depends upon the degree of alveolar hypoventilation. One hundred percent oxygen quickly produces atelectasis under conditions of hypoventilation unless other measures are taken to maintain alveolar volume (i.e., positive expiratory pressure breathing).

Carbon Dioxide Exchange

Carbon dioxide is approximately twentyfold as diffusible as oxygen. Under conditions of equal diffusion rates for oxygen and carbon dioxide, the carbon dioxide tension difference required is about one twentieth of that required for oxygen. It would appear that the Bohr effect of hemoglobin-releasing or binding cations accounts for about 80 percent of carbon dioxide transport and accounts significantly for the small arteriovenous carbon dioxide tension difference of 4 to 5 mm Hg. Because of this as oxygen reacts with hemoglobin, bicarbonate is converted to H_2CO_3 and then to CO_2 via carbonic anhydrase, so that the carbon dioxide tension rises within the alveolar capillary and increases carbon dioxide diffusion from the alveolar capillary blood to the alveolar gas. The removal of carbon dioxide from the alveolus depends upon the rate of expiratory ventilation and the concentration of carbon dioxide in the alveolar gas. As the carbon dioxide concentration rises secondary to hypoventilation, the rate of carbon dioxide removal from the alveolus increases.

The rate at which mixed venous carbon dioxide tension rises following hypoventilation depends in large part on the body's capacity to store carbon dioxide. This capacity is quite large so that the mixed venous carbon dioxide tension rises slowly following hypoventilation. In contrast to the slow rise of carbon dioxide tension with hypoventilation, the arterial carbon dioxide tension drops almost instantly with hyperventilation because the rate of carbon dioxide removal by expiratory ventilation from the alveolar gas is the major controlling factor.

In transition from hypoventilation to hyperventilation the arteriovenous carbon dioxide tension difference may increase dramatically. Alveolar hyperventilation is thus very effective in removing carbon dioxide from the blood, while it has only a very slight effect on oxygen transport related to the increase in alveolar oxygen tension.

These normal considerations regarding carbon dioxide tension and transport all depend upon an active carbonic anhydrase system to convert H_2CO_3 to CO_2. A number of carbonic anhydrase inhibitors are known and used.

Under conditions of carbonic anhydrase inhibition the conversion of H_2CO_3 to CO_2 may proceed slowly enough so that equilibrium is not attained in the alveolar capillary, and the carbon dioxide tension continues to rise after the blood leaves the lung. Under these conditions the body's carbon dioxide stores increase, and the mixed venous carbon dioxide tension rises until carbon dioxide transport through the lungs once again equals the rate of production. Carbonic anhydrase inhibition leads to an increase in the arteriovenous carbon dioxide tension difference.

Summary. Carbon dioxide transport from the blood under normal conditions is almost exclusively a property of alveolar ventilation. However, the arterial carbon dioxide tension rises slowly with the onset of alveolar hypoventilation but drops rapidly with alveolar hyperventilation.

The Lung as a Whole

The lung consists of approximately 300 million alveoli which operate in parallel. To achieve appropriate distribution of air flow and blood flow so that each alveolus receives the proper ventilation relative to blood flow is an enormously complicated task. This appears to be achieved largely by "design" and not by active controls of flow.[4] Parallel flow systems in general are acutely sensitive to changes in the resistance to flow in one parallel element versus another. In an electrical circuit this is avoided in part by placing a much larger common resistor in series with the parallel resistors. In the air flow system of the lung this same arrangement appears with the larynx, mouth, and nose having approximately 45 to 55 percent of the total resistance to air flow. The smaller airways and their subdivisions appear ideally designed to minimize resistance to air flow. Further because the airways (especially the smaller ones) are attached to the parenchyma, the airways expand as the lung expands and the resistance to air flow decreases as inspiration continues.

The air flow system of the lung may be con-sidered essentially a series of parallel tubes and balloons. The flow in such a system depends upon the resistance to air flow in the tube, the compliance of the balloon, and the pressures applied. The pressures applied must be subdivided into the pressure drop along the tube $(P_1 - P_2)$ and the transmembrane balloon pressure $(P_2 - P_3)$. The pressure drop along the tube is related to the volume rate of air flow and the size of the tube. The size of the tube, as previously discussed, varies with the volume of air in the lung and thus has a variable resistance. The transmembrane balloon pressure may be equated in vivo to the alveolar ventilating pressure. The compliance in the alveolus is a function of volume, starting at a small value in the small alveolus where the radius of curvature and surface active forces are dominant, increasing to a maximum at middle values, and decreasing to a minimum at large alveolar volumes where the fibrous elements in the alveolar wall become dominant.

The volume of the alveolus and its compliance are not only functions of the transmembrane pressure but also of the volume of blood and its pressure in the alveolar capillaries. The volume of blood and its pressure in the capillaries depend, because of certain hydrostatic considerations to be developed, upon the vertical position of the alveolus relative to the most dependent versus the most superior segment of the lung, versus the level of the mitral and pulmonary valves.

Capillary Pressure

The pulmonary vascular tree begins at the pulmonary valve and ends at the mitral valve (Figure 2–12). The vascular loops between these points may be considered a series of U-shaped loops. The alveolar capillaries in the most dependent segments are supplied with blood via the most dependent loops which therefore have the greatest vertical height. These may be equated with the U manometer utilized in the laboratory. The pressure at the most dependent segment of the U (i.e., alveolar capillaries) is therefore equal under conditions of zero left atrial pressure and zero flow to the vertical height of a column of blood from the most dependent capillary to the level of the pulmonary-mitral valve. The pressure in the U loops connecting the horizontal pulmonary and mitral valves will be zero, and the pressure at the apex of the inverted Us going to the most superior segment of the lung will be negative by the height of a column of blood from the pulmonary mitral valve level to the most superior alveolar capillary. In cardiac output the mean left atrial pressure is 4 to 5 mm Hg and may oscillate from

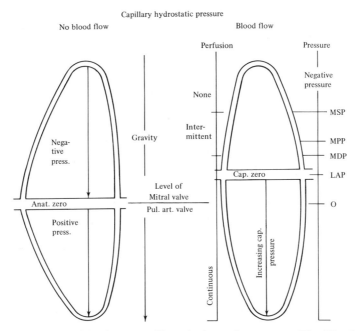

Figure 2–12. Normal upright lung—capillary hydrostatic pressure. The U tube capillary hydrostatic pressure is important in matching pulmonary ventilation to perfusion. In the lung, because of the lack of active controls of blood flow, the capillary hydrostatic pressure at any point is equal to the height of a column of blood parallel to the pull of gravity. The zero point, when there is no flow of blood, is the level of the mitral and pulmonary arterial valves. With blood flow, the zero point is the blood volume above the valves required to provide the left atrial pressure (*LAP*) for cardiac output. When there is no flow of blood, the capillary hydrostatic pressures above the valves are increasingly negative (inverted U tube). Between the mean pulmonary diastolic pressure and the peak systolic pulmonary arterial pressures (*MSP*) there is flow only when the pulmonary arterial pressure exceeds the height of a column of blood parallel to gravity. At this time the waterfall effect occurs, and the left atrial pressure has no significant effect on flow. In between periods of flow the pressure in the capillaries is negative. Above this level is a region with continuous negative pressure and no blood flow.

0 to 12 mm Hg. Under these conditions the height at which zero pressure occurs on a mean basis is the height of a column of blood equal to 4 to 5 mm Hg above the pulmonary-mitral valve level, and the pressure in the most dependent segment is increased by this amount. The pulmonary capillary blood flow in contrast to systemic capillaries has been established to pulsate with the cardiac cycle. This is in keeping with a very low arterial precapillary resistance. Because of the pulsatile capillary flow it is probable that the pulsatile pressure in the left atrium during the cardiac cycle is reflected in a variable zero hydrostatic pressure point so that this varies during each cardiac cycle.

As we have seen, there is a variable point above the mitral-pulmonary valve level above which in the absence of flow a negative capillary pressure would exist. Under conditions of cardiac output the mean pulmonary artery pressure is 12 to 15 mm Hg with a systolic of 20 to 30 mm Hg and a diastolic of 7 to 12 mm

Hg.[18] Since the zero point has a mean value of 4 to 5 mm Hg equivalent of blood above the mitral valve, it is apparent that the region above this will be perfused during systole to the extent and for the duration that the systolic pressure exceeds 4 to 5 mm Hg. Thus this region is intermittently perfused. Because perfusion occurs and the vessels are collapsible, the effective pressure of perfusion is pulmonary artery pressure minus the vertical height above the zero point. Because of the intermittent perfusion it is apparent that additional capillary bed may be recruited if the left atrial pressure rises or the pulmonary artery pressure rises. Further since all of these considerations have been related to gravity, it is apparent that the zero of maximal hydrostatic pressure, although in the bases of the lungs in the erect position, changes to the most posterior segment of the lungs in the supine position, the most anterior in the prone position, and the most dependent lateral in the lateral decubitus position. Further since the vertical distance of the lungs changes with position, it is apparent that the most non-uniform distribution of pressures occurs in the erect position and the most uniform in the supine and prone positions.

Pressure Flow Relationships

Pulmonary vascular blood flow appears to be primarily controlled by transmural pressures and to be very little affected by vasomotor activity.[4,18] The transmural pressure is the difference in pressure between the intravascular and extravascular pressures. The extravascular pressure, although a definite concept, is difficult to measure practically. It is, under conditions of quiet respiration, a function of intrapleural pressure and its oscillations because the intra-alveolar pressure changes only slightly with inspiration-expiration. Under abnormal conditions large changes in intra-alveolar pressure may occur with respiration (e.g., ventilation with positive expiratory pressure), and the transmural

extravascular pressure may become in major part a function of intra-alveolar total gas pressure.

The pulmonary vascular tree has, compared to the systemic vasculature, a minor muscular component with the pulmonary artery having a compliance for blood volume changes roughly equivalent to that of a large systemic vein. The pulmonary vascular tree has no muscular component equivalent to the systemic arteriole but instead has a much smaller muscular coat which terminates on much larger vessels than the systemic arteriole. Thus in general the pulmonary distribution of blood flow is determined by transmural pressures distending vessels and opening new capillaries so that recruitment of additional capillaries occurs but not by arteriolar vasomotor activity. The calculations of Roughton show a total alveolar capillary blood volume of about 60 ml at rest, which increases to about 95 ml with hard physical work. This suggests that at rest only about two thirds of the capillary bed is perfused

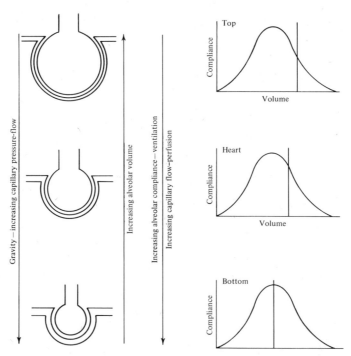

Figure 2–13. Normal lung—blood flow matches ventilation by design. Blood flow matches ventilation by design because the U tube effect on capillary hydrostatic pressure interacts with alveolar capillary blood flow and alveolar volume-compliance. This occurs because as capillary hydrostatic pressure increases, the alveolar capillary perfusion increases and the alveolar capillary hydrostatic pressure increases as the alveolar gas volume decreases. The alveolar gas volumes are located at or above the peak alveolar compliance. The alveoli are ventilated in parallel by expansion of the thoracic cage. Thus, because of the effect of U tube capillary hydrostatic pressure on perfusion and alveolar gas volume, plus the location of normal alveolar volumes at or above peak compliance, ventilation matches perfusion by design and the alveoli of greater volume have both decreased ventilation and perfusion.

and that another one third is available for recruitment[4] (Figures 2–3 and 2–4).

Regional atelectasis, regional fluid-filled alveoli, and regional areas of hypoventilation are associated with a decrease in blood flow (derecruitment). The evidence for regional areas of decrease in perfusion secondary to a decrease in alveolar oxygen tension is rather clear. This appears to be a very weak vasomotor phenomenon that depends upon the parasympathetic nervous system and that may be reversed by acetylcholine.[18] This is one of the few clear vasomotor phenomena available in the lung in spite of the fact that the lung is well innervated by the parasympathetic system and less well innervated by the sympathetic nervous system.[20,27]

Obviously if less than one third of the lung is involved in a decrease in blood flow (derecruitment), then this may not be apparent at all in overall tests of pulmonary function, since the blood flow may be diverted to areas that were not previously perfused (recruitment).

The relationship of transmural capillary pressure to flow and the previously described hydrostatic considerations of pressure suggest that the most dependent sections of the lung will always be the best perfused. This appears to be the case in all experimental observations. Alveolar gas volume is also related to alveolar capillary blood volume which is a direct function of capillary blood flow and therefore capillary blood pressure (Figure 2–13). These considerations suggest, and it has been observed experimentally, that the alveolar volume will be less in the dependent segments of the lung than in the most superior segments. In fact the dependent alveoli have a volume that places them in the most compliant portion of the alveolar volume compliance curve, while the highest alveoli have volumes great enough so that their compliance is decreased.[4] This means that for the same alveolar ventilating pressure the basal alveoli with the greatest blood flow will also receive the greatest ventilation, and thus the ventilation perfusion match is improved by these physical relationships.

Effect of Lung Weight on Ventilation

The lung has weight. This is transmitted vertically within the lung parenchyma. Because of this the effective pleural pressure decreases vertically by about 0.25 cm H_2O per centimeter of distance for the normal lung.[4]

Thus the effective negative pressure to keep the lung expanded by approximating the pleural membranes decreases as one moves from the highest to the most dependent segment of the lung. Obviously the effect will be greater in the fluid-filled lung (e.g., pulmonary edema, pneumonia, pulmonary contusion). The magnitude of the effect will depend on where the fluid is located relative to the most dependent segment of the lung. Fortunately the pulmonary edema produced by an increased left atrial pressure will be localized to the most dependent segments by virtue of the hydrostatic pressure considerations developed, and thus the increased weight will not involve significant portions of the superior lung. In addition the increased left atrial pressure will recruit capillaries in the superior segment of the lungs. In contrast pneumonia and pulmonary contusions may increase the weight of the lung above the bases. In order for ventilation to occur in the segments below this weight a sufficient pressure must be generated either by increased negative pressure in the pleura during inspiration or by external pressure to support the weight of fluid on the cushion of air beneath it.

This consideration of lung weight and its support by a cushion of air largely explains why air trapping with regional hypoventilation on expiration occurs in the dependent segments of the lung. The same effect occurs with the heavy thorax of obesity and fluid-filled areas of lung above the most dependent ventilated lung.

Because of these considerations regarding the weight of the lung the effective alveolar ventilating pressure decreases by about 0.25 cm H_2O per centimeter/vertical distance of the normal lung ongoing from the highest to the most dependent area.

Total Pulmonary Blood Volume Relative to Systemic Blood Volume

As previously stated, the pulmonary vascular blood volume and distribution of blood flow are primarily controlled by the transmural pressure which is a direct function of left atrial pressure and an indirect function of pulmonary artery pressure. It is also a function of systemic vasoconstriction, particularly venous vasomotor tone. As pointed out, the mean circulatory pressure depends upon blood volume and venous vasomotor tone. The mean circulatory pressure characterizes the circulation as a whole. The pulmonary vasculature and the systemic vasculature have very different vasomotor activity. Because of the difference it is apparent that a mean systemic circulatory pressure and a mean pulmonary circulatory pressure should be defined and that in principle they will be under different controls or the same control with a different magnitude of response (Figure 2–4). This consideration is strengthened by the knowledge that the volume compliance of the pulmonary artery is about equal to that of a systemic vein. Thus it may be expected that increases in the mean systemic circulatory pressure (as occurs with an increase in cardiac output) will be associated with shifts of blood from the systemic system to the pulmonary system until the mean pulmonary circulatory pressure equals the mean systemic pressure. This shift of blood from one circulation to the other appears to be well documented with a variety of maneuvers.[18] It is clear that exercise increases the pulmonary blood volume, as do immersion in water, infusion of norepinephrine, and negative intrathoracic pressure (Mueller maneuver). Further it is clear that increasing intrathoracic pressure decreases intrathoracic blood volume. Thus in general increases in cardiac output by mobilizing blood from the systemic circulation increase pulmonary pressure, blood volume, and thus capillary recruitment and oxygen uptake. The same phenomenon occurs due to increased pressures in a single lung when the blood flow is stopped to the other lung. Under these conditions pulmonary artery pressure rises about 30 to 40 percent while the vascular resistance of the perfused lung drops 40 to 50 percent.[18]

Summary: Control of Blood Flow Through Lung

The preceding considerations suggest that transmural pressure is the dominant factor in the lung controlling the distribution and the magnitude of blood flow through it. However, the exact circumstances under which the transmural pressure is considered may mean that the extravascular pressure may be chiefly related to intrapleural pressure or to intra-alveolar gas pressure. Vasomotor activity under many conditions in the lung appears minimal except for the weak reponse of regional alveolar hypoxia. The proper distribution of ventilation to perfusion in the millions of parallel units in the lung therefore appears to be more a matter of proper mechanical design than of active controls.

Expiratory Ventilation

The smaller airways clearly vary in size with the air volume of the lung because they are supported by attachments to the lung parenchyma and thereby the pleura. During quiet respiration expiration occurs passively with the force provided by the elastic energy stored in the alveolar surface active forces and the elastic elements of the lungs by the preceding active inspiration. During forced expiration the muscles actively constrict and the pleural pressure rises above atmospheric pressure. Under these conditions this increase in pleural pressure is transmitted not only to the alveoli but to all elements of the lung including the airways. The airways as well as the alveoli are therefore compressed. At large lung volumes in the normal lung, because of the relative forces supporting the alveoli versus the airways and the energy stored in surface active forces, the rate of expiratory air flow is proportional to the force applied by muscular contraction. This occurs from 75 to 100 percent of total lung capacity. In the normal lung below 75 percent of total lung capacity the rate of forced expiration becomes independent of the force applied.[4] This occurs because in the range of total lung capacity from 75 percent to zero (residual volume) the force applied by the muscles via a rise in pleural pressure is equally applied to the alveoli and terminal airways. Under these conditions the rise in intra-alveolar total gas pressure, which occurs because of the increased muscular effort, is counteracted by increased resistance to air flow in the terminal airways because of terminal airway compression with diminished size of the airways. Further increases in the applied pleural pressure do not produce increases in air flow. We have previously considered the effect of lung weight and its vertical transmission on the effective intrapleural pressure. In the normal lung the effective intrapleural pressure diminishes at the rate of 0.25 cm H_2O per centimeter of vertical distance. Thus the effective pleural pressure in the dependent segments of the lung is more positive than in the highest segments. Because of this the volume of the alveoli and the airways is smaller in the dependent segments of the lungs, and the increased resistance to air flow occurs predominantly in these segments.

There are many conditions under which the lung as a whole operates at a reduced air volume, in which the elastic elements are reduced, or in which there is increased lung weight. All of these conditions operate to produce increased resistance to expiratory air flow. Thus in the aged, because of loss of elastic elements to support the airways, the airway resistance in the dependent segments may routinely increase to such a point that air trapping occurs in the bases of the lungs at the end of each tidal volume. This means that it occurs at a point on the total lung capacity normally designated the functional residual capacity instead of the much smaller lung volume in the normal healthy man designated the residual volume and that it occurs at a much smaller positive pleural pressure. Many critically ill patients have a grossly reduced functional residual capacity and a reduced tidal volume.[39] Their lungs are operating around a grossly reduced lung volume. Further these lungs are commonly edematous and thus have a further increase in the effective positive pleural pressure in the dependent segments. Increased resistance to air flow and air trapping during expiration are particularly likely to occur in these lungs.

Physiology of Pulmonary Failure

Pulmonary failure may be defined as an increase in the volume of blood that passes through the lungs without picking up oxygen[18] (Figure 2–2). This may be quantitated by calculating the shunt on the basis of the measured mixed venous oxygen content, measured arterial oxygen content, and estimated alveolar capillary blood oxygen content on the basis of the assumption that it has the same 2-3 DPG, pH, and hemoglobin as arterial blood and the oxygen tension of alveolar gas. In addition the assumption that arterial blood is composed of a mixture of alveolar capillary blood and mixed venous blood leads to the equation previously developed.

1. $CaO_2 = CAO_2 + Y(CvO_2 - CAO_2)$

This equation is mathematically correct but physiologically incorrect, since there are several different blood oxygen contents that contribute to the oxygen content of arterial blood and not just mixed venous blood and alveolar capillary blood. This difficulty is accommodated by a further analysis of the calculated shunt Y in physiologic terms. Equation 1, when analyzed, reveals that arterial hypoxia may occur on the basis of circulatory failure (decreased mixed venous oxygen content) or pulmonary failure (increased calculated pulmonary shunt Y) or both. It also reveals that arterial hypoxia secondary to pulmonary failure may be alleviated or reversed by increasing the mixed venous oxygen content. This is done by increasing cardiac output relative to the rate of oxygen consumption and by the peripheral maldistribution of blood flow (physiologically compatible with systemic arteriovenous shunts).[10] Both of these compensatory mechanisms may in time become exhausted or lead to other life-threatening consequences, at which time severe arterial hypoxia occurs and death ensues.

Blood may pass through the lungs without picking up a normal amount of oxygen because of diffusion limitations, areas of regional hypoventilation, or by passing through collapsed or fluid-filled areas that are not ventilated at all.[40]

Thus the following equation may be written:

2. $\underset{\substack{\text{calculated} \\ \text{total}}}{Y} = \underset{\substack{\text{diffusion} \\ \text{limitations}}}{Y} + \underset{\substack{\text{regional} \\ \text{hypo-} \\ \text{ventilation}}}{Y} + \underset{\substack{\text{perfused} \\ \text{nonventilated} \\ \text{alveoli}}}{Y}$

Analysis of this equation in physiologic and thus clinical terms allows rational management of the patient in pulmonary failure. The following statement on the basic processes may be made:

1. Diffusion limitations

The basic law of diffusion states in essence that the rate of movement of substance by diffusion increases as the concentration difference between the two sides of the membrane increases.

The lung is commonly discussed as though oxygen transfer occurred only through the alveolar wall. It is apparent that by progressively increasing the inspired oxygen content significant oxygen transfer could be made to occur through progressively thicker areas of lung from the gas to blood phase. This possibility has been demonstrated by showing a sudden increase in small pulmonary artery oxygen content on switching from room air to 100 percent oxygen. At a constant rate of oxygen transfer through a membrane, the oxygen tension difference between the two sides directly depends upon the thickness of the membrane. It is apparent from knowledge of the thickness of the membrane and oxygen tension difference in the normal lung that the most severe interstitial pulmonary edema (short of a fluid-filled alveolus) could produce only 20 to 50 mm Hg difference in oxygen tension from alveolar gas to blood. It is probable in view of the basic principles and a multitude of observations that interstitial pulmonary edema seldom contibutes significantly to arterial hypoxia and that what little contribution is made can be easily overcome by a rise in the inspired oxygen content and serum albumin (see discussion under blood volume controls).

Regional Hypoventilation

The critically ill or acutely injured patient usually has arterial hypoxia (relative to the inspired oxygen), arterial hypocarbia (decreased carbon dioxide tension), and mouth hyperventilation. The decreased arterial carbon dioxide tension is compatible only with overall alveolar hyperventilation. However, overall alveolar hyperventilation does not mean that regional hypoventilation is not present. In fact the two commonly coexist, with the area of regional hypoventilation (Figure 2–14) being partially counterbalanced in terms of carbon dioxide transport but not oxygen transport by areas in the lungs with a regional hyperventilation greater than the overall alveolar hyperventilation (Figure 2–15). The discrepancy between the effects of regional alveolar hypoventilation and hyperventilation on carbon dioxide and oxygen transport is related largely

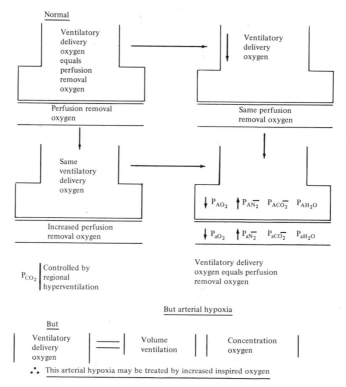

Figure 2–14. Regional hypoventilation. Regional hypoventilation as utilized here means regional oxygen hypoventilation. This occurs when oxygen is delivered by ventilation at a lower rate than it is taken away by perfusion. This may occur because of decreased ventilatory delivery of oxygen or increased removal of oxygen by perfusion. This results in a fall in alveolar gas oxygen tension, a rise in alveolar gas nitrogen tension, and a decrease in perfusion oxygen removal until it equals the rate of ventilatory oxygen delivery in association with an arterial hypoxia responsive to increased inspired oxygen.

to the properties of oxygen binding by hemoglobin and the relationship of blood oxygen content to blood oxygen tension.

Under normal conditions the percent of oxyhemoglobin at an oxygen tension of 90 to 100 is 95 to 98 percent and the oxygen content with 14 gm of hemoglobin per 100 ml of blood about 20 volumes percent. Mixed venous blood under the same conditions may have an oxygen tension of 40 and oxygen content of 15 volumes per 100 ml (Figure 2–2). Regional changes in ventilation in the presence of an inert gas (usually nitrogen) produce a change in the alveolar gas oxygen tension directly proportional to the degree of hypoventilation or hyperventilation. However, because of the shape of the hemoglobin oxygen binding curve with its sharp break at 90 to 100 mm Hg, a decrease in alveolar gas oxygen tension of 60 mm Hg (100 to 40 mm Hg) in one area of the lung will produce a far greater decrease in alveolar blood oxygen content in that area than an increase in alveolar gas oxygen tension of 60 mm Hg in

another area (100 to 160 mm Hg) will produce an increase in oxygen content. In fact alveolar gas on room air normally has a great enough oxygen tension, except in areas of regional hypoventilation, that the hemoglobin is 100 percent oxygen saturated. Thus regional hypoventilation produces arterial hypoxia that cannot be counterbalanced by the corresponding area of regional hyperventilation.

Oxygen hypoventilation has been previously defined as a condition under which the rate of oxygen supply by ventilation is less than the rate at which oxygen is removed by the blood. Further it has been pointed out that breathing air leads to an accumulation of nitrogen so that for each mm Hg decrease in alveolar gas oxygen tension a mm Hg increase in nitrogen tension occurs. The increase in nitrogen tension helps stabilize the gas volume of the alveolus, while the decrease in oxygen tension decreases the rate at which blood removes oxygen until the rate of oxygen supply by ventilation once again equals the rate of oxygen removal. The rate

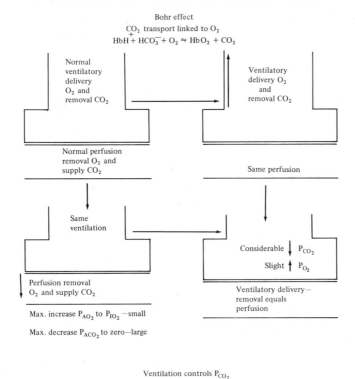

Bohr effect
CO_2 transport linked to O_2
$HbH + HCO_3^- + O_2 \rightleftharpoons HbO_2 + CO_2$

Normal ventilatory delivery O_2 and removal CO_2

Ventilatory delivery O_2 and removal CO_2

Normal perfusion removal O_2 and supply CO_2

Same perfusion

Same ventilation

Considerable ↓ P_{CO_2}

Slight ↑ P_{O_2}

Perfusion removal O_2 and supply CO_2

Ventilatory delivery— removal equals perfusion

Max. increase P_{AO_2} to P_{IO_2} —small

Max. decrease P_{ACO_2} to zero—large

Ventilation controls P_{CO_2}

Figure 2–15. Regional hyperventilation. Regional hyperventilation may be defined as occurring when the ventilatory delivery of oxygen and removal of carbon dioxide exceed the rate at which oxygen is consumed and carbon dioxide is delivered. The alveolar gas oxygen tension rises and the carbon dioxide tension falls until once again the rate of delivery of oxygen by ventilation equals the rate of removal by perfusion and the rate of removal of carbon dioxide by ventilation equals the rate of supply by perfusion.

There are two major restrictions on these processes. In the alveolus with normal ventilation the oxygen tension is already sufficient to produce almost 100 percent saturation of hemoglobin with oxygen so that oxygen transport away from the alveolus cannot be significantly increased. The alveolar gas oxygen tension can at most be increased from its normal value of 120 to 135 to the inspired value of 147 mm Hg so that with maximal regional hyperventilation the alveolar gas oxygen tension can only increase a slight amount. In contrast, the alveolar gas carbon dioxide tension may be lowered from its normal value of 35 to 40 mm Hg to that of inspired carbon dioxide tension which is close to zero, so that large percentage changes in carbon dioxide tensions are possible with hyperventilation.

The second restriction is the Bohr effect. This links carbon dioxide transport and oxygen transport in such a way that as oxygen is taken up in the alveolar capillary, carbon dioxide is evolved from bicarbonate so that a local rise in carbon dioxide tension occurs in the alveolar capillary. Thus in regionally hypoventilated areas with little oxygen transport there is also only a small amount of carbon dioxide transport. This link in hyperventilated areas provides maximal carbon dioxide transport with maximal oxygen transport.

The net result is that regional hyperventilation areas are very effective in carbon dioxide transport and largely control arterial carbon dioxide tension whereas regionally hypoventilated areas largely limit and control oxygen transport and arterial oxygen tension. Therefore limitations of carbon dioxide transport seldom present as a clinical problem except for total lung hypoventilation, but limitations of pulmonary oxygen transport are commonly a clinical problem and occur with reduced carbon dioxide tension.

of oxygen supply depends upon the volume of gas movement into and out of the alveolus and the concentration of oxygen in the gas moved. Therefore hypoventilation (regional or generalized) as a mechanism of arterial hypoxia may in general be overcome by increasing the inspired oxygen content. Further since the major mechanism of arterial hypoxia depends upon the accumulation of nitrogen, a normal arterial oxygen tension for 100 percent oxygen will be obtained when 100 percent oxygen is administered. However, unless this increases the rate of oxygen supply by ventilation to equal or exceed the rate of oxygen removal by the blood, the alveolar gas volume will be progressively reduced until it collapses and atelectasis occurs.

Blood Perfusion of Nonventilated Areas

The pulmonary artery may perfuse nonventilated segments of the lung because the alveoli are fluid-filled or collapsed (atelectatic). Alveoli may be fluid-filled because of end-stage pulmonary edema, pulmonary contusions with blood, or various septic processes. Atelectatic alveoli may occur because of compressive forces with expulsion of the air from the alveolus, a decrease in surfactant with a decrease in alveolar compliance, or regional hypoventilation especially with 100 percent oxygen. Regional hypoventilation may occur because of airway obstruction, a decrease in the alveolar ventilation pressure, a decrease in compliance, or because of an increased capillary blood flow relative to ventilatory air movement.

The point has been made that the arterial hypoxia of regional hypoventilation can be overcome by increasing the inspired oxygen concentration and that this is not true of the arterial hypoxia that occurs secondary to perfused nonventilated alveoli. A common observation in the days before effective pulmonary support was that day after day the patient required a higher inspired oxygen in order to achieve the same arterial oxygen tension.[1,8] This can only be interpreted as a progressive conversion of areas of regional hypoventilation to areas of perfused nonventilated alveoli. Regional hypoventilation probably leads to atelectasis for the following reasons:[43]

1. Surfactant is synthesized by the giant alveolar cell situated on the alveolar gas side of the alveolar membrane. Surfactant controls the compliance of the alveolus.

2. The giant alveolar cell is highly aerobic and metabolically active.

3. A consideration of relative oxygen tensions suggests that most of the oxygen required by the giant alveolar cell is obtained from alveolar gas.

4. The oxygen tension of the alveolar gas depends upon ventilation and perfusion.

5. Regional hypoventilation by decreasing the oxygen supply to the giant alveolar cell probably limits the rate of surfactant synthesis.

6. Surfactant has a half-life of 12 to 16 hours. Therefore if the regional hypoventilation is not corrected, the alveolus will become progressively less compliant and ventilation will further decrease until atelectasis occurs.

7. The giant alveolar cell obtains its oxygen from alveolar gas but its other nutrients from the blood.

8. Therefore fat emboli, microthromboemboli, and pulmonary thromboemboli by decreasing the supply of nutrients other than oxygen may also lead to a regional decrease in compliance, regional alveolar gas hypoxia, and eventually atelectasis just as do the lesions which primarily involve ventilation.

The shunting secondary to perfusion of nonventilated areas in the lung is much less or not at all responsive to increases in the inspired oxygen content as compared to areas of regional hypoventilation. The only sensitivity can be due to diffusion through rather large distances as compared to the alveolar membrane with interstitial edema and under conditions of rather small volume shunts with high mixed venous oxygen contents where sufficient oxygen can be placed in solution by the ventilated alveoli to saturate the hemoglobin in the shunt blood.

Summary: Mechanisms of Arterial Hypoxia

The hallmark of shunting through perfused nonventilated alveoli is the essential lack of response of the arterial oxygen tension to changes in inspired oxygen. The hallmark of pure regional hypoventilation is that the arterial oxygen tension does not respond much to increased inspired oxygen until an oxygen concentration is achieved that overcomes the regional hypoventilation limitation of alveolar oxygen delivery. At this time with regional hypoventilation the arterial oxygen tension rapidly increases until at 100 percent oxygen a normal arterial oxygen tension is achieved for 100 percent oxygen. Most pulmonary failure involves both perfused nonventilated alveoli and regional hypoventilation. The conversion of areas of regional hypoventilation to perfused nonventilated alveoli represents advancing pulmonary failure even though the calculated shunt does not change.

Definition of Arterial Hypoxia

Arterial hypoxia may be utilized either in terms of the body's metabolic needs or in terms of pulmonary function. Arterial oxygen tension less than 45 probably interferes with the body's metabolic needs, and arterial hypoxia is commonly used in this sense. Arterial hypoxia in pulmonary terms means an arterial oxygen tension less than would be expected for the inspired oxygen, assuming a normal mixed venous oxygen tension (Figure 2–16). In the perfect lung (i.e., zero shunt) a mm Hg increase in arterial oxygen tension would be expected for each mm Hg increase in alveolar gas oxygen

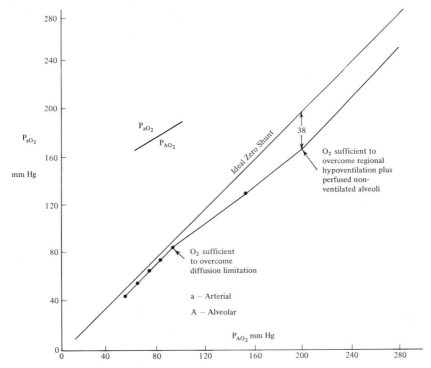

Figure 2–16. Normal lung—ideal versus observed relationship of arterial oxygen tension to alveolar gas oxygen tension. In the presence of zero pulmonary shunt, the arterial oxygen tension equals the alveolar gas oxygen tension. The difference between ideal and observed occurs on the basis of three mechanisms (Rahn and Farhi). Diffusion gradients become maximal at low alveolar oxygen tensions, ventilation-perfusion mismatches are dominant in normal lungs at middle oxygen tension, and perfused nonventilated alveoli are dominant at higher oxygen tensions.

In the normal lung, the relationship of alveolar gas to arterial oxygen tension deviates so slightly from the ideal that no detectable difference can be found with clinical measurements. Therefore, the normal arterial oxygen tension can be predicted in the presence of adequate overall ventilation (normal or low P_{aCO_2}) by multiplying the normal arterial oxygen tension at 100 percent by the measured inspired oxygen fraction. The normal arterial oxygen tension on 100 percent oxygen is in the range 500 to 650 mm Hg. Thus 20 percent oxygen should give an arterial oxygen tension of 100 to 120 mm Hg; 50 percent oxygen should give an arterial tension normally of 250 to 300 mm Hg. Using this relationship an expected arterial oxygen tension may be calculated and compared with the observed oxygen tension.

tension so that the two are always equal. The normal lung has a shunt of 2 to 5 percent of cardiac output. This may cause arterial oxygen tension to be as much as 40 to 80 mm Hg less than alveolar oxygen tension at about 200 mm Hg alveolar oxygen tension. This, however, is a maximum and declines on either side of an alveolar oxygen tension of about 200 mm Hg, according to Rahn and Farhi.[40]

Apart from this deviation in the normal lung without hypoventilation a mm Hg increase in alveolar oxygen tension does produce a mm Hg increase in arterial oxygen tension with 600 to 650 mm Hg arterial oxygen tension occurring on 100 percent oxygen. The inspired oxygen actually achieved can be accurately determined only under research conditions. Clinically inspired oxygen, even though directly analyzed with the usual small paramagnetic analyses, is seldom known so accurately that the 40 mm Hg difference previously discussed can be accurately picked up. Therefore we utilize 500 to 600 mm Hg as the ideal oxygen tension on 100 percent oxygen and simply multiply by the fraction of the inspired oxygen in order to calculate the expected ideal arterial oxygen tension. This if combined with an arterial carbon dioxide tension of 40 or less predicts the expected arterial oxygen tension accurately enough for the clinical setting. Thus on 50 percent oxygen tension one would expect an arterial oxygen tension of about 250, on 30 percent about 150 mm Hg, and on 20 percent about 100 mm Hg. While not quite correct these give an easily available reference point. Arterial oxygen tensions less than these are considered arterial hypoxia in terms of pulmonary function.

Figure 2–17 presents a graph of the preceding comments on arterial hypoxia. Line 1 is the basic equation summing the components of the pulmonary shunt in the presence of a normal mixed venous oxygen and absence of hypoventilation.

Line 2 shows the effects of pure increasing

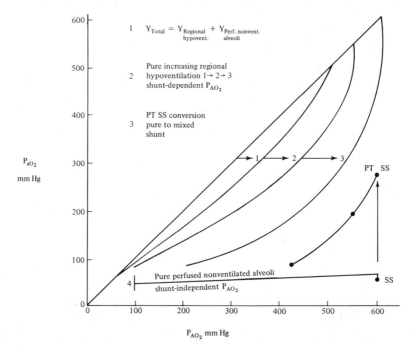

1   $Y_{Total} = Y_{Regional \atop hypovent.} + Y_{Perf. nonvent. \atop alveoli}$

2   Pure increasing regional hypoventilation $1 \rightarrow 2 \rightarrow 3$ shunt-dependent P_{AO_2}

3   PT SS conversion pure to mixed shunt

4   Pure perfused nonventilated alveoli shunt-independent P_{AO_2}

P_{aO_2} mm Hg

P_{AO_2} mm Hg

Figure 2–17. Pulmonary failure—relationship of arterial oxygen tension to alveolar gas oxygen tension. The difference between alveolar gas oxygen tension and arterial oxygen tension occurs mainly because of regional hypoventilation and the presence of perfused nonventilated alveoli. With regional hypoventilation nitrogen tension rises as the oxygen tension in the alveoli falls. This allows total pressure to remain constant. Therefore pure regional hypoventilation is associated with a normal oxygen tension when 100 percent oxygen is provided and after all nitrogen is washed out of the lungs.

There are varying degrees of regional hypoventilation. When sufficient oxygen is supplied by ventilation to equal the rate at which oxygen is removed by perfusion, the arterial oxygen tension should equal the ideal (curves 1, 2, and 3). The more severe the regional hypoventilation, the greater the inspired oxygen required to achieve ventilatory delivery equal to perfusion removal. Pure regional hypoventilation therefore has, as its major characteristic, a period of increasing inspired oxygen in which only small increases in arterial oxygen tension occur, followed by a second period of increasing inspired oxygen in which arterial oxygen tension very rapidly increases. This form of arterial hypoxia responds to an increased inspired oxygen.

The second type of arterial hypoxia (perfused nonventilated) is associated with only slight changes in arterial oxygen tension for large changes in inspired oxygen (line 4). The blood passing through perfused nonventilated alveoli is not exposed to the inspired oxygen, and such little increase in arterial oxygen tension as does occur is due to increased diffusion of oxygen over long distances.

With curve 3 patient SS appeared to have adequate ventilatory support. She achieved an arterial oxygen tension of 50 on 100 percent oxygen with an external dead space that had gone from 300 cc to 50 in association with a rising arterial carbon dioxide tension (65) in spite of a minute ventilatory volume of 15 liters. She was known to have a right pulmonary contusion. She therefore had massive shunting through perfused nonventilated alveoli plus alveolar hypoventilation. The conclusion was therefore drawn that she must have major airway obstruction with the ventilatory volume being distributed to only a small portion of the lung and probably at high enough pressures to impede perfusion in the ventilated alveoli. After removing secretions from the left main stem bronchus, the arterial oxygen tension was 270 on 100 percent oxygen with an arterial carbon dioxide tension of 35. The arterial oxygen tensions were then 190 on 90 percent oxygen and 66 on 60 percent oxygen.

regional hypoventilation. Note that arterial oxygen tension rises very slowly as the alveolar oxygen tension increases until a given inspired oxygen where it rises very rapidly to reach the normal line at 100 percent oxygen.

Line 4 shows the effects of shunting through perfused nonventilated alveoli. Note that large changes in inspired oxygen have very little effect on arterial oxygen.

Patient SS shows the effects of a combined shunt through areas of both regional hypoventilation and perfused nonventilated alveoli. Note that the arterial oxygen tension on 100 percent oxygen is considerably less than the expected 600 mm Hg, but that arterial oxygen tension does rise rapidly when the inspired oxygen is sufficient to overcome the limited ventilatory oxygen delivery.

Mechanisms of Regional Hypoventilation

Regional hypoventilation occurs because of limited ventilatory oxygen delivery relative to perfusion. This may go awry because of regional factors that limit ventilation relative to perfusion or enhance perfusion relative to ventilation. The factors that regionally limit ventilation may be intrapulmonic or extrapulmonic. The factors that enhance perfusion are always intrapulmonic.

Extrapulmonic Causes of Regional Hypoventilation

The extrapulmonic factors that produce regional hypoventilation are based upon the normal shape match that occurs with growth between the lung and its thoracic-diaphragmatic envelope (Figure 2–18). This shape match allows the expansion of the thoracic diaphragmatic envelope to be evenly transmitted throughout the lung so that this factor plus the intrapulmonic factors previously described assures that each alveolus has the proper ventilation for its perfusion. Any extrapulmonic factor that interferes with the shape match produces areas of regional hypoventilation and corresponding areas of regional hyperventilation.

Regional hypoventilation on the basis of extrapulmonary shape mismatches may occur by the following mechanisms:

1. Pneumothorax
2. Hemothorax
3. Flail chest
4. Elevated diaphragms
   a. Obese supine individual
   b. Gastrointestinal distention
   c. Ascites
   d. Patient in traction

Elevated diaphragms are common and in general involve a much greater volume of

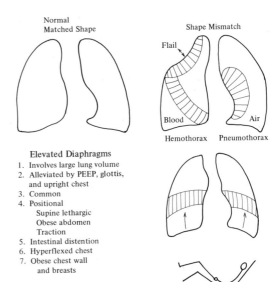

Elevated Diaphragms
1. Involves large lung volume
2. Alleviated by PEEP, glottis, and upright chest
3. Common
4. Positional
   Supine lethargic
   Obese abdomen
   Traction
5. Intestinal distention
6. Hyperflexed chest
7. Obese chest wall and breasts

Figure 2–18. Regional hypoventilation—extrapulmonic. Anything that interferes with the matched shape of the chest tends to produce regional hypoventilation. Elevation of the diaphragms can be treated by using the upright position, deep breathing, and proper use of the glottis to cough. However, in the obese, lethargic, supine patient, the elevated diaphragms may lead to pulmonary failure.

the lungs than the other mechanisms. This mechanism of regional hypoventilation with its corresponding threat of conversion to perfused nonventilated alveoli is therefore a particularly serious problem. The patient in traction who is thin and alert may, by using his glottis and respiratory muscles, treat the problem effectively by himself. The obese and lethargic patient in traction is particularly apt to develop progressive pulmonary failure. The problem is compounded if in addition he develops intestinal distention or has direct thoracic trauma producing compressive atelectasis or a pulmonary contusion.

Flail chests produce an area of regional hypoventilation that may be very effectively managed with the ventilator. The major problem with flail chests lies in lack of effective treatment with conversion of the area of regional hypoventilation to one of perfused nonventilated alveoli and in underlying pulmonary contusions, compressive atelectasis, or pneumonia.

Hemothorax and pneumothorax are generally treated because they appear on x-ray without thought being given to their causing regional hypoventilation. However, when one starts from the arterial blood gases in the critically ill patient on the ventilator, it is necessary to search for pneumothorax and hemothorax as common causes of regional hypoventilation by getting appropriate chest x-rays.

Intrapulmonic Causes of Regional Hypoventilation

Regional hypoventilation secondary to intrapulmonic causes may occur because of the following mechanisms (Figure 2–19):

1. Retained secretions
2. Aspiration of irritants with mucosal edema
   a. Gastric contents
   b. Smoke and irritant gases
3. Aspiration of blood
4. Aspiration of foreign bodies
5. Pulmonary edema
6. Embolic phenomena

Retained secretions are by far the most common cause of intrapulmonic regional hypoventilation. Almost every morning the patient will be found to have increased arterial hypoxia which responds to suctioning. Retained secretions in the absence of adequate humidification may become very thick and difficult to suction. It is most important that the air delivered be essentially 100 percent humidified so that the secretions remain as liquid as possible. This is best done by using a heated humidifier. One may then simply measure the temperature of the inspired air to determine humidity. This should be maintained at about 95°F (35°C) to ensure close to 100 percent humidity.

Retained secretions may exist in the presence of repeated suctioning if a straight catheter is utilized. The straight catheter tends to suction only the right main stem bronchus. In general adequate suctioning is much more difficult with a nasotracheal tube and orotracheal tube than with a tracheostomy tube. The patient in whom retained secretions are a real problem should have a tracheostomy tube and should be suctioned with a curved Caude catheter. Caude catheters are commonly misused. The patient with increasing arterial hypoxia should be personally suctioned by the physician with the Caude catheter turned so that it enters both main stem bronchi. If any doubt still remains about retained secretions, the patient should be bronchoscoped with a fiberoptic scope while being ventilated. In general this requires a 3-mm scope and a large tracheostomy tube in place so that the bronchoscope does not obstruct ventilation. It is most unwise to disconnect the patient with severe pulmonary failure from the ventilator for bronchoscopy or for movement to the operating room for tracheostomy. Our tracheostomies are all done in the intensive care unit on the original ventilator.

The aspiration of a large variety of irritants

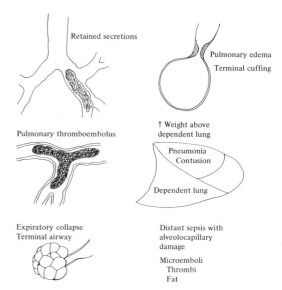

Figure 2–19. Regional hypoventilation—intrapulmonic. Most of the intrapulmonic causes of regional hypoventilation, with the single exception of those that produce pulmonary infiltrates, cannot be diagnosed by x-ray. Retained secretions most often affect the left main bronchus because a suction catheter most commonly enters the right main stem bronchus. Pulmonary edema results in dependent regional hypoventilation and responds quickly to positive end expiratory pressure. Pulmonary thromboemboli, fat emboli, and microthromboemboli may cause regional hypoventilation if they obstruct flow to sufficient pulmonary capillaries to increase flow to the remaining capillaries. If the pulmonary capillary blood flow is increased more than about three times, a further increase in cardiac output may decrease arterial oxygen content because there is insufficient time in the pulmonary capillary for oxygen to react with hemoglobin.

Pneumonia and pulmonary contusion produce pulmonary shunting directly through perfused nonventilated alveoli and indirectly by the increase in weight above dependent ventilated lung.

In sepsis there is pulmonary shunting as a result of alveolocapillary damage with interstitial edema, intra-alveolar edema, and congestive atelectasis.

may cause regional hypoventilation by producing mucosal edema as well as by the physical presence of the irritant. If these actually enter the alveoli, they may also produce perfused nonventilated alveoli. Smoke inhalation has now been recognized to produce this process in the subglottic area. Fortunately most particulate matter aspirated does not reach the alveoli or small airways and causes most of its damage in the large airways. The most effective treatment for gastric aspiration is not steroids but rather removal of the irritant with subsequent proper ventilatory support as for any pulmonary failure.

Patients with severe thoracic trauma may have massive bleeding into these airways. This may also occur secondary to tumors, tuberculosis, or even pulmonary thromboemboli in patients who receive too much anticoagulant. Such patients may then effectively drown in their own blood. It is most important that they be placed in the Trendelenburg position so that the blood leaves the airways and does not become impacted in the pulmonary parenchyma. Trauma patients, by the same token, commonly have severe pulmonary failure and require ventilatory support. In these patients each tidal volume is followed by the need to aspirate blood. The trauma patient with massive airway bleeding must be considered to have a bronchial, tracheal, or laryngeal rupture until proven otherwise by examination.

Pulmonary edema has, as its major mechanism of arterial hypoxia, regional hypoventilation of the dependent lung secondary to edema cuffing of the terminal airways. This may be effectively treated by positive end expiratory pressure.

Embolic phenomena, to the extent that they occlude the pulmonary vasculature, do not produce arterial hypoxia but rather an increase in the physiologic dead space. Embolic phenomena give rise to arterial hypoxia by producing an increase in blood flow to the unobstructed lung. They may be treated by increasing the inspired oxygen just as any other regional hypoventilation. Normally arterial hypoxia may be relieved by increasing cardiac output and thus the mixed venous oxygen. When emboli occlude most of the pulmonary vasculature, further increases in cardiac output by decreasing further the time available for the reaction of oxygen with hemoglobin may worsen the arterial hypoxia. The large pulmonary thromboembolus is the most common cause of this problem, although the same phenomenon may occur from fat emboli and microthromboemboli. Pulmonary contusions, pneumonia, or heavy thoracic walls produce regional hypoventilation in the lung beneath them by interfering with expiratory ventilation. This may be overcome by increasing airway pressure.

Perfusion of Nonventilated Alveoli (Atelectasis, Fluid-Filled Alveoli)

Atelectasis may occur because of regional hypoventilation (Figure 2–20). In normal man this has been called the progressive atelectasis

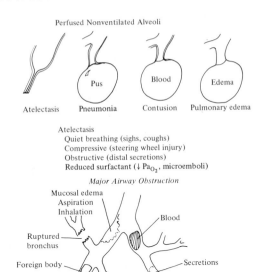

Figure 2–20. Intrapulmonic pulmonary failure—perfused nonventilated alveoli. Alveolar causes of pulmonary failure are atelectasis, blood, pus, edema, and quiet breathing. Blunt trauma expels air from the alveoli and immediately produces atelectasis. This also occurs with blunt trauma to the abdomen since the major response is a sudden rise of the diaphragm. The effects are less if the trauma occurs during inspiration when the glottis is closed so that the intra-alveolar air pressure is increased and the thoracic viscera are wrapped in a cushion of air.

of quiet breathing.[38] Normal man several times an hour sighs, coughs, talks, and, utilizing his glottis in one way or another, hyperinflates his lungs and reexpands atelectatic areas. The absence of significant glottis control, as with coma or severe lethargy, or the absence of the glottis in the airway, as with a tracheostomy, are associated with the absence of these hyperinflation maneuvers and the progressive atelectasis of quiet breathing. The problem is made worse if in addition, because of traction, patients are placed in the Trendelenburg position, are supine, have obese abdomens, and are comatose. These individuals must have their chest as upright as possible.

The patient with blunt chest trauma may have arterial hypoxia without pulmonary infiltrates or circulatory failure. He will be found, on close examination of his x-rays, to have several signs suggestive of a decreased intrapulmonic air volume. In fact, he probably has compressive atelectasis in that the blunt trauma expelled air from his alveoli and caused them to collapse.[9] This sort of atelectasis has occurred without any loss of surfactant and is generally easily re-expanded by the patient himself as he becomes conscious and begins to cough. If, however, he remains lethargic or comatose, the atelectasis is not reexpanded, the surfactant is depleted, and then arterial hypoxia is recognized. After 24 to 48 hours it may not be possible to reexpand the atelectasis and death may eventually occur.

The individual who presents immediately after trauma with a pulmonary infiltrate, severe arterial hypoxia, and no circulatory failure has a pulmonary contusion plus compressive atelectasis. Commonly he also has massive tracheal bleeding so that on top of his other problems, if he is not placed in the Trendelenburg position and vigorously aspirated of blood, he may drown in his own blood or at least develop severe obstructive atelectasis. This patient has arterial hypoxia due to perfused nonventilated areas for several reasons. The pulmonary contusion can only be reversed by absorption of the blood. However, the various kinds of atelectasis can be reversed or prevented if therapy begins early and correctly.

Fluid-filled alveoli as a cause of perfused nonventilated alveoli may also occur because of pus or severe pulmonary edema with regional hypoventilation in the dependent lung. One of the major objectives in the early treatment of pulmonary failure is the prevention of pneumonia by mobilizing the energetic substrate required for bacterial growth. This may be considered a physiologic debridement of the lung and is achieved by adequate suctioning so that retained secretions are not present to support bacterial growth and airway obstruction does not occur and provide an isolated area for bacterial growth of atelectasis and edema fluid. Ventilatory support by preventing atelectasis and mobilizing fluid from the lung can only prevent pneumonia. In contrast ventilatory support also means enhanced bacterial delivery of the organisms that grow well in stagnant water. These are the coliforms, pseudomonas, and certain fungi. It is therefore most important that the heated humidifier be frequently changed and sterilized and that the water-containing tubes be frequently changed.

Summary: Regional Hypoventilation, Perfused Nonventilated Alveoli

The perfused nonventilated alveoli except for acute atelectasis and the pulmonary edema-filled alveolus cannot be significantly affected by ventilatory support. These mechanisms of arterial hypoxia are reversed over relatively long periods of time by the endogenous processes which reabsorb blood and pus and reexpand chronically atelectatic alveoli. In con-

trast, all the mechanisms of regional hypoventilation except retained secretions may be effectively treated by proper ventilatory support. Ventilatory support is very poor treatment for retained secretions, and this differentiation must be made.

The essence of treating pulmonary failure is ventilatory treatment of regional hypoventilation, so that it is not converted to perfused nonventilated alveoli, in order to buy time for the natural body processes to reverse the perfused nonventilated shunt originally present.

Functional Residual Capacity

Regional hypoventilation and perfused nonventilated alveoli both decrease the lung's air volume and therefore the functional residual capacity (Figure 2–21). Powers has made extensive use of this property in correlation with the calculated shunt to investigate the effects of ventilatory support regimes on pulmonary failure.[39] As might be expected, an increased functional residual capacity correlates well with

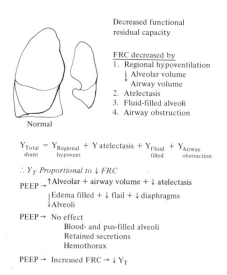

Decreased functional residual capacity

FRC decreased by
1. Regional hypoventilation
   $\downarrow$ Alveolar volume
   $\downarrow$ Airway volume
2. Atelectasis
3. Fluid-filled alveoli
4. Airway obstruction

Normal

$$Y_{Total} = Y_{Regional} + Y\,atelectasis + Y_{Fluid} + Y_{Airway}$$
$$\phantom{Y_{Total} = }{}_{shunt}{}_{hypovent}{}_{filled}{}_{obstruction}$$

$\therefore Y_T$ *Proportional to* $\downarrow FRC$

PEEP $\rightarrow$ $\uparrow$Alveolar + airway volume + $\downarrow$ atelectasis
      $\downarrow$Edema filled + $\downarrow$ flail + $\downarrow$ diaphragms
      $\downarrow$Alveoli

PEEP $\rightarrow$ No effect
      Blood- and pus-filled alveoli
      Retained secretions
      Hemothorax

PEEP $\rightarrow$ Increased FRC $\rightarrow$ $\downarrow Y_T$

Figure 2–21. Pulmonary failure—functional residual capacity. Processes that produce pulmonary failure by regional hypoventilation as a result of perfusion through nonventilated alveoli reduce the pulmonary air volume. This may be measured at a given point in the ventilatory pattern as a reduction in functional residual capacity. Thus, in general, a reduction in functional residual capacity correlates with an increase in the calculated pulmonary shunt and pulmonary failure.

PEEP (positive end expiratory pressure), by increasing alveolar volume generally, increasing terminal airway volume, reversing acute atelectasis, and helping clear edema-filled alveoli both increases functional residual capacity and decreases the calculated pulmonary shunt.

a decreased calculated shunt and therefore decreased pulmonary failure. This work would be expected to pick up much more the effects of regional hypoventilation than those of perfused nonventilated alveoli. One of the interesting findings is that reduced effective pulmonary compliance is primarily related to the reduced functional residual capacity and that the compliance is relatively normal when functional residual capacity returns to normal. This again can only reflect regional hypoventilation and probably patients not in severe pulmonary failure.

Regional Hyperventilation

All patients in pulmonary failure have an increase in their calculated physiologic dead space (Figure 2–15). This calculation is based upon the arterial carbon dioxide tension and the quantity of carbon dioxide expired in a single tidal volume plus the volume of the tidal volume. The assumption is that a tidal volume contains one volume of air which has the carbon dioxide tension of arterial blood and another volume which has the carbon dioxide tension of the inspired air. An underlying assumption is that all alveolar air has the same carbon dioxide tension. This assumption is not valid for embolic phenomena or regional hyperventilation. Pulmonary thromboemboli were at one time thought to have an increase in the alveolar-arterial carbon dioxide tension difference, which is normally zero. However, this characteristic represents nothing more than heterogeneous ventilation in which the ventilation from the nonperfused thromboembolic areas is expired last so that the alveolar air apparently has a lower carbon dioxide tension than the arterial blood. In effect emboli, by creating a nonperfused ventilated area, increase the calculated physiologic dead space and produce an expiratory disorder in which this alveolar gas is expired last.

Millions of alveoli operate in parallel to obtain their ventilation. Granted the same tidal volume, any intrapulmonic factor that limits ventilation in one area must necessarily increase it in other areas. Thus regional hypoventilation produced by any of the intrapulmonic factors must necessarily produce regional hyperventilation in the uninvolved areas (Figure 2–22). As previously discussed, the areas of regional hypoventilation are particularly the dependent areas and the bases of the lungs. Therefore the areas of regional hyperventilation must be the superior lung and the apices.

The removal of carbon dioxide from the blood depends particularly on alveolar ventilation. Thus areas of regional hyperventilation may be expected to be efficacious in removing carbon dioxide and lowering carbon dioxide tension. The total in vivo picture then is that regional hyperventilation removes carbon dioxide to such an extent that the areas of regional hypoventilation and perfused nonventilated alveoli have little effect on arterial carbon dioxide tension. Thus regional hyperventilation is able to overcome the effects of regional hypoventilation on carbon dioxide transport but not on oxygen transport.

The pulmonary alveolus has a compliance-volume relationship in which compliance rapidly increases to a peak at low volumes but decreases as volume further increases. Thus there is a bell-shaped curve when compliance is plotted against volume. Regional hypoventilation, however, produces decreased alveolar volume and therefore compliance. Regional hyperventilation in effect means an alveolar volume at which compliance is maximal and therefore close to the peak of the bell-shaped curve.

Any factor that uniformly increases the volume of all alveoli may be expected to increase the compliance of the regionally hypoventilated area by moving them up the curve and decrease the compliance of the regionally hyperventilated area by moving them past the peak of the curve into the area where compliance decreases with further increases in alveolar volume. The point is that the proper uniform increase in all alveolar volumes would tend to equalize compliance of the regionally hypoventilated and hyperventilated areas and equalize ventilation and therefore match ventilation and perfusion.

This effect may be in part achieved by positive end expiratory pressure for expiratory ventilation.

Physiologic Dead Space

The major therapeutic implication of the increased physiologic dead space produced by regional hyperventilation and ventilated nonperfused areas secondary to emboli is that larger minute volumes of ventilation are required to achieve a given arterial carbon dioxide tension. Treating regional hypoventilation by simultaneously treating the regional hyperventilation also decreases the minute volume required for a given arterial carbon dioxide tension.

Because of the effects of tidal volume on pulmonary failure secondary to atelectasis, we routinely run our adult patients at tidal volumes of 1000 cc (minute volumes of 14 to 15 liters) and control arterial carbon dioxide tension by varying a dead space inserted between the ventilator and the patient. This dead space may be 50 to 300 cc. A standard observation in the patient whose pulmonary failure in terms of oxygen transport is getting worse is that a

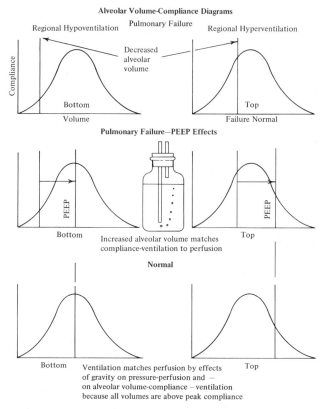

Figure 2–22. Pulmonary failure–alveolar volume–compliance diagrams. Ventilation matches perfusion by design in the normal lung because capillary hydrostatic pressure influences alveolar capillary perfusion and alveolar volume. As the alveolar volume decreases secondary to increasing capillary hydrostatic pressure (going from top to bottom), the compliance and ventilation increase so that perfusion matches ventilation.

The upper panel shows the effects of pulmonary failure if no change occurs other than a generalized decrease in alveolar volume so that on the alveolar-compliance diagram all alveolar volumes are located in the volume range from peak compliance down. In this range, as alveolar volume decreases, the compliance decreases rather than increases as it normally does. Again, increasing capillary hydrostatic pressure in going from the superior to the dependent lung is associated with increasing perfusion and decreasing alveolar volume. However, under these conditions, decreasing alveolar volume is associated with decreasing alveolar compliance and therefore decreased ventilation.

Positive end expiratory pressure not only affects alveolar volume but also affects pulmonary capillary perfusion and, if transmitted through the lung to the heart, diastolic cardiac filling. The greatest positive end expiratory pressure usable is that which does not interfere unduly with these elements of circulation. The normal patient can easily tolerate in terms of the circulation 5 to 10 cm H_2O of PEEP. The hypovolemic patient may have trouble in terms of circulation with 5 cm H_2O. The patient with severe pulmonary failure may require 15 cm H_2O PEEP but will simultaneously require a high central venous pressure.

progressively smaller dead space is required to achieve the same carbon dioxide tension at the same minute volume. The patient whose pulmonary failure is getting better in terms of oxygen transport requires a progressively larger dead space to achieve the same carbon dioxide tension. The changes in the external dead space are the reciprocal of the changes in intrapulmonic physiologic dead space. Thus, even

by this simple measure, regional hypoventilation and regional hyperventilation are strongly associated processes.

Interaction of Pulmonary Failure with the Rest of the Body

The work of Clowes and various associates has demonstrated that severe sepsis anywhere in the body releases bloodborne agents that induce pulmonary multifocal congestive atelectasis and thus can produce pulmonary failure.[7,14] In general severely septic patients have not only several varieties of systemic circulatory failure but also pulmonary failure.

The lung has a number of important endocrine functions. These include conversion of angiotensin 1 to angiotensin 2, clearance of norepinephrine but not epinephrine, clearance of bradykinins and the prostaglandins E and F.[19] Thus pulmonary failure may well affect the neuroendocrine regulation of metabolism and blood flow.

Pulmonary failure to the extent that it requires an increase in central venous pressure can influence hepatic function. All of our patients who have remained in severe pulmonary failure for any period of time have developed several signs of hepatic dysfunction. This is probably also because of the prolonged use of pure intravenous glucose and the prolonged stress catabolic state as described in the metabolic response to sepsis, starvation, and trauma.

Management of Pulmonary Failure

Pulmonary failure may be diagnosed with an arterial oxygen tension 70 mm Hg or less on room air or an oxygen tension less than that expected for the inspired oxygen [$(F_{I_{O_2}})$ (500 mm Hg)] when the central venous oxygen tension is close to 40 mm Hg, and the arterial carbon dioxide tension is normal. This pulmonary failure may be acute or chronic, and the differentiation may be determined from the history. However, in trauma patients our greatest near tragedies have occurred in those who were assumed to have chronic lung disease. We therefore routinely treat such patients for acute pulmonary failure until they prove, by being stable over a period of time, to have chronic lung disease.

Pulmonary failure if not present initially may be expected to occur in the multiple trauma patient; the severely septic patient; the patient in prolonged shock; the lethargic to comatose patient, particularly if in traction or supine; the patient with a flail chest, and the depleted patient such as the fractured hip patient who is in pain and supine (Figure 2–23; Table 2–1). These patients commonly begin with relatively normal blood gases which deteriorate over a period of days to severe arterial hypoxia.

Progressive pulmonary failure means the progressive conversion of regional hypoventilation to perfused nonventilated alveoli. The patient with the advanced pulmonary failure characterized by massive shunting through areas of perfused nonventilated alveoli is almost certainly going to die. The essence of

Table 2–1. SEVERE SEPSIS

(Commonly Leads to Pulmonary Failure by Multiple Mechanisms)

Lethargy	Inadequate use of glottis and muscles of inspiration
Supine position	Made worse by obesity Elevated diaphragm Heavy chest wall
Intestinal distention	Elevated diaphragm
Septic areas	Release bloodborne agents producing direct pulmonary alveolo-capillary damage
Pneumonia	From bloodborne or airborne bacteria in the presence of edema fluid, atelectasis, and congestive atelectasis Also results in direct pulmonary failure consequences

Hepatic metabolic consequences of sepsis and support
    Catabolic setting metabolism
    Pure glucose support
    Direct consequences peritonitis
    Decreased protein synthesis

treatment is therefore treating regional hypoventilation to prevent its conversion to perfused nonventilated alveoli. It is much easier to prevent severe pulmonary failure than to treat it. Therefore the use of increased inspired oxygen to treat pulmonary failure is rational only when used simultaneously with maneuvers to treat regional hypoventilation.

Regional hypoventilation from extrapulmonic causes, with the exception of the flail chest, is best treated by measures to lower the diaphragm and thoracostomy tubes for pneumohemothorax. Gastrointestinal distention is best handled by an early nasogastric tube to prevent it. The patient who has a laparotomy with distended bowel should have it decompressed at surgery to prevent his subsequent pulmonary failure. The patient in traction for proximal shaft fractures should have them internally fixed early so that he may be removed from traction and his chest placed in the upright position. If this cannot be done, a Thomas splint with countertraction should be utilized so that the patient's chest can be placed upright. The patient with a hip fracture should be operated upon as early as possible so that his chest can be placed upright.

Flail chests produce regional hypoventilation easily corrected by ventilatory support. The magnitude of the flail chest has no necessary relationship to the magnitude of the underlying

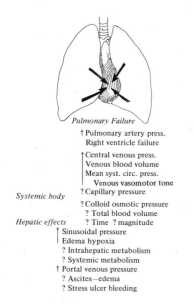

Pulmonary Failure

↑ Pulmonary artery press.
    Right ventricle failure

↑ Central venous press.
    Venous blood volume
    Mean syst. circ. press.
    Venous vasomotor tone
? Capillary pressure

Systemic body

? Colloid osmotic pressure
? Total blood volume

Hepatic effects   ? Time ? magnitude

↑ Sinusoidal pressure
    Edema hypoxia
? Intrahepatic metabolism
? Systemic metabolism
↑ Portal venous pressure
? Ascites—edema
? Stress ulcer bleeding

Figure 2–23. Severe trauma—commonly leads to pulmonary failure.

1. Compressive atelectasis—blow to chest or abdomen.
2. Pulmonary contusion—immediate infiltrate with arterial hypoxia.
3. Lethargic comatose state—progressive atelectasis of quiet breathing without appropriate use of glottis and muscle.
4. Intestinal distention—elevated diaphragm.
5. Supine position—traction, obese abdomen, and chest.
6. Pneumonia.
7. Fat and microthromboemboli.
8. Hypovolemic circulatory failure.
9. Direct cardiac trauma.
10. Pneumohemothorax.
11. Flail chest.
12. Metabolic consequences—dead tissue and hematomas.
13. Hepatic metabolic consequences—catabolic state, nutritional support, high central venous pressure.

pulmonary damage. Thus some of our most massive flail chests have had essentially no pulmonary failure as soon as they were placed on the ventilator. In contrast we have had minimal flail chests associated with severe underlying pulmonary damage and failure, particularly in young patients.

Essentially all of our patients in traction have regional hypoventilation. However, the young, healthy, alert patient who has his traction arranged so that his chest is upright easily overcomes this problem, probably by producing with the glottis his own positive end expiratory pressure. This does not happen even in the young patient who remains supine or is not alert and conscious. Bilateral femoral shaft traction with the chest essentially in the Trendelenburg position is particularly apt to be associated with progressive pulmonary failure. This problem is worsened if, in attempting to raise the chest, the bed is angulated and then the traction pulls the patient down in bed so that the chest is hyperflexed at the diaphragm. The upright chest with a functioning diaphragm and glottis is of the utmost importance in preventing pulmonary failure.

The intrapulmonic causes of pulmonary failure, except retained secretions, and the extrapulmonic causes of pulmonary failure affecting the diaphragm that cannot be corrected are treated with ventilatory support. This is very poor therapy for retained secretions, and these are by far the most common cause of pulmonary failure.

Ventilatory therapy has as its keystone the use of positive end expiratory pressure because of its effect on equalizing alveolar compliance, distending the small airways during expiration when they have a great tendency to collapse, and expanding atelectatic areas and mobilizing fluid from the alveoli. Positive end expiratory pressure is generally used in a range of 5 to 15 cm H_2O. The magnitude of the pressure to be used is that which maximally improves oxygen transport without interfering significantly with the circulation. Arterial hypoxia unresponsive to maximal positive end expiratory pressure is treated with an increase in inspired oxygen. More than 60 percent oxygen is seldom required.

The arterial oxygen tension desired varies somewhat with the pathology involved. In patients with head injuries, those in whom infection would be a life- or limb-threatening catastrophe, or in patients already infected, we attempt to maintain an arterial oxygen tension of 120 to 130 mm Hg so that we are absolutely certain that maximal oxygen delivery can occur. We do not do this if inspired oxygens greater than 60 to 80 percent are required. In other patients we are satisfied with arterial oxygen tensions of 90 to 100 mm Hg.

The conscious alert patient with arterial hypoxia, if sufficiently encouraged, can generally clear his pulmonary failure by coughing and deep breathing if his chest can be maintained upright and he does not have wound pain. This patient is treated with 5 cm H_2O positive end expiratory pressure with a face mask or mouthpiece without a ventilator at the inspired oxygen for an adequate arterial oxygen tension. While this is going on, he is vigorously and repeatedly encouraged to cough and deep breathe. If no improvement has occurred in one hour, he is placed on intermittent positive pressure breathing at 25 cm H_2O for 10 minutes each hour in addition to the positive end expiratory pressure.

If the patient does not improve, gets worse, or cannot cooperate, he requires intubation. The lethargic or comatose patient with arterial hypoxia requires immediate intubation. The patient who is operated upon following severe trauma or with severe sepsis should remain on the ventilator postoperatively until he proves via repeated arterial and central venous blood gases that it is not required. After removal from the ventilator these patients should continue to be observed with blood gases over several days since they are highly likely to go back into pulmonary failure. The patient with severe head trauma is placed on the ventilator and given maximum cardiopulmonary support because of his great tendency to go into cardiopulmonary failure and expand his area of cerebral damage.

Ventilatory support is begun with nasotracheal intubation if this can be done easily. If not, the patient has an oral endotracheal tube placed with Pentothal and succinylcholine. Both of these tubes provide much less satisfying endotracheal suction than the tracheostomy tube. Therefore patients with copious secretions, or in whom another type of tracheal tube has been present two to three days, have tracheostomies done for intubation. We have had a number of fatalities occur while moving patients to the operating room for tracheostomy; therefore all tracheostomies are done in the intensive care unit. All tracheostomies are done with vertical incisions which come down on the lower end of the larynx. This allows a finger to be slipped down the anterior surface of the trachea so that all structures anterior to it may be divided between the fingers and all bleeders controlled by them. The tracheal wall is then incised at the second to third cartilage for the tracheostomy tube.

The tracheostomy cuff should be very soft and flexible and inflated to create a 200- to 300-cc air leak. This allows the patient to talk and prevents tracheal stenosis. The inability to talk for a prolonged period can only produce severe anxiety and contribute to the stress catabolic state. The tidal volume of importance is not the one set on the machine but the one expired by the patient. Therefore any ventilator without an expiratory spirometer should not be used.

The tidal volume is set at 15 cc per kilogram. For normal adults this approximates 1000 cc. This volume is selected to help prevent the progressive atelectasis of quiet breathing and to help keep the lung filled with air. Also to prevent atelectasis a sigh, set at twice the tidal volume

(1600 cc to 2000 cc), is delivered by the machine 45 times each hour.

All critically ill patients should be managed on volume-cycled ventilators. The pressure-cycled machines allow the tidal volume to decrease as the compliance decreases. The patient should, in general, be allowed to trip the ventilator. The exceptions to this lie in the patient who ventilates too rapidly or fights the ventilator. This cannot be allowed since it interferes with proper ventilation and circulation. To prevent this in the patient without head trauma, 10 to 20 mg of morphine IV every hour is given if he is unable to cooperate with the ventilator. It should be pointed out that morphine under these conditions is used more for anesthesia than analgesia. The patient with head trauma receives succinylcholine 2 to 4 gm per liter at a rate that allows ventilator cooperation with a minidripper.

Positive end expiratory pressure is applied with a glass tube submerged in a chest bottle (Table 2–2). This method has been chosen so that considerable effort is required to change it; therefore it is not changed casually. A major problem with ventilators is the tendency of some individuals to twist the knobs. The chest bottle prevents this since every important knob is taped down.

Positive end expiratory pressure affects only expiration, by increasing both pressure and duration. Regional hypoventilation in severe pulmonary failure may also be treated by manipulating inspiration. In general under

Table 2–2. POSITIVE END EXPIRATORY PRESSURE

PEEP alleviates
 1. High diaphragms
 2. Regional hypoventilation and hyperventilation
 3. Flail chest
 4. Obese chest and breasts
 5. Improper weight distribution in lung—pneumonia, contusion
 6. Terminal airway collapse
 7. Terminal airway pulmonary edema cuffing
 8. Acute atelectasis
 9. Edema-filled alveoli
10. Mucosal edema
11. Consequences of distant sepsis
12. Gastric aspiration when contents removed

PEEP no effect
 1. Retained secretions with obstruction
 2. Hemothorax

PEEP may make worse
 1. Hypovolemic circulatory failure
 2. Pneumothorax
 3. Hepatic problems

these conditions the compliance is so poor that inspiratory pressure cannot be further increased. The problem may be managed by increasing the time of inspiration. This may be done by decreasing the rate of inspiratory air flow or by utilizing, at the peak of inspiration, an inspiratory hold. Both allow more time for air to go from the large airways to the alveoli just as positive expiratory pressure allows more time for air to leave the alveoli.

The rate of inspiratory air flow is generally set at 50 to 60 liters per minute. This may be reduced to 40 liters per minute. Positive expiratory pressure prolongs expiration, and this maneuver prolongs inspiration. The result is that the respiratory rate must be decreased. Under these conditions we have gone as low as a respiration rate of seven to eight.

The patient with arterial hypoxia requires a definite monitoring plan. This must include arterial and central venous blood gases, inspired oxygen, plasma albumin, urine output, and vital signs. The frequency of monitoring depends upon knowledge of the patient's stability. Rapidly changing patients should be monitored hourly. This requires arterial and central venous blood catheters plus a Foley catheter. When the patient has proved stable, the frequency of monitoring may be decreased. This monitoring should begin in the emergency room and be carried through surgery, exactly as it is in the intensive care unit but more often.

Increasing arterial hypoxia on the ventilator with positive end expiratory pressure commonly means retained secretions, hemopneumothorax, pneumonia, or the endotracheal tube in the right main stem bronchus. These diagnoses must be considered separately. Retained secretions may occur with frequent suctioning if the endotracheal tube is too far in, a straight catheter has been utilized, or a Caude catheter improperly used. The position of the endotracheal tube must be established. If the position is proper, then the physician should personally utilize the suction catheter. If no improvement occurs, then fiberoptic bronchoscopy with a 3-mm tube through a large endotracheal tube should be done while the patient is on the ventilator. Removal from the ventilator for bronchoscopy in these patients can be extremely hazardous.

If fiberoptic bronchoscopy for secretions is negative and there is no x-ray evidence for hemopneumothorax, then in general the diagnosis is either pneumonia or some other intrapulmonic disorder. The diagnosis of pneumonia in chest trauma patients on the ventilator is particularly difficult. In general a pneumonia is diagnosed with bacteria and pus in the sputum, an infiltrate on the chest x-ray, fever, and leukocytosis. The chest trauma patient may have all of these findings without necessarily having pneumonia. In general if the pulmonary failure is getting better and all of these findings are present, the patient is not treated for pneumonia. In contrast, if the pulmonary failure is getting worse and these findings are present, or if some well-known pulmonary pathogen such as the pneumococcus is present, the patient is treated with antibiotics for pneumonia.

Death from progressive pulmonary failure in our previous experience occurred when arterial oxygen tension on 100 percent oxygen fell to about 50 mm Hg and simultaneously the arterial carbon dioxide tension began to rise after the external dead space had been reduced to zero. This always occurred on minute ventilatory volumes of 15 to 20 liters with very poor compliance and was not improved with repeated suctioning. All such patients died. The advent of the Caude catheter and the more sophisticated analysis of pulmonary failure now available has changed this problem considerably. Analysis of the preceding information with a rising carbon dioxide tension and falling external dead space reveals alveolar hypoventilation in the presence of a minute ventilatory volume of 15 to 20 liters, a grossly increasing physiologic dead space, and severe pulmonary failure due to perfused nonventilated alveoli. This combination can only mean severe pulmonary damage in one area and major airway obstruction to another area plus, in all probability, the whole tidal volume being shunted to a third area of the lung with such pressures that it interferes with blood flow.

This analysis was first made on a young girl who appeared to be dying. Proper persistent use of Caude catheter was associated with an increase in arterial oxygen to 271 mm Hg within the hour and survival. We have since seen a few more such cases where for one reason or another our protocols were not followed and severe pulmonary failure was present. The problem will probably disappear now that fiberoptic bronchoscopy is available.

The patient is ready for weaning when he has been alert, stable, with an upright chest for several days, and has an arterial oxygen tension of 90 to 100 on 30 percent oxygen (Figure 2–24). Progressive atelectasis is particularly apt to occur during weaning because of the functional absence of the glottis and the unstable condition of the lungs. The first steps in weaning therefore are the use of short periods of positive end expiratory pressure without the ventilator. The Briggs adaptor, a tee piece commonly used, allows increased oxygen and humidity but also

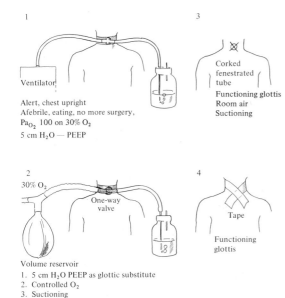

1

Ventilator

Alert, chest upright
Afebrile, eating, no more surgery,
Pa_{O_2} 100 on 30% O_2
5 cm H_2O — PEEP

3

Corked
fenestrated
tube

Functioning glottis
Room air
Suctioning

2

30% O_2

One-way
valve

Volume reservoir

4

Tape

Functioning
glottis

1. 5 cm H_2O PEEP as glottic substitute
2. Controlled O_2
3. Suctioning

Figure 2–24. Weaning sequence. During weaning it is essential to maintain pulmonary air volume spontaneously or by mechanical aids. It should not begin (*1*) until the chest can be maintained upright, the patient is alert, and can generate an oxygen tension of 100 mm Hg on 30 percent oxygen with 5 cm H_2O PEEP.

The first step in weaning is the use of positive end expiratory pressure (5 cm H_2O) with 30 percent oxygen without the ventilator (*2*). This requires a volume reservoir (anesthesia bag) on a tee piece and a one-way valve. However, it allows spontaneous ventilation while providing the most effective measure for preventing the progressive atelectasis of quiet breathing and at the same time allowing a controlled inspired oxygen together with the possibility of suctioning. The Briggs tee piece commonly used at this stage allows the progressive atelectasis of quiet breathing in lungs particularly prone to this problem.

When the patient's arterial oxygens are stable for about two days on PEEP without the ventilator and adequate oxygen tensions can be achieved on room air, the patient is ready for the next stage of weaning. This consists of the use of corked fenestrated tube (*3*). This restores a functioning glottis while yet allowing suctioning. If he remains stable and shows an adequate cough to raise secretions he is ready for the next stage (*4*). The fenestrated tube is removed and the tracheostomy tube taped tightly in place, thus again immediately providing a glottis to allow glottic manipulation of pulmonary air volume and effective coughing.

allows ventilation without a glottis and therefore progressive atelectasis. This is almost routinely used during weaning and is opposed to all principles of basic pulmonary physiology.

Positive end expiratory pressure without the ventilator requires a one-way valve but also allows known inspired oxygen and increased humidity plus a glottic substitute that should help prevent atelectasis.

When the patient can tolerate ventilation with positive end expiratory pressure for about 48 hours and remains stable, he is ready for the next stage of weaning. Again the key is the use of the glottis to maintain the lungs expanded. Thus the next step is the insertion of a corked fenestrated tracheostomy tube. It allows the patient to use his own glottis to prevent atelectasis while simultaneously still allowing suctioning if the patient cannot satisfactorily raise his own secretions.

When the patient has been stable on this regime and coughs up his own secretions for about 48 hours, the fenestrated tracheostomy tube may be removed. The tracheostomy wound is then tightly closed with an occlusive dressing so that once again the glottis is immediately active to prevent atelectasis. The normal role of the glottis in preventing atelectasis cannot be overemphasized.

Summary: Pulmonary Failure

The introduction recounts the hopelessness and despair that progressive pulmonary failure produced prior to 1969. The physiologic discussion presents the normal physiology required to understand the physiology of pulmonary failure, which is then analyzed so that specific treatment and, even more important, specific maneuvers to prevent pulmonary failure can be undertaken. The section on management then offers specific routines designed to prevent and treat pulmonary failure. Understanding this material together with that on circulatory failure and metabolic management has made a dramatic difference in the management of the critically ill patient. It is very unusual these days for a previously healthy patient who could be resuscitated in the emergency room to die of cardiopulmonary failure in spite of our best efforts. Key to this change is the recognition that severe pulmonary failure can be present and not be recognized clinically. In fact, clinically recognized pulmonary failure is normally terminal; therefore all critically ill patients should have arterial blood gases whether they are thought to be needed clinically or not.

Pulmonary failure recognized at the stage of regional hypoventilation is easy to treat, while in the stage of perfused nonventilated alveoli treatment is very difficult. Recognizing the interrelation between pulmonary failure, circulatory failure, and the metabolic changes subsequently discussed provides a rational framework for management. This management begins in the emergency room and must be carried out during surgery just as it is in the intensive care unit. All critically ill patients being operated upon should be getting arterial and central venous blood gases just as arterial and central venous pressures are taken. In addition, hourly urine volumes and specific gravities should be taken just as they are in the intensive care unit. The emergency room and operating room should be just as sophisticated as the intensive care unit in terms of the care delivered.

CITED REFERENCES

1. Alfano, G. S., and Hale, H. W., Jr.: Pulmonary contusion. *J. Trauma*, 5:647–58, 1965.
2. Ashbaugh, D. G.: Effect of ventilatory methods and patterns on physiologic shunt. *Surgery*, 68:99–104, 1970.
3. Ashbaugh, D. G.; Petty, T. L.; Bigelow, D. B.; and Harris, T. M.: Continuous positive-pressure breathing (CPPB) in adult respiratory distress syndrome. *J. Thorac. Cardiovasc. Surg.*, 57:31–41, 1969.
4. Bates, D. B.; Macklem, P. T.; and Christie, R. W.: *Respiratory Function in Disease*. W. B. Saunders, Philadelphia, 1971.
5. Berk, J. L.: Use of beta blockers in shock. In Forscher, B. K.; Lillehei, R. C.; and Stubbe, S. S. (eds.): *Shock in Low and High Flow States*. Excerpta Medica Foundation, Amsterdam, pp. 282–92, 1972.
6. Border, J. R.: Advances and newer concepts in shock. In Cooper, P. (ed.): *Surgery Annual*. Appleton-Century-Crofts, New York, pp. 79–123, 1969.
7. Border, J. R.: Changes in cardiopulmonary function in the severely stressed patient. In Hershey, S. G.; Del Guercio, L. R. M.; and Conn, R. (eds.): *Septic Shock in Man*. Little, Brown, Boston, pp. 239–54, 1971.
8. Border, J. R.; Tibbetts, J. C.; and Schenk, W. G.: Hypoxic hyperventilation and acute respiratory failure in the severely stressed patient: Massive pulmonary arteriovenous shunts. *Surgery*, 64:710–19, 1968.
9. Border, J. R.; Hopkinson, B. R.; and Schenk, W. G., Jr.: Mechanisms of pulmonary trauma. An experimental study. *J. Trauma*, 8:47–62, 1968.
10. Border, J. R.; Gallo, E.; and Schenk, W. G., Jr.: Systemic arteriovenous shunts in patients under severe stress. A common cause of high output cardiac failure. *Surgery*, 60:225–31, 1966.
11. Braunwald, E. (ed.): *The Myocardium: Failure and Infarction*. HP Publishing Co., New York, 1974.
12. Burke, J. F.; Pontoppidan, H.; and Welch, C. E.: High output respiratory failure: An important cause of death ascribed to peritonitis or ileus. *Ann Surg.*, 158:581–95, 1963.
13. Clowes, G. H. A.; O'Donnell, T. F.; Ryand, N. T.; and Blackburn, G. L.: Energy metabolism in sepsis: Treatment based on different patterns in shock and high output stage. *Ann. Surg.*, 179:684–96, 1974.
14. Clowes, G. H. A.; Zuschneid, W.; Turner, M.; Blackburn, G.; Rubin, J.; Toala, P.; and Green, G.: Observations on the pathogenesis of the pneumonitis associated with severe infections in other parts of the body. *Ann. Surg.*, 167:630–50, 1968.
15. Davis, J. O.: The physiology of congestive failure. In Hamilton, W. F. (ed.): *Handbook of Physiology*. Vol. 3, Section 2. Williams & Wilkins, Baltimore, pp. 2071–127, 1965.
16. Epstein, S. E.; Kent, K. M.; Goldstein, R. E.; Borer, T. S.; and Redwood, D. R.: Reduction of ischemic injury by nitroglycerin during acute myocardial infarction. *N. Engl. J. Med.*, 292:29–35, 1975.
17. Fine, T.: Shock and peripheral circulatory insufficiency. In Hamilton, W. F. (ed.): *Handbook of Physiology*. Vol. 3, Section 2. Williams & Wilkins, Baltimore, pp. 2037–71, 1965.
18. Fishman, A. P.: Dynamics of the pulmonary circulation. In Hamilton, W. F. (ed.): *Handbook of Physiology*. Vol. 2, Section 2. Williams & Wilkins, Baltimore, pp. 1667–1745, 1963.
19. Fishman, A. P., and Pietra, G. G.: Handling of bioactive materials by the lung. *N. Engl. J. Med.*, 291:884–89 and 953–59, 1974.
20. Fishman, A. P., and Hecht, H. H. (eds.): *The Pulmonary Circulation and Interstitial Space*. University of Chicago Press, Chicago, 1969.
21. Greene, P. O.: Pulmonary edema. In Fenn, W. O., and Rahn, H. (eds.): *Handbook of Physiology*. Vol. 2, Section 3. Williams & Wilkins, Baltimore, pp. 1585–1601, 1965.
22. Gump, F. E.; Price, J. B.; and Kinney, J. M.: Whole body and splanchnic blood flow and oxygen consumption measurements in patients with intraperitoneal infection. *Ann. Surg.*, 171:321–28, 1970.
23. Guyton, A. C.: A concept of negative interstitial pressure based on pressures in implanted perforated capsules. *Circ. Res.*, 12:399–414, 1963.
24. Guyton, A. C.; Coleman, T. G.; and Granger, H. J.: Circulation: Overall regulation. *Annu. Rev. Physiol.*, 34:13–46, 1972.
25. Guyton, A. C.; Jones, G. E.; and Coleman, T. G.: *Circulatory Physiology: Cardiac Output and Its Regulation*. W. B. Saunders, Philadelphia, 1973.
26. Guyton, A. C.: *Textbook of Medical Physiology*. W. B. Saunders, Philadelphia, 1966.
27. Hirsch, E. F., and Kaiser, G. C.: *The Innervation of the Lungs*. Charles C Thomas, Springfield, Ill., 1969.
28. Hopkinson, B. R.; Border, J. R.; Heyden, W. C.; and Schenk, W. G., Jr.: Interstitial fluid pressure changes during hemorrhage and blood replacement with and without hypotension. *Surgery*, 64:68–74, 1968.
29. Landis, F. M., and Papenheimer, J. R.: Exchange of substances through the capillary walls. In Hershey, S. G.; Del Guercio, L. R. M.; and Conn, R. (eds.): *Septic Shock in Man*. Vol. 2. Little, Brown, Boston, pp. 961–1035, 1971.
30. Lillehei, R. C., and Dietzman, R. H.: Circulatory collapse and shock. In Schwartz, S. I. (ed.): *Principles of Surgery*. 2nd ed. McGraw-Hill, New York, pp. 133–65, 1969.
31. Lillehei, R. C.; Motsay, G. J.; and Dietzman, R. H.: The use of corticosteroids in the treatment of shock. *Int. Z. Klin. Pharmakol. Ther. Toxik.*, 5:423–33, 1972.
32. MacLean, L. D.: Shock: Causes and management of circulatory collapse. In Sabiston, D. C. (ed.): *Textbook of Surgery*. W. B. Saunders, Philadelphia, pp. 65–94, 1972.
33. Majno, G.: Ultrastructure of the vascular membrane. In Hershey, G. S.; Del Guercio, L. R. M.; and Conn, R. (eds.): *Septic Shock in Man*. Vol. 3. Little, Brown, Boston, pp. 2293–377, 1971.
34. Markello, R.; Schuder, R.; and Border, J.: Arterial-alveolar N_2 differences documenting ventilation-perfusion mismatching following trauma. *J. Trauma*, 14:423–26, 1974.
35. Mayerson, H. S.: The physiologic importance of lymph. In Hershey, S. G.; Del Guercio, L. R. M.; and Conn, R. (eds.): *Septic Shock in Man*. Vol. 2. Little, Bown, Boston, pp. 1035–75, 1971.
36. Moore, F. D.; Lyons, J. A.; Pierce, E. C.; Morgan, A. P.; Drinker, P. A.; MacArthur, J. D.; and

Dammin, G. J.: *Post-Traumatic Pulmonary Insufficiency*. W. B. Saunders, Philadelphia, 1969.

37. Moore, F. D.: *The Body Cell Mass*. W. B. Saunders, Philadelphia, 1963.

38. Pontoppidan, H.; Laver, M. B.; and Geffin, B.: Acute respiratory failure in the surgical patient. *Adv. Surg.*, **4**:163–255, 1970.

39. Powers, S. R.; Mannal, R.; Neclerio, M.; English, M., et al.: Physiologic consequences of positive end-expiratory pressure (PEEP) ventilation. *Ann. Surg.*, **178**:265–72, 1973.

40. Rahn, H., and Farhi, L. E.: Ventilation, perfusion and gas exchange. In Fenn, W. O., and Rahn, H. (eds.): *Handbook of Physiology*. Vol. 1, Section 3. Williams & Wilkins, Baltimore, pp. 735–67, 1964.

41. Ramp, J. M.; Hankins, J. R.; and Mason, G. R.: Cardiac tamponade secondary to blunt trauma. A report of two cases and review of the literature. *J. Trauma*, **14**:767–72, 1974.

42. Said, S. I.; Longacher, J. W.; Davis, R. K.; Banerjee, C. M.; Davis, W. M.; and Wooddell, W. J.: Pulmonary gas exchange during induction of pulmonary edema in anesthetized dogs. *J. Appl. Physiol.*, **19**:403–407, 1964.

43. Said, S. I.: The lung as a metabolic organ. *N. Engl. J. Med.*, **279**:1330–34, 1968.

44. Sasahara, A. A., and Stein, M. (eds.): *Pulmonary Embolic Disease*. Grune & Stratton, New York, 1965.

45. Shoemaker, W. C.: *Shock, Chemistry, Physiology, Therapy*. Charles C. Thomas, Springfield, Ill., 1967.

46. Siegel, J. H.; Goldwyn, R. M.; and Friedman, H. P.: Pattern and process in the evolution of human septic shock. *Surgery*, **70**:232–45, 1971.

47. Stein, L.; Beraud, J. J.; Cavanilles, J.; da Luz, P.; Weil, M. H.; and Shubin, H.: Pulmonary edema during fluid infusion in the absence of heart failure. *JAMA*, **229**:65–68, 1974.

48. Swan, H. J. C.; Ganz, W.; Forrester, J.; Marcus, H.; Diamond, G.; and Chonette, D.: Catheterization of the heart in man with use of a flow-directed balloon-tipped catheter. *N. Engl. J. Med.*, **283**:447–51, 1970.

49. Thal, A. P.: *Shock: A Physiologic Basis for Treatment*. Year Book Medical Publishers, Chicago, 1971.

50. Torteson, D. C.: Regulation of cell volume by sodium and potassium transport. In Hoffman, T. F. (ed.): *The Cellular Function of Membrane Transport*. Prentice Hall, Englewood Cliffs, N. J., pp. 3–23, 1964.

51. Weil, M. H., and Shubin, A.: *Diagnosis and Treatment of Shock*. Williams & Wilkins, Baltimore, 1967.

52. Weil, M. H., and Shubin, H.: The "VIP" approach to the bedside management of shock. *JAMA*, **207**:337–40, 1969.

53. Whittam, R., and Wheeler, K. P.: Transport across cell membranes. *Annu. Rev. Physiol.*, **32**:21–60, 1970.

SUGGESTIONS FOR FURTHER READING

Bates, D. B.; Macklem, P. T.; and Christie, R. W.: *Respiratory Function in Disease*. W. B. Saunders, Philadelphia, 1971.
This book is particularly valuable for its section on normal pulmonary physiology.

Fishman, A. P.: Dynamics of the pulmonary circulation. In Hamilton, W. F. (ed.): *Handbook of Physiology*. Section 2. Williams & Wilkins, Baltimore, pp. 1667–1745, 1963. Vol. II.
An exceptionally valuable discussion of normal pulmonary blood flow and its controls.

Guyton, A. C.; Jones, C. E.; and Coleman, T. G.: *Circulatory Physiology: Cardiac Output and Its Regulation*. W. B. Saunders, Philadelphia, 1973.
A valuable discussion of the normal regulation of cardiac output. There is no hope of understanding circulatory physiology without understanding the normal.

MacLean, L. D.: Shock: Causes and management of circulatory collapse. In Sabiston, D. C. (ed.): *Textbook of Surgery*. W. B. Saunders, Philadelphia, 1972, pp. 65–94.
A good discussion of shock from the point of view of an able clinician and investigator.

Pontppidan, H.; Laver, M. D.; and Gaffin, B.: Acute respiratory failure in the surgical patient. *Adv. Surg.*, **4**:163–255, 1970.
A very valuable discussion of the observations on pulmonary failure but with rather difficult terminology.

Siegel, J. H.; Goldwyn, R. M.; and Friedman, H. P.: Patterns and processes in the evaluation of human septic shock. *Surgery*, **70**:232–45, 1975.
A multidimensional point of view of septic shock such as presented in this chapter, but utilizing the aid of computers.

Chapter 3

FLUID, ELECTROLYTE, AND ACID-BASE BALANCE

John A. McCredie

CHAPTER OUTLINE

Basic Considerations
   Atomic Structure
   Milliequivalent
   Hydrogen Ion Concentration
     Henderson-Hasselbalch Equation
   Buffer
     Buffering Action of Hemoglobin
   Fluid Compartments
The Surgical Patient
   Water Balance
     Clinical Manifestations of Overhydration
       and Underhydration
   Electrolytes
    Sodium
    Potassium
    Magnesium
   Nutrition
    Calories

    Protein
    Fat
    Vitamins
   Intravenous Fluids
   Intravenous Orders
    Past Deficit
    Concurrent Losses
Metabolic Acidosis and Alkalosis
   Hydrogen Ion Balance
    Metabolic Acidosis
    Metabolic Alkalosis
   Simple and Mixed Acid-Base Disturbances
Respiratory Acidosis and Alkalosis
   Respiratory Acidosis
   Respiratory Alkalosis
Determination of Acid-Base Balance
   Total Carbon Dioxide Content
   Astrup Equilibration Method

It is critical for cellular function that fluid, electrolyte, and acid-base balance be maintained within a narrow range. Complex mechanisms are available to maintain the normal internal environment through the endocrine system, kidneys, lungs, and skin.

During the development of a fluid-deficient state, compensatory mechanisms are called into play, especially the secretion of antidiuretic and salt-retaining hormones. Thus care should be exercised to permit balanced readjustment as fluid replacement proceeds; otherwise injurious retention of salt and water may occur.

A rational approach to fluid and electrolyte therapy requires a knowledge of the volume and composition of body fluids and reliable methods to quickly determine any deficiencies. Certain changes in fluids and electrolytes regularly follow the stress of an operation or injury. Special problems are present in patients with intestinal fistulas or obstruction and with renal, cardiac, and pulmonary disease. Fluid and electrolyte replacement should proceed cautiously and always with frequent clinical observa-

tion monitoring the therapeutic effects. Few patients fit exactly into one of the theoretical categories of electrolyte and fluid disturbances. Each patient therefore presents an individual challenge.

BASIC CONSIDERATIONS

Atomic Structure

The atomic nucleus contains positively charged protons and neutrons. The number of protons (Z number) is the atomic number and determines the properties of the element, while the number of protons and neutrons (A number) determines the atomic weight. Isotopes of the element have the same number of protons, but the number of neutrons varies. Extremely light and rapidly moving negatively charged electrons, or beta particles, equal in number to the protons, orbit the nucleus. They are arranged in orbital paths or shells K, L, M around the nucleus; the maximum number in K, the innermost shell, is 2, in L 8, and in M 18. The closer the shell to the nucleus the greater the attractive force of the nucleus for the electron. The number of electrons in the outermost shell determines the reactivity of the element which is least when the full complement is reached. When an element or molecule loses one or more electrons, it is positively charged; on gaining one or more it becomes negative. A solution containing charged particles is said to be ionized. On placing a positive and negative electrode in the solution, positively charged particles pass to the cathode (cations H^+, K^+, Na^+, Mg^{++}, Ca^{++}), and negatively charged particles go to the anode (anions Cl^-, HCO_3^-, HPO_4^{--}).

Mendeleev observed that when elements were arranged in order of increasing atomic weight they formed groups which reflected a periodicity in their properties (the periodic table). Later it was recognized that placing the elements in order of increasing Z number was more accurate. The columns in the periodic table are groups 0 to VIII, representing the valency or combining power of the element. Valency is the gram atomic weight determined by the gram equivalent weight. Groups 0 and VIII are the stable, nonreactive noble gases with the maximum number of electrons in the outermost shell. Elements in the intervening groups are unstable and tend to lose or gain electrons in their outermost shell to reach the stable state. Thus elements in group I, the alkali metals, have to lose only one electron to reach the stable ionic state, for Na^+. The alkaline-earth metals in group II lose two electrons, for example Ca^{++}, and in group IV four electrons, C^{++++}. Elements in subsequent groups gain electrons in the outermost shell and become negatively charged to reach the most stable state: group V, N^{---}, group VI, O^{--}, and group VII, Cl^-. The shells K, L, M, etc., are in rows in the periodic table and express the increasing atomic numbers. Elements react according to their valency; thus Na^+ in group I readily combines with Cl^- in group VII since Na^+ is more stable with one less electron and Cl^- requires an additional electron. This is an example of ionic bonding.

Milliequivalent

Since substances react according to the number of electrons in the outermost shell and not according to their mass, it is better to speak of reactions in terms of equivalent weights. The equivalent weight is the weight in grams of any ion that will react directly or indirectly with 1 gm of hydrogen; the milliequivalent is one thousandth of the equivalent weight. If the atom is monovalent, for example Na^+, the equivalent weight is the same as the atomic weight. For divalent atoms, such as Ca^{++}, the equivalent weight is half the atomic weight. Concentra-

tions of ions are expressed as milliequivalents per liter.

$$mEq/liter = \frac{mg \text{ per } 100 \text{ ml} \times 10 \times valency}{Atom \text{ weight}}$$

Hydrogen Ion Concentration

An acid is a substance that provides hydrogen ions and a base accepts hydrogen ions. HNO_3 and H_2SO_4 are acids and NO_3^- and SO_4^{--} are bases. A strong acid or base is almost completely ionized (H_2SO_4, $NaOH$), while a weak acid or base is only partly ionized ($H_2CO_3 \rightleftharpoons H^+ + HCO_3^-$). A salt is formed from the combination of an acid with a base; it is almost completely ionized if it is derived from a strong acid ($NaCl \rightleftharpoons Na^+ + Cl^-$).

In pure water the concentrations of H^+ and OH^- are 10^{-7} gm per liter at 23°C (equivalent weights are 1 gm of H^+ and 17 gm of OH^- per liter). The product of the equivalent weights of the ions, 10^{-14}, is the ionization constant of water (K_{H_2O}) and applies to all aqueous solutions regardless of the presence of other ionic material.

The pH nomenclature is employed to avoid using the negative logarithm to the base 10—pH $= -\log [H^+]$. An increase of one in the pH represents a tenfold decrease in the hydrogen ion concentration. The normal pH of arterial blood is 7.37 to 7.43.

Henderson-Hasselbalch Equation. In any buffer solution in equilibrium the product of the dissociated forms over the undissociated form is a constant specific for that system when applied to the dissociation of carbonic acid:

$$\frac{[H^+][HCO_3^-]}{[H_2CO_3]} = K_{H_2CO_3}$$

$$[H^+] = K_{H_2CO_3} \frac{[H_2CO_3]}{[HCO_3^-]}$$

Applying the negative logarithm, this becomes:

$$-\log [H^+] = -\log K_{H_2CO_3} - \log \frac{[H_2CO_3]}{[HCO_3^-]}$$

Let pH $= -\log [H^+]$ and pK $= -\log K_{H_2CO_3}$

$$pH = pK + \log \frac{[HCO_3^-]}{[H_2CO_3]}$$

The pH therefore varies according to the numerator HCO_3^- and the denominator $[H_2CO_3]$ of the equation. The numerator is the metabolic component and can be expressed as the carbon dioxide content minus the amount of carbon dioxide in solution in blood. The denominator is related to the partial pressure of carbon dioxide in arterial blood (P_{CO_2}). The equation then becomes:

$$pH = 6.1 + \log \frac{CO_2CT - 0.03P_{CO_2}}{P_{CO_2}}$$

If the CO_2CT and P_{CO_2} are known, the pH and HCO_3^- can be determined using a nomogram.

Control mechanisms attempt to keep the ratio of the numerator HCO_3^- to the denominator H_2CO_3 at 20:1. When there is a primary change in the HCO_3^- or metabolic component, as occurs in metabolic acidosis or alkalosis, there is a compensatory decrease or increase in the respiratory component H_2CO_3. For example, in metabolic acidosis there is a primary decrease in HCO_3^- because of the decrease in bicarbonate buffer. This is compensated for by increased respiration to provide a compensatory decrease in the respiratory component. When there is a primary change in the respiratory component, as in respiratory acidosis or alkalosis, renal compensation results in an increase or decrease in the plasma bicarbonate. It should be noted that HCO_3^- is decreased in metabolic acidosis and is increased in respiratory acidosis.

Buffer

On adding acidic or basic radicals to the mixture of a weak acid and its salt, there is little change in the pH. In the blood the acid radicals are buffered by anions, HCO_3^-, hemoglobin, and protein.

$$H_2CO_3 \rightleftharpoons H^+ + HCO_3^-$$

In metabolic acidosis there is an increased H^+ in the blood in the form of carbonic acid, lactic acid, pyruvic acid, or ketone bodies or there is an excessive loss of base (HCO_3^-), for example, from intestinal secretions in diarrhea or intestinal fistula. The bicarbonate ion, HCO_3^-, combines with the acids resulting in a decrease in HCO_3^-, and the reaction moves to the left providing less bicarbonate.

There are two main buffer systems in the blood, the bicarbonate and nonbicarbonate. The bicarbonate system is the more important and is mostly in the plasma; the nonbicarbonate system is mostly in the erythrocytes:

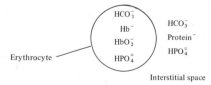

When a strong acid or base is added to blood, it is buffered by both systems; the amount

contributed by each depends upon the amount of each buffer present.

From a practical point of view the erythrocyte membrane can be ignored and the total buffer base be considered:

Buffer   Bicarbonate   Nonbicarbonate
base = buffers + buffers
(BB)   (HCO_3^-)   (Buf$^-$)

More often the term "base excess" (BE) is used:

BE = Observed buffer base − Normal buffer base

If 10 mEq/liter H^+ is added to whole blood containing 48 mEq/liter buffer base, there is a 10 mEq/liter decrease in buffer base and the BE is −10 mEq/liter. The normal buffer base depends upon the hemoglobin concentration. The normal buffer base at 15 gm hemoglobin per 100 ml of blood is 48 mEq/liter and 45 mEq/liter at a hemoglobin of 8 gm.

The numerator of the Henderson-Hesselbalch equation may be expressed as the amount of bicarbonate buffer, the total buffer base, or as base excess.

Buffering Action of Hemoglobin. The heme molecule contains four imidizole rings attached to a centrally placed ion molecule (Fe^{++}). When oxygen is taken up by Fe^{++}, the affinity of the imidizole ring for hydrogen is decreased and H^+ is liberated. The reverse occurs when oxygen is given up by hemoglobin in the lungs and the strong acid $HHbO_2$ is formed:

In Lungs

$$HHb + O_2 \rightleftharpoons HHbO_2 \rightleftharpoons H^+ + HbO_2^-$$
Weak   Strong
acid   acid

On reaching the tissues, oxygen is given up and the reduced hemoglobin has an increased affinity for H^+. The acid HHb is weak; therefore the hemoglobin buffers the H^+.

In tissues $HbO_2^- + H^+ \longrightarrow O_2 + HHb$

$$\uparrow\downarrow$$

$$H^+ + Hb^-$$

Fluid Compartments

The total body water is 0.6 liter per kilogram with 0.4 liter per kilogram intracellular and 0.2

liter per kilogram extracellular. The intracellular fluid is mainly in cells outside the blood circulation (0.37 liter per kilogram) while that in the circulation is mostly in the erythrocytes (0.03 liter per kilogram). The extracellular fluid is mostly in the interstitial space (0.15 liter per kilogram) and only 0.05 liter per kilogram in the plasma.

TBW =			
Total body water (0.6 L/kg)			
ICF		+	ECF
Intracellular fluid (0.4 L/kg)			Extracellular fluid (0.2 L/kg)
Intracellular (0.37 L/kg)	Erythrocytes (0.03 L/kg)	Plasma (0.05 L/kg)	Interstitial fluid (0.15 L/kg)

In the 70-kg man there are 14 liters of water in the interstitial space. A portion of this fluid, about 3 percent of total body weight or 2 liters, is in sites that do not communicate freely with the circulation in a manner similar to the remainder of the interstitial fluid. This is known as transcellular water and consists of fluid in the pleural and peritoneal cavities, joints, cerebrospinal space, and within the eyes. The gastrointestinal secretions, about 9 liters per 24 hours, are also included in this space and abnormal collections of fluid at sites of trauma. Transcellular water may be increased to volumes such as 8 percent of total body weight, as in the patient with ascites or multiple injuries, and seriously decrease the amount of water in the other compartments. The patient with gastrointestinal losses of secretions by vomiting, diarrhea, or intestinal fistulas will have a decrease in transcellular water and also a decrease in water in the other spaces.

The distribution of water in the idealized intracellular and extracellular spaces depends on hydrostatic pressure, oncotic pressure, and distribution of ions in the spaces. Starling's law states that fluid is driven out of the arteriolar end of the capillary with a force of about 40 mm Hg. The relatively higher oncotic pressure of the plasma proteins compared with that in the interstitial space results in fluid being drawn back into the vessels at the venular end of the capillary bed. This is aided by the hydrostatic pressure of tissue turgor in the interstitial space. The normal effect is that there is normally excessive interstitital fluid which is returned to the blood circulation through the lymphatics. The volume of intracellular water is 28 liters and is mainly in skeletal muscle cells.

The distribution of water in the body compartments depends on the oncotic pressure produced by the ions and proteins in the spaces. Ions pass freely through the vascular capillary walls. Proteins, however, are larger molecules and are mainly distributed in the vascular space. Ions are therefore distributed according to Donnan's law, which states that the total number of cations must equal the total number of anions on each side of the capillary membrane. Gibbs further developed this relationship and showed that the product of cations and anions on one side of the semipermeable membrane is equal to their product on the other side. Since the protein anions are high in the circulation, the concentration of other anions such as HCO_3^- and Cl^- is lower, and the concentration of cations, Na^+, K^+, Ca^{++}, and Mg^{++}, is slightly higher than in the interstitial space.

There is considerable difference in the distribution of ions in the interstitial and intracellular spaces. The concentration of K^+ is high in the intracellular space while that of the Na^+ is high in the interstitial space. This is not a passive phenomenon as determines the distribution of cations in the intravascular and interstitial spaces but is an active process involving the utilization of energy. The most popular theory is that there is a cation pump in the cell membrane that maintains a high level of K^+ within the cell and of Na^+ in the interstitial space. Function of the cation pump is inhibited by hypoxia, cold, and metabolic inhibitors. In stored blood there is passage of K^+ into the plasma and Na^+ into the erythrocytes. With cell death the concentration of the cations becomes the same in both compartments. Darrow and Yannet (1935) made an observation that has important clinical application. They found that the addition of sodium chloride to the interstitial space resulted in a decrease in intracellular water and that withdrawal of sodium chloride led to an increase in intracellular water.

THE SURGICAL PATIENT
Water Balance

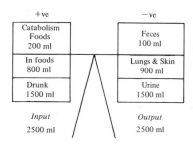

The normal adult ingests and loses about 2500 ml of water per 24 hours. The amount of water drunk, about 1500 ml per day, varies according to habits, foods eaten, and the environmental temperature and humidity. There is about 800 ml of water in foods eaten per day. Complete catabolism of carbohydrates and fats results in the formation of mainly water and carbon dioxide. The water from this source is about 200 ml per day.

The amount of urine excreted per day, about 1500 ml, is adjusted by aldosterone and antidiuretic hormone to maintain a zero body water balance. About 35 gm of solids are excreted in the urine each day in a minimum volume of 500 ml of urine and specific gravity of 1.030. A larger volume is necessary when it is not possible to attain this specific gravity because of poor renal function, as frequently occurs in geriatric patients. Loss of water in sweat, by evaporation from the skin, and in the expired air is about 100 ml per day. Insensible loss from the skin is increased in the postoperative period and in febrile and debilitated patients. Although water loss is negligible in the gastrointestinal tract under normal circumstances, about 100 ml, this becomes important in patients with persistent diarrhea, vomiting, prolongated nasogastric suction, or continuous drainage from an ileostomy or fistula. Third-space loss of water at the site of trauma or operation is often underestimated. It may be necessary to provide additional fluid in various kidney diseases, such as chronic nephritis, nephrosclerosis, and the diuretic recovery phase following acute tubular necrosis, when the ability to concentrate urine is impaired.

Clinical Manifestations of Overhydration and Underhydration. Clinically overhydration occurs as a result of giving excessive intravenous fluids, especially in cardiac, renal, or hepatic failure. It is also liable to occur after severe stress such as a major operation or injury. Secretion of antidiuretic hormone and aldosterone is decreased. Overhydration results in headache, drowsiness, and, if extreme, seizures and coma. There is an increase in body weight, blood pressure, and urinary output. Pulmonary ventilation is impaired as a result of intrapulmonary edema, and cardiac failure may occur. The interstitial fluid and plasma volume increase. The blood volume is therefore increased and the hematocrit decreased. Treatment is to decrease intake of water and sodium and, if marked, to remove 500 to 1000 ml of blood.

Causes of dehydration are inadequate oral intake, diabetes mellitus and insipidus, and hyperpyrexia. Clinically dehydration is often secondary to hyponatremia from vomiting, diarrhea, intestinal fistula, or less often Addison's disease. Compensation is by increasing secretion of antidiuretic hormone and aldosterone and movement of intracellular fluid to the extracellular compartment. Underhydrated patients have a lowering of extracellular fluid and have decreased skin turgor, sunken eyes, and may or may not be thirsty. The urinary output and blood pressure are decreased as is the blood volume, and the hematocrit is increased. Treatment consists of administering water along with electrolytes. Generally, but not always, the urine volume is a reliable indicator of the adequacy of water replacement. For greater accuracy determination should be made of the central venous pressure, daily body weight, serum and urine osmolality, and the serum sodium, chloride, potassium, and bicarbonate levels.

Sodium is a major determinant in fluid movement. Patients with depleted intravascular and extravascular fluids compensate by preserving sodium at the renal tubular level. Hence dehydrated patients have a small amount of sodium in the urine. The serum sodium may be high, normal, or low. Under special circumstances, especially after head injury, ADH can be produced inappropriately. There is continued retention of water in spite of a low serum osmolality. The osmoreceptors in the hypothalamus do not respond normally by decreasing the production of ADH. The urinary sodium may therefore be normal or increased. Treatment consists of fluid restriction.

Of prime importance in the surgical patient is an accurate record of the quantity and source of the fluid loss if proper replacement is to be given. However in critically ill patients it is often difficult to determine accurately fluid losses. Under such circumstances weighing the patient several times per day is of great value. Surgical patients maintained on parenteral fluids, unless on hyperalimentation, do not gain weight unless they are overhydrated. Indeed properly hydrated adult patients lose up to 0.5 kg daily until they resume a normal diet. A patient should be presumed to be dehydrated if rapid weight loss occurs. On the other hand, the risk of keeping a seriously ill patient in an overhydrated state cannot be overemphasized.

During the immediate postoperative period increased secretion of antidiuretic hormone, aldosterone, and cortisol results in increased sodium and water retention. The urinary output may therefore be a poor guide in estimating fluid replacement, and oliguria at this time may be a normal physiologic response. Additional fluid administered under such circumstances will not only be ineffective but could result in serious overhydration with its sequelae.

On the other hand, extracellular fluids may be depleted by losses into newly created spaces such as injured and burned tissues, the serous cavities in infections, and intestine during ileus. Such losses are termed third-space losses or internal hydration and must be treated by giving additional fluids.

Electrolytes

It is important to recognize the difference in electrolyte composition between intracellular and extracellular fluid. The principal anions are phosphate in the cell and chloride in the extracellular space. The principal cations are potassium in the cell and sodium in the extracellular space. There is more intracellular than extracellular protein.

Sodium. Sodium is the most important element in maintaining the volume of the extracellular fluid. Frequent estimations of the serum sodium are essential in seriously ill surgical patients, since these measurements give important information about the status of water and acid-base balance. The normal value is about 140 mEq per 100 ml of plasma. The values, however, do not necessarily give information about the total body sodium because the amount of water affects the concentration of plasma electrolytes. Serum sodium concentrations therefore must be interpreted in the light of clinical findings and the degree of hemoconcentration as determined by the hematocrit. Thus a serum sodium may be "low" in the presence of high, normal, or low total body sodium. In edematous states, regardless of the apparent concentration of serum sodium, the total body sodium is increased. A low serum sodium in the presence of a known normal total body sodium indicates an excess water load, so-called "dilutional hyponatremia." The patient with a high serum sodium is usually water-depleted; water is then indicated to bring the serum sodium to a normal value. Clinically this presents as acute water intoxication. In patients with chronic hyponatremia there is a sufficient time for a decrease also to occur in the intracellular electrolytes. The low serum sodium level can then often be tolerated without symptoms. Hyponatremia in surgical patients is most often from intestinal loss due to vomiting, diarrhea, or fistula. Another important cause is the intake of especially the chlorothiazide diuretics, and postoperatively it is most often the result of poor intravenous therapy. Excessive sweating and Addison's disease are uncommon causes. The symptoms and signs are similar to those of underhydration. Treatment consists of administration of salt and water.

Hypernatremia most often results from giving excess saline intravenously, especially in patients with cardiac or renal disease. Primary aldosteronism and Cushing's disease also are associated with hypernatremia. Hypernatremia may occur from a marked loss of water either as a result of osmotic diuresis or lesions of the central nervous system. Hyperalimentation and gastrostomy feedings rich in carbohydrate and protein can produce a marked urinary loss of water and hypernatremia. There is a decrease in aldosterone and ADH secretion. As a result of movement of water between the intracellular and extracellular spaces nervous symptoms develop such as stupor, seizures, and coma. The signs are those of overhydration. Treatment is restoration of the normal fluid and electrolyte balance.

Potassium. Potassium is almost entirely intracellular, and its level does not necessarily reflect the total body potassium. The normal value is 3 to 4.5 mg percent. A high serum potassium may indicate release of potassium from damaged cells or impaired renal excretion as in renal failure, shock, or dehydration. Hyperkalemia may occur if potassium is administered too rapidly. There are often no clinical manifestations of hyperkalemia prior to the occurrence of cardiac complications. Occasionally muscular irritability is present. Electrocardiographic changes are the presence of extrasystoles, increase in the T wave, widening of the QRS complex, and ultimately cardiac arrest in systole. The electrocardiographic changes occur when the serum level is about 6 mg percent. Treatment depends on the level of the serum potassium and renal function. Insulin and glucose may be necessary to rapidly reduce a dangerously high level, and treatment of renal shutdown is then indicated (see Chap. 32).

Hypokalemia usually indicates true total potassium depletion. It must be emphasized that an intracellular deficit may be present with normal serum levels. Potassium deficiency develops rapidly when solutions low in potassium are given intravenously for more than three days. The patients are often in negative nitrogen and caloric balance with the result that potassium is lost from the cells and excreted in the urine. Potassium depletion can also occur from loss of gastrointestinal fluids as a result of prolonged nasogastric suction, fistula, or severe diarrhea. Hypokalemia also occurs in those with healing burns, Cushing's disease, primary aldosteronism, and in those given mercurial and chlorothiazide diuretics. There is continued loss of potassium in the urine in hypokalemia. Potassium leaves the cells to compensate for the decrease in extracellular potassium and sodium enters the cells. This results in intracellular edema and is a factor in muscular weakness. Hypokalemic alkalosis is accentuated by loss of chloride ion. It is important to appreciate that there is increased sensitivity to digitalis in the hypokalemic patient.

Clinical manifestations of hypokalemia are weakness of cardiac, voluntary, and smooth muscles. The effect on the cardiac muscle results in characteristic changes in the electrocardiogram, prolongation of the Q-T interval, and flattening or inversion of the T wave. There are marked weakness and intestinal ileus. Treatment is to give potassium chloride and to manage any associated alkalosis.

Magnesium. The cation magnesium, Mg^{++}, has only recently been given attention in surgical patients. Normally the ratio of that within cells to that in the extracellular fluid is 20:1. The normal level in the serum, 1.5 to 2.5 mEq/liter, is maintained mainly through secretion of cortisol. The highest concentration is in the gastric secretion. The most frequent clinical condition giving rise to magnesium deficiency is postoperative administration of fluids that do not contain this cation. Chronic alcoholics are especially prone to a low serum magnesium. Clinical signs of deficiency are often mistaken for those of calcium deficiency. These are twitchings, tremor, disorientation, and convulsions similar to those seen with hyponatremia and hypokalemic alkalosis. Special care should be taken when administering magnesium to patients with impaired renal function.

Nutrition

Calories. The daily resting requirements are 30 kilocalories per kilogram, or 1400 kilocalories per square meter. One liter of 5 percent glucose contains 50 gm of carbohydrate yielding 170 calories (Table 3-1). Four liters per day, equivalent to 680 calories, is not sufficient to inhibit gluconeogenesis. A minimum of 100 gm of glucose per day is necessary to prevent ketosis. To provide a larger number of calories using carbohydrate solutions alone, concentrations of 10 to 50 percent sugar must be used. These solutions are irritating to the peripheral veins and cause thrombosis. It is therefore necessary to deliver concentrations above 10 percent directly into the superior vena cava (see Chap. 14). Intravenous alcohol, 5 percent alcohol in 5 percent dextrose, may be given as a source of calories and as a means of sedation in chronic alcoholics.

Protein. An attempt may be made to increase protein synthesis and prevent excessive breakdown of tissues by giving intravenous proteins. An adequate number of calories must be supplied as carbohydrate; otherwise the amino acids are metabolized as a source of calories. The number of calories that must be supplied to minimize gluconeogenesis depends upon the patient's catabolic state (see Chap. 1). The sources of protein are blood, plasma, and albumin. Protein hydrolysates and synthetic amino acids may also be given to increase the amino acid pool (Table 3–1).

Fat. Small-molecular-weight fat solutions have been prepared that can be given intravenously. They consist of mainly medium- and short-chain triglycerides and are directly absorbed into the blood vessels and not into the lacteals as are the fatty acids. The advantages are the high calorie content, 1.1 calories per milliliter, and that the solution can be administered through a peripheral vein. Occasionally there is a severe hypersensitivity reaction to the intravenous fat. Patients on intravenous hyperalimentation require about 2 units (1000 ml) Intralipid per week to prevent fatty acid deficiency. Excess administration of fats results in fatty infiltration of the liver and tendency to bleed.

Vitamins. The accessory food factors of the vitamin B group are essential for normal carbohydrate metabolism. Increased amounts are needed when food is supplied solely as carbohydrate and in febrile states as often occurs after operation. Vitamin C is important in wound healing. Both vitamins can be given intravenously. Vitamin K must be given to jaundiced patients and (Chap. 19) patients receiving elemental diets and on prolonged oral antibiotics.

Intravenous Fluids

The water and saline systems include glucose in water, glucose in saline, isotonic saline, supplementary potassium, Ringer's solution, Ringer's lactate, M/6 sodium lactate, M/6 ammonium chloride, and 5 percent sodium bicarbonate (Table 3–2). Ringer's solution may be described as isotonic saline with calcium and potassium added at the concentrations

Table 3–1. CALORIE AND AMINO ACID CONTENT OF INTRAVENOUS FLUIDS

	CONSTITUENTS	CALORIE CONTENT
5% glucose in water	Glucose	170C/liter
10% Travert	5% glucose + 5% fructose	375C/liter
Intralipid	Small fat droplets—mainly medium-chain triglycerides	1100C/liter
Casein hydrolystate (Amigen)	Essential amino acids and electrolytes in maintenance dose	——

Table 3–2. COMMONLY USED INTRAVENOUS FLUIDS

	Na^+	K^+	Ca^{++}	Mg^{++}	Cl^-	LACTATE$^-$
Normal plasma	142	5	5	2	103	5
Isotonic saline (0.9%)	154	—	—	—	154	—
Ringer's solution	147	4	6	—	157	—
Ringer's lactate (Hartmann)	130	4	4	—	111	27
Darrow's K lactate	122	35	—	—	104	53
Na lactate M/6 (1.9%)	167	—	—	—	—	167

present in normal plasma. In Ringer's lactate the Cl^- has been reduced to the level present in plasma and lactate added; the Na^+, K^+, Ca^{++}, and Cl^- are therefore present in the concentrations of normal plasma and lactate is added to be metabolized to bicarbonate to combat a mild acidosis.

Organs responsible for homeostasis—the kidney, adrenals, pituitary, and parathyroids—control the amount of each electrolyte retained, and this differs markedly from the electrolyte content of fluids given using the water and saline system. The homeolyte solutions were therefore introduced to provide a more physiologic fluid; they contain about one half the milliequivalents of isotonic saline or Ringer's lactate, have a "relatively" high water content, and contain carbohydrate.

Intravenous Orders

There are many different ways that intravenous orders may be written. The aim is to correct any past deficiencies, to provide for basal requirements, and to give adequate fluids to compensate for anticipated losses. The orders shown in Table 3–3 are suggested for a 70-kg man using the simpler nonhomeolytic solutions.

Past Deficit. A patient who has been vomiting for 24 hours from acute obstruction of the terminal ileum without strangulation should be given rapid fluid replacement within about two hours. Ringer's lactate, 2000 to 3000 ml, may be administered according to clinical signs of dehydration, blood pressure, pulse, and urinary output.

Concurrent Losses. A patient with paralytic ileus with 2000 ml of gastric aspirate per 24 hours would besides his basal daily requirements need 2000 ml of water, 300 mEq Na^+, 300 mEq Cl^-, 80 mEq K^+, and preferably more than 1000 calories, proteins or amino acids and vitamins. A useful approximation is to consider that 1000 ml of gastric aspirate should be replaced with isotonic saline and that each 1000 ml contains 40 mEq of potassium chloride. Additional orders would then be 2000 ml of isotonic saline in 5 percent dextrose, 80 mEq of potassium chloride, and albumin or amino acids.

The patient with persistent paralytic ileus would require additional calories either using the 10 percent homeolyte solution or Intralipid solution so that the administered proteins should be utilized as proteins and not be catabolized to produce energy.

METABOLIC ACIDOSIS AND ALKALOSIS

Acid or base entering the blood is initially buffered by the bicarbonate and nonbicarbonate buffer systems to minimize changes in the hydrogen ion concentration. Their excretion in the urine is known as renal correction. Pulmonary hyperventilation or hypoventilation occurs to decrease or increase the denominator

Table 3–3. BASAL DAILY REQUIREMENTS

		VOLUME	mEq	SOLUTION
1.	Water	3000 ml	—	2500 ml in 5% dextrose
2.	Na^+	—	75	500 ml isotonic saline in 5% dextrose
3.	Cl^-	—	75	Contained in No. 2
4.	K^+	—	40	40 mEq potassium chloride ampule added to 5% dextrose in water solution if urinary output adequate
5.	Calories	1400/sq m	—	Above solutions provide only 510 calories
6.	Protein	70 gm	—	Albumin, amino acids (as in Amigen solution) require adequate calorie intake
7.	Vitamins	—	—	Vitamins B and C given in ampule daily in dextrose and water solution.

of the Henderson-Hesselbalch equation and decrease or increase the change in pH (pulmonary compensation). Compensation always occurs through the system that is not primarily affected. For example, respiratory compensation occurs in metabolic acidosis.

The range of pH of the urine is 4 to 8 and the H^+ at pH 4 is 0.1 mEq/liter. Since the body produces about 50 mEq H^+ per day, only a small amount can be excreted in an uncombined state in the urine.* Two additional renal mechanisms are available to buffer the large amount of H^+ which is excreted in the urine:

$$HPO_4^{--} + H^+ \rightarrow H_2PO_4^-$$
$$NH_3 + H^+ \rightarrow NH_4^+$$

The ammonia is produced by the renal tubular cells. For each atom of H^+ excreted in the urine one molecule of HCO_3^- is retained in the circulation. The renal correction in patients with metabolic acidosis due to loss of the base HCO_3^- is similar to that due to addition of H^+.

In patients with metabolic alkalosis the urine becomes alkaline due to increased excretion of HCO_3^-. Synthesis of ammonia and formation of titratable acids are decreased. There may be paradoxical aciduria because of increased tubular loss of K^+ and H^+, the result of an increase in renal tubular reabsorption of Na^+. This occurs in an attempt to preserve blood volume.

Hydrogen Ion Balance

It is useful to consider the acid-base status of a patient in the form of a balance:

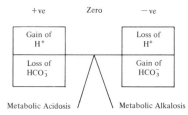

Metabolic Acidosis. This is the most common acid-base abnormality in surgical patients and results from addition of excess hydrogen ion or loss of base. Gain of metabolic H^+ occurs in patients given ammonium chloride, as a result of normal metabolism of proteins, in patients with inadequate kidney function, and in those with incomplete catabolism of carbohydrate and fat. The high content of sulfur, nitrogen, and phosphorus in proteins results, on incomplete catabolism, in the production of sulfuric,

nitric, and phosphoric acids. It is therefore important in those with renal shutdown to stop intake of protein and to inhibit gluconeogenesis by the administration of carbohydrate. In any patient with poor peripheral tissue blood flow, as occurs in hypovolemic shock, hypothermia, and often cardiac arrest, there is an increase in anaerobic glycolysis. This results in an increase in hydrogen ions from lactic and pyruvic acids. Failure of carbohydrate metabolism to enter the Krebs cycle produces accumulation of fatty acids, amino acids, and ketones in the blood. The failure of ADP to combine with phosphoric acid to form ATP as a result of the energy released in the Krebs cycle gives rise to an increase in phosphoric acid. In the patient with uncontrolled diabetes mellitus, starvation, or vomiting with ketosis acetoacetic acid, beta-hydroxybutyric acid, and acetone increase. In the patient with cardiac, renal, and hepatic failure, there is also a tendency to metabolic acidosis. Since bicarbonate is in all the alimentary secretions except the gastric juice, metabolic acidosis therefore tends to occur in those with intestinal fistulae or diarrhea. It also occurs in certain forms of renal disease when a large amount of base is lost.

There are a decrease in plasma pH and bicarbonate and a decrease in P_{CO_2} as a result of compensatory pulmonary hyperventilation (Kussmaul respiration). Renal correction is through excretion of a large amount of acid urine and activation of the renal ammonia and phosphate buffering systems.

Treatment consists of correcting any associated water or electrolyte deficit. A small amount of base, 27 mEq per liter, can be given using Ringer's lactate. A more advanced metabolic acidosis is treated using M/6 sodium bicarbonate.

Metabolic Alkalosis. Metabolic alkalosis is the result of excessive loss of hydrogen ion or an increase in base. Loss of hydrogen ion occurs in patients vomiting gastric secretions and in those with hypokalemia. The loss of K^+ in the secretions into the stomach depletes the K^+ in the cells and interstitial space. The cellular cation deficit is compensated for by passage of the cations H^+ and Na^+ into the cells. The H^+ was derived from the ionization of water; therefore a surplus of OH^- is present in the interstitial space. The loss of K^+ therefore produces a metabolic alkalosis and its correction requires administration of K^+ rather than H^+.

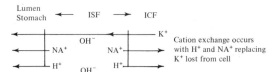

---

* The primary buffering system in the kidney is the bicarbonate system.

An increase in base occurs as a result of increased intake of HCO_3^- either in the inorganic form, $NaHCO_3$, or as salts of organic acids, such as Ringer's lactate and sodium citrate, which on complete oxidation form H_2O, CO_2, and HCO_3^-. Metabolic alkalosis occurs in Cushing's disease as a result of renal tubular loss of potassium. There is an increase in plasma bicarbonate and pH, and compensatory pulmonary hypoventilation results in an increased plasma P_{CO_2}. The urine is alkaline, and the renal buffering ammonia and phosphate systems are not utilized. Treatment is by correction of any fluid and electrolyte deficits. A more severe metabolic alkalosis is treated by giving M/6 ammonium chloride.

The diagnosis of metabolic acidosis or alkalosis describes an abnormal physiologic state and cannot be made on a single measurement of some constituent in blood. There must be an abnormal clinical state combined with some objective change in the blood electrolytes. Metabolic acidosis occurs when there is gain of H^+ or loss of HCO_3^- and metabolic alkalosis when there is gain of HCO_3^- or loss of H^+. The exact cause of metabolic disorder can only be determined from the history. A respiratory disorder must also be considered. A base excess of $+15$ could, for example, follow intake of HCO_3^- or OH^- or loss of H^+, but could also be due to renal compensation for respiratory acidosis. Respiratory acidosis occurs when there is a primary decrease in respiration relative to the rate of CO_2 production. In respiratory alkalosis there is a primary increase in alveolar ventilation relative to the rate of CO_2 production.

Simple and Mixed Acid-Base Disturbances

A simple disturbance affects one of the four possible abnormalities in acid-base balance: metabolic acidosis, metabolic alkalosis, respiratory acidosis, or respiratory alkalosis. Each is compensated for by changes in the other component. In a mixed disturbance a primary disturbance affects each component, for example, metabolic acidosis and respiratory acidosis or alkalosis. Metabolic acidosis and respiratory acidosis are additive in their effect on the pH, while metabolic acidosis and respiratory alkalosis have opposite effects on blood pH.

RESPIRATORY ACIDOSIS AND ALKALOSIS

Respiratory Acidosis

Respiratory acidosis occurs when the output of CO_2 by alveolar ventilation is less than that produced by the tissues. The primary defect is therefore a high P_{CO_2}.

1. Central respiratory depression from excessive sedation or use of muscle relaxants.

2. Impaired chest movement as in the patient with a staved-in chest, pneumothorax, or hemothorax.

3. Blockage or congestion in the respiratory tract from aspiration, emphysema, asthma, shock lung, or congestive heart failure.

4. Excessive retention of carbon dioxide as may occur during general anesthesia.

Renal compensation occurs after about six hours by excretion of an acid urine with a high content of $H_2PO_4^-$ and NH_4^+. The plasma HCO_3^- is therefore increased. The pH is down and the P_{CO_2} is increased. The bicarbonate or metabolic component is increased in respiratory acidosis to compensate for the increase in the respiratory component or denominator of the Henderson-Hesselbalch equation. Both the metabolic and respiratory components are therefore increased. Treatment of respiratory acidosis is that of the underlying cause.

Respiratory Alkalosis

This disorder occurs when loss of CO_2 by alveolar ventilation is greater than that produced by tissue metabolism. The plasma P_{CO_2} is therefore low. The causes are:

1. Direct stimulation of the respiratory center by salicylates, emotion, and certain diseases of the central nervous system. Respiratory alkalosis may occur in patients with ammonia intoxication from hepatic failure.

2. Reflex stimulation of the respiratory center by hypoxia acting on the peripheral chemoreceptors.

3. Reflex stimulation of the respiratory center by lung disease such as pneumonia.

4. Excessive ventilation using a respirator.

Tetany may occur because of the decrease in ionized calcium. Output of HCO_3^- in the urine is increased to compensate for the decrease in the respiratory component of the Henderson-Hesselbalch equation. The plasma bicarbonate and P_{CO_2} are both decreased, while the pH is increased. Treatment is that of the cause.

DETERMINATION OF ACID-BASE BALANCE

Since physicochemical considerations determine the interrelationships among the three parameters of the Henderson-Hesselbalch equation, it is only necessary to make two measurements, the third being readily estimated. Either HCO_3^- or BE can be used to determine the metabolic component and P_{CO_2} to obtain the respiratory component.

The acid-base balance is best determined on arterial blood. The findings in capillary blood obtained from the warm finger or earlobe (arterialized capillary blood) are sufficiently accurate for a P_{O_2} less than 150 mm Hg. The pH is lower, and the HCO_3^- and P_{CO_2} are higher in venous than arterial blood.

Total Carbon Dioxide Content

The metabolic component alone is often used to screen for an abnormality in acid-base balance. It is useful in metabolic acidosis and alkalosis and in partially or completely compensated respiratory acidosis and alkalosis. It is inaccurate in acute respiratory acidosis or alkalosis; however, clinical state is usually obvious.

When a strong acid is added to blood, carbon dioxide is liberated:

$$[CO_2]_T = HCO_3^- + H_2CO_3 + CO_2(d) = HCO_3^- + 0.03\ P_{CO_2}$$

Since 95 percent of the $CO_2(g)$ is derived from HCO_3^-, the $[CO_2]_T$ is a good estimate of the metabolic component HCO_3^-. The normal value is 25 mm/liter.

Astrup Equilibration Method

The total CO_2 content is only a screening procedure and does not give details of all the components determining acid-base status. Exact data can be obtained from the pH alone using the Astrup equilibration method. The CO_2 titration curve of whole blood in vitro is linear; therefore if two pHs are known at given CO_2 pressures, an unknown P_{CO_2} can be determined from the pH alone.

The slope of the curve varies with the hemoglobin concentration since Hb is the main non-bicarbonate buffer. A low Hb results in a low pH and vice versa. A decrease in base as in acidosis shifts the buffer base line to the left, and alkalosis causes a shift to the right.

A curved nomogram can be produced by calculating the pH and P_{CO_2} for different amounts of base, and from this the values of BB, BE, and standard bicarbonate can be obtained (Figure 3–1). The pH is determined on the sample of blood at two known values of P_{CO_2}; then the pH is determined on the sample. This value must lie on the line connecting the first two readings; therefore the P_{CO_2} of the sample can readily be obtained and the values of the other parameters from the points of

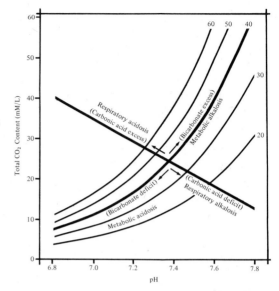

Figure 3–1. Evaluation of acid-base balance.

intersection of this line on the appropriate curves. The BB varies with the Hb—it is 48 mEq/liter when the Hb is 15 gm percent. The normal buffer base line is shifted to the left when blood is well oxygenated because HbO_2 is a stronger acid than reduced Hb. A correction can therefore be introduced for a decrease in O_2 saturation.

SUGGESTIONS FOR FURTHER READING

Davenport, H. W.: *The ABC of Acid-Base Chemistry*, 4th ed. The University of Chicago Press, Chicago, 1965. An excellent presentation of the physiologic basis of acid-base chemistry.

Frisell, W. R.: *Acid-Base Chemistry in Medicine.* Macmillan Publishing Co., Inc., New York, 1968. A clearly written account on the subject emphasizing the chemical reactions.

Shires, G. T.: Fluid and electrolyte therapy. In *Manual of Preoperative and Postoperative Care.* W. B. Saunders, Philadelphia, pp. 42–74, 1971. A short but clear description of the important aspects of fluid and electrolyte balance in the surgical patient.

Shires, T.: The role of sodium-containing solutions in the treatment of oligemic shock. *Surg. Clin. North Am.,* **45** (2):365–76, 1965. The role of sodium in resuscitation is fully presented.

Winters, R. W.; Knud, E.; and Dell, R. B.: *Acid-Base Physiology in Medicine,* 2nd ed. The London Company of Cleveland and Radiometer A/S of Copenhagen. 1969. This is probably one of the best self-instruction texts that has been produced on the subject.

Chapter 4

IMMUNE RESPONSE IN TISSUE TRANSPLANTATION AND CANCER

Nicholas R. St. C. Sinclair and *John A. McCredie*

CHAPTER OUTLINE

Immune Response
  Development of Immune Competence
  Structure of Antibody
  Complement System
  Components of the Immune Response
  Primary and Secondary Responses
  Immunologic Tolerance
  Immunologic Surveillance
  Autoimmune Disease
  Immunologic Enhancement
  Major Theories to Account for the Immune Response
Hypersensitivity
  Anaphylactic Shock
  Immune Complex Reactions
  Delayed Hypersensitivity Reaction
Tissue Transplantation
  Terminology

Histocompatibility Tests
Rejection
  Means of Inhibiting Rejection
Tissue and Organ Transplantation
  Skin
  Kidney
  Liver
  Other Tissues
Immunity in Cancer
  Evidence for an Immune Response in Patients with Cancer
  Latent Metastases
  Spontaneous Regression
  Mononuclear Cell Infiltration
  Decreased Immune Response
  Cancer-Specific Antigens and Antibodies
  Immunotherapeutic Studies

IMMUNE RESPONSE

Immunobiology has become increasingly important to surgical disciplines because of the roles it plays in our understanding of many aspects of infection, hypersensitivity reactions, healing processes, organ transplantation, and cancer. Initially interest was concentrated on humoral immune responses to infections with microorganisms. The classic example is the administration of tetanus antitoxin to patients with potentially infected wounds. It was only recognized in the 1940s that a cell-mediated immune response is important in patients with tuberculosis and fungal and viral infections. More recently a role for cell-mediated immune responses has been realized in tissue transplantation and cancer. It is now recognized that humoral and cellular immune responses contribute to tissue healing in surgical wounds.

Examples of natural humoral agents that help in combating infection are lysozymes, opsonins, properdin system, and complement. Examples of natural cellular resistance are phagocytosis of particles by granulocytes and macrophages. In contrast, acquired humoral and cellular immune responses require previous sensitization to the foreign organism or substance. The humoral or antibody-mediated immune response may be cytotoxic, causing death of bacteria, fungi, or virally infected cells. On the other hand, it may also enhance their growth. Lymphocytes and large mononuclear cells are responsible for acquired cell-mediated immunity. Macrophages of the lymphoreticular system are important in mediating the protective effects in both antibody and cell-mediated immunity. Illustrative examples of cell-mediated immunity are the skin reactions following the injection of specific antigens in patients with tuberculosis and a number of fungal and viral infections, the rejection of an allogeneic organ transplant, and the response of patients to certain types of cancer.

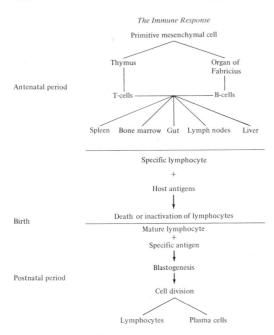

Figure 4–1. The development of lymphoid tissues. Lymphoid stem cells from the bone marrow grow in the primary lymphoid organs and then in the secondary lymphoid tissues. Contact between host antigens and specific lymphocytes leads to inactivation or death of the lymphocytes. After the neonatal period interaction of a foreign antigen with its specific lymphocyte is followed by transformation of the sensitized lymphocyte to a large mononuclear cell that divides to form lymphocytes or plasma cells.

Development of Immune Competence

Primitive mesenchymal stem cells from the bone marrow enter and populate two primary lymphoid organs, namely, the thymus and the equivalent of the bursa of Fabricius (thought to be a subpopulation of the bone marrow in mammals) (Figure 4–1). Lymphocytes then leave these two organs and seed secondary lymphoid tissues in the spleen, lymph nodes, bone marrow, and intestinal submucosa. Lymphocytes responsible for cell-mediated immunologic response are derived from the thymus and are known as thymus-derived lymphocytes or T-cells. Those responsible for the production of antibody emanate from the equivalent of the bursa of Fabricius and are bursal-dependent or B-cells. There is considerable interaction of T-cells and B-cells during a humoral immune response. In the human infant the thymus is a large organ and after the first decade decreases with age. In animals thymectomy at birth causes loss of weight, weakness, lymphopenia, and inability to produce cell-mediated and

humoral immune responses. The outcome is generally death from infection. This phenomenon is referred to as wasting disease. The deep cortical thymic-dependent zone in lymph nodes does not develop. However, immunoglobulin synthesis is impaired only slightly (Figure 4–2).

The bursa of Fabricius is a distinct organ in the cloacal region of birds. Its removal from chickens in early life leads to failure to produce immunoglobulins, absence of plasma cells in the medullary cords and primary follicles of lymph nodes, inability to elaborate all humoral immune responses, and a normal or slightly impaired cell-mediated immune response. Death often occurs from bacterial infection. Various investigators have suggested that in the human the bursa is in the tonsil, vermiform appendix, or Peyer's patches in the intestine. Its equivalent may not be a discrete organ in mammals but rather a stem cell population in the bone marrow which gives rise to the precursors of antibody-forming cells.

In animal studies the evidence for roles of the thymus gland and bursa of Fabricius has been obtained by observing the effects of their removal. It is interesting that a number of rare conditions have been recognized in man that are similar to the models produced in animals. For example, in patients with the DiGeorge syndrome the thymus and parathyroid glands are absent. T-cells are reduced and cell-mediated

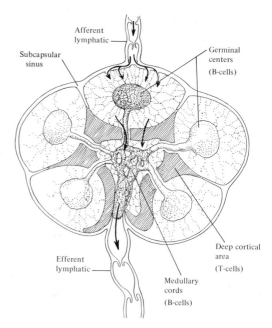

Figure 4–2. The T- and B-cell zones in a lymph node. T-cells are in the deep cortical area. B-cells are located in the germinal centers of the primary follicles and in the medullary cords.

immune responses are deficient. Individuals with the Bruton-type of agammaglobulinemia have findings similar to those in birds which have had the bursa of Fabricius removed with a defect in the ability to produce antibodies. Further, in individuals with the Swiss type of agammaglobulinemia the findings are consistent with an impairment in both antibody and cell-mediated responses.

Structure of Antibody

Antibodies are recognized by their reaction with specific antigens and by their physical and chemical properties. Plasma proteins can be fractionated by electrophoresis into albumin and the globulins α_1, α_2, β, γ. Gamma globulin contains the immunoglobulins and can be subdivided into the major classes IgG, IgA, IgM, IgD, and IgE. The immunoglobulin G (IgG) has two antigen-binding sites, is present in the largest amount in man, activates complement, crosses the placenta from mother to fetus, and plays an important part in conferring immunity against bacteria. Immunoglobulin M (IgM) has five to ten antigen-binding sites, activates complement, and is important in resistance to infections especially by gram-negative organisms. Immunoglobulin A (IgA) is found in respiratory and gut secretions and counteracts infections in these systems. Immunoglobulin D is found on the surface of immunocompetent cells where it serves as a specific antigen receptor. Immunoglobulin E (IgE) is responsible for allergic reactions as in asthma and hay fever. A beneficial role for IgE is its ability to induce rapid vascular alterations in the inflammatory response.

The antibody molecule contains a Fab portion (fragment antigen binding) that determines its immunologic specificity, and a Fc portion (fragment crystalline) that is more constant and is responsible for many of the biologic properties of antibody, such as complement fixation and placental transfer (Figure 4–3). Immunoglobulins are made of short (light) and long (heavy) peptide chains. The monomeric unit of immunoglobulin has two light and two heavy chains. IgG, IgD, and IgE contain one monomeric unit, IgM has five monomeric units, and IgA is made up of one or two units and in addition has other peptide chains. The heavy chain determines the class of immunoglobulin (IgG, IgA, etc.). The light chains are either kappa (K) or lambda (λ) and are present in all classes of immunoglobulins. One end [the carboxy (C) terminal] of each light chain is attached to the central portion of a heavy chain. The site of antigen-antibody binding is in the amino-(N)-terminal halves of the light chain and the adjacent heavy chain. Thus the unique arrangement of amino acids in the N-terminal region determines the specificity of antibody.

The reaction occurring on combination of an antibody with its specific antigen varies with the immunoglobulin class, whether the antigen is soluble or particulate, whether or not complement is activated, and with the relative concentrations of antigen and antibody.

Complement System

In the 1880s it was recognized that a substance in the serum aided killing of bacteria by antibodies. This is a complex system of 11 proteins, Clq, Clr, Cls, C4, C2, C3, C5 → C9, that are

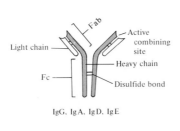

IgG, IgA, IgD, IgE

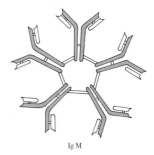

Ig M

Figure 4–3. Structure of antibody molecule. Antigen interacts with the ends of probably the long and short chains of the Fab (fragment antigen binding) portion of the immunoglobulin molecule.

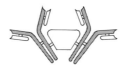

Ig A with secretory piece

activated sequentially to form a complex that can cause cell death. The role of antibody is to identify the foreign material and activate the complement system. In addition to causing destruction of cells and organisms, activation of the system results in the release of histamine from leukocytes, mast cells, and platelets, production of chemotactic factors causing leukocytes to migrate to the region, and attachment of C3 to antigen resulting in immune adherence which facilitates phagocytosis of the antigen. The IgG and IgM antibodies are the only classes with the capacity to activate the complement system. Complement may also be activated by the properdin system beginning at C3 (alternate pathway).

Components of the Immune Response

The steps in an immune response to a foreign antigen may be subdivided into afferent, central, and efferent components (Figure 4–4). These have no rigid boundaries and overlap extensively.

The afferent component is approach of antigen to and its recognition by the lymphoid system. Antigen approaches the lymphoid system through the blood vessels and afferent lymphatics. Macrophages ingest the antigen, present antigen on their cell surfaces, and play a role in the sensitization of specific lymphocytes. The macrophages are essential for initiating the humoral thymus-dependent response but may not be as obligatory for induction of cell-mediated immune responses. Afferent lym-

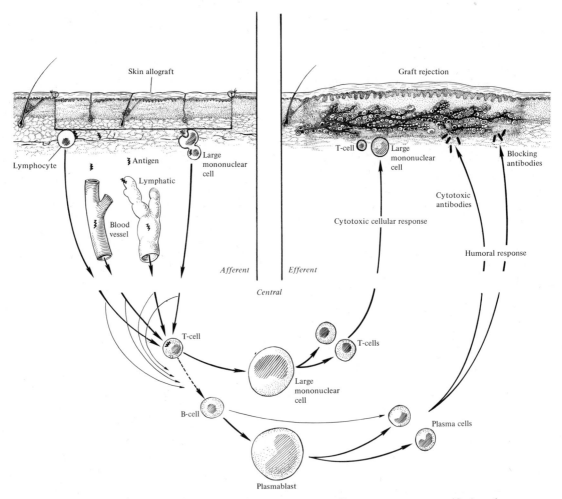

Figure 4–4. Components of the immune response. In the afferent component specific lymphocytes are sensitized to antigen. The major role is played by the macrophages that process the antigen. In the central component cell replication occurs with the production of lymphocytes, large mononuclear cells, and plasma cells. The efferent component is deposition at the site of the antigen of cytotoxic or enhancing immunoglobulins (humoral) or mononuclear cells and lymphocytes (cellular).

phatics are essential for the initiation of the afferent component of cell-mediated immune responses when the antigen is implanted in the skin or subcutaneous tissues. Barker and Billingham[3] demonstrated that an allograft placed on a skin pedicle is not rejected as long as afferent lymphatics do not reach the graft. Yet if a portion of the pedicle is in contact with tissues such that the afferent lymphatics enter the pedicle, then the graft is rejected. When an organ is attached by large vessels and lymphatic channels are absent, afferent sensitization may occur by entry of antigen into the veins. A few lymphocytes in the population are capable of recognizing antigen (because they have the specific antigen-receptors on their surface) and on contact with antigen become triggered.

In the central component antigen-triggered lymphocytes transform into large pyroninophilic (rich in RNA) mononuclear cells in regional lymph nodes or other parts of the lymphoreticular system. Two separate lines of lymphocytes (T and B) proliferate and differentiate to form lymphocytes and plasma cells. The lymphocytes are specific and are responsible for immunologic memory and cell-mediated immune responses, while the plasma cells and some lymphoblastic cells produce specific immunoglobulins. The lymphocyte responsible for the cell-mediated resistance of the host is the T-cell and that responsible for plasma cell formation is the B-cell. There is considerable interaction between T-cells and B-cells in the generation of many humoral immune responses. However, B-cells can be sensitized directly by antigen without the cooperation of T-cells; these are the thymus-independent antibody responses.

The T-cells appear to produce humoral factors that aid in the recruitment of B-cells. The B-cells may then proliferate and become large lymphoblastic cells. These lymphoblastic cells undergo further differentiation to become mature plasma cells found in the medulla of lymph nodes.

There are probably many families of T-cells with life-spans varying from days to years. The B-cells, however, are produced continuously in the bone marrow and appear to be more rapidly dividing. The B-cell has on its surface a heavy density of immunoglobulin that can be demonstrated by immunofluorescence, while the T-cells and thymocytes have little immunoglobulin on their surfaces and contain a surface antigen (theta). Two families of lymphocytes can, therefore, be recognized in the peripheral blood of a normal adult: *one third* are B-cells and *two thirds* are T-cells.[18] The nonactivated T-cells that move through the tissues recognize specific foreign antigens and play the major role in the anamnestic response and are known as "memory" T-cells. They may have a life of 10 years. Effector cells are known as "killer" T-cells. T-cells may also inhibit the production of antibody and other activated cells and are then known as suppressor cells. Other T-cells are "helper" and aid B-cells to produce antibodies. The "killer" T-cells also produce factors that specifically sensitize macrophages, such as a cytophilic antibody, which then become cytotoxic A-cells (adherent, activated, armed, or angry). In addition, cytophilic antibody may become attached to target cells or organisms, rendering them more easy to attack by A-cells. This is a form of opsonization. The lack of correlation of response of T-cells to prognosis in patients with cancer may be the result of the test not identifying the "killer" T-cells that specifically attack the cancer cells.

In the efferent component the cellular reaction consists of accumulation of large lymphoblasts and small lymphocytes at the site of the foreign antigen. The lymphocytic cells are referred to as effector or "killer" lymphocytes. Also, macrophages are essential and under certain conditions account for 80 percent of the cells in the graft. They may cause death or inhibit growth of bacteria, fungi, or virus-infected cells. Cells that have undergone mutation may be recognized and destroyed by effector lymphocytes or macrophages. The accumulation of mononuclear cells in and around a cancer and in the regional nodes may represent a beneficial immune response by the host. Their presence in allografted tissues, however, is an attempt at rejection of the foreign tissues. In graft-versus-host disease injected donor mononuclear cells recognize and attack the foreign tissues of the recipient.

The humoral reaction is deposition of specific immunoglobulins at the site of the specific antigens. These may be cytotoxic or protective (causing enhancement). There is now general agreement that cytotoxic antibody belongs to the IgM and IgG classes, and blocking antibody is restricted to IgM. The reaction between antibody and antigen may result in inactivation of antigen by sterically interfering with the active site on the antigen (as in the case of toxin-antitoxin reactions); or, if complement is also activated, a form of inflammatory reaction may ensue. When the antigen is on the surface of a target cell, the interaction with antibody and the activation of complement or cells with receptors for the Fc portion of antibody may cause target cell death. Examples include acute rejection of allografts and death of microorganisms, cells infected by microorganisms, and allogeneic cancer cells. Acute rejection most likely involves attachment of antibody to the antigens of endothelial cells, activation of complement, and other inflammatory intermediates, and these result in vascular damage and thrombosis.

The interaction of antibody with antigens on cell surfaces may enhance growth of the cells, either acting peripherally by masking antigens from killer lymphocytes or centrally by inactivating specific lymphocytes.

The distinction between cellular and humoral immunity is likely not complete. The specificity of lymphocytes may be due to the presence of immunoglobulins produced by the lymphocytes which are bound to and not released from their surfaces. In addition, fractions of lymphocytes can induce a cell-mediated immune response. Lawrence[11] demonstrated that a subcellular fraction of lymphocytes, transfer factor, could cause transformation of uncommitted lymphocytes, a finding that may be incompatible with the classic form of clonal selection.

Primary and Secondary Responses

In the adult, interaction between a foreign antigen and its mature specific lymphocyte results in lymphocytic transformation, division, and the production of antibody-forming cells, plasma cells, effector or "killer" cells, and memory cells. During the primary response, those memory cells, which are both B- and T-cells, are produced in the antigen-stimulated lymphoid tissues and colonize other lymphoid tissues that did not receive antigen, so that all regions of the body become sensitized. On second challenge with the same antigen this enlarged memory cell population produces cellular and humoral responses larger and more rapid than in the primary response. These increased and more rapid immune responses are referred to as secondary or anamnestic responses.

In the secondary response there are more rapid localization of antigen in the secondary follicles formed during the primary response, a larger burst of mitoses in various parts of the lymph node, and the production of a larger number of mature plasma cells in the medulla which produce a larger amount of antibody.

The cell-mediated immune responses also display primary and secondary forms. The activity in the primary responses depends on whether or not antigen remains at the time of production of effector or "killer" lymphocytes. If the antigen persists, as in a foreign transplant, first set rejection occurs later than after a second exposure to the antigen (second set rejection). If the antigen disappears rapidly from the site of injection, there is no visible reaction. The secondary response evolves over a number of days and has been referred to as the delayed hypersensitivity reaction.

Immunologic Tolerance

When a foreign antigen is injected during neonatal life, the host may not respond to a second challenge of the same antigen given during later life. To maintain tolerance it is essential that the foreign antigen persists in the animal either as a replicating cell or that a chemical is repeatedly administered. Natural tolerance was first detected in cattle,[14] in which nonidentical twins with one placenta were found to have two blood groups and to allow permanent "takes" of skin grafts interchanged in adult life. The passage of hematopoietic stem cells with allogeneic histocompatibility antigens across the placenta in intrauterine life led to nonresponsiveness to these antigens in adult life. The continued presence of cells from the opposite twin is referred to as chimerism. Tolerance is easily induced in the neonatal period but with greater difficulty in adults, and depends on the number of immunologically active lymphocytes.

The lymphocyte population can be reduced by total-body irradiation or chemotherapy to obtain tolerance in adults. Allogeneic bone marrow cells injected intravenously repopulate the bone marrow and render the host tolerant (immunologically nonreactive) to tissues of the allogeneic donor. This phenomenon only occurs when the differences in histocompatibility antigens between donor and recipient are minor and is unlikely when there are major genetic differences, as in the strong H-2 locus in the mouse and the HLA locus in man. Immunologic tolerance can be induced in the adult by administration of small or large amounts of soluble antigen, so-called "low-zone" or "high-zone" tolerance.

Immunologic tolerance can be cited to explain immunologic nonreactivity to host tissues. Lymphocytes that code for destruction of host antigens are removed or inactivated during intrauterine life, obviating postnatal host destruction by its own lymphoid tissues. Perhaps such lymphocytes do persist but do not respond to their antigens because of the presence of serum factors, most likely blocking antibodies, antigens, or antigen-antibody complexes.

Immunologic Surveillance

Mutations probably occur frequently in cells of dividing tissues. Lethal mutations cause cell death; mutations of less severity result in cell repair. A few mutations may persist, and a cancer with an altered antigenic structure may develop. It has been postulated that specific lymphocytes passing through tissues recognize the altered antigens on a mutated cell and kill that cell. In addition, macrophages activated by T-cells may kill cancer cells.

Autoimmune Disease

Secluded normal tissue antigens, as those from the lens and uvea, cartilage, or the brain, may not enter the general circulation in neonatal life to interact with their specific lymphocytes and lead to their consequent inactivation. Lymphocytes are therefore present in the adult that can be stimulated into activity on contact with these secluded antigens when they are released for some reason. The ensuing antibody-antigen interaction results in tissue death, release of more antigen, and further stimulation of lymphocytes. Very few of the autoreactive processes can be explained by the release o secluded antigens. Other theories must be invoked, such as an induced change in a tissue antigen or the emergence of initially autoreactive lymphocytes that cannot be inactivated by tolerance or enhancement mechanisms. A popular theory is that a viral infection may alter the antigenicity of normal tissue cells resulting in a delayed hypersensitivity reaction. An experimental model for autoimmune disease has been the injection of allogeneic lymph node or bone marrow cells into animals given total body irradiation or chemotherapeutic drugs. The recipient is unable to recognize antigens on the injected lymphocytes (this may be facilitated by using parental cells and an F_1 host). Frequently the adult cells repopulate the bone marrow and react against the tissues of the host. This reaction, referred to as graft-versus-host (GVH) reaction, gives rise to runt disease which is severe and often fatal. GVH reactions are not strictly autoimmune, and experimental models where an animal has been immunized *by* its own tissues *against* its own tissues have been established.

Immunologic Enhancement

Enhancement is increased survival or growth of a foreign tissue and occurs when the tissue-destroying, cell-mediated immune response is depressed by nondestructive antibody. Enhancement may be induced by passive transfer of immune serum or actively by injection of antigen. Specific lymphocytes may not respond to the antigen because the antibody has coated the antigens in the tissues (peripheral blocking). Alternately, the immunocompetent T-cell may contact antigen but may not be able to respond (central blocking); however, T-cells appear to be quite resistant to the feedback suppressive effects of antibody, whereas B-cells and T-B collaboration are highly sensitive.

Major Theories to Account for the Immune Response

These immunologic phenomena can best be accounted for by the clonal selection theory of Burnet: A small proportion of cells within the lymphoid system is capable of recognizing and responding to a given antigen.[4] When antigen comes in contact with specific T- or B-cells, the cells proliferate to form clones of cells. The cells produce antibody, develop the capacity to kill (as in cell-mediated immune responses), or serve as an increased population of "memory" cells for subsequent secondary or anamnestic immune responses on further contact with antigen. Thus antigen reacts with a small population of cells possessing a predetermined ability to recognize the given antigen and, through a process of proliferation, these cells form larger collections or clones of cells that specifically react to the antigen.

The instructional theory postulates that antigen instructs a population of lymphoid cells, which do not recognize a specific antigen, to produce the specific products of the immune response. The antigen could act on DNA altering the genome, vary the messenger RNA formed on a constant genome, or change the protein antibody formed on a constant messenger RNA. The final result is synthesis of a specific immunoglobulin.

The clonal selection theory postulates the presence of many different lymphocytes with capacities to recognize a restricted range of antigens, whereas the instructional theory postulates that the starting immunocompetent cells have the ability to recognize any antigen and that antigen confers on these cells the particular immune reactivity. Because of the improbability of having a vast array of different lymphocytes which are required to recognize the various antigens, the clonal selection theory was considered less likely than the instructional theory. However, because clonal proliferation was demonstrated directly and could be fitted into our understanding of the mechanisms for the synthesis of proteins—which cannot be done with the instructional theory—the clonal selection theory is favored at present.

HYPERSENSITIVITY

Hypersensitivity is a heightened tissue reaction that may occur after one or more exposures to a foreign antigen. The reaction may be beneficial, as in inflammation leading to removal of organisms, or harmful if a state of shock (anaphylaxis), uncomfortable reaction, or tissue damage ensues.

Anaphylactic Shock

A patient sensitized to penicillin by prior exposure may exhibit a violent reaction when given the drug. Generalized edema and spasm of smooth muscle may result in respiratory collapse. An interaction of the antigen (allergen) with preformed (by prior exposure to allergen) IgE antibody on the surface of certain cells results in the liberation of chemical mediators such as histamine, bradykinin, serotonin, and slow-reacting substance of anaphylaxis (SRS-A). Eosinophils are increased in the circulating blood at the site of a local reaction. The concentration of histamine is greatest in the mast cells, and to a lesser extent in the platelets, and in smaller amounts in most tissue cells. The release of histamine increases capillary permeability, causes smooth muscle in the intestine and bronchioles to contract, and reduces the blood pressure by dilating arterioles and increasing the size of the capillary bed. Enzymes liberated from damaged cells interact with α_2 globulins to produce a bradykinin with almost the same properties as histamine. The origin of SRS-A has not been established; its main action is to cause bronchial constriction.

The presence of an allergic state can be detected from the history and by performing skin tests. A minute amount of the suspected allergen is injected intracutaneously. The region is examined for a wheal and flare reaction occurring within a few minutes. The IgE antibodies in the blood of an allergic individual can be demonstrated by injecting serum from the allergic individual into the skin of a normal person. The allergen is injected hours or days later. If the wheal and flare of an indirect cutaneous anaphylactic reaction appear, then the serum must have contained IgE antibodies. This test is called the Prausnitz-Kustner (PK) test. The IqE antibodies in the injected serum become fixed to cells in the skin of the non-allergic individual, and, when the allergen is given in that region, the allergen attaches to the cell-fixed IgE antibodies and releases chemical mediators which lead to the wheal and flare reaction. Radioimmune assays for detection of specific IgE antibodies have been developed recently.

Seasonal allergies, reactions to many chemicals, uticaria or hives, and some forms of asthma are other IgE allergies.

Immune Complex Reactions

Repeated injections of a foreign antigen into the skin or subcutaneous tissues may result in increasing reactions at the injection sites. The antigen interacts with preformed IgG to form an immune complex that activates complement and results in destruction of endothelial cells and hemorrhage into the tissues (the Arthus phenomenon). Enzymes liberated from polymorphonuclear leukocytes are responsible for much of the local reaction. The cellular infiltration is best seen about 24 hours following administration of the antigen. Serum sickness and acute poststreptococcal glomerulonephritis are immune complex reactions.

Delayed Hypersensitivity Reaction

The local swelling fully developed at 48 hours and occurring after injection of a foreign antigen into a sensitized person is a delayed hypersensitivity reaction. Initially the cellular response is polymorphonuclear, but at four hours the predominant cell is mononuclear. Delayed hypersensitivity reactions do not require antibody nor the release of histamine but depend on the presence of specific T-cells which become cytotoxic and activate macrophages. Examples of delayed hypersensitivity reactions are contact allergies, Mantoux test for tuberculosis, Casoni test for hydatid disease, and possibly the Kveim test for sarcoidosis.

TISSUE TRANSPLANTATION

The scientific basis for transplantation of foreign tissues was established in 1945 by Medawar.[13] He showed that skin grafted onto an outbred rat was rejected and that, on repeating the transplant from the same donor, rejection occurred more rapidly. He called the two rejections "first set" and "second set." The second is an anamnestic response. Both reactions are mediated by T-cells. Measures to inhibit these phenomena have led to the development of tissue transplantation.

Terminology

Greek and Latin prefixes, auto-, homo-, and hetero-, were used to describe the sources of transplanted tissues. It has now been agreed that only the Greek prefixes syn-, allo-, and xeno- should be used. *Syn-*, together, means that the donor and recipient belong to the same inbred strain of animals or are identical human twins. *Iso-*, identical, was discarded because transplantation workers used the term to mean *syn-* and hematologists used it to mean *allo-*. *Allo-*, other, is used when the strains are different. The prefix *xeno-*, stranger, means that the donor and recipient belong to different species, for example, when mouse tissues are transplanted to the rat.

A *vital* graft consists of living cells and a *static* graft contains dead cells. A graft is *isotopic* when it is placed in the same position, *orthotopic* when it is surrounded by the same tissues but situated elsewhere, and *heterotopic* when it is placed in a different tissue.

Histocompatibility Tests

The time of a graft rejection is related mainly to the degree of difference in the histocompatibility genes between the donor and recipient. Generally the greater the incompatibility the more rapidly the tissue is rejected. Snell[16] showed that there are about 15 histocompatibility loci (H-1 to H-15) in the mouse and that mismatching at the most powerful locus (H-2) resulted in early rejection of allografted skin. He also showed that the H-2 locus provided the genetic information for at least 40 antigens. The histocompatibility genes are inherited from each parent. In man the major genetic locus coding for the histocompatibility antigen system for tissue transplantation is the human leukocyte antigen system (HLA) and corresponds to the H-2 locus in the mouse. Mismatching here signifies dissimilarity and a high likelihood of tissue rejection. There are two HLA subloci linked together on the same chromosome. Each has 10 or more alleles which code for different HLA antigens. Since there are two subloci and two chromosomes (maternal and paternal), there are usually four HLA antigens expressed in each individual. Other weaker loci are almost certainly present. The specificity of HLA antigens in each person is the same on leukocytes and on other nucleated cells, but the amount varies in different cell types. The HLA antigens are probably glycoproteins situated on the cell membranes.

Tissue typing can be carried out using antibodies directed against the histocompatibility antigens. The most widely used technique is to add lymphocytes from the peripheral blood of a patient to about 50 known antisera and observe cell death following the addition of rabbit complement.[17] The antisera are obtained from women who have had many pregnancies and have developed antibodies to the fetuses or from individuals who have had multiple transfusions. Cytotoxicity, determined by lysis of the lymphocytes and indicated by uptake of a vital dye, denotes a positive test. Histocompatibility antigens of the lymphocytes from the donor are then compared with those of the recipient and the "best fit" donor selected. Donors may possess antigens not expressed on recipient cells. Because of the two-loci and two-chromosomes nature of the HLA system this means that donors may differ from recipients by 0, 1, 2, 3, or 4 antigens. Various transplantation centers have reported different results with respect to clinical graft survival on transplanting across the varying transplantation antigen barriers.

Immunologic factors other than the degree of similarity in HLA antigens between donor and host are important in determining the likelihood of graft survival. These include (1) the amount of cross-reactivity between antigens typed as different; (2) presence of a sensitized state against histocompatibility antigens present on donor tissue. This is not always detectable with direct crossmatching (looking for circulating cytotoxic antibodies in recipient which are active against donor tissue); (3) presence of noncytotoxic antibodies that may help or hinder graft survival; (4) presence of antibody that can induce cells with Fc receptors to display cytotoxic properties. It is not known whether this type of effect or mechanism is associated with increased or decreased graft survival; and (5) ability of the recipient to react generally to histocompatibility antigens. There appear to be "low" and "high" responders. The "low" responders may be able to tolerate histocompatibility antigen differences whereas the "high" responders cannot.

In addition to determining the histocompatibility genes of peripheral blood lymphocytes, preformed cytotoxic antibodies are also looked for in the recipient's blood. These are likely to be present in patients who have had a previous organ transplant, multiple transfusions, or multiple pregnancies or infections. Serum from the patient is tested for antibodies against cells of the prospective donor. The presence of cytotoxic antibodies indicates an F match and a high likelihood that hyperacute rejection of a tissue allograft will occur. An agglutination test should also be done to determine the presence of noncytotoxic antibody. Its presence may enhance the likelihood of "take" of an allograft.

The mixed lymphocyte culture test (MLC) is due to a series of antigens expressed on the surface of B-cells. The antigens are coded for by genes next to those that code for the serologically defined antigens but are clearly distinct from them. The test is done by adding radioactive thymidine and measuring its incorporation into DNA. The lymphocytes of the donor are generally killed, using radiotherapy or mitomycin-C prior to the test, so that the response of the recipient's lymphocytes are assessed to donor antigens (the one-way mixed lymphocyte test).[2] The antigens determined by anti-HLA antibodies and the MLC test are coded for by different but closely linked genes. Graft survival depends on these and other unknown genetic systems which are responsible for the production of cell surface antigens.

Rejection

Rejection may be hyperacute, occurring within minutes to hours; acute, within about one week; or delayed, in months to years. In hyperacute rejection the tissues do not function, the endothelial cells become damaged, the small vessels are occluded by platelet and fibrin thrombi, and there are edema, infiltration with neutrophil leukocytes, and extravasation of blood. Endothelial damage and vessel occlusion are due to the presence of preformed antibodies that interact with antigen in the presence of complement. Mismatching in the ABO blood groups and the presence of antibodies cytotoxic to the donor tissue can result in a hyperacute rejection. In the patient with acute rejection organ function is lost, the endothelium of blood vessels is damaged, and mononuclear cells and neutrophils infiltrate the graft tissue. A cellular response and cytotoxic antibodies probably both contribute to the rejection. Chronic rejection features progressive loss of function of the transplanted organ, perivascular cuffing with mononuclear cells, and partial or complete occlusion of the lumen of vessels by endarteritis. Antibodies and the cell-mediated response both contribute to this form of rejection. The likelihood of rejection and rejection episodes may be predicted by the demonstration of specific antibodies and cytotoxic cells.

Means of Inhibiting Rejection. *Adrenocortical Steroids.* Prednisone inhibits rejection by its anti-inflammatory properties and by decreasing the number of lymphocytes in the peripheral blood, thymus, spleen, and lymph nodes. The number of neutrophils in the peripheral blood is increased. Undesirable side effects are the development of a cushingoid appearance, hypertension, breakdown of tissue proteins, and an increase in infections.

Purine Antagonists. Azathioprine is converted to the purine antagonist 6-mercaptopurine in the liver and inhibits DNA and RNA synthesis. Azathioprine is a powerful inhibitor of the central component of the immune response by interfering with nucleic acid synthesis required for the production of immunoblasts. Because of bone marrow depression, azathioprine decreases all of the white cells and the platelets in the peripheral blood. Common complications therefore are infections and hemorrhage. Liver damage occurs in about 20 percent of patients.

Alkylating Agents. Nitrogen mustard is immunosuppressive by alkylating and cross linking the guanine bases in DNA and interferes with the generation of lymphoblasts. All the white cells and the platelets are decreased in the peripheral blood. Recently cyclophosphamide has been used because it is less toxic.

Antilymphocytic Serum (ALS). As immunosuppressants, antilymphocytic serum and globulin (ALG) are less toxic than any of the previously described agents. The action of ALS is not clear, but it probably kills the T-cells. ALS and ALG are prepared by giving repeated injections of human lymphocytes to horses, removing blood, and isolating heterologous ALS or by precipitation with ammonium sulfate of the globulin fraction of serum giving ALG. When lymphocytes from the peripheral blood are injected, antibodies are also produced to the platelets and cause a thrombocytopenia and often bleeding. A pure preparation of lymphocytes can be obtained from lymph in the thoracic duct. Thymocytes from the thymuses of fetuses have been used extensively as the source of antigen to produce ALS or ALG for use in patients. The patient may become sensitized to antigens in the horse serum and develop a painful swelling at the site of injection. This is most likely to occur when employing ALS that contains more antigens than ALG. Antibodies directed against glomerular basement membrane antigens may cause renal damage. There is considerable difficulty in assaying the potency of an ALS or ALG preparation. Other forms of immunosuppressive therapy are given with ALS or ALG. Smaller doses of the standard immunosuppressive agents can be given when ALS or ALG is included in the treatment regime.

Radiotherapy. Radiotherapy has been given to the whole body or locally to destroy the extremely radiosensitive lymphocytes. Treatment to the whole body is hazardous in man because there is a small margin of safety between the dose which kills lymphocytes and that which causes serious symptoms. Local radiotherapy can be given at the time of operation to inhibit the afferent component of the immune response. The transplanted organ may be irradiated at a dose that does not impair its function to remove donor lymphocytes in the graft which serve as a major source of antigen. The graft may be irradiated when signs of rejection are present, especially in patients who are having reactions from immunosuppressive agents. Blood has been irradiated while passing through an isotope source (for example, using radioactive cesium in an extracorporeal circuit) to destroy lymphocytes in the blood circulation. Irradiation of the spleen or thymus is of no value in patients.

Specific Immunologic Tolerance and Enhancement. The cell-mediated immune attack on a transplanted organ may be reduced or eliminated either by removing the cells responsible for generating the specific "killer" cells or by preventing the "killer" cells from functioning with the use of specific blocking agents. The removal of the T-cells that can recognize the graft antigens is attained by giving animals antigen in such a way that the antigen will inactivate or kill the specific T-cells rather than trigger them into an activated state. This is specific immunologic tolerance. The problem is that tolerance is not attained frequently enough to make it suitable for clinical use. Another approach is to generate or to place in the recipient antibodies or antigen-antibody complexes that interfere with the function of the "killer" cells. Again, this procedure is potent in a limited number of allogeneic donor-recipient combinations but requires much more investigation to increase its applicability.

Tissue and Organ Transplantation

Skin. Much of the experimental work on tissue transplantation was done using skin in animals. The results were applied to organ transplantation in patients (see Chapter 33). The reaction of the host to a skin graft is more severe and more difficult to present than to other tissue grafts. Measures to inhibit rejection are therefore more effective when tissues other than skin are transplanted. The regional nodes are the important central component of the immune response when a graft is placed on the skin or in the subcutaneous tissues. Fetal and porcine skin are often used as a temporary dressing for burns (see Chapter 15).

Kidney. Renal transplantation is now an established operation and is no longer considered experimental (see Chapter 32). Longest survival is more likely when the kidney is obtained from an identical twin. A consanguineous transplant, with a good match for histocompatibility antigens and consequently MLC system whose locus is near the HLA loci, is more likely to survive than one from an unrelated donor.

The clinical signs of chronic rejection are pain in the transplanted kidney, pyrexia, decrease in urinary output, increase in blood creatinine and urea nitrogen, decreased creatinine clearance, leukocytosis, and the presence of lymphocytes and gamma globulin in the urine. Narrowing of the renal vessels is seen on angiography, and the changes of chronic rejection are seen in a renal biopsy. Rejection can be inhibited by increasing the dose of immunosuppressive drugs or by local radiotherapy. Glomerulonephritis may occur in the transplanted kidney and cause renal damage. The likelihood of this is lessened by maintaining immunosuppressive treatment at a reasonably high level. It is also advisable to remove both diseased kidneys in patients with glomerulonephritis. Nephrectomy should also be performed when the kidneys are causing hypertension or are infected.

Liver. Liver transplantation has proved to be much more difficult than kidney transplantation. Early failure is frequent because of the occurrence of vascular thrombosis or the development of liver abscesses. Most liver transplants have been done in patients with congenital biliary atresia or with malignant hepatoma in a cirrhotic liver. Best results have been obtained when the liver is transplanted isotopically.

Other Tissues. *Heart.* Cardiac transplantation must still be considered experimental. The main problems are that it is a single and not a paired organ and that cessation of function leads to immediate death. There are fewer histocompatibility antigens on myocardial cells than on the cells of other organs that have been transplanted (see Chapter 30). Signs of rejection are congestive heart failure, leukocytosis, fever, increase in LDH, and changes in the ECG.

Vascular Grafts. Vascular grafts have been used extensively, most often with autografts. The saphenous vein has been used extensively to bridge arterial defects, especially in the limbs and heart (see Chapter 31).

Corneal Grafts. Corneal allografts are among the first tissues that were successfully grafted. Corneal allografts survived because they were transplanted into an eye that did not contain blood vessels or lymphatics.

Cartilage and Bone. These grafts have been used as a static, nonliving, tissue.

IMMUNITY IN CANCER

Interest in the immunologic treatment of cancer has dated from the time of Koch when it was recognized that a number of infections could be prevented or cured by active or passive immunization. The results of immunizing animals against cancer were extremely encouraging but were not confirmed in patients. This difference stemmed from the fact that the experimental animal tumors were injected into allogeneic hosts. The resistance induced was similar to that to a tissue allograft and not to the presence of tumor-specific antigens. When inbred strains of mice and syngeneic tumor systems became available, it was much more difficult to demonstrate tumor immunity. In 1953 Foley[7] showed that the mouse could be immunized against a chemically induced syngeneic tumor. Others have confirmed his results using spontaneous, chemical, physical, or virally induced tumors. The tumor was grown in the animal, excised, and the animal subsequently challenged with a small number of tumor cells. Animals were also immunized with low doses of nonirradiated or high doses of irradiated tumor cells, then challenged with a lethal dose of tumor cells. The resistance was relatively weak and was similar to that of a tissue allograft when there are minor differences in the histocompatibility antigens between the two tissues. The results of challenge with autologous (autochthonous) tumors were the same as those found in patients.

Growth or nongrowth of a tumor is the result of a balance between the immunologic surveillance and growth-promoting reactions of the host. Cytotoxic cellular reactions are mediated by "killer" T-cell lymphocytes, by macrophages activated by T-cells, and by macrophages and monocytes acting on cancer cells that have been coated with specific antibodies (antibody-mediated cell dependent and opsonic antibody). Cancer growth is increased by blocking factors. Free antigen may block the action of lymphocytes (central inactivation), or antibody may cover the cancer cell and prevent the recognition of cancer-specific antigens by the lymphocytes (peripheral inactivation). The most important blocking factor is probably the formation of antigen-antibody complexes which act at both the lymphocyte and the cancer cell level. Blocking factors can be inactivated by an unblocking factor which is probably a specific cytotoxic antibody. The three cell-mediated components of immunologic surveillance then inhibit cancer growth. This balance between growth-inhibiting and growth-enhancing factors probably varies with tumor growth and probably explains the inability of the host to destroy a clinically recognized tumor. Initially immunologic surveillance is dominant but for some unknown reason is not sufficient to destroy the cancer cells. Blocking factors predominate when the tumor is large.

Evidence for an Immune Response in Patients with Cancer

There is increasing evidence that an immune response is present in patients with cancer. The response may be cellular or humoral and probably varies with the amount of tumor present.

Latent Metastases. Metastases sometimes develop many years after treatment of the primary tumor and then grow rapidly. The sudden rapid growth after a slow progression suggests that host resistance has been depressed. Severe stress following operation, infection, or injury may decrease the cellular immunity

through release of corticosteroids from the adrenal cortex.

Spontaneous Regression. Everson and Cole[5] have collected more than 200 cases of spontaneous regression of cancer, including Wilms' tumor, neuroblastoma, hypernephroma, choriocarcinoma, malignant melanoma, and Burkitt's lymphoma. The regressions have occurred spontaneously after incomplete removal of the tumor, after termination of pregnancy, or blood transfusion. Many of the tumors, such as neuroblastoma, choriocarcinoma, and Burkitt's lymphoma, were infiltrated with mononuclear cells. The occurrence of regression in association with mononuclear cell infiltration suggests that the host produces a cellular immune response that under certain circumstances can lead to tumor regression.

Mononuclear Cell Infiltration. Mononuclear cell infiltration is present in many tumors and is associated with an improved prognosis. This was first demonstrated in patients with carcinoma of the stomach. It was later recognized that patients with medullary carcinoma of the breast with lymphoid infiltration had a much better prognosis than those in whom it was absent. Patients with Hodgkin's disease with lymphoid-rich infiltration of the lesions have a better prognosis than those with lymphocyte depletion. Prognosis is also improved when there is mononuclear cell infiltration of carcinomas of the esophagus and cervix, and in neuroblastomas, seminoma testis, and certain embryonal tumors.

Decreased Immune Response. Cancer is increased in patients with a congenital or acquired depression in the immune response. Many of the congenital immune deficiency states are associated with tumors which are, in the main, neoplasms of the lymphoreticular system. Patients with DiGeorge syndrome (T-cell deficiency), Bruton type of agammaglobulinemia (B-cell deficiency), and Swiss-type agammaglobulinemia and hereditary telangiectasia (both have B- and T-cell deficiencies) have an increased incidence of cancer. Patients with kidney transplants were first found to have an increase in reticulum cell sarcomas but later were also found to have an increase in epithelial tumors, especially of the skin, lip, and cervix.[15] The average age of the patients was 36 years, and the mean time of appearance of the tumors was 28 months. The increase in lymphatic malignancy may have been the result of damage to the lymphoreticular system by the immunosuppressants, especially azathioprine. A number of kidneys from cancer patients have been used as transplants. The same type of cancer has developed in the recipient while on immunosuppressant therapy and has regressed after treatment was stopped. Normally cancer cells from another individual will not grow on transplantation. This is important evidence that a decrease in immune response enhances allogeneic cancer "takes" and growth. An increase in lymphomas also occurs in patients with celiac disease with damage to the lymphoreticular system and from infection with chronic malaria resulting in Burkitt's lymphoma. The increase in epithelial tumors may be the result of decrease in immunologic surveillance due to immunosuppressive therapy. It has also been reported that the patients with Hodgkin's disease treated by extended field radiotherapy and chemotherapy have an increase in cancer.[1]

Cancer-Specific Antigens and Antibodies. Cancer-specific antigens may be classified as reversionary, tissue specific, or viral. They may be released into the circulation or secretions or be confined to the tumors. Some of the antigens are on the surface of the cell, but antigens have also been demonstrated in the cytoplasm. Some of the antigens in virally transformed cells are very specific, while others are widely distributed among other related viruses which transform cells. The RNA-dependent DNA polymerase (reverse transcriptase) antigen appears to be interspecies specific.

The presence of antigens similar to those found in the fetus is of particular interest. A fetal sulfoglycoprotein, closely allied to type A substance, is present in the gastric secretions of about 80 percent of patients with carcinoma of the stomach. The high incidence of carcinoma of the stomach in patients with blood group A may be the result of the host being unable to react against cancer cells with antigens similar to group A substance. The sulfoglycoprotein is also present in the gastric secretions in 10 percent of people who do not have cancer.

An α-fetoprotein, a glycoprotein, occurs in large amounts in the serum of about 80 percent Negro and 40 percent Caucasian patients with malignant hepatoma of the liver and in about about 25 percent of those with malignant teratomas. The values are higher in children than adults, and the percentages are much greater using a more sensitive radioimmunoassay. The antigen is present in the serum of the fetus and disappears after birth. Its function is to transport estrogens and protect the fetus from excessive amounts of maternal estrogens. Occasionally α-fetoprotein is found in the serum of patients with hepatocellular necrosis, as for example with infectious hepatitis, and rarely with metastases from carcinoma elsewhere, especially of the stomach.

Carcinoembryonic antigen (CEA) is present in minute amounts, about 2 nanograms, in the serum of patients with carcinoma of the gut and gut-derived organs.[6] It increases as the site of the primary tumor approaches the rectum and also with the size of the tumor. Recently it has been confirmed that false positives are frequent in patients with chronic ulcerative colitis, carcinoma of the breast, and chronic renal and liver disease. The test is of no value in screening for cancer but may be useful in determining the development of metastases. A value of above 20 nanograms in a patient with carcinoma of the colorectum, who previously had a lower value, is highly suspicious of metastases.

In animal studies embryonic antigens have also been demonstrated in virally transformed cells and chemically induced tumors. Specific cancer cell antigens have been recognized in animals and in patients. Evidence for the presence of virus-associated antigens in patients is indirect. Different tumors caused by the same virus have a common virus-induced transplantation antigen. A common antigen is present in cancers of the same site in different patients. Patients with soft tissue sarcomas have a common antigen and also patients with neuroblastomas and their families.[8] This suggests that the tumors may be induced by viruses, or that tissue-specific antigens are being detected.

Cancer-specific antibodies have been demonstrated in the serum of patients with Burkitt's lymphoma, melanoma, neuroblastoma, choriocarcinoma, soft tissue sarcomas, osteogenic sarcoma, bladder tumors, and Hodgkin's disease. Their relation to prognosis has not been established. Anti-CEA antibodies are present after removal of the tumor in the serum of about 70 percent of patients with carcinoma of the colon.[6]

Immunotherapeutic Studies. The results of immunotherapeutic studies have not been highly successful. There have been, however, enough partial regressions to suggest that changing the immunologic status of the host can affect cancer growth. Active immunotherapy has been attempted by generalized nonspecific stimulation of the mononuclear cells using BCG by scarification[12] or orally in patients with carcinoma of the lung and colorectum. Localized, active, nonspecific cellular immunotherapy using BCG, vaccinia vaccine, pertussis vaccine, or dinitrochlorobenzene (DNCB)[10] injected into cutaneous metastases, especially of malignant melanoma, has resulted in a marked local reaction followed by tumor regression. It is highly suggestive that the responses were the result of a delayed hypersensitivity reaction induced by the agents. Some attempts to increase the antigenicity of the cancer cells using neuraminidase or radiotherapy have been successful in animals but have not been confirmed in patients.[9] Isolated reports of partial regressions following passive or adoptive immunotherapy giving large numbers of treated or untreated lymphocytes from the same patient or allogeneic lymphocytes have been published. Interchange of tumors followed by exchange "buffy coats" between patients (active immunization followed by adoptive immunization) has produced partial regressions in about 20 percent of patients.[9] It is clear that immunotherapeutic approaches have not yet met with overwhelming success, but that this field holds promise.

CITED REFERENCES

1. Arseneau, I. C.; Sponzo, R. W.; Levin, D. L.; Schnipper, L. E.; Bonner, H.; Young, R. C.; Canellos, G. P.; Johnson, R. E.; and DeVita, V. T.: Nonlymphomatous malignant tumors complicating Hodgkin's disease. *N. Engl. J. Med.*, **287**:1119–22, 1972.
2. Bach, F. H., and Kisken, W. A.: Predictive value of results of mixed leukocyte cultures for skin allograft survival in man. *Transplantation*, **5**:1045–52, 1967.
3. Barker, C. F., and Billingham, R. E.: The role of regional lymphatics in the skin homograft response. *Transplantation*, Part 2, **5**:962A–66, 1967.
4. Burnet, F. M., and Fenner, F.: Genetics and immunology. *Heredity*, **2**:289–324, 1948.
5. Everson, T. C., and Cole, W. H.: *Spontaneous Regression of Cancer.* W. B. Saunders, Philadelphia, 1966.
6. Gold, P., and Freedman, S. O.: Demonstration of tumor-specific antigen in human colonic carcinomata by immunological tolerance and absorption techniques. *J. Exp. Med.*, **121**:439–62, 1965.
7. Foley, E. J.: Antigenic properties of methylcholanthrene-induced tumors in mice of the strain of origin. *Cancer Res.*, **13**:835–37, 1953.
8. Hellstrom, I.; Hellstrom, K. E.; Pierce, G. E.; and Bill, A. H.: Demonstration of cell bound and humoral immunity against neuroblastoma cells. *Proc. Natl. Acad. Sci. USA*, **60**:1231–38, 1968.
9. Humphrey, L. J.; Murray, D. R.; and Boehm, O. R.: Effect of tumor vaccines in immunizing patients with cancer. *Surg. Gynecol. Obstet.*, **132**:437–42, 1971.
10. Klein, E.: Hypersensitivity reactions at tumor sites. *Cancer Res.*, **29**:2351–62, 1969.
11. Lawrence, H. S.: Transfer factor and cellular immunity. *Hosp. Pract.*, Dec., pp. 40–58, 1969.
12. Mathe, G.: Approaches to the immunological treatment of cancer in man. *Br. Med. J.*, **4**:7–10, 1969.
13. Medawar, P. B.: Second study of behaviour and fate of skin homografts in rabbits: reports to war wounds committee of Medical Research Council. *J. Anat.*, **79**:157–76, 1945.
14. Owen, R. D.: Immunogenetic consequences of vascular anastomoses between bovine twins. *Science*, **102**:400, 1945.
15. Penn, I., and Starzl, T. E.: Immunosuppression and cancer. *Transplant Proc.*, **5**:943–47, 1973.
16. Snell, G. D., and Stimpfling, J. H.: Genetics of tissue transplantation. In: *Jackson Laboratory: Biology of the Laboratory Mouse.* McGraw-Hill, New York, p. 457, 1966.
17. Terasaki, P. I., and McClelland, J. D.: Microdroplet assay of human serum cytotoxins. *Nature*, **204**:998, 1964.
18. Wilson, J. D., and Nossal, G. J. V.: Identification of human T and B lymphocytic leukaemia. *Lancet*, **2**:788–91, 1971.

SUGGESTIONS FOR FURTHER READING

Alexander, J. W., and Good, R. A.: *Immunobiology for Surgeons.* W. B. Saunders, Philadelphia, 1970.
An excellent basic description of cellular and humoral immunity.

Cinader, B.: The future of tumor immunology. *Med. Clin. North Am.*, **56**:801–36, 1972.
A stimulating overview of present status and possible future developments in tumor immunology.

Mathiew, A., and Kahan, B. D.: *Immunologic Aspects of Anesthetic and Surgical Practice.* Grune & Stratton, New York, pp. 1–400, 1975.
An excellent survey of immunology relevant to clinical practice.

Miller, J. F. A. F., and Mitchell, G. F.: Thymus and antigen reactive cells. *Transplant. Rev.*, **1**:3–42, 1969.
Deals with evidence for the distinction between B- and T-cells.

Moller, G.: Experiments and the concept of immunological surveillance. *Transplant. Rev.*, **28**:3–97, 1976.
A multiauthored review covering various recent contributions to the field of tumor immunology.

Najarian, J. S., and Simmons, R. L.: *Transplantation.* Lea & Febiger, Philadelphia, 1972.
A comprehensive review of the subject of tissue transplantation.

Vyas, G. N.; Stiles, D. T.; and Brecher, G.: *Laboratory Diagnosis of Immunologic Disorders.* Grune & Stratton, New York, pp. 1–289, 1975.
A practical survey of the clinical uses of immunologic data.

Chapter 5

TISSUE HEALING

Walter J. Pories and *Fred R. Plecha*

CHAPTER OUTLINE

Physiology and Chemistry of Healing
  Phases of Healing
  Local Changes
    Hemostatic Response
    Vascular Response
    Cellular Invasion and Phagocytosis
    Chemical Debridement
    Cellular Repair
    Fibroblasts
    Connective Tissue
    Humoral Factors
  Systemic Factors
  Healing in Specialized Tissues
    Epithelium

Nerves
Muscle
Blood Vessels
Bones
Tendons
Treatment of Wounds
  Care of the Acute Wound
    Hemostasis
    Cleansing and Debridement
    Delayed Wound Closure
    Transplantation of Tissues
    Foreign Bodies
    Drainage
    Dressing Care

Healing has always been the primary objective of medical care. The pneumonic lung, the heart with infarction, and the colon dotted with multiple ulcers pose problems similar basically to those encountered in the treatment of an infected laceration, a comminuted tibia, and a brain abscess. The basic physiologic phenomena are the same in each instance and successful management depends on restoration of function with a minimum of deformity and scar.

PHYSIOLOGY AND CHEMISTRY OF HEALING

Phases of Healing

Although the healing process is a continuum that begins immediately after injury and persists for years, it has been divided arbitrarily into two phases: an initial or substrate phase and a second or collagen phase. The *initial phase*, also called lag, autolytic, catabolic, or inflammatory, is generally considered to include the first five days of healing. All of the names are partially correct. It is a period of intense activity, including outpouring of tissue fluids, autolysis, invasion by leukocytes, phagocytosis, development of new vessels, and accumulation of substrate. The wound quickly becomes shallow, the edges invert, and its size may be reduced by 50 percent during the 48 hours after injury, perhaps due to dehydration. From the time of injury a healthy, cared-for wound closes at first due to wound collapse and later by contraction. The gain in strength of a wound increases exponentially.

The *second phase*, also called collagen, proliferate, or anabolic, begins about the sixth day and is the period of collagen accumulation, wound contracture, and scar remodeling.

Local Changes

Hemostatic Response. The injured region fills with blood clot containing dead and injured cells from traumatized tissues. In most wounds bleeding is controlled by the clot formation and vascular constriction. The transected vessels are soon plugged with platelet aggregates and later by a thrombus. The clot becomes dehydrated and hardens into a scab which protects and binds the wound edges tenuously with young, polymerized fibrin strands. Under this fragile roof the intricate process of healing begins (Figure 5–1, *A*).

Vascular Response. The clot and probably the injury to the local nerve endings then initiate a vascular response. Within a few seconds the surrounding vessels constrict, but

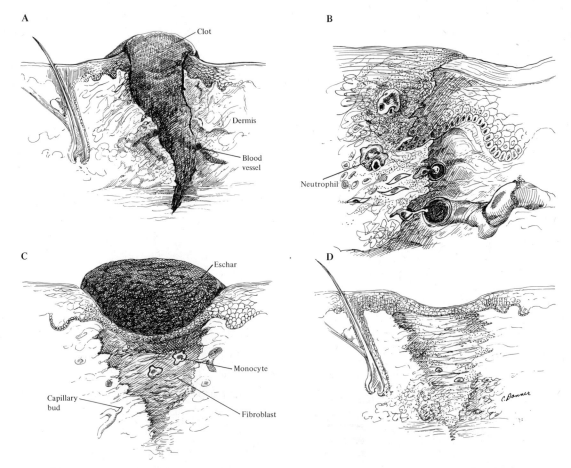

Figure 5–1. *A*. Wound healing begins with a clot. Immediately after injury, the wound is filled with a coagulum of fibrinogen, other serum proteins, erythrocytes, leukocytes, cellular debris, and usually bacteria and other foreign material.

   B. Within 24 hours, the initial or inflammatory phase of healing is well under way. Vessels dilate, neutrophils diapedese from the edematous tissues, epithelial cells slide in as active mitosis begins in the basal cell layer. Phagocytosis of necrotic debris begins amid the network of fibrin strands.

   C. Two to four days later, the second or collagen phase begins. A new generation of inflammatory cells, the monocytes, have invaded the wound. Capillary buds form, branch, and develop lumina. Fibroblasts begin to lay down collagen. A thin sheet of epithelium has migrated under the scab and joined with cells from the other site.

   D. One to two weeks after the injury, the scab has separated and a thickening scar replaces the previous area of imflammation. Initially the area is more vascular than the surrounding dermis, but later the scar becomes almost avascular. The epithelium remains thin and, because of the inability to re-form epithelial appendages, is poorly attached to the dermis.

within minutes they dilate, producing marked local stasis. Arterioles dilate, capillary shunts open, and the efferent venules fail to handle the increased volume of blood in the area. With increasing pressures venous endothelial cells separate, and the vascular walls become more permeable, first to proteins and later to cells. Serum leaks into the wound, and globulins, fibrin, albumin, nutrients, substrates, enzymes, antibodies, and hormones flood the area to resist invading organisms and to sustain the phagocytes and reparative cells which will soon follow. As a result of the vascular changes and the local edema, hypoxia and acidosis occur with a local fall in pH and P_{O_2} and a rise in P_{CO_2}. Combinations of the vasoactive amines and polypeptides, such as histamine, serotonin, and bradykinin with epinephrine, probably serve as some of the chemical mediators producing these changes (Figure 5–1, *B*).

Although a clot is essential for initiating the process of healing and for providing a fibrin framework, an excessive amount of clot may interfere with healing. It acts as a foreign body, enlarges the wound volume, serves as a culture medium for bacteria, and interferes with fibroplasia. Avoidance of a hematoma, or excessive clot, is one of the basic tenets of surgery.

Cellular Invasion and Phagocytosis. *White blood cells* play an important role in the early stages of healing. Most wounds are contaminated by bacteria and foreign material that interfere with healing and predispose to infection. The *polymorphonuclear cells* migrate by diapedesis through the vessel walls within two to eight minutes of injury. The neutrophils phagocytose bacteria and foreign materials and transport them to the respiratory or gastrointestinal tracts for elimination. Acid hydrolases, antibacterial substances, phagocytin, and lysozymes are released when the cells disintegrate and cleanse the wound.

The function of other white blood cells is not well understood. *Eosinophils* take part in antigen-antibody reactions and act as antagonists to serotonin, bradykinin, and histamine. *Lymphocytes* can be divided into several populations; the larger act as phagocytes within the wound, while the smaller take part in the cell-mediated immune response and others mature into immunoglobulin-forming plasma cells. *Monocytes and macrophages*, laden with hydrolases, appear later than the polymorphonuclear cells and phagocytoze wound detritus and dead neutrophils. *Epithelioid and giant cells* are later found in wounds containing foreign materials, such as sutures or metal fragments, and in chronically infected wounds. *Mast cells* contain mucopolysaccharides for the formation of ground substance and collagen and also release histamine, chymotrypsin, and trypsinlike enzymes, cytochrome oxidase, lipase, and probably heparin.

Phagocytosis can be stimulated or delayed by changes in the cellular environment. Opsonins and antibodies from the serum increase the rate of ingestion, while elevated concentrations of urea, glucose, or sodium cause a decrease. Deviations from the normal pH and osmolality inhibit phagocytosis. Rough particles are more easily engulfed than smooth, but large numbers of particles, such as follow the injection of colloids or fat emulsions, interfere with phagocytosis.

Chemical Debridement. Lysosomes in the cytoplasm of leukocytes contain a wide variety of hydrolytic enzymes and basic proteins and participate in intracellular digestion. At cell death the lysosomes rupture and cause autolysis of the cell and digestion of necrotic tissues. The lysosomes also contain a number of substances that produce the changes of inflammation such as proteases, pyrogens, and phagocytin, an antibacterial substance.

Lysosomes are labilized by antigen-antibody interaction, radiation, streptolysis, bacterial toxins, shock, oxygen poisoning, viruses, and a low pH. Conversely, they are stabilized by cortisone, chloroquine, aspirin, chlorpromazine, antihistamines, and cholesterol.

Cellular Repair. As the wound is cleaned and the inflammatory response subsides, other cells rebuild the damaged tissues. The *epithelial cells* enter first and in largest numbers. In the skin they appear as if squeezed out of the layers of the intact epidermis and slide into the wound at the interface between viable tissues and clot. When epithelial integrity is restored, the epithelium thickens, but rarely to its full depth, and gradually with time may resume some of its specialized functions.

The stimuli that begin and stop this remarkable process of epitheliazation are poorly understood. Wounding results in a breach in cell-to-cell contact with loss of surface inhibition and induces changes in humoral factors, energy levels, surface potentials, protein concentrations, P_{O_2}, P_{CO_2}, and pH. Changes in the wound surfaces greatly influence epithelial migration. Epithelium grows best on a moist wound rather than a dry one and at body temperature. The attraction of like cells and the contact disaffinity of unlike cells help in sorting out the various layers.

Within 72 hours *endothelial buds* sprout from adjacent blood vessels and invade the wound in the form of syncytia and solid cords. These branches soon develop lumens and form the network of fragile and permeable capillaries of granulation tissue. Most of these vessels regress during the later stages of healing, but a few remain to differentiate into mature arteries and veins.

Fibroblasts. Fibroblasts and, to a lesser extent, osteoblasts and chondroblasts restore the strength of the wound by building collagen and probably elastin. They enter the wound before capillary buds appear. Connective tissue fibers appear four to five days later. Initially, isolated fibroblasts establish connections with other fibroblasts and form a syncytium with remarkable cytoplasmic movement and massive protein synthesis. Labeled *l*-proline is taken up by the fibroblasts, passes from the ribosomes to the Golgi apparatus, and finally in 24 hours is present as hydroxyproline in the extracellular collagen. Fibroblasts also incorporate sulfate into chondroitin sulfate, heparin sulfate, and other heparinlike material (Figure 5–1, *C*).

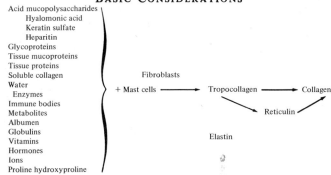

Figure 5–2. The synthesis of collagen is an extremely complex process requiring a rich, varied substrate. Even small changes in pH and concentrations interfere with synthesis and the subsequent coiling of the collagen molecule. Hydroxyproline is of special importance in surgical research because it is an amino acid utilized only in collagen and therefore serves as an excellent biologic marker.

Connective Tissue. The connective tissues are polymerized from a gel-like *ground substance* that surrounds the cells. The ground substance contains acid mucopolysaccharides, glycoproteins, tissue mucoproteins, tissue proteins, soluble collagen, water, enzymes, immune bodies, metabolites, albumin, globulins, vitamins, hormones, and ions. The mucopolysaccharides, which are probably synthesized locally from glycoproteins originating in the liver, include hyaluronic acid, the chondroitins, keratin sulfate, and heparin. These large-complex polymers are then incorporated into the large fibers of connective tissues, collagen, reticulin, and elastin.

The basic framework of connective tissue consists of collagen. Collagen accounts for 30 percent of total body protein and is a polymer of three left-handed polypeptide chains wound into a right-handed helix. At least 100 ribosomes are needed to synthesize tropocollagen (M. wt. 300,000, $10 \text{ Å} \times 2800 \text{ Å}$), the basic building block of collagen, from hydroxyproline amino acid radicals. The tropocollagen is then transported across the cell wall and polymerized into the superhelix in the extracellular space.

Collagen fibers are assembled from aggregates of macromolecules and form a continuously changing net, which is repeatedly assembled and disassembled in a constant process of remodeling. The fibers align themselves in the direction of lines of tension and can effectively change chemical energy into powerful mechanical forces. Changes in pH, salt concentration, and ionization alter the coiling and retraction of these giant chains. The changes are rapid and have been timed at 150 mm per second. The unique helical structure of collagen has been attributed to the large moieties of glycine, proline, and hydroxyproline in the molecule.

Collagen provides the strong force of wound contraction and is thus a major cause of reduction in wound volume. It provides tensile strength and structural integrity. Without collagen wounds would take much longer to heal and tissues would not knit. On the other hand, collagen can also deform, cripple, and kill. The heavy scar contractures after a severe burn, the obstructing stricture of the esophagus after ingestion of dye, and the fibrous septae in the cirrhotic liver are but a few examples. The deformities of rheumatoid arthritis, the epilepsy following a cerebral scar, and the formation of hyalin, amyloid, and fibrinoid are all instances of uncontrolled or abnormal collagen production or failure of collagen lysis (Figure 5–1, *D*, and Figure 5–2).

Humoral Factors. A number of hormones, trace elements, and other compounds affect the rate of wound healing. *Cortisone* in large doses blocks the process, perhaps by stabilizing the lysosomes. This effect has recently been reported to be reversed by the administration of vitamin A. Hypervitaminosis A, however, causes increased lysis of lysosomes.

Inflammation is mediated by a number of hormones such as the *protease kallikrein*, the *polypeptide bradykinin*, and the *amine histamine*. *Epinephrine* and *norepinephrine*, on the other hand, are anti-inflammatory hormones. Thyroid hormone and growth hormone do not influence wound healing.

The *trace elements* are essential for healing through their actions as metal moieties or cofactors of enzymes essential for protein synthesis and cellular respiration. *Zinc* is required for epithelial replication and collagen synthesis, while *copper* is needed for the polymerization of elastin. Deficiencies of these and other trace elements cause delay in healing and loss of wound tensile strength.

Numerous compounds influence healing, and many have still probably not been identified. *Vitamin C* is essential for the fibroblast for synthesis of collagen; deficiency produces scurvy with failure of healing and breakdown of previously healed wounds. The breakdown of intact scars is particularly interesting, because it reaffirms that collagen is not an inert tissue and that lysis and synthesis of the scar tissue continue for years. Nitrogen mustard and methotrexate reduce granulation tissues, collagen concentration, and wound contraction. It is likely that other cytotoxic agents such as azathioprine and antilymphocytic globulin have similar effects.

Systemic Factors

The patient's general health greatly influences the quality of healing. A young, healthy, well-nourished boy will handle his injury much better than an old, malnourished diabetic man with advanced cancer. Many of the systemic factors that interfere with healing have not been identified. Despite the clinical impression that anemia, cancer, paralysis, sepsis, and many other diseases slow healing, none has been shown to slow tissue repair. Animals with hemoglobin levels as low as 4.0 gm percent heal at the same rate as controls. Wound healing is inhibited in those with scurvy, certain coagulation defects including hemophilia, lack of factor 13, and Danlos' syndrome, severe protein deficiency, advancing age, zinc deficiency, and certain chronic diseases, including rheumatoid arthritis, lupus erythematosus, myositis ossificans, periarteritis nodosa, and thromboangiitis obliterans.

HEALING IN SPECIALIZED TISSUES

Epithelium

Epithelium provides protective cover for all tissues and produces a number of secretions that digest, lubricate, and excrete. It is a thin layer in the pharynx, the respiratory system, the intestinal tract, the genitourinary system, and the vagina. Epithelium heals rapidly if the wound is properly dressed and protected from infection. The epithelial cells flatten and slide into the defect as a fragile single cell layer which thickens as new epithelial cells divide during later stages of repair. Until the wound is completely covered, scabs form, fall off, and form again; capillaries protrude as edematous granulations or as "proud flesh," and fibroblasts continue to lay down collagens with increasingly heavy scarring and contracture.

Cutaneous epithelium is capable of covering a defect about 10 cm, but it takes a long time and the wound remains a continuing source of pain, discharge, odor, protein loss, and bacteremia. In addition, the regenerated layer is not fully functional. The new epidermis lacks rete pegs and therefore slides off even with minimal trauma. A scar from a burn on the shin, for example, can be repeatedly injured with repeated epithelial loss until a thick, avascular layer of dermis is formed. Eventually normal epitheliazation ceases, and the wound may be transformed into a squamous cell carcinoma (Marjolin's ulcer).

It is evident that epithelial healing is vitally important. Careful wound closure, skin grafting, rotation of flaps, layer-by-layer anastomosis of the esophagus, plastic repair of a through-and-through laceration of the cheek, and the immediate maturation of an ileostomy are all directed toward the goal of immediate epithelial integrity.

Nerves

In contrast to epithelium, the nervous system does not regenerate. Postganglionic fibers regrow at the rate of 1 mm per day if the cell is intact, preganglionic fibers grow less rapidly, and sympathetic fibers may regrow for only short distances. Nerves can be repaired with moderate success. It is apparent that optimal end-to-end approximation of the nerve sheaths with a minimum of scar is essential if the nerve fibers are to be reunited with their end organs. Repair of nerves therefore is usually only carried out in clean wounds and is usually delayed for several weeks if the injury is accompanied by contamination and crushing. With meticulous technique nerve grafts can be interposed between the severed ends of a nerve.

Muscle

Divided muscle bundles heal by scar formation and normally regain their function, but individual muscle fibers do not regenerate. Excessive scar formation can be avoided by careful debridement of necrotic tissue, avoidance of hematoma, and accurate approximation of investing fascia. The excellent vascularity and high healing potential of muscle make it a good tissue to cover bone, nerves, and vessels. Also, muscle provides an excellent base for application of skin grafts. For example, a deep wound of the groin requiring repair of the femoral artery can be closed by mobilizing the sartorius muscle and placing it over the arterial suture line. A split-thickness skin graft can then be placed on the muscle.

Blood Vessels

A transected artery or vein generally retracts, thromboses, scars, and becomes occluded up to the next proximal branch. Flow is reestablished rapidly around the injury by a net of collaterals. A lateral injury, on the other hand, presents a much more dangerous situation, because the orifice is held open by the elasticity of the vessel and a thrombus may not be able to occlude the flow. Exsanguination may result unless the intrinsic pressure of the accumulating hematoma arrests the flow. These injuries will also, if the bleeding stops, be healed by an investing scar. A thrombosed vein may eventually recanalize, but arteries in general remain occluded. Vessels can be sutured with maintenance of patency. Arteries can be replaced by arterial autografts, arterial homografts, vein autografts, plastic prostheses, and denatured bovine carotid arteries. Autogenous vein grafts are presently preferred. Vein grafts remain viable and undergo characteristic changes of thickening and rarely even atherosclerosis. These alterations are increased by slow blood flow, trauma, and infection.

Dacron grafts are held in place for years by the investing scar and sutures. The endothelium does not cover the inner surface completely but grows in for only 1 to 2 cm from the suture lines. The remainder is lined by a pseudointima which may eventually separate and form an embolus. The failure of dacron to heal was first recognized when patients, whose grafts had been sutured in place with silk, returned with false aneurysm at the suture lines. The silk sutures had fragmented a year or two after implantation and allowed the dacron to loosen and break the anastomosis. Permanent plastic sutures prevent this complication.

Atherosclerosis may be a manifestation of poor arterial healing. When systemic conditions are optimal, arteries heal with a fine scar. When these conditions are changed, however, by hypercholesterolemia in an experimental animal, arterial injuries do not heal readily and an atherosclerotic plaque results. Atherosclerotic lesions are characteristically seen in areas of chronic vascular trauma such as bifurcations, stenoses, and fistulas, and atherosclerotic lesions can be produced easily by the local application of electric current, freezing, infection, crushing, and cautery.

Bones

The healing of bone is similar to that of other tissues except that it has a third phase and is slower. After a substrate and collagen phase, there is a maturation phase when callus is replaced by new bone.

The fracture is followed by a hematoma which becomes the matrix for repair. During the first five days leukocytes invade the clot, fibroblasts appear, and new vessels are formed. New collagen and organic matrix are produced after about 10 days, and after 15 days osteoblasts produce new bone. In bone, as in collagen, there is a continuous process of modeling and remodeling along lines of force.

Tendons

Tendons are almost pure collagen and heal well. The concern is not whether the tendon will regain its strength, but if it will maintain its mobility within the tendon sheath.

TREATMENT OF WOUNDS

Wounds heal best if the optimum environment is provided for each cell. Cells thrive in normothermic, isotonic, clean surroundings at normal pH, provided with adequate substrate, and protected from infection and trauma. On the other hand, cells die quickly if they dry out, if they are exposed to foreign and toxic chemicals, surrounded by necrotic debris, and overwhelmed by bacteria.

Wounds heal by first, second, or third intention. *First intention* refers to the ideal situation of a "primary union" following a clean incision, excellent approximation of tissues, and healing with a minimal scar. Surgical incisions usually heal in this manner. *Second intention* is the term applied to healing by the slow process of filling in with granulation tissue, scar, and the gradual coverage by epithelium. Most ulcers fill in by second intention and form a thick, poorly epithelialized scar. Healing by *third intention* or delayed suture should be called "intermediate intention." Some wounds are not suitable for primary closure because of possible infection but may be closed on the fourth or fifth day after injury. Such wounds heal as well and as quickly as those closed by first intention but form a thicker scar.

Care of the Acute Wound

Hemostasis. Bleeding, even arterial, can usually be controlled by pressure, and hemostats can then be applied to individual vessels. Clamping should be precise and limited to the vessel, and the ties should be fine and cut close to the knot, leaving a minimum of foreign material. Occasionally wounds are encountered in which clamping and ligation of individual vessels are not possible. In such situations, suture ligatures, electric cautery, or packing may have to be used. For example, the bleeding of scalp lacerations is best handled by a through-and-through approximating stitch, the ooze from large masses of muscle is frequently best avoided by transecting them with cautery, and a bleeding nose can usually be controlled by anterior or posterior nasal packing.

Cleansing and Debridement. Wounds must be cleaned of foreign material and necrotic tissue. Traumatized globules of fat, bacteria, and clots must be flushed out using large volumes of isotonic saline. Antiseptic solutions should not be used because there is no evidence that they aid healing and they may damage normal tissues.

All foreign material must be removed and dead tissues completely excised.

Delayed Wound Closure. Possibly contaminated wounds should not be closed. A laceration from a pitchfork, a traumatic amputation from a battlefield explosion, and an abdominal incision fouled by stool are examples of such wounds. Even with the most meticulous technique these wounds cannot be adequately cleansed and remain excellent culture media for bacteria.

Delayed wound closure offers an excellent approach to such problems. After the wound has been debrided, it is covered with a layer of fine mesh gauze, filled with loosely fluffed gauze, and covered with an occlusive dressing. The dressing is only changed if indicated by excessive drainage, pain, or odor. Four or five days later the dressing is removed and, in almost all cases, the wound edges are found to be clean, red, and ready for secondary closure. The wound edges can under such circumstances be sutured loosely and will heal as well, although with a slightly wider scar, than if primary suture had been done.

Transplantation of Tissues. All wounds cannot be closed by the simple approximation of the edges. A large segment of pretibial tissue may be avulsed with a tibial fracture, a melanoma of the face may require sacrifice of a large volume of tissue, and a deep burn results in loss of skin. In such situations tissue transplantation offers an excellent approach for wound closure (see Chapter 33).

Foreign Bodies. Foreign bodies interfere with healing. Hematomas, seromas, collections of pus, dead tissue, glove talcum, cauterized surfaces, and lost instruments or sponges must be removed or they will form a nidus for continuing inflammation and bacterial invasion. Even if healing occurs, it is generally delayed and associated with a high incidence of infection, heavy scarring, greater deformity, and eventually rejection. Foreign materials are, however, often used, such as dacron grafts, hip nails, Kirschner wires, and silastic breast prostheses. Because of risk of chronic infection special care is taken during their implantation.

When infection occurs in the presence of a foreign material, it is generally necessary to remove the prosthesis. Infected arterial grafts, for example, eventually rupture at their anastomoses and cause massive hemorrhage. Occasionally an exposed dacron graft can be preserved by careful dressing technique and 0.1 percent neomycin drip, but in most cases the infected graft must be removed and blood flow rerouted with another graft through clean tissue.

The tensile strength of a wound is greater even after one to two months if the sutures have been left in position. Skin stitches are generally removed before the dermis regains its strength to minimize and avoid "railroad track" scars. They can generally be removed from the head and neck in two to three days, the thorax and abdomen in five to seven days, and the extremities in two to three weeks. Sutures can be removed earlier in younger patients and in those who are healthy rather than debilitated. Other techniques to reduce skin scarring are the use of fine suture material, placement of the sutures in close apposition and near the skin edge, provision of perpendicular wound edges, minimum tension, and observance of wrinkle lines.

Drainage. Collections of fluid interfere with healing and must be evacuated. Hematomas, seromas, and collections of lymph, pus, or bile will usually re-form and require a continuous route of escape. Drainage can be open or closed. A collection of fluid may be removed through a large incision or allowed to escape more slowly along a drain. Drains are generally of soft rubber but have been made of a variety of materials and occasionally contain a gauze wick. Open drainage carries the serious disadvantage of providing an easy route of entry for bacteria. A catheter, used for closed drainage, has usually several holes and is attached to a water seal or suction. Its advantages are ease of wound care and less risk of infection, but it is likely to obstruct with clots and other debris. Drains should be radiopaque, fixed to wound edges, and gradually removed as soon as drainage decreases.

Dressing Care. Open wounds generally require dressings. When such wounds are not covered, exposed cells die of dehydration and a scab with underlying infection soon forms. Pus leaks intermittently from beneath the scab.

Undressed and exposed wounds, even if closed by primary suture, are usually ugly to the patient and sensitive to touch. Almost all wounds are more comfortable and heal more quickly if dressed. Initially a dry, thin gauze layer absorbs any serosanguineous fluid. After about two days a piece of microporous or non-allergenic tape applied directly to the wound protects the skin edges.

SUGGESTIONS FOR FURTHER READING

Dunphy, J. E.: The fibroblast—a ubiquitous ally for the surgeon. *N. Engl. J. Med.*, **268**:1367–77, 1963.

In the Shattuck Lecture at the 182nd Anniversary of the Massachusetts Medical Society, the importance of the fibroblast in wound healing is eloquently reviewed.

Dunphy, J. E., and Van Winkle, W., Jr.: *Repair and Regeneration*. McGraw-Hill, New York, 1969.

An excellent review and reference source by 38 authorities.

Peacock, E. E., Jr., and Van Winkle, W., Jr.: *Surgery and Biology of Wound Repair*. W. B. Saunders., Philadelphia, 1970.

A comprehensive review of the basic concepts of wound repair and its clinical applications.

Shilling, J. A.: Wound healing. *Physiol. Rev.*, **48**:374–423, 1968.

A collation of the important contributions to the understanding of wound healing.

Chapter 6

SURGICAL INFECTIONS

G. William Odling-Smee

CHAPTER OUTLINE

Etiology, Diagnosis, and Surgical Management
Factors Predisposing to Infection
Local Factors
  Contamination
  Inflammatory Response
General Factors
Diagnosis of Infection
  Clinical Diagnosis
  Laboratory Diagnosis
Surgical Management
  Debridement of Wounds
Antibiotics
Mechanism of Action
Choice of an Antibiotic
  Types of Antibiotics
  Hypersensitivity
Prophylactic Antibiotics
Misuse of Antibiotics

Antiseptics and Disinfectants
  Classification
Types of Infections
  Cellulitis
  Lymphangitis and Lymphadenitis
  Abscess
  Ulceration
  Gangrene
  Septicemia
Specific Infections in Surgery
  Tetanus
    Treatment
    Prophylaxis
  Gas Gangrene (Clostridial Myonecrosis)
    Treatment
  Anaerobic Clostridial Myositis
  Streptococcal Myositis
  Diabetic Necrotizing Cellulitis

ETIOLOGY, DIAGNOSIS, AND SURGICAL MANAGEMENT

Infections continue to be a major problem in surgery. Hippocrates recognized in the third millennium B.C. that cleanliness was important. Surgeons, however, were still ignoring this during most of the nineteenth century. Semmelweis in Vienna and Holmes in Boston stressed the importance of cleanliness; Semmelweis was derided, dismissed from his post, and died insane, while Holmes lived to see his views vindicated. Most surgeons preferred to believe that infection was an act of God rather than the result of their unclean habits. In the late nineteenth century Pasteur showed that disease was caused by microscopic organisms. Lister then introduced antiseptic surgery using phenol and later aseptic technique. In 1928 Fleming noticed that a mold, *Penicillium notatum*, that accidentally contaminated plates containing *Staphylococcus aureus* microorganisms inhibited their growth. Florey, Chain, and Fleming later extracted penicillin.

Severe cases of erysipelas, moist gangrene, and uncontrolled case-to-case wound infection are rarely seen in hospital wards. However, wound infections on a lesser scale are disturbingly common. Wound infection is the result of implantation of pathogenic organisms through a breach in the epithelial lining of the skin or alimentary tract. The portal of entry through the skin may be a surgical incision, wound, or burn. Infection in a viscus, as in the lung, liver, or gut, may extend to the overlying serosa and infect a serous cavity. Surgical infections are now only occasionally the result of blood spread. The response of the host is both local and systemic. The factors determining establishment of the infection include the organism and conditions at the site of injury.

The general principles governing the sources,

diagnosis, and treatment of infections will be discussed in this chapter. Specific infections will be dealt with in their appropriate chapters.

Factors Predisposing to Infection

Susceptibility to infection depends on the infecting organism, and local and constitutional factors of the host.

Avirulent organisms are unable to multiply in the tissues and are phagocytosed by macrophages and polymorphonuclear leukocytes or killed by humoral mechanisms. If the organism is capable of producing disease (i.e., pathogenic), it may invade the tissues and produce toxins. Organisms that are normally present on the skin and in the bowel may multiply in the tissues and produce infection at the extremes of life and in malnourished and immunosuppressed patients. They are sometimes called opportunistic organisms. Some organisms, such as *Staphylococcus aureus*, tend to cause localized infection with marked tissue reaction and formation of pus. The production of staphylocoagulase and leukocidin by the organisms may be important. Others readily spread in the tissues and into the blood stream, such as *Streptococcus hemolyticus*. This organism produces toxins, leukocidins, fibrinolysin, and hyaluronidase to counteract the body's attempt at localization. *Treponema pallidum* produces a lesion at the site of entry long after the organism has spread throughout the body.

Some organisms secrete exotoxins which act locally or at a distance. *Clostridium perfringens* secretes a powerful exotoxin that causes severe local tissue damage, while *Clostridium tetani* produces a toxin that acts mainly at a distance. The exotoxin produced by *Clostridium tetani* is highly specific and can be used to immunize the patient against tetanus. Endotoxins responsible for septic shock are lipopolysaccharides derived from the breakdown of the cell membranes of gram-negative bacteria.

A minimum number of organisms is necessary in the tissues for an infection to become established, and this varies with the organism. Experimentally in calves a small number produced minor local lesions, while large numbers resulted in spreading infections.[2] One million organisms had to be injected into healthy tissues for an infection to become established. Several hundred may be adequate when introduced into an operative wound and a smaller number in a wound in a patient with oligemic shock.

The combined effect of two infecting agents may be greater than the sum of the two. The anaerobic organisms *Fusobacterium nucleatum* and *Borrelia vincentii* act synergistically to

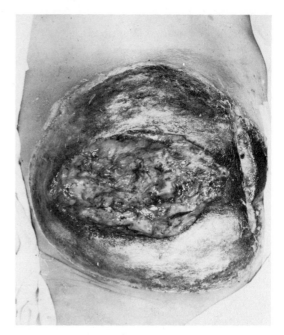

Figure 6–1. Meleney's gangrene. This is a patient 12 days after operation for a perforated colonic carcinoma. There is gangrene caused by anaerobic streptococci acting in concert with *Staphylococcus aureus* and *Proteus vulgaris* organisms.

produce an ulceromembranous stomatitis, Vincent's angina. Meleney's postoperative bacterial synergistic gangrene (Figure 6–1) is a spreading gangrene of the skin of the anterior abdominal wall caused by anaerobic streptococci acting in concert with other bacteria, usually *Staphylococcus pyogenes*, hemolytic streptococci, or *Proteus* organisms. Aerobic and anaerobic infections may occur together and act synergistically as in gas gangrene. In those mixed infections the anaerobic component may be missed, because the organisms are killed by exposure to oxygen for four minutes and adequate measures may not have been taken to check for their presence.

Local Factors

Contamination. The skin, including the sweat glands and hair follicles, normally contains pathogenic and nonpathogenic organisms. It is virtually impossible to kill all the organisms by preparing the hands before operation or at the site of an operative incision. Antiseptics applied for skin preparation preoperatively kill bacteria on the surface but have no effect on those in the hair follicles and sebaceous and sweat glands. Vigorous rubbing may be harmful by bringing pathogens to the surface from these deep sites. Care must be taken to keep their number to a minimum and to decrease the risk of contaminating an incision. Most of the pathogens from the skin are gram positive while those from within the patient are more often gram negative.

An infective process, such as an abscess or gangrenous tissue, may be opened into by the surgeon and the wound contaminated with pathogenic bacteria, as in appendicitis and diverticulitis. Contents of the upper gastrointestinal tract are less likely to contain virulent organisms. Operation for repair of a perforated duodenal ulcer is uncommonly complicated by wound infection.

Foreign Bodies. Foreign bodies provide a focus for initiation and propagation of infection and are commonly introduced as a result of injury. Following traffic accidents small pieces of grit and clothing are often left in a wound. Bullets are usually sterile, but they often carry pieces of clothing into the wound and provide a nidus for infection. Bullet tracks and all potentially infected wounds should be carefully inspected and explored to ensure that no foreign material is left.

Necrotic tissue acts as a foreign body and inevitably leads to infection. All dead tissues must therefore be carefully excised.

It is essential that foreign materials introduced at operation be inserted without introduction of pathogenic organisms or devitalization of tissues. Examples of materials so inserted are nails, plates, Teflon prostheses, and cardiac pacemakers covered with siliconized rubber. When infection occurs, it is usually necessary to remove the foreign material. Nonabsorbable sutures often act as foci for infection and produce a discharging wound that will not heal until they have been removed.

Location of the Wound. Regions with a good blood supply are less likely to become infected. A wound on the face, for example, is less likely to become infected than one on the foot. Wounds on the perineum are especially liable to infection.

Inflammatory Response. The local reaction to injury or infection is inflammation,[5,11] which depends on alterations in the capillary bed, the arrival of humoral substances and phagocytic cells, the removal of necrotic tissues, and finally tissue repair (see Chapter 5).

Vascular Response. The inflammatory response begins with the release of vasoactive mediators. These substances cause constriction of the venous sphincters at the junction of the veins and venules, which results in an increase in venular and capillary pressures, stasis in the vessels, hypoxia and acidosis, and exudation of fluid into the extravascular space. Lymphatic flow is increased. Arteriolar-venular shunts open up and divert blood from the region. The decreased rate of flow in the affected area results in leukocytes adhering to the capillary endothelium.

Cellular Response. Leukocytes adhere to the vascular endothelium and pass through the wall by diapedesis. Erythrocytes may also pass through the wall at the same site as the leukocytes. Later monocytes enter the interstitial spaces by passing between the endothelial cells while lymphocytes pass through and not between the endothelial cells. Locally produced chemicals attract monocytes and probably leukocytes.[6,7]

The main function of white cells in inflammation is phagocytosis of foreign particles, bacteria, and cell debris and the production of antibodies. Commensals are readily ingested by polymorphs.[8] Virulent organisms, however, can only be phagocytosed in the presence of opsonins and complement. Opsonin coats the surface of the organism rendering it more acceptable to the phagocyte. A number of pathogenic organisms require specific antibodies before they can be ingested. The more virulent the organism the more "unpleasant" are its surface antigens, and only "tailormade" or specific antibodies will render it suitable for phagocytosis. After ingesting particles, polymorphs show degranulation and liberate phagocytin. Pyrogen is secreted and is probably responsible for fever. Lactic acid is produced and results in a low intracellular pH. The high acidity and lactic acid both inhibit bacterial growth. A polymorph that has successfully destroyed an organism is itself destroyed in the process and has therefore been called a "suicide" cell. Macrophages phagocytose organisms, necrotic tissues, and small foreign bodies, but their main role is probably removing dead polymorphs. They contain lactic acid and a lysozyme and are not inhibited by a low pH.

Granulocyte function is probably the single most important factor in determining the outcome of a bacterial infection and is decreased after severe stress as following trauma, a major operation, treatment with immunosuppressant drugs, and burns. There is a normal unexplained cycling in the function of granulocytes with the cycle recurring every 20 days in the human.

The initial polymorph reaction is later replaced by one that is mainly mononuclear. The macrophages engulf foreign and dead material and sometimes fuse to form giant cells. When the tissue damage has been slight, the macrophages remove the exudate and the tissue returns to normal. This is known as resolution, the most common result of inflammation.

When the pathogens produce much necrosis, the necrotic material softens and forms pus, a process known as *suppuration*. Abscesses usually rupture or are drained, but occasionally they remain sequestrated in the tissues and are surrounded by dense fibrous tissue. The pus thickens as the water is absorbed and eventually may become calcified.

Chronic Inflammation. Chronic inflammation is the simultaneous presence of inflammation and healing. Polymorphs, large mononuclear cells, lymphocytes, and fibroblasts are present. A common feature is endarteritis obliterans, when the small arteries are gradually obliterated by a proliferation of the intima.

General Factors

The patient's general state of health is important in resisting infection.[1,12] Protein deficiency inhibits the formation of immunoglobulins, complement, and opsonins. A congenital or acquired deficiency in any of the cells involved in the inflammatory response predisposes to infection. The following states and conditions also predispose to infection: (1) nutritional—avitaminosis, protein-calorie malnutrition (kwashiorkor), and starvation; (2) chronic disease—diabetes mellitus (uncontrolled), chronic nephritis and uremia, leukemias, and carcinomatosis; (3) endocrine—Cushing's disease, Cushing's syndrome, and steroid therapy; (4) therapy—immunosuppression, cancer chemotherapy, and radiation. Patients given immunosuppressant drugs after renal transplantation or chemotherapeutic agents in the treatment of cancer are especially liable to develop infections and often by organisms that are normally present. Organisms commonly causing "opportunistic" infections are *Candida albicans* and *Bacteroides*. Since gentamicin appears to predispose to growth of the yeast *Candida albicans*, it should be discontinued and the patient given amphotericin B. Patients with a humoral immune deficiency are especially liable to develop bacterial infections, and those with a cell-mediated immune deficiency are vulnerable to fungal and viral infections.

Diagnosis of Infection

The diagnosis of infections is mainly clinical, but the laboratory can assist here and in assessing the response to treatment.

Clinical Diagnosis. In the first century A.D. Celsus described the four cardinal signs of inflammation, and Galen in the second century added a fifth. They are: (1) increased heat, the result of a local increase in metabolism and not an increase in blood flow; (2) redness, caused by the dilated arterioles and capillaries; (3) pain, caused by the tension in the tissues following the increase in permeability. This accounts for the throbbing nature of the pain, particularly when the part is dependent. Toxins also contribute to the pain; (4) swelling, caused by the increased microvascular permeability which allows protein-rich fluid to escape into the tissues; (5) loss of function, mainly the result of pain, although edema may play some part.

All exudates and pus should be carefully examined. The unpleasant smell of gram-negative infections is often characteristic, for example, the fecal smell of *Escherichia coli* infection. Streptococcal exudates tend to be watery, staphylococcal to be thick and purulent, and those produced by *Pseudomonas aeruginosa* to be greenish-blue.

In addition to local signs of inflammation there are general symptoms and signs of infection. The patient appears ill and looks flushed, the pulse rate is increased, and body temperature is raised.

The endogenous pyrogen produced is a protein with a molecular weight between 10,000 and 20,000. It acts centrally on the hypothalamus where stimulation of certain nuclei increases body temperature and stimulation of others causes a decrease. Anorexia occurs with a decrease in metabolism and temperature. When the temperature of the blood flowing through the hypothalamic nuclei is lower than a threshold, muscular activity is initiated in the form of rigors and results in a temperature increase.

Laboratory Diagnosis. The laboratory can assist in diagnosing and determining the progress of an infection. The hemoglobin value and erythrocyte count are decreased in patients with acute infections, associated with hemolysis (especially streptococcal), and in those with chronic infections. The total white blood cell count is a useful nonspecific test to aid the diagnosis and to follow the progress of an infection. The differential count may help in diagnosing the type of infection. Acute pyogenic infection produces a polymorphonuclear leukocytosis; chronic infection, a lymphocytosis; and those associated with an immune response, an eosinophilia. The erythrocyte sedimentation rate can be used to monitor the course of a chronic infection. A sample of exudate or pus should be taken via aseptic technique and examined for organisms and their sensitivity to antibiotics. Anaerobic culture of pus from infected wounds is important, especially if tetanus, gas gangrene, or actinomycosis is suspected. In the pus from a patient with actinomycosis "sulfur" granules may be seen consisting of mycelia and calcium phosphate. Blood cultures, aerobic and anaerobic, are

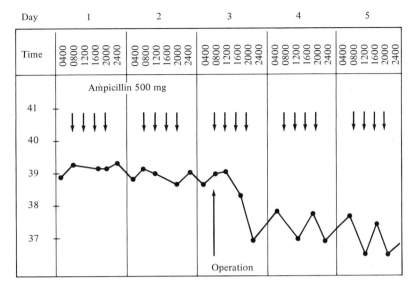

Figure 6–2. Effect of abscess drainage on temperature. The temperature chart is that of a patient with a wound infection following an appendectomy. A dramatic fall in temperature occurs when the wound is drained. The prophylactic use of antibiotics has not affected the temperature.

essential in patients with severe infections. The cultures are most likely to be positive before a rise in temperature.

Surgical Management

The dictum attributed to Rutherford Morison, "pus about, let it out," is still important in the management of surgical infections. Any infection, whether it be a wound infection, abscess, or peritonitis, is generally treated by evacuating the pus and establishing adequate drainage. The dramatic fall in temperature that occurs after drainage demonstrates the importance of operation in managing wound infections (Figure 6–2). The wound is drained by removing the skin sutures, laying it open, and later performing a delayed primary or secondary closure or

allowing healing to occur by secondary intention. Necrotic tissue acts as a foreign body and must be carefully removed along with any other foreign bodies such as sutures. This is especially important in dealing with neglected wounds and with accidental wounds containing foreign bodies and necrotic tissue. In contaminated operative wounds the tissues may die as a result of the infection. A chronic infection then develops and persists until the necrotic tissue is removed and adequate drainage established.

Debridement of Wounds. Prophylaxis of wound infections depends on good surgical technique. Careful preoperative preparation, gentle treatment of the wound edges, careful excision of necrotic material, careful approximation of tissues without tension, and establishment of

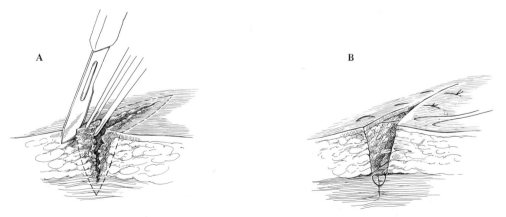

Figure 6–3. Debridement. Steps in the treatment of a contaminated or contused wound. *A.* After the wound has been cleaned and the foreign bodies removed, the jagged edges are excised and dead tissue removed. *B.* The wound is now clean and can be closed.

adequate drainage, if indicated, minimize the chance of wound infection. Good hemostasis is also essential as blood clot is an excellent growth medium for microorganisms.

The operative care of traumatic wounds is debridement (Figure 6–3). All devitalized tissues and foreign materials are removed, and optimum conditions are produced for healing without infection. Adequate debridement is the most important factor in preventing infection of contaminated traumatic wounds.

The patient's general condition must first be evaluated. An adequate airway and control of hemorrhage are essential. Pain is relieved by immobilizing the injured part. The nature of the injury, the time since the accident, and the presence of tendon, bone, and nerve injuries must be determined. The wound is examined using an aseptic technique and covered with a sterile towel. Intravenous blood, fluids and electrolytes, analgesics, and antibiotics are given as indicated. Tetanus immune globulin or tetanus toxoid is injected intramuscularly. X-rays may help detect foreign bodies, air entrapment, a ruptured viscus, or an unsuspected fracture.

Using regional or general anesthesia, the skin around the wound is cleaned with a non-irritative soap and antiseptic solution. The wound is irrigated with isotonic saline, hemostasis is obtained, and foreign bodies, such as grit, dirt, pieces of clothing, are removed. The wound is inspected for injuries to blood vessels, tendons, bones, and nerves. It may be necessary to extend the wound to make an adequate exploration. Jagged skin edges are excised. The amount removed depends on the degree and location of damage. Dead and traumatized fat is freely excised because it is the layer most likely to become infected. Torn fascial edges and devitalized muscle are also excised. The management of injuries to blood vessels (see Chapter 31, pp. 549–51), nerves (see Chapter 28, pp. 498–99), tendons (see Chapter 28, p. 498), and bones (see Chapter 29, pp. 512–16) are described elsewhere. Primary, delayed primary, or secondary closure of the wound is then performed (see Chapter 5, pp. 122–23). Debridement and delayed primary closure should be performed in wounds likely to become infected and in those from high explosive injuries. Human bites are particularly liable to infection, especially with staphylococci, fusiform bacilli, spirochetes, and anaerobic streptococci, and should never be closed by primary suture.

ANTIBIOTICS

Antibiotics are chemicals produced by microorganisms that suppress the growth of (bacterio-static) or kill (bactericidal) microorganisms. Some are semisynthetic or completely synthetic. Ideally an antibiotic should be effective against a wide range of microbes, be bactericidal rather than bacteriostatic, and should not easily induce bacterial resistance. The largest dose required for long periods should not cause toxic or allergic side effects, and its efficacy should not be reduced by body fluids, exudates, plasma proteins, or tissue enzymes.

Mechanism of Action

Antibiotics may be classified by their action on the microorganism.[14]

1. Agents impairing oncotic properties of the cell membrane. Penicillin, cephalothin, cycloserine, vancomycin, ristocetin, and bacitracin prevent the incorporation of certain nucleotides into the cell wall and lead to changes in the oncotic pressure on the two sides of the membrane. These agents are bactericidal.

2. Agents impairing the barrier function of the cell membrane. The polymyxins, nystatin, and amphotericin act on the cytoplasmic membrane, damage the cell membrane by a detergent action, and allow intracellular contents to escape. They are bactericidal.

3. Agents interfering with protein synthesis. Chloramphenicol, novobiocin, the tetracyclines, kanamycin, gentamicin, neomycin, the streptomycins, erythromycin, and oleandomycin alter RNA and interfere with protein synthesis of essential enzyme systems. When treatment is stopped, recovery can occur. These agents inhibit bacterial proliferation. Cellular and humoral host defenses must kill the remaining organisms. These agents are therefore bacteriostatic except for the aminoglycosides, kanamycin, gentamicin, neomycin, and the streptomycins which are bactericidal.

4. Agents impairing base synthesis in DNA. Griseofulvin causes metaphase arrest in dividing cells by interfering with purine nucleotide synthesis at the prepolymerization stage. It is only effective against fungal hypha and is fungistatic.

5. Drugs affecting intermediary metabolism. Sulfonamides, isoniazid, and para-aminosalicylic acid compete with microorganisms for para-aminobenzoic acid and probably interfere with other enzyme systems.

A classification of antibiotics according to their clinical effectiveness is the basis of the "spectrum" of microorganisms that they attack. Thus penicillin G is considered to have a "narrow spectrum" because in the doses usually employed it affects only gram-positive bacteria and *Neisseria*. On the other hand, tetracyclines are "broad-spectrum" because they attack both gram-positive and gram-negative organisms and are also effective in the treatment of rickettsial infections.

Choice of an Antibiotic

An exudate or pus is cultured for organisms and their sensitivities to antibiotics determined. The increasing incidence of anaerobic infections, as for example with *Bacteroides*, makes it often essential to obtain anaerobic cultures. Adequate drainage of pus is often all that is necessary to treat an infection. Antibiotics should be given if the patient's general health is poor or when a severe infection is present, as for example in fecal peritonitis and septicemia. A broad-spectrum antibiotic may be used until the antibiotic sensitivities of the organism are available. The nature of the illness also affects the choice of agent. For example, an orally administered drug should not be given to a patient who is vomiting, or an intramuscular injection to a patient with a bleeding dyscrasia. In critically ill patients combinations of antibiotics may be given to broaden their spectrum and guard against an organism being resistant to a particular agent. The combination of carbenicillin and gentamicin is particularly effective in treating infections with *Pseudomonas aeruginosa*. Previous history of hypersensitivity or serious side effects will affect the choice of an antibiotic, and such a history should be carefully sought.

Types of Antibiotics. *Sulfonamides.* Sulfonilamide was the first antibiotic used and was introduced by Domagk in 1935. It acts by competitive inhibition with *p*-aminobenzoic acid in the synthesis of folic acid and is bacteriostatic. It is effective against gram-positive and gram-negative infections, but its use is largely confined to urinary tract infections by *Escherichia coli* and prophylaxis of rheumatic fever. Toxic effects include skin reactions, methemoglobinemia, aplastic anemia, and renal and hepatic damage. Sulfasuxidine, which is insoluble in water, may be used orally to sterilize the colon before operation, often in combination with neomycin sulfate. Sulfisoxazole (Gantrisin) is frequently used for urinary tract infections and mafenide (Sulfamylon) in the treatment of burns.

The Penicillins. Penicillin G (benzyl penicillin) is effective against most gram-positive pathogens. It must be given by the intramuscular or intravenous routes because it is inactivated by stomach acid. It is excreted in the urine and is not toxic even at high doses. Unfortunately it frequently induces sensitization leading to urticaria or anaphylactic shock.

Penicillin V (phenoxymethyl penicillin) can be taken by mouth, is more resistant to penicillinase produced by a number of organisms, but especially by certain strains of *Staphylococcus aureus*, and it is more slowly excreted in the urine than penicillin G.

Semisynthetic penicillins are prepared by adding side chains to naturally occurring penicillin. They can be given orally and are effective against penicillinase-producing staphylococci and a number of gram-negative as well as gram-positive organisms. Methicillin (Staphcillin) must be given parenterally, while oxacillin, cloxacillin, and dicloxacillin are acid-resistant and can be given by mouth. These semisynthetic penicillins are now the initial treatment of choice for penicillinase and nonpenicillinase-producing staphylococcal infections. Ampicillin should not be used for staphylococcal infections because it is destroyed by penicillinase but is more effective than methicillin, oxacillin, cloxacillin, or dicloxacillin in treating enterococcal infections. Ampicillin can be given by mouth. Carbenicillin is effective against *Pseudomonas aeruginosa* and *Proteus*.

Cephalothin. Cephalothin is not effective orally and has much the same antibacterial spectrum as the semisynthetic penicillins. It can be given to patients who are allergic to penicillin; however, there is a cross-sensitivity in about 10 percent of patients. Another antibiotic should preferably be used in those sensitive to penicillin.

Vancomycin. Vancomycin is indicated in patients with severe gram-positive infections that are resistant or allergic to penicillin or cephalothin. It must be given intravenously. It does not cause drug resistance but may result in deafness.

The Tetracyclines. The tetracyclines are effective against most gram-positive and gram-negative organisms and can be given by mouth. Tetracyclines are deposited in bone and developing teeth and may produce a yellowish-brown pigmentation of teeth when given to children. They may also cause gastrointestinal upsets due to interference with the normal bacterial flora in the bowel and may induce photosensitivity of the skin.

Erythromycin, Lincomycin, and Clindamycin. Erythromycin is effective against a number of gram-positive infections and can be used as a substitute for penicillin G in patients who are sensitive to penicillin. Lincomycin and clindamycin resemble erythromycin in most ways but are especially effective against *Bacteroides*. Clindamycin is effective against gram-positive and gram-negative anaerobic and also gram-positive aerobic infection. It has little effect on gram-negative aerobic infections. Since gentamicin is most useful against gram-negative aerobic infection, administration of clindamycin with gentamicin is particularly effective in treating most gram-positive and gram-negative aerobic and anaerobic infections.

The Aminoglycosides. The aminoglycosides kanamycin, gentamicin, and neomycin are potent bactericidal antibiotics that are effective in severe gram-negative infections. Kanamycin is given intramuscularly or intravenously and is effective especially in *Pseudomonas pyocyanea* and *Proteus* infection. The dose has to be carefully monitored in renal insufficiency. A serious toxic effect is ototoxicity.

Gentamicin is also only effective given intramuscularly or intravenously. It can cause renal damage and ototoxicity especially in those with renal disease. The drug is especially effective in *Pseudomonas aeruginosa, Proteus,* and *Escherichia coli* infections.

Neomycin should not be given parenterally because of its marked toxicity. Its main use is to sterilize the colon when given orally preoperatively and in patients with hepatic failure. Generally the colon is so effectively sterilized that only yeasts remain. Neomycin may also be applied locally as a powder or ointment.

The Polymyxins. Polymyxin B and colistin (polymyxin E) are sensitive to most gram-negative infections except for *Proteus.* They can be nephrotoxic and cause respiratory paralysis.

Chloramphenicol. This broad-spectrum antibiotic, formerly used extensively, should be confined to typhoid and paratyphoid infections because of the occasional occurrence of aplastic anemia and, in infants, respiratory collapse ("gray baby syndrome").

Streptomycin. Streptomycin is effective against infections by *Mycobacterium tuberculosis, Staphylococcus aureus, Pseudomonas aeruginosa,* and *Proteus* species. It is not effective when given by mouth. Ototoxicity and skin reactions may occur.

Antifungal Antibiotics. Nystatin is used to treat infections by *Candida albicans* in skin, mouth, and bowel. It may be used orally or topically as a powder or cream. Griseofulvin is effective orally against *Epidermophyton, Trichophyton,* and chronic fungal nailbed infections. Amphotericin B is the only agent effective against systemic fungal infections such as those caused by *Candida albicans, Histoplasma,* and *Sporotrichum.*

Hypersensitivity. Hypersensitivity to antibiotics can occur in susceptible individuals. The drug may induce antibody formation and on subsequent administration result in a hypersensitivity reaction. The antibiotic may act as a hapten and combine with a protein to produce sensitization. Hypersensitivity should not be confused with allergic contact dermatitis. Hypersensitivity reactions are manifested by immediate collapse, bronchospasm, diarrhea, and exudative urticarial skin rashes. Eosinophilia may occur in the blood. Contact dermatitis is an eczematous eruption and is not accompanied by eosinophilia. Patients with drug hypersensitivity often give a family history of similar reactions. The initial sensitization may be from a small amount of the drug and be forgotten by the patient. A nurse who spills streptomycin on her fingers may develop a skin rash on subsequent contact with the drug. If hypersensitivity is suspected, a scratch test or intradermal injection will confirm its presence. Generally it is possible to avoid giving the drug to the sensitized patient. Desensitization can be undertaken by injecting very small doses of the drug over a period of some days. The desensitization is often of short duration. Antihistamines, both systemically and locally, should be given when a reaction occurs. If bronchospasm is a feature, cortisol or epinephrine should be administered.

Prophylactic Antibiotics

Antibiotics have been used to protect healthy persons against specific organisms to which they have been exposed, to prevent secondary bacterial infection in acutely ill individuals, to reduce the risk of infection in patients with various types of chronic illness, and to inhibit the spread of disease from areas of localized infection. The routine use of antibiotics after operation usually does more harm than good.[13] The antibiotics do not decrease the incidence of infections but merely change their nature.

Antibiotics should be given prophylactically before operation in patients who are likely to develop infection. To be effective they should be present in the tissues prior to bacterial contamination, and they can be discontinued early after operation because there is no benefit from their prolonged administration. Patients at risk are:

1. Those in whom there is a definite risk of bacterial contamination, for example, peritonitis from perforation of the appendix, colon, or gallbladder, drainage of an abscess involving opening of tissue planes, excision of a brain abscess, and excision of infected lymph nodes.

2. Patients with diseases that decrease host resistance, such as malnutrition from prolonged intestinal obstruction or fistulas, impaired liver function or advanced malignancy, diabetic acidosis, congenital or acquired immune deficiency, hemolytic or aplastic anemia, hypersplenism, and myeloproliferative diseases. Prophylactic antibiotics are more frequently indicated in geriatric patients because of the

decrease in host resistance. They are often malnourished, have chronic diseases, such as diabetes mellitus and atherosclerosis, and have impaired function of the cells involved in healing and resistance to infection. Recently it has been suggested that prophylactic antibiotics should be given to all elderly patients who have operation on the biliary tract.

3. Those with congenital or acquired disease, valvular disease of the heart.

4. Patients who have a prosthesis inserted, such as replacement arthroplasties, are generally given prophylactic antibiotics.

There is some evidence[9] that antibiotic powder instilled into a wound may reduce the infection rate, but this needs more study before it can be accepted as a general principle.

Weinstein[15] showed that the following generalizations apply when antibiotics are administered prophylactically:

1. When a single potent drug is used to avoid infection by a specific organism or to eradicate it immediately after it has become established, chemoprophylaxis is, with uncommon exceptions, highly successful.

2. If the aim of prophylaxis is to prevent colonization or infection by all and any organisms that may be present in a patient's internal or external environment, failure is the rule.

Misuse of Antibiotics

Although there are clear indications for the use of antibiotics in surgical infections, it must be stressed that they can never be used as a substitute for the establishment of adequate drainage. They rarely result in removal of established pus and usually under these circumstances do no more than slow down the progress of the infection. Other misuses are in the treatment of viral infections and of fevers of undetermined origin. Improper doses, using too high or too small a dose, constitute misuse as does an improper duration of therapy and failure to discontinue treatment in the presence of reactions. An area of important and widespread abuse is self-medication by patients. These drugs, like any other therapeutic compound, may produce serious and even fatal reactions and must never be taken without medical supervision. Antibiotics have been employed commercially to increase the weight of meat animals, and their use has been forbidden in many countries.

Antiseptics and Disinfectants

Antiseptics are substances that, when applied to tissues, kill or prevent the growth of microorganisms. Their ability to remain active in the presence of protein-containing fluids is an asset.

The therapeutic index is a relationship between the concentration effective against microorganisms and one producing harmful effects.

Disinfectants are agents that prevent infection by destroying pathogenic microorganisms. They are usually harmful to tissues. Their usefulness is related to their spectrum against microorganisms, their ability to penetrate into crevices and cavities, and their ability to remain active in the presence of organic matter such as blood, sputum, and feces.

Classification. These agents are best classified by their chemical nature:

Phenols. Phenol, cresols, resorcinol, picric acid, thymol, and hexachlorophene are mainly disinfectants and are widely used in surgical practice.

Alcohols. Ethyl alcohol is widely employed as an antiseptic but is not very effective against spores.

Aldehydes. Formaldehyde is the most used of this group. It is effective in a concentration as low as 1 in 200 but needs to be more concentrated to act on spores. It is a valuable detoxifying agent, capable of converting toxins to toxoids. Formerly it was used for fumigation, but other more effective agents are now available.

Acids. Benzoic acid, boric acid, mandelic acid, and nalidixic acid. Benzoic acid is used as a food preservative; boric acid is an antiseptic with a low therapeutic index, while mandelic and nalidixic acids are concentrated and excreted by the kidney and are effective against a wide range of microorganisms. Resistance is developed easily. Mandelic acid acts only in an acid urine.

Halogens. Iodine- and chlorine-containing compounds are old, established, and effective antiseptic agents with a high therapeutic index.

Oxidizing Agents. Hydrogen peroxide and permanganates, the most commonly used of this group, are used for cleaning wounds.

Heavy Metals. Mercuric chloride, merbromin (Mercurochrome), thimerosal (Merthiolate), silver nitrate, zinc sulfate, and copper sulfate are all used in weak solutions as antiseptics. Mercury is absorbed and can cause poisoning if the salts are used frequently.

Surface-Active Compounds. These commonly used substances are bactericidal to a very wide spectrum of microorganisms, but their mechanism of action is unknown.

Dyes. Many are antiseptic, but their therapeutic index is not high.

TYPES OF INFECTIONS
Cellulitis

Cellulitis strictly means an infection of the cells but is used to mean a spreading infection

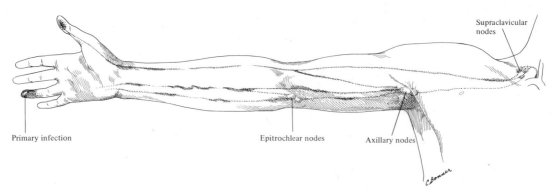

Figure 6–4.   Cellulitis with lymphadenitis. A primary infection in the finger may cause secondary infection in the lymphatic vessels. The infection may be arrested at the next lymph nodes (the epitrochlear group) but may bypass them and affect those at a higher level.

in the subcutaneous tissues, usually superficial to the deep fascia. It is most often caused by the beta-hemolytic streptococcus which produces the enzymes hyaluronidase and streptokinase that promote rapid diffusion of the infection in the loose tissues. Operation is only required to treat the more chronic condition when abscess formation has occurred. The treatment of choice is penicillin.

Lymphangitis and Lymphadenitis

Infection can spread along lymphatic vessels to the regional nodes or bypass the first nodes and enter those at a higher level. Lymphangitis is the establishment of infection within the lymphatic and is characterized by the develop-

ment of red, warm, tender streaks in the skin (Figure 6–4). The regional nodes are almost invariably enlarged and tender. The infection often complicates cellulitis caused by the beta-hemolytic streptococcus. Toxemia may be severe.

Abscess

When a noxious agent produces much necrosis, resolution is impossible. The combination of necrotic tissue and dead cells, mainly polymorphonuclear leukocytes, forms pus. Autolytic enzymes released from the "pus" cells cause liquefaction. The cavity containing the pus is lined by a pyogenic membrane consisting of a fibrin heavily infiltrated by polymorphs. As

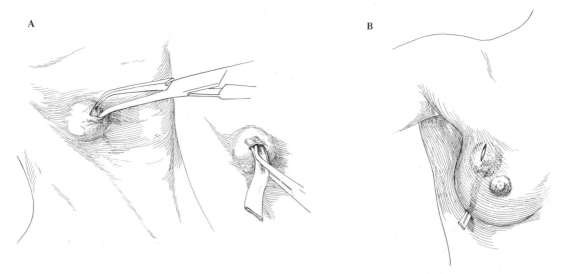

Figure 6–5.   Treatment of an abscess. *A.* An incision is made over the most fluctuant part, and sinus forceps inserted to break down locules. A drain is inserted and the wound left open or sutured loosely. *B.* The effect of gravity in the drainage of an abscess is important. Drainage is instituted at the lowest point.

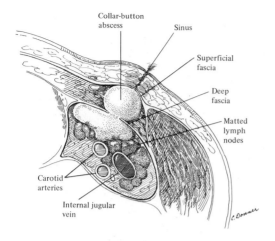

Figure 6–6. A "collar-button" abscess. An abscess in a lymph node, lying below the deep fascia, perforates the fascia to form a locule in the superficial fascia.

the pressure increases, the pus takes the line of least resistance and discharges through the skin or into a cavity or hollow viscus. An abscess should be drained while it is still localized. This ensures more rapid resolution of toxicity, prevents rupture in a direction that could be dangerous for the patient, and permits filling of the cavity with granulation tissue and healing by second intention.

To institute proper drainage an incision is made over the most fluctuant part, sinus forceps or a finger is inserted to break down the locules, a soft rubber or gauze drain is inserted and the skin left open or sutured very loosely (Figure 6–5, *A*). Dependent drainage should be established when possible, as for example when draining a breast abscess (Figure 6–5, *B*). An undrained or improperly drained abscess may become the source of chronic inflammation.

An abscess below the deep fascia with an extension in the subcutaneous tissues is a

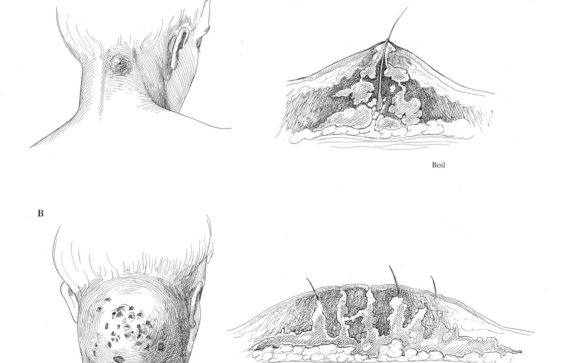

Figure 6–7. *A.* A boil. This is an abscess that forms in a hair follicle or a sebaceous gland. *B.* A carbuncle. This is a honeycomb mass of abscesses in the subcutaneous tissues containing pus and necrotic tissue, with areas of healing and fibrosis.

"collar-button" abscess (Figure 6–6). In the neck the deep portion generally has its origin in a suppurating lymph node. In the web space in the hand infection is introduced into the deep component by a puncture wound. The significance of this abscess lies in recognizing the need to enlarge the track between the deep and superficial portions and to drain adequately the deep part.

A furuncle is an abscess arising in a hair follicle or a sebaceous gland (Figure 6–7, *A*). A painful indurated swelling develops in the skin, the center softens after two to three days, and pus is discharged. A "blind boil" is one that subsides without suppuration. They are particularly common on the back of the neck and in other hairy areas. A hordeolum (synonym, sty) is an infection in an eyelash follicle. A furuncle should be drained when it becomes fluctuant. The infecting organism is generally *Staphylococcus aureus*.

A carbuncle is a honeycomb abscess in the subcutaneous tissues containing pus and necrotic tissues (Figure 6–7, *B*). It commonly occurs on the nape of the neck, especially in male diabetics, where the skin is coarse and ill-nourished. The infecting organism is usually *Staphylococcus aureus*. The patient complains of pain, tenderness, and stiffness. The subcutaneous tissues become indurated and the overlying skin red. After a few days areas of softening appear and pus is discharged at several points. Necrotic tissue should be excised and antibiotics given.

Hydradenitis is a bacterial infection of apocrine sweat glands in the axilla, the anogenital region, and below the breasts in women. It occurs more frequently in women than in men. The lesions present as inflammatory nodules which superficially resemble furuncles but do not come to a distinct head. The discharge is thick, purulent, and frequently bloody fluid rather than the thick, creamy pus seen in the furuncle. After discharging for a short time, the lesion tends to subside and heal temporarily only to recur in days or weeks. Hydradenitis of less than two months' duration usually responds to high doses of antibiotics given for a minimum of 10 days. Infections present for longer than two months seldom respond to antibiotics, because fibrosis walls off the organisms in the deeply seated coils of the apocrine glands and places them beyond reach of a systemically administered antibiotic. Treatment is then excision of the entire inflammatory mass and closure of the defect by a skin graft.

Other abscesses are described elsewhere: intraperitoneal abscess (Chapter 14), brain abscesses (Chapter 34), osteomyelitis (Chapter

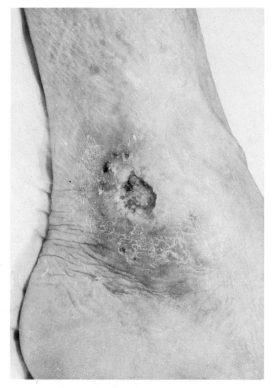

Figure 6–8. An ulcer. There is suppuration of an epithelial surface, followed by its destruction. When the dead tissue separates, an ulcer remains. This is an ulcer in the leg in a patient with chronic venous stasis.

29), parotid abscesses (Chapter 16), empyema and lung abscesses (Chapter 30), hand and finger abscesses (Chapter 28), perianal abscesses (Chapter 22), and liver abscesses (Chapter 19).

Ulceration

When an active suppurative infection involves an epithelial surface, necrosis of the superficial tissues occurs and produces a slough. When the slough separates, it leaves a bare area, called an ulcer (Figure 6–8).

Meleney's ulcer results from infection with microaerophilic nonhemolytic streptococci often associated with *Staphylococcus aureus*. It arises spontaneously or at an operative site and is characterized by the development of an extremely painful, diffuse, undermining ulcer with marked tissue necrosis.

Gangrene

Gangrene is tissue necrosis with superadded putrefaction, "wet" gangrene (Figure 6–9, *A*).

B

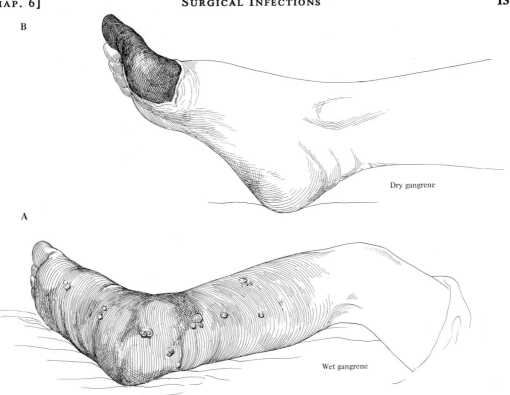

Dry gangrene

A

Wet gangrene

Figure 6–9. Gangrene. Necrosis of tissue with superadded putrefaction is gangrene. *A.* "Wet" gangrene means that there is a progressive tissue destruction. *B.* "Dry" gangrene is an infarction with minimal putrefactive change.

"Dry" gangrene is infarction with minimal or no putrefactive change. It is really necrosis followed by mummification and is not "true" gangrene (Figure 6–9, *B*) (see Chapter 1).

Septicemia

Septicemia is the persistence and growth of organisms in the blood. Bacteremia, when organisms are present in the blood but do not multiply, is much more frequent and occurs after dental extraction, tonsillectomy, and instrumentation of the male urethra. Septicemia may occur after infection with a virulent organism in a previously healthy individual. Organisms generally considered to be nonpathogenic may cause septicemia in patients who have a congenital or acquired immune deficiency, as in advanced cancer, and in those given immunosuppressive drugs after kidney transplantation. Septic shock is described in Chapter 1.

Around 1950 about two thirds of the organisms causing septicemia were gram positive, but now the same percentage are gram negative. This is largely the result of the widespread use of antibiotics.

A number of special "invasive techniques" now in use are especially liable to septicemia. Ill patients are monitored using catheters placed in large vessels. Hyperalimentation has proven an extremely useful means of improving nutrition in the severely ill but requires the presence of a catheter in a large vein for days or weeks. Aseptic technique must be used when inserting these catheters and special measures must be taken to prevent the catheter from becoming infected (see Chapter 14). If the patient develops a fever, a blood culture is taken and if found to be positive, the catheter must be removed. A careful check must be made on the sterility of intravenous fluids.

SPECIFIC INFECTIONS IN SURGERY

Tetanus

The spores of *Clostridium tetani* are frequently present in wounds. A reduced oxygen tension plus ionizable calcium salts are essential for their germination. This reduced tension is present especially in contused and puncture wounds that have an impaired blood supply and contain necrotic tissues and when there is an associated infection with aerobic organisms.

Foreign bodies such as bullets or pieces of clothing predispose to infection. Contamination with soil is particularly dangerous because it contains the tetanus spores, commensal organisms, and ionized calcium. Tetanus infections may occur after injury, especially in battle casualties and agricultural accidents, and may also complicate burns. Not infrequently the wound is considered trivial and may be healed when symptoms of tetanus occur. It may occasionally be latent, developing in old wounds containing the spores that have germinated following surgical intervention. *Tetanus neonatorum* results in death of many babies in communities where dung is used as a dressing.

The spores germinate and secrete a neurotoxin that travels in the motor trunks of the spinal nerves in the spaces between the fibers and may also reach nerve cells by the blood stream. In the spinal cord the neurotoxin stops the inhibitory impulses from the reticular formation from acting on the anterior horn cells, thus causing a general increase in tone and a tendency to spasm following the slightest stimulus.

The incubation period is usually 5 to 10 days but may be as long as 30 days. Prodromal symptoms are stiffness and tingling of the jaw muscles, muscular twitchings, and restlessness. Later stiffness and muscle spasm develop at the site of infection accompanied by headache and yawning. This is soon followed by trismus from spasm of the masseter muscle (lockjaw) and the development of the characteristic risus sardonicus from facial muscle spasm. Retention of urine is frequent. Painful general spasms then occur, and death results from respiratory failure following spasm of the respiratory muscles.

Treatment. Treatment consists of giving large doses of antitoxin to destroy any circulating exotoxin, administering penicillin or oxytetracycline, and debriding wounds to eliminate infection. Muscle spasm is treated by sedation and administration of muscle relaxants. A tracheostomy with controlled respiration may be necessary to maintain respiration during muscle relaxation. If the patient can be kept alive and all the exotoxin eliminated, the effects of the exotoxin wear off after about three weeks and the patient makes a complete recovery.

Prophylaxis. The best prophylaxis for tetanus is active immunization. Three injections of precipitated tetanus toxoid (PPTD), 0.5 ml, are injected intramuscularly, the second at four weeks and the last at six months. A booster injection should be given every 5 to 10 years. It is only necessary to give 0.5 ml of toxoid at the time of injury if toxoid has not been given for 12 months. Allergic reactions are uncommon following its administration. Passive immunization consists of giving antibodies produced in other individuals to nonimmunized patients. Human tetanus immune globulin (TIGH), 500 units, should be injected intramuscularly and active immunization commenced by injection of 0.5 ml of toxoid in a different syringe and needle and at a distant site.[4,10] The decision to give TIGH for passive immunization must be made for each patient by the physician. Passive immunization with antitetanus serum (ATS) prepared in horses carries a great risk of anaphylaxis and serum sickness[3] and is no longer used (Table 6-1).

Contaminated wounds should be carefully debrided with all devitalized tissues and foreign bodies removed. If infection is considered likely, the incision should be left open. Penicillin or oxytetracycline should be given prophylactically to patients with grossly contaminated wounds. The overall mortality approaches about 30 percent.

Gas Gangrene (*Clostridial Myonecrosis*)

Gas gangrene may follow the contamination of a wound with spores of pathogenic clostridia. Considering the ubiquitous presence of the spores and the rarity of gas gangrene in civilian practice, it is evident that healthy incised wounds do not develop this infection. As with tetanus the essential factor for spore germina-

Table 6-1. PROPHYLACTIC TREATMENT OF ACCIDENTAL WOUNDS POSSIBLY INFECTED WITH TETANUS

	IMMUNIZED PATIENT	NONIMMUNIZED PATIENT	DOUBTFUL
Debridement*	Yes	Yes	Yes
Tetanus Toxoid	Booster dose	Tetanus course	Toxoid course
Tetanus Immune Globulin (Human)	No	If wound potentially infected	If wound potentially infected
Penicillin or Oxytetracycline	Penicillin	Penicillin	Penicillin

* Debridement means excision of all devitalized tissues and foreign materials and the establishment of adequate drainage.

tion is a reduced oxygen tension. An associated infection with saccharolytic and proteolytic organisms is always present for gas gangrene to occur. The pathogens *Cl. perfringens*, *Cl. septicum*, and *Cl. novyi* produce an endotoxin that causes marked tissue necrosis and profound toxemia. The proteolytic saphrophytes, *Cl. sporogenes* and *Cl. histolyticum*, multiply in and further break down the dead tissues. The process proceeds rapidly with a progressive necrosis of muscle fibers due to the exotoxins of the saccharolytic clostridia, which ferment the muscle carbohydrate and liberate gas. The increased intramuscular pressure causes ischemia and necrosis. The process spreads primarily within muscles, often to involve all in a fascial compartment. The region is painful, tense, edematous, and crepitant, and the necrotic muscle is brick-red. As putrefaction proceeds, the typical odor of "sweet rotting hay" appears with the onset of gangrene. Circulating endotoxin produces a profound toxemia with increase in the pulse more than anticipated from the rise in temperature. Lecithinase is probably the most lethal exotoxin produced and is largely responsible for the cardiovascular collapse. Microscopically the muscle fibers are dead and contain few if any inflammatory cells.

Treatment. Operative excision is most important in treating a patient with gas gangrene. All necrotic tissue is excised back to healthy, well-vascularized tissues. An involved limb is amputated. Penicillin and tetracycline are given in large doses intravenously and measures taken to treat septic shock.

A high P_{O_2} in the tissues may inhibit growth of the anaerobic clostridia. Patients have therefore been treated in a chamber with hyperbaric oxygen. When pure oxygen is breathed, the partial pressure of oxygen in the arterial blood rises from 100 mm Hg to about 670 mm Hg. If the atmospheric pressure is increased to four atmospheres absolute pressure, the P_{O_2} is increased to above 2000 mm Hg. Treatments are usually given for one hour twice daily. Oxygen toxicity may result in muscular weakness and incoordination and may progress to monoplegia and paraplegia and terminate in major epileptiform convulsions. Thickening may occur in the alveolar walls and produce focal collapse, massive atelectasis, and pulmonary edema.

Growth, in vitro, of clostridial organisms and toxin production do not occur at a partial pressure of oxygen of 2280 mm Hg. In the patient, however, the organisms are growing in avascular tissues, and they may not be exposed to such an increase in oxygen tension. The value of hyperbaric oxygen has yet to be demonstrated. Polyvalent serum is of no value.

Anaerobic Clostridial Myositis

Anaerobic clostridial myositis is a gas-producing infection of wounds unassociated with the marked toxemia seen in clostridial myonecrosis. The infecting organism is usually *Clostridium perfringens*, and the condition is frequently mistaken for the more serious clostridial infection. The infection is primarily a cellulitis and does not primarily involve muscle. Treatment is less radical than for clostridial myonecrosis and consists of antibiotics and adequate drainage but not wide excision of infected tissues. Radical operative excision or limb amputation is not necessary.

Streptococcal Myositis

An anaerobic streptococcal gas-forming infection of subcutaneous tissues and muscle may occur that is readily mistaken for clostridial myonecrosis. Profound toxemia does not develop. Antibiotics should be given and the area drained adequately.

Diabetic Necrotizing Cellulitis

A crepitant necrotizing cellulitis may develop in the diabetic as a result of infection with multiple organisms, aerobic and anaerobic. It is important to recognize that crepitation may be present in streptococcal and coliform infections as well as in those caused by clostridia.

CITED REFERENCES

1. Annotation: The body's underground defences. *Lancet*, **2**:908–909, 1954.
2. Cobbett, L.: The causes of tuberculosis. *Cambridge Public Health Series*. Cambridge University Press, Cambridge, 1917.
3. Cox, C. A.; Knowelden, J.; Sharrard, W. J. W.: Tetanus prophylaxis. *Br. Med. J.*, **2**:1360–66, 1963.
4. Ellis, M.: Human antitetanus serum in the treatment of tetanus. *Br. Med. J.*, **1**:1123–26, 1963.
5. Florey, Lord (H. W.): Inflammation. In H. W. Florey, (ed.): *General Pathology*. W. B. Saunders, Philadelphia, p. 22, 1970.
6. Harris, H.: The role of chemotaxis in inflammation. *Physiol. Rev.*, **34**:529–62, 1954.
7. Harris, H.: The mobilization of defensive cells in inflammatory tissue. *Bacteriol. Rev.*, **24**:3–15, 1960.
8. Howard, J. G.: Natural immunity. In Cruickshank, R. (ed.): *Modern Trends in Immunology*. Vol. 1. Butterworth, London, pp. 86–106, 1963.
9. Longland, C. J.; Gray, J. G.; Lees, W.; and Garrett, J. A. M.: The prevention of infection in appendicectomy wounds. *Br. J. Surg.*, **58**:117–19, 1971.
10. Rubbo, S. D., and Suri, J. C.: Passive immunisation against tetanus with human immune globulin. *Br. Med. J.*, **2**:79–81, 1962.
11. Robbins, S. L. (ed.): *Pathology*, 3rd ed. W. B. Saunders, Philadelphia, pp. 31–73, 1968.
12. Smith, W.: Host and tissue specificity in infective disease. *Proc. R. Soc. Med.*, **42**:11–18, 1949.
13. Taylor, G. W.: Preventative use of antibiotics in surgery. *Br. Med. Bull.*, **16**:51–54, 1960.

14. Weinstein, L.: Chemotherapy of microbial diseases. In Goodman, L. S., and Gilman, A. (eds.): *Pharmacological Basis of Therapeutics*, 4th ed. Macmillan Publishing Co., Inc., New York, p. 1154, 1970.

15. Weinstein, L.: The complications of antibiotic therapy. *Bull. N. Y. Acad. Med.*, 31:500–518, 1965.

SUGGESTIONS FOR FURTHER READING

Goodman, L. S., and Gilman, A. (eds.): *The Pharmacological Basis of Therapeutics*. 5th ed. Macmillan Publishing Co., Inc., New York, 1975.
  This is probably the best-known and most clearly presented description of antibiotics for the physician.

Meleney, F. R.: *Surgical Infections*. W. B. Saunders, Philadelphia, 1949.
  A review of the problems of infection in surgery written early in the antibiotic era with some excellent descriptions of the natural history of abscesses.

Topley and Wilson's *Principles of Bacteriology and Immunity*. Wilson, G. S., and Miles, A. A. (eds.), 5th ed. Arnold, London, 1964.
  A standard two-volume reference work on microbiology with a wide bibliography.

Williams, R. E. O.; Blowers, R.; Garrod, L. P,; and Shooter, R. A.: *Hospital Infections: Causes and Prevention*. Lloyd-Luke, London, 1960.
  A review of the problems that infection presents in a hospital, how they arise, and their prevention.

Chapter 7

CANCER: SPREAD AND PRINCIPLES OF TREATMENT

John A. McCredie and *W. Rodger Inch*

CHAPTER OUTLINE

Spread of Cancer
  Spread in Continuity
    Local
    Lymphatic
    Hematogenous
    Transluminal
    Transserous
  Spread by Metastasis
    Lymphatic
    Hematogenous
    Transluminal
    Transserous
Treatment by Surgery
  Surgery to Establish Diagnosis
    Excisional Biopsy
    Incisional Biopsy
    Needle Biopsy
    General Considerations
  Surgery to Attempt Cure
    Selection of Patients
    Operative Technique
    Regional Lymph Nodes

Surgery to Provide Palliation
  Tumor Excision
  Tumor Bypass
Treatment by Radiotherapy
  Principles of Radiotherapy
    Methods
    Other Considerations
  Attempted Curative Radiotherapy
    Radiotherapy Alone
    With Chemotherapy
    With Operative Excision
  Palliative Radiotherapy
Treatment by Chemotherapy
  Classification
    Source or Chemical Action
    Effect on Generation Cycle
  Adjunct to Surgical Excision
    Preoperative
    Operative
    Postoperative
  Palliative Chemotherapy
  Combined Treatments

SPREAD OF CANCER

The properties of the cancer cell that distinguish it from the tissue of origin are (1) its growth is not under normal control by the host, and (2) it tends to spread to distant regions and form metastases. Growth may still be under some control, as in a hormone-dependent tumor. Local recurrence after excision is not an adequate criterion since it can occur after incomplete removal of a benign tumor, such as a mixed parotid tumor. The presence of cells where they are not normally found, for example, uterine muscle cells in the lungs, is not an adequate criterion for metastasis. It is necessary for the cells to grow at the new site to be called malignant. The distinction between a benign and malignant tumor is often difficult, as in the bladder, thyroid, bone, and lymph nodes.

It is not known why the cancer cell tends to leave a tumor. Increase in ameboid movement, production of diffusible enzymes such as hyaluronidase, decrease in calcium content of the cell membrane, and decrease in the electrical charge on its surface causing loss of contact inhibition have been suggested. Local factors that inhibit spread are mechanical barriers and infiltration with mononuclear cells; general factors that can increase or decrease the growth rate are age, sex, diet, stress, and administration of hormones and drugs. Immune factors are discussed in Chapter 4. Cancer cells readily enter lymphatics through the stomata in the walls; they penetrate small blood vessels more easily than large vessels (Figure 7–1). The walls of ducts are relatively resistant to cancer cell passage.

141

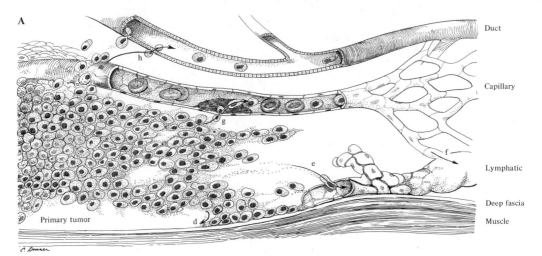

A

Duct

Capillary

h

g

f

Lymphatic

e

Deep fascia

Muscle

d

Primary tumor

C. Donner

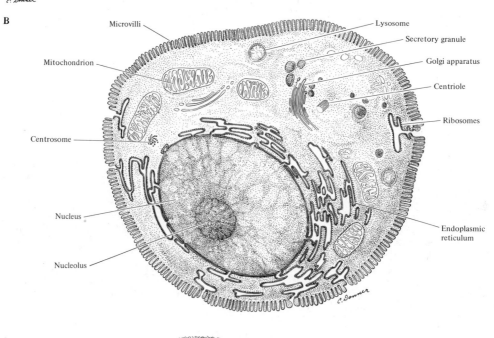

B

Microvilli

Mitochondrion

Centrosome

Nucleus

Nucleolus

Lysosome

Secretory granule

Golgi apparatus

Centriole

Ribosomes

Endoplasmic
reticulum

C. Donner

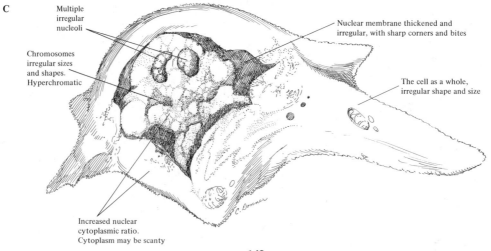

C

Multiple
irregular
nucleoli

Chromosomes
irregular sizes
and shapes.
Hyperchromatic

Nuclear membrane thickened and
irregular, with sharp corners and bites

The cell as a whole,
irregular shape and size

Increased nuclear
cytoplasmic ratio.
Cytoplasm may be scanty

C. Donner

Cancer may spread in continuity with the primary tumor, interstitially (by permeation of a lymphatic, blood vessel, or duct, or by permeation into a serous cavity), or by formation of metastases (lymphatic, hematogenous, transluminal, or through a serous cavity).[16]

Spread in Continuity

Local. Cancer cells tend to spread locally in the interstitial space in the direction of least mechanical resistance (Figure 7–2). Fascia, bone, and cartilage inhibit local growth, whereas less dense tissues, such as the submucosa of the bowel, are readily invaded. A carcinoma in the fundus of the stomach, for example, may extend in the loose submucosal tissues into the esophagus and be recognized only on microscopic examination. Occasionally cancer cells enter normal tissue cells, especially those of striated muscle, and grow within the cytoplasm. The basal cell carcinoma of the skin spreads locally into the deeper tissues and if untreated can grow into bone. It does not spread by any other route. Tumors that are infiltrating and have irregular margins, as occurs in two thirds of patients with cancer of the breast, are more likely to produce metastases than those that grow by expansions and have smooth or nodular margins.

A number of tumors grow by expansion and do not infiltrate the local tissues. Their peripheries tend to be round or nodular.

Lymphatic. Extensive lymphatic permeation occurs only in patients who have large metastases in the regional lymph nodes. Cancer cells pass readily, by ameboid movement, through the openings in the walls of lymphatics, are carried in the lymph to the subcapsular sinus of a regional lymph node, and enter the cortex, where some may remain, proliferate, and establish subcapsular metastases. The foci ultimately coalesce and largely replace the substance of the node. Flow of lymph becomes sluggish, cancer cells proliferate and accumulate within the vessel, and retrograde permeation may occur from the node to the primary tumor. Extensive lymphatic permeation is important because it signifies that the regional nodes are extensively infiltrated with tumor and the prognosis is bad. Spread by permeation can

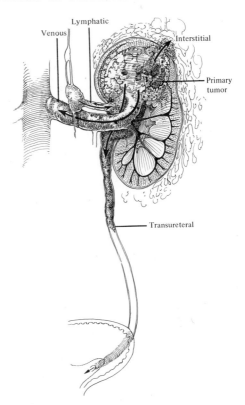

Figure 7–2. Local spread of cancer cells by permeation. Spread of a renal carcinoma in continuity with the primary tumor into the interstitial tissues by permeation of a lymphatic, the renal vein, and the ureter.

occur in patients with abdominal cancer into the large abdominal lymphatics, the receptaculum chyli, and along the thoracic duct into the neck. Perivascular and perineural lymphatics are often permeated by tumor tissue. In patients with carcinoma of the parotid salivary gland, perineural lymphatic spread into the cranium may lead to local recurrence after parotidectomy.

Hematogenous. Cancer cells may pass by ameboid movement between the endothelial cells in the wall of a capillary, sinusoid, or thin-walled vein; damage the endothelium and produce thrombus-containing platelets and fibrin; invade the clot, generate and occlude the

---

Figure 7–1. [OPPOSITE] *A*. The local spread of cancer cells. *B*. Electron microscopic features of a normal cell. *C*. The cancer cell. As seen in *A*, cancer cells (*d*) spread readily in the loose interstitial tissues; their passage is inhibited by fascial layers. (*e*) They readily enter lymphatics through openings in the walls. (*f*) Cells can enter and leave small vessels through numerous communications between the lymphatics and blood vessels. (*g*) Small blood vessels, capillaries, and sinusoids are more readily penetrated than those that are large. A thrombus is produced at the site of entry of the cancer cells. (*h*) The walls of ducts are relatively resistant to passage by cancer cells.

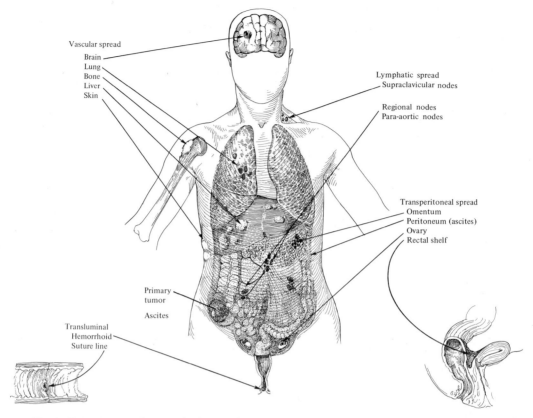

Vascular spread
Brain
Lung
Bone
Liver
Skin

Lymphatic spread
Supraclavicular nodes

Regional nodes
Para-aortic nodes

Transperitoneal spread
Omentum
Peritoneum (ascites)
Ovary
Rectal shelf

Primary
tumor

Ascites

Transluminal
Hemorrhoid
Suture line

Figure 7–3.   Metastatic spread of a carcinoma. Spread by metastasis of a carcinoma of the cecum by the lymphatic, vascular, transperitoneal, and transluminal routes.

lumen; and extend by permeation into the vessel for a considerable distance. A renal carcinoma may extend in continuity along the renal vein into the inferior vena cava, right atrium, and right ventricle.

Transluminal.   The wall of a duct is relatively resistant to spread of cancer cells. A primary tumor within a hollow viscus may spread by permeation along the lumen of the duct draining the organ. Carcinoma of the renal pelvis may grow along the ureter and project into the bladder; a carcinoma of the breast may grow along the mammary ducts and be expressed as caseous material from the sectioned operative specimen (the "comedo" carcinoma).

Transserous.   The visceral peritoneum and pleura inhibit spread of cancer cells into the peritoneal and pleural cavities. Penetration eventually occurs, and viable cells pass freely through the spaces.

Spread by Metastasis (Figure 7–3)

Lymphatic.   Cancer cells that enter the afferent regional lymphatics are carried in the lymph to a regional node, where they may establish metastases in the cortex. They may, however, pass through or bypass the closest nodes and enter the efferent lymphatics and establish metastases, "skip" metastases, at more distant nodes (Figure 7–4). Carcinoma of the colon and breast tend to metastasize first to adjacent nodes, while carcinoma of the tongue and malignant melanoma often produce "skip" metastases. The cells are then carried in the thoracic or jugular lymph ducts to the systemic venous circulation. Metastases in the regional lymph nodes are primary, and those developing from cancer cells that have left nodal tumor are secondary. The importance of anastomoses between small lymphatic and blood vessels has recently been stressed. Their presence means that lymphatic and hematogenous spread often occur at the same time. In patients with abdominal cancer, cells may pass along the thoracic duct, establish metastases on the valves at the termination of the thoracic duct, occlude the jugular lymph ducts, and extend by retrograde permeation to produce metastases in the lymph nodes in the left supraclavicular triangle (Figure 7–5). Alternatively, the supraclavicular

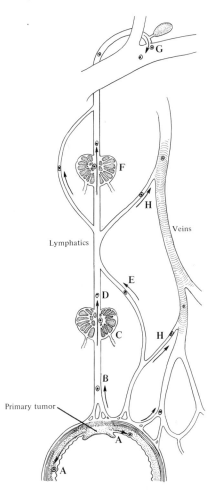

Figure 7–4. Lymphatic spread of cancer cells. Cells of a carcinoma of the gut grow along the submucosal lymphatics (*A*), they enter afferent lymphatics (*B*), establish metastases in the adjacent regional nodes (*C*), and pass through the nodes (*D*). They may also bypass the closest nodes (*E*), enter more distant nodes, and establish "skip" metastases (*F*). They then enter the thoracic duct and reach the systemic circulation at the root of the neck (*G*). It should be noted that the cells can enter the blood circulation through numerous small lymphovascular communicating vessels (*H*).

domyosarcoma, and osteogenic sarcoma not infrequently spread by this route.

Hematogenous. In the nineteenth century metastases from carcinomas were thought to develop first in the regional nodes and later at a distance from cancer cells that had entered the blood from a locally advanced primary tumor or the nodal metastases. More recently cancer cells were detected in the blood of patients with small tumors and especially after the lesion had been handled.[2] Host resistance was then

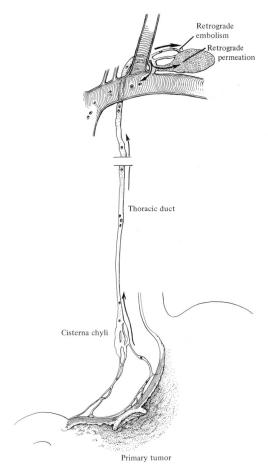

Figure 7–5. Supraclavicular nodal metastasis from abdominal tumor. Carcinoma cells may enter the lymphatics from any abdominal tumor and reach the neck through the thoracic duct. They may then spread in a retrograde direction along small lymphatics entering the cervical portions of the duct and establish metastases in the supraclavicular nodes; or they may grow on the valves of the jugular lymphatics, occlude the lumen, and grow by retrograde permeation to the nodes. Metastases are established in the left supraclavicular triangle in 90 percent of patients; in the remainder they occur on the right side.

metastases may develop from cancer cells that have travelled in a retrograde direction from the thoracic duct along small lymphatic vessels directly to the nodes. The first presentation of abdominal cancer may be the development of a tumor in the left supraclavicular triangle. Occasionally the enlarged node is on the right side. Carcinomas tend to metastasize to nodes more frequently than do sarcomas; however, neuroblastoma, synovioma, fibrosarcoma, rhab-

considered to be the important factor in determining the development of metastases. Many of the cells thought to have been malignant were large atypical mononuclear cells which are often present in the peripheral blood of patients with cancer. The time of entry of cancer cells and the role of host resistance are not known.

Cancer cells enter the blood through the wall of a capillary or sinusoid and less often a vein or artery. Many enter directly through communications with small lymphatics. They circulate singly or in clumps and often in a platelet and fibrin thrombus. Some are filtered out in the first capillary bed in the lungs or liver, but they may pass through and implant elsewhere.

The method of establishing hematogenous metastases is not known. The surface of the malignant cell may be "sticky," causing it to adhere to the endothelium of small vessels where the rate of flow is slow. Platelets are deposited, a thrombus forms, and the cancer cell passes by ameboid movement between the endothelial cells into the interstitial space where it generates and produces a metastasis. Wood[17] constructed an ear chamber in the rabbit and watched the method of arrest and penetration through the capillary wall of V_2 allogeneic tumor cells. He observed the "sticky" carcinoma cells adhering to the endothelium and the formation of a thrombus. A leukocyte then passed through the wall between the endothelial cell. The carcinoma cell then passed through the wall at the same site and was accompanied by thrombus. He stressed the importance of clot formation in the arrest and vascular penetration by the carcinoma cells. There are two explanations for the distribution of metastases.

Soil Theory. Metastases often develop in liver, lungs, bones, and adrenals and infrequently in muscles, spleen, and gut. The soil theory suggests that the cells are distributed to tissues according to the blood flow and that they grow where there is poor tissue resistance. At some sites, such as muscle, the nature of the reaction is not known, but at others, such as the spleen and Peyer's patches in the intestine, mononuclear cell infiltration may be important. The presence of mononuclear cells improves the prognosis in patients with carcinomas of the breast, stomach, esophagus, and testis, and in those with choriocarcinoma, neuroblastoma, Hodgkin's disease, and Burkitt's lymphoma. The host response to cancer is similar to that to an allograft when there are minor differences in the histocompatibility genes between the donor and recipient. Confirmation of this hypothesis is that lympholytic agents, such as prednisone, increase metastases in the spleen and small

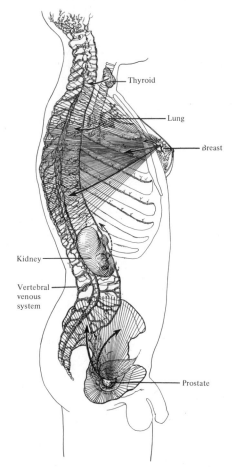

Figure 7–6. Spread of cancer cells through the vertebral venous system. Cells from carcinoma of the prostate and breast enter the vertebral venous system and form metastases in adjacent bones. This may also occur in patients with carcinoma of the thyroid, lung, and kidney.

intestine and that there is an increase in cancer in patients who have been on immunosuppressive therapy after kidney transplantation.

Mechanical Theory. Metastases may develop in organs that receive a large number of cancer cells, as for example the liver and lungs. The vertebral venous system could explain the high incidence of metastases in bones close to the primary tumor in patients with cancers of the prostate and breast (Figure 7–6). The veins extend from the base of the skull to the coccyx, communicate freely with the bodies of the vertebrae and ribs, and have few valves. Flow of blood is sluggish and is reversible on straining and coughing. Cancer cells can therefore be carried directly to the red bone marrow without passing through the pulmonary circulation.

Transluminal. Cancer cells can leave the ulcerated surface of a tumor, be carried along the lumen of a tube or the gut, and implant at a distance, especially at a site of tissue damage. In patients with carcinoma of the colon metastases may develop on the surface of an internal hemorrhoid, in an anal fistula, or on the pectinate line in the anal canal. Recurrence often occurs at the intestinal anastomosis in patients after resection of a colon carcinoma.[9] This is probably the result of cancer cells being carried into the wall on sutures used for the anastomosis. Other explanations are that the recurrence has arisen from cancer cells present in the wall, especially the lymphatics, at the time of operation, by infiltration from metastases in adjacent lymph nodes, by development of a new primary tumor, or by malignant change in a benign polypus.

Transserous. Gravity predisposes to localization of cancer cells in the costovertebral region in patients with carcinoma of the lung and in the pelvis in those with abdominal carcinoma. The pelvic metastases can be felt on vaginal or rectal examination (the "rectal shelf"). It is often impossible to determine whether the rectal shelf is the result of transserous or lymphatic spread. Metastases frequently develop in the omentum and on the surface of the ovary (the "Kruckenburg" tumor). Widespread metastases cause exudation of ascitic fluid or a pleural effusion that contains cancer cells and is often blood stained.

TREATMENT BY SURGERY

Surgery to Establish Diagnosis

The diagnosis of cancer can frequently be made by clinical, radiologic, or biochemical investigation. However, when the organ or tissue is readily accessible or if the definitive operation has a significant mortality or morbidity, diagnosis by microscopic examination is desirable. Willis[15] found that in a series of 1000 autopsies on patients supposed to have died from cancer the diagnosis based on clinical examination alone was wrong in one third of the cases.

Excisional Biopsy. Excisional biopsy is the best procedure when the tumor is small and mobile. It provides a large amount of tissue for microscopic examination and causes minimal contamination with cancer cells (Table 7–1, Figure 7–7). The tumor should not be enucleated but be surrounded by a rim of normal tissues.

Incisional Biopsy. Incisional biopsy is indicated when tumors are large or fixed and when the site of an excisional biopsy might be opened into during definitive excision. In patients with

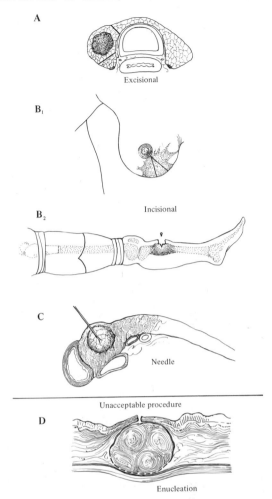

Figure 7–7. Types of biopsy.

breast cancer incisional biopsy is indicated when the tumor is large or medially placed, because it can be performed through a smaller and less deep incision than that required for an excisional biopsy. There is therefore less chance of opening into this region during the definitive excision and causing contamination with cancer cells.

A modified incisional biopsy is sometimes used in patients with bone tumors who might be treated by a limb amputation. Two tourniquets are applied proximally before taking the biopsy and, if diagnosis of malignancy is confirmed by frozen section, the limb is amputated between the tourniquets. Cancer cells that may have entered the blood vessels or lymphatics as a result of taking the biopsy are included in the operative specimen.

Needle Biopsy. A small piece of tumor is removed by inserting a hypodermic needle and aspirating, or by coring out a larger amount with

Table 7–1. TYPES OF BIOPSY

	ADVANTAGES	DISADVANTAGES	SITES
A. Excisional	Provides whole specimen surrounded by normal tissues for the pathologist. An incision is not made into the primary tumor; therefore, there is less likelihood of disseminating cancer cells.	The large exposure may make it difficult to avoid opening into the biopsy site during the definitive excision.	Thyroid Breast Lung Malignant melanoma Lymph nodes
B. Incisional	a. Definitive excision can be performed clear of the biopsy site.	Provides only a portion of the tumor for microscopic examination. The incision into the tumor may cause lymphatic or hematogenous spread of cancer cells.	Breast Pancreas Lung Gut Liver
	b. Prevents dissemination of cancer cells during biopsy.	None.	Bone
C. Needle	Easy to perform.	Some false negatives.	Lymph nodes Pancreas Breast, Liver
D. Enucleation	None	Should not be performed.	

a trochar. The procedure is simple; however, it provides only a small piece of tissue for microscopic examination and this may be normal rather than tumor tissue. There is a possibility, therefore, of making a false negative diagnosis.

A portion of a tumor can be removed readily during sigmoidoscopy, esophagoscopy, bronchoscopy, or gastroscopy. The pathologist is provided with a smaller specimen than that from incisional biopsy but larger than that from needle biopsy.

General Considerations. The effect of biopsy on local recurrence and distant metastasis is not known. Precautions should be taken to avoid leaving cancer cells at the operative site and to prevent their spread elsewhere. The interval between biopsy and definitive excision should be as short as possible. Animal studies show that local recurrence increases as the interval between biopsy and excision is increased. Diagnosis should, if possible, be made by microscopic examination of the frozen section and definitive excision performed while the patient is under the same anesthetic. Fresh gowns, gloves, drapes, and instruments should be used after taking the biopsy to prevent contamination of the operative site with cancer cells. The biopsy site should be included and not opened into during the definitive excision. The needle track should be included in the specimen at the time of definitive excision because tumor has been observed growing along the needle path.

Surgery to Attempt Cure

Selection of Patients. An attempted curative operation should be performed when it is considered possible to remove the primary tumor completely with or without the regional nodes and distant metastases. Incomplete removal of the primary tumor, without postoperative radiotherapy, is usually followed by early local recurrence. Survival is often less than following treatment by radiotherapy or chemotherapy.

The origin of many cancers is multicentric. It is therefore important to remove all the tissues that may be involved, if possible. In the patient with a carcinoma arising in a scar, patch of leukoplakia in the mouth or vulva, or irradiated tissues, all the tissues at risk should be excised. Carcinoma of the breast is frequently multicentric. The whole breast should therefore be excised.

Operative Technique. The tumor should not be handled during operation to minimize lymphatic and vascular spread of cancer cells. The blood supply should be divided as early as possible before mobilizing the tumor. If possible, a wide margin of normal tissues should be included with the operative specimen to include spread into the interstitial tissues. The amount of normal tissue that can be removed depends upon the method of spread, involvement or proximity of vital organs, and operative mortality and morbidity. In patients with cancer in the distal stomach mortality and morbidity contraindicate total gastrectomy. The proximity of vital structures limits the amount of normal tissues that can be removed in patients with esophageal cancer. In patients with carcinoma of the kidney the operative specimen should include the kidney surrounded by fat, the renal vein up to the inferior vena cava, the whole length of the ureter, and the tissues surrounding the vessels and pelvis along with the para-aortic lymph nodes. Special precautions are taken when resecting a carcinoma of the colon (see page 384).

Regional Lymph Nodes. Opinions differ as to whether regional lymph nodes should be removed prophylactically at the time of removing the primary carcinoma or whether they should be excised therapeutically when they contain clinically recognizable metastases. It is agreed that in patients with carcinoma of the lip, which metastasizes slowly, prophylactic excision should not be done. Where metastases rapidly occur in the nodes there is a stronger case for their prophylactic excision.

Metastases from carcinoma were thought to develop first in the regional nodes and later to occur at a distance as a result of hematogenous spread. Their excision at the time of treating the primary tumor appeared logical. The "mono-bloc" technique, removing the primary tumor and regional nodes in continuity, was then performed when it was recognized that spread could occur by embolism or permeation of the lymphatics.

The free communication between small lymphatic and blood vessels means that spread may occur by both routes at the same time. Superficial regional nodal metastases are recognized earlier than those in a deep tissue such as the liver, lung, bone, or brain. The time of detection of deep metastases will therefore depend upon their rate of growth. Few patients with malignant melanoma who have metastases in the nodes in the operative specimen survive for more than 10 years. In patients with breast carcinoma prognosis is worse when the regional lymph nodes contain metastases than when they are absent. Prolonged observation is necessary because survival decreases exponentially with time. Few patients are alive at 20 years who had metastases in the regional nodes. In contrast cervical nodal metastases often occur in patients with primary tumor in the head and neck without the development of distant metastases. The simultaneous occurrence of regional nodal and hematogenous metastases therefore depends mainly on the site of the primary tumor. They probably occur at the same time in patients with malignant melanoma, perhaps less frequently in

patients with breast carcinoma; however, nodal metastases occur earlier than hematogenous in patients with carcinoma of the head and neck.

Recently considerable interest has been focused on the role of the regional nodes in host resistance to cancer and speculation that their removal may cause a decrease (see page 466).

Opinions differ on the relative efficacy of radiotherapy and surgical excision in treating nodal metastases. Metastases in the cervical and inguinal nodes are best dealt with by surgical excision when the primary tumor is a well-differentiated squamous cell carcinoma. In breast carcinoma it has generally been believed that surgical excision is superior; however, controlled studies show that radiotherapy is as effective as excision (see page 469).

Surgery to Provide Palliation

Tumor Excision. Best palliation can often be obtained by removing the primary tumor even in the presence of distant metastases. Excision of an infected, bleeding carcinoma of the stomach or colon in a patient with liver metastases relieves symptoms and improves the general condition. The liver metastases will eventually cause death, but their rate of growth is not predictable.

Tumor Bypass. When a locally advanced tumor is causing obstructive symptoms, a bypass operation may produce marked relief. Examples are anastomosis of afferent to efferent bowel in a patient with a locally advanced carcinoma of the colon; diversion of urine, by ureteric transplantation into an isolated segment of ileum or skin in a patient with advanced carcinoma of the bladder; and anastomosis of the gallbladder or common bile duct to the stomach, duodenum, or jejunum in a patient with pancreatic carcinoma obstructing the common bile duct.

TREATMENT BY RADIOTHERAPY

Principles of Radiotherapy

Several types of ionizing radiation are used to treat patients with cancer. Nonparticulate forms, such as x-rays or gamma-rays, are used most widely, but high-energy particles, such as electrons, have a number of physical advantages and are being used more frequently.

Methods. The methods of giving radiotherapy include:

Teletherapy. The source of radiation is placed at a distance from the patient, and a beam-defining collimator controls the amount of tissues irradiated. High-energy x-rays, gamma-rays from the artificially produced isotope of cobalt, or high-energy electrons are used.

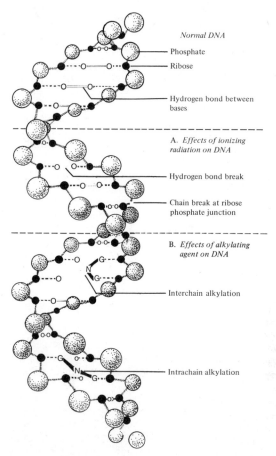

Normal DNA

— Phosphate
— Ribose

— Hydrogen bond between bases

A. *Effects of ionizing radiation on DNA*

— Hydrogen bond break

— Chain break at ribose phosphate junction

B. *Effects of alkylating agent on DNA*

— Interchain alkylation

— Intrachain alkylation

Figure 7–8. The effects of radiotherapy and nitrogen mustard on DNA. Radiotherapy damages DNA by breaking the chains at the ribose phosphate junctions and hydrolyzing the interchain hydrogen bonds. The two ethylenimine radicals, N—CH_2·CH_2, alkylate guanine bases in the same or complementary chains of DNA.

Deep-seated lesions are usually treated by this method.

When high-energy x-rays or gamma-rays are used, the dose decreases little on passing through the tissues and absorption by different tissues is almost the same. There is less reaction in the skin than occurs with a low-energy source, because the maximal dose is several millimeters below the epidermis. Less radiation is absorbed by bone than is the case with a low-energy source. Pathologic fracture of bone is therefore uncommon. When high-energy electrons are used, the depth of maximal dose is determined by the voltage, and a well-defined volume of tissue is treated.

Short-Range and Contact Therapy. A low-energy source, generating x-rays or electrons, is occasionally used to treat superficial skin lesions. The dose to the deep tissues is small because the intensity of the radiation decreases rapidly with depth.

Endotherapy. An isotope may be placed within a cavity such as the bladder or a serous cavity to treat diffuse superficial lesions (intracavitary therapy). Radioactive colloidal gold, ^{198}Au, in the peritoneal or pleural cavity provides good palliation in patients with ascitic or pleural effusions due to diffuse carcinomatosis. Radium needles or radioactive gold grains placed in the tissues, interstitial therapy, deliver a large dose at a low-dose rate to a well-localized small volume of tissue. The dose rate for radium needles is about 8.4 R/mCi-hour and for ^{198}Au grains 2.2 R/mCi-hour, 1 cm from the source. The radium needles are removed when the desired dose has been given, while the grains are left in the patient because the half-life of radiogold is short.

Intracellular Therapy. Radioactive isotopes of some elements are preferentially taken up by certain cells in sufficient amounts to be used for treatment. Examples are the uptake of radioactive iodine by the thyroid, radioactive phosphorus by the red bone marrow and some lesions of the brain, and colloidal radioactive gold by lymph nodes.

Other Considerations. Electrons are produced when tissues absorb x-ray or gamma-ray photons. The distance that they travel depends on the energy of the incident photons and the number of interactions with atoms in the absorbing medium. The electrons may enter a cell and interact with a sensitive site that is vital for survival, or they may react with molecules of water and oxygen to produce oxidizing OH and HO_2 radicals that can also damage the cell. The

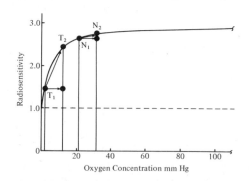

Figure 7–9. The relation of oxygen tension to radiosensitivity. An increase of 10 mm Hg in the oxygen tension increases the radiosensitivity of hypoxic cancer cells by about two but that of the relatively well-oxygenated tumor bed by only 0.3. *T* represents a carcinoma cell and *N* a normal tissue cell.

sensitive site or target within the cell is deoxyribonucleic acid (DNA). Direct damage by electrons produces breaks at the sugar phosphate junction; indirect damage by radicals is mainly by oxidation of the hydrogen bonds between the purine and pyrimidine bases (Figure 7–8).

A single dose of x-rays to an established tumor and its bed produces changes within a few hours in the water content, electrolytes, and DNA and, depending on the dose, causes greater damage after several days.

Radiosensitivity and cell oxygen tension follow a hyperbolic relation (Figure 7–9). A small increase in oxygen tension allows radiotherapy to produce considerable damage to hypoxic cancer cells but little damage to well-oxygenated normal cells.[6] Attempts have therefore been made to improve the oxygenation of tumors during radiotherapy. Inhalation of 95 percent oxygen and 5 percent carbon dioxide at atmospheric pressure or pure oxygen at 3 atmospheres absolute pressure increases the tension of oxygen in solution in the blood and interstitial fluid. The oxygen diffuses into hypoxic areas containing radioresistant cancer cells and increases their radiosensitivity.

Cells in a number of tumors, such as bronchogenic carcinoma, are arranged in columns with the blood supply in the periphery and few vessels within the nodules (Figure 7–10).[12] There is therefore a tendency to develop central necrosis at a critical diameter. The well-oxygenated cells in the periphery are damaged by radiotherapy and lose their reproductive integrity and, although appearing normal, do not divide again, or divide several times and die. Cells adjacent to necrotic areas are hypoxic and are damaged only one third as much; they maintain their nutrition largely by anaerobic glycolysis, and subsequently, when nutrition and oxygenation improve, they divide again. The radiosensitivity of benign and malignant cells under similar growth conditions does not differ greatly. Repair processes, however, are better developed in normal tissues and permit recovery of the tumor bed.

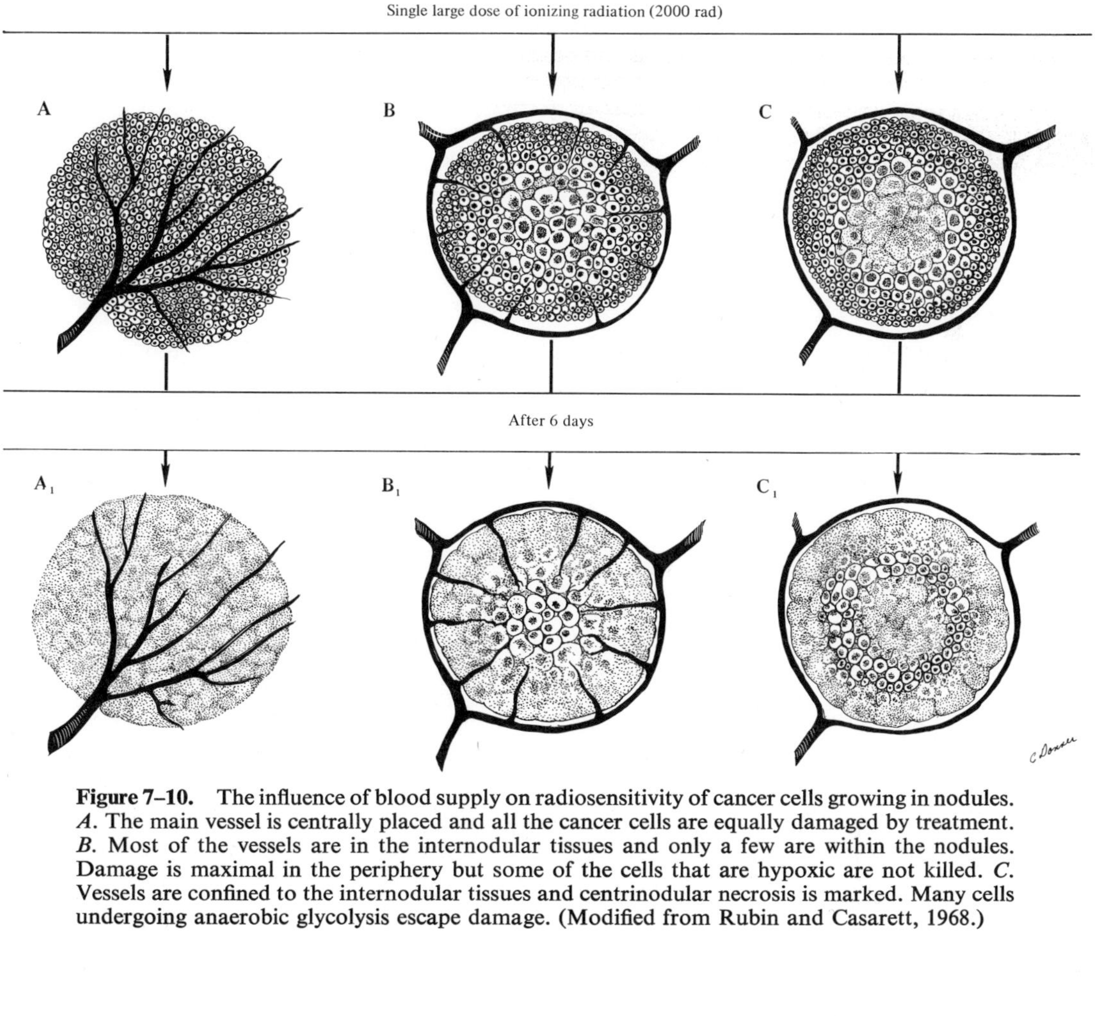

Figure 7–10. The influence of blood supply on radiosensitivity of cancer cells growing in nodules. *A.* The main vessel is centrally placed and all the cancer cells are equally damaged by treatment. *B.* Most of the vessels are in the internodular tissues and only a few are within the nodules. Damage is maximal in the periphery but some of the cells that are hypoxic are not killed. *C.* Vessels are confined to the internodular tissues and centrinodular necrosis is marked. Many cells undergoing anaerobic glycolysis escape damage. (Modified from Rubin and Casarett, 1968.)

Fractionating the dose of radiation increases the therapeutic ratio because recovery is more rapid in normal than in malignant cells. The first fractions kill the well-oxygenated tissues. There is an increase in blood supply after removal of the dead cells, and those that were previously hypoxic are damaged by later fractions.

Attempted Curative Radiotherapy

Radiotherapy may be used to attempt cure. A large dose, about 6000 rad, may be given in a number of fractions during four to five weeks.

Radiotherapy Alone. Radiotherapy is often the only treatment necessary for patients with rodent ulcer, squamous carcinoma of the skin, mouth, pharynx, larynx, and cervix uteri, and lymphomas.

With Chemotherapy. The value of combining the two treatments has not been established. Dactinomycin has been given with radiotherapy to patients with Wilms' tumor of the kidney and is probably of value. It is important not to interfere with a well-established treatment, such as radiotherapy, whose biologic effects are well known and whose dosage can be given to a well-defined volume of tissue, by giving a less localized treatment such as chemotherapy. Chemicals may be given before radiotherapy to produce partial tumor regression. However, their administration a number of months after radiotherapy is seldom effective. The decrease in blood flow, from endarteritis and perivascular fibrosis, after large doses of ionizing radiation, may reduce delivery of the drug to the cancer cells. The role of chemotherapy and radiotherapy in the treatment of lymphomas is well established (see Chapter 24).

With Operative Excision. Radiotherapy is used frequently before or after operation, especially in patients with locally advanced tumors and in those likely to have local recurrence.

Preoperative Radiotherapy. Preoperative radiotherapy has been confined largely to patients with locally advanced tumors. There are a number of theoretic considerations, and results from animal studies suggest that it may be of value in patients with mobile tumors. Preoperative therapy should be more effective than postoperative treatment because oxygenation is better, the decrease in tumor size may facilitate excision, and cells close to vessels that may be disseminated at the time of operation are killed. Excessive tissue reaction and impairment of healing should not occur using modern high-energy therapy.

Conventional Fractionated Radiotherapy. This is most frequently used because it gives an opportunity to observe a gradually increasing response. Fractionation gives the maximum therapeutic response with minimal damage to the normal tissues, and the aim is to kill all the cancer cells. Roswit and coworkers[11] found that it was of no value and was possibly harmful in a trial, using randomized controls, in patients with bronchogenic carcinoma. They found that survival at 30 months was 14 percent in those given radiotherapy and 20 percent in those untreated. At 12 months after entering the study there was a 16 percent better survival in those who were not irradiated.

Concentrated Preoperative Radiotherapy. Administration of a biologically large dose of radiation in one or several fractions to a tumor and its regional lymphatics several days before operation may increase survival in selected patients. Results from animal studies support the use of concentrated preoperative radiotherapy.[8] Treatment is given to kill the well-oxygenated, and therefore radiosensitive, cancer cells in the periphery and must be followed by surgical excision to remove the more centrally located and often radioresistant cells. Concentrated preoperative radiotherapy should therefore be confined to patients with "operable" cancers in whom all gross tumor is removed at operation and there is the possibility of residual microscopic foci of malignant cells. The total dose of radiotherapy should approach the maximum that normal tissues can safely tolerate and should be given probably about six days before operation. Patients who are treated by block dissection of the neck and those with carcinoma of the rectum and sigmoid colon are most likely to benefit. A controlled clinical trial in patients with carcinoma of the colon and rectum shows that mortality and morbidity are not increased by treatment and that survival is increased in those with positive nodes.[7]

Postoperative Radiotherapy. A large, well-localized dose of ionizing radiation can be given therapeutically to residual tumor marked by clips at the time of operation. Examples are patients treated by block dissection of the neck and abdominoperineal resection for carcinoma of the rectum.

There is now considerable controversy concerning the prophylactic use of radiotherapy after operation. Theoretic advantages are that treatment to small foci of cancer cells is more effective than to a large mass of tumor-containing hypoxic areas, and that it may prevent distant metastases developing as the microscopic foci grow to clinically detectable tumor. The disadvantages are that treatment is given unnecessarily to a number of patients who would not develop a local recurrence, that there is increased morbidity from the combined use of excision and radiotherapy, and that it may decrease host resistance to cancer cells.

Paterson and Russell,[10] in a study using randomized controls, showed that survival of patients with breast carcinoma treated by radical mastectomy was the same when radiotherapy was given prophylactically after operation as when given therapeutically to locally recurrent disease. Fisher and his coworkers[5] reported the results of a controlled clinical study by the National Surgical Adjuvant Breast Project on the prophylactic use of postoperative radiotherapy in patients treated by radical mastectomy for breast carcinoma. Survival at five years was 56 percent in those given prophylactic postoperative radiotherapy and 62 percent in those treated by radical mastectomy. Total recurrence, local and distant, was the same in both groups. Recurrence in the regions treated by radiotherapy, however, was decreased. The first presentation of distant metastases tended to be earlier in patients treated by radiotherapy. This suggested that radiotherapy might impair the host's immune response (see page 115).

Palliative Radiotherapy

Ionizing radiation is often given for palliation in patients with locally advanced tumors or metastases. The primary is treated to make the tumor smaller, to decrease ulceration and pain, and to prevent pressure on or infiltration of adjacent structures. Metastases are treated to relieve pain, to decrease their size, or to improve function of an involved organ. The dose is usually lower than for curative therapy, the fractionation shorter, and the biologic reaction less.

TREATMENT BY CHEMOTHERAPY

The present interest in chemotherapy started in the late 1940s with the use of nitrogen mustard in patients with Hodgkin's disease. A number of effective anticancer agents were discovered, but all were toxic and damaged normal cells almost as much as the cancer cells. The use of chemotherapy as an adjunct to operation or radiotherapy proved disappointing. We now have a number of effective agents and better understanding of the best treatment regimes and of the choice of agent.

Chemotherapy may be used alone to treat tumors that show marked response. More frequently it is used to provide palliation in patients with advanced local or generalized disease. It may also be used as an adjunct to surgical excision or radiotherapy. Its main role is in the treatment of acute and chronic forms of leukemia. Generally a combination of drugs has been found to be more effective than a single agent.

Chemotherapy can produce cure in choriocarcinoma of the uterus, some lymphomas and leukemias, and Burkitt's lymphoma. Immunologic factors may be important in the response of tumors to chemotherapy. There is mononuclear tissue infiltration of the tumor in many of those that regress following treatment. Stewart and his coworkers[14] found that the response of squamous cell carcinoma of the skin to methotrexate was related to mononuclear infiltration. The anticancer drug decreases the cell mass. The cell-mediated immune response of the host then destroys the remaining cancer cells. A good response to chemotherapy is often obtained in patients with lymphomas using many agents, Wilms' tumor using dactinomycin, pleural and peritoneal effusions using thioTEPA, and squamous cell carcinoma with amethopterin (methotrexate).

Most chemicals used to treat cancer impair protein synthesis by damaging DNA or RNA or act directly on the proteins synthesized in the cytoplasm. Their action is often the same in normal and cancer cells. Cancer cells are damaged more because they are generating more rapidly than normal tissue cells, their membranes may be more permeable, permitting a higher concentration of the agent within the cell, or their repair processes may be less developed than those in normal tissues. Cells in the bone marrow and the gastrointestinal tract, and well-nourished leukemic cells that are growing exponentially, are maximally damaged. Many cancer cells, however, in the inhomogeneous mass of cells in carcinomas and sarcomas are not affected. The agents have a number of undesirable side effects. They often cause leukopenia, stomatitis, diarrhea, and sometimes loss of hair.

Classification

Source or Chemical Action. Chemicals were initially grouped according to their biochemical action or their source.

Alkylating Agents. Alkylating agents damage cells by forming firm bonds between the guanine bases in DNA and to a lesser extent by damaging the cytoplasm and cell membrane (Figure 7–8). There are one, two, or three alkylating ethylenimine groups ($=N-CH_2-CH_2$) in each molecule; potency tends to increase with the number of groups. If the DNA is sufficiently damaged, the cell is killed immediately or after several divisions; lesser damage may produce carcinogenic mutations. Repair can occur provided that the corresponding portion of the complementary strand in DNA is intact. The agents of special interest to surgeons are:

1. Nitrogen mustard, $CH_3N(CH_2CH_2Cl)_2$. This agent was used locally and intravenously as an adjunct to operation. Animal studies suggested that it would be of value, but this has not been confirmed in patients. It is still used occasionally in advanced Hodgkin's disease.

2. ThioTEPA. This drug has three ethylenimine radicles. It is now mainly used for the palliative treatment of patients with hormone-resistant metastases from carcinoma of the breast. Cystitis occurs in 5 to 10 percent.

3. Cyclophosphamide. Nitrogen mustard combines with plasma proteins and has a half-life in the systemic circulation of less than 30 seconds. Cyclophosphamide is an inert carrier form of nitrogen mustard that is activated in the liver by phosphatase enzymes forming a hydrophilic compound. Cancer cells have more permeable cell membranes and take up a greater amount of the drug than normal cells. Intracellular phosphatase enzymes act on the phosphamide portion and free active nitrogen mustard within the cell. Cyclophosphamide does not affect the platelets and rarely produces a persistent leukopenia; it often causes a temporary or permanent loss of hair. Its main use is in the treatment of patients with metastases from carcinoma of the ovary and hormone-resistant metastases from carcinoma of the breast. Cystitis occurs in 5 to 10 percent.

Antimetabolites. Antimetabolites differ in molecular structure from their normal cell counterparts but have similar biochemical properties. They are therefore taken up and form abnormal metabolites, or they inactivate enzymes and block essential metabolic pathways. Commonly used agents are amethopterin (methotrexate), which interferes with folic acid metabolism, and 5-fluorouracil (5-FU), which interferes with DNA and RNA synthesis. Amethopterin is frequently given by intra-arterial infusion in patients with advanced carcinoma of the head and neck. The pyrimidine 5-FU produces good palliation in many patients with advanced primary or metastases from carcinomas of the bowel. Recently massive doses of methotrexate followed by citrovorum factor "rescue" have been used successfully in children to reduce metastases from osteogenic sarcoma following removal of the primary.

Antibiotics. Dactinomycin has been used extensively as an adjunct to surgery and radiotherapy in children with Wilms' tumor of the kidney. Adriamycin, doxorubicin hydrochloride, is an anthracycline antibiotic isolated from a culture of *Streptomyces peucetius*. It is the chemotherapeutic agent of greatest interest because of its potency against a great variety of tumors, a number of which did not respond to any other agent. Following intravenous administration it is rapidly cleared from the plasma, metabolized by the liver, extensively bound to tissues, and slowly excreted in the bile and urine. Unfortunately it is extremely toxic. It causes myelosuppression, mucositis, loss of hair, liver damage, and extensive tissue necrosis when injected into the subcutaneous tissues. The most serious toxic effect is cardiotoxicity when the total dose exceeds 400 mg/m^2. This may result in death or chronic cardiac failure. The dose that is most often used is 60 to 75 mg/m^2 injected into an intravenous infusion every three weeks until the total dose is 400 mg/m^2. It is now the treatment of choice for soft tissue sarcomas, oat cell carcinoma of the lung, and histiocytic lymphomas and should be used alone or in combination in Hodgkin's disease after failure to respond to MOPP. In osteogenic sarcoma, survival has markedly improved following treatment with methotrexate and adriamycin. It plays a major role in the palliative treatment of carcinoma of the breast. Objective remission occurs in about 50 percent treated by adriamycin and up to 80 percent with combination chemotherapy such as 5-fluorouracil, adriamycin, and cyclophosphamide. It is also of value in thyroid carcinoma, neuroblastoma, carcinoma of the bladder and stomach, Wilms' tumor, and gynecologic malignancies. Unfortunately it is not effective in carcinoma of the colon or malignant melanoma.

Plant Extracts. Colchicine is often used in animal studies but is too toxic for clinical use. Vincristine is used mainly in the treatment of advanced lymphomas and certain types of leukemia.

Effect on Generation Cycle. Chemotherapeutic agents have recently been classified according to how they act on generating and nongenerating cells (Figure 7–11).[13] Cells that are generating or "cycling" are described as being in the G_1, S, G_2, or M phase. In G_1, the first gap phase, the chromosomes are extended and poorly defined. In the S phase the amount of DNA is doubled. The second gap or G_2 phase is another rest period with little nuclear activity, but there is some condensation of the chromosomes near the end of this period. Cell division, mitosis, occurs in the M phase. Many cells do not generate or have long generation times as, for example, nerve cells and the stem cells in the bone marrow. These nongenerating or noncycling cells are in the G_0 phase. Agents can be classified as affecting cells that are:

Generating and Nongenerating. X-rays and nitrogen mustard damage generating and non-

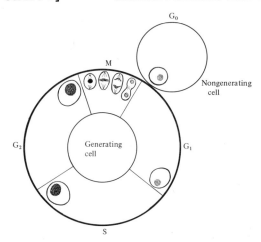

Figure 7–11. The cell generation cycle. The generation cycle can be divided into the first gap (G_1), DNA synthesis (S), gap 2 (G_2), or mitotic (M) phases. Cells that are not dividing or have a long generation time are noncycling and in G_0.

generating cells. X-rays produce greatest damage to cells in the M phase and have three times greater effect on well-oxygenated than on hypoxic cells. The effect of nitrogen mustard depends upon the blood supply and its ability to diffuse in active form into the cells.

Cycling. Cyclophosphamide, dactinomycin, and 5-fluorouracil (5-FU) damage generating cells.

Phase Specific. Amethopterin (methotrexate) damages cells that are in the S phase; vincristine those that are in the M phase.

The recognition that damage to cancer cells depends upon their state in the generation cycle is important when arranging treatment. An agent, such as cyclophosphamide, that affects generating cells kills those that it reaches in adequate concentration and in addition white blood cells in the peripheral blood and red bone marrow. The stem myeloid cells in the bone marrow in G_0 phase are then stimulated to generate. If a second dose of the agent is given before the stem cells have reverted to the G_0 phase, they are damaged and severe leukopenia occurs. Intermittent large doses at intervals of four to six weeks should therefore be given rather than daily treatments. Phase-specific agents should be given for a prolonged time because the generation cycles of cancer cells are not synchronous. Combination therapy is often effective in the treatment of solid tumors using agents in different groups, such as vincristine, 5-FU, cyclophosphamide, and adriamycin.

Adjunct to Surgical Excision

Preoperative. A chemotherapeutic agent should be more effective before than after

operation because the blood supply is intact. The tumor becomes smaller and can be removed more readily. In addition, viable cancer cells are less likely to be disseminated at surgery. On the other hand, the agents now available decrease the white cell count and may impair wound healing, and it has recently been suggested that they may decrease host resistance and increase local recurrence and metastases.

Operative. There has been considerable interest in the use of chemotherapeutic agents at the time of operation to kill cells that have entered the lymphatics or blood circulation and to prevent local recurrence (Figure 7–12). Their use, however, must still be considered experimental.

Postoperative. It has been suggested that chemotherapy should be given after operative excision to treat small numbers of cancer cells rather than a large tumor mass. Such postoperative use must still be considered experimental. A National Surgical Adjuvant Breast Project clinical trial has been completed on the adjunctive intravenous use of thioTEPA on the day of operation and the two subsequent days.[4] The drug was of no value in postmenopausal women but decreased local recurrence in premenopausal women who had four or more positive axillary nodes (see Chapter 26). Farber[3] has shown that survival increases when dactinomycin is given postoperatively along with radiotherapy to children with Wilms' tumor of the kidney.

Palliative Chemotherapy

The use of 5-fluorouracil sometimes provides good palliation in bowel cancer, as do thioTEPA in breast carcinoma and amethopterin in advanced squamous cell carcinoma. Bateman and his coworkers,[1] in a trial using randomized controls, found an objective response in 20 percent of patients with metastatic carcinoma of the bowel given 5-FU intravenously and a 40 percent response when it was given orally.

Most drugs now available are toxic at therapeutic doses; therefore the general effect on the patient must be considered in addition to their action on the tumor.

Combined Treatments

Surgery, radiotherapy, and chemotherapy can be used in different combinations in the primary treatment of a number of cancers. In Hodgkin's disease surgery and radiotherapy are used to treat those in stages I, II, and IIIA. In the treatment of a rhabdomyosarcoma the five-year survival has been increased from about 20 percent when treatment was by excision alone to 80 percent when treatment consists of excision,

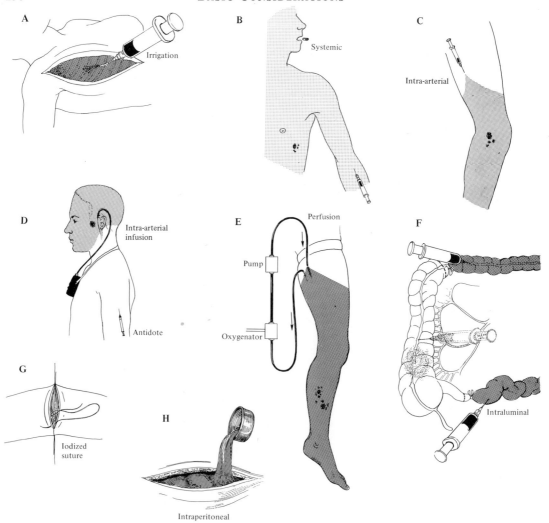

Figure 7–12. Chemotherapy of cancer.

A. Local irrigation. The operative site is irrigated with the agent. There is a high local concentration with almost no systemic effect.

B. Systemic. Parenteral administration results in the concentration of the drug being the same in the cancer as in the normal tissue and there is marked systemic effect.

C. Intra-arterial. A high concentration at the site of the tumor can be obtained by regional arterial injection. There is little systemic effect if the agent has a short biologic half-life. The agent can only be given for a short time.

D. Intra-arterial infusion. Intra-arterial infusion, through a catheter placed in the regional artery, delivers a high concentration of the drug to the tumor for days or weeks. When the antifolic agent amethopterin is given, the portion that reaches the systemic circulation can be neutralized by the antifolinic acid (citrivorum factor) given every 6 hours by the intramuscular route. Infusion of the liver through the hepatic artery is of special interest because the blood supply to liver metastases is by hepatic arterial and not portal venous blood.

E. Perfusion. The agent can be given for about one hour by perfusion of the regional artery. The regional artery and vein are cannulated and attached to an extracorporeal circulation containing a pump and oxygenator. When the limb is perfused, a tourniquet is placed proximally and there is little escape of the agent into the systemic circulation. Local damage to the tissues limits the dose when a limb is perfused; leakage to the systemic circulation limits the dose when a regional artery in the torso is perfused.

F. Intraluminal. Perchloride of mercury, nitrogen mustard, chlorpactin XCB, or 5-fluorouracil has been placed in the gut to kill cancer cells within the lumen. Tapes are placed proximal and distal to the tumor to prevent intraluminal dissemination of cancer cells during manipulation.

radiotherapy, and chemotherapy. The three treatments also improve survival in the treatment of neuroblastoma.

CITED REFERENCES

1. Bateman, J. R.; Pugh, R. P.; Cassidy, F. R.; Marshall, G. J.; and Irwin, L. E.: 5-Fluorouracil given once weekly: comparison of intravenous and oral administration. *Cancer*, 28:907–13, 1971.
2. Cole, W. H.: Recent advances in treatment of the cancer patient. *JAMA*, **174**:1287, 1960.
3. Farber, S.: Chemotherapy in treatment of leukemia and Wilms' tumor. *JAMA*, **198**:826–36, 1966.
4. Fisher, B.; Ravdin, R. G.; Ausman, R. K.; Slack, N. H.; Moore, G. E.; and Noer, R. J.: Surgical adjuvant chemotherapy in breast cancer: results of a decade of cooperative investigation. *Ann. Surg.*, **168**:337–56, 1968.
5. Fisher, B.; Slack, N. H.; Cavanagh, P. J.; and Ravdin, R. G.: The worth of postoperative irradiation for breast cancer: results of the National Surgical Adjuvant Breast Project Clinical Trial. *Ann. Surg.*, **172**:711–32, 1970.
6. Gray, L. H.; Conger, A. D.; Ebert, M.; Hornsey, S.; and Scott, O. C. A.: Concentration of oxygen dissolved in tissues at time of irradiation as factor in radiotherapy. *Br. J. Radiol.*, **26**:638, 1953.
7. Higgins, G. A.: Preoperative irradiation for colorectal carcinoma: The V.A. National Study. In Rush, B. S., Jr., and Greenlaw, R. H. (eds.): *Cancer Therapy by Integrated Radiation and Operation*. Charles C Thomas, Springfield, Ill., Chap. 18, pp. 107–10, 1968.
8. McCredie, J. A.; Inch, R. W.; and Watson, T. A.: Concentrated preoperative radiotherapy. *Rev. Surg.*, **25**:2, 80–86, 1968.
9. Morgan, C. N., and Lloyd-Davies, O. V.: Restorative resection of the rectum. *Proc. R. Soc. Med.*, **43**:701, 1950.
10. Paterson, R., and Russell, M. H.: Clinical trials in malignant disease. Part III. Breast cancer: evaluation of postoperative radiotherapy. *J. Fac. Radiol.*, **10**:175–80, 1959.
11. Roswit, B.; Higgins, G. A.; Shields, W.; and Keehn, R. J.: Preoperative radiation therapy for carcinoma of the lung: report of a national VA controlled study. In Vaeth, J. M. (ed.): *Frontiers of Radiation Therapy and Oncology*, Vol. 5. S. Karger, Basel, pp. 163–76, 1970.
12. Rubin, P., and Casarett, G. W.: *Clinical Radiation Pathology*. Vol. II. W. B. Saunders, Philadelphia, p. 941, 1968.
13. Skipper, H. E.: The cell cycle and chemotherapy of cancer. In Baserga, R. (ed.): *The Cell Cycle and Cancer*. Marcel Dekker, Inc., New York, pp. 365–87, 1971.
14. Stewart, T. H. M.; Klaassen, D.; and Crook, A. F.: Methotrexate in the treatment of malignant tumors:

evidence for the possible participation of host defense mechanisms. *Can. Med. Assoc. J.*, **101**:191–99, 1969.
15. Willis, R. A.: *Pathology of Tumours*. Butterworth and Co., London, p. 76, 1967.
16. Willis, R. A.: *Ibid.*, p. 163.
17. Wood, S., Jr.: Pathogenesis of metastases formation observed in vivo in the rabbit ear chamber. *Arch. Pathol.*, **66**:550–68, 1958.

SUGGESTIONS FOR FURTHER READING

SPREAD OF CANCER

Engell, H. C.: Cancer cells in the circulating blood. *Acta. Chir. Scand.*, Suppl. 201, Stockholm, 1955.
First major publication suggesting that cancer cells enter the blood in large numbers in patients with "early" tumors.

Willis, R. A.: *Pathology of Tumours*, 4th ed. Butterworth and Co., London, 1967.
A classic for clarity and content.

SURGERY

Cole, W. H.: Factors important in the growth and spread of cancer. In Cole, W. H. (ed.): *Dissemination of Cancer*. Appleton-Century-Crofts, New York, pp. 1–20, 1961.

Griffiths, J. D., and Salsbury, A. J.: Entry of malignant cells into the blood. In Kugelmass, I. N. (ed.): *Circulating Cancer Cells*. Charles C Thomas, Springfield, Ill., pp. 3–15, 1965.

RADIOTHERAPY

Rubin, P., and Casarett, G. W.: *Clinical Radiation Pathology*. W. B. Saunders, Philadelphia, 1968.
The principles of radiobiology and their application to radiotherapy are clearly reviewed.

Rush, B. F., and Greenlaw, R. H.: *Cancer Therapy by Integrated Radiation and Operation*. Charles C Thomas, Springfield, Ill., 1968.

Vaeth, J. M.: *Frontiers of Radiation Therapy and Oncology: The Interrelationship of Surgery and Radiation Therapy in the Treatment of Cancer*. S. Karger, Basel, 1970.
Two reviews on the preoperative and post-operative use of radiotherapy in the treatment of cancer.

CHEMOTHERAPY

Baserga, R.: *The Cell Cycle and Cancer*. Marcel Dekker, Inc., New York, 1971.
This is an up-to-date review on the use of chemotherapy in relation to the cell cycle.

Cline, M. J., and Haskell, C. M.: *Cancer Chemotherapy*. W. B. Saunders, Philadelphia, 1975.
Describes chemotherapeutic agents and their clinical application, including their use for solid tumors.

Cole, W. H.: *Chemotherapy of Cancer*. Lea & Febiger, Philadelphia, 1970.
A review of the status of chemotherapy, including a description of adjuvant clinical trials using chemotherapy with surgery.

Placing the agent outside the tapes kills cancer cells that may be carried into the wall on sutures. It has been suggested that the agent should be placed between the tapes at an early stage during the operation so that it is absorbed and destroys cancer cells that enter the circulation.

G. Iodized sutures. Iodized sutures have been used to kill cancer cells that may be carried into the wall on their surfaces and produce a recurrence at the suture line.

H. Into serous cavity. The chemical may be placed in the peritoneal cavity prior to closing the abdomen to kill free cancer cells.

Chapter 8

CONTROLLED TRIALS IN SURGERY

Richard B. Welbourn

CHAPTER OUTLINE

Introduction
False Claims
Controlled Trials
Principles
Ethical Objections
Preliminary Considerations
  Resources
  Number of Patients
  Number of Treatment Groups
  Controls
  Pilot Experiments

Multicenter Trials
Telling the Patient
Standardization of Operations
Protocol
Allocation of Patients
Assessment of Results
Analysis of the Data
Stopping the Trial
Outcome of the Trial
Conclusion

"Ignorance is preferable to error and he is less remote from the truth who believes nothing, than he who believes what is wrong."

Thomas Jefferson

INTRODUCTION

Very occasionally in medicine and in surgery new methods of treatment are introduced whose results are outstandingly superior to any that have been achieved before. In medicine, for example, hormones, vitamins, sulfonamides, and antibiotics have restored to health millions of patients who would have died without them. In surgery antisepsis and asepsis, appendectomy, internal fixation of fractures of the femoral neck, operations on the heart, and renal transplantation have changed completely the prospects for many thousands more. The new procedures were not always accepted immediately, but the results were so good that it was apparent to anyone who examined the facts objectively that, although the details needed to be investigated further, the general principles had been established and should be implemented without delay.

Much more frequently, however, new methods are not obviously superior to those in use already, even though their originators strongly advocate them. Indeed, physicians and surgeons are often embarrassed by the number of procedures from which to choose and by the wide range of opinion as to which is best. They are usually influenced in their choice by what they were taught as students, what they read in books and articles, what they hear in lectures and discussion, and by their own experience.

FALSE CLAIMS

Claims that one procedure is better than another often fail to stand up to critical examination for various reasons. The following examples are mostly surgical, but similar considerations apply to the whole of medicine, and surgeons are no more culpable than other clinicians.

1. A surgeon may advise a particular operation because he has a general impression that the results are good or simply because he thinks that he has a good idea. Inquiry, however, reveals that he has not analyzed his operative mortality nor followed all (or even many) of his patients long enough to discover the long-term results.

2. A careful retrospective study of a series of patients will reveal fairly accurately the operative mortality, the cure rate (and recurrence rate) of the disease, and the morbidity rate. These results may then be compared with others (a) performed by the same surgeon or other surgeons in the same hospital at the same time; (b) performed by the same surgeons at an earlier period (a "consecutive" comparison); or (c) published by

other surgeons elsewhere. All such comparisons are open to serious objections.

i. Diseases often change in their character and behavior at different times and in different places.

ii. Criteria for selecting patients for operation vary greatly, and individual surgeons adopt different criteria (perhaps unconsciously) at different times. The criteria may be defined carefully by agreed definitions, but observers differ in their subjective assessments and in the thoroughness with which they investigate patients. For instance, there is considerable observer error in estimating the size and fixity of tumors and in recognizing the involvement of lymph nodes. Moreover, while some surgeons undertake mastectomy for breast carcinoma without even surveying the skeleton for secondary deposits by conventional radiography, others use isotopes and a gamma camera to exclude patients with occult advanced disease. Similar differences are found in the criteria used for assessment after operation.

iii. Even objective measurements made in the laboratory leave room for error and may suggest differences, more apparent than real, between different series. Simple estimations of the hemoglobin concentration, for instance, may vary regularly by as much as 20 percent between different laboratories, and the presence or absence of anemia may depend on whether or not patients have been encouraged to take iron tablets.

iv. Surgeons often become interested in particular diseases and start to pay special attention to all their patients who suffer from them, so that their results improve. They may attribute the improvement to new specific therapeutic measures that they have introduced, when it is really due to the extra general care, both physical and psychologic, that they have provided.

v. Surgeons are often biased in favor of one procedure and against another, often unconsciously and for quite irrational reasons, and this fact influences their assessment, particularly of subjective phenomena.

vi. Retrospective studies often have the disadvantage that essential observations were not made at the appropriate times in some or all of the patients or that, if made, they were not recorded or the records have been lost.

CONTROLLED TRIALS

It is clear that while many studies provide accurate accounts of the progress of groups of patients, they can rarely be used for valid comparisons with other groups. Even when differences are found, it is rarely possible to be certain that they are due to the operative procedures and not to other factors. What, then, is the solution? It must be recognized that problems in medicine and surgery, even though they concern human beings, are of precisely the same nature as those in biologic science as a whole. Consequently the precepts and methods of biologic science must be used for their solution. A comparison of two or more treatment methods can be valid only if a proper experimental design is used as in an investigation in the laboratory. As in any other scientific experiment, a hypothesis must be proposed—in this case that one method of treatment is better than others—and its truth must be tested by observations planned prospectively. This is the basis of the controlled prospective therapeutic trial.

The first controlled trial on record is that of Dr. James Lind, a surgeon in the British Navy, who observed in 1747 that oranges and lemons cured scurvy rapidly while other remedies failed to do so. The controlled trial as we understand it today had been used on several occasions before it was refined and popularized in the early 1950s by the British statistician Sir Austin Bradford Hill, mainly as a method of testing the relative efficacy of different drugs. The first *surgical* controlled trial to be reported was that undertaken by Sir Hedley Atkins and his colleagues at Guy's Hospital, London, and published in 1957, to compare the effects of adrenalectomy and hypophysectomy for the relief of advanced cancer of the breast.

PRINCIPLES

The principles of a prospective controlled therapeutic trial are:

1. Similar patients are randomly divided into two or more groups for treatment by two or more different methods.

2. The results of the operations or other methods of treatment are assessed as far as possible by objective quantitative methods, and the numerical differences are analyzed statistically.

3. As a result of the findings decisions are made about the relative merits of the procedures and their implications for surgical practice.

ETHICAL OBJECTIONS

Some surgeons are worried by the fact that the treatment is decided by random allocation and feel that they are failing in their responsibilities if they do not themselves decide on the best method for each patient. This argument is understandable but fallacious, because it presupposes that the best method is known. If it *were* known, it would be quite wrong not to use it and there would be no need for a controlled trial. The essential prerequisite for a trial is a genuine doubt in the face of the available evidence about the relative merits of different forms of treatment. If the best method is *not* known, it is entirely ethical to use such a method of selection. Usually all the procedures under comparison are being advocated and used widely by other surgeons, all of whom are claiming comparable results. If a controlled trial is not undertaken, it will often (as in the past) take many years, and perhaps two or three generations of surgeons, before the truth is known and all patients are able to benefit from the best form of treatment. In medical practice if one form of treatment is ineffective, it is often possible, without detriment, to try another. It is much more difficult and hazardous to undo a surgical operation and perform another. It is surely *more* ethical for a surgeon to undertake a controlled trial, which will provide an answer within a few months or years, than it is for him to pretend to a knowledge that he does not possess. In practice the ethics of a particular trial are decided by thorough discussion by all those concerned with it and finally by submission of the plan to the hospital's ethical committee.

PRELIMINARY CONSIDERATIONS

Resources

Ample resources for a trial must be assured before it is started. The people involved must be enthusiastic, devoted to the task, disciplined, capable of organizing, and patient. There must be sufficient manpower (including secretarial help), money, and materials. The cooperation of a statistician should be enlisted at the outset. Responsibility for the trial must be in the hands of one individual, who can be relied upon to stay the course and see the work completed. A trial that may be completed in a few weeks or months (e.g., a comparison of methods for the prevention of early postoperative complications) can be undertaken by junior staff. On the other hand, a trial that will require several years to complete (e.g., a comparison of the long-term results of operations for cancer or peptic ulcer) must be in the charge of a permanent staff member.

Number of Patients

A reasonable forecast must be made before the start of the trial of the number of patients who will be required for its successful completion. This must be discussed with the statistician. The number will depend on the size of the difference that is likely to emerge and on the variability of quantitative data within each group. An adequate number of patients must be available for the work to be completed within a reasonable period.

Number of Treatment Groups

In general it is best to have two different groups only. Sometimes three or more are used, but the conduct of the trial is then more complicated and a longer time is required for completion. Multiple groups may be desirable when there are plenty of suitable patients and when the trial is expected to take several years. Two groups are better when there are fewer patients and when the trial is likely to be finished quickly. Under these circumstances a succession of trials, each involving two groups, may be undertaken.

Controls

In a scientific experiment involving animals it is usual for a control group to be compared with a test group. If the test involves a surgical operation, a sham operation is used in the controls. In drug trials it is usual to employ a placebo for comparison with the drug to be tested. Surgical operations in patients do not lend themselves to the use of controls in this way. It is possible to compare a surgical operation with a nonsurgical method, but sham operations are not justifiable. Most trials therefore involve the comparison of two or more operations.

Pilot Experiments

If a new operation is to be compared with an established one, it must be tried out on a few carefully selected patients first, to discover whether or not it is a practicable and desirable form of treatment. A full-scale trial should be undertaken only when the results of the pilot experiment are favorable.

Multicenter Trials

Sometimes two or more medical centers may agree to pool their resources in a joint trial with the object of obtaining sufficient patients quickly. Such a scheme can be successful but is fraught with difficulties. The more people involved in planning a trial, the longer it will take to agree about its details and the more difficult it will be to ensure uniformity of the selection criteria, of the procedures to be undertaken, and of the assessment of results.

Telling the Patient

Opinions differ about whether a patient should be told that his treatment will be decided by random selection. If he is knowledgable and wants to know the details, he must be told and his cooperation obtained. If he has a preference (as may happen, for instance, if he is a physician or the relative of one), it must of course be respected, but he cannot then be included in the trial. If the patient is content to accept any treatment that the surgeon advises, it is probably better not to tell him.

Standardization of Operations

The precise details of the operations to be performed must be decided before the start of the trial, and all the surgeons must do them in the same way. If any of the surgeons is not experienced in one or more of them, he should spend sufficient time learning to do them well before taking part in the trial.

Protocol

Before a trial is started, a complete protocol should be drawn up and agreed upon by all concerned, including the statistician. The protocol should state the precise purpose, the types of patient to be included and excluded, the method of allocation, the forms of treatment to be employed, the methods and times of assessment, the end point of the trial, and all other important details.

ALLOCATION OF PATIENTS

It is essential that the patients in each group should be similar and that they be distinguished only by the method of treatment. To ensure this the types of patient to be treated and the indications for operation are decided first. Then the patients who fulfill the criteria are allocated at random to one of the treatment groups. No other system of allocation may be used, and clearly all the patients must be suitable for all the treatment forms being compared. The decision that a patient is suitable for the trial is best taken jointly by two or more members of the team. If there are special reasons (including the patient's wishes) for preferring one form of treatment to another, it should of course be used and the patient excluded from the trial. It is not admissible to include him if the system of randomization selects the preferred operation and to exclude him if it selects another.

The simplest form of randomization is to prepare a series of well-shuffled, sealed envelopes containing cards labeled "operation A" or "operation B" in equal numbers, and to draw a card immediately before the operation. Sometimes the allocation cannot be made until the operation has been started and the surgeon is satisfied by the pathologic findings that any one of the treatment forms would be feasible. Under these circumstances the anesthesiologist or a nurse may be asked to draw the card. Once it has been drawn, the decision is binding. Other methods of selecting the operation to be undertaken, such as operation A on even dates and operation B on odd dates, are used sometimes but are not truly random and are open to objections.

As pointed out, often other factors, besides the nature of the operation, influence the result. Age, sex, the severity of the disease, and so on are often important and must be represented equally in the different groups. If the numbers are large enough, say 50 or more in each group, the system just described can usually be relied upon to ensure an approximately equal distribution. When the numbers are small, the technique of "paired stratification" is very helpful. The patients are divided into subgroups, defined by the factors known to influence the result. The first member of each pair of patients (if two operations are being compared) in each subgroup is treated by one procedure and the second patient by the other. A random method is used to decide which patient in each pair undergoes operation A and which operation B. The allocation of each patient to a subgroup should usually be made by agreement between two or more members of the team.

An example will make this clear. Suppose that radical mastectomy (R) is being compared with simple mastectomy plus radiotherapy (S) for the treatment of mammary cancer. Whatever method is used, the result will be influenced by the patient's age, by her menstrual or menopausal status, and by the clinical staging of the disease. (For the purposes of the trial it has been decided that patients staged T_4, N_2, or M_1 will be excluded; those with T_3 will be included if the size of the tumor is the only reason for placing them in this category.) The patients may therefore be classified as follows:

---

1. *Age* (years)
   a. 21–30
   b. 31–40
   c. 41–50
   d. 51–60
   e. 61–70
   f. 71–80
   g. 81–90
2. *Menopausal status* (natural or artificial)
   a. Menstruating
   b. Menopause within past 10 years
   c. Menopause more than 10 years previously
3. *Clinical staging*
   a. T_1 N_0
   b. T_1 N_1
   c. T_2 N_0
   d. T_2 N_1
   e. T_3 N_0
   f. T_3 N_1

Theoretically there are $7 \times 3 \times 6$ or 126 sub-groups. In practice it is rare for a postmenopausal patient to be under 30 or a premenopausal patient over 60, so that the effective number of subgroups is 78.

In each subgroup (e.g., 1a, 2b, 3c—patients aged 51–60, less than 10 years postmenopausal, and with $T_2 N_0$ lesions), the pairs may be arranged as follows:

	PATIENT	
Pair I	1	S
	2	R
Pair II	1	S
	2	R
Pair III	1	R
	2	S
Pair IV	1	S
	2	R
Pair V	1	R
	2	S
Etc.		

It should be emphasized that radical mastectomy and simple mastectomy plus radiotherapy are represented in each pair and that their order is decided at random, for example by the toss of a coin. The appropriate lists are prepared beforehand and are consulted as each patient enters the trial to determine the treatment to be used.

ASSESSMENT OF RESULTS

After all the operations have been completed, the results must be assessed by accurate observation. Every effort must be made to follow all the patients for as long as is needed to determine the outcome and, when necessary, until they die. If patients are lost to follow-up, the comparisons can rarely be conclusive.

The observations must be complete. It is essential to prepare a checklist of the data to be recorded at certain predetermined times and to have a form prepared for each patient in which the findings are recorded. The investigator keeps this, but the relevant information should be recorded in the patient's case sheet also. The observations must be as objective as possible. Objectivity is achieved in three ways: (1) by making measurements, (2) by using independent observers, and (3) by employing "blind" techniques.

The measurements may be simple clinical ones, such as the patient's height and weight, the size of a lump measured with calipers, the circumference of a limb, the range of movement of a joint, and so on. Quantitative laboratory tests should be undertaken whenever possible, and to minimize errors all the tests in all groups of patients should be done in the same laboratory by the same methods.

Independent observers, who have no vested interest in the forms of treatment used, can usually assess the results of treatment more objectively and accurately than the surgeon who undertakes them; but they should be people who are thoroughly familiar with the clinical problems involved. Two or more working together should reach an agreed assessment.

The double-blind technique involves neither the patient nor the observer knowing what form of treatment was used. It provides the best possible insurance against subjective bias and should be used whenever possible. With the single-blind technique the observer, but not the patient, knows. A double-blind procedure is quite feasible when, for instance, drugs and placebos or different types of operation for peptic ulcer are being compared. It is obviously impossible when an operation is being compared with a drug or when two operations under trial require different incisions (e.g., hypophysectomy and adrenalectomy). Such limitations must sometimes be accepted.

The detailed attention that is paid to each patient ensures a very high standard of medical care, higher perhaps than that provided in any other circumstances.

ANALYSIS OF THE DATA

When the data have been collected, they must be analyzed by appropriate statistical methods, and each characteristic or measurement should be analyzed separately. This will usually be the statistician's responsibility. If the patients have been paired, complete pairs only should be used for analysis. If the subgroups are large enough, comparisons may be made between them. If pairing has not been used, factors such as age, sex, and the severity of the disease, which may influence the outcome, must be examined to ensure that they are represented similarly in the different treatment groups.

The purpose of a statistical test is to discover how likely it is that observed differences between groups of patients could have arisen by chance alone. The result can never be a definite "yes" or "no," but only that once in, say, 20, 100, or 1000 times it might have done so. Such differences are described as being "significant" at the 5 percent, 1 percent, and 0.1 percent levels, respectively, and the smaller these "probability" or P values are, the more likely it is that the differences are real. The fact that a difference is statistically significant does not necessarily imply that it is *important*. Its importance depends on how large it is and on whether or not it matters enough for other reasons for it to be taken into account.

Two main types of statistical test are used. The first is *qualitative*, in which the patients in each group who have a particular characteristic are counted. Examples are the number who die or whose disease recurs within a certain time. The "incidences" of these characteristics are then compared by means of the χ^2 test.

The second type of test is *quantitative*. The measurements made on each patient allow arithmetical means and standard deviations for each variable to be calculated and compared by means of Student's *t*-test. This type of test, in which every patient contributes a numerical value instead of only a "0" or a "1," is usually more informative than the χ^2 and allows significant differences to emerge from smaller numbers of patients.

A simple and elegant method of keeping a running account of the statistical score in paired trials is a *sequential analysis*, in which the critical observations about each pair of patients are recorded on a prepared diagram as they are made. The diagram is drawn so that it can be seen at a glance when the data reveal a significant difference (at any desired and previously agreed level) between the two forms of treatment or when they indicate that no significant difference is likely to emerge, at least for a very long time. This form of test can be used for both qualitative and quantitative data so that, for practical purposes, it provides the equivalent of a χ^2 test or of a *t*-test with the results of a running analysis always readily available. It may be used to advantage when the results will be available quickly, as in an investigation of the treatment of a condition with a high early mortality rate (e.g., acute pancreatitis) or of the prevention of early postoperative complications. It is not suitable for analysis of long-term results.

Other more sophisticated statistical methods are required sometimes, especially when more than two forms of treatment are being compared or when quantitative data are not distributed normally. The statistician will advise on the appropriate techniques.

The storage and analysis of data are helped greatly by the use of a computer, especially if the numbers of patients and observations on each patient are large. Suitable programming allows tabulation and analysis of the data to be written out on demand at any time.

STOPPING THE TRIAL

A very important decision, which must be made in every clinical trial, is when to stop it. The criteria for the end point must be decided before the trial begins, and its progress must be kept under review constantly as the work proceeds. Clearly the trial must be stopped *either* when a significant *and important* difference has emerged between the groups *or* when it is apparent that no large and significant difference is likely to appear within a reasonable period of time. It is usually advisable (as in any scientific experiment) to work to a 1 percent level of significance, but there are sometimes occasions when a 5 percent (or even a 10 percent) level is acceptable, as when a new method of treatment is apparently giving worse results than an accepted one. If a trial is stopped before these conditions are met, no conclusion will be reached and it might as well never have been started.

OUTCOME OF THE TRIAL

When the trial is completed, the whole situation must be reviewed. Often one method of treatment is better in some respects and worse in others. One operation, for instance, may cure the disease more effectively than another but produce more unpleasant side effects. All the similarities and differences, however, will have been established in statistical terms, and information will therefore be available on which a responsible judgment may be made. It is important to remember that the results are valid only for the types of patient who were studied. If, for instance, one procedure was found to be better than another in a trial in men with advanced disease, it cannot be inferred that it would be better also in men with early disease or in women. As a result of the trial those who conducted it may change their surgical practice, and when the results are published, others may be persuaded to do so too. A new trial may then perhaps be planned in which the better procedure is compared with another.

CONCLUSION

References are given below to some controlled trials that have been undertaken in surgery. A study of the papers will show that they have been at least as valuable in refuting claims that some procedures are better than others as in establishing clear differences. It is also clear from the paper by Lionel and Herxheimer that many so-called controlled trials have not been undertaken properly and that their conclusions are therefore invalid.

The controlled trial is so vital and fundamental a method of clinical research that, except in the rare circumstance when a new method is clearly and overwhelmingly better than any that has been used before, no surgeon should presume to advocate one operation or other form of treatment over another unless it has been submitted to the type of disciplined observation that has been described.

SUGGESTIONS FOR FURTHER READING

GENERAL REVIEWS

Chalmers, T. C.; Black, J. B.; and Lee, S.: Controlled studies in clinical cancer research. *N. Engl. J. Med.*, **287**:75–78, 1972.
Ingelfinger, F. J.: The randomized clinical trial. *N. Engl. J. Med.*, **287**:100–101, 1972.
Lionel, N. D. W., and Herxheimer, A.: Assessing reports of therapeutic trials. *Br. Med. J.*, **3**:637–40, 1970.

BREAST CANCER—EARLY

Atkins, H. J. B.; Hayward, J. L.; Klugman, D. J., *et al.*: Treatment of early breast cancer: a report after 10 years of clinical trial. *Br. Med. J.*, **2**:423–29, 1972.

BREAST CANCER—ADVANCED

Atkins, H. J. B.; Falconer, M. A.; Hayward, J. L., *et al.*: Adrenalectomy and hypophysectomy for advanced cancer of the breast. *Lancet*, **1**:489–96, 1957.
Dao, T. L.: Early compared with late adrenalectomy. In Joslin, C. A. F., and Gleave, E. N. (eds.): *The Clinical Management of Advanced Breast Cancer*. Second Tenovus Workshop, 1970. Cardiff: Alpha Omega Alpha.

DEEP VENOUS THROMBOSIS

Hills, N. H.; Pflug, J. J.; Jeyasingh, K., *et al.*: Prevention of deep vein thrombosis by intermittent pneumatic compression of calf. *Br. Med. J.*, **1**:131–35, 1972.

GASTRIC SURGERY

Goligher, J. C.; Pulvertaft, C. N.; De Dombal, F. T., *et al.*: Five to eight year results of Leeds/York controlled trial of elective surgery for duodenal ulcer. *Br. Med. J.*, **2**:781–87, 1968.

UNIT II

TOTAL CARE OF THE SURGICAL PATIENT

Chapter 9

MODERN CONCEPTS IN THE CARE OF THE CRITICALLY INJURED

David R. Boyd

CHAPTER OUTLINE

General Principles
  Initial Resuscitation
    Establishment of an Airway
    Ventilatory Failure
    Cardiopulmonary Arrest
    Treatment of Shock
  Clinical Evaluation
    Physical Survey

History
Regional Anatomic Evaluation
  Head and Neck
  Thoracic Chest and Thoracic Cavity
  Abdominal Injuries
  Extremity Injuries
  Special Investigations
Summary

The initial identification and early care of a critical injury are crucial to a successful outcome after major trauma. The responsibility for proper early care belongs to all health professionals and others, including law enforcement officers, who commonly attend the acutely injured. Programs to upgrade patient care by providing a ready availability of optimal medical care for the injured are now being initiated statewide in Illinois[4] and in selected communities across the nation.[2,12] A statewide comprehensive total systems approach must extend from the scene of the accident and on through the rehabilitation phase after major injury. Ambulance attendants, allied health personnel, nurses, and physicians will need to participate in this new approach.

With the mechanization of our society the number of serious injuries from vocational and recreational activities has increased. In 1972 the National Safety Council reported 11 million injuries from all types of accidents.[15] Wage losses, medical expenses, and insurance administrative costs resulting from trauma totaled $13½ billion. The estimated overall cost of this pandemic is over $30 billion annually.[6,14] There are about 100,000 civilian accidental deaths annually, of which one half are due to vehicular accidents.[17] The one-millionth traffic fatality occurred in 1951, and if the present rate continues, the two-millionth victim will die by 1976.[8] Accidents are currently the third most common cause of death in the United States, being only slightly less than death from cardiovascular disease and cancer.[13] Trauma is our leading cause of death in individuals under 40 years. There are over 15 million injuries to children under 14 years annually and of these 16,000 are fatal.[7] Trauma is the commonest cause of death in children, the peak incidence being from 2 to 3 years. One third of all hospital admissions, approximately two million a year, are the result of accidents.[11] In one study pediatric patients accounted for 47 percent of all emergency room visits, and of these one quarter were treated for trauma.[7]

Presently there is much interest in this previously neglected surgical and community health problem.[6] A significant improvement in the care of the critically injured can only be achieved by improving the clinical skills of all professionals and allied health workers involved with the accident victim. Physician training must begin with the medical student and continue to postgraduate education in emergency medicine, trauma surgery, and critical care medicine.

GENERAL PRINCIPLES

A satisfactory outcome after severe traumatic injury depends on two basic factors: the availability of initial medical care and the adequacy of early treatment. Delays in proper resuscitation and evaluation in life-endangering injuries are critical for survival. Injudicious or inadequate emergency management can cause unnecessary fatalities and permanent disabilities. A reevaluation and reeducation of the priorities and techniques of trauma patient care are essential. New developments in the surgical specialties and biomedical disciplines have been responsible for major progress in trauma management.

The physician's first objective in examining an injured person is to preserve life. When dealing with acute trauma, it is impossible to separate diagnostic and therapeutic measures. The techniques for resuscitation do not depend on the etiology. Airway obstruction, shock, and cardiorespiratory failure are treated similarly without knowing the precipitating cause. When stabilized, the patient is rapidly and thoroughly evaluated for the cause of the derangements.

Although the steps in management are inseparable and performed simultaneously, it is convenient to discuss them separately under the headings Initial Resuscitation and Clinical Evaluation. Resuscitation consists of those procedures that must be instituted to maintain life; evaluation is the diagnostic measures necessary after the patient has been stabilized. The principles and techniques are based on experience gained since 1966 at the Trauma Unit of Cook County Hospital in the care of over 28,000 seriously injured patients. The Trauma Unit is a specialized facility staffed and equipped to cope with life-threatening emergencies. It is a centralized area where all essential resources are concentrated for the patients' comprehensive resuscitation, evaluation, and perioperative needs, but the principles can be effectively utilized in the emergency department of any hospital. The trauma patient, because of the possible complexity and severity of his injuries, should be separated from other patients in any emergency room by "streamlining" his evacuation through the admitting and the x-ray departments into an intensive care area. In this specialized area the patient is recognized as a special problem. Shock, aspiration, respiratory distress, and cardiopulmonary arrest can be avoided by close surveillance for the warning signs of these catastrophes. Should such a complication occur, adequately trained physicians, nurses, and paramedical personnel are available to institute effective therapy. Many patients go into shock during transport or in regions where trained personnel are not in attendance. The main operative room of a small community hospital is the best place to observe the seriously injured patient.[1] After adequate resuscitation a complete and systematic evaluation is made for all possible injuries. The patient can then be moved safely to other areas in the hospital or transported to another hospital better equipped to handle complex traumatic problems. In a specialized area the magnitude and urgency of the patient's illness command the attention of the Trauma Unit staff. This is possible through the use of *triage*, the sorting of patients based on priorities. Implicit in the design of this system is a chain of command. Patients with complex multiple-systems injuries require the skills of many specialists, but a successful final outcome depends on one physician remaining in charge during the entire course of the illness. Most often this is the surgeon with the broadest training and interests.

After resuscitation and evaluation a priority list is established and definitive management is undertaken. It is possible that not all the injuries will be treated during the acute period. However, knowledge about their presence and their supportive management is necessary to prevent progressive damage while attention is given to more urgent problems.

The initial evaluation at the accident scene, during transport, or at the trauma treatment area must begin with a rapid overall examination. While this is primarily visual and auditory, much information can be gained by quick but thorough palpation. The rapid assessment of the vital life functions and a quick survey of gross deformities and injuries will set the stage for further diagnosis, priority setting, and treatment. This initial evaluation must begin before the patient is moved or disrobed (Figure 9–1, *A*). Injudicious or aggressive manipulation may aggravate some undetected injury or worsen an already compensated vital function. The proper evaluation of the acutely injured requires a series of repeated examinations starting with the most superficial and progressing to the more sophisticated, as life-threatening problems are identified and satisfactorily resolved. The necessary reevaluation process starts immediately and continues for an extended period, usually hours, and, not uncommonly, over several days.

When immediate life-threatening problems have been controlled, a complete evaluation is then possible to assess the full extent of injuries. This is the time to document all those preexisting medical conditions that will influence the course of management. Patient resuscitation is then directed to the adequacy of ventilation, circulation, and the control of blood loss. Other injuries lead to slower deterioration of the patient's condition and therefore have a lower initial priority in the emergency management. They will be discussed in the section on Clinical Evaluation.

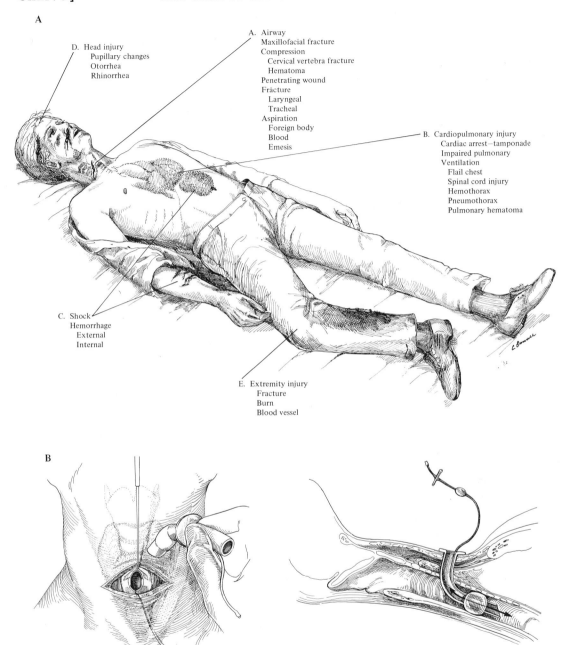

A. Airway
      Maxillofacial fracture
      Compression
          Cervical vertebra fracture
          Hematoma
      Penetrating wound
      Fracture
          Laryngeal
          Tracheal
      Aspiration
          Foreign body
          Blood
          Emesis

D. Head injury
      Pupillary changes
      Otorrhea
      Rhinorrhea

B. Cardiopulmonary injury
      Cardiac arrest—tamponade
      Impaired pulmonary
      Ventilation
          Flail chest
          Spinal cord injury
          Hemothorax
          Pneumothorax
          Pulmonary hematoma

C. Shock
      Hemorrhage
      External
      Internal

E. Extremity injury
      Fracture
      Burn
      Blood vessel

Figure 9–1. *A*. A critically injured patient following an automobile accident may have an obstructed airway, abnormal cardiopulmonary dynamics, external bleeding, and grossly distorted extremities.

B. Technique of performing a tracheostomy. A tracheostomy is only performed as an emergency procedure on the rare occasion when it is not possible to insert an endotracheal tube.

The head is well extended and the trachea is approached through a transverse incision. Part of a tracheal ring is removed below the isthmus of the thyroid and the tracheostomy tube is inserted. Care is taken not to insert too long a tube or it may pass beyond the bifurcation of the trachea and enter one of the main bronchi.

Initial Resuscitation

Establishment of an Airway.   The first priority in any trauma patient is to establish and maintain the airway by inserting an oropharyngeal airway or an endotracheal tube. Only rarely is a tracheostomy needed as an emergency procedure (see Figure 9–1, *B*; Chapter 12). An oropharyngeal airway is easy to insert but does not prevent aspiration of blood or gastric content. The most effective and safest procedure is to insert a cuffed endotracheal tube.

Patients with depressed consciousness from intoxications, cerebral injury, or shock are most likely to aspirate foreign material such as blood, food, vomitus, or dentures. A pharyngeal block with adequate aspiration and removal of foreign materials is mandatory. The patient must be closely observed and suctioned frequently. He must not be allowed to lie flat on his back, unattended and restrained in this position. The semiprone position is satisfactory. Some common causes of upper airway obstruction are edema of the mouth, tongue, posterior pharyngeal wall, and epiglottis. Hemorrhage and penetrating wounds of these parts are particularly dangerous. A cervical spine injury with vertebral subluxation and hematoma formation can cause obstruction of the upper airway. Severe maxillofacial trauma with obliteration of the nasal passage will contribute to the obstruction. A history of steering wheel injury, respiratory distress with stridor, and a contusion of the neck must alert one to the possibility of a fracture of the larynx, trachea, or cervical vertebra. Endotracheal intubation is not possible, and an emergency tracheostomy may be necessary (see Chapter 2, pages 42–43). When manipulating the head and neck for such procedures, one must be aware of the state of the cervical spine. A patient with only abdominal breathing may have a cervical vertebral dislocation with injury to the spinal cord. Rough manipulation may complete a partial transection of the spinal cord. Vascular injuries of the neck with hematoma formation may be troublesome and require control of the airway. Combative patients with hypoxia from airway obstruction or major chest injuries can be safely intubated after a rapidly acting neuromuscular depolarizing agent has been given (see Chapter 12, pages 228–29).

Ventilatory Failure.   Trauma patients can rapidly develop respiratory embarrassment from an obstructed airway, when the central nervous system stimuli to the respiratory muscles fail, or when the mechanical ventilation is restricted. Ventilatory arrest with asphyxia can only be tolerated for generally less than four minutes, after which irreversible brain damage occurs. Thus ventilatory failure from whatever cause must be directly and aggressively corrected and has the highest priority for initial evaluation and reevaluation in every trauma or seriously ill surgical patient.

Chest injuries must be evaluated immediately and correctly because of the severe impairment that may occur. Penetrating injuries, rib fractures, and major blunt forces can disrupt pleura, lung parenchyma, trachea, or bronchial structures, or cause major vascular injuries. Subsequent pulmonary collapse with hemothorax, pneumothorax, or even a tension pneumothorax, as well as major hemorrhage, can produce catastrophic results immediately or at almost any time in the acute posttraumatic period. An open pneumothorax from a penetrating wound of the chest must be covered with a moist dressing (see Chapter 30, pages 530–31). A tension pneumothorax must be treated immediately by insertion of a large-bore needle in the midclavicular line anteriorly in the second or third intercostal space (see Chapter 30, page 531).

Cardiopulmonary Arrest.   After the upper airway is secure, attention must be directed to cardiopulmonary dynamics (see Chapter 2, pages 42–90). Severe hypoxia, acidosis, and direct chest trauma are responsible for cardiac arrest. When arrest has occurred, mouth-to-mouth resuscitation, or in-hospital "ambuing or bagging," must be employed immediately, followed by endotracheal intubation. Closed chest massage is preferred and is effective unless the chest wall is unstable. An emergency thoracotomy and manual cardiac compression are seldom necessary (see Chapter 14, pages 255–56). Adequate ventilation with an "Ambu" bag supplying extra oxygen is provided simultaneously. Intravenous injection of sodium bicarbonate corrects the associated metabolic acidosis. Initial and periodic arterial blood gases and pH analyses and electrocardiographic monitoring are essential. Cardiac defibrillation may be necessary because the heart is hypoxic and acidotic and is prone to arrhythmias, fibrillation, and asystole.

Treatment of Shock.   External hemorrhage can be controlled readily by direct manual pressure. Continued gentle pressure is often all that is necessary until the patient is taken to the operating room where vascular repair may be possible. There is no place for application of a tourniquet or clamping and ligation of bleeding vessels. After hemostasis has been obtained, blood volume should be restored. Blood should be given after a major blood loss.

The magnitude of blood loss can be estimated by clinical observation. Keen observation of

Table 9–1. CATEGORIES OF TRAUMA-HEMORRHAGE ASSESSMENT AND TREATMENT

Grade I—Minor Blood Loss:
    10–15% of blood volume (500–750 ml)
Clinical findings
    Well compensated
    Dizziness
    Tachycardia (100/min)
Etiology
    External loss
        Blood donation
        Laceration
    Internal loss
        Hematoma
        Extremity fractures
        Hemothorax
Treatment
    Control hemorrhage
    Crystalloid infusion

Grade II—Moderate Blood Loss:
    15–30% of blood volume (750–1500 ml)
Clinical findings
    Partial compensation
    Cool, sweating skin
    Thirst, anxiety
    Tachycardia (110/min)
    Tachypnea (24/min)
    Slight hypotension (90–100 mm Hg)
    Decrease in pulse pressure
Etiology
    External loss
        Major laceration
    Internal loss
        Visceral injury, e.g., spleen
        Fractured femur
Treatment
    Control hemorrhage
    Crystalloid and colloid infusion
    Oxygen administration
    Evaluate obscure bleeding

Grade III—Major Blood Loss:
    30–45% of blood volume (1500–2250 ml)
Clinical findings
    Decompensation
    Pale, cold, clammy skin
    Restless, agitation
    Tachycardia (120/min)
    Tachypnea (32/min)
    Hypotension (less than 80 mm Hg)
    Oliguria (30 ml/hr)
    Metabolic acidosis
Etiology
    External loss
        Vascular injury
    Internal loss
        Visceral injuries, e.g., liver rupture
        Pelvic fracture
Treatment
    Control hemorrhage
    Crystalloid, colloid, and blood infusion
    Oxygen and bicarbonate administration
    Physiologic monitoring

Grade IV—Massive Blood Loss:
    Over 45% of blood volume (over
    2250 ml)
Clinical findings
    Marked pallor, cyanosis
    Semiconscious
    Tachycardia (over 200/min)
    Respiratory distress
    Profound hypotension (less than 50 mm Hg)
    Anuria
    Metabolic acidosis
Etiology
    External loss
        Traumatic amputation
    Internal loss
        Vascular or aortic rupture
        Multiple injuries
Treatment
    Control hemorrhage
    Oxygen administration
    Blood, colloid, and crystalloid infusion
    Bicarbonate administration
    Cardiac monitoring
    Antibiotics

physiologic signs and an accurate assessment of all potential injuries can provide a working basis for initiating shock therapy and blood replacement. The severity of traumatic hemorrhage can be effectively graded or categorized into minor (I), moderate (II), major (III), and massive (IV) for initial assessment and to anticipate immediate treatments (Table 9–1). Subsequent patient improvement or failure of an adequate treatment response can be measured and reassessed in relation to these trauma-hemorrhage categories (see Table 9–1).

The normal circulating blood volume in a 150-lb (70-kg) adult is approximately 5 liters. Small injuries with minor (grade I) blood loss of less than 10 to 15 percent (500 to 750 ml) may cause no apparent physiologic changes. This type of hemorrhage may be caused by blood donation venisection, a laceration, or bleeding into a distal extremity fracture site. The treatment is simply control of further hemorrhage and blood replacement by crystalloid solution.

A moderate (grade II) hemorrhagic loss of 15 to 30 percent of the circulating blood volume (750 to 1500 ml) should be well compensated for in most otherwise healthy individuals. The injured patient with this degree of injury should demonstrate many of the visible signs of physiologic compensation (see Table 9–1): cool skin, slight tachycardia (110/min), tachypnea (24/min), a fall in pulse pressure, and possibly a small decrease in systolic blood pressure. These effects are caused by significant injuries such as ruptured spleen or a major femoral shaft fracture. Treatment is hemorrhage control and the rapid infusion of blood substitutes, crystalloid and colloid solutions (plasma or albumin). Oxygen should be administered by mask. If hemorrhage is controlled, blood replacement is not necessary, and 2 to 3 liters of crystalloid-colloid infusates will suffice.

Major (grade III) hemorrhage with a loss of 30 to 45 percent of the effective circulating blood volume (1500 to 2250 ml) will cause marked physiologic decompensation. This classic "shock" patient has cold, clammy skin, is restless, and has a tachycardia (120/min), tachypnea (32/min), and hypotension (less than 80 mm Hg); he will also be oliguric and have a marked metabolic acidosis.

Obvious points of external loss from a major vessel or severe internal injuries (lacerated liver or pelvic fractures) should be the suspected lesions. Whole blood replacement for resuscitation must be included in addition to those measures discussed above. Bicarbonate ($NaHCO_3$) must be administered to combat the metabolic acidosis of shock, and these patients will need repeated physiologic monitoring of systolic blood and central venous pressures, urinary output, hematocrit, and arterial blood gases. The seriously ill patient can be effectively resuscitated if therapy is appropriate to a sound diagnosis, a correct interpretation of the physiologic derangements, and those pathophysiologic signs readily detectable by the astute clinician.

Massive (grade IV) blood loss is a catastrophic situation in which the extent of loss (over 45 percent) has gone uncorrected and the patient is first seen in extremis. The physiologic compensatory mechanisms have failed, and now many of these have become pathologic and are effecting further detriment to the patient.

This patient may be cyanotic, with marked pallor, have a severe and irregular tachycardia, respiratory distress, marked hypotension (less than 50 mm Hg), and complete anuria. Patients with catastrophic losses of over 45 percent of their effective circulating blood volumes are severely prostrated, hypoxic, and unresponsive. If not vigorously resuscitated, they will progress to cardiopulmonary arrest.

Multiple severe trauma will cause these effects, but, more important, such injuries and even lesser trauma can deteriorate to this state if hemorrhage is not initially controlled and "physiologic" therapy is not correctly administered. These patients, unfortunately, often represent a "systems failure" or a "patient management failure," where the proper trauma care was not given early enough to prevent this deteriorated state.

Blood Volume Replacement. For initial volume replacement intravenous infusion of moderate volumes of a buffered saline solution (lactated Ringer's) is satisfactory. It is necessary to replace approximately two to three times as much of this crystalloid solution as the amount of estimated blood loss. The oxygen-carrying capacity of hemoglobin is diminished by the hemodilution. It is safe in most patients without previous cardiovascular disease to maintain the hematocrit at 30 to 35 percent. There has been considerable argument about the equilibration period for blood after hemorrhage. The hematocrit determination has certain limitations during acute changes, but serial measurements provide valuable information about hypovolemic shock. No other parameter, including blood volume determinations, has proved more helpful during this acute period.[18] The management of shock is facilitated by repeated observations of blood pressure, heart rate, respiratory rate, skin temperature, central venous pressure, and urinary output. An increase in systolic blood pressure and a decrease in pulse and respiratory rates herald successful resuscitation. A return of normal skin temperature and urinary output and improved state of consciousness attests to the restoration of adequate tissue perfusion.

There is little place for the use of plasma expanders such as low-molecular-weight dextran in treating hemorrhagic shock, but they are still important in treating burns. The best treatment for a major blood loss is the administration of cross-matched, type-specific whole blood. The time for grouping and cross matching varies from 30 to 60 minutes. The patient who has had a major hemorrhage and in whom lactated Ringer's solution would result in excessive hemodilution should receive RH-negative, type O blood. Vasopressors or steroids should not be given to patients in hemorrhagic shock.

Central venous pressure (CVP) monitoring is one of the most significant advances in managing shock patients. An intravenous catheter is inserted into the superior vena cava. A venous blood sample is taken for type and cross match, blood counts, and biochemical tests, and an infusion of lactated Ringer's solution is started. The central venous pressure is monitored intermittently through the catheter in the superior vena cava using a simple water manometer.[19]

The pressure readings are not a measure of "blood volume" as previously interpreted but reflect a dynamic state between the adequacy of the venous return and the pumping action of the right ventricle. Absolute values are not as important as relative changes observed over time. Typically in hypovolemic shock the CVP is below normal values of 4 to 8 cm of saline. With adequate volume replacement a rise in CVP and systolic blood pressure occurs. A persistently low CVP after adequate volume replacement should stimulate a search for occult bleeding. Blood losses into fracture sites, especially the major long bones or pelvis, occult rupture of the liver or spleen, and collections in silent areas such as the pleural cavity and the retroperitoneal space must be considered. An elevated central venous pressure and low systemic blood pressure suggest a pericardial tamponade, myocardial infarction, or acute congestive heart failure. Changes in the quality of the heart tones, cardiac rhythm, electrocardiographic findings, and the response to volume loading are helpful in these patients.

Clinical Evaluation

Physical Survey. After successful resuscitation the critically ill trauma patient must be continually evaluated for possible deterioration of any vital function. This assessment includes careful observation of the level of consciousness, spontaneous motion of the extremities, chest excursion, abdominal habitus, and injured regions. All patients are disrobed and totally examined, including a complete physical examination. Deformities or asymmetry of body parts, lacerations, and contusions demand special attention. A rapid assessment of the extent of injuries is performed by gentle but firm palpation of all body parts, especially where injuries are suspected. Palpation of the scalp, facial bones, trachea, and vertebral column, as well as gentle compression of the thorax, ribs, pelvis, and extremities, will elicit hidden fractures and dislocations and lead to intelligent and precise requests for x-rays. Local tenderness, crepitation of subcutaneous air, and grating of bony parts will suggest a diagnosis. The chest is auscultated for signs of pleural collapse, rub, and effusion. Changes in heart tones and the occurrence of murmurs in the chest or over extremities will be diagnostic of vascular injuries. A careful abdominal examination for peritoneal irritation and distention is mandatory. Rectal and pelvic examinations are routinely performed. Checking the palpable pulses, temperature, and the neuromuscular tone of all extremities is necessary.

This initial rapid physical examination must be followed by an in-depth evaluation of each regional anatomic area and its relevant physiologic systems. Those with obvious injuries will be carefully scrutinized, but this must not cause the examiner to concentrate only on the most apparent injuries. A continual search for the less obvious hidden occult injuries must complete the examination.

A patient with multiple injuries from an automobile accident will require such a rapid and repeated examination. As shown in Figure 9-1, much information can be obtained by simple observation. One can observe cranial, facial, and laryngeal injuries. This observation, along with the respiratory noises caused by blood and aspirated materials, is enough to appraise initially the adequacy of the upper airway. High-pitched and rattling breath sounds will dictate the obvious, necessary first resuscitative steps.

A quick appraisal of the state of consciousness, arousal, and pupillary reflexes will give one an advantage in evaluating the frequency, depth, and adequacy of spontaneous ventilatory efforts. Thoracic contusions, bony irregularities, open wounds, asymmetric paradoxical movements, or lack of intercostal muscle activity will provide adequate information for instituting the proper life-saving measures.

Hemorrhage may be obvious, as demonstrated in the forearm laceration. However, unexplained shock may be due to an occult injury, and blood loss may be occurring into the pleural space (hemothorax), into the peritoneal cavity from a ruptured viscus (hemoperitoneum), or into the soft tissue around fractures or major burn sites.

The obvious external rotation and shortening provide the necessary preliminary diagnosis and allow one to assign a lesser priority of care while simultaneously positioning the injured limb to prevent unnecessary further injury. Simple identification, dressing, and splinting of all soft tissue and extremity injuries of scalp, forearm, and leg are all that are necessary initially. To attempt more definitive care at this juncture will probably give less than optimal results and may detract the physician from other and possibly less obvious critical injuries. This initial evaluation and care can and should be performed at the accident scene or in the emergency department before the patient is transported. At this time as much information as possible is obtained from clinical examination and interviewing. All critical information must be gained as soon as possible.

The patient is shown as observed in an emergency department or trauma care hospital (Figure 9-2). He is completely disrobed for adequate observation and care. The airway has been established and maintained by an

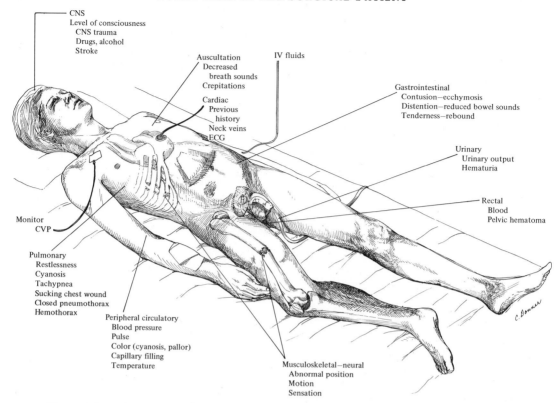

CNS
Level of consciousness
CNS trauma
Drugs, alcohol
Stroke

Auscultation
Decreased
breath sounds
Crepitations

IV fluids

Cardiac
Previous
history
Neck veins
ECG

Gastrointestinal
Contusion—ecchymosis
Distention—reduced bowel sounds
Tenderness—rebound

Urinary
Urinary output
Hematuria

Rectal
Blood
Pelvic hematoma

Monitor
CVP

Pulmonary
Restlessness
Cyanosis
Tachypnea
Sucking chest wound
Closed pneumothorax
Hemothorax

Peripheral circulatory
Blood pressure
Pulse
Color (cyanosis, pallor)
Capillary filling
Temperature

Musculoskeletal—neural
Abnormal position
Motion
Sensation

Figure 9–2. After the patient is disrobed, multiple injuries may be found by observation, palpation, and auscultation. A steering wheel imprint in the chest and upper abdomen suggests the diagnosis of ruptured aorta, fractured liver, or ruptured duodenum or pancreas. Initial resuscitation, including establishment of an adequate airway and management of shock, is instituted. More sophisticated emergency diagnostic procedures such as paracentesis, thoracentesis, pericardicentesis, and proctoscopy are performed as indicated by clinical findings.

endotracheal tube. This is the most direct and sure way and should be among the skills of every physician. In many communities rescue emergency medical technicians are becoming skilled in this and other life-saving techniques. The appropriate form of ventilatory support, open airway, enhanced oxygen supply, ventilatory assist, and blood volume replacement must be started.

Additional information can be readily obtained at this time. Clinical findings must be reevaluated and recorded in order to recognize treatment progress or clinical deterioration. Repeated examination should be performed by the same individual or team of trauma specialists so that reliable and correct management decisions can be made.

History. As thorough a history as possible is obtained. The preinjury health status, factors causing the accident, and the conditions at the scene of the accident are important. Previous medical problems, allergies, medications, or diseases must be elicited prior to operation. This

information must be sought from any source possible as it may be crucial for survival. During this acute period patients have an established airway, two large intravenous catheters (one in the superior vena cava), and a Foley catheter in the urinary bladder. The initial bladder urine specimen and subsequent specimens are sent for analysis. A nasogastric tube is inserted. Any aspirate is inspected and the stomach emptied and kept decompressed by intermittent suction. Fractures and dislocations are immobilized to prevent further injury and relieve pain. Open wounds are inspected, cleaned, and covered with sterile dressings.

Regional Anatomic Evaluation

After the patient is initially evaluated and life-support measures have been instituted, an in-depth regional anatomic and systems examination is performed. This starts at the head and proceeds down the neck, torso, and extremities, and is followed by examination of all body orifices and potential anatomic cavities.

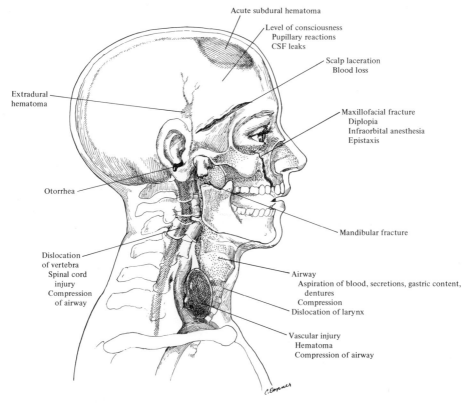

Acute subdural hematoma

Level of consciousness
Pupillary reactions
CSF leaks

Scalp laceration
Blood loss

Extradural
hematoma

Maxillofacial fracture
Diplopia
Infraorbital anesthesia
Epistaxis

Otorrhea

Mandibular fracture

Dislocation
of vertebra
Spinal cord
injury
Compression
of airway

Airway
Aspiration of blood, secretions, gastric content,
dentures
Compression
Dislocation of larynx

Vascular injury
Hematoma
Compression of airway

Figure 9–3.   Severe injuries to the head, face, and neck may affect the upper airway and ventilatory dynamics. These important injuries can be diagnosed or suspected by careful clinical observation and palpation. Because of their significance to overall patient management, they rate a high priority.

Head and Neck (see Plates II and III). Trauma to the head and neck is common and unfortunately many times poorly managed (Figure 9–3). A scalp laceration can account for massive blood loss from the very vascular galea. The location of scalp injuries may relate to cranial fractures. A fracture of the temporal bone at the pterion may tear the middle meningeal vessels and cause an epidural hematoma. Other severe closed head injuries may cause subdural or intracerebral hemorrhage. Otorrhea and rhinorrhea are signs of basilar skull fractures. Pupillary changes and level of consciousness recorded serially accurately indicate cerebral injury.

Pain over the vertebral spinous process should be considered a positive sign of subluxation, and impaired extremity sensation confirms this diagnosis. A simple cross-table spinal x-ray is mandatory in this situation.

Facial contusions, distortion, and asymmetry should alert one to the diagnosis of maxillofacial fracture with resulting significant soft tissue injuries. Diplopia, squint, and infraorbital anesthesia are objective evidence of maxillary fracture with disruption of the visual apparatus and orbit. These injuries can be diagnosed early and must be followed carefully and managed electively in the postresuscitation period.

Soft tissue injuries to the floor of the mouth, hypopharynx, and neck may obstruct the upper airway and may even prevent the passage of an endotracheal airway. Under these circumstances a primary tracheostomy may be indicated to maintain adequate ventilation. All penetrating wounds of the neck should be explored.

Thoracic Chest and Thoracic Cavity (see Plates IV and V). The thoracic cavity and the adequacy of cardiopulmonary function are then evaluated (Figure 9–4). Air and bony crepitus on the hemithorax and a steering wheel contusion suggest severe injuries. A thorough physical, radiographic, biochemical, and electrocardiographic evaluation is needed of the lungs, heart, and aorta. Pulmonary collapse (pneumo-, hemothorax), pulmonary contusion, cardiac injury (ischemia), and a widened mediastinum (ruptured thoracic aorta) are all critical diagnoses

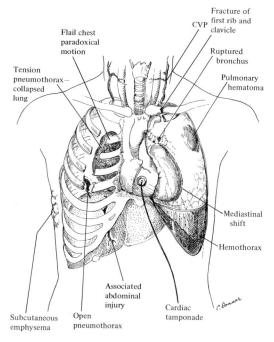

Figure 9–4. Serious chest injuries include hemothorax, pneumothorax, cardiac contusion, and ruptured aorta. If not ascertained early and corrected, they can rapidly result in death. All can be diagnosed or suspected with a high degree of confidence by clinical examination, x-ray, or electrocardiogram.

and demand immediate resolution. Most of the injuries can be diagnosed by clinical evaluation upon first examination. In fact, x-rays and other sophisticated evaluation may not add to the diagnosis and may lose valuable time. After a complete clinical evaluation with observation, palpation, auscultation, and monitoring vital signs (blood pressure, central venous pressure, ECG, and blood gases), the patient can be moved for further x-ray and arteriographic studies.

Most patients with penetrating chest wounds require thoracotomy. In closed chest injuries thoracotomy is only required if there is continued bleeding or decreasing respiratory function (see Chapter 30).

Direct injury to the chest is not necessary for the patient to develop respiratory complications. Acute respiratory distress may occur following injuries to the abdomen or extremities (see Chapter 2). Signs generally do not occur until more than 24 hours after the injury.

Abdominal Injuries (see Plates IV, V, and VIII). A complete abdominal examination is performed and repeated often during the acute post-traumatic period. Peritoneal irritation, splinting

rebound, distention, and hypoactive bowel sounds are significant findings. Abdominal x-rays (posterior, anterior, lateral, and upright) and chest x-rays (posterior, anterior, and lateral) are obtained.

In evaluating abdominal injuries it is important to remember the upper limits of the abdominal cavity and the lower limits of the thoracic cavity (Figure 9–5). The abdominal cavity extends as high as the nipple line anteriorly and the angle of the scapula posteriorly. Injury to the thorax below these levels is liable to result in an injury to the spleen, liver, or kidneys. Since the diaphragm originates from the lower border of the bony thorax, any wound that penetrates the trunk above the level of the rib margin may involve the pleural cavity. The umbilicus is at the level of the posterior pleural sulcus; therefore a penetrating wound above the

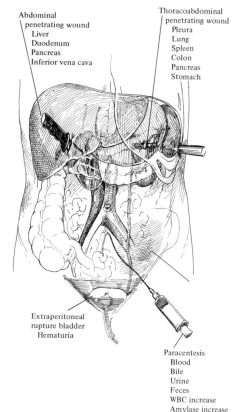

Figure 9–5. Abdominal injuries are the result of blunt or penetrating wounds. Repeated examinations are essential using palpation and auscultation. Abnormal signs in the right upper quadrant suggest injuries to the liver, biliary system, head of the pancreas, duodenum, and inferior vena cava. A penetrating wound in the left upper quadrant may damage the lung, diaphragm, and intra-abdominal organs.

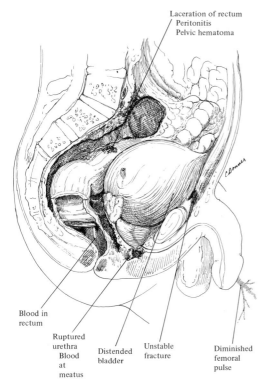

Laceration of rectum
Peritonitis
Pelvic hematoma

Blood in rectum

Ruptured urethra
Blood at meatus

Distended bladder

Unstable fracture

Diminished femoral pulse

Figure 9–6. Extraperitoneal abdominal injuries are often missed. Rectal and vaginal examination and insertion of a catheter are important in establishing the diagnosis.

umbilicus and passing directly backward through the body is likely to involve the pleural cavity.

Rectal and intra-abdominal (extraperitoneal) injuries must also be evaluated as abdominal injuries (Figure 9–6). They often involve the peritoneal cavity and are often confused preoperatively with intra-abdominal injuries. Rectal and vaginal examinations are essential, with special attention paid to possible injuries to the urinary system (see Chapter 32). The possibility of injury to the major pelvic vessels must always be considered.

Types of Injuries. Abdominal injuries may be classified as penetrating or nonpenetrating. Penetrating wounds are most often produced by a knife or bullet and usually involve solid viscera or supporting structures because the hollow organs such as the intestine tend to roll away. Those in the esophagus, stomach, and rectum are often self-inflicted. Shotgun blasts at close range result in massive tissue destruction and numerous intra-abdominal injuries and are often fatal. Shotgun pellets fired at a distance may cause multiple perforations of bowel. High-velocity missiles cause widespread lateral damage because of their enormous kinetic energy

released in the tissues as an explosive force. Wide debridement is necessary because the amount of devitalized tissue is often not immediately apparent. The tissues or organs damaged can be classified as:

1. Solid organs: liver, spleen, kidneys, and pancreas.
2. The hollow organs: esophagus, stomach, small and large bowel, rectum, ureters, and bladder.
3. Supporting structures: mesentery, peritoneal reflections, blood vessels, and the abdominal wall.

PATHOPHYSIOLOGY. Abdominal injuries may be fatal, the result of shock or infection. The most immediate danger is hypovolemic shock from blood loss accompanied by fluid loss from vomiting, ileus, fluid collecting in the peritoneal cavity, and edema in the injured tissues. The hemorrhage from solid organs may be profuse and tends to be continuous because of poor retraction of the blood vessels. Gastrointestinal contents in the peritoneal cavity cause peritonitis by chemical and bacterial irritation. The severity of the peritonitis depends on the amount of fluid and its nature. Colonic contents cause a particularly virulent peritonitis.[5] On ascending the alimentary tract perforation results in less severe infections. Bile and urine seldom contain organisms but produce chemical peritonitis.

On abdominal examination there are generally no signs of skin or soft tissue damage in those with blunt abdominal injuries. Splinting of the abdomen with respiration is a valuable localizing sign. Paradoxical movement of the upper abdomen indicates rupture of the corresponding side of the diaphragm. Tenderness, guarding, rigidity, distention, and a mass are looked for. Peritoneal sounds may be decreased or absent in those with peritonitis. Rectal and vaginal examinations are essential in looking for blood and in detecting pelvic fractures and a pelvic hematoma or peritonitis.

MANAGEMENT. Successful management depends on accurately evaluating the patient, aggressively treating shock, and early operation when indicated. Patients with penetrating wounds should be operated on to prove that the wound has not entered the abdominal cavity. Recently it has been suggested that in units with extensive experience of abdominal injuries many penetrating wounds may be treated conservatively and only operated on if there are signs of internal bleeding or peritoneal irritation and a negative peritoneal tap.[10] In nonpenetrating injuries the decision is more difficult and depends on the demonstration of intra-abdominal injury from the physical signs. The patient may have minimal abnormal signs in the early stages and must be examined repeatedly.

A nasogastric tube is passed to prevent vomiting and abdominal distention and permit observation of the gastric contents for the presence of blood. An indwelling catheter is inserted to determine the presence of blood in the urine and to measure the urinary output. A central venous pressure catheter is inserted to monitor the blood volume and to administer fluids.

Special Investigations. A peritoneal tap is indicated in patients who are comatose after a head injury, in those with multiple injuries, and in those with suspected abdominal injuries who are being treated conservatively. Blood, bile, urine, or feces signifies a positive and early laparotomy. Negative tap should not deter exploration when other positive signs are present. Tap is carried out using a syringe and a No. 18 intravenous needle, a spinal needle with a stylet in place, or an Intracath or peritoneal dialysis catheter. The needle is inserted through a small incision in the skin in the midline, 2 to 5 cm below the umbilicus. Alternatively, a peritoneal dialysis catheter may be used. A slight snapping sensation is felt as the needle passes through the peritoneum. The patient may be turned on his side to aid accumulation of the fluid in one region. If initial aspiration is negative, 500 ml of isotonic saline is infused and then aspirated. The fluid is examined microscopically for erythrocytes, leukocytes, bile, and amylase.

Free gas may be found on an upright or lateral decubitus x-ray of the abdomen. It means that a hollow viscus has been ruptured and that early laparotomy is indicated. A pelvic fracture suggests an injury to the bladder or urethra, while lower rib fractures may be associated with injury to the spleen or liver. Fracture of lumbar vertebrae suggests an associated abdominal injury. Elevation of the diaphragm may be the result of rupture of the diaphragm or its upward displacement by a hematoma. Displacement of organs may be seen and suggests a hematoma. Foreign bodies such as bullets or those used for self-inflicted injuries may be seen on x-ray. Barium studies are generally not indicated in the investigation of acute abdominal injuries. An intravenous pyelogram is especially useful in those with suspected renal injuries, retroperitoneal hematomas, and lumbar spine fractures.

The indications for laparotomy may be described as absolute or relative.

Absolute:

1. Evidence of continued bleeding or peritonitis.

2. Aspiration of blood, intestinal contents, bile, or urine by peritoneal tap.

3. X-ray demonstration of free air in the abdominal cavity.

Relative:

1. Persistent vomiting, abdominal pain, and tenderness.

2. Recovery of blood from the stomach, bladder, or rectum.

Laparotomy is performed through a large midabdominal incision which may be extended upward or downward and, if necessary, into the right or left chest. Bleeding is controlled and a thorough laparotomy always performed looking for more than one injury. Massive hemorrhage from the aorta, inferior vena cava, or iliac vessels is initially controlled by direct pressure, bleeding from the liver by pressure on the hepatic artery and portal vein as they lie in the free border of the lesser omentum, and bleeding from the spleen by direct pressure on the structures forming the splenic pedicle. A retroperitoneal hematoma in the upper abdomen should be explored because of the possibility of a retroperitoneal rupture of the duodenum. Hematomas in the lower abdomen and pelvis are best not explored unless they are large or increasing in size. Injuries to the liver (see Chapter 19), spleen (see Chapter 24), stomach (see Chapter 20), small intestine (see Chapter 21), colon and rectum (see Chapter 22), and urinary system (see Chapter 32) are looked for and appropriately treated.

Thoracic injuries are described in Chapter 30, head injuries in Chapter 34, burns in Chapter 15, peripheral vascular injuries in Chapter 31, genitourinary injuries in Chapter 32, hand injuries in Chapter 28, and fractures and soft tissue injuries in Chapter 29.

Extremity Injuries.   Injuries to the extremities generally assume a lower priority in the management of the critically injured patient. Care must be taken to prevent further damage, continuing injury, and contamination. Control of hemorrhage, preservation of soft tissue parts, and "splint them where they lie" constitute the most appropriate approach (Figure 9–7). The common injuries are fractures, soft tissue laceration, vascular and nerve injuries, and burns. Such injuries will require complex management with fixation and splinting of bone and soft tissues, revascularization procedures, and release of tissue compression. Many of the treatments are best staged. All require gentleness, cleansing, and debridement with expert initial and follow-up care.

Special Investigations.   An aggressive diagnostic approach to the trauma patient is necessary for proper evaluation. The decision as

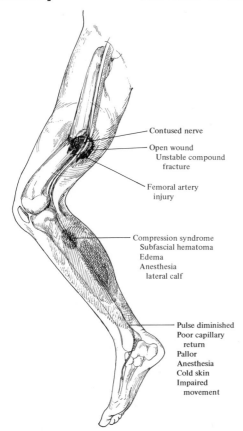

- Contused nerve

- Open wound
  Unstable compound
  fracture

- Femoral artery
  injury

- Compression syndrome
  Subfascial hematoma
  Edema
  Anesthesia
  lateral calf

- Pulse diminished
  Poor capillary
  return
  Pallor
  Anesthesia
  Cold skin
  Impaired
  movement

Figure 9–7. Combinations of injuries to the skin, soft tissues, vessels, nerves, and bones are common. Although the specific injuries independently have a low priority in the management of the critically injured patient, the adequacy of their initial care is important for successful recovery.

to how many x-rays to order is based on the clinical situation and the patient's status. X-rays take valuable time and are performed under conditions that are not ideal for continuous observation. Often a few routine views are adequate. The unconscious patient is more difficult to evaluate and may require additional studies. Single views of possible fractures and dislocations and standard views of chest and abdomen are obtained. Special studies such as tomograms of facial fractures can be done later. The intravenous pyelogram (IVP), cystogram, and arteriography are often useful. The patient with traumatic hematuria from any cause and with suspected renal trauma must have an IVP. To identify injuries to the bladder, pelvic fractures are evaluated by cystography visualizing the full and empty bladder in the PA and lateral views (see Chapter 32).

Arteriography is particularly useful when

circulation in an extremity is impaired, in abdominal and chest trauma, and in closed head injuries. There is no significant morbidity from these studies and they are often of great value. An incidental excretory nephrourogram is obtained 15 minutes after the arteriogram.

Paracentesis is helpful to rapidly evaluate intra-abdominal injuries. If fluid is obtained, it is tested for bile, examined microscopically for white and red blood cells, and a portion sent for determination of amylase. If no fluid is obtained, a plastic catheter may be inserted through the lower abdominal area in the midline and 300 ml of peritoneal dialysis solution slowly infused.[16] The fluid is then aspirated after five minutes and tested. A positive tap is a definitive indication for laparotomy.

Thoracentesis may be used to rapidly evaluate the patient with a possible chest injury. Blood and air, especially if under pressure, are immediate indications to establish tube drainage even prior to taking x-rays. These findings prompt investigation for other underlying visceral injuries.

Direct laryngoscopy and bronchoscopy are performed when injury of the upper airway, trachea, or major bronchi is suspected. Proctoscopy is done in all suspected rectal injuries prior to operation.

Since the introduction of ultrasonic techniques by Leksell,[9] the usefulness of echoencephalography in acute head injuries has been established. Rapid and repeatable examinations are of great value, especially in children. Repeated echo and neurologic examinations are effective and reliable ways to observe head trauma patients safely.

Routinely ordered biochemical tests include serial serum and urine amylase determinations, especially in those with blunt abdominal injuries. A high amylase suggests major injury to the pancreas. Complete blood counts are also serially performed. Changes in hematocrit reflect the status of the circulating red cell mass. Leukocyte counts are elevated in those with visceral injuries, especially when serosal irritation is present. Osmolality by freezing point depression is useful in monitoring fluid and electrolyte problems and defining the status of renal function after severe injury.[3] It is more useful than measurements of the specific gravity of the urine.

SUMMARY

Resuscitation is the initial approach to managing the severely injured. Only after all life-threatening problems have been adequately stabilized can the physician direct his attention to diagnostic evaluation. The need for continued and intensive observation of critically ill patients is emphasized. The clinical response to resuscitative measures gives additional clues and provides a basis for further diagnostic and therapeutic measures. Orderly management, planned at leisure to be executed promptly in an emergency, yields the greatest survival and minimizes the duration and extent of disability.

CITED REFERENCES

1. Baker, R. J.; Boyd, D. R.; and Condon, R. E.: Priorities of the management of patients with multiple injuries. *Surg. Clin. North Am.*, **50**:3–11, 1970.
2. Boyd, D. R.: Introduction: a controlled systems approach to trauma patient care. In A Symposium on the Illinois Trauma Program: a systems approach to the care of the critically injured. *J. Trauma*, **13**:275–76, 1973.
3. Boyd, D. R., and Baker, R. J.: Osmometry: a new bedside laboratory aid for the management of surgical patients. *Surg. Clin. North Am.*, **51**:241–50, 1971.
4. Boyd, D. R.; Dunea, M. M.; and Flashner, B. A.: The Illinois plan for a statewide system of trauma centers. *J. Trauma*, **13**:24–31, 1973.
5. Chilimindris, C.; Boyd, D. R.; Carlson, L. E.; Folk, F. A.; Baker, R. J.; and Freeark, R. J.: A critical review of management of right colon injuries. *J. Trauma*, **11**:651–60, 1971.
6. Committee on Trauma and Committee on Shock, National Academy of Sciences, National Research Council: *Accidental Death and Disability: The Neglected Disease of Modern Society.* N.A.S.-N.R.C., Washington, D.C., 1966.
7. Izant, R. J., Jr., and Hubay, C. A.: The annual injury of 15,000,000 children: a limited study of childhood accidental injury and death. *J. Trauma*, **6**:65–74, 1966.
8. Keeton, R. E., and O'Connell, J.: *The Basic Protection for the Traffic Victim: A Blueprint for Reforming Automobile Insurance.* Little, Brown, Boston, 1965.
9. Leksell, L.: Echoencephalography. II. Midline echo from the pineal body as an index of pineal displacement. *Acta Chir. Scand.*, **115**:255, 1958.
10. Lowe, R. J.; Boyd, D. R.; Folk, F. A.; and Baker, R. J.: The negative laparotomy for abdominal trauma. *J. Trauma*, **12**:853–61, 1972.
11. Manegold, F. R., and Silver, M. H.: The emergency medical care system. *JAMA*, **200**:300–304, 1967.
12. Nagel, E. L.; Hirschman, J. C.; Nussenfeld, F. R.; Rankin, D.; and Lundblade, E.: Telemetry-medical command in coronary and other mobile emergency care systems. *JAMA*, **214**:332–38, 1970.
13. National Institute of General Medical Science, National Institutes of Health: *Report Conference on Trauma*, Feb. 24, 25. N.I.G.M.S., N.I.H., Bethesda, 1968.
14. National Institutes of Health: *1968 Annual Report.* U.S. Government Printing Office, Washington, D.C.
15. National Safety Council: *Accidental Facts 1969.* N.S.C., Chicago.
16. Perry, J. F., Jr.; DeMeules, J. E.; and Root, H. D.: Diagnostic peritoneal lavage in blunt abdominal trauma. *Surg. Gynecol. Obstet.*, **131**:742–44, 1970.
17. Report Conference on Trauma. *J. Trauma*, **8**:113, 1968.
18. Shoemaker, W. C.; Lim, L.; Boyd, D. R.; Corley, R. S.; Reinhard, J. M.; Dreiling, D. A.; and Kark, A. E.: Sequential hemodynamic events after trauma to the unanesthetized patient. *Surg. Gynecol. Obstet.*, **132**:651–56, 1971.
19. Stahl, W. M.: Resuscitation in trauma: the value of central venous pressure monitoring. *J. Trauma*, **5**:200–212, 1965.

SUGGESTIONS FOR FURTHER READING

Ballinger, W. F.; Rutherford, R. B.; and Zuidema, G. D.: *The Management of Trauma.* W. B. Saunders, Philadelphia, 1968.

This book describes the latest techniques for immediate diagnosis and care in almost any kind of life-threatening injury. It is recommended for residents, practicing physicians, and all who deal with trauma.

Committee on Injuries, American Academy of Orthopaedic Surgeons: *Emergency Care and Transportation of the Sick and Injured.* A.A.O.S., Chicago, 1971.

Expert emergency medical care must be started at the scene of an emergency and maintained to prevent deterioration of the patient's condition during transportation to a hospital. To better equip the ambulance technician and all who work with the emergency ill and injured at the scene and during transportation, and to enable them to serve as the most valuable lay members of the medical care team outside the hospital, the A.A.O.S. has developed this textbook which is being used in conjunction with the nationally accepted 82-hour course for emergency medical technicians.

A Symposium on the Illinois Trauma Program: a systems approach to the care of the critically injured. *J. Trauma*, **13**:275–320, 1973.

Current progress in the field of trauma care is exemplified by the Illinois Trauma Program which is featured in this symposium. A systems approach to resuscitation and management techniques has demonstrated that expert care, previously available only at university centers, can now be effectively and efficiently provided throughout the state, especially in the rural community. Some of the articles are: "A Systems Approach to Statewide Emergency Medical Care"; "Organization and Function of Trauma Care Units"; "New Health Specialists for Trauma Patient Care"; "Special Centers for the Care of the Injured"; and "A Profile of the Trauma Registry."

Chapter 10

MANAGEMENT OF PAIN

Donald H. Pearson and *John F. Mullan*

CHAPTER OUTLINE

Introduction
The "Pain Patient"
Theories of Pain
  Specificity Theory
  Pattern Theory
  Gate Theory
  Psychologic Theories
Anatomy of Pain
  Peripheral Reception and Transmission
  Posterior Roots
  Lateral Spinothalamic Tract
  Quintothalamic Tract
  Other Cranial Nerve Tracts
  "C" Fiber System
  Anatomy of Referred Pain
Therapy of Pain
  Nonsurgical Treatment of Pain
    Hypnotics and Sedatives
    Psychoaffective Drugs
    Narcotic Analgesic Agents
    Analgesic and Antipyretic Drugs

Local Anesthetic Agents
Surgical Treatment of Pain
  Peripheral Nerve Sections
  Posterior Rhizotomy
  Spinal Cord Tractotomy
  "Paraphysiologic" Treatment of Pain
Chronic Pain Syndromes
  Intractable Pain from Cancer
    Head and Neck Cancer
    Cancer of the Thorax
    Gastrointestinal Cancer,
      and Tumors of Other Abdominal
      Viscera
  Intractable Pain from Benign Disease
    Cephalic Neuralgias
    Visceral Pain
    Pain Following Peripheral Injuries
    Postinfectious Pain
  Psychologic Pain
Summary

INTRODUCTION

The concept of pain has not been satisfactorily defined, yet its meaning is readily understood and it is one of the commonest symptoms that physicians treat. In its simplest form pain may be thought of as the appreciation of injury that is present in all phyla. The clinician must, however, think of it also as an attribute of humanity. It is sometimes useful to divide pain into sensation and the reaction to sensation with the clear realization that the two can set up a reverberating cycle.

THE "PAIN PATIENT"

The following case history demonstrates some of the problems faced in dealing with what is sometimes carelessly referred to as the "pain patient."

An industrial laborer, 38 years old, began to have recurrent abdominal pains in his early 20s. Although initially no diagnosis was made, he was eventually found to have a peptic ulcer that did not respond to conservative management, and he was then treated by partial gastrectomy. He remained asymptomatic until age 34 and then fell at work, sustaining a fractured femur. An open reduction was complicated by osteomyelitis necessitating a number of operations. His hip joint became ankylosed and caused persistent pain. Exploration of the sciatic nerve and lysis of adhesions resulted only in transient relief of pain. A subsequent lumbar sympathectomy afforded relief for only three months. He then took large amounts of narcotics. Following a posterior rhizotomy from T_{10} to L_2 he was able to return to work for nine months. The pain then recurred. A percutaneous cervical cordotomy, making the patient semianesthetic from C_3 to the sacral area, was necessary because the pain involved a wide area by this time. Six months later he developed pain in his opposite shoulder which remained refractory to diagnosis and does so till the present time. At present he obtains relief of pain for variable intervals ranging from hours to days by the intermittent application of an external nerve stimulator over the ulnar nerve in his painful arm. In addition, he uses frequent doses of mild nonnarcotic analgesic agents and undergoes daily physiotherapy. He remains unemployed.

This case demonstrates several features commonly observed in patients with prolonged, severe pain. The first is that frequently the etiology of the pain is obscure. Second, they pass through the hands of numerous physicians, exhausting themselves and each physician in turn. Third, it demonstrates the variety of surgical procedures that are frequently performed in an effort to relieve the patient. Last, it shows how the varying theories of pain are commonly utilized in an attempt to rationalize treatment. These will be detailed further below.

THEORIES OF PAIN

There is no entirely satisfactory theory to describe pain. None includes all the sensations that are described as painful. The anatomic theories deal primarily with pain as a sensation, and the physiologic theories deal primarily with the suffering caused by pain.

Specificity Theory

The specificity theory, one of the older theories, considers pain a specific sensation such as sight and hearing. Pain therefore has its own receptors, is carried by special tracts in the central nervous system, and reaches conscious perception in the thalamus. Much of the surgical relief of pain is built on this theory.

Pattern Theory

The pattern theory and specificity theory are mutually exclusive. The pattern theory suggests that painful impulses are produced by the spaciotemporal patterns of nerve impulses and are not transmitted along specific tracts. These patterns are recorded as pain in higher centers. The essential difference between this theory and the specificity theory is the claim that there are no tracts that transmit only painful impulses. While the specificity theory primarily emphasizes peripheral receptors and their pathways, most versions of the pattern theory emphasize central reverberating mechanisms.

Gate Theory

Neither pattern theories nor specificity theories account for all types of pain. Furthermore they make no provision for affective modulation of pain. A recent theory that attempts to embrace all types of pain perception borrows from both and centers upon recent physiologic evidence demonstrating spinal integrating mechanisms combined with evidence demonstrating central, i.e., higher, control over afferent input. Briefly

the gate theory postulates a gating system within the substantia gelatinosa of the spinal cord, acted upon by volleys from afferent fibers in the peripheral nerves and modulated by descending impulses in the spinal cord from brain stem, thalamus, and cortical systems. The output of this gating system reascends the spinal cord in an "action system" to provoke appropriate physiologic responses of the organism to peripheral stimulation, one of which is the perceptual awareness of pain. Thus the gate may be "opened" or "closed" in varying degrees by the summation of excitatory and inhibitory impulses both from the periphery and from higher centers.

There are two readily apparent consequences from such a theory. The first is that the "set" of the gate, and thus the conscious perception of pain, may vary widely independently of the force of the external stimulus. Second, such a pain mechanism may be manipulated in many ways by altering both the peripheral stimuli and the central "feedback" mechanisms. It thus provides a satisfactory substrate for understanding many of the "problem" pains not adequately accounted for by previous theories, such as cutaneous hyperalgesia, spontaneous pain, and the long latency period between stimulus and perception characteristic of some pathologic pain syndromes.

The gate theory has led to the development of new methods to control pain. The nervous input into the spinal cord or within spinal tracts may be altered by stimulation either of peripheral nerves or of sensory tracts in the posterior columns. It is thought that pain is reduced by altering either the input to the gate system or by modulating its reflex pathways with the higher centers. It is too early yet to evaluate definitively these new methods of "closing the gate."

Psychologic Theories

The purely psychologic theories of pain deal with the patient's reaction or attitude to pain rather than to the painful stimulus. This is an important distinction. These attitudes range largely from the statement by Spinoza that pain is a form of intense melancholia and can be treated by rationally understanding its causes to the more modern theories that pain and anxiety are closely related. Threats to the ego both in infancy and adulthood by physical damage and by emotional disturbances are felt to intensify the painful syndrome.

ANATOMY OF PAIN

Surgical interruption of pain pathways from the integument to the brain has long been known to control some types of pain. In the peripheral nerve and nerve root sensations are mixed; in the spinal cord there is some division into well-defined groups or columns. Advantage can be taken of this separation to divide only those fibers carrying pain and spare those serving useful functions such as touch and proprioception. The best-defined of these long sensory tracts is the lateral spinothalamic tract.

Peripheral Reception and Transmission

Since the total body surface appreciates pain (and touch) readily, it would appear that free nerve endings which are found everywhere are the receptive organs for pain. They belong either to unmyelinated or to myelinated fibers of less than 6 microns in diameter. They connect with dorsal roots of the spinal cord. It is possible that these free endings transmit a sensation of touch when they are gently deformed and a sensation of pain when the contact is a more violent one or when acted upon by the metabolites of cell injury, ischemia, or inflammation. Nerve fibers are classically divided into three types: "A," myelinated afferent and efferent somatic; "B," myelinated preganglionic sympathetic; and "C," unmyelinated somatic afferent and unmyelinated sympathetic fibers. We therefore consider the "A" and "C" fibers in the transmission of pain. It is well known that there are at least two types of pain, a rather precise, rapidly conducted pain and a slow, diffuse, longer lasting pain. The function of these nerve fibers has been determined by selective electrical blocking, by asphyxia and local anesthesia. The rapid, more precise type of pain and discrete temperature sensations are carried by fibers in the upper ranges, and diffuse burning pain is carried by those in the "C" range. It is also probable that the smaller "A" fibers carry touch and that "C" fibers carry touch, pressure, and temperature.

Posterior Roots

As the posterior roots enter the cord they divide into medial and lateral segments. The larger medial fibers branch into long ascending and short descending fibers. Some of these fibers synapse in the posterior horn at the various levels; some are continued into the well-known gracilis and cuneate nuclei. The lateral fibers of the posterior root, which carry pain, also branch as they enter the horn. These branches ascend or descend one or more segments to form the tract of Lissauer. One or more synapses occur in the substance of the substantia gelatinosa which caps the posterior horn. From cells in the body of the horn fibers arise which carry pain and temperature sensation across the anterior commissure into the contralateral anterior quadrant. Fibers carrying "C" responses (which are presumed to be painful) may be found in the fasciculus proprius of both sides and in the posterior commissure. It is thus possible that pain could be transmitted up both sides of the spinal cord.

Lateral Spinothalamic Tract

Although many older anatomic textbooks have portrayed a rather small and well-defined lateral spinothalamic tract presumed to carry pain, it is well known clinically that pain and temperature are transmitted throughout a wide area of the anterior quadrant of the spinal cord between the dentate posteriorly and the emergence of the anterior roots anteriorly. There is an anteromedial segmental arrangement of the fibers, the most lateral and posterior fibers representing the lowest portion of the body, whereas the more medial and anterior fibers are related to the upper extremity and neck. It should be noted also that the area anterior to the arm fibers and close to the anterior horn transmits efferent respiratory fibers. Also the area between the leg region and the pyramidal tract has to do with bladder function. Note must be taken of these relationships in performing surgical procedures on this tract. In addition, it is thought there is lamination of the sensory modalities within this tract; that is, fibers concerned with thermal sensation lie more deeply and posterior, while pain fibers are thought to be located more anteriorly. Lesions made surgically in the area of this tract produce hemianesthesia of the opposite side of the body below the level at which the lesion is produced. There is a profound sensory loss if the lesion is complete, and this can result in gratifying reduction in pain. A primary disadvantage is that the sensory loss seems to depend on lesion size with sensation returning to a greater or lesser extent within one or two years. The reason for this is not clear.

As it ascends, the tract is located at medullary levels dorsolateral to the inferior olivary nucleus, while in the pons and midbrain it is lateral to the medial lemniscus. Many of the fibers of the anterior lateral quadrant are distributed into the medullary and pontine reticular formation. Others are distributed to the lateral region of the mesencephalic gray matter and the deeper layers of the superior colliculus. A small number of fibers, about 10 to 12 percent in the monkey, enter the thalamus to be distributed in the posterior ventral nucleus and other thalamic nuclei. All these terminations from the medulla to the thalamus are bilateral. Those in the ventral posterior nucleus predominate on the side ipsilateral to the tract (contralateral to the side of origin of the pain). Thus it is clear that

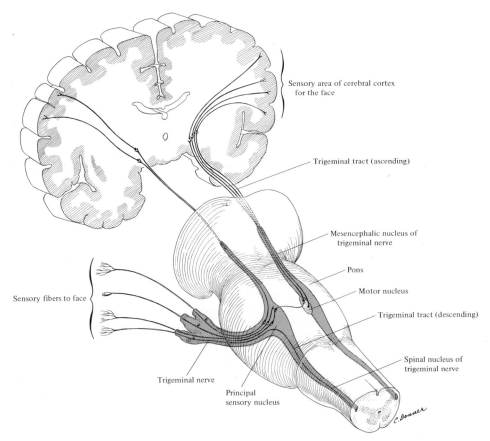

Sensory area of cerebral cortex
for the face

Trigeminal tract (ascending)

Mesencephalic nucleus of
trigeminal nerve

Pons

Motor nucleus

Trigeminal tract (descending)

Spinal nucleus of
trigeminal nerve

Sensory fibers to face

Trigeminal nerve

Principal
sensory nucleus

C. Bonner

Figure 10–1. The nucleus and tract of the fifth cranial nerve. The descending spinal trigeminal tract may lie as low as C_2.

there is a progressive termination of neurons at and above the medulla and that this termination occurs bilaterally. In the thalamus there is a prominent representation of large fibers in the ipsilateral ventral posterior nucleus which is called the classic spinothalamic system.

Quintothalamic Tract

The homologue to the spinothalamic tract, which subserves sensation to the body, is the quintothalamic tract, which subserves sensation to the face (Figure 10–1). This nerve, the trigeminal nerve, is, like the spinal nerves, a mixed motor and sensory structure. The three well-known major branches of the trigeminal nerve each enter the skull cavity through separate apertures and join together to synapse in the main sensory ganglion, the gasserian ganglion. The motor fibers of course do not synapse in the ganglion but pass beneath it to join the main trunk prior to its entry into the brainstem in the midportion of the pons. The sensory ganglion is located in Meckel's cave at the medial edge of

the temporal bone, and is covered by a pocket of dura formed at the tentorial margin. At the entry zone of the fifth cranial nerve there is, as with the posterior roots, a separation into fibers that carry pain and those that do not. Fibers ascend and descend in the mesencephalon, pons, medulla, and upper spinal segments. It is usually held that the mesencephalic portion of the nucleus subserves primarily touch and proprioceptive impulses, while the spinal nucleus subserves pain and thermal sensations. Considerable clinical use is made of this division, particularly since the spinal trigeminal tract and nucleus are near the surface of the medulla. The skin representation of this tract and nucleus is one of which much has been written. If we take the classic three divisions of the fifth nerve, we find the third division situated dorsimedially, the first ventrolaterally. There is another lamination to be considered. If we take an onionskin map of the face with three concentric semicircles based upon the midline, extending from mouth to ear, we find that the area between the outer and middle lines (forehead and posterior face) is represented caudally and the circumoral area (lips) is represented rostrally. Destruction of the spinotrigeminal tract and nucleus at the level of the obex or slightly below produces relief of pain and thermal anesthesia of the face, while touch and proprioception are largely untouched. This is a factor in diminishing the possibility of corneal ulceration in an analgesic face.

From the spinal nucleus fibers sweep across the midline and reach the opposite side between the olive and the pyramid. In the midbrain they are lateral to the medial lemniscus and run with it into the ventroposterior medial portion of the thalamus. In addition, fibers project bilaterally to the midbrain reticular formation and to other areas of the thalamus.

Other Cranial Nerve Tracts

Sensory fibers from the soft palate, pharynx, ear, and contiguous structures run with the seventh, ninth, and tenth cranial nerves. These are sometimes implicated in troublesome neuralgias similar to the trigeminal neuralgia. These fibers are distributed to the nucleus and tractus solitarius which is situated dorsimedially to the descending trigeminal tract at low pontine and medullary levels. However, it is supposed that a considerable part of these fibers does not enter the tractus solitarius but instead passes down along the spinal nucleus of the fifth nerve, located between it and the cuneate nucleus. This has been proved in humans by section of this area to relieve pain in the ear and pharyngeal area.

"C" Fiber System

The ubiquitous small nerve endings found everywhere in the integument are thought to represent the mechanism that subserves pain. Similar small unmyelinated "C" fibers are represented widely in the spinal cord. These may be responsible for the slow-response, burning, disagreeable pain common to many of the pathologic pain syndromes. It has been shown that "C" fiber responses may be recorded in the propriospinal fasciculi and in the posterior commissure of the cord and may also be picked up in the medulla and inferior reticular area of the ventral tegmentum. Appropriate electrical stimulation will set up repetitive discharge in these areas. It should be noted that repetitive stimulation of "C" fibers in the peripheral nerve of man is associated with pain. This widespread small fiber system is one that cannot be obliterated by localized surgical ablation in the cord, and it is probably responsible for postcordotomy

dysesthesia and other failures of surgical cordotomy.

Anatomy of Referred Pain

It is of historical interest that the original theory of referred pain denied the possibility that painful impulses could originate in viscera. Weight was given to this idea when it was noted that cutting, crushing, or burning the intestine did not hurt during laparotomies performed under local anesthesia. It was soon discovered that distention was the physiologic stimulus producing pain for hollow viscera, and some years later it was found that cardiac pain was evoked by ischemia of the myocardium. The fact that diseased organs produced pain referred to somatic areas was explained as follows. Impulses from a diseased organ ascended no further than the posterior horn of spinal gray matter, where they set up an "irritable focus." This was thought to lower the threshold of cutaneous stimulation at that dermatome level to the point of permitting the constant stream of sensory impulses, normally below threshold, to ascend to the sensorium and be recorded as pain. Henry Head in 1893 employed maps of the superficial nerve distribution for each intervertebral level to direct attention to specific painful diseases of various viscera, thus systematizing the well-known clinical syndromes of referred pain from diseased viscera.

It is now known that afferent impulses from the viscera run centripetally through autonomic nerves and pass through the paravertebral sympathetic ganglia, their communicant rami, and posterior roots of the spinal nerves to the posterior horn of the spinal cord. It has been shown, on the basis of fiber counts, that there are more pain-conducting axons in the posterior roots than in the spinothalamic tracts. Therefore many of the secondary spinal axons must carry both somatic and visceral sensation. This fact and the inability to localize visceral sensation explain why it is referred to cutaneous areas related to the same segment of the spinal cord. Thus, for example, pain from the heart enters the middle cervical to the fifth thoracic sympathetic ganglia and enters the cord in the upper five thoracic roots. Since the dermatomes of these roots include the chest wall and the medial aspect of the arm, the classic referred pain pattern of angina pectoris can be predicted. Gastrointestinal pain is carried through the splanchnic nerves and ramifies over the entire thoracic inflow. Fibers conveying pain sensation from the pancreas are carried on the right and left splanchnic nerves and the celiac plexus. The right splanchnic trunk transmits pain from the head of the pancreas, and sensation from the tail is conveyed mainly by the left splanchnic trunk. These visceral afferent fibers pursue an uninterrupted course through autonomic ganglia to reach the posterior sixth through the twelfth thoracic nerve roots. It should be noted that painful conditions of the pancreas, because of its retroperitoneal position, frequently involve the somatic nerves of the posterior abdominal wall as well. Therefore surgical relief of pancreatic pain frequently must take into account both sympathetic and somatic pathways. Pain from the gallbladder and biliary ducts is mediated by sensory fibers running in plexuses along the ductal system. The majority of these fibers are conveyed by the right greater splanchnic nerve and pass to the seventh and eighth posterior nerve roots. The sensory innervation of the kidney and ureter passes from the dorsal root ganglia of the tenth thoracic to the second lumbar nerves. These fibers accompany the lesser and least splanchnic nerves to reach the aorticorenal and celiac ganglia from which sensory fibers form a fine network surrounding the renal vessels and extending to the hilum of the kidney. Pain from pelvic structures such as the uterine cervix and the rectum is transmitted via sacral parasympathetic fibers to the second, third, and fourth sacral roots.

It should be noted that the sensory nerves that supply internal viscera are not autonomic nerves but merely accompany the splanchnic nerves and the sacral parasympathetic. These unmyelinated fibers that convey visceral sensation pass in an uninterrupted course through the autonomic ganglia without synapse to reach their cell bodies in the posterior root ganglion, their central processes entering the spinal cord via the posterior root. Although most referred pains can be understood on a segmental basis, their widespread manifestations , and relatively poor localizations can be accounted for by recognizing upward and downward ramification of afferent fibers both within the sympathetic chain and also in the spinal cord, spreading afferent impulses over several levels.

Since the final common pathway of referred pain is the spinal cord, spinothalamic tractotomy seems to be an attractive method of relieving these pains. However, since most viscera have bilateral innervation, the added risks of bilateral cordotomy must be considered.

THERAPY OF PAIN

It is difficult to fit all pains into clearly defined patterns, but certain patterns are helpful when considering treatment. Pain may be useful and symptomatic or of no value and debilitating. Each may be of short duration lasting for hours to weeks or prolonged lasting for months to years. An acute pain may lead to the diagnosis of a disease. Its treatment is usually well defined if not simple. The acute pains without an obvious cause tax the physician's diagnostic ingenuity and are often difficult to control. It is the prolonged pains that tax the therapeutic resources of the physician, both those with an obvious cause such as cancer and those with no obvious stimulus.

The treatment of pain falls into two general categories. These are the surgery of pain, which deals primarily with interruption of pathways subserving pain or thought to modify pain, and the nonsurgical or pharmacologic approach, which attempts to minimize the pain perception and to alleviate the emotional response to pain. A third approach, one which is poorly appreciated or understood but frequently unwittingly used, may be termed the "paraphysiologic" manipulation of pain patterns.

Nonsurgical Treatment of Pain

Almost every drug known to have some action upon the central or peripheral nervous system has been used for attempted relief of pain at one time or another. A few drugs have proved by continued use to be effective in altering pain patterns. The drugs used to modify pain fall into four general classifications: hypnotics and sedatives, psychoaffective drugs, narcotic analgesics, and the analgesic and antipyretic group.

Hypnotics and Sedatives. Most widely used in this class are the barbiturates. These have a wide effect on most organ systems including the central nervous system, which is exquisitely sensitive to them, and are used primarily as general depressants. They have little analgesic action and are most effective only as adjuncts to more direct means of relieving pain. They are useful in providing relaxation and assistance at night or when there is little opportunity for the normal stimuli of life to distract the patient from his painful symptoms. Their danger is that, although not addictive, they lend themselves to habitual abuse. Overdosage may occur with these drugs but is usually heralded by the onset of lethargy. There are numerous barbiturate compounds and they are classified by their length of action. Other drugs whose action is similar to the barbiturates include chloral hydrate, paraldehyde, glutethamide, and, at least within the context of this chapter, ethyl alcohol. It is important to bear in mind that these and many other drugs, such as the phenothiazines, either have an additive depressant effect or are potentiated and thus when used in combination their dosage must be reduced accordingly.

Psychoaffective Drugs. Drugs used primarily for their psychologic effects have great use in painful syndromes by altering the affective response to pain. The most useful of these are probably the phenothiazines and related compounds. These drugs again have little or no analgesic property but alter the emotional feeling-tone associated with pain. They have often been likened to a chemical frontal lobotomy. They produce an apparent indifference or slowing of responses to external stimuli without a change in the state of consciousness or of intellectual function, at least in normal dosage. This psychomotor slowing, emotional quieting, and affective indifference constitute the "neuroleptic syndrome." The drug that has achieved the widest use for this purpose is chlorpromazine. This class of drugs should be considered part of the therapeutic approach to any chronic pain syndrome and is particularly useful in assisting with the withdrawal from narcotic or alcoholic addiction. Other drugs closely related in action to the phenothiazine drugs and used to treat anxiety include meprobamate, chlorprothixene (Taractan), chlordiazepoxide (Librium), and diazepam (Valium). The choice of drug largely depends upon the physician's preference, which in turn depends upon his familiarity with the drug and its side effects. The most troublesome side effect of all these compounds, aside from their rare toxic effect on other organ systems when given in normal dosage, is the production of extrapyramidal motor disorders. These are usually reversible on withdrawal of the medication. The psychologic effect of these drugs has proved of real benefit in managing chronic pain, and their use should be seriously considered in every disabling pain syndrome, or until more definitive therapy is effective.

There is a group of drugs used primarily to treat depression and less valuable in the treatment of pain. However, pain and depression frequently coexist, and certainly suffering can be alleviated by lifting depression. They are inconvenient to use since their therapeutic effect may take several weeks to become manifest. The commonly used drugs of this type include the monoamine oxidase inhibitors, such as isocarboxazid (Marplan) and tranylcypromine (Parnate), and the dibenzodiazepine compounds, such as imipramine (Tofranil) and amitriptyline (Elavil). The drugs in the last group are held to be less toxic than the former and to act somewhat more rapidly. MAO inhibitors can markedly enhance the excitatory or depressant effects of other drugs and may cause hypertensive crises when given in conjunction with sympathomimetic amines and related compounds, or tyramine-containing substances such as cheese.

Narcotic Analgesic Agents. The prototype of the narcotic analgesics and the most useful one is morphine. These drugs are truly analgesic in that their primary action is to reduce painful sensations. However, they all as well have wide psychologic effects. They have the following disadvantages: First, they are addictive; second, they produce tolerance to their analgesic effect; and third, they are respiratory depressants. For this reason in spite of their excellent analgesic properties they cannot be used in the management of long-term pain. The potent analgesic effect of morphine is well appreciated, but poorly understood. Physiologic evidence suggests it exerts its pain-relieving qualities upon several levels of the central nervous system. It seems to have a direct depressive effect on central summation mechanisms within the spinal cord; for example, polysynaptic reflexes are inhibited while monosynaptic reflexes seem untouched. In addition, it produces a variety of mental effects such as drowsiness, mental clouding, and changes in mood. When analgesia occurs euphoria frequently follows. Experience has shown that pain syndromes may be intensified rather than relieved by the prolonged use of narcotics, thus making the pain more difficult to treat as long as their compulsive use persists. This problem is so sufficiently widespread as to lead most authorities to consider the use of narcotics absolutely contraindicated in the management of chronic pain. Such use only compounds the patient's problems of physical discomfort, depression, and anxiety with problems of dependence and addiction. Indeed in the authors' experience little progress can be made in the treatment of pain until the patient's addiction is relieved by either withdrawal of the narcotic or treatment of his physical dependence by substitution of another drug with less euphoric and hypnotic effects, such as methadone. Most other opium alkaloids or their congeners such as hydromorphone, oxycodone, and meperidine are not qualitatively different from morphine. Codeine deserves special mention since it is much less addictive, and when combined with aspirin seems to exhibit with it a mild but definite potentiation of the analgesic effect.

A number of semisynthetic opiate alkaloids have been developed with the goal of producing analgesia with little of the addictive effects of morphine. In general their analgesic effects are low, paralleling their addictive effects, and while they may be used judiciously to treat chronic pain, milder analgesics are probably just as efficacious. Among these drugs are propoxyphene (Darvon) and ethoheptazine (Zactirin).

Analgesic and Antipyretic Drugs. Probably the most useful of all analgesic agents are the salicylates, as common experience testifies. Their effectiveness is shown by the vast quantities consumed annually. Their locus of action is thought to be not supraspinal but subcortical as no depression of higher mental function occurs; the thalamus has been suggested. Part of their analgesic effect may be due to their potent anti-inflammatory action in connective tissue, particularly since they seem most effective in relieving musculoskeletal and integument pain and less useful in visceral pain; however, this must be of adjunctive value only. This group of drugs share antipyretic action as well as central effect. Closely related drugs are acetaminophen and phenacetin. They have essentially the same action as the salicylates.

Because of their relative safety and efficacy these drugs should probably be included in any regimen for the treatment of the chronic pain syndrome, barring individual contraindications. Although effective for only mild to moderate pain, their additive effect with other methods of pain control is useful. They have no significant organ toxicity in usual doses and do not exhibit tolerance or addiction. Their major problem is one of gastric irritation with occasional erosion and hemorrhage in susceptible individuals.

Local Anesthetic Agents. Local anesthetic agents such as cocaine, procaine, and their relatives are also of use in treating the chronic pain patient, particularly when there is irritation of local cutaneous nerves or in musculoskeletal pain with well-defined "trigger" areas. The framework of action involves reversible blocking of the conduction of nerve impulses. This is used most effectively in peripheral nerves, but such drugs also have a widespread effect on conduction within the central nervous system. Both the generation and the production of the nerve impulse are prevented by altering the membrane permeability of the axon and inhibiting passage of sodium and potassium ions. Smaller fibers, such as unmyelinated and small myelinated fibers, are first to be blocked and last to recover. Both motor and sensory fibers are blocked equally. Since the blockade persists as long as the anesthetic agent is in direct contact with nervous tissue, prolonged pain relief may be effected by including in the anesthetic mixture a small proportion of epinephrine to cause local vasoconstriction and to slow the absorption of the compound from surrounding tissues. Although the duration of action of most local anesthetics is short and measured only in minutes to hours, it has been empirically shown that the repeated blockade of an irritable focus producing pain may afford lasting relief of chronic pain for days or months. Physiologic mechanisms for allowing such relief are not understood.

In an attempt to produce more prolonged blockade of peripheral nerves other agents are occasionally injected for local pain relief. The most common of these are ammonium sulfate, phenol in a dilute solution (5 percent), and absolute alcohol, all of which have a neurolytic action. They must be used with caution because of their corrosive effect on other tissues, but when used judiciously, partial destruction of peripheral nerves provides temporary relief. Phenol in a hyperbaric solution is sometimes injected into the sacral thecal sac to relieve pain in the pelvis and extremities. Because of poor control over the amount of nervous tissue destruction that thus can be accomplished, this is usually reserved for patients who have lost sphincter control from their primary pathologic process, such as a pelvic tumor.

Surgical Treatment of Pain

Surgical section of the long sensory tracts of the body still remains one of the most useful methods of dealing with chronic pain. Unfortunately not all pain syndromes lend themselves to this form of treatment, but for the many that do it remains one of the most effective. Nervous tracts may be sectioned at any level of the central nervous system beginning at the peripheral nerve and extending all the way to the cerebral cortex. Certain sites, such as the lateral spinothalamic tract within the cord, have shown by experience to be safe and of lasting value. Figure 10–2 shows diagrammatically some of the sites for interruption of nervous pathways subserving pain.

Peripheral Nerve Sections. Certain well-localized pains due to irritation of a cutaneous nerve, such as meralgia paresthetica secondary to damage or compression of the lateral femoral cutaneous nerve, are well treated by simple section of the appropriate nerve. It should be recognized, however, that pain covering a wider area than that subserved by a simple peripheral nerve cannot be so treated, and that there are pains which, even though well-localized, respond poorly to simple nerve section, if there is no obvious etiology.

One pain of uncertain etiology which is helped by a peripheral neurectomy is trigeminal neuralgia. If the trigger area is denervated by the avulsion of the appropriate cutaneous facial nerve, relief will be afforded until nerve regeneration occurs.

It is appropriate to mention here the treatment of painful neuromas of peripheral nerves caused by injury or amputation. If such neuromas are

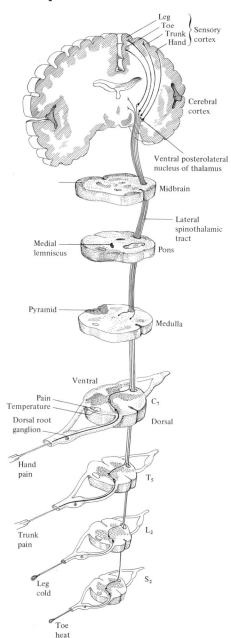

Leg
Toe
Trunk } Sensory
Hand } cortex

Cerebral
cortex

Ventral posterolateral
nucleus of thalamus

Midbrain

Lateral
spinothalamic
tract

Medial
lemniscus   Pons

Pyramid

Medulla

Ventral

Pain
Temperature   C₇

Dorsal root
ganglion   Dorsal

Hand
pain

T₅

Trunk
pain   L₂

Leg
cold   S₂

Toe
heat

Figure 10–2. The figure demonstrates areas where surgical interruption has been attempted for the control of pain. Not all have been successful. Prefrontal lobotomy has been refined to bilateral cingulumotomy and remains under investigation. Resection of the sensory cortex has been abandoned. Thalamotomy remains a research topic. Spinothalamic tractotomy in the midbrain is technically difficult and carries a high risk. Trigeminal tractotomy is occasionally done for intractable facial pain. Medullary tractotomy is also a high-risk operation. Spinal cordotomy is the most

found at exploration or by palpation, careful excision or higher transection of the damaged nerve is worthwhile. Unfortunately in such cases a certain percentage will re-form further neuromas at the site of surgery, and probably only one such trial is justified. If pain recurs, interruption of pain pathways at higher levels is recommended. Some surgeons suggest several trials of blocking the painful neuroma with a local anesthetic to see if pain relief is complete before proceeding with surgery.

Posterior Rhizotomy. For those pains of obvious etiology that cover a wider area than is subserved by a peripheral nerve, section more centrally in the nervous system may be of some help. The next level to be considered is the posterior roots as they exit from the spinal cord. Several posterior roots in sequence may be sectioned to denervate a wide area of the body. Because of cutaneous overlap it is necessary to section at least one root above and one root below the pain level. Because sectioning the posterior roots abolishes all sensory modalities to the body, those roots responsible for important joint sensations in the extremities cannot be sectioned widely. A denervated extremity is useless and cannot function normally due to its proprioceptive loss, although sometimes with impunity one or two subserving an extremity may be sectioned. Similarly, the second, third, and fourth sacral roots must be left intact on both sides to preserve potency in the male and on one side to preserve bladder function and rectal sensation. These limitations restrict the usefulness of this procedure.

Another limitation is the fact that the denervated part is entirely without sensation, even touch, and the cutaneous anesthesia may be as distressing to some patients as their original pain. Again, blocking of the appropriate roots with local anesthetic is often performed to test the adequacy of pain relief and to allow the patient to experience the anesthesia. The "all-or-none" theory of denervation is well demonstrated here, since if insufficient levels are sectioned, or if even a single rootlet is missed during the surgery, debilitating pain may remain after operation. Nevertheless, despite these limitations, posterior rhizotomy remains a valuable technique with one striking advantage: Unlike sections at higher levels the anesthesia is never lost, and thus it is excellent treatment for pain in benign disease.

successful of the tractotomies. Posterior root section can be useful in restricted pain. Sympathectomy is used in the sympathetic dystrophies and sometimes to relieve splanchnic pain.

Spinal Cord Tractotomy. As previously mentioned, within the spinal cord the sensations of pain and temperature are separated from the sensations to touch and proprioception. Thus by judicious section of the anterolateral quadrant wide areas of analgesia can be produced without loss of useful sensation (Figure 10–3). Because of its great utility and wide application the method will be described in some detail.

This procedure is performed either open, that is by direct visualization of the spinal cord, or closed, by stereotactic placement of an electrode within the cord.

In the open method under general anesthesia a laminectomy is performed, the dura is opened, and the cord is visualized. The dentate ligaments are cut, permitting the cord to be rotated about 45° for visualization of the anterolateral quadrant. A sharp knife is then inserted at a point midway between the exit of the anterior and posterior rootlets to a carefully measured depth 2 mm from the midline, in order to spare the anterior spinal artery. The anterior quadrant is then incised. At this point some surgeons recommend awakening the patient briefly to test the adequacy of the incision and pain relief. The cordotomy should be performed at a sufficiently high level to provide adequate pain relief. This is usually a high thoracic level for trunk and leg pain and a high cervical (C_2–C_3) level for upper extremity pain.

For unilateral pain a unilateral incision suffices, but for midline or visceral pain, a bilateral incision is needed. The two incisions should be made at least 2 cm apart along the longitudinal axis of the cord to minimize the potential of vascular damage to the cord, necessitating a larger laminectomy.

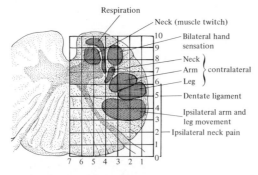

Figure 10–3. The authors' experiences in performing percutaneous high cervical cordotomy are summarized on a map overlying a cross section of the spinal cord. The exploring electrode seeks to find the arm or leg area in the lateral spinothalamic tract. A well-controlled lesion then denervates the appropriate body quadrant.

In the stereotactic method the level is confined to the area between C_1 and C_2, since this is the only area of spinal cord sufficiently uncovered by bone to allow for easy manipulation of the needle. The procedure is performed with the patient awake, supine, with his head supported in a biplane x-ray or fluoroscopy unit. With local anesthesia and under x-ray control, a No. 22 spinal needle is placed in the subarachnoid space between the laminae of C_1 and C_2, entering laterally from a point just below and behind the mastoid tip. Once a free flow of cerebrospinal fluid is obtained, the anterior surface of the cord and/or the dentate ligament is outlined either by air or by an emulsion of Pantopaque and cerebrospinal fluid. With the anterior quadrant of the cord thus identified, the needle is manipulated so a very fine electrode, insulated except for its tip, can be passed into the cord substance through the needle. From this point the portion of the lateral spinothalamic tract subserving the painful area, usually either arm or leg, can be identified by passing a stimulating current and asking the patient to report the peripheral locus of sensation. Once the electrode has been appropriately placed, the tract can be destroyed in successive steps by making lesions with a radiofrequency current, testing for the adequacy of sensory loss and pain relief between them. The procedure can be terminated if motor loss due to inappropriate placement of the electrode too near the cortical tract seems imminent.

One disadvantage of both types of cordotomy is the transitoriness of pain relief. The majority of patients experience return of pain within one to two years, presumably because other cord pathways have "taken over" crude painful sensations since there is no evidence of tract regeneration in an adequate lesion. This does not restrict its value in patients with malignant disease and limited longevity. In patients with benign disease this is a severe restriction, since a cordotomy cannot be repeated unless the first procedure was inadequate.

Cordotomy receives its major use in ipsilateral somatic pain, since bilateral cordotomy at any level may impair normal urinary function and sexual potency (providing these remain in spite of the primary malignant disease). In addition bilateral high cervical cordotomy is generally contraindicated for any condition, since respiratory fibers may be included in the lesion, especially if the analgesic level is carried high. Mortality from such respiratory failure is insidious, since respiration may appear normal while the patient is awake, but during sleep he may successively hypoventilate and remain unstimulated by increasing CO_2 levels because of

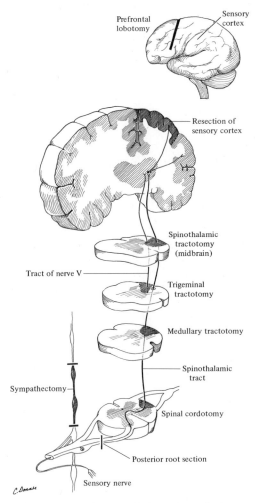

Prefrontal lobotomy

Sensory cortex

Resection of sensory cortex

Spinothalamic tractotomy (midbrain)

Tract of nerve V

Trigeminal tractotomy

Medullary tractotomy

Spinothalamic tract

Sympathectomy

Spinal cordotomy

Posterior root section

Sensory nerve

C. Donati

Figure 10–4.   Sites at which neurosurgical procedures may be performed for the relief of intractable pain.

the neurologic lesion. During the early days of cordotomy nocturnal death was a major reason for mortality until this mechanism was discovered. With judicious placement of the stereotactic electrode in the appropriate patient levels of analgesia may be kept low enough to allow bilateral cordotomy without causing mortality.

Ipsilateral paresis due to encroachment of the lesion on the corticospinal tract below the dentate is an occasional complication in the open method but is absent from the stereotactic method, since needle placement can be checked prior to lesion making.

The advantage of the stereotactic method over the open method is obvious. The procedure does not entail major surgery, is easier on the patient, and precludes the complications of anesthesia,

blood loss, and surgical trauma. Pain relief by this method can thus be offered to older and more debilitated patients. There remains a place for open cordotomies, however, primarily for bilateral, midline, or visceral pain of the lower trunk and extremities in selected patients.

Brain Stem Tractotomy.   Since the level of high cervical cordotomy may not completely eradicate pain in the neck and shoulder, still higher levels of interruption of the spinothalamic tract have been sought (Figure 10–4). In the medulla the tract lies ventral to the spinal tract and nucleus of the fifth nerve, and sections have been made here to treat high-lying pain. Respiratory difficulty is a possibility. This procedure is rarely done, since there are relatively few patients who require it and the surgery is technically difficult in that the tract is difficult to localize at the operating table.

As mentioned, the spinal trigeminal tract lies just posterior to the spinothalamic tract at medullary levels, and this is frequently sectioned to produce facial analgesia. Since touch is spared, satisfactory analgesia can be maintained without fear of distressing anesthesia or the danger of corneal ulceration. The same complications exist as with spinothalamic tractotomy in this area.

Worthy of note is the fact that sensory tracts of the seventh, ninth, and tenth cranial nerves lie just dorsal to the trigeminal tract at medullary levels, between it and the cuneate nucleus. Section of this tract, frequently performed at the same time as trigeminal tract section, will relieve pain in the palate, pharynx, and ear.

In the midbrain the spinothalamic tract is still superficial. It is close to the inferior colliculus and here one may perform mesencephalic tractotomy. The procedure is technically difficult and because of the closeness of neighboring tracts and the frequent production of disagreeable dysesthesias, frequently worse than the original pain, this operation is little done at present and is of historical interest only.

Thalamotomy.   Since the thalamus is thought to be the lowest way station in the perception of pain in the cerebral hemispheres and is a well-localized nuclear group, thalamotomy has been considered at various times as an appropriate target for surgical pain relief. At present it is clear that stereotactic lesions made in the main sensory nuclei of the thalamus produce extensive sensory loss but do not relieve pain. Lesions made in parafascicular–centrum medianum regions, alone or in combination with lesions in the intralaminar nuclei, have been reported to produce good subjective pain relief in some cases without sensory loss. The types of pain that may be relieved and the exact sites and extent of the lesions needed remain an active area of investigation.

Lesions in the dorsal medial and anterior nuclei produce effects similar to frontal lobe lesions, described below.

Cortical and Subcortical Sections. Resection of the sensory cortex has proved of no value in the management of chronic pain syndromes. Other cortical resections deal primarily with the control of the affective response to pain.

Section of various portions of thalamocortical radiations in the white matter of the frontal lobe produces pain relief but in proportion to the disturbance of personality. For this reason if the personality disturbance is short-lived, so is usually the pain relief. The operation is still occasionally used for patients with a limited life-span and intense mental anguish secondary to pain. In some individuals the response is remarkable. They apparently continue to experience pain but appear indifferent to it.

In an attempt to relieve the intense suffering associated with pain without altering personality, recent experiments on lesions made in the limbic system, particularly the cingulate gyrus, have appeared promising. This also remains under investigation.

Activation of Pain Inhibitory Mechanisms. With the description of the "gate" theory of pain a theoretical mechanism became available to explain the so-called counterirritant method of pain relief. It has been known that some patients discover serendipitously that they may provoke periods of pain relief through some form of stimulation. The authors are acquainted with several cases demonstrating this phenomenon. In one, a patient with intense burning pain secondary to a median nerve injury found he could be relieved of his pain for several hours after vigorously massaging his arm with an electric vibrator. In another, a patient with a painful amputation stump similarly sought relief by vigorously pounding it with a rubber hammer he bought for the purpose. These are not rare experiences.

Using evidence from experiments on pain conduction and central summation within the spinal cord and at higher levels, inhibition of pain by stimulation of various areas is under investigation. The sites stimulated include peripheral nerves, posterior columns in the cord, and various cerebral structures including the thalamus and the septal area of the frontal lobes. Promising results have been obtained in some cases, primarily with stimulation of peripheral nerves and posterior columns. It is too early to state definitively whether these will be useful techniques.

"Paraphysiologic" Treatment of Pain. The control of the unconscious mind over the conscious is little understood but has tremendous value in pain control, both in the control of the affective response to pain and also on the penetration and expression of painful impulses arising from lower nervous elements into the conscious level. For the purposes of discussion this may be divided into three topics to be considered in the treatment of pain. The first is the well-known placebo effect, the second hypnosis, and last, more formally organized social and cultural phenomena such as acupuncture.

Placebo Effect. Nearly every physician has administered an innocuous or perhaps totally ineffective preparation and observed a dramatic though usually temporary clinical effect. This is widely known as the placebo effect, but it has much wider implications than just the administration of medications. The placebo effect of surgery cannot be underestimated and should be taken into account when evaluating any surgical procedure for pain control. The medical literature contains sufficient examples of dramatic relief of pain by sham operations (e.g., angina pectoris) for this not to be a well-documented experience. Any concerned physician who approaches his patient enthusiastically with a new method for pain relief should recognize that he is also making use of the placebo effect in his treatment. The placebo effect expresses itself in three areas: in the physician's concern and desire to help his patient which is reflected in the patient's desire to be helped, in the complex and prolonged preparations undergone in performing any surgical procedure, and in the administration of any drug.

Hypnosis. An attempt to manipulate the affective response to pain is carried on by those physicians who are acquainted with and skillful in the technique of hypnosis. It may be termed a conscious attempt to alter the affective response to pain. In those patients susceptible to the technique, autohypnosis may be useful in teaching them to manipulate their own pain responses. A firm line cannot be drawn between the use of suggestion, perhaps unwittingly, that operates in the placebo effect and the conscious attempt with the use of hypnosis to alter pain, and one is tempted to think they are parts of a continuum.

Hypnosis has been outstandingly successful in the management of short-term pain with well-known etiology about to occur on a predictive basis, such as dental and obstetric pains. It has been much less successful in chronic pain syndromes.

Acupuncture and Other Phenomena. In the past have arisen many formally organized and culturally associated disciplines which in whole or in part claim pain relief as their goal. Currently, one of these, the field of acupuncture, has been "discovered" by the Western world which had largely ignored it for centuries. As yet no clear physiologic explanation of this phenomenon can be drawn, but its effectiveness is undeniable. Its most remarkable success seems to be in acute pain control, particularly surgical analgesia. That suggestion or autohypnosis plays an important part seems likely, since most patients are prepared for several days with explanations and demonstrations prior to undergoing surgery. This does not explain its seeming effectiveness in reducing pain in animals and infants, however.

Recent experiments reported in China, if confirmed, suggest that acupuncture sites are close to proprioceptors, muscle spindle organs, and related stretch and pressure receptors. Vigorous proprioceptive discharges induced by manipulation of the acupuncture needle in various ways are thought to block painful impulses arising in other pathways by means of central inhibitory mechanisms. Deep massage of certain areas is said to produce similar effects. In addition, by the use of cross-profusion experiment with animals, humoral substances inhibiting pain are said to have been demonstrated.

CHRONIC PAIN SYNDROMES

Chronic pain can be profitably discussed in terms of certain patterns or syndromes, together with principles for management proved useful by experience. Pain from malignant disease is conveniently separated from "benign" pain, since the patient's expected longevity may dictate the mode of therapy. As a general principle it may be stated that in benign disease section of nerves distal to the central nervous system is preferable, as the denervation is permanent. In malignant disease section of central nervous system tracts subserving pain but sparing the other modalities of sensation may be both more convenient and more effective even though pain relief is not necessarily permanent. This is a matter of little consequence if the expected life-span is also known to be limited.

Intractable Pain from Cancer

Cancer does not produce pain as a primary symptom, a fact that has been well advertised. It is only when cancer bursts the bounds of its primary locus and compresses or infiltrates nerves and tracts or reactively inflames and irritates tissues that it becomes a significant problem. Pain at this point fulfills no useful purpose and causes needless suffering. The approach to such pain consists of three phases: treatment directed toward the tumor itself, pharmacotherapy of pain, surgical intervention on pain pathways.

Surgery for pain is not recommended until the other methods are exhausted, that is, until all possible palliation through reasonable surgical decompression of the tumor itself or surgical diversions around obstructed hollow organs has been performed. Many tumors, even though considered "nonoperable," can still be treated through chemotherapeutic or hormonal techniques. Examples are ovariectomy followed by hypophysectomy or adrenalectomy in breast carcinoma, diethylstilbestrol therapy in carcinoma of the prostate, chemotherapy for multiple myeloma and other solid hematopoietic tumors, and ^{131}I in thyroid cancers. Because of the occasional dramatic relief and prolonged survival in selected cases no patient should go unevaluated for such therapy.

The palliative effects of radiation for pain relief should not be overlooked in the treatment of primary tumors or metastatic masses. It has long been recognized that ionizing radiation frequently has a dramatic analgesic effect. Since very little reduction of the tumor mass is needed to significantly reduce pressure, this form of therapy should be attempted on all painful primary or secondary tumors, even though the tumor is not known to be extremely radiosensitive. The radiotherapist will recognize the aim of therapy as merciful palliation and avoid a massive dose with all its own attendant problems in a vain attempt to "cure." By the same token there is no point in radiating a metastatic mass "because it's there," unless some expected palliative benefit is sought.

Every patient with prolonged pain, except those with individual contraindications, should be placed on the simple, safe salicylates or related drugs. It is surprising how many patients with prolonged pain can be carried with these alone. For their maximum effectiveness the physician should invest a little of himself in their use and, recognizing their real pharmacologic worth as analgesic agents, avoid communicating to his patient indirectly his fear that "they aren't strong enough." If he disbelieves the efficacy of his own therapy, why should his patient contradict him? We make such medications readily available to the patient at frequent intervals when he feels his pain, not doled out parsimoniously on a rigid time schedule. We also intersperse aspirin with one of the milder narcotic analogues, such as propoxyphene (Darvon) or ethoheptazine (Zactirin), so the patient can take some medication as often as every two hours if he feels the need.

Barbiturates, because they can produce habituation, should probably not be used in benign pain but are useful in malignant disease as mild sedatives or to produce nighttime relaxation, especially in the hospitalized patient in unfamiliar, perhaps noisy surroundings.

Every pain produces its counterpoint in suffering, and advantage should be taken of the tranquilizing agents available to subdue this symptom. Our routine has been to give chlorpromazine, 25 mg, three or four times a day as an initial dose, increasing as needed unless sedation becomes troublesome. If depression is a serious symptom, antidepressives are obviously in order and should not be withheld. A recent tranquilizer-antidepressant regime has become available that we have used with good success—in some pains as the only medication needed for control. This consists of chlorprothixene (Taractan), 10 to 25 mg three times a day, coupled with amitriptyline (Elavil), 25 to 50 mg at night.

Some of these drugs have toxic effects that must be watched for, but they are nevertheless preferable to narcotic addiction or surgical procedures if such can be avoided.

The use of the true narcotic drugs is contraindicated unless the patient has a soon-to-be fatal disease. Their ability to produce tolerance severely limits their usefulness, and while they are the best short-term analgesics and should not be withheld on this basis, their sedative and addictive effects outweigh their analgesic benefits as doses gradually increase. It is doubtful that any patient can be carried longer than four months on narcotics, sinking toward the end of this time into somnolence, unable to communicate with his friends and relatives or take adequate nourishment, and arousing only briefly enough to cry piteously for more medicine for his pain. One has only to witness one or two such cases to eschew the chronic use of narcotics forever.

Codeine is the only opiate alkaloid which has a place in the chronic control of pain. In combination with aspirin it is sometimes used to "give an extra punch" to pain relief during particularly stressful situations. It is maximally effective at a dose of 60 mg every four hours, and larger doses or chronic long-term use should be guarded against.

With this background in the general treatment of pain from malignant disease we turn to the surgical approach to cancer pain.

Head and Neck Cancer.   Unlike the spinal nerves, there is little overlap in the distribution of the major trunks of the trigeminal nerve, and their exit is above spinal cord levels. The surgical treatment of pain in head and neck cancer is discussed under benign pain.

Cancer of the Thorax.   Fundamentally tumors of the thorax have similar pain problems. Breast carcinoma, considered as a prototype, frequently involves the brachial plexus by lymphatic spread or metastasizes to ribs, vertebrae, or other bones. After appropriate hormonal therapy, both surgical and pharmacologic, and if x-ray therapy fails, neurosurgical intervention may be sought.

Tumor infiltrating the brachial plexus produces intense arm pain. Posterior rhizotomy is not appropriate, as a totally denervated arm is useless and distressing. Standard surgical cordotomy frequently does not provide a high enough level to completely obliterate pain. It was for this type of pain that the higher tractotomy in the medulla was designed, but its complication rate was too high for general use. With the advent of percutaneous stereotactic cordotomy the lesion can be raised to high levels by incremental increase with careful testing for motor function in between, and in most cases adequate pain relief can be obtained without major surgery. Frontal leukotomy is reserved for those patients totally incapacitated by their emotional response to their disease.

Locally advanced breast cancer resistant to other treatment responds to unilateral cordotomy. Bilateral cordotomy for bilateral pain may be performed, remembering its attendant risks to respiration and bladder function. In general widely diffused cancer is better treated by chemotherapy, hormone therapy, or radiotherapy than by cordotomy.

Pain from spinal metastases, which is a bilateral or midline pain, may sometimes be treated with the intrathecal injection of 5 percent phenol in Pantopaque, manipulated under fluoroscopic control to bathe the appropriate roots. Although it is possible to obtain relief without significant loss of motor function or sphincter control, the patient should be informed of such risks. Pain relief is probably produced by selective destruction of "C" fibers, although pathologic material demonstrates that all size fibers may be destroyed.

What has been said about the relief of pain from distant metastases of breast cancer applies equally well for other types of metastatic disease and will not be repeated.

Tumors of the lung commonly present the same pain problems as tumors of the breast. As the life-span is short, there is rarely any problem associated with wearing-off of the cordotomy analgesia.

Gastrointestinal Cancer and Tumors of Other Abdominal Viscera.   Tumors of intra-abdominal organs are rarely painful until they have spread beyond the confines of the abdominal wall and involve sciatic or lumbar plexi, intercostal nerves, splanchnic nerves, or bone. Injection of the celiac ganglion by alcohol or phenol is effective for some upper abdominal cancers of limited spread. In the rare case where intercostal nerves are involved, a posterior rhizotomy will give lasting relief. If the upper filaments of the lumbar plexus are involved, they may be sacrificed without symptomatic deficit. Lower sacral and coccygeal nerves may be sectioned in those instances where bladder and rectal sphincters are already lost ($S_{2,3,4}$ supply the bladder and S_{3-4} the rectum). However, most pain due to visceral cancer will respond best to spinothalamic tractotomy if unilateral.

In summary, most pain secondary to tumors of the thorax and trunk is best treated, after all other palliative efforts have failed, by spinothalamic tractotomy. For midline, pelvic, and bilateral lower extremity pain, intrathecal phenol may be effective, especially in those who have already lost bladder control from their primary disease.

Surgical relief should be offered to the patient when narcotic medication is needed to control pain in spite of all other efforts and before addiction becomes a possibility.

Intractable Pain from Benign Disease

Spinothalamic tractotomy, so useful in malignant disease, is much less satisfactory in benign disease, since its effectiveness is limited to one or two years in the vast majority of cases. It should be resorted to only when no other form of pain relief seems adequate. The principles of emotional and pharmacologic support, detailed in the previous section, should be vigorously pursued in this type of pain and will work in a surprising number of patients. The surgical therapy of benign pain presents some special problems.

Cephalic Neuralgias. Trigeminal neuralgia, or tic douloureux, is the classic benign facial pain. This is a specific pain syndrome, although its etiology remains obscure. Other types of facial pain, lumped under the loose heading of "atypical facial pain," respond poorly to most attempts for control.

Five hallmarks of tic douloureux are the character of the pain, described as frequent flashes of "lightning-like" or lancinating pain, absence of continuous pain, its characteristic distribution along one of the three major branches of the trigeminal nerve, the absence of abnormal neurologic signs, and the presence of a "trigger area," whose manipulation by touch or facial motion precipitates the pain.

Pharmacologic therapy is useful in many cases of trigeminal neuralgia and should be tried before resorting to surgery. Dilantin, in doses of 300 or 400 mg per day, occasionally is effective. Tegretol is a specific agent for trigeminal neuralgia and is supplied in 200-mg tablets. Dosage should be started at three tablets a day and increased tablet by tablet until relief occurs or a maximum of six tablets a day is reached. The dose should not be increased beyond this level, and a check on white cell count and on hepatic and renal function should be made periodically, as this drug has significant toxicity.

Surgery on nerves subserving facial pain can be performed at several levels. If the pain is restricted to a small area, the appropriate cutaneous nerve—supraorbital, infraorbital, or mandibular—has in the past been avulsed. This procedure is now rarely performed, as its results are only slightly more long-lasting than the simpler alcohol injection. It still has a position for milder first division neuralgia where alcohol block is technically less satisfactory. The second division can be blocked at the infraorbital foramen or farther back for longer duration and more complete denervation in the pterygoid fossa. The third division is sometimes blocked by dentists in the mandible but is done more satisfactorily at the foramen ovale. When more than one division is affected, blocking in Meckel's cave, reached by passing a needle from the lower face lateral to the maxilla through the foramen ovale, is very satisfactory. It is technically difficult but if well performed it can permanently destroy the ganglion cells. A more recent innovation consists of destroying the cells by a radiofrequency electric current.

The most consistently satisfactory form of relief can be obtained by retrogasserian fiber section, reached either through a craniectomy along the floor of the temporal fossa or via a posterior fossa approach to the nerve as it leaves the brain stem. These last are major surgical approaches. The posterior fossa approach takes advantage of the fact that touch and pain nerves separate as they enter the brain stem, and partial section of the nerve abolishes pain but not all touch, thus preserving corneal reflexes.

Denervation of the cornea, if the first division is involved, may cause trouble—some corneal ulceration if the eye care is not excellent. To avoid a completely anesthetic area of the face which can be as distressing to some patients as the pain itself, a medullary section of the spinal trigeminal tract has also been devised, which spares touch and thus corneal sensation. This again is a major procedure and technically difficult. A recent innovation is localization of the tract by stimulating the three trigeminal branches in the face and recording evoked potentials in the medulla before making a section. Medullary tractotomy carries some risk of dysesthesias and is therefore more suited to cancer of the oropharynx than to trigeminal neuralgia.

Paroxysmal pain of other cranial nerves is also known. Accompanying the seventh nerve there is the tiny nervus intermedius which supplies some sensation to the ear. This may be subject to pain of a character similar to trigeminal neuralgia. The pain may be precipitated by touching the external auditory canal. Division of the nervus intermedius does not usually give an area of analgesia because of overlapping fibers from other sensory sources but does cure the pain.

Glossopharyngeal and upper vagal neuralgia are considered together. They are rare but slightly more common than nervus intermedius pain. The pain of glossopharyngeal neuralgia exists at the root of the tongue, radiating down the throat to the ear. It can be precipitated by touching the pharynx and is diagnosed by abolishing the trigger zone by cocainization of the pharynx. The pain is relieved by section of the glossopharyngeal and upper few vagal rootlets in the posterior fossa.

Cancer of the head and neck produces pain carried in the sensory fibers of the cranial nerves described above. The mouth, pharynx, and larynx are innervated by the fifth nerve, the nervus intermedius of the seventh nerve, the ninth nerve, and the upper part of the tenth nerve. To produce analgesia for carcinoma in this area by nerve section, division of all these nerves must be complete. Poor results in some cases may be attributed to leaving the nervus intermedius intact. A carcinoma involving the neck may also require division of the second, third, and fourth posterior nerve roots of the cervical region. If carcinoma involves both sides of the pharynx, complete division of all these nerves is impossible. Bilateral division of the motor root of the fifth nerve results in the paralyzed mechanism of mastication, while bilateral division of the ninth nerve eliminates control of the carotid pressure regulatory mechanism, with intense rise of blood pressure. Medullary tractotomy which includes the descending pain fibers of the fifth, seventh, ninth, and tenth nerves in one small section is therefore the procedure of choice. It requires a very precise technique.

Visceral Pain. As mentioned, the sensory afferents from the viscera travel in splanchnic nerves, pass through the sympathetic chain, and enter posterior roots. Rarely benign intractable pain from the viscera may be best treated by splanchnicectomy and sympathectomy. Psycho-somatic complaints often masquerade as visceral pain and must be avoided. Since most visceral pain on careful investigation is found to arise from unrecognized pathologic conditions which have their own appropriate therapy, only the most desperate cases should be considered for denervating surgery. Pancreatitis has been variously treated by splanchnic alcohol injection, splanchnicectomy, bilateral rhizotomy, and bilateral cordotomy without unanimous consensus as to the best method.

Anginal Pain. Sympathetic denervation for angina pectoris has in the past been performed. Pain fibers are carried in the sympathetic nerves and travel via the superior, middle, and inferior cardiac nerves together with a few direct cardiac nerves from the upper thoracic sympathetic chain. Their connection with the spinal cord is through the first three intercostal nerves, and division of the communications between the sympathetic chain and these three nerves does provide relief from cardiac pain.

Liver and Biliary Tracts. Ordinarily pain from these structures can be corrected by standard surgical procedures. In persistent pain resection of the splanchnic nerves and lower thoracic ganglia on the right side has been effective after satisfactory response to a preliminary diagnostic block.

Pain of Kidney and Ureter. Renal and upper ureteral afferents pass through the minor and least splanchnic trunks to reach the lower thoracic and first lumbar ganglia. Section of these has occasionally resulted in prolonged pain relief. A posterior rhizotomy of T_{10} to L_2 may also give permanent pain freedom.

Pain of Spinal Origin. Intractable pain of spinal origin usually results from scarring and arachnoiditis consequent to spinal infection, trauma, or multiple surgical procedures. Incapacitating lower back pain after multiple discectomies, laminectomies, and fusions is unfortunately not rare and is one of the most difficult pains to treat. Cordotomy has rarely been effective in such cases, although if the pain is well lateralized it may give one or two years of relief. Posterior rhizotomy when only one root is involved seems most effective, but unfortunately usually several are implicated. Limited section of L_5 or S_1 has been carried out, producing pain relief without disability in some cases.

Pain Following Peripheral Injuries. Several well-defined pain patterns are known after traumatic peripheral injuries.

Causalgia. Following partial peripheral nerve injuries an intense burning pain occurs in the peripheral distribution of the nerve. The median nerve is the most commonly involved.

There may be sensory loss but rarely motor loss. The pain is accompanied by a variety of alterations in the autonomic nervous system of the area. The skin is usually cold, pale, dry, and shiny but it may be moist, cyanotic, or red. Pain is precipitated by touch of the affected area or even by the jarring produced by someone walking across the room. It is also aggravated by emotional factors, and for that reason the pain was ascribed at one time to psychologic causes. This does not seem to be the case. It is supposed that efferent sympathetic tonic impulses, continuously flowing out to the peripheral blood vessels, join up directly to the afferent pain fibers so that there is a constant pain related to the tonic sympathetic innervation of the peripheral area. Such junctions have never been demonstrated, but this is a plausible explanation for the fact that some patients with causalgia are relieved by sympathectomy.

Painful Amputation Stumps. Any amputation stump may be painful, mainly because the end neuromata which form at the divided nerves may be pressed upon by an ill-fitting prosthesis. Sometimes Novocain block of these end bulbs over a short period may be all that is required. Reoperation produces more bulbs, and neither reoperation nor alcohol injection of the neuromata can be guaranteed to relieve pain, but they are worth trying. Cordotomy is usually effective, but it must be recognized that the patient cannot tolerate any iatrogenic weakness of the unamputated extremity.

Painful Phantoms. After an amputation almost every patient has a phantom limb. This within a few months or years shortens and disappears into the stump. It is obvious that when a limb is removed the portion of the brain concerned with the appreciation of that limb in space takes some time to forget about it. Some phantoms, however, may be painful, and such patients are aware of their phantom in a crushed or distorted position such as it assumed at the time of injury. It is difficult to understand why cordotomy should benefit these people, but if performed early in many cases it does. It is more effective in lower limb amputations than in upper limb amputations. It is likely to be effective if phantom pain can be produced by manipulating the stump and unlikely if it is totally unrelated to such activity.

Postinfectious Pain. Two types of postinfectious pain are worth mentioning. The first is postherpetic neuralgia, which is a continuous, intense, burning pain following herpetic infection of peripheral nerves, including the cranial nerves, and occurring usually in the elderly. It is thought that the causative virus enters the posterior root ganglion via the spinal nerves or cranial nerves, but it is also possible that it enters the spinal cord and sets up irritable foci there. For this reason posterior rhizotomy has not been an effective treatment. Good results of anterolateral cordotomy are less than 50 percent.

The pain of tabes dorsalis is fortunately much less frequent now than formerly. In patients who have frequent gastric crises of lightning pains, bilateral anterolateral cordotomy will provide relief in the majority of cases.

Psychologic Pain

There remains a small residuum of patients with pain which has no discoverable etiology and who fit into none of the known patterns of idiopathic pain. Before consigning such patients to prolonged psychiatric treatment, it is well to remember that a portion of these will in time develop disease that had escaped previous diagnostic efforts. The criteria of psychiatric diagnosis must be fulfilled before one can rest assured that such treatment is appropriate.

Similarly the psychology of pain itself should be appreciated. The advantage of "knowing one's patient" in determining the severity of a pain syndrome cannot be overemphasized. The appreciation of pain varies from patient to patient and from time to time within the same patient. It has long been noted in warfare that soldiers may experience severe and mutilating injuries without subjective feelings of pain while on the battlefield, only to complain after being taken back to hospitals in rear areas. Thus one can appreciate the intensification of pain in the carcinoma patient faced with the inevitability of his own death and the consequent dislocation of his plans. The physician then must treat the entire syndrome of pain, not only by interrupting nervous pathways to reduce painful stimuli but also by calm and patient understanding of the patient's difficulties.

SUMMARY

The problems engendered in the care of the acute and chronic pain patient need to be managed in three areas. These are (1) the affective control of the responses to pain; (2) pharmacologic agents for deafferentation; (3) surgical approaches for section of pain-carrying nerve tracts. Physicians will obtain their greatest degree of success if they bear in mind that all pain problems must be approached through these three avenues. Which of the three to rely on primarily can be understood in terms of a knowledge of the pain patterns that are common to the human organism.

SUGGESTIONS FOR
FURTHER READING

Goodman, L. S., and Gilman, A. (eds.): *The Pharmacologic Basis of Therapeutics.* 5th ed. Macmillan Publishing Co., Inc., New York, 1975.
A superior discussion of drugs used in the treatment of pain is included in this standard text.

Melzock, R., and Wall, P. D.: Pain mechanisms, a new theory. *Science,* **150**:971, 1965.
A bit dated in this rapidly expanding field but still a good short introduction to the "gate" theory of pain.

Mullan, S.: The transmission and central projection of pain. *Med. Clin. North Am.,* **52**:15, 1968.
A discussion by one of the authors of the anatomy of pain tracts. The volume containing this article also has several excellent reviews of other topics on pain.

White, J. C., and Sweet, W. H.: *Pain and the Neurosurgeon.* Charles C Thomas, Springfield, Ill., 1969.
This is the most complete treatise on the surgical control of pain, written by neurosurgeons for other neurosurgeons.

Chapter 11

PREOPERATIVE ASSESSMENT AND CARE

Robert E. Madden

CHAPTER OUTLINE

History
    Biographic Data
    History of Present Illness
    Past History
    Family History
    Review of Systems
    Social and Occupational History and
      Habits
Physical Examination
    Vital Signs
    Inspection
    Head and Neck
    Thorax and Lungs
    Abdomen
Basic Laboratory Examination
Problem-Oriented Record Keeping
Further Considerations by System
    Cardiovascular System
    Respiratory System

Genitourinary System
Gastrointestinal System and Nutrition
Neurologic System
Musculoskeletal System
Endocrine System
Special Considerations
    Blood Coagulation and Fibrinolysis
    Evaluation of Hemostasis
    Clinical Defects
Blood Transfusion
    Complications
    Frozen Blood
    Problems with Massive Whole-Blood
      Transfusion
Nonobstetric Surgery in Pregnancy
Surgery in the Aged
Psychologic Preparation for Surgery
Preoperative Monitoring in the Critically
    Ill Patient

The successful outcome of an operation depends largely on accurate preoperative assessment and preparation. The integrity and functional reserves of the major organ system should be known before operation. The extent of this evaluation depends upon the type of procedure contemplated and the findings from the history, physical examination, and laboratory tests. The results of the initial assessment reveal the extent and nature of the patient's disease and determine the operative management. Detection of additional diseases may delay, modify, or result in cancelling the operation. When early operation is necessary, the preoperative preparation must be rapid. For an elective procedure the preparation may take days or even weeks.

HISTORY

A detailed history should be obtained of the present illness and of previous symptoms, treatments, and operations. All data from the admitting or referring physician should be made available. Language difficulties may require the services of an interpreter, and knowledge of the local or cultural idiom is helpful. Parents or other responsible adults will be required in history taking from a child or an incompetent.

An adequate history outline for the surgical patient would include:

1. Biographic Data. Name, age, sex, nationality, occupation, marital status, number of previous admissions.

2. History of Present Illness. A good starting point is "when were you last entirely well?" or "what brought you to the doctor?" As the story unfolds one or more disease processes will suggest themselves to the interviewer which can be either reinforced or eliminated by further questioning. The principal symptoms should be developed and characterized. *Establish the approximate date of onset.* Was it a day ago, a month ago, a year ago? Of course a precise onset may not be remembered but any approximation will be helpful. *Characterize the chief*

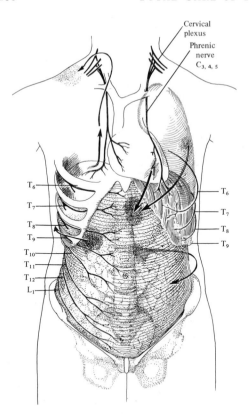

Cervical
plexus
Phrenic
nerve
$C_{3, 4, 5}$

T_6
T_7
T_8
T_9
T_{10}
T_{11}
T_{12}
L_1

T_6
T_7
T_8
T_9

Figure 11–1. The afferent fibers of the parietal peritoneum are somatic and pass back to the cord in the seventh to tenth intercostal nerves. The innervation of the diaphragm is also somatic with the fibers traveling in the phrenic nerve. Pain is then referred by the supraclavicular nerves to the top of the shoulder. Myocardial and pleuritic pain may be referred to the epigastrium and pain from a retroperitoneal source may be referred anteriorly in the abdomen.

complaint. Pain is the most frequent complaint. Is it steady, cramping, localized, radiating, progressive? What is the relationship with time of day, meals, body position? Pain can frequently be referred from another area. Examples are epigastric pain referred from the chest (pleuritis, pneumonia, myocardial ischemia) or from the duodenum (perforated ulcer), shoulder pain referred from the abdomen (subphrenic abscess), and intrascapular pain referred from the biliary tract or pancreatic bed (Figure 11–1). *Were there other symptoms?* Fever, chill, anorexia, malaise, weight loss are all constitutional symptoms. *What is the progress of the symptom?* Were there exacerbations and remissions or has it been progressive? *Has there been any treatment?* The patient could have been self-medicated or have consulted a physician. Questioning must be

complete, careful, and considerate.[19] The patient has his own personal disease problem, although a rushed house officer may have eight or ten others to see that day. Patients are nearly always frightened, sometimes terrified.[18,28] Will it be cancer? Will I lose a breast? Will I live? Illness may also portend a financial or business disaster to the breadwinner. A considerate attitude is welcome. The injection of personal feelings and prejudices into the interview or the hospital record is to be avoided. The hospital record of today can become the court evidence of tomorrow. The house officer may disagree with the opinions of his attending surgeons, but he or she would be encouraged to voice these privately and they should not become part of the record.

3. Past History. For most surgical problems the past history has its greatest value in assessing present surgical risk. Other problems may be uncovered, and the discovery of coincidental disease is a dividend of the workup and helps assess the surgical risk. Many people with surgical problems have not seen a physician in years; for some it is the first time. This encounter could be very beneficial to the patient in terms of total health.

Any past surgical procedures should be recorded in detail since it may affect the technique or approach of reoperation. Of particular importance is a past history suggestive of diabetes, coronary artery disease, or hypertension.

The dose of any medication being taken and the duration of therapy should be noted. A previous history of phlebitis or embolism with the use of anticoagulants may predict a postoperative problem. Previous use of corticosteroids or ACTH may have produced adrenal atrophy, and postoperative collapse may result. Intravenous steroid replacement is essential (Chapter 27). Patients receiving rauwolfia derivatives have depletion of catecholamines and may require vasopressors during operation.[1] Phenothiazine tranquilizers depress general endocrine function and may precipitate hypotension under anesthesia.[2] Diuretics may have depleted potassium reserves which can potentiate the action of muscle relaxants or the dosage of digitalis.[14] A number of drugs interfere with platelet aggregation ranging from aspirin and antihistamines to phenylbutazone and many tranquilizers. This effect, which can last for several days after taking the drug, has been responsible for many postoperative bleeding problems previously not understood. Other drugs including methyldopa, penicillin, cephalothin, quinine, sulfonamides, and others form weak, reversible protein bonds. These immunogens can result in a positive Coombs test and even hemolytic anemia. Most important, if their usage is not known, they can cause difficulty in the cross-matching of blood.[11] The patient must always be asked about a history of drug or other allergies.

Some diseases of surgical interest are endemic. Examples include the fungal diseases of the lungs and soft tissues, amebic infestations, and the parasites of both blood and reticuloendothelial systems. A previous history of endocrine disease, such as Addison's disease, diabetes mellitus or insipidus, and thyroid dysfunction, is important because of the high risk that surgery entails.

4. Family History.   There are many diseases with familial tendencies. They include disorders of the endocrine system, hemolytic disorders, hypertension and arteriosclerosis, enzyme deficiencies, and neoplasms. Communicable diseases are also important to note and may be prevalent in lower socioeconomic populations.

5. Review of Systems.   This is really a checklist supplementing the present illness and past history to ensure completeness. The surgeon's main concern is the integrity of the three major organ systems: cardiovascular respiratory (CVR), gastrointestinal (GI), and genitourinary (GU). A series of standard questions is asked. These include inquiry for cough, dyspnea, hemoptysis, chest pain, orthopnea, ankle edema (CVR); nausea, vomiting, diarrhea, weight loss, abdominal pain, itching (GI); or flank pain frequency, fever, burning, hematuria, discharge (GU); excessive thirst could mean kidney disease or diabetes. Inquiry for symptoms common to the integument, the head, eye, ears, nose, throat, the peripheral vascular system, the nervous system (such as convulsions, vertigo, sensory and motor losses), the musculoskeletal disabilities, and a menstrual and gynecologic history is part of a thorough system review. Each specialty would emphasize its own area, but it is essential to cover the three major support systems.

6. Social and Occupational History and Habits.   Alcohol, tobacco, and drug use can produce serious operative and postoperative complications. The patient may, however, deny or minimize their use. The chronic alcoholic has reduced hepatic function and postoperatively he may go into delirium tremens or bleed. Smoking reduces respiratory reserve, predisposes to postoperative secretions, and it adversely affects peripheral vascular flow. Its use is to be discouraged in the preoperative period. Users of "hard drugs," such as heroin and morphine, commonly have hepatitis and parasites and are predisposed to cardiovascular instability and the acute withdrawal syndrome in the postoperative period. Drug users can often be recognized by their furtive appearance, state of anxiety during examination, and the presence of phlebitis, chronic abscesses, and scars. Many, however, are discovered by the appearances of acute withdrawal in the immediate postoperative period.

The patient's occupation may help in the diagnosis and assessment of risk. Exposure to industrial dust and nitrous oxide produces bronchitis and reduced pulmonary function. Specific dusts produce pneumoconioses, cancer, or fungal lung diseases. Some occupations are thought to cause hypertension and early coronary heart disease.

PHYSICAL EXAMINATION

The scope of the physical examination should be thorough but may be limited by the urge for treatment, as in the severely traumatized patient requiring emergency surgery. The physical examination, more so than the history, results in the detection of hidden or unsuspected disease. Hypertension, organomegaly, aneurysms, tumors, enlarged lymph nodes, nodules of the thyroid gland, the prostate and the breast, rectal polyps, and cystic ovaries may all be discovered during a careful examination.

The properly organized physical examination starts with determination of vital signs, then a general inspection, and finally a systematic coverage of the body.

1. Vital Signs.   Vital signs on admission form the preoperative baseline for anesthetic and postoperative management. The detection of preoperative abnormalities is therefore most important. Hypertension itself is usually essential but occasionally results from hyperthyroidism, adrenal tumor, renal artery stenosis, or aortic insufficiency. Hypotension is usually associated with shock but could mean an endocrine deficiency. Cardiac irregularities are due usually to primary heart disease, coronary, valvular, or myocardial, but could be metabolic or endocrine, as, for example, hyperkalemia or thyrotoxicosis. Dyspnea is seen in primary parenchymal lung disease, atelectasis, pleural disease, and obesity. It is also seen in metabolic acidosis and early heart failure.

2. Inspection.   Some conditions can be recognized immediately on inspection. The cachectic patient is wrinkled and has general wasting, dry skin, and prominent cheekbones. Muscles are stretched over and between bony prominences, and the fingers, arms, and legs resemble spindles (Figure 11–2). Important causes are advanced cancer, severe cardiac disease, chronic infection, renal disease, Addison's disease, psychic depression, and starvation. Severe weight loss results in a reduction of body protein, a decrease in blood volume, and alterations in electrolytes.

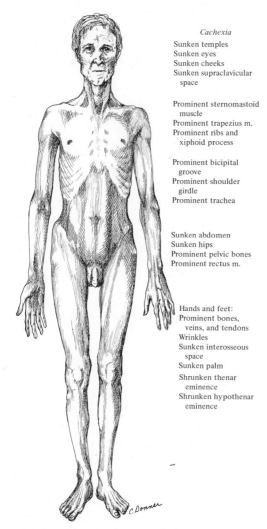

Cachexia

Sunken temples
Sunken eyes
Sunken cheeks
Sunken supraclavicular
space

Prominent sternomastoid
muscle
Prominent trapezius m.
Prominent ribs and
xiphoid process

Prominent bicipital
groove
Prominent shoulder
girdle
Prominent trachea

Sunken abdomen
Sunken hips
Prominent pelvic bones
Prominent rectus m.

Hands and feet:
Prominent bones,
veins, and tendons
Wrinkles
Sunken interosseous
space
Sunken palm
Shrunken thenar
eminence
Shrunken hypothenar
eminence

Figure 11–2. Cachexia can be the result of a number of advanced conditions, including malignancy, cardiac, renal, or endocrine disease, psychotic states, or starvation.

Edema and ascites should be looked for. Dehydration is seen in the sunken eyes, dry lips and tongue, and a parchmentlike skin. Obesity is usually due to overeating but may result from Cushing's disease or corticosteroid medication. The obese patient represents as great a surgical risk as one who is cachectic.

Loss of blood, acute or chronic, produces pallor of the skin and conjunctivae (Chapter 2). In acute blood loss the patient may have a pale, cold, clammy skin. If it is chronic blood loss, as from an hiatal hernia or gastrointestinal malignancy, the peripheral vasoconstriction is missing, and it is difficult to rule out other causes of anemia such as pernicious anemia or chronic

infection. Jaundice may accompany anemia or be mistaken for pallor. Pain is recognized in the patient's face, gait, habitus, and in protective reactions during examination.

3. Head and Neck. The chief surgical problems are tumors of the intraoral cavity and pharynx, including hypopharynx and nasopharynx, enlargement of lymph nodes of the neck and supraclavicular fossae, skin and scalp lesions, and thyroid enlargements (Chapters 16 and 27). Other findings suggest unsuspected disease. Occular changes in both hypothyroidism and hyperthyroidism would be examples. Periorbital edema could mean nephritis. Shifts in the trachea, retractions, flaring nostrils, and prominent neck veins reflect cardiorespiratory disease or perhaps vascular obstructions in the thorax or pleural effusion. A supple neck is needed for uncomplicated intubation. Special tests, such as ophthalmodynamometry in evaluating carotid artery stenosis, could be obtained on consultation.

4. Thorax and Lungs. Well-developed skills in inspection, palpation, auscultation, and percussion are required in the examination of the chest. A complete discussion will be found in Chapter 30. Proper examination of the breast is described in Chapter 26.

5. Abdomen. Of most frequent interest to the general surgeon are the organ systems in the abdomen. The abdomen is topically divided into four quadrants.

With the patient supine, relaxed, and comfortable, the abdomen is inspected under adequate light. Bulging flanks, spider nevi, and distended veins combine to give the picture of liver disease with ascites and portal hypertension. An abnormal distribution of hair or its absence may indicate a liver disease. In the distention of mechanical bowel obstruction peristalsis may be visible. A pulsating mass could mean an aortic aneurysm.

Palpation should be performed with the head elevated on a pillow and the knees flexed, bringing the pelvis and the costal margins closer. The examination begins away from the region of suspected pathology. The principal findings of surgical disease are masses and tenderness. Pathologic masses within or between organs may displace them. In health the bare edge of the liver may be felt, the lower pole of the right kidney, and perhaps the fecal-containing left colon. Percussion of the abdomen should also be systematic. It will confirm the outlines of liver or spleen or of tumor masses, and distinguish between gas and fluid. Auscultation of the abdomen is most valuable in characterizing the bowel sounds and discovering vascular bruits. Vascular bruits are heard in renal artery stenosis, occasionally in aneurysms of the aorta or splenic artery, and in arteriovenous fistulas. A thorough search for abdominal aneurysm should be made in patients with occlusive arterial disease in the legs. Rectal and vaginal examinations are essential in every complete physical examination. Examination of the extremities is necessary to detect orthopedic and peripheral vascular problems (see Chapters 29 and 31).

BASIC LABORATORY EXAMINATION

Complete blood count (CBC), including platelet estimation, and a midstream urinalysis are essential in all patients, except in extreme emergencies. Sickle cell preps should be done in Negroes. Partial thromboplastin time (PTT) is the most widely used screening test for clotting deficiency. The prothrombin time, however, also considered routine in many centers, will detect the presence of anticoagulant drugs and other acquired coagulopathies. Blood chemistries are determined today in most centers by automated multichannel analyzers. Unsuspected problems may be detected such as hypercalcemia (parathyroid disease, cancer), hyperuricemia (leukemia, gout, polycythemia, or patients taking drugs such as Diuril and aspirin), and raised enzyme levels (liver disease, myocardial infarction). When multichannel analysis is not available, a minimal requirement would include blood sugar (diabetes mellitus) and blood urea nitrogen or creatinine (kidney disease). The chest x-ray and ECG should be performed in all patients over 40.

Two screening tests for cancer are now often routine: the cervical Pap smear for all female admissions between certain ages and examination of the stool for blood as obtained on the examination finger. Their value cannot be overestimated.

PROBLEM-ORIENTED RECORD KEEPING

Medical record keeping has traditionally been oriented to the source of the information. A system, oriented to the patient's problem or problems, named for its author the Weed System, has gained usage in a number of centers.

The information obtained from the history, physical examination, and laboratory investigations forms the data base. The physician can then proceed in several ways. The patient may be treated immediately, the data base may be expanded, or corrective measures may be initiated. Other possibilities are that the patient may be discharged without treatment, be so ill as to preclude further treatment, or may die. Audit of the data base for reliability and completeness usually results in requests for further data. Additional history may be obtained from the patient or family, consultations may be requested, or further laboratory investigations may be required. The process ends with the formulation of a problem or list of problems. A problem is defined as one or more abnormalities in the history, physical examination, or laboratory investigations. The problem may be a simple diagnosis, such as an uncomplicated inguinal hernia in a healthy young male. Frequently, however, the problem may be difficult, e.g., the patient with severe abdominal pain and few abnormal physical signs. Examples are porphyria, mesenteric occlusion, or drug withdrawal. Here a definite diagnosis cannot be made. "Diagnosis" should be used only when it is felt to be accurate. Otherwise the term "problem" is used. Problems may be multiple, as in a patient with an embolus in the axillary artery complicated by cancer, hypertension, electrocardiographic evidence of a recent myocardial infarction, and hyperglycemia. The problems may converge on one diagnosis or diverge producing two or more diagnoses. During the assessment new problems may arise or others may resolve or become inactive. For example, a patient with uncontrolled diabetes may respond to treatment, but his vascular insufficiency may progress to gangrene. Diagnoses with question marks or preceded by the phrase "rule out" are not used. The word "impression" is reserved for discussion or assessment of the problem. A current problem or flow sheet is prepared, and a plan is developed for diagnosis and therapy.

In problem-oriented record keeping, progress notes are organized into a format: S, subjective changes; O, objective changes; A, assessment; P, plan. In this way the patient's chief problem or problems are reviewed and updated until therapeutic resolution or failure.

FURTHER CONSIDERATIONS BY SYSTEM

1. **Cardiovascular System.** A careful history should always be obtained of any possible cardiac disease, such as myocardial infarction, congestive failure, or unexplained chest pain.[13] In addition, as stated above, an ECG is essential in every patient over 40 who will have a general anesthetic. About one third of patients over this age will be found to have some cardiovascular abnormality. Special attention should be paid to drugs that are taken, such as diuretics, cardiac glycosides, tranquilizers, rauwolfia, and anticoagulants (pages 211–12). Any abnormalities of the cardiovascular system should be corrected

as rapidly as possible (see Chapter 2). Treatment may be needed for congestive heart failure, fibrillation, or arrhythmias. A history of myocardial infarction within nine months should lead to postponing an elective operation. If it is necessary to operate on a patient with recent myocardial infarction, special care should be taken to prevent hypoxia and hypotension during and after surgery and to monitor the patient for extrasystoles and signs of cardiac ischemia. Special care is necessary in the patient with complete or incomplete heart block. Temporary artificial electrical pacing may be necessary. Arteriosclerosis is a generalized disease. The detection of arterial disease means that the patient could develop coronary thrombosis, a cerebrovascular complication or thrombosis, or embolism of a peripheral artery postoperatively. The patient with venous disease may develop phlebitis and pulmonary embolism.

2. Respiratory System.   The site of operation is a major factor in the production of postoperative pulmonary complications. The incidence of such complications is as high as 10 percent after operation in the upper abdomen in men. Other factors are obesity, smoking, age, and type, depth, and duration of anesthesia and the presence of oral sepsis. Elective operations should not be performed in patients with acute respiratory infections. The assessment of pulmonary function is most often determined by sound clinical judgment.[31] In patients with known pulmonary disease, however, specific pulmonary function testing, including blood gas studies, is indicated particularly if a thoracic procedure is contemplated. A reduced ventilatory reserve is present when the maximum ventilatory capacity is two thirds of calculated normal. Chronic infection, emphysema, and neoplasm are the chief causes of concern. Without proper preoperative preparation serious postoperative problems of atelectasis, pneumonia, pulmonary insufficiency, and heart failure may occur. Breathing exercises and the use of aerosols and intermittent positive pressure breathing are very useful in preoperative preparation. Special measures under anesthesia must be taken to prevent hypoxia and respiratory acidosis that may cause cardiac arrest. Pulmonary fibrosis in the patient with chronic lung disease may lead to pulmonary hypertension and congestive cardiac failure (see Chapter 30).

3. Genitourinary System.   Abnormalities in the urinary system are particularly liable to be missed before operation and can cause serious complications in the postoperative period. The presence of renal disease, often without symptoms and indicated only by albuminuria and elevation of serum creatinine, may lead to renal failure after operation (see Chapter 32). When renal function is impaired, a greater volume of urine than normal is required to maintain a proper acid-base, water, and electrolyte balance. The presence of leukocytes and organisms in the urine indicates the need for careful search for the source. Any obstructive uropathy should, if possible, be treated prior to operation on other organs. Urinary infections should be treated with appropriate antibiotics. A pregnancy test should be done in women with amenorrhea. The bladder must be emptied before operation. An indwelling catheter is used in most major surgical procedures today in order to monitor urinary output. It is always used in operations involving the pelvis to prevent injury to the bladder and to avoid postoperative retention.

4. Gastrointestinal System and Nutrition.   It is essential to have an empty stomach in every patient given a general anesthetic (see Chapter 12). A minimum of six hours should elapse between the last meal and giving the anesthetic or between the meal and occurrence of an injury. In those who do not have an empty stomach and who need immediate operation administration of regional anesthesia and intubation performed while the patient is awake can prevent aspiration. The colon should be emptied prior to operation to avoid fecal impaction in the postoperative period. Severe catharsis, however, should be avoided because of the fluid loss that it induces. It is important to remove all barium from the bowel after an upper gastrointestinal x-ray or barium enema because of its marked tendency to produce impaction.

Special precautions are necessary in the patient with liver disease. Albumin is synthesized only in the liver and is a good indicator of hepatic function. A level of below 3 gm per 100 ml could be an important contributing factor to edema and inhibition of wound healing. Most of the clotting factors such as prothrombin and fibrinogen are synthesized in the liver. Their deficiency could result in bleeding. Treatment of prothrombin deficiency is especially important in the jaundiced patient (see Chapter 19). Severe protein deficiencies are seen in (a) certain chronic diseases of the gastrointestinal tract (ulcerative colitis, regional or granulomatous enteritis, chronic pancreatitis); (b) partial loss of function of the gastrointestinal tract (gastric, biliary, small bowel, or colonic fistulas, short-gut syndrome); (c) accelerated metabolic states (multiple trauma, burns and infection, long-bone fractures); (d) simple starvation (food deprivation, brain injury); (e) malignancy; and (f) renal disease. Hypoproteinemia leads to decreased gastrointestinal motility, decreased antibody production, infection, and wound dehiscence. Although the daily requirements for the nonactive adult male may be the nitrogen equivalent of only 40 gm of protein, the requirements for the same individual after major surgery may exceed the equivalent of 200 gm of protein. Although a substantial cumulative protein loss cannot ordinarily be replaced, partial replacement and the attainment of preoperative positive nitrogen balance are desirable. This goal can be aided by hyperalimentation (Chapter 14) or the use of elemental diets.[33] These diets, which are bulk-free and low-fat, are designed to provide essential nutrition with adequate calories and high protein. They effectively reduce pancreatic and biliary secretions and produce a low stool volume. Supplied in dry powder form, they are L-amino acid mixtures derived from acid hydrolysis of casein to which are added tryptophan, carbohydrate, electrolytes, vitamins, trace minerals, and flavoring. Suitably mixed in water, elemental diets can be either ingested or tube fed. When needed, they can be given via gastrostomy or jejunostomy. Excessive osmolality, which could result in diarrhea, is controlled by volume dilution and rate of administration. Small doses of codeine are also helpful. Nausea and vomiting are other complications when these diets are given orally. Changing of flavors, washing down with water, and administering with cracked ice are useful in increasing patient acceptance. Gastric retention and aspiration can be a serious problem. Frequent abdominal examinations should be performed and night feedings avoided. If water retention develops, diuretics are employed. Other complications to be watched for include hypertonic dehydration and hypertonic, nonketotic coma. These usually are seen when sustained hyperosmolar mixtures are administered. Patients who are unsuspected diabetics may develop hyperglycemia and glycosuria, and will require insulin. Finally patients on sustained elemental dietary support should receive added vitamin K since this fat-soluble factor is not supplied. In spite of the foregoing problems, elemental diets have definite indications as a diet or a dietary supplement in preoperative preparation.[9] They have been used for periods up to six months or longer.

5. Neurologic System. The status of cerebral function may influence the choice of anesthetic agent and pose special problems both preoperatively and postoperatively. Patients with stroke, chronic brain syndromes, or encephalopathies are prone to pulmonary complications related to the inability to effectively ventilate and cough. Since they are often bed-bound, hypostatic pneumonias and decubitus ulcers are frequent dangers. Previous history of a stroke predisposes to its recurrence with the stress of a surgical operation, and hypoxia, hypotension, and hypertension must be avoided.

Mentally ill or retarded patients pose special problems. Many are on tranquilizers and tolerate deeper planes of anesthesia poorly. About half such patients have serious complicating respiratory or urinary tract problems, and tenacious constipation is the rule. Preoperative evaluation is made difficult by the absence or unreliability of the history. Cleansing enemas and preoperative tracheal suctioning may avert postoperative problems.

Patients with peripheral neuropathies also tend to form decubitus ulcers and have ventilatory problems. They also become hypotensive more easily than other patients. Heating and cooling blankets must be used with extreme caution.

6. Musculoskeletal System. Patients should be kept active up to the time of operation. Good musculature results in the patient being able to cough better in the postoperative period and helps in early ambulation.[27] Muscular dystrophics present a problem quite similar to that of patients with peripheral neuropathies. Ambulation is delayed and difficult, and pulmonary ventilation is frequently inadequate. A rigid arthritic neck will make endotracheal intubation difficult and severe kyphoscoliosis will prevent esophagoscopy with a rigid instrument. Joint deformities and fusions affect positioning on the operating table. Severe injury could result if these are neglected. Pathologic fractures could result if the patient with metastatic bone disease is not transferred carefully.

7. Endocrine System. The detection of occult endocrine disease is important in surgical patients. Latent hyperthyroidism may precipitate a thyroid crisis after operation. A previously undetected pheochromocytoma may secrete large amounts of catecholamines during and after operation and cause malignant hypertension, coma, and death. Patients with malignant disease of nonendocrine tissues may have excess of ACTH, steroids, parathormone, or inappropriate secretion of antidiuretic hormone (paraneoplastic syndromes).[5]

Diabetes Mellitus. Diabetes mellitus may present special problems during and after operation.[32] The diagnosis may not be known, and the stress of operation may cause hyperglycemic coma while the patient is still in the recovery room. It is therefore essential that at least the urine be examined for sugar in all patients before operation. If the patient is a known diabetic, he should be given regular insulin before operation and the blood and

Table 11–1. FORMS OF ADDISONIAN DISORDERS

CLINICAL ENTITY	CAUSE
Adrenogenital syndrome	Congenital impairment of cortisol secretion
Acute addisonian crisis	Severe trauma, sepsis, or burns
	Hemorrhage after anticoagulants
	Postablative states—untreated adrenalectomy, hypophysectomy
	Thyroid storms
	Acute withdrawal after glucocorticoid administration
	Drug sensitivities
Chronic Addison's disease	Idiopathic autoimmune atrophy
	Adrenal tuberculosis
	Metastatic destruction
	Hypopituitarism
	Fungus infections
	Amyloidosis

urine regularly examined after operation.[17] A diabetic may be in ketosis before operation because of infection, such as a perforated appendix, a carbuncle, or moist gangrene of a limb. The diabetic tends to be refractory to insulin while pus is present but responds and is liable to go into hypoglycemic coma after treatment.

The diabetic is also likely to have a higher incidence than normal of vascular complications after operation, such as coronary and cerebral thrombosis because of the high incidence of atherosclerosis in diabetics. Wound healing is slow and infections are more frequent, especially if the diabetes is not well controlled.

Addison's Disease. Addison's disease, although a relatively rare disorder (0.03 per 100,000 population), presents problems that are important in surgery, because it can easily escape detection. The cause may be located in the hypothalamic-pituitary axis, the pituitary gland, the adrenal gland, or may result from

Table 11–2. METABOLIC CONSEQUENCES OF ADRENOCORTICAL DEPRIVATION AS PART OF ADDISON'S DISEASE

GLUCOCORTICOIDS	MINERALOCORTICOIDS
Hypoglycemia	Salt loss
Fatigue	Potassium retention
Hypotension	Decreased blood volume
Wasting	Hypotension
Hypochlorhydria	Muscle cramps
Skin pigmentation (due to pituitary feedback loss)	Contractures
	Dental caries

excessive demand upon a normal gland (Table 11–1).

To understand the addisonian state, two classes of adrenocortical secretions and the metabolic consequences of their deprivation must be considered (Table 11–2). These glucocorticoid and mineralocorticoid deprivations are more important in the production of symptoms than the androgenic-anabolic and estrogen groups. Disorders of the hypothalamic-pituitary axis are less apt to produce mineralocorticoid deprivation, since aldosterone secretion largely depends on the renin-angiotensin mechanism. Primary hypofunction of the adrenal gland and excessive demand produce deficiency states of both gluco- and mineralocorticoids.

Although there are several causes of the adrenogenital syndrome, the most common is a congenital block in hydroxylation at the C_{21} position. Cortisol production is deficient and leads to excessive ACTH production. This results in oversecretion of androgens with virilization, while the cortisol deficiency produces a latent addisonian state. The condition may not be recognized in the male and may lead to a crisis after stress by trauma, sepsis, or operations. An additional block in aldosterone synthesis produces severe mineralocorticoid deprivation with salt-losing crisis. Prepubertal and adult forms of adrenogenital syndrome occur with virilization and are usually due to the presence of an adenoma or carcinoma in the adrenal cortex.

The acute addisonian crisis is due to acquired disease and has a number of etiologies (Table 11–1). The most common is acute withdrawal following previous steroid therapy, as in corticoid administration for arthritis, allergies, and advanced cancer. Should these patients receive sudden stress, such as surgery, an addisonian crisis could develop within hours. There may be signs that the patient has been on steroid therapy, such as a Cushinglike appearance of the face, acne, striae, and hirsutism. The history of drug therapy, however, is most important. Laboratory findings during steroid therapy include hypernatremia, hypokalemia, and hyperglycemia, but these may be normal if the patient has discontinued medication. The onset of the crisis is abrupt. Anorexia and nausea are quickly followed by vomiting, diarrhea, hypotension, and finally prostration, lethargy, and death. The laboratory findings include hypoglycemia, hyponatremia, and hyperkalemia. A low circulating plasma cortisol level can be determined by radioimmunoassay. Urinary salt is excessive.

If Addison's disease is suspected, an elective operation should be postponed and the condition investigated. When early operation is necessary, steroids should be given to those who have been given steroids within two years and those in whom the disease is suspected.[21] Cortisone, 100 mg, is given intravenously every six hours before, during, and after operation. The drug is then given by mouth and the dose slowly reduced. In the event of a crisis 1000 mg of cortisone should be given intravenously and vasopressors administered.

Originally tuberculosis of the adrenals was the common cause of acquired chronic Addison's disease. Today it is most often idiopathic and probably a form of autoimmune disease (Table 11–1). It rarely occurs in those with chronic infection or in those with metastases in the adrenals, as for example from a bronchogenic carcinoma, carcinoma of the breast, or malignant melanoma. Primary hypopituitarism following infection, infarction, or tumor is also a cause of Addison's disease which can be either acute or chronic. Chronic Addison's disease causes hypotension, anorexia and nausea, weakness, easy fatigability, and weight loss. There are also loss of libido and in the female amenorrhea. Hyperpigmentation of the skin occurs, especially in the axillae, palms, and about the mouth. Unopposed hyperactivity of the anterior pituitary from absence of negative feedback of adrenocorticoids results in oversecretion of both ACTH and the melanophore-stimulating hormone (MSH) of the anterior pituitary. Laboratory tests will show hyponatremia, hyperkalemia, hypoglycemia, and an increased salt loss in the urine. Plasma cortisol and 17-hydroxycorticosteroids are decreased as are urinary 17-ketosteroids. The ECG shows a reduced voltage, and on the chest x-ray the heart may be small. Abdominal x-rays may show adrenal calcifications in tuberculosis. Direct confirmation of chronic adrenal insufficiency is obtained from the plasma cortisol or by the ACTH stimulation test. In the normal subject the absolute eosinophil count should decrease 50 percent after intramuscular injection of 25 USP units of ACTH. After an eight-hour infusion of 25 USP units of ACTH, both plasma 17-hydroxycorticoids and urinary 17-hydroxycorticoids and 17-ketosteroids should rise.

SPECIAL CONSIDERATIONS

Blood Coagulation and Fibrinolysis. Special assessment and care are necessary in patients with a history of bleeding or excessive tendency to bruise. Disorders of coagulation and fibrinolysis are important at all stages of care of the surgical patient.

Hemostasis depends for its integrity on an intact vascular endothelium, vasoconstriction,

platelets, and a complex series of enzyme reactions leading to the formation of blood clot. A firm fibrin clot in a narrowed vessel stops loss of blood (Figure 11–3). The fibrinolytic system prevents excessive intravascular clotting. Disorders of these processes can result in a tendency to bleed or in intravascular coagulation in intact vessels.

The normal response of blood vessels to injury is vasoconstriction. This is primarily a neurogenic response, but the pressor amines, serotonin and epinephrine released from platelets, are also involved. The platelets adhere to the subendothelial tissues of the damaged endothelium and to exposed tissue collagen. The initial adherence is reversible but is quickly followed by platelet fusion, called viscous metamorphosis, that plugs the capillaries for several hours. Serotonin and epinephrine are released at this time. In addition, a phospholipid, platelet factor 3, becomes available for participation in the intrinsic pathway of coagulation. Platelets also contain or absorb certain procoagulant and

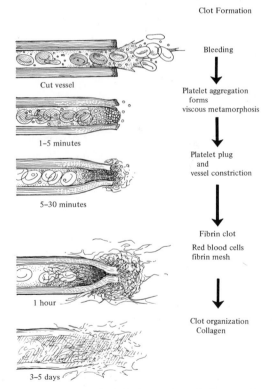

Clot Formation

Cut vessel

Bleeding

1–5 minutes

Platelet aggregation forms viscous metamorphosis

5–30 minutes

Platelet plug and vessel constriction

1 hour

Fibrin clot
Red blood cells fibrin mesh

3–5 days

Clot organization Collagen

Figure 11–3. Initially vasoconstriction and platelet adhesion stop blood flow from a severed vessel. The coagulation sequence is then activated, resulting in the fibrin clot. Fibrous organization completes the obliteration of the bleeding site.

anticoagulant factors: I, V, XI, XII, XIII, plasminogen, antiplasmin, and antiheparin. The coagulation sequence is rapidly activated leading to formation of a firm fibrin clot. Clot retraction is then produced by thrombasthenin, a contractile protein in platelets.

The coagulation mechanism is best described as a series of dominos of increasing size.[12] Initial and exceedingly small amounts of intrinsic activator result in a relatively enormous amount of fibrin blood clot. The original theory of blood coagulation as presented by Morawitz[25] in 1905 remains valid today. Although numerous additions have been made, it is likely that our knowledge of the event sequence remains incomplete.

Table 11–3 lists the coagulation factors known today with their common literature synonyms. Factor VI was originally known as activated factor V. The term is no longer in use. The sequence of activity is shown in Figure 11–4. Inactive factors present in platelets and plasma are converted to active forms. Intrinsic activity occurs when factor XII comes in contact with a wettable surface (in vitro), or with damaged intima, connective tissue, a vascular prosthesis, artificial organs, etc. (in vivo). Extrinsic activity occurs when tissue factor (complete thromboplastin), a lipoprotein found in many tissues,

Table 11–3.   COAGULATION FACTORS

FACTOR NUMBER	SYNONYMS
Factor I	Fibrinogen; Fs: urea-soluble fibrin Fi: urea-insoluble fibrin
Factor II	Prothrombin; IIa: thrombin Thromboplastin Ca^{++}
Factor V	Labile factor (Quick), proaccelerin (Owren)
Factor VII	Proconvertin (Owren)
Factor VIII	Antihemophilic globulin (AHG)
Factor IX	Christmas factor (Biggs) Plasma thromboplastin component or PTC (Aggeler) Autoprothrombin II (Seegers)
Factor X	Stuart factor (Hougie)
Factor XI	Plasma thromboplastin antecedent (PTA) (Rosenthal)
Factor XII	Contact or Hageman factor (Ratnoff, Haanen)
Factor XIII	Fibrin-stabilizing factor (Laki-Lorand); profibrinase (Loewy) Fletcher factor (prekallikrein)

enters the vascular space. Burns, trauma, sepsis, and poor surgical technique (as in vascular anastomosis) produce extrinsic activation. The

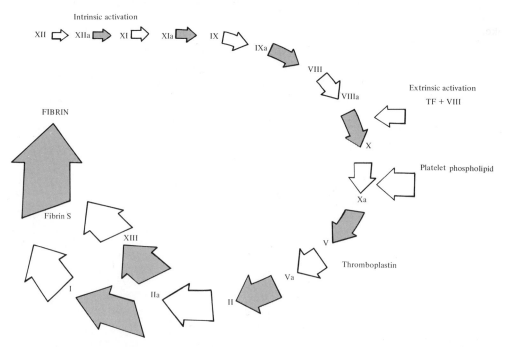

Figure 11–4.   The sequence of the coagulation mechanism. Intrinsic activation occurs when blood contacts a wettable surface (damaged intima, connective tissue, a vascular prosthesis, artificial organ, etc.). Extrinsic activation occurs when tissue factor enters the vascular space, as in burns, trauma, sepsis, and poor surgical technique. The final product is insoluble fibrin I.

terminal event is formation of the fibrin clot, which may be either protective or harmful. Ionized calcium and platelet phospholipid are required. The rate of the first two steps, of the intrinsic system, are relatively slow, and those of the last four, those shared by both intrinsic and extrinsic systems, are rapid. All of the protein clotting factors except VIII (antihemophilic globulin) are probably manufactured in the liver.

Both intrinsic and extrinsic systems lead to the formation of thrombin, the enzyme that cleaves small polypeptides from two of the three molecules in fibrinogen. Fibrin monomers are produced which polymerize to a large protein aggregate which is acted upon by fibrinase (factor XIII) to form the stable fibrin molecule. Fibrin monomers may complex with adjacent fibrinogen molecules or fibrin degradation products to form soluble fibrin monomer complexes (SFMCs). This could produce one of the hypercoagulable states.

The fibrinolytic system protects against excessive coagulation. The protein plasminogen in the globulin fraction of plasma is activated to plasmin by naturally occurring and pathologic substances, e.g., plasma and tissue activators, trypsin, urokinase, streptokinase and staphylokinase, by common pharmacologic agents such as protamine, nicotinic acid, epinephrine or acetylcholine, and in patients with hypoxia, prostatic cancer, leukemia, shock, or after stroke. It has also been observed to be activated after extensive pulmonary, cardiac, hepatic, and prostatic operations. Plasmin hydrolyzes both fibrinogen and fibrin to fibrin degradation products (FDPs) that delay clot formation and platelet aggregation, which in turn inhibits formation of fibrin. Naturally occuring inhibitors in alpha$_1$ and alpha$_2$ globulin fractions of serum limit plasmin activity to the site of clot formation. Thus free or generalized plasmin activity is rarely seen. Several synthetic inhibitors of the fibrinolytic mechanism have been developed such as epsilon aminocaproic acid and kalikrein inhibitor.

Evaluation of Hemostasis. The patient should be asked about a family history of bleeding.[7] The patient may give a history of excessive bleeding after circumcision, tonsillectomy, dental extractions, or trauma. Easy bruising, frequent epistaxis, or excessive menstrual flow may be present. Vascular defects or platelet abnormalities generally give rise to petechiae, mucosal bleeding, or spontaneous ecchymosis. A coagulation deficiency is associated with epistaxis, prolonged bleeding after operation, the development of a large hematoma after injury, and spontaneous hemarthrosis (Figure 11–5). This type of bleeding is difficult to control

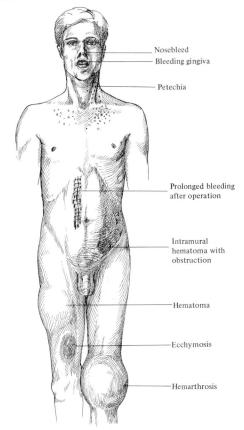

Figure 11–5. A composite of features seen in hemorrhagic diatheses. Petechiae, epistaxis, and surgical bleeding are associated with platelet or vascular deficiencies. Deep bleeding (into muscle spaces, joints, and bowel wall) and postsurgical bleeding suggest congenital or acquired coagulation defects. Ecchymoses and hematuria are nonspecific.

with pressure and often recurs. Other important points in the history are the presence of liver disease, use of anticoagulants, intake of steroids (which affect the vascular endothelium), and the use of drugs that interfere with platelet function.

Screening tests can be done to check (1) the platelets and vascular integrity, (2) the clotting mechanism, and (3) fibrinolysis. *Platelet count* is obtained in all patients. The number of platelets may be low due to decreased production or increased consumption. The *tourniquet test* is done by applying a blood pressure cuff inflated to occlude veins in the arm for five minutes. The development of petechiae indicates a platelet or vascular defect. *Clot retraction* is poor if the platelet count or function is deficient. *Bleeding time* is prolonged in patients with platelet deficiency. This test is most valuable, however, in diagnosing deficiency of factor VIII as in hemophilia. Of the screening tests for clotting the *partial thromboplastin time* (PTT) is the most valuable and is more sensitive than the whole blood clotting time. This test assays the entire clotting sequence and is abnormal if any of the factors is significantly decreased. Some feel that the activated recalcification time (ART) is the most valuable screening test.[20] The *prothrombin time* (PT) measures the extrinsic pathway and does not detect deficiencies of factors VIII, IX, XI, or XII. The third screening test for clotting is the *thrombin time*. Its main value is detecting hypofibrinogenemia, circulating anticoagulants, inhibition of fibrin monomer polymerization, or of abnormal fibrinolysins. Preformed thrombin is added to normal plasma and the patient's plasma to form a fibrin clot. In a positive test, if protamine sulfate does not correct the prolonged thrombin time, fibrinolysins or anticoagulants are present. A final screening test is the *factor VIII assay*. This test diagnoses factor VIII deficiency but is also positive when there is excessive fibrinolysis. Fibrinolysis is measured by the clot lysis time. Whole blood clot is incubated at 37°C, and the time for lysis to occur is compared with that of normal blood. More sophisticated tests are available for platelet function, clotting mechanism, and fibrinolysis (Table 11–4).

Clinical Defects. The deficiency states are congenital or acquired.[22] Hemophilia is the most important congenital bleeding defect. It is a sex-linked recessive trait carried by the female and expressed by the male and results from deficiency in function or level of factor VIII. Symptoms occur in infancy or early childhood. There is prolonged bleeding after circumcision, trauma, or dental extraction. The family history may also be positive. The patient may present with epistaxis, intestinal bleeding, or hemarthrosis. Bleeding time is normal, and clotting time is normal unless factor VIII is decreased to below 5 percent of normal. The PTT, however, detects even a slight deficiency. The normal PTT is 65 to 85 seconds but in the hemophiliac may be over 250 seconds. The factor VIII assay is practically diagnostic. When operation is required, bank cryoprecipitates or fresh normal plasma is administered, 1 mg per kilogram of body weight, until the PTT reaches 120 seconds and factor VIII is above 30 percent of normal. Operations should be performed promptly.

Christmas disease or factor IX deficiency (also known as hemophilia B) is the second most common congenital bleeding disorder. Its clinical manifestations are similar to those of true hemophilia and it is detected by an abnormal PTT. The amount of factor VIII in the blood is normal. Treatment is to give whole blood or the plasma concentrate Konyne. Other less common congenital bleeding disorders are factor V deficiency (parahemophilia) and von Willebrand's disease (vascular hemophilia), in which there are loss of platelet adhesiveness and factor VIII deficiency. Fresh blood or plasma will control the bleeding preoperatively.

Most acquired defects in hemostasis are the result of decrease in the number or function of platelets, impaired coagulation, vascular endothelial damage, or the presence of anticoagulants. The number of platelets is reduced in a variety of autoimmune, neoplastic, traumatic, and iatrogenic states (Table 11–5). In thrombocytopenia of uncertain origin preoperative assessment may include, in addition to the screening tests already described, a bone marrow and lymph node biopsy, the Coombs' test, a lupus erythematosus cell test, and selective drug elimination. Specific treatment of the primary disease is indicated. Steroid therapy and platelet transfusions may be necessary before a surgical procedure, and platelet transfusions are used during splenectomy for idiopathic thrombocytopenia purpura.

The platelet count may be increased after fractures, splenectomy, infections, rheumatic fever, and in patients with neoplasms and myeloproliferative diseases. Thrombocytosis itself

Table 11–4.   TESTS USED IN THE DIAGNOSIS OF BLEEDING DISORDERS

PLATELET TESTS	CLOTTING TESTS	TESTS FOR FIBRINOLYSIS
Platelet count	PTT	Plasma clot lysis time
Clot retraction	Protime	Euglobulin clot lysis time
Bleeding time	Thrombin time	Plasminogen concentration
Tourniquet test	Factor VIII assay	
Platelet adhesiveness		
Platelet factor III activity	Factor VIII assay	Plasminogen activator activity
ADP aggregation test	Fibrinogen	Antiplasmin concentration
	Cryofibrinogen	
Platelet life-span	Prothrombin consumption	FDP concentration
Platelet morphology	Factor analysis (IX, XIII, etc.)	

Table 11–5. SOME CAUSES OF
THROMBOCYTOPENIA

TYPE	SPECIFIC
Metabolic, toxic	Uremia
	Burns
	Massive infection
Autoimmunity	Lupus erythematosus
	Sarcoidosis
	Idiopathic thrombocytopenic
	purpura
	Platelet isoantibodies
Drugs	
Sedatives	Barbiturates, meprobamate
Alkaloids	Quinine, quinidine
Antibiotics	Tetracyclines,
	choramphenicol, mycins
Antibacterials	Sulfanilamindes (most types)
Sulfanilamide	Tolbutamide,
derivatives	chlorothiazide,
	chlorpropamide,
	actozolamide
Antineoplastics	Nitrogen mustard, Cytoxan,
	methotrexate,
	dactinomycin,
	5-fluorouracil
Others	Acetylsalicylic acid, PAS,
	estrogens, dinitrophenol,
	digitoxin, KI, mercurials,
	arsenicals
Increased	Burns
consumption	Massive transfusions
	Prosthetic devices
	Hypersplenism
	Disseminated intravascular
	clotting

can cause a bleeding tendency because the platelets are defective and they absorb several clotting factors, leading to their functional deficiency

Defects in platelet function, or thrombopathies, may occur in a variety of congenital or acquired conditions (Table 11–6). Both bleeding time and clot retraction are abnormal, but the platelet count is adequate. This combination indicates impaired platelet function, and further studies are indicated to determine the specific defect.

Most coagulation defects are acquired. All the protein clotting factors except VIII are probably produced in the liver. Advanced liver disease is the most common cause of an acquired clotting disorder. Fresh frozen plasma contains all these factors and should be administered to patients with liver disease who are bleeding. Stored plasma may be used as a substitute but does not contain factor V. Patients with liver disease with thrombocytopenia and fibrinolysis should be given platelets or fresh blood and epsilon aminocaproic acid (EACA, see below). Plasminogen,

which is the precursor of the fibrinolytic protease plasmin, is found in many tissues, such as the prostate gland. In prostatic carcinoma there is increased fibrinolytic activity, and this predisposes to bleeding after prostatic surgery.

Vitamin K deficiency occurs in patients with obstruction and fistula of the biliary tract, mild liver disease, intestinal malabsorption, during prolonged use of antibiotics, starvation, after trauma, and during the use of coumarin anticoagulants. There is a deficiency of prothrombin and also factors VII, IX, and X. The PT is always prolonged, as is the PTT. Oral or intramuscular vitamin K replacement is effective. Intravenous replacement may also be used in urgent situations. Although conversion of vitamin K to prothrombin is hepatocellular-dependent, sufficient prothrombin is produced except in those with advanced liver disease. Hypoprothrombinemia is the most frequent cause of bleeding in the newborn.

Anticoagulants can cause bleeding. Heparin is strongly electronegative, and in the presence of a plasma cofactor has antithrombin activity. It also impairs activation of factors IX and X, and it interferes with platelet function. Heparin prolongs the whole blood clotting time, and this test is dose-dependent. If the clotting time exceeds 30 minutes, spontaneous bleeding may occur. The thrombin time is prolonged and is brought to normal by adding small amounts of protamine sulfate to the test mixture. If this does not occur, either there is increased fibrinolysis, or other circulating anticoagulants are present. Heparinlike substances have been reported in disseminated lupus erythematosus and after massive transfusions. After cardiopulmonary

Table 11–6. THROMBOPATHIES:
CONGENITAL AND ACQUIRED

CONDITION	DEFICIENCY
Glanzmann's disease	Nonadhesion (also factors VII and IX deficiency)
von Willebrand's disease	Nonadhesion (also factor VIII deficiency)
Thrombasthenia	Nonaggregation due to platelet enzyme deficiencies
	Platelet factor 3
Uremia	Platelet factor 3
Multiple myeloma	Nonaggregation
Lupus erythematosus	Nonaggregation
Renal or liver disease	Platelet factor 3
Drug administration	Nonaggregation
Acetylsalicylates	
Antihistamines	
Dextrans	
Phenylbutazone	
Reserpine	

bypass or prolonged vascular procedures excess heparin used in the procedure may also be present. Cautious parenteral treatment with protamine is then necessary when excess heparin substances are demonstrated. Protamine "overtitration" is dangerous since this substance can itself act as an anticoagulant.

Dicumarol and Coumadin are the most widely used prothrombinopenic agents and can be given orally for months or years. They deplete factors II, VIII, IX, and X. The PT is prolonged and is the best index of the effect of the drugs. The PT level should be kept between two and three times normal to prevent embolism after myocardial infarction, prosthetic heart valve implantation, and phlebitis. Vitamin K, 25 to 50 mg, is given intravenously if bleeding occurs or if operation is necessary. If the treatment is not urgent, the agents can be stopped and the liver allowed to produce the clotting factors in two to three days. Salicylates, oral antibiotics, phenylbutazolidine, and quinidine potentiate the effect of dicumarol and Coumadin. Barbiturates induce or stimulate liver enzymes which can increase production of clotting factors and reduce the effect of these anticoagulants.

Massive blood transfusions cause bleeding disorders by depleting the clotting factors and platelets, and by producing anticoagulants.[24] Ionized calcium is rarely reduced to a level sufficient to cause bleeding. Warm fresh blood or platelet transfusion is the appropriate therapy in this situation.

Disseminated intravascular coagulation (DIC) may be acute or chronic.[15] Some common causes are listed in Table 11–7. There is intravascular formation of fibrin, consumption of clotting factors and platelets (consumptive coagulo-

Table 11–7. CLINICAL CAUSES OF DISSEMINATED INTRAVASCULAR COAGULATION

ACUTE	CHRONIC
Hemorrhagic shock	Atherosclerosis
Endotoxic shock	Malignancy
Soft tissue trauma	Systemic lupus
Acute hemorrhagic	erythematosus
pancreatitis	Cyanotic heart disease
Incompatible or massive	Prosthetic heart valves
blood transfusions	Cirrhosis
Abruptio placentae, dead	Periarteritis
fetus syndrome	Giant hemangiomata
Extracorporeal circulation	
Organ graft rejection	
Fat embolism	
Snake bites	
Viral and rickettsial	
infection	
Vascular prosthesis	

pathy), and an activation of the fibrinolytic system. This fibrinolysis is secondary and must be differentiated from primary fibrinolysis. Multiple organ failure and generalized bleeding may occur with a high mortality unless treatment is prompt. The initiating mechanism is probably entry of a tissue factor into the blood or contact activation of the intrinsic mechanism. Microcirculatory occlusions produce ischemic damage to the brain, liver, kidneys, lungs, adrenals, gastrointestinal tract, and to muscle and soft tissue. Finally, when clotting factors are depleted, a hemorrhagic diathesis ensues. Common clinical manifestations include cerebral insufficiency, uremia, hyperkalemia, hyponatremia, abnormal liver function, thrombocytopenia, gastrointestinal hemorrhage, pulmonary insufficiency, right heart strain, and peripheral gangrene. Early suspicion, the use of screening and confirmatory tests, and prompt treatment are necessary if the patient is to survive. A slight prolongation of the PT and PTT together with thrombocytopenia and a rapidly developing anemia should alert the surgeon to the possibility of DIC in a patient with acute onset of unexplained hypotension or bleeding. A differential diagnosis at this early stage may be between DIC and major pulmonary embolism. The thrombin time is prolonged, suggesting hypofibrinogenemia or presence of FDPs. Protein precipitation when protamine is added to plasma (protamine paracoagulation precipitation, PPP) indicates the presence of fibrin monomer. Clot lysis may be accelerated, suggesting plasmin activation. A low plasma fibrinogen should confirm the diagnosis of DIC. Cryoglobulin can be demonstrated in vitro. In summary therefore, the patient with fully developed DIC displays an absence of clot formation, a markedly reduced fibrinogen (normal 200 to 400 mg/100 ml), an increased PPT (normal 70 to 85 seconds), a markedly decreased platelet count, a decreased serum calcium, and a normal or nearly normal PT.

Treatment is aimed at restoring the depleted clotting factors and treating the underlying cause. Intravenous heparin is indicated even though the patient is bleeding. Fibrinogen should be given if the level is low. Transfusions may be needed to correct anemia. Platelets may be administered only with caution since they could aggravate clotting. In patients with liver failure, repeated transfusions of fresh whole blood may be necessary. The use of EACA, steroids, or adrenergic agents is to be avoided. Although these agents are indicated in other bleeding states, they enhance the deposition of fibrin and aggravate DIC. When successfully treated, acute DIC will ordinarily disappear in 24 to 48 hours.

Table 11–8. SCREENING TEST PATTERNS IN COMMON HEMORRHAGIC DISORDERS

DISORDER	BLEEDING TIME	NUMERICAL PLATELETS	PT	PTT	THROMBIN TIME	CLOT RETRACTION
Thrombocytopenia	Long	Decreased	Normal	Normal	Normal	Poor
Thrombopathy	Long	Normal	Normal	Normal	Normal	Normal or poor
von Willebrand's disease	Normal or long	Normal	Normal	Normal or long	Normal	Normal
Hemophilia A	Normal	Normal	Normal	Long	Normal	
Hemophilia B	Normal	Normal	Normal	Long	Normal	
Vitamin-K deficiency, oral anticoagulants	Normal	Normal	Long	Long	Normal	Normal
Chronic liver disease	Normal or long	Normal or mod. decreased	Long	Long	Normal or slightly long	Normal
Acute massive hepatic necrosis	Long	Normal or decreased	Long	Long	Long	Normal
Massive intravascular coagulation	Long	Decreased	Normal to long	Long	Long	Poor
Heparinemia	Normal	Normal	Normal or long	Long	Long	Normal

In the chronic form of DIC symptoms and hematologic abnormalities are minimal. Both anemia and thrombocytopenia occur, and low fibrinogen levels are present. Initial treatment is with heparin, but following control of acute symptoms, long-term anticoagulant therapy is continued with Coumadin. Chronic DIC is seen in patients with atherosclerosis, prosthetic heart valves, and malignancy with generalized thrombosis.

Should primary fibrinolysis be present rather than consumptive coagulopathy, the platelet count will be normal, but FDP level will be high and the thrombin time prolonged. Anemia does not occur. This rare condition seen after shock, sunstroke, or major surgery is caused by excessive amounts of activator and/or plasmin and is treated by plasmin inhibitors: aminocaproic acid and trasylol. Consumptive coagulopathy with secondary fibrinolysis should, however, be ruled out since these inhibitors would be damaging if such were the case. The correlation of screening test findings with some common abnormalities of hemostasis is summarized in Table 11–8.

Blood Transfusion

The basis for blood transfusion is largely the result of the recognition by Landsteiner of the ABO and later the Rh blood groups. He also described the MN and P groups, but these are mainly of genetic interest. More recently numerous other groups have been recognized such as the Lewis, Kell, Vel, and Duffy systems.

Blood transfusion is indicated when the oxygen-carrying capacity of the blood must be increased in those in whom there has been external or internal loss, excessive hemolysis, or impairment of red cell production by the bone marrow. It is not indicated for blood volume replacement because other fluids such as electrolytic solutions, albumin, and low-molecular-weight dextran are available. It is not necessary to give one or possibly two units of blood to any patient. At present about one third of blood is given in these amounts. This represents loss of much blood and in addition exposes the patient to many complications that may even result in death. A number of constituents of blood are now available, including packed red cells, plasma, platelets, and cryoprecipitate. In many hospitals whole fresh blood is no longer available and the constituent that the patient requires must be ordered. Packed red cells should be given when it is only necessary to increase the oxygen-carrying capacity of blood. The complications of hepatitis, reactions to donor serum, and overloading the circulation are markedly decreased.

Grouping and cross-matching are essential to exclude ABO and Rh incompatibilities. These tests include (1) grouping of the patient's red cells; this can be done in a matter of minutes so that the use of ungrouped blood, i.e., O negative cells, should not really be necessary; (2) a major cross-match, testing the recipient's serum with the donor red cells, will detect antibodies that might produce a hemolytic transfusion reaction; (3) testing the serum of the donor with the recipient's red cells, a minor cross-match, is not done in many blood banks; (4) testing the patient's serum against a panel of cells to detect other antibodies which might not react with the donor's red cells but might cause difficulty in subsequent transfusions, or in pregnancies.

Blood grouping takes a few minutes, cross-matching 30 to 60 minutes. Male Rh-negative patients may be given Rh-positive blood if the supply of Rh-negative blood is inadequate. Rh-positive males may be given Rh-negative blood. It is most important not to give Rh-positive blood to Rh-negative females who may have a subsequent pregnancy. If an Rh-negative patient, who may be in the childbearing age, receives Rh-positive blood by mistake, Rh sensitization may be preventable with the use of large amounts of Rh immune globulin. In emergencies it may occasionally be necessary to give group O Rh-negative blood. Harmful iso-antibodies may be present and result in reactions. It may then be necessary to continue to give group O Rh-negative blood.

Acid citrate dextrose (ACD) has been used most extensively for the storage of blood. Recently it has been found that the addition of phosphate (CPD solution) increases the level of 2,3-diphosphoglycerate (2,3-DPG) in the erythrocyte and decreases the shift to the left in the oxygen dissociation curve. In addition the time during which the blood can be used can be increased from about 21 to 35 days.

A number of changes occur in stored blood with aging. The platelets are no longer viable, and the granulocytes are markedly decreased within 24 hours. Potassium leaves the erythrocytes, and the level in the serum may reach 30 mEq per liter by 21 days. The normal life of red cells is about 120 days. When fresh ACD blood is given within 24 hours of collection, about one half of the red cells survive for 60 days, while if ACD blood stored 21 days is given, only about one quarter survive to 60 days. Hemolysis is not a problem in stored blood unless it has been brought to 37°C several times or infection is present. Only about 1 percent of the red cells are hemolyzed at 21 days.

Patients who are bleeding before or after operation must have an accurate coagulation assessment to try to determine which particular factors need replacing. For instance, if the platelets are low and the bleeding is on this basis, platelet transfusions may be ordered. On the other hand, if a clotting deficiency is present, a specific factor or fresh whole plasma may be given. After open heart surgery, overuse of heparin or protamine may cause bleeding.

Complications. Complications of blood transfusion are common. Signs of a reaction often appear within minutes of starting the transfusion. The patient must therefore be carefully observed, especially during the first 20 minutes. The complications are greatest with whole blood. It is therefore important that, having decided that a blood transfusion is definitely required, consideration should be given to replacement with one of the constituents of blood such as packed red cells. The complications of a transfusion are discussed below.

Hemolytic Reactions. Mismatched hemolytic transfusion reactions are, fortunately, extremely rare and are almost entirely due to errors in taking the blood or labeling rather than errors in the blood bank. Since these reactions can be fatal, the physician or surgeon is ultimately responsible for making sure that no clerical errors occur during taking and labeling of the blood sample.

The rate at which red cells become hemolyzed and removed from the circulation depends upon the anticoagulant solution used, how long the blood has been stored, and the presence or absence of an incompatibility. A gross mismatch will cause immediate extensive hemolysis of red cells. If the mismatch is less severe, hemolysis may occur in hours or days. The patient may become flushed, develop headaches, loin pain, or a constrictive feeling in the chest. The temperature may be elevated and the patient may become hypotensive and tend to bleed. In the anesthetized patient a tendency to bleed, hypotension, tachycardia, and hemoglobinuria may be the only signs of an incompatible transfusion.

Free hemoglobin in the circulation combines with haptoglobin and is normally removed by the lymphoreticular system. In excessive hemolysis the heme combines with albumin to form methemalbumin, and in addition the patient develops hemoglobinuria. There are a marked increase in the serum bilirubin and jaundice. Renal hypoxia from the hypotension, aciduria, and hemoglobinuria result in tubular necrosis and deposit of hemoglobin within the renal tubules.

The blood should be immediately discontinued and a sample of the patient's blood and the remaining blood sent to the blood bank for further examination. Bicarbonate is given to increase the pH of the urine and 100 ml of 20 percent mannitol to induce a diuresis. Urinary output is carefully monitored and if anuria occurs, it will be necessary to treat the patient for renal shutdown. Intravenous fluids are necessary to treat the hypotension.

Nonhemolytic Reactions. Most reactions not associated with excessive hemolysis are mainly the result of incompatibilities involving substances in the serum, platelets, or white blood cells. The patient usually develops a fever and sometimes an itchy, urticarial skin rash. Pyrogenic or allergic transfusion reactions are rarely fatal or serious, and if the blood is really necessary it need not be discontinued. Urticarial or allergic reactions can be treated with antihistamines or if necessary intravenous corticoids. It may be necessary to stop the transfusion and check the patient for hemolysis if there is doubt concerning the cause of the reaction. Occasional severe anaphylactic reactions to serum are rare. Psychologic reactions, such as pallor, sweating, vague pains, are quite common.

Disease Transmission. Serum hepatitis is one of the most serious complications of blood transfusion and occurs in about one half of 1 percent of patients. The mortality is as high as 25 percent in patients in renal dialysis units. The virus is transmitted in the serum, so that the incidence of infectious hepatitis is extremely low when packed red cells and frozen red cells are given and is particularly high with pooled serum. The incubation period is 50 to 150 days. Blood is now routinely checked for hepatitis antigen; unfortunately, however, the test is positive in only about 30 percent of infected donors.

Malaria may be transmitted by infected erythrocytes. Syphilis may be transmitted only if fresh blood is given. A temperature of 4°C kills the organism in about four days.

Septicemia. Gram-positive organisms grow readily in blood at 37°C, while a number of gram-negative organisms can grow at 4°C. It is therefore important not to heat blood for several hours and then store it again at 4°C.

Citrate Toxicity. This is a rare complication in patients receiving a large volume of blood. The citrate in the ACD solution combines with ionized calcium in the blood and induces a hypocalcemia which if severe results in myocardial asystole. Calcium gluconate, 10 ml of 10 percent solution, should be given for every liter of blood in patients who have already been given a large volume of blood.

Pulmonary Edema and Congestive Heart Failure. Care must be taken when giving whole blood to patients with incipient heart failure. It is often not appreciated that 25 gm albumin has an oncotic pressure of 500 ml and could readily result in overloading of the circulation. Careful monitoring of pulse, blood pressure, urinary output, and, when indicated, the central venous or pulmonary wedge pressures should prevent overtransfusion.

Frozen Blood. Frozen blood is increasingly used. The erythrocytes are separated from the serum and suspended in glycerol. The blood is then kept in liquid nitrogen at about −190°C or refrigerated at less than −80°C. Glycerolization

and freezing decrease the metabolic processes within the cells so that they remain viable for several years. The blood is then thawed, washed in isotonic saline, and reconstituted in saline and glucose. The blood can be given after crossmatching with the recipient's serum within 45 minutes of its removal from the frozen state. It is important to remove the glycerol completely by washing the cells several times with saline to prevent hemolysis. There are a number of advantages to the use of frozen blood.

1. Virtually all the blood can be used since it can be stored for years. Probably about one third of ordinary blood bank blood is not used due to outdating. On the other hand, only about 2 percent of the erythrocytes are lost during freezing.

2. There is a marked decrease in the incidence of serum hepatitis. The virus responsible for serum hepatitis is present in the serum and not in the erythrocytes and is removed during the processing of frozen blood. In the United States there are about 5,000 deaths per year from serum hepatitis in patients given whole blood.

3. There are few allergic reactions because most of the granulocytes have been removed with the serum, both of which are rich sources of foreign antigens. This is of special value in patients on renal dialysis and on cardiopulmonary bypass.

4. The incidence of shock lung may be decreased. One of the factors responsible for shock lung is embolization of pulmonary vessels with macroaggregates of white cells, platelets, and proteins in the plasma.

5. Citrate intoxication cannot occur.

Cadaver blood has been extensively used in Russia but seldom in the Western world.

Problems with Massive Whole-Blood Transfusion. The administration of more than about 5 liters of blood in several hours often results in serious complications.

1. There is a marked tendency for the patient to develop a bleeding diathesis because of lack of platelets and disseminated intravascular coagulopathy. Deficiency of the labile factors V and VIII has been incriminated. Very gross deficiency, however, must be present for them to be responsible for bleeding. Fresh blood should be given to correct the condition because it is rich in platelets and in these factors.

2. Pulmonary complications are shock lung and pulmonary edema. In shock lung, white cell platelet and protein aggregates in the blood block the pulmonary arterioles. Blood should be filtered to remove those large particles. Pulmonary edema may readily occur from overloading of the circulation.

3. Body temperature may fall when large

volumes of cooled blood are given. This causes a shift of the oxygen dissociation curve to the left which is more marked if aged blood is given because of increase in pH. Blood should be brought to 37°C just before use.

4. Electrolyte abnormalities may occur. Hyperkalemia occurs because potassium ion is lost from the erythrocytes into the serum on storage. This, however, is usually a transient disturbance because the potassium ion moves intracellularly again when the hemoglobin is reoxygenated. Hypocalcemia may occur if large volumes of ACD blood are given. In addition, the citrate in ACD solution causes myocardial irritability.

5. Reactions, such as fever, chills, urticaria, dyspnea, pain, nausea, hematuria, and shock, are increased, as well as the risk of hepatitis. Hemosiderosis is a late complication. There are also an unexplained increase in infections and impairment of wound healing.

Nonobstetric Surgery in Pregnancy

The rate of major nonobstetric surgical intervention in pregnancy is 232 per 100,000. Unique problems are presented by the presence of a large abdominal mass, the risk to the fetus by anesthesia and surgery, and altered hemodynamic and electrolyte patterns in the mother.

Because of the enlarged uterus, clinical signs may be obscured or located in abnormal regions, and there may be less response to peritoneal irritation. Abdominal masses may be difficult to palpate. Nonsurgical conditions may be present, e.g., urinary tract obstruction or infection, stretch or hemorrhage into the broad ligament, or premature labor. It is most important to delineate whether a true surgical condition exists or an obstetric problem is mimicking a surgical condition.[23]

When a true surgical condition is diagnosed, the pregnant patient's special anesthetic requirements must be considered. Adequate blood volume is difficult to assess because of hemodilution. In late pregnancy a hypotensive syndrome consisting of low blood pressure, tachycardia, pallor, and sweating may occur, the result of the occlusive pressure of the gravid uterus on the inferior vena cava. There is also a hormone-induced hyperventilation resulting in a decrease in total acid and base. The most dangerous period for anesthesia and surgery is at 12 weeks of gestation when uterine irritability and the danger of abortion are greatest. At any period of gestation both hypotension and hypoxia can lead to fetal distress and/or fetal death. The inhalation agent chosen should produce a rapid induction and permit delivery of a high concentration of oxygen. Agents that are fat soluble and of low molecular weight exchange rapidly with the fetus and are rapidly removed. Halothane has all these features and in addition relaxes uterine muscle.[26] X-ray studies in the pregnant patient should be avoided if possible because of the increased incidence of leukemia and carcinoma in the offspring. If absolutely necessary careful fetal shielding and limiting of fluoroscopy should be employed.

Red degeneration with torsion of a fibroid and of an ovary can simulate appendicitis. Classic appendicitis is altered because of the displacement of the appendix by the enlarged uterus and by the physiologic leukocytosis of pregnancy. If perforation occurs, severe toxemia results because of the increased blood and lymphatic supplies. The most important physical sign is point tenderness unrelieved by position change, as would occur in genital tract disease. Fetal mortality is 4 percent on removing a normal or locally inflamed appendix but rises to 10 percent when the appendix is perforated.[6]

Although pregnancy predisposes to cholelithiasis from bile stasis and increased cholesterol concentration, acute cholecystitis is rare during pregnancy. Since the appendix is displaced upward, acute appendicitis may simulate gallbladder disease. If the diagnosis is in doubt, laparotomy should be performed.

Since secretion of gastric acid is decreased during pregnancy, more than three quarters of women with duodenal ulcer history become symptom free. Rarely will the complications of perforation and hemorrhage require operative treatment. Intestinal obstruction is usually due to adhesive bands. Although symptoms and physical and x-ray findings are similar to those in a nonpregnant female, abdominal distention is difficult to assess. Pancreatitis is rare, but women with a previous history tend to have exacerbations during pregnancy. The treatment is nonoperative, but if the diagnosis is uncertain, exploration should be carried out.

The ideal time to repair a hernia is before pregnancy. If detected early in pregnancy, it can be safely repaired to remove the danger of later strangulation. In the last trimester, however, it should be watched closely and repaired after delivery. Hiatal hernias are aggravated by pregnancy and frequently bleed. Surgery for varicose veins and hemorrhoids should be deferred since both conditions tend to improve after delivery. Surgery for cancer, as for example, a breast mass or cervical lesion, must be performed when the lesion is discovered and without regard to the pregnant state. Figure 11–6 illustrates a number of these conditions.

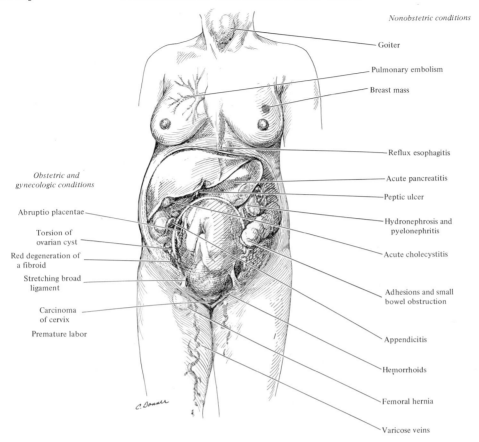

Nonobstetric conditions

Goiter

Pulmonary embolism

Breast mass

Reflux esophagitis

Acute pancreatitis

Peptic ulcer

Hydronephrosis and
pyelonephritis

Acute cholecystitis

Adhesions and small
bowel obstruction

Appendicitis

Hemorrhoids

Femoral hernia

Varicose veins

*Obstetric and
gynecologic conditions*

Abruptio placentae

Torsion of
ovarian cyst

Red degeneration of
a fibroid

Stretching broad
ligament

Carcinoma
of cervix

Premature labor

C. Donner

Figure 11–6. Some diseases occur only in pregnancy (abruptio placentae, broad ligament hemorrhage), and others are aggravated (varicose veins, hemorrhoids, and pyelitis). A large abdominal tumor modifies or obscures the picture of intra-abdominal inflammatory disease.

Surgery in the Aged

Surgical disorders in the aged must be treated differently than in the young.[10] Elderly patients tolerate some surgical procedures as well as the young, e.g., thyroidectomy and herniorrhaphy, but radical surgery and emergency procedures are withstood much more poorly. Some surgeons may feel that when life expectancy is reached the time of natural death is at hand; a relaxation of efforts could develop. On the contrary, when average life expectancy is reached, life tables will show several more years of life expectancy at that attained age (Table 11–9). The surgeon therefore should redouble his efforts to understand the differences in the aged patient and to do what he can to save him.

A number of physiologic impairments are associated with aging. The development of arteriosclerosis is the most universal change in the cardiovascular system and certainly has the greatest impact. Yet these changes are highly variable with respect to chronologic age. Many aged patients show only the slightest evidence of arteriosclerosis, while others develop crippling sequelae such as myocardial ischemia, aneurysm, and peripheral vascular occlusions in early middle age. Severe atherosclerosis when present reduces the elasticity of the vascular tree and increases the likelihood of shock after moderate blood loss. More predictable cardiovascular changes with age include a slight drop in the hematocrit, a moderate increase in blood pressure, and a decrease in cardiac work.

Table 11–9. LIFE EXPECTANCY AT ATTAINED AGES
(U.S. Vital Statistics, 1967)

AGE	YEARS REMAINING MALE	YEARS REMAINING FEMALE
Birth	67.0	74.2
60	16.0	20.2
65	13.0	16.4
70	10.4	13.0
75	8.3	10.0
80	6.4	7.3

Myocardial reserve is reduced, resulting in a higher incidence of heart failure following the demands of major surgery.

Progressive changes in renal function with age include a reduced ability to concentrate, reduced renal plasma flow and glomerular filtration, and diminished tubular excretory and resorptive powers. This loss of regulatory powers to cope with shock and acid-base disorders probably comes from a loss of nephrons. Careful anesthetic management becomes important. Prostatic hypertrophy with residual urine after voiding is a common cause of increased blood urea nitrogen and bladder infection in elderly males.

Pulmonary complications are the most common cause of postoperative death in the elderly.[8] Pulmonary function is reduced and emphysema is common. Inadequate ventilatory and diffusion capacities often result in peripheral oxygen desaturation. Preoperative instructions in deep breathing, the use of bronchodilators, and refraining from smoking are helpful. General metabolic changes with age include a reduction in basal metabolic rate, increase in the total body sodium-to-potassium ratio, and a relative increase in extracellular fluid. Unsuspected diabetes is sometimes discovered during preoperative assessment in the elderly.

Preoperative preparation in the elderly requires a certain technique and should not be hurried. The "routine" tests may need to be supplemented with renal, pulmonary, or other function tests. Blood volume determination may be indicated. If preoperative transfusions are required, packed cells are preferred. Excessive bed rest is to be avoided since this can result in pressure ulcers, hypostatic pneumonia, and a negative nitrogen balance. Preoperative digitalization or the use of quinidine has been suggested before thoracic prodecures because of the high incidence of arrhythmias in the elderly. Finally a high incidence of psychotic breakdown, 2 to 3 percent, might be anticipated among elderly patients.

Psychologic Preparation for Surgery

Pope has said, "The proper study of mankind is man." Nevertheless surgeons have a reputation for ignoring their patients' emotional state. Although his craft is concerned with the challenge of surgical correction, the surgeon should be concerned with the entire patient. Managing duodenal ulcer thus becomes managing the *patient* with a duodenal ulcer. A major problem for the surgeon is understanding what the patient really needs or wants. Thus some complaints may not express a symptom but rather a demand for care, a misplaced anxiety.[29]

Unrealistic expectations could cause postoperative psychologic problems.[3] Unless the surgeon understands what is troubling the patient, he is in a poor position to deal with him. Fears of anesthesia, of cancer, of loss of earning power, or of mutilation may be under the surface and may or may not be realistic.[18] In some cases, however, the exact diagnosis should be withheld and be given to a family member.

The surgeon should spend time explaining the proposed procedure, postoperative care, and possible disabilities.[30] Anticipated use of tubes, intravenous fluids, tracheostomy, etc., is included in the discussion, as well as the anticipated time of hospitalization.

Psychiatric consultation is rarely requested but is probably frequently indicated.[4] It should be sought in patients with a previous history of psychotic decompensation, in patients refusing essential procedures, those with fantasies or lack of affect, and when relationships with the staff deteriorate. Intersex surgery always requires psychiatric consultation.

Patients requiring ostomies must be instructed or even trained preoperatively. Many hospitals now have stomal therapists. Ostomy clubs provide very helpful pre- and postoperative visits by their members. Topics covered include type and use of bags, enemas, skin care, and medications to remove fecal odor (bismuth subgalate). Preoperatively the patient is reassured that the ostomy is compatible with a full active life. Physician and nursing assistance must be carried through postoperatively.[16]

Some procedures are mutilating. Women undergoing mastectomy need special attention since the breast may represent anything from a sex symbol to a respiratory organ. Mastectomy clubs have been organized and their members help in preoperative preparation. Amputation of an extremity, head and neck procedures, and staged procedures, such as esophagectomy and reconstruction, are other examples of surgery in which psychologic preparation is important.

Preoperative Monitoring in the Critically Ill Patient

The developments of pharmacologic and biophysical control of body processes must be considered at least as equally important to surgery as advances in surgical technique. Such control has not only extended the scope of surgery but has permitted timely surgical operations upon patients otherwise at prohibitive risk. Nowhere is this illustrated better than in the handling of the critically ill patient. The proper preoperative assessment and care of critically ill patients will require monitoring of certain vital body functions. Critically ill patients may be broadly

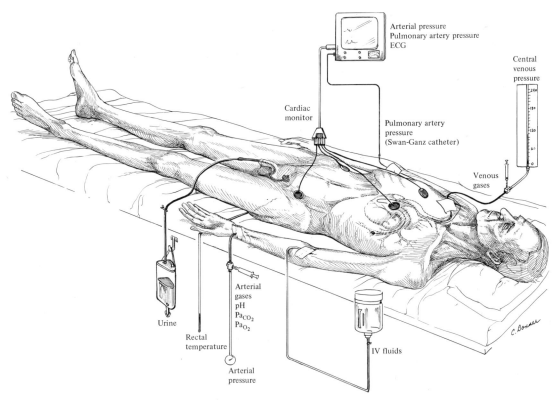

Figure 11–7. The survival of the critically ill patient depends on adequate monitoring of the vital support systems—cardiovascular, pulmonary, and renal.

Table 11–10. MONITORING IN THE CRITICALLY ILL PATIENT

PARAMETER MONITORED	BODY PROCESS MEASURED
Arterial pressure	Peripheral resistance
	Myocardial function
	Circulating volume
Central venous pressure	Circulating volume (right ventricular function)
Central venous saturation (S_vO_2)	Peripheral perfusion (cardiac output)
Urine volume	Renal perfusion
	Tubular function
ECG	Myocardial perfusion
	Electrolytes—K^+, Ca^{++}, alkalosis
Arterial P_{O_2}	Pulmonary perfusion diffusion
Arterial P_{CO_2}	Pulmonary ventilation
Arterial pH	Tissue perfusion
Pulmonary artery pressure	Left ventricular function
Rectal temperature	Heat production and loss

classified as having (1) pump failure (myocardial infarction, arrhythmias, congestive heart failure); (2) a rapidly developing third space (trauma, burns, sepsis); (3) pulmonary insufficiency (shock lung, advanced pulmonary disease, pulmonary embolus); or (4) fluid and electrolyte instability (hemorrhage, diabetic acidosis, kidney disease). Shock may or may not be present. Specific problems are discussed in detail elsewhere (Chapters 1, 2, and 3).

Figure 11–7 illustrates in composite form the commonly employed measurements of vital function. Table 11–10 lists the parameters and the most important body processes that are measured.

CITED REFERENCES

1. Alper, M. H.; Flacke, W.; and Krayer, O.: Pharmacology of reserpine and its implications for anesthesia. *Anesthesiology*, **24**:524–42, 1963.
2. Anton, A. H.: Psychopharmacology: A review. In Gravenstein, J. S. (ed.): *Pharmacology for the Preoperative Visit.* Int. Anesthesiol. Clin., **6**:65–96, Little, Brown & Co., Boston, 1968.
3. Baudry, F., and Weiner, A.: Preoperative preparation of the surgical patient. *Surgery*, **63**:885–89, 1968.

4. Baudry, F.; Weiner, A.; and Hurwitt, E. S.: Indications for psychiatric consultation on a surgical service *Surgery*, 60:993–1000, 1966.
5. Bhattacharya, S. K., and Sealy, W. C.: Paraneoplastic syndromes. *Current Problems in Surgery.* Year Book Med. Pub., Chicago, 1972.
6. Black, W. P.: Acute appendicitis in pregnancy. *Br. Med. J.*, 1:1938–41, 1960.
7. Bowie, E. J. W.: The hemorrhagic patient. *Hosp. Med.* 111–23, May 1971.
8. Burnett, W., and McCaffrey, J.: Surgical procedures in the elderly. *Surg. Gynecol. Obstet.*, 134:221–26, 1972.
9. Bury, K. D.; Stephens, R. V.; and Randall, H. T.: Use of a chemically defined, liquid, elemental diet for nutritional management of fistulas of the alimentary tract. *Am. J. Surg.*, 121:174–83, 1971.
10. Cole, W. H.: Medical differences between the young and the aged. *J. Am. Geriatr. Soc.*, 18:589–614, 1970.
11. Croft, J. D.; Swisher, S. N.; Gilliland, B. C.; Bakemeier, R. F.; Leddy, J. P.; and Weed, R. I.: Coombs'-test positivity induced by drugs. *Ann. Intern. Med.*, 68:176–83, 1968.
12. Davie, E. W., and Ratnoff, O. D.: Waterfall sequence for intrinsic blood clotting. *Science*, 145:1310–13, 1964.
13. Gazes, P. C.: Noncardiac surgery in cardiac patients. *Postgrad. Med.*, 49:170–75, 1971.
14. Early, L. E., and Orloff, J.: Thiazide diuretics. *Annu. Rev. Med.*, 15:149–66, 1964.
15. Fletcher, A. P., and Alkjaersing, N.: Blood hypercoagulability, intravascular coagulation, and thrombosis: New diagnostic concepts. *Thromb. Diath. Haemorrh.*, Suppl. 45, p. 389, 1970.
16. Gallagher, A. M.: Body image changes in the patient with a colostomy. *Nurs. Clin. North Am.*, 7:669–76, 1972.
17. Gastineau, C. F., and Molnar, G. D.: The care of the diabetic patient during emergency surgery. *Surg. Clin. North Am.*, 49:1171–75, 1969.
18. Graham, L. E.; and Conley, E. M.: Evaluation of anxiety and fear in adult surgical patients. *Nurs. Res.*, 20:113–22, 1971.
19. Helberg, D. H.: Communicating under stress. *J Assoc. Oper. Rm. Nurs.*, 16:46–50, 1972.
20. Hill, N. O.; Ridgway, N. J.; and Speer, R. J.: Coagulation testing in the surgical patient. *Tex. Med.*, 66:54–57, 1970.
21. Hume, D. M.: Surgery of the adrenals. In Kinney, J. M.; Egdahl, R. H.; and Zuidema, G. D. (eds.): *Manual of Preoperative and Postoperative Care.* W. B. Saunders, Philadelphia, pp. 529–58, 1971.
22. Louis, J.: Management of the bleeding patient. *Hosp. Med.*, 97–116, April, 1971.
23. Mersheimer, W. L., and Kazarian, K. K.: The acute abdomen in pregnancy. In Barber, H. (ed.): *Complications of Pregnancy.* W. B. Saunders, Philadelphia. In press.
24. Miller R. D.; Robbins, T. O.; Tong, M. J.; and Barton, S. L.: Coagulation defects associated with massive transfusions. *Ann. Surg.*, 174:794–801, 1971.
25. Morawitz, P.: *Blutgerinnung Ergebnisse der Physiologie*, 4:307, 1905.
26. Moya, F., and Spicer, A. R.: An appraisal of halothane in obstetrics. In Greene, N. M. (ed.): *Clinical Anesthesia.* F. A. Davis Co., Philadelphia, 1968.
27. Nichols, P. J.: Routine preoperative and postoperative physiotherapy. Replies to a questionnaire. *Ann. Physiol. Med.*, 9:264–69, 1968.
28. Ramsay, M. A.: A survey of preoperative fear. *Anesthesia*, 27:396–402, 1972.
29. Rynearson, R. R., and Stewart, W. L.: The dependency problem: The most common surgical risk. *Surg. Clin. North Am.*, 52:459–95, 1972.
30. Schmitt, F. E., and Wooldridge, P. J.: Psychological preparation of surgical patients. *Nurs. Res.*, 22:108–16, 1973.
31. Schwaber, J. R.: Evaluation of respiratory status in surgical patients. *Surg. Clin. North Am.*, 50:637–44, 1970.
32. Steinke, J.: Management of diabetes mellitus and surgery. *N. Engl. J. Med.*, 282:1472–74, 1970.
33. Winitz, M.; Graff, J.; Gallagher, N.; Narkin, A.; and Seedman, D. A.: Evaluation of chemical diets as nutrition for man-in-space. *Nature*, 205:741–43, 1965.

SUGGESTIONS FOR FURTHER READING

Comroe, J. H.; Forster, R. E.; Dubois, A. B. II; Briscoe, W. A.; and Carlsen, E.: *The Lung, Clinical Physiology and Pulmonary Function Tests.* 2nd ed. Year Book Med. Pub. Chicago, 1962.
The concepts of ventilation, diffusion, and pulmonary blood flow together with blood gases are fully discussed. Clinical applications and practical aspects of therapy are presented in a most useful manner.

Delp, M. H., and Manning, R. T.: *Major's Physical Diagnosis*, 7th ed. W. B. Saunders Co., Philadelphia, 1968.
We have found this the most useful of the several texts available in physical diagnosis. The illustrations, although in black and white, are excellent.

Gans, H.: Hemostasis and the surgical patient. In: *Current Problems in Surgery.* Year Book Medical Publisher, Chicago, 1969.
This is probably the most in-depth presentation in the recent surgical literature.

Griffen, W. O., Jr.; Dilts, P. V., Jr.; and Reddick, J. W., Jr.: Non-obstetric surgery during pregnancy. In: *Current Problems in Surgery.* Year Book Medical Publisher, Chicago, 1969.
"The pregnant patient can have any disease that any other woman can have—except sterility." Surgical problems, however, have unique aspects in the pregnant patient, and this monograph, written by a surgeon and two gynecologists, more than adequately discusses nonobstetric surgical problems.

Kinney, J. M.; Egdahl, R. H.; and Zuidema, G. D. (eds.): *Manual of Preoperative and Postoperative Care.* W. B. Saunders, Philadelphia, 1971.
This is the standard reference of the Committee on Pre- and Postoperative Care of the American College of Surgeons. The appendix is an excellent reference for standard values.

Mitty, W. F., Jr.: *Surgery in the Aged.* Charles C Thomas, Springfield, Ill., 1966.
There are only a small number of books covering this subject. Dr. Mitty's is both concise and easily readable.

Stahl, W. M.: *Supportive Care of the Surgical Patient.* Grune & Stratton, New York, 1972.
The systems of the body are described in this very excellent treatise as exchange, transport, and regulatory. The subject matter, although not in depth, is most extensive; it is recommended to any student of surgical physiology.

Stephens, R. V., and Randall, H. T.: Use of a concentrated, balanced, liquid elemental diet for nutritional management of catabolic states. *Ann. Surg.*, 170:642–67, 1969.
Use of elemental diets as a surgical adjuvant is covered in depth in this classic paper. Case presentations

illustrate the current usefulness of these diets in pre-operative preparation.

Weed, L. L.: *Medical Records, Medical Education, and Patient Care: The Problem-Oriented Record as a Basic Tool.* Cleveland, The Press of Case Western Reserve University, 1969.

Dr. Weed presents his thinking on the subject of medical records and its impact on medical education and patient care. This is a new and controversial approach to record-keeping and promises to be much discussed for a long time.

Chapter 12

OPERATIVE ANESTHESIA

Gordon D. Glennie

CHAPTER OUTLINE

Preoperative Assessment and Medication
  Preanesthetic Medication
    Sedatives
    Drugs Affecting the Autonomic Nervous
    System
Regional Anesthesia
  Topical Anesthesia
  Local Infiltration
  Nerve Block
    Brachial Plexus Block
  Intravenous Regional Anesthesia
  Epidural Anesthesia
  Spinal Anesthesia
  Action of Local Anesthetics
  Local and Regional Anesthetics
    Cocaine
    Procaine
    Amethocaine
    Lidocaine
    Mepivacaine
    Bupivacaine Hydrochloride
General Anesthesia
  Stages of Anesthesia

Volatile Anesthesia Agents
  Nitrous Oxide
  Halothane
  Methoxyflurane
  Other Volatile Anesthetic Agents
Intravenous Agents Used in Anesthesia
  Thiopental
  Narcotics
  Innovar
  Ketamine
  Diazepam
  Propanidid
Muscle Relaxants
  Endotracheal Anesthesia
Anesthetic Apparatus
Anesthetic Complications
  Vomiting and Regurgitation
  Cardiac Arrest
  Drug Reactions
  Malignant Hyperthemia
  Unsuspected Endocrine Disorders
Recovery Room

General anesthesia for surgical operations was introduced in the middle of the nineteenth century. Despite the discovery of nitrous oxide many years earlier, it was not until 1844 that Horace Wells demonstrated its usefulness for dental extractions. Two years later William Norton rendered a patient insensible with ether. In the following year James Simpson of Edinburgh advocated chloroform to relieve labor pain. In 1934 Lundy showed that intravenous injection of the barbiturate thiopental (Pentothal) rapidly produced unconsciousness. Perhaps the greatest landmark in the development of anesthesia in the present century was the introduction of curare to produce muscular relaxation by Griffiths and Johnson in Montreal in 1942. More recently, nonexplosive inhalational agents such as halothane and methoxyflurane have supplanted ether and cyclopropane. For intravenous anesthesia the anesthesiologist's armamentarium has been extended by the addition of such drugs as diazepam (Valium), the phencyclidine derivative ketamine, the narcotic analgesic fentanyl, and the neuroleptic agent droperidol. A combination of fentanyl and droperidol (Innovar) is frequently used. A number of synthetic muscle relaxants have been elaborated such as succinylcholine, gallamine, and pancuronium.

At first a physician without any special training (or in North America a nurse) administered the anesthetic. The role of the anesthesiologist has now extended into the preoperative period when he examines the patient and plays an active part in the preparation for surgery. Proper selection of anesthesia requires correct preoperative assessment of the patient's psychologic, physiologic, and pharmacologic status. Thus he is often called on to see the critically injured patient to establish the airway and maintain adequate respiration.

Rapid progress in applied physiology and pharmacology during the past three decades, to which anesthesiologists have made significant contributions, has increased the scope and safety of surgery and has led to increasing commitment of the anesthesiologist in critical care medicine. It was during the 1952 poliomyelitis epidemic in Copenhagen that the use of intermittent positive pressure ventilation was first used on a large scale as a therapeutic measure, and due to successful cooperation between surgeon and anesthesiologist many lives were saved.

The anesthesiologist takes an active part in the patient's postoperative care, especially in the intensive care unit. He is also involved in the care of patients who have not received an anesthetic, such as the comatose patient, multiple trauma patient, and those with chest disease resulting in varying degrees of respiratory insufficiency. In many institutions he supervises a pain clinic for the treatment of intractable pain. This chapter attempts to present the basic knowledge about anesthesia that every physician should have.

PREOPERATIVE ASSESSMENT AND MEDICATION

Every patient who is to receive an anesthetic should have a history and physical examination. If general anesthesia is contemplated, it is mandatory that no food or drink be taken for a minimum of six hours previously. This rule is broken only in the most critical circumstances. Particular attention should be paid to respiratory and cardiovascular status. Patients should be carefully questioned about any drugs they are presently taking and any to which they believe they are allergic. A hemoglobin estimation and urinalysis are necessary in all patients prior to operation. A consent for anesthetic and operation must be properly signed and witnessed.

Preanesthetic Medication

The purpose of administering drugs to patients before they enter the operating room is (1) to allay anxiety and induce drowsiness; (2) to reduce the amount of general anesthetic required; (3) to diminish undesirable reflex activity such as nausea, vomiting, or bradycardia; and (4) to prevent excessive secretion by the mucous membrane of the respiratory tract. Drugs for premedication should be given intra-

muscularly at least three quarters of an hour before operation.

Sedatives. Morphine is a time-honored drug, producing euphoria in most patients. The dose in the average adult is 10 mg by intramuscular injection. Higher doses contribute little further sedation and may produce undesirable side effects such as nausea and vomiting.

The synthetic narcotic Demerol produces less sedation and respiratory depression and acts for a shorter time than morphine. It may be given every three hours postoperatively for pain relief. The usual dose in the adult is 75 to 100 mg intramuscularly and 1 mg per kilogram in the child.

In the aged, poor-risk patient a preoperative narcotic should not be given. Some sedation may be obtained with a small intramuscular dose of diazepam (Valium), 5 mg. If thought desirable diazepam may be substituted for narcotics in other age groups.

Drugs Affecting the Autonomic Nervous System. The belladonna alkaloids are used mainly to inhibit the autonomic nervous system. By their parasympathetic blocking action they decrease secretions in the mouth and respiratory tract. Atropine and scopolamine (hyoscine) are the two drugs mainly employed. Atropine is more effective in its vagolytic action on the heart, while scopolamine has a greater effect on secretions and also produces amnesia. Both decrease heat loss by causing depression of the sweat glands. Atropine is satisfactory in all age groups, while scopolamine is best avoided in children and the aged since it occasionally produces restlessness and confusion. The adult dose of both drugs is 0.4 to 0.6 mg intravenously or intramuscularly.

REGIONAL ANESTHESIA

Regional anesthesia is usually employed for minor operations and reduction of fractures. When used for more major procedures the advantages over general anesthesia include patient cooperation, a reduced risk of aspiration, a decreased incidence of pulmonary complications and postoperative vomiting, together with a more rapid recovery. The agent may be applied topically, given by local infiltration, or injected to produce nerve block, epidural, or spinal anesthesia (Figure 12–1).

Topical Anesthesia

Certain anesthetic agents applied to mucous membranes produce local anesthesia. They are also effective when applied to inflamed skin. Their main use is in the eye, mouth, upper respiratory tract, anus, and urethra.

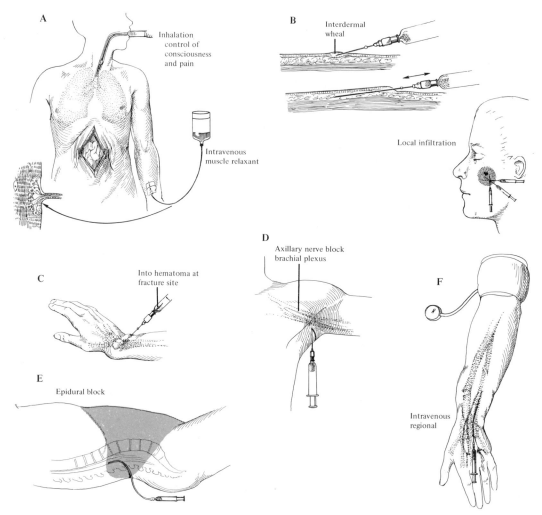

Figure 12–1.   Types of anesthesia. *A.* Inhalation. *B.* Local infiltration. *C.* Into hematoma. *D.* Axillary nerve block. *E.* Epidural. *F.* Intravenous regional.

Local Infiltration

Local infiltration is useful at the site of a laceration or fracture.

Nerve Block

A peripheral nerve block may be produced by infiltrating around a nerve with a local anesthetic, for example at the base of a finger. In the case of fingers and toes vasoconstrictor agents should not be added to the local anesthetic. The agent may also be injected beside a major nerve or plexus to produce a greater region of anesthesia.

Brachial Plexus Block. A brachial plexus block may be performed by a supraclavicular or axillary approach. A disadvantage of the supra-clavicular route is the possibility of inducing a pneumothorax, and this is avoided by the axillary technique. The arm is abducted at right angles to the body. A light venous tourniquet is placed around the upper arm to keep the anesthetic solution localized beneath the fascia surrounding the neurovascular bundle. The axillary artery is palpated as high in the axilla as possible where it lies in the groove beneath the coracobrachialis muscle. The median and ulnar nerves lie on either side of the artery and the radial nerve slightly posterior. A No. 22 needle introduced close to the artery transmits pulsations that are felt in the hub. About 15 ml of 1.5 percent mepivacaine is injected on either side of the artery. Anesthesia is complete in about 25 minutes.

Intravenous Regional Anesthesia

A No. 21 butterfly needle is inserted into a small vein in the limb near the operative site. The limb is elevated and blood evacuated using an esmarch bandage. A tourniquet is placed around the upper limb and inflated above the arterial blood pressure. For the arm 40 ml of 0.5 percent lidocaine is injected and 80 ml for the lower extremity. Anesthesia and muscle paralysis develop rapidly. At the end of the procedure the tourniquet is deflated gradually to prevent sudden flooding of the circulation with the anesthetic solution. It is more comfortable for the patient if two tourniquets are applied, inflating the more distal one when the region beneath it is analgesic.

Epidural Anesthesia

Local anesthetic solution may be injected into the epidural space in the lumbar region through a needle passed between adjacent vertebral spines to pierce the ligamentum flavum but not the dura. Caudal epidural anesthesia is produced by injecting local anesthetic into the sacral canal through the sacrococcygeal membrane. Postanesthesia headache is not a problem unless the dura has been inadvertently punctured. Continuous epidural anesthesia is particularly useful in obstetric patients.

Spinal Anesthesia

Spinal anesthesia is produced by injecting a local anesthetic into the subarachnoid space below the termination of the spinal cord. The anesthetic mixes with the cerebrospinal fluid and produces reversible blockade of sensory, motor, and autonomic nerve fibers. Sterile technique is essential. The dura is punctured by passing a needle between the third and fourth lumbar vertebrae. The anesthetic solution may be either heavier or lighter than cerebrospinal fluid. The patient is positioned to achieve blockade of the desired segments of the cord. In general, spinal anesthesia is most suited for procedures below the umbilicus. Serious complications do not usually occur in experienced hands. Hypotension resulting from involvement of the sympathetic nervous system is best treated with oxygen by mask and intravenous infusion to which may be added if necessary a small dose of a vasopressor.

Postoperative spinal headache may occur from escape of cerebrospinal fluid through the site of dural puncture. In order to minimize this possibility, a fine-bore needle (22 gauge or smaller) should be employed, and the patient should remain flat for 24 hours postoperatively. Established headache is difficult to treat, but increased hydration, abdominal binders, and other measures to increase spinal fluid pressure may be tried.

Action of Local Anesthetics

Anesthetics injected locally block conduction through myelinated nerve fibers by interfering with the passage of ions through the neuronal sheath. The effect is reversible and does not damage the nerve fibers or cells. Toxic reactions can occur when an overdose is given or when the drug is injected intravenously. Overdosage may result in convulsions followed by respiratory and circulatory failure. Convulsions may be controlled with small intravenous doses of thiopental or with a short-acting muscle relaxant. Respiratory failure is treated with endotracheal intubation and artificial ventilation and hypotension by administration of a vasopressor. Cardiac arrhythmias and garrulousness may also occur. A vasoconstrictor such as epinephrine may be used to delay absorption.

Local and Regional Anesthetics

Cocaine. Cocaine is an alkaloid obtained from the leaves of *Erythroxylon coca*, a plant growing in the Andes Mountains of South America. Peruvian Indians chew the leaves to increase endurance and produce euphoria. Cocaine is too toxic to be given by injection. Today it is used mainly to produce topical anesthesia in the nose and throat (10 to 15 percent solution).

Procaine. Procaine (Novocaine), a synthetic derivative of para-aminobenzoic acid, is destroyed more rapidly than cocaine and is about one quarter as toxic. Procaine may be used for infiltration, regional, and spinal anesthesia but is not employed topically. Since it is hydrolyzed in the liver by plasma cholinesterase, a deficiency of this enzyme may lead to toxicity.

Amethocaine. Amethocaine (Pontocaine), a derivative of para-aminobenzoic acid, is ten times more toxic than procaine after intravenous injection. It is used mainly for topical and spinal anesthesia (10 to 20 mg).

Lidocaine. The acetanilide derivative lidocaine (Xylocaine) has a more rapid, powerful, and longer action than procaine. It is used for infiltration, regional, spinal, epidural, and topical anesthesia. Epinephrine may be added to delay absorption.

Mepivacaine. Mepivacaine (Carbocaine) resembles lidocaine chemically and in its clinical effects and is possibly less toxic. It is ineffective topically.

Bupivacaine Hydrochloride. Bupivacaine hydrochloride (Marcaine) was synthesized in 1957 and is a homolog of mepivacaine. Although slower in onset its action lasts longer than other local anesthetics with no increase in toxicity. It is relatively short acting in the subarachnoid space, longer acting when given extradurally, and very long acting in peripheral nerve blocks. It is available in 0.25 percent and 0.5 percent solutions.[1]

GENERAL ANESTHESIA

Anesthetics may be divided into those causing central depression of the sensorium (general anesthetics) and those blocking afferent stimuli from peripheral regions (local, regional, and spinal anesthesia).

General anesthetics are introduced into the body by direct injection into the blood stream or by absorption from the tissues, lungs, or gastrointestinal tract. A concentration must be achieved sufficient to depress transmission of impulses through the synapses of the reticular system in the brain stem. General anesthetics are eliminated unchanged by the lungs or kidneys or are broken down in the liver and their degradation products eliminated in the urine.

The depth of general anesthesia depends on the partial pressure or tension of the anesthetic agent in the brain cells and is closely related to the tension in the arterial blood. The time of induction or recovery depends on the rate of increase or decrease of the tension of the agent in arterial blood. Agents highly soluble in blood, such as ether or methoxyflurane, take longer to achieve a satisfactory tension than less soluble agents, such as nitrous oxide and halothane.

Stages of Anesthesia

In 1920 Guedel described the stages of anesthesia in patients given ether. Although not so readily applicable today they are of considerable help when an inhalational agent is the sole anesthetic used. The four stages are (1) analgesia, (2) delirium, (3) surgical anesthesia, and (4) respiratory paralysis.

The third stage is divided into four planes of increasing depths of anesthesia. At the onset of stage 3 (surgical anesthesia) respirations are regular and "automatic," while as stage 4 is approached respirations diminish in amplitude and the blood pressure falls.[1]

When muscle relaxants are used, respiratory signs are of no value. It is essential, therefore, to monitor carefully the pulse and blood pressure and observe the patient's reflex responses to determine the depth of anesthesia. Adequacy of oxygenation and ventilation must be ensured at all times.

Volatile Anesthetic Agents

Nitrous Oxide. Nitrous oxide is sweet smelling, colorless, nonirritating, nonflam-

mable, nonexplosive, and nontoxic. However, it is a weak anesthetic and is generally used as a vehicle for delivering more potent anesthetics such as halothane or in combination with narcotics and muscle relaxants. It is seldom used alone except to produce analgesia and amnesia in dentistry and labor. Nitrous oxide is usually given with oxygen in the proportion of three parts of the gas to one of oxygen. It may adversely affect the course of a patient with bowel distention or a pneumothorax or one who has had an air encephalogram.

Halothane. Halothane is a sweet-smelling, colorless, nonflammable liquid introduced into clinical practice in 1956. It is a fluorinated hydrocarbon.

$$F-\overset{\displaystyle \overset{F}{|}}{\underset{\displaystyle \underset{F}{|}}{C}}-\overset{\displaystyle \overset{Br}{|}}{\underset{\displaystyle \underset{Cl}{|}}{C}}-H$$

The fluorine atoms are attached by strong bonds to the carbon atoms and cannot be split off. Fluorine toxicity therefore does not occur. Halothane is compatible with soda lime, used for absorption of carbon dioxide, and is frequently administered with a partial rebreathing technique in a circle system. Respiration is decreased mainly as a result of a diminution in tidal volume while the respiratory rate tends to increase. Halothane decreases cardiac contractile force, causes peripheral vasodilatation, a fall in arterial blood pressure, and slowing of the pulse. Compensatory vasoconstriction is minimal. It is stored in dark glass bottles because exposure to light causes decomposition.

Halothane is a powerful anesthetic and requires administration in precise dosage using calibrated vaporizers. A concentration of 2.5 percent is required for induction and 0.5 to 1 percent for maintenance. Since it is a poor analgesic, halothane is usually given with nitrous oxide and oxygen, part of the gas flow being deflected through the vaporizer. It is moderately soluble in blood; therefore a high arterial tension is soon achieved. Induction and recovery are rapid. There is only a minimal degree of muscular relaxation. In abdominal procedures supplementation of the anesthetic with muscle relaxants is required. Halothane should not be used with epinephrine because halothane sensitizes the heart to the effects of epinephrine, and arrhythmias and even ventricular fibrillation may result. Postoperatively halothane causes minimal nausea and vomiting. Shivering may occur in the recovery room, and since this is accompanied by increased oxygen utilization, oxygen should be administered.

Is halothane toxic? This possibility has occurred to many workers because halothane is chemically related to other toxic halogenated hydrocarbons such as chloroform and carbon tetrachloride. The National Halothane Study conducted over a five-year period by the National Research Council of the United States found no evidence of hepatotoxicity and concluded that halothane was safer than other anesthetics and had a lower mortality. However, it has been shown that hypersensitivity and liver damage do rarely occur in patients to whom the anesthetic is repeatedly administered.[2]

Methoxyflurane. Methoxyflurane (Penthrane) is a clear liquid with a characteristic fruity odor. It is stable when used with soda lime and, although an ether, is nonflammable except at high concentrations and temperatures. It is stored in amber bottles to prevent decomposition and has the formula:

$$
\begin{array}{ccc}
\mathrm{Cl} & \mathrm{F} & \mathrm{H} \\
| & | & | \\
\mathrm{H-C-C-O-C-H} \\
| & | & | \\
\mathrm{Cl} & \mathrm{F} & \mathrm{H}
\end{array}
$$

Because of the extreme solubility of the drug in blood, induction and recovery are relatively slow. As the concentration in the body increases, respiration is depressed and there is a progressive decline in ventricular contractile force. Hypotension is not, however, usually significant. Methoxyflurane has good analgesic properties and produces marked muscular relaxation during deep anesthesia. Elimination occurs through the lungs over a prolonged period. Postoperative nausea and vomiting are commoner than with halothane. The drug can occasionally cause kidney damage producing high-output renal failure and should not be given to patients with renal disease. The mechanism of its toxicity is unclear, but it appears to be dose related.[3]

Other Volatile Anesthetic Agents. *Ether.* Ether (diethyl ether) is seldom used because it is flammable and explosive. It has been considered safe in unskilled hands because it is the only general anesthetic which increases respiration and cardiac output.

Cyclopropane. Cyclopropane (Trimethylene) is a sweet-smelling, colorless, extremely potent anesthetic gas. It is very explosive and has been displaced by the new nonflammable agents. It may cause hypertension and myocardial irritability.

Trichlorethylene. Trichlorethylene (Trilene) is a colorless liquid with a chloroformlike odor, which does not burn or explode. It is an excellent analgesic but suffers from the drawback of forming the poison dichloracetylene when brought in contact with soda lime. It therefore cannot be used in rebreathing systems when soda lime is used.

Intravenous Agents Used in Anesthesia

When a drug is injected into the blood stream, its effect cannot be reversed as readily as when it is delivered and excreted through the lungs. The heart and vital centers are immediately subjected to a high concentration of the agent. Intravenous agents should therefore be administered slowly. Inhalational anesthesia produces its effects more gradually.

Thiopental. The short-acting barbiturate thiopental (Pentothal) is dispensed as a pale yellow powder and used as a 2.5 percent solution in sterile water. In the adult an intravenous injection of 250 mg in 10 ml produces sleep in about 30 seconds. The dose required decreases with age. When used alone the effect wears off rapidly due to its distribution in many tissues. The drug is slowly detoxified in the liver. It is used mainly to induce anesthesia. Great care should be exercised in its administration to old or feeble patients because of its depressant actions on the myocardium and respiration. Barbiturates have no analgesic properties and thiopental should not be used alone for painful procedures. As soon as sleep has been produced, anesthesia is continued using other agents.

Local complications from thiopental are sloughing of tissues due to perivenous injection and gangrene of the arm from intra-arterial injection. If the drug is injected outside a vein, the patient usually complains of local pain. When injected into an artery, there is severe burning pain. To minimize local complications solutions stronger than 2.5 percent should not be used.

Narcotics. Narcotics such as Demerol or morphine may be combined with nitrous oxide and oxygen. Satisfactory anesthesia with relatively rapid awakening is produced, but there is not the degree of control obtained with the inhalational agents. The dose of Demerol is 1 mg/kg with small additional doses as required.

Innovar. A combination of fentanyl (Sublimaze), a potent narcotic analgesic, and droperidol (Inapsine), a neuroleptic agent with antiemetic properties, can be used as an adjunct to nitrous oxide-oxygen anesthesia. It produces good cardiovascular stability and is therefore especially suitable for geriatric and poor-risk patients. The narcotic component may cause marked respiratory depression. Means of artificial ventilation should therefore be at hand. Conscious patients may become apneic but will breathe on command. Some increase of muscle tone usually occurs which may be counteracted by muscle relaxants. Extrapyramidal symptoms have been reported postoperatively and are readily reversed with antiparkinsonism agents. Each component of Innovar may be administered separately.

Ketamine. The recently introduced anesthetic ketamine produces "dissociative anesthesia" resembling a cataleptic trance. The patient is unconscious but has open eyes and does not respond to painful stimuli. Pharyngeal and laryngeal reflexes are preserved. Following intravenous injection anesthesia is produced within 60 seconds, respiratory depression is minimal, and the heart rate and mean arterial blood pressure increase. It may be used as the sole anesthetic agent for short diagnostic and operative procedures in children. There is a high incidence of postoperative hallucination in adults. The dose is 2 mg/kg intravenously or 8 mg/kg intramuscularly.

Diazepam. Diazepam (Valium) produces sedation and a slight degree of muscular relaxation. It may produce local irritation and should be diluted with blood on injection. If diluted with water or saline a precipitate is formed. It may be used intravenously to induce anesthesia and to tranquillize unruly patients.

Propanidid. This compound is a eugenol derivative, which is rapidly broken down in the blood and is useful for short procedures in ambulatory patients. It depresses the cardiovascular system in much the same manner as thiopental but stimulates the respiratory system. The initial dose is 4 to 6 mg/kg.

Muscle Relaxants

No drug should be given to produce muscle paralysis unless an adequate means of artificial ventilation is at hand. These agents block transmission of nerve impulses at the nerve-muscle junction.

The depolarizing muscle relaxants prolong the normally brief depolarizing effect of acetylcholine. Succinylcholine (Anectine) is a short-acting muscle relaxant. A dose of 40 mg causes complete paralysis for one to two minutes. It is used mainly to facilitate intubation of the trachea but may also be administered as a slow intravenous drip (0.1 percent solution) for prolonged relaxation. It is more potent in the hypothermic than the normothermic patient. There is no antidote available, and adequate blood levels of serum pseudocholinesterase must be present; otherwise prolonged apnea may occur. It can produce hyperkalemia and dangerous arrhythmias, particularly in patients with recent burns and muscle denervation.

Nondepolarizing muscle relaxants act by displacing acetylcholine from its receptor sites on the muscle cell membrane. D-Tubocurarine chloride (curare) and gallamine are long-acting muscle relaxants, curare having the longer effect. Curare may cause a fall in blood pressure due to release of histamine and ganglion blockade. Gallamine causes a pronounced tachycardia which may persist in the postoperative period. Muscle paralysis resulting from the action of nondepolarizing agents may be reversed by the anticholinesterase neostigmine (Prostigmine). Atropine is given before the neostigmine to minimize muscurinic effects.

Endotracheal Anesthesia. *Indications.* (1) To secure an airway when difficulty is encountered using a mask, (2) to control or assist breathing during abdominal or thoracic operations, (3) to prevent aspiration in emergencies when the stomach may contain food, (4) to permit greater freedom of access to the surgeon as, for example, in operations involving the head and neck.

Technique. A rubber or plastic endotracheal tube is passed through the nose or mouth. In most cases intubation is performed under direct vision using a laryngoscope held in the left hand while the blade is advanced into the pharynx between the base of the tongue and the epiglottis. The vocal cords are exposed by lifting the mandible upward and forward avoiding angulation on the upper incisors.

Endotracheal tubes are equipped with inflatable cuffs which when filled with air ensure a seal between the walls of the tube and the trachea. For orotracheal intubation a suitable sized tube is selected, lubricated, and threaded onto a curved copper wire stillette. For ease of withdrawal the stillette should also be lubricated, and its tip should reach as far as the end of the tube but not protrude beyond it. Laryngoscopy is performed. The tube is then passed between the vocal cords, the stillette is withdrawn and the tube advanced until the cuff lies below the level of the cords. The cuff is inflated, an airway inserted, the tube anchored in position with adhesive tape, and the end of the tube connected to the corrugated breathing tubes of the anesthetic apparatus.

When nasotracheal intubation is performed, it is advisable to spray the nasal cavity with a 10 percent cocaine solution to anesthetize the region and shrink the vascular nasal mucosa. A nasotracheal tube, which is slightly longer than an orotracheal tube, is passed through a nostril parallel to the floor of the nasal cavity beneath the inferior concha. A laryngoscope is inserted and as the tube enters the oropharynx, it is grasped by intubating forceps (e.g., Magill's forceps) and guided to the laryngeal inlet. In addition to its usefulness in oral operations nasotracheal intubation is the method of choice in comatose patients whose airway is endangered.

The tube is less readily obstructed by kinking or biting and is more readily tolerated for prolonged periods.

Complications. The complications of intubation are mostly due to faulty technique. Breath sounds should be checked after intubation. If air entry is diminished or absent on one side of the chest it should be assumed that the tube has been passed too far and has entered a main bronchus, usually the right. The tube is then partially withdrawn. Other complications are damage to the lips or teeth, nasal hemorrhage, kinking of the tube, or passage of the tube into the esophagus. When an old tube is used, it is possible for the inflated cuff to override and obstruct the lumen of the tube. Prolonged intubation can result in tracheal or laryngeal stenosis.

Anesthetic Apparatus

Most gas machines are variations of the Boyle gas-oxygen apparatus introduced in 1917 (Figure 12–2). The gas is stored in a reservoir bag during expiration and flow is continuous. The Boyle-type machine consists of:

1. Gas cylinders. The pressure is modified by reducing valves.

2. Rubber or metal tubes connecting the cylinders with the flow meters.

3. Vaporizing bottles. With the introduction of halothane and methoxyflurane these have been replaced by more precise metal vaporizers.

4. A reservoir bag which fills during expiration and empties during inspiration. The bag is compressed manually when respiration is assisted or controlled.

5. Corrugated rubber tubing of sufficiently wide bore to minimize resistance to respiration.

6. Expiratory valve which opens during expiration and closes during inspiration.

7. Mask connected to the expiratory valve by an angle piece.

Inspired gas composition and volume of ventilation must be adjusted to satisfy the patient's requirements for oxygenation and carbon dioxide elimination. Anesthesia and surgery cause abnormal ratios of alveolar ventilation to pulmonary capillary blood flow, so that at least 30 percent oxygen is required in the inspired gas mixture to ensure adequate oxygenation.

The volume of ventilation required to eliminate carbon dioxide is influenced by the amount of dead space in the patient's respiratory tract and anesthetic apparatus. Physiologic dead space may be increased during anesthesia. In controlling ventilation most anesthetists tend to err on the side of overventilation. Underventilation causes carbon dioxide accumulation and a tendency to bleeding, hypertension, cardiac arrhythmias, and increased muscle tone.

Adequate carbon dioxide elimination is achieved in properly designed anesthetic circuits,

A

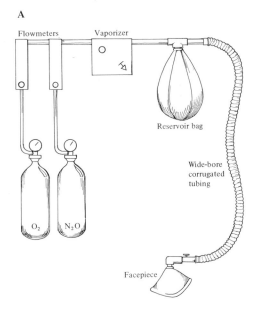

B

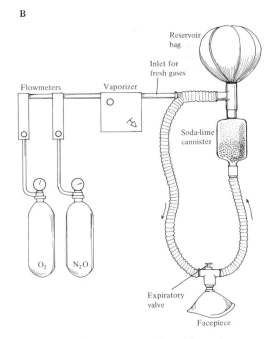

Figure 12–2. Types of anesthetic equipment. *A.* Single circuit anesthetic system (Magill attachment). *B.* Circle circuit anesthetic system with carbon dioxide absorption.

either by high flows of fresh gas with elimination of rebreathing by suitably placed unidirectional or nonrebreathing valves, or by absorption of carbon dioxide with soda lime. Semiclosed systems with carbon dioxide absorption and low flows of fresh gases are advantageous when economy of anesthetic agents is important. In a completely closed system dependence is placed solely on the soda lime to ensure elimination of carbon dioxide. Sufficient oxygen is given for basal requirements, normally about 300 cc per minute.

Anesthetic Complications

Vomiting and Regurgitation. Vomiting is an active process involving contraction of the abdominal muscles and diaphragm and is most likely to occur during induction and recovery from anesthesia. Regurgitation is a passive process occurring when a pressure gradient exists sufficient to overcome the valvular and sphincteric mechanisms of the gastroesophageal junction (Figure 12–3). It is less likely to occur when the head is elevated but more liable when the patient is in the Trendelenburg position. Reflex pylorospasm may occur in the nervous or injured patient and delay gastric emptying. In emergency operations an interval of six hours since eating does not assure that the stomach is empty. Narcotics used for preanesthetic medication sometimes cause nausea and vomiting in sensitive patients.

Regurgitation occurs without warning but vomiting is usually preceded by breath holding and contractions of the abdominal muscles. An observant anesthetist may have a few seconds warning that vomiting is going to occur. In addition the glottis closes by reflex action and affords initial temporary protection. The patient should be placed immediately in the steep Trendelenburg position. If possible a laryngo-

scope blade is inserted between the teeth and suction applied to the mouth and pharynx. When the teeth are tightly clenched, a rubber suction catheter may be inserted through the nose.

If tracheal aspiration is suspected, an endotracheal tube is inserted and a suction catheter is immediately passed. After inflation of the lungs with oxygen, further treatment is influenced by the severity of the aspiration. Bronchial lavage may be performed using about 50 ml of istotonic saline, rapidly removed with suction to permit prompt reoxygenation. When acid gastric contents have been aspirated, the patient becomes cyanotic and dyspneic and has a high respiratory rate and bradycardia (Mendelson's syndrome). Auscultation of the chest usually reveals signs of bronchospasm. X-ray shows irregular, patchy consolidation scattered through both lungs. The picture may progress rapidly to pulmonary edema and death from cardiac failure. Treatment includes administration of aminophylline, hydrocortisone, and antibiotics. Positive pressure ventilation may be necessary to prevent the development of pulmonary edema. Patients who have aspirated solid material require bronchoscopy.

Cardiac Arrest. Sudden cessation of the heart may be caused by direct surgical stimulation of the heart or by reflex stimuli arising during manipulation of structures in the chest or abdomen. More frequently it is caused by hypoxia resulting from obstruction of the airway or hypoxia and hypercarbia from hypoventilation (see Chapter 2). Oxygenated blood must reach the brain within four minutes or irreversible brain damage will result.

Drug Reactions. With the increasing complexities of treatment it is important for the anesthesiologist to be familiar with the patient's medical history.

Steroids. Steroids may have been prescribed

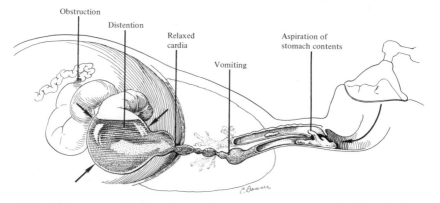

Figure 12–3. Pulmonary aspiration of stomach contents occurs as a result of intestinal obstruction, relaxation of the cardia, and the presence of food in the stomach.

for arthritis, ulcerative colitis, collagen disease, skin conditions, asthma, or pulmonary disease. They suppress endogenous steroid secretion and decrease the patient's reaction to the stresses of anesthesia and operation. Hypotension may occur out of proportion to blood loss, respiration be depressed, and return of consciousness delayed. Any patient who has been given steroids within three months of operation is liable to have suppression of the adrenocortical system. Steroids should be given prior to, during, and after operation. Hydrocortisone, 100 mg, is given at six-hour intervals intramuscularly and if necessary later by mouth.

Antihypertensive Medication. Drugs used in the treatment of hypertension reduce peripheral vascular tone. This effect is augmented by general anesthesia. The patient may therefore develop severe hypotension.

Rauwolfia Compounds. The rauwolfia compounds lower blood pressure by depleting tissue catecholamines. A normal level of catecholamines does not return until about two weeks after stopping the drug. Patients recently treated with resperine (Serpasil) may develop hypotension and bradycardia under anesthesia. In most cases the effects can be controlled by atropine and a peripherally acting vasopressor such as Neo-synephrine.

Diuretics. Diuretics lower the serum sodium and potassium. The hypokalemia may result in cardiac arrhythmias and increased sensitivity to nondepolarizing muscle relaxants. When potassium chloride is given intravenously, it is important to ensure an adequate urine output and to monitor the patient with an electrocardiogram. A low serum sodium may cause weakness, drop in blood pressure, and coma in the postoperative period.

Monoamine Oxidase Inhibitors. Tranylcypromine sulfate (Parnate) and similar drugs used to treat mental depression prevent deamination of naturally occurring amines. This may result in a hypertensive crisis developing after a small dose of a vasopressor, such as ephedrine, or possibly from the addition of epinephrine to a local anesthetic solution. Also the action of anesthetic agents may be potentiated by MAO inhibitors and result in profound cardiovascular and respiratory depression. Elective operations should be postponed for three weeks in patients under treatment with MAO inhibitors to allow their effects to be dissipated. Hypertension associated with the use of a MAO inhibitor should be treated with an alpha-adrenergic blocking agent such as phentolamine (Regitine), 5 mg intravenously. Hypotension can be counteracted with hydrocortisone, 100 mg intravenously. Meperidine hydrochloride (Demerol)

should not be given to patients undergoing treatment with MAO inhibitors.

Alcohol. Heavy drinking results in an increase in enzymes in the liver and rapid metabolism of anesthetics. Chronic alcoholics therefore require larger doses of anesthetic agents. Alcoholism may also impair the ability of the liver to break down anesthetic drugs and decrease synthesis of serum pseudocholinesterase that is responsible for terminating the action of succinylcholine.

Antibiotics. Most antibiotics, with the exception of penicillin, have weak neuromuscular blocking activity. Streptomycin, neomycin, gentamicin, and kanamycin produce their effect by decreasing release of acetylcholine from the nerve endings or by acting as nondepolarizing blocking agents. The effects of nondepolarizing muscle relaxants are enhanced and may result in profound respiratory depression. "Topical" administration of the antibiotic into the peritoneal cavity can result in respiratory depression.

Epinephrine and Halothane. Halothane sensitizes the myocardium to the action of epinephrine and may result in abnormalities of cardiac rhythm. This is not likely to occur in man providing the patient is well ventilated and has a normal arterial P_{CO_2}. However, if the surgeon wishes to inject a dilute solution of epinephrine, it is advisable not to use a halogenated hydrocarbon.

Malignant Hyperthermia. The cause of this pharmacogenetic disease is not known.[4] It is commoner in men than women and rare in infants and the elderly. In susceptible subjects it does not necessarily develop during the first anesthetic but may occur during the second, third, or fourth administration.

The following clinical features are characteristic:

1. Associated with the use of muscle relaxants and potent inhalational agents.

2. Failure to relax after the injection of succinylcholine and the development of skeletal muscle rigidity.

3. Rapid temperature rise to 40°C or more (rate of rise varies between 1 and 4°C per hour).

4. Cardiac arrhythmias and tachypnea.

5. Respiratory and metabolic acidosis.

The treatment consists of early recognition and terminating the anesthetic, hyperventilation with 100 percent oxygen, and cooling with ice bags, fans, and intravenous refrigerated lactated Ringer's solution. To prevent acidosis intravenous sodium bicarbonate (4 ml/kg of 7.5 percent solution) is given and repeated according to the blood gas measurements. To relieve the rigidity an intravenous solution of 1 percent procaine hydrochloride may be given. The loading dose is 30–40 mg/kg followed by an infusion of 0.2 mg/kg per minute.

Unsuspected Endocrine Disorders. *Diabetes Mellitus.* The patient with undetected diabetes may lapse into hyperglycemic coma, especially if anesthetic agents, such as ether, are used. The patient with infection does not respond normally to insulin and may go into hypoglycemic coma during an operation to remove a septic focus (see Chapter 11).

Addison's Disease. The patient with undetected Addison's disease may develop hypotension during operation and has a low serum sodium (see Chapter 27).

Primary Aldosteronism. An undetected aldosterone-secreting tumor may give rise to cardiac arrhythmia and possible arrest.

Pheochromocytoma. A catecholamine-secreting tumor of the adrenal medulla may produce hypertension that may lead to cerebral edema, hemorrhage, and death.

Hyperthyroidism. Hyperthyroidism is especially liable to be missed in the patient who has a toxic nodule that is producing cardiac arrhythmias or fibrillation and who has few neurologic or other system abnormalities.

RECOVERY ROOM

The introduction of the recovery room in the 1950s has been a major factor in reducing operative mortality. Recovery room care is directed toward support of respiratory and cardiovascular function in the immediate postoperative period. Protective reflexes may be suppressed by anesthesia and respiratory function by residual neuromuscular blockade.

Unconscious patients are placed in the lateral decubitus position with the lower thigh and knee flexed and the head extended. The airway should be continuously monitored by an experienced nurse until the occurrence of purposeful movements indicates that consciousness is returning. At this stage the nurse should be especially watchful in case of vomiting. Blood pressure, pulse, and respiration are recorded initially every five minutes, and the patient should be closely observed for signs of bleeding. The patient's color and level of consciousness are regularly noted.

The nursing staff should be especially trained and not rotated through other departments in the hospital. The recovery room should be designed so that every patient can be kept under continuous observation. Each bed should be provided with suction and oxygen outlets. Equipment must be available to treat emergencies such as cardiac arrest and respiratory complications. Special care should be taken in the ordering of analgesics. An anesthesiologist must always be available to treat any complications and to discharge the patient from the unit when consciousness is fully regained, bleeding has ceased, and vital signs have remained stable for at least 30 minutes.

CITED REFERENCES

1. Bromage, P. R., and Gertel, M.: An evaluation of two new local anesthetics for major conduction blockade. *Can. Anaesth. Soc. J.*, **17**:557, 1970.
2. Klatskin, G., and Kimberg, D. V.: Recurrent hepatitis attributable to halothane sensitization in an anesthetist. *N. Engl. J. Med.*, **280**:515–22, 1969.
3. McIntyre, J. W. R., and Russell, J. C.: Renal function and methoxyflurane anesthesia. *Can. Anaesth. Soc. J.*, **18**:131–36, 1971.
4. Relton, J. E. S.; Steward, D. J.; Creighton, R. E.; and Britt, B.: Malignant hyperpyrexia: a therapeutic and investigative regimen. *Can. Anaesth. Soc. J.*, **19**:200–202, 1972.

SUGGESTIONS FOR FURTHER READING

Dripps, R. D.; Eckenholt, J. E.; and Vandam, L. D.: *Introduction to Anesthesia*, 4th ed. W. B. Saunders Co., Philadelphia, 1972.
An excellent book covering all the basic principles.

Goodman, L. S., and Gilman, A. (eds.): *The Pharmacological Basis of Therapeutics*, 5th ed. Macmillan Publishing Co., Inc., New York, Chaps. 2–10, 1975.
This is a standard and most comprehensive textbook of pharmacology which will be readily understood by any physician.

Gray, T. C., and Nunn, J. F.: *General Anaesthesia*. 3rd ed. Appleton. New York, 1971.
The first volume deals with basic sciences and the second with clinical practice. It is primarily designed for the practicing anesthesiologist and those engaged in seeking higher qualifications in the specialty.

Ostlere, G., and Bryce-Smith, R.: *Anaesthetics for Medical Students*, 7th ed. Williams & Wilkins, Co., Baltimore, 1972.
An excellent and well-written book for those wanting an elementary and dogmatic presentation of the subject.

Chapter 13

OPERATING ROOM MANAGEMENT

John A. McCredie and *Gerard P. Burns*

CHAPTER OUTLINE

Immediate Preoperative Assessment
Identification of the Patient
Aseptic Procedures
    Transport to the Operating Room
    Air
    Personnel
    Skin Preparation
Conduct of Operation
    Positioning of the Patient
    Application of Drapes
    Assistants
    Intraoperative Hazards
    Special Precautions

Visitors to the Operating Room
Surgical Technique
    Incision
    Control of Bleeding
    Dissection and Exposure
    Sutures
    Prostheses
    Drains
    Topical Irrigation
    Wound Closure
    Application of Dressings and Appliances
    Classification of Wounds
Immediate Postoperative Management

The operation is a critical event in the total care of the surgical patient but only part of the total management. Good preoperative and postoperative care have resulted in major procedures being performed with a decreasing morbidity and mortality as greater attention is paid to total care. During the operation special attention is paid to avoiding introduction of infection, using careful surgical technique, and adhering to the principles of the basic sciences as practiced pre- and postoperatively.

IMMEDIATE PREOPERATIVE ASSESSMENT

In the preoperative period the patient should be brought to the optimal general condition and be informed of the nature of the operation and how he will be treated postoperatively. The surgeon must check that all preoperative orders have been carried out, such as insertion of an indwelling catheter and administration of prophylactic antibiotics. He should also ensure that the operating room staff are familiar with the proposed operation and aware of any special requirements such as instruments, prostheses, and intraoperative x-rays (see Chapters 11 and 14). The anesthesiologist should see the patient before operation to assess his general condition, to determine the most suitable type of anesthesia, and to arrange preoperative medication (see Chapter 12). The chart must be inspected for completion of the history and physical examination and also for essential laboratory data, such as the hemoglobin value and urinalysis. Pertinent x-rays should accompany the patient.

IDENTIFICATION OF THE PATIENT

The patient's identity should be confirmed from the name tag on the wrist and from the consent form on the chart. The type of operation must also be checked on the consent form and operating list. This is particularly important when a paired organ is to be removed, such as kidney, lung, or eye. When operation is performed on a limb or on one side of the body, the disease may be obvious such as gangrene of the foot, but often the diseased side is normal externally, for example a torn meniscus or a small inguinal hernia. It is therefore essential to have marked the site of operation with a skin pencil and confirm it from the patient's chart.

When blood is to be given, the group and

number on the container should be compared with the wrist tag on the patient and the cross-matching report in the chart.

ASEPTIC PROCEDURES

Transport to the Operating Room. Measures are taken to decrease the likelihood of infection being carried into the operating room on the patient or his clothing. The wheels of the cart are passed through an antiseptic solution on entering the operating suite or the patient is transferred to another cart. When possible, bed linens should not be taken into the operating room.

Air. The air delivered into the operating room is kept at a relative humidity of 50 to 60 percent and at a temperature of about 22°C and is filtered to remove particles and bacteria. An average of four bacteria are present on each particle in the air and the number of particles in the air varies from about 1000 per cubic foot when there is no activity in the operating room, as in the early hours of the morning, to about 10,000 per cubic foot when the room is used for a major procedure. The use of laminar air flow with a high pressure inside the operating room and a low pressure outside allows passage of air in one direction from a sterile to a nonsterile region with a complete change every 5 to 10 minutes. Laminar air flow systems may decrease wound infection from exogenous sources. Laminar flow results in removal of particulate matter, helps in maintenance of a constant temperature, and can be applied to existing facilities at relatively low cost. Charnley found that the laminar air flow reduced infection in patients with total hip replacement from 4 percent to 0.8 percent. Others, however, feel that the simpler and cheaper procedure of removing particles in the air by good filtration may be more important. Ultraviolet radiation has been used to sterilize the air already in the operating room. Its use has been shown to decrease bacterial counts by 50 percent. Care must be taken to protect the eyes of personnel from damage by the ultraviolet ray. The staff are instructed to move as little as possible during the operation and to open and close doors only when absolutely necessary. Conversation should be kept to a minimum.

Personnel. Members of staff with significant respiratory infections should not be allowed to enter the operating room. Periodic bacteriologic swabs should be taken from the nasopharynx of staff members to identify asymptomatic carriers of *Staphylococcus aureus*. The carriage of pathogens in droplets from the nose is more important than from the mouth. About one third of operating room personnel have *Staphylococcus aureus* in the nose, and about 3 percent have beta-hemolytic streptococcus in their throat. It is essential that clothing be changed on entering and leaving the operating suite. Hair must be covered because it frequently contains *Staphylococcus aureus*. A number of people shed this organism in large numbers from their hair. A mask worn over the nose and mouth should have a layer impervious to water, for example fiberglass, because materials that readily become moist permit passage of organisms from the mouth and nose to the air.[2] There is no place for the use of cloth masks. The preoperative hand and forearm preparation must be adequate and special attention paid to cleaning the nails. The skin cannot be completely sterilized because of the presence of organisms in the sweat and sebaceous glands (see Chapter 6). The organisms on the surface, however, can be removed. Hexachlorophene (pHisoHex) and iodophors (Betadine) are particularly effective in killing superficial organisms.[3] A proper technique should be used when putting on gowns and gloves. About 50 percent of gloves are punctured during an operation, and pathogenic organisms can escape from sweat glands and hair follicles and readily contaminate the operative site.[5] It is important, especially during prolonged operations, to make certain that gloves remain intact. About one half of scrubbed hands still have *Staphylococcus aureus* on their surface.

Skin Preparation. The patient should have had a bath, preferably with hexachlorophene soap, on the evening before operation. Opinions differ on the method for removal of hair. Shaving produces minute lacerations, thereby predisposing to bacterial contamination. Close cutting of hair with scissors or clippers or the use of depilatory creams may be preferable. Cruz found the incidence of wound infection to be 2.3 percent after shaving, 1.9 percent after clipping, and only 0.9 percent when the hair was left in position.

In the operating room the skin antiseptic must be applied for an adequate time to allow it to act. Iodophors (Betadine) kill gram-positive and gram-negative organisms and rarely cause reactions in the skin. An adequate area of skin is prepared to allow for possible extensions of the incision. For example, patients treated by laparotomy have the total abdomen, lower chest, and upper thighs prepared. The use of an adherent plastic sheet or stain towels around the incision may decrease the likelihood of pathogenic organisms contaminating the operative site.

CONDUCT OF OPERATION

Positioning of the Patient. The patient should be securely placed in the position that gives

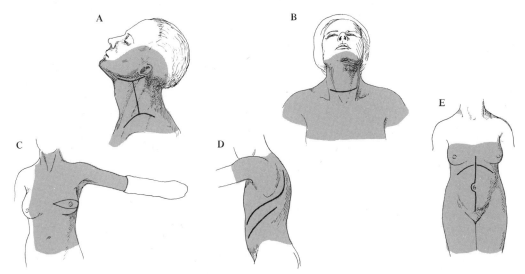

Figure 13–1. Areas of skin prepared as well as incisions for common operations. *A.* Block dissection of neck. *B.* Thyroidectomy. *C.* Mastectomy. *D.* i. Thoracoabdominal. ii. Renal. *E.* Abdominal. i. Bilateral subcostal. ii. Midabdominal.

optimal exposure (Figure 13–1). Exposure in the pelvic cavity can be improved by raising the foot of the table (the Trendelenburg position) and kidney exposure improved by placing the patient on his side and "splitting" the table. Pressure points should be protected by padding to prevent pressure sores and nerve palsies, for example of the radial and lateral popliteal nerves. When the patient is placed in the lithotomy position, careful padding of the legs is essential to prevent pressure by the stirrups. Overextension of the arm during operations on the breast or thorax may produce a traction injury to the brachial plexus. In elderly patients who often have cervical spondylosis care should be taken not to hyperextend the neck, as for example during operations on the thyroid and trachea. Patients with respiratory deficiency may not tolerate the prone position because of upward displacement of the diaphragm. Conversely, the prone position may be beneficial in operation on the spine when it decreases bleeding by increasing blood flow to the dependent abdomen.

Application of Drapes. Drapes should be placed to adequately expose the operative site and cover the remainder of the patient. A waterproof layer in the drapes prevents organisms passing through moist drapes into the operative field. Disposable drapes are now being used in some centers.

Assistants. The first assistant should stand opposite the surgeon during a laparotomy and the second generally on his left. It is essential that strong retraction be avoided to prevent tissue damage. The use of the proper incision of adequate size should minimize the necessity for retraction. The assistant should avoid leaning on the patient's chest.

Intraoperative Hazards. Special care should be taken to avoid producing burns of the skin when diathermy is used. Burns occur when the electrode touches an instrument that is in contact with the skin. They also occur when the patient is not properly grounded, and the current leaves the patient at a site where the skin is in contact with metal. Flammable anesthetic gases should not be used, as suitable nonflammable anesthetic agents are now available. An instrument, sponge, swab, and needle count must be made before the conclusion of every operation. Only sponges containing a radiopaque thread should be used. If the count is incorrect, an x-ray taken in the operating room will demonstrate the retained sponge.

Special Precautions. A number of special precautions are necessary in the patient who has been on chronic renal dialysis. This type of patient should have been dialyzed preferably on the day before operation. During operation it is essential not to give excessive intravenous fluids because of loss of the regulatory functions of the kidney. Because of the difficulty in giving blood, it is often necessary for the operation to be performed with a low hemoglobin (e.g., 7 gm). There is danger of reactivating muscle relaxants during the postoperative period.

In the patient whose blood is known to have the Australia antigen care should be taken that none of the staff has a skin abrasion or punctures a glove during operation. The anesthetist is especially at risk because the particle can be transmitted by air. Disposable materials should be used as much as possible. Gamma globulin is of questionable value. Recently a hyperimmune globulin has been used.

Visitors to the Operating Room. All personnel entering the operating room should have changed clothes and should understand operating room procedure. When the pathologist is asked to report on a frozen section, it is usually not necessary for him to enter the operating room. However, it is sometimes helpful for him to be present to view the gross pathology, as for example when selecting a lymph node for biopsy. The surgeon may wish to have a consultation, for example, with a gynecologist, urologist, or hematologist if there is an unexpected finding during the operation. The hematologist may help in diagnosing and managing a hemorrhagic diathesis occurring during the operation. The increasing use of electronic measuring devices often by technicians poorly instructed in operating room procedures increases the risk of infection. A breach in asepsis is especially liable to occur when radiologic procedures are performed. It is essential that radiographic technicians observe aseptic technique.

SURGICAL TECHNIQUE

Incision. The incision should give optimal exposure for the most difficult part of the operation and should allow for extension in the event of a greater than expected procedure being required. For example, an upper abdominal midline incision does not give optimal exposure for elective removal of the spleen, nor a lower midline abdominal incision give the best exposure for removal of the appendix. In certain upper abdominal diseases, provision should be made for extending the incision into the chest, for example when doing a total gastrectomy. Midline abdominal incisions can be made and closed rapidly, extended readily, and are of particular value for abdominal injuries (Figure 13–2). Oblique and transverse incisions placed over the diseased organ give excellent exposure and usually heal well with a low incidence of herniation (see Chapter 14, page 251).

Control of Bleeding. Hemostasis should be adequately controlled to facilitate exposure and prevent shock and hematoma formation. Temporary arrest of bleeding can be obtained by pressure using a finger, sponge, or a hemostat (Figure 13–3). Definitive control can be obtained by a ligature or a hemoclip, or the vessel may be repaired by suture, application of a patch graft or a graft. Occasionally bleeding is diffuse and has to be controlled by packing often supplemented by applying a fibrin sponge.

Dissection and Exposure. Damage to tissues is minimized by using sharp dissection with the scalpel rather than blunt dissection. Gentle handling of tissues decreases the possibility of tissue damage and the likelihood of infection.

Before bowel is opened, the peritoneal cavity is excluded from the operative site by packs to avoid peritoneal contamination. In abdominal operations exposure can often be improved by the proper use of packing.

Sutures. There is now a wide choice of absorbable and nonabsorbable suture materials. The suture should have adequate tensile strength and produce minimal reaction in the tissues. It may be threaded onto a needle or swedged on by the manufacturer.

Absorbable Sutures. Catgut is derived from collagen of the intestinal submucosa of the sheep, and polyglycolic acid is synthetic. Plain catgut causes a marked reaction in the tissues and is absorbed in about one week. Its use is confined almost entirely to tying small blood vessels and approximating subcutaneous fat. Catgut may be treated with chromic acid to produce a material that causes less reaction in

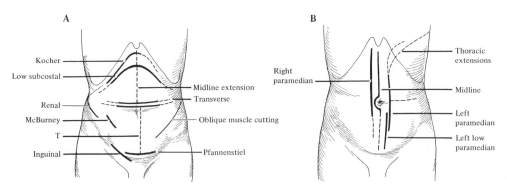

Figure 13–2. *A.* Transverse and oblique abdominal incisions with possible directions of extension. *B.* Vertical abdominal incisions with possible directions of extension.

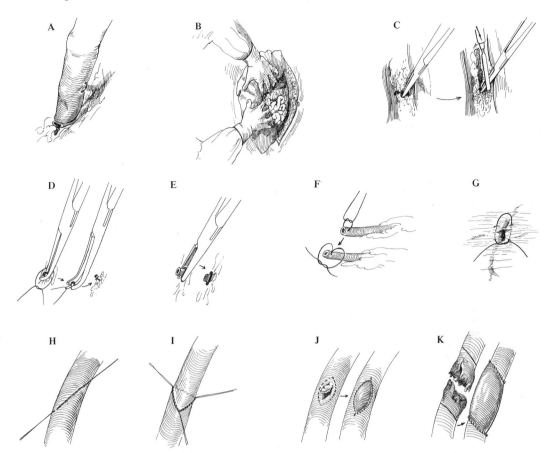

Figure 13–3. Methods of controlling bleeding. *A*. Direct digital pressure. *B*. Pressure using a sponge. *C*. i. Hemostat to bleeding spot. ii. Coagulation using diathermy. *D*. Hemostat to vessel and ligation. *E*. Application of hemoclip. *F*. Transfixion. *G*. Underpinning of vessel. *H*. Suture of laceration in vessel. *I*. End-to-end suture of completely divided vessel. *J*. Excision of part of damaged wall and application of patch graft. *K*. Excision of badly traumatized vessel and insertion of a graft.

the tissues, has a greater tensile strength, and persists for two to three weeks in the tissues. It has a wide use in general surgery, for example in bowel and urinary tract anastomoses and for wound closure. Polyglycolic acid has slightly greater tensile strength than catgut, produces less tissue reaction, and remains in the tissue for about six weeks before complete absorption. It is now often used in place of catgut.[4]

Nonabsorbable Sutures. These are made from the naturally occurring fibers silk, cotton, and linen, the synthetic polymers nylon and dacron, and stainless steel wire. There is less tissue reaction to nonabsorbable sutures, but since they remain in the tissues they can serve as the nidus for persistent infection. In the event of a sinus developing in a wound it is necessary to remove nonabsorbable sutures. Monofilamentous nonabsorbable sutures can readily be sterilized but are more difficult to handle than multifilamentous or braided sutures, and the knots tend to slip. There are a number of reports that infections are less frequent when monofilamentous, rather than multifilamentous, sutures are used. A "surgeons' knot" and an additional throw must be used. Multifilamentous nonabsorbable sutures are particularly popular because of their ease of handling.

Silk was originally introduced by Halsted and is still frequently used. It is strong, cheap, easy to handle, and induces only a moderate tissue reaction. Cotton resembles silk but is not as strong as either catgut or silk. The synthetic materials now commonly used are nylon, dacron, polypropylene, and Tevdek. Synthetic fibers are stronger than silk, cotton, or catgut and produce less tissue reaction. Stainless steel wire is popular because it induces the least reaction within the tissues. The monofilamentous form is difficult to use; braided wire is much easier to handle. Care must be taken when cutting the suture to avoid leaving a sharp point projecting toward the surface. The knots should be covered with an adequate layer of fat so that they do not become palpable and cause discomfort.

In certain situations special suture materials may be required, such as floss silk or a strip of autogenous fascia lata. To repair large hernial defects, foreign materials such as Marlex mesh or tantalum gauze may be used.

The sizes of catgut sutures range from 6-0 for ophthalmic sutures to 2 for heavy tension sutures. Nonabsorbable sutures range from 10-0 ophthalmic to 4. Needles may be threaded on the needle or swedged to the sutures to produce less tissue damage. Needles may be cutting for approximating strong tissues, such as deep fascia, or round for use in the peritoneal cavity. The needles may be straight, half circle, one quarter, or five eighths and are provided in a variety of sizes. Most are made from stainless steel.

Prostheses. Foreign materials are frequently used to hold structures together, to fill defects, and to provide artificial joints. Stainless steel, and vitallium screws are used for the internal fixation of bones. Intramedullary metallic rods provide excellent fixation for fractures of the long bones. Defects in the skull and face can be filled with acrylic resins. Joint replacement can be successfully accomplished with stainless steels and synthetic polymers. Large hernial defects can be repaired using tantalum mesh. Breast enlargement has been accomplished with silicone and plastic devices.

The use of prostheses predisposes to infection; therefore great care must be taken not to introduce infection when they are used. In the event of infection it is usually necessary to remove the foreign material.

Drains. Drains have been used to prevent abnormal collections of fluid such as blood, air, pus, gastrointestinal content, and urine. A drain is often inserted in the subcutaneous fat to prevent accumulation of blood and serous fluid in obese patients. The neck should be drained for 24 to 48 hours after operations on the thyroid to prevent possible pressure by blood on the trachea. After thoracotomy a drainage tube is usually left in the pleural space to permit escape of blood and air and to allow the lung to expand.

The types commonly used are open drains which allow escape of fluid into the dressings. These include a Penrose drain, a semiclosed sump drain, such as a double-lumen plastic tube with one limb connected to suction and the other acting as an air inlet, and closed drainage using a plastic tube attached to a bag or low-pressure suction machine. Another form of closed drainage is a Hemovac with a plastic tube attached to a suction reservoir. Closed drainage using the Hemovac system is effective in removing collections of fluid and is less likely to introduce infection than an open or semiopen system.

Before the introduction of antibiotics drains were extensively used in patients operated on for peritonitis. It is now realized that the drain is sealed off in less than 24 hours. Established intraperitoneal abscess such as appendiceal or subphrenic abscess should be drained. Most surgeons drain the site of cholecystectomy to permit drainage of bile which occurs to a variable extent from the gallbladder bed. A Penrose drain, with or without central wick, is most frequently used. A soft plastic tube drain attached to suction or a plastic bag provides a closed drainage system and reduces the risk of infection.

Topical Irrigation. Wounds are often irrigated with isotonic saline to remove free fat globules, blood clots, and foreign particles and to decrease the likelihood of infection. Antibiotic powders have been applied but are probably of less importance than a good surgical technique for wound closure.

Views differ on the value of irrigating the peritoneal cavity with isotonic saline in a patient with possible contamination of the peritoneal cavity. Irrigation may help remove bacteria or pus but could possibly spread infection to non-infected regions. Fluid containing antibiotics, such as kanamycin (1 gm per 500 ml of isotonic saline), has been placed in the peritoneal cavity in patients with peritonitis. Care must be taken when using antibiotics such as neomycin and kanamycin of causing muscle paralysis that may necessitate artificial ventilation for even hours after operation. Aspiration of pus and good intravenous electrolyte and antibiotic therapy are of much greater importance.

Wound Closure. Abdominal incisions are closed in layers with careful approximation of the tissues (Figure 13–4). In patients in whom poor wound healing is anticipated, as in the elderly, cirrhotic, infected, or cachectic patient, it may be preferable to close the incision in a single layer with through-and-through retention sutures. Devitalized tissues are excised. Fat is carefully approximated to avoid leaving a dead space that may become infected. Care should be taken when tying the sutures to avoid excessive tension on the skin edges. Michelle clips are sometimes used, especially for thyroid incisions. Recently tape closure of skin with steri-strips has been found to produce a better cosmetic effect and less wound infection for some incisions.

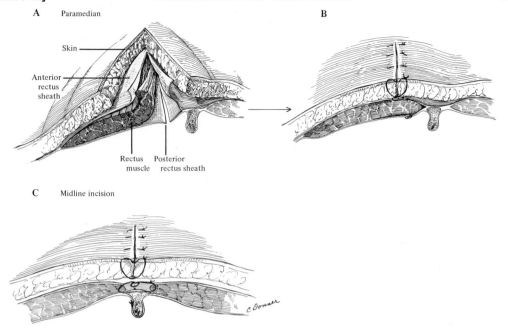

A   Paramedian   B

Skin

Anterior
rectus
sheath

Rectus   Posterior
muscle   rectus sheath

C   Midline incision

Figure 13–4.   Closure of midabdominal incisions. *A.* Layers in paramedian incision. *B.* Sutures inserted to close paramedian incision. *C.* Completed midline incision.

When a wound infection is anticipated, primary closure should not be performed. The skin and subcutaneous tissues are dressed open and usually closed later (see Chapter 6, page 130).

Application of Dressings and Appliances.   A dressing should absorb any serous discharge from a wound and not permit the operative site to become moist. A plastic tape, preferably nonallergic, is applied that does not damage the skin. Dressings on the abdomen should be taped vertically so that respiration is not impaired. Special care is taken when a pressure dressing is applied to avoid damage to the skin. A plaster slab may be incorporated in the dressing to maintain a limb in the correct position, for example after repair of a tendon in the forearm. At a number of sites that tend to become moist, such as the face and perineum, no dressing is applied.

Ileostomy and colostomy bags should be fixed in position in the operating room to avoid fecal contamination of the skin.

Wounds that are packed are sealed off carefully to avoid introduction of infection.

Classification of Wounds.   Wounds should be classified at the conclusion of the operation according to the likelihood of infection.[1]

Type I: Clean.   Endogenous contamination is nil or minimal; a wound that should not become infected, for example cholecystectomy and herniorrhaphy.

Type II: Clean Contaminated.   Bacterial contamination may have occurred from endogenous sources. For example bowel was opened during the operation, there was a minor break in surgical technique, the biliary or urinary tract was entered in the presence of infected bile or urine, or the oropharyngeal cavity was entered but there was no unusual contamination.

Type III: Contaminated.   Definite contamination has occurred. For example there was spillage from the gastrointestinal tract into the peritoneal cavity or an open emergency cardiac massage was performed. The wounds are infected but pus is not present.

Type IV: Dirty.   There is gross infection; for example traumatic wounds of more than 12 hours or from a dirty source, peritonitis from a perforated viscus such as the appendix or colon, perforation of a peptic ulcer complicated by purulent peritonitis or gangrene of the gut, or drainage of an abscess.

The incidence of infection should be less than 1.5 percent for type I wounds and is about 30 percent for type IV wounds. Hospitals should maintain a continuous record of their wound infection rates.

IMMEDIATE POSTOPERATIVE MANAGEMENT

Postoperative orders must be written immediately after operation. They include fluid and electrolyte therapy, pain medications, antibiotics, specific instructions for the care of drainage tubes and catheters, special investigations such as a postoperative chest x-ray, electrocardiogram, hematocrit, and blood gases.

It is most important for the surgeon to speak to the relatives after the operation. The patient's condition, the nature and extent of the operation, and the prognosis should be described in simple terms. If a procedure that was not anticipated had to be performed, such as a colostomy, the reason should be carefully explained.

A precise operative report must be completed at the conclusion of every operation.

CITED REFERENCES

1. Cooperative Study Group: Postoperative infections. *Ann. Surg.*, Supp., **160**:35, 1964.
2. Ford, C. R.; Peterson, D. E.; and Mitchell, C. R.: An appraisal of the role of surgical face masks. *Am. J. Surg.*, **113**:787–90, 1967.
3. Joress, S. M.: A study of disinfection of skin: a comparison of povidone-iodine with other agents used for surgical scrubs. *Ann. Surg.*, **155**:296–304, 1962.
4. Katz, A. R., and Turner, R. J.: Evaluation of tensile and absorption properties of polyglycolic acid sutures. *Surg. Gynecol. Obstet.*, **131**:701–16, 1970.
5. Miller, J. M.; Collier, C. S.; and Griffith, N. M.: Permeability of surgical rubber gloves. *Am. J. Surg.*, **124**:57–59, 1972.

SUGGESTIONS FOR FURTHER READING

Cooperative Study Group: Postoperative infections. *Ann. Surg.*, Supp., **160**:1–192, 1964.
    An excellent comprehensive review of the major aspects of operating room management with emphasis on prevention of infection.
Hermann, G.: Intraperitoneal drainage. *Surg. Clin. North Am.*, **49**:1279–88, 1969.
    Review of types and principles of abdominal drainage.
Jenkins, H. P.; Hrdina, L. S.; Owens, F. M.; and Swisher, F. M.: Absorption of surgical gut. III. Duration in the tissues after loss of tensile strength. *Arch. Surg.*, **45**:74–102, 1942.
    The reaction in the tissues and microscopic changes are described in detail.

Chapter 14

POSTOPERATIVE CARE AND COMPLICATIONS

Arthur E. Baue and *Alexander S. Geha*

CHAPTER OUTLINE

Preoperative and Operative Care
Postanesthetic Care
  General Principles
  Routine Care
  Surgical Intensive Care Unit
Postoperative Nutrition
  Basic Methods of Nourishment
  Intravenous Hyperalimentation
Postoperative Complications
  Postoperative Fever
    Atelectasis and Pulmonary Complications
  Venous Thrombosis: Thrombophlebitis
    and Pulmonary Embolism
    Prevention
    Recognition
    Treatment
  Fat Embolism
  Parotitis
  Pancreatitis
  Stress Ulcer
  Abdominal Distention
    Treatment
  Wound Disruption (Dehiscence) and
    Evisceration
  Intraperitoneal Abscesses
    Pelvic
    Subphrenic
  Wound Hematoma
  Urinary Retention and Infection
  Psychiatric Complications
  Decubitus Ulcer

Diabetes
Adrenal Insufficiency
Gout
Organ Failure After Operation
  Cardiac Arrhythmias
    Prevention
    Recognition
    Treatment
  Congestive Failure; Pulmonary Edema
    Prevention
    Recognition
    Treatment
  Myocardial Ischemia and Infarction
    Prevention
    Recognition
    Treatment
  Cardiac Arrest
    Prevention
    Recognition
    Treatment
  Decrease in Cardiac Output
  Renal Failure
    Prevention
    Recognition
    Treatment
    High-Output Renal Failure
  Ventilatory Failure
    Prevention
    Recognition
    Treatment

Proper postoperative care provides a safe and supportive environment to assist the patient's homeostatic mechanisms in maintaining the internal environment, to promote rapid recovery, and to prevent complications. Effective postoperative care must be anticipated before operation, continue during the procedure, and be maintained until recovery is complete.[10,26] Failure to appreciate the continuum of care increases postoperative difficulties and hazards.

A good background in human biology and an understanding of the stresses of disease, injury, and operation on all organ systems will best provide for complete recovery. In the patient we deal with the interface of normal physiology and pathologic physiology. This is preventive medicine in surgery.

PREOPERATIVE AND OPERATIVE CARE

An adequate preoperative evaluation of the integrity and reserve of all body systems is essential. Knowledge about a deficiency permits complications to be anticipated and treated early. This evaluation requires a detailed history, physical examination, and routine laboratory tests. When some abnormality is suspected, more sophisticated studies may be required, such as creatinine clearance measurement, pulmonary function tests, or a coronary arteriogram.

Timing of the operation is important. Postponing an elective operation for several days to improve pulmonary function by exercises, postural drainage, and medications may be lifesaving. In a patient with a large incisional hernia preoperative decompression of the gastrointestinal tract may make the repair easier and prevent ventilatory embarrassment and wound separation after operation. On the other hand, allowing intraperitoneal sepsis to continue without operation for even a few hours may contribute to death in the postoperative period.

During the operation perhaps the most important detail bearing on postoperative care is the proper conduct of anesthesia to maintain alveolar inflation, oxygenation, cardiac output, and renal function.

The operation should be performed so as to minimize blood and fluid loss, prevent tissue necrosis and infection, and assure proper healing of anastomoses and incisions.

POSTANESTHETIC CARE

General Principles

The need for a recovery room became evident from the findings of an Anesthesia Study Commission[27] inquiring into the causes of death after anesthesia: half the deaths were judged preventable. Recovery rooms were found to be useful in armed forces hospitals for the treatment of patients in shock; they provided an area where trained nursing personnel and expensive equipment could be used more efficiently.[16] Their use has been one of the most important factors in decreasing postoperative morbidity and mortality (see Chapter 12).

A recovery room provides specialized surveillance for patients recovering from the acute effects of anesthesia and operation. The unit should be close to the operating suite to minimize the hazards of transporting unconscious patients. It should be readily accessible to surgeons and anesthesiologists and be fully equipped to handle all emergencies. The recovery room should have permanent equipment for oxygen therapy, endotracheal intuba-tion, assisted ventilation, bronchoscopy, blood gas measurement, electrocardiographic monitoring, external cardiac massage, electrical defibrillation, and drugs needed for resuscitation.

Patients should be kept in the recovery room with a trained person in close attendance until they are fully conscious and free from potential immediate complications of the operation. A few hours is generally adequate. If further close observation is required, the patient should be transferred to the intensive care unit.

Routine Care

Recovery from the immediate effects of the anesthetic consists of awakening and regaining normal spontaneous ventilation and the protective reflexes that guard the airway. Hypoxia and cardiovascular instability are the main problems encountered. These may be prevented by the following systematic approach.

1. An open airway must be maintained. During most operations an endotracheal tube is used for ventilation. This should be left in place after operation until spontaneous ventilation is adequate. When it is removed, an oropharyngeal tube should be inserted to prevent the tongue from falling back and blocking the airway. The tube should be left in place until the patient can no longer tolerate it, has regained gag and swallowing reflexes, and has control of his tongue.

2. Secretions in the mouth and throat must be removed by suction.

3. Aspiration of gastric contents into the trachea should be prevented by keeping the stomach empty. A nasogastric tube is helpful but does not completely eliminate the possibility of vomiting and aspiration. The semiconscious patient should be placed on his side with head down so that secretions and emesis drain away or can be removed easily. If aspiration occurs, immediate bronchoscopy with cleaning and washing of the bronchial tree is mandatory. An endotracheal tube should be left in place until the possibility of further aspiration is gone. Steroids are given to prevent tracheobronchial edema and pneumonitis.

4. Adequacy of ventilation must be assured by close observation of the patient and by use of an endotracheal tube with mechanical ventilation until continued spontaneous ventilation is demonstrated. The causes of inadequate ventilation in the recovery room are persistent effects of the anesthetic and muscle-relaxing drugs, overdose of narcotics, and a long operation in an ill or wasted patient. Inadequate ventilation is defined as not moving enough air in and out of the alveoli to maintain a normal arterial P_{CO_2} (Pa_{CO_2}). Such a condition produces classic signs

of CO_2 retention or respiratory acidosis: the patient is obtunded, does not regain consciousness as expected, has a rising blood pressure and slowing of the heart rate. Respiratory acidosis may or may not be associated with hypoxia; the only certain way to diagnose it is by measuring the arterial blood gases. This measurement should be taken whenever there is doubt about the adequacy of ventilation, as cardiac arrest may occur if the endotracheal tube is removed before the return of adequate spontaneous ventilation.

Causes of hypoxia in the immediate postoperative period are massive atelectasis, pulmonary edema, and hemo- or pneumothorax. Examination and a portable chest x-ray will provide the diagnosis.

Laryngospasm and bronchospasm are serious problems in the immediate postanesthetic period. There is inspiratory difficulty and stridor (laryngospasm) or difficult, prolonged, or noisy wheezing expiration (bronchospasm). Severe laryngospasm with cyanosis is treated by giving a muscle-paralyzing drug and inserting an endotracheal tube. Bronchospasm is treated by giving warm moist air, isoproterenol in a nebulizer, and intravenous or rectal aminophylline.

5. Supplemental oxygen in inspired air will help to eliminate hypoxia. The arterial P_{O_2} of patients is often as low as 60 to 70 mm Hg after prolonged general anesthesia. This degree of hypoxia may not be evident from the patient's color and can be determined only by measuring arterial P_{O_2}. Oxygen given by face tent or nasal catheter increases the amount of oxygen from 20 percent in room air to about 40 percent and should be used routinely for several hours after a major operation.

6. Cardiac arrest and serious arrhythmias most often result from hypoxia and are preventable.

7. Hypotension is most frequently the result of blood loss, narcotics, bradycardia due to vasovagal reflexes, and sequestration of fluid at the operative site. The most common causes of hypotension in the first 48 hours after operation are an inadequate blood volume or an inadequate fluid replacement due to loss into the operative site or bowel.[2] Less frequent causes, which may occur at any time postoperatively, are inadequate ventilation, gastric dilatation, adrenal insufficiency, hyponatremia, myocardial infarction, pulmonary embolism, gram-negative septicemia, and cerebral damage.

8. Hypertension in a previously normotensive patient suggests hypervolemia due to overtransfusion, respiratory acidosis, or rarely a pheochromocytoma or hyperthyroidism.

9. Failure to awaken promptly after a general anesthetic is most often due to persistent effects of the anesthetic agent. Other causes are hypothermia, a low cardiac output, brain damage from a cerebrovascular accident, or hypoxia with or without hypotension.

10. Pain is one of the leading factors in postoperative atelectasis and pneumonitis. Frequent small doses of narcotics in the early postoperative period relieve pain and improve respiratory function,[14,15] but the depressant effect of large doses of analgesics on the respiratory center must also be recognized.

Surgical Intensive Care Unit

The surgical intensive care unit provides specialized nursing, monitoring, and treatment of patients who need close supervision for more than a few hours. It should be located close to the recovery room and be staffed and equipped to detect and care for circulatory, respiratory, and other complications. The facilities required are oxygen and suction outlets, solutions for parenteral administration, endoscopic and bronchoscopic equipment, mechanical ventilators, electrocardiographic monitoring equipment with a central monitoring station, capabilities for direct measurement of intravascular arterial and venous pressures, pacemakers and defibrillators, drugs for respiratory or circulatory emergencies, and facilities for measuring blood gases and carrying out other simple laboratory tests.[6] Subunits may be provided within the intensive care area for treating cardiothoracic or neurosurgical patients.

A radial design with rooms built around a central nursing station gives privacy and permits observation through large glass windows or doors. Medical help should be available continuously. The unit should be under the direction of a surgeon or anesthesiologist.

POSTOPERATIVE NUTRITION

Since many postoperative developments are likely to increase basal metabolic requirements, nutrition becames an important, even crucial, aspect of later postoperative care.[25]

Basic Methods of Nourishment

Oral intake of food is of course the ideal means to adequate nutrition, but if this is not possible, alternatives may be instituted with some success. Nasogastric gastrostomy or jejunostomy tube feeding of a standard liquid diet may be quite satisfactory for patients with adequate gastrointestinal tract function. Elemental diets, typically composed of purified amino acids, simple sugars, and vitamins, may also be desirable; taken by mouth or by tube, they can supply as many as 5000 calories per day.[32]

Intravenous Hyperalimentation

Standard intravenous fluids provide nutrition but only at near starvation levels; a more effective but more demanding procedure established in recent years is intravenous hyperalimentation.

Developed from studies by Dudrick and associates,[8,9] it provides sufficient nutrients to promote or maintain positive nitrogen balance and an anabolic state. It may be beneficial in a variety of clinical situations which preclude the functioning of the gastrointestinal tract.[34,35] Early recognition of the need for this procedure, however, is essential to its success.

Intravenous hyperalimentation requires infusion of a hypertonic solution through a catheter which passes through a large central vein into the superior vena cava. (Infusion through a catheter in a peripheral vein increases the likelihood of chemical phlebitis.) Venipuncture of the subclavian vein or the internal jugular vein are the two routes that have proved most satisfactory and are of equal technical difficulty. Percutaneous venipuncture of the subclavian vein can lead to pneumothorax, but once the catheter is in place it can remain for several weeks or more. Conversely, the internal jugular vein catheter is harder to maintain for long periods of time (due to motion of the neck), but pneumothorax is less likely and central placement of the catheter more certain.

For percutaneous puncture of the subclavian vein[34] the patient is placed in Trendelenburg position, with a small rolled towel between the scapulae and the head turned to the opposite side. The area is shaved, cleaned with acetone and povidone-iodine (Betadine), and draped. Gloves are worn and sterile technique used. A point beneath the midclavicle is infiltrated with 1 percent lidocaine (Xylocaine). A 14-gauge needle is attached to a 5-ml syringe. The needle is introduced bevel-down beneath the clavicle and over the first rib in the horizontal plane, aiming at the posterior aspect of the suprasternal notch. As the needle is advanced, mild negative pressure is maintained on the syringe until the vein is punctured and a free flow of blood is obtained. The patient then performs a Valsalva maneuver to prevent air embolus as the syringe is removed from the needle. A 12-inch, 16-gauge, radiopaque catheter is introduced approximately 8 to 9 inches. The inner cannula is removed from the catheter and intravenous fluids attached. Rapid forward and backward flow of blood from the catheter must be demonstrable.

The needle is removed and moved proximally to the hub and covered with the needle guard. The catheter is secured to the skin with a 4-0 silk suture. An ointment containing a mixture of polymyxin B sulfate, bacitracin, and neomycin sulfate (Neosporin Ointment) is placed over the puncture site which is covered with sterile gauze secured with benzoin and tape. The needle with tubing is also secured to the anterior part of the chest wall with benzoin and tape. The position of the catheter must be verified by chest x-rays.

For percutaneous puncture of the internal jugular vein,[34] the patient is placed in the Trendelenburg position, and the side of the neck (preferably the right side) is cleaned and draped. The triangle bound by the clavicle, sternal head of the sternocleidomastoid muscle, and clavicular head of the sternocleidomastoid muscle is located, and a 14-gauge needle with attached syringe is introduced at the apex, which is formed by the two heads of the sternocleidomastoid muscle. This is usually about 3 cm above the clavicle. The needle is advanced parallel to the long axis of the body and 30 degrees to the vertical plane. After blood flows into it, the syringe can be lowered so that the needle is at 70 degrees with the vertical plane. The syringe is removed and the 12-inch catheter is inserted. The remainder of the procedure is identical to that of subclavian venipuncture.

After the catheter is in place, it must be properly looked after to prevent local and systemic infection. Every three days[7,9] the dressing around the catheter is removed, and the area is carefully cleaned and treated with acetone and povidone-iodine. An ointment containing polymyxin B sulfate, bacitracin, and neomycin sulfate is applied to the puncture site, and a new sterile dressing is applied. There should be strict instructions prohibiting withdrawal of blood samples or administration of blood or medications through the central catheter, so as to avoid infectious complications. The intravenous infusion set attached to the catheter should be changed daily.

The intravenous hyperalimentation solution may be hospital-manufactured, but parenteral stock solutions are available commercially. A typical commercial solution consists of 500 ml of 10 percent protein hydrolysate injection and 500 ml of 50 percent dextrose, which are mixed before use. One liter of such a solution contains 38 gm protein, 6.8 gm nitrogen, 25 mEq sodium, 18 mEq potassium, 5 mEq calcium, 5 mEq magnesium, 18 mEq chloride, and 25 mEq phosphate, with a total of 1000 calories.

If supplementary measures are needed, vitamin B_{12} and folic acid may be added in the form of a mixture of ascorbic acid, thiamine mononitrate, niacinamide, riboflavin, folic acid, and cyanocobalamin (Folbesyn). If the prothrombin time is prolonged, phytonadione (Aquamephyton) is given intramuscularly or intravenously. For iron deficiency, iron dextran injection (Imferon) may be given by deep intramuscular injection.

In the average patient 1000 ml are given over 12 hours on the first day; 1000 ml in each of two 10-hour periods on the second day; and 1000 ml in each of three 8-hour periods on the third day. Other intravenous fluids which have been given are decreased and stopped as the amount of hyperalimentation fluid is increased.

To ensure adequate monitoring the following measurements should be made: daily weight, accurate caloric intake and output, temperature four times daily, urine samples for glucose and acetone four times daily, serum electrolyte values three times a week, and hemoglobin level, hematocrit reading, white blood cell count, prothrombin time, blood urea nitrogen level, and protein values, all weekly. A flow sheet with the above data helps to eliminate serious metabolic complications.

The common complications of subclavian vein puncture include pneumothorax, hemothorax, hydrothorax, puncture of the subclavian artery, air embolus, septicemia (particularly with fungi), phlebitis, lost catheter, brachial plexus injury, and thoracic duct injury. In good part these should be avoidable, particularly if subclavian vein puncture is performed and cared for by experienced house officers and if chest x-ray is obtained after insertion of the catheter to determine its location before fluid is administered.

Less common complications are those arising from dextrose intolerance or overloading. Utilization of dextrose varies from 0.5 gm/kg/hr in the normal adult to 1.2 gm/kg/hr in infants. However, in periods of stress these amounts may not be tolerated; hyperglycemia and osmotic diuresis will result. On the other hand, dextrose overloading may produce persistent glycosuria leading to osmotic diuresis followed by dehydration, azotemia, and hypernatremia. Usually the pancreas responds to a large dextrose stimulus by increasing insulin output, and the amount of dextrose given can be gradually increased. Nonetheless, diabetic patients, certain postoperative patients, some patients just beginning intravenous hyperalimentation, and patients with pancreatic insufficiency are prone to develop hyperglycemia and an osmotic diuresis. Because of the severity of complications that may occur during the hyperosmolar state, it is best to begin infusion of hypertonic

dextrose slowly and increase the dextrose load over several days. Frequent monitoring of blood glucose, serum electrolyte, and urine glucose levels is essential in these patients. With a persistent glycosuria (3+ to 4+) the rate of infusion must be decreased, or insulin injection administered, or both.

Infusion by gravity drip without an infusion pump is usually satisfactory, although close nursing attention is necessary; in infants and young children an infusion pump may be required. If the infusion falls behind the prescribed infusion rate by more than 250 ml, the prescribed rate should be maintained and the remaining solution discarded at the end of the day—a rapid infusion of large volumes of this hypertonic solution, to catch up, may quickly precipitate an osmotic diuresis and dehydration.

Electrolyte imbalance may occur. Commercial solutions generally supply about 25 mEq/liter of sodium; a maintenance amount can be provided by adding 30 mEq sodium chloride to each of 2 liters of solution a day. (Low sodium concentration may not be appreciated and hyponatremia could develop.) Inadequate potassium replacement could produce both decreased potassium content and increased carbon dioxide. Potassium requirements will usually be between 100 to 150 mEq per day rather than the usual 40 to 80 mEq per day.

When hyperalimentation is to be discontinued, it is advisable to decrease the infusion slowly and conclude it with 5 percent dextrose in water to prevent "rebound" hypoglycemia from the high levels of endogenous insulin secretion produced by the previous large dextrose load. Patients should be weaned gradually from intravenous to oral feedings.

Intravenous hyperalimentation can best be carried out by an institutional program that includes a standardized protocol and a hyperalimentation team familiar with the solutions, catheter insertion and care, and possible complications.

POSTOPERATIVE COMPLICATIONS

Although complications may be related to previous coincidental disease or entirely fortuitous, they are principally either general or brought on by the specific operation. General complications are discussed here, complications related to specific operations in the appropriate chapters.

Postoperative Fever

The major causes of postoperative fever are atelectasis and pulmonary infection, urinary tract and wound infections, anastomotic leaks and peritonitis, empyema following thoracic operations, and venous thrombosis. Less common causes are drug reactions, increased osmolar concentration from lack of water or salt excess, infection at site of intravenous injection or from catheterization, bacterial enterocolitis, deep abscesses, septicemia, adrenal insufficiency, thyroid crisis, relapse of malaria, and an inaccurate or factitiously heated thermometer. The cause of postoperative fever should be sought by examination of the patient, appropriate x-rays, laboratory studies, and fluid cultures. Hyperpyrexia stresses the cardiovascular system and increases energy needs. The temperature should be reduced by applying a cooling blanket, water-alcohol sponging, and inserting aspirin suppositories.

Atelectasis and Pulmonary Complications. Atelectasis, the most common cause of fever in the first 24 to 48 hours after operation, is defined as collapse of part of the lung from failure to maintain normal alveolar inflation. The process may be patchy or involve a segment, a lobe, or an entire lung (Figure 14–1). Normally there is a cycle of alveolar collapse followed by reinflation when the same tidal volume is inhaled with each breath. Periodic sighs or deep breaths reinflate collapsed alveoli.[4,36] Continuous ventilation

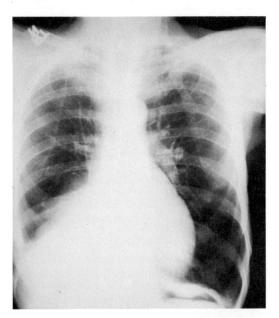

Figure 14–1. Chest x-ray that demonstrates atelectasis of the right middle lobe and a portion of the right lower lobe. There may be a small amount of fluid as well. Note that the major fissure is seen, indicating that the superior segment of the lower lobe is probably still inflated. This is a classic example of lobar atelectasis that may occur after operation.

during operation without occasional hyperinflation contributes to alveolar collapse. Pain, medications, immobility, and depression of the central nervous system impair respiration. A mild state of dehydration and the drying effect of premedication on bronchial secretions, inhibition of the cough reflex and bronchial ciliary motion predispose to obstruction of the smaller bronchi with inspissated mucus. Bronchial obstruction from foreign bodies (food particles, dentures, teeth) are less frequent causes.

Atelectasis can be prevented by preparing the patient before operation, by restoring normal breathing patterns after the operation, and by early ambulation. Preoperative preparation consists of cessation of smoking, institution of breathing and coughing exercises, and treatment of respiratory infections. During operation frequent suction of secretions is essential. After operation breathing and coughing exercises should be started immediately to clear secretions and restore the normal cycle of periodic sighing and deep breathing. Patients often do not move after an operation to avoid pain and therefore have shallow breathing. They must be given medication to relieve pain and encouraged to breathe deeply and cough frequently. Rebreathing tubes and intermittent positive pressure breathing systems are useful aids. Breathing exercises, chest percussion, and postural drainage may be indicated. The administration of humidified air or 40 percent oxygen prevents drying of the secretions.

Tachycardia, tachypnea, and fever suggest atelectasis. Fever, however, may be the only sign. Cyanosis indicates that a large amount of lung tissue is not aerated with blood flowing through it; this has the effect of a right-to-left cardiac shunt. Dyspnea occurs when a large segment of the lung is airless. The trachea and mediastinum move toward the affected side. Breath sounds are diminished and are bronchial over atelectatic segments in contact with the chest wall but may be normal when atelectasis is centrally placed. Rales, rhonchi, and wheezes almost always accompany obstructive atelectasis. Compression atelectasis may occur from pressure on the lung by fluid or air within the thoracic cavity or by distended viscera in the peritoneal cavity. The pathophysiology and physical signs are the same as in obstructive atelectasis. Deviation of the mediastinum and trachea, however, does not occur or is to the opposite side. A chest x-ray is essential in the investigation of most patients with postoperative fever. The Pa_{O_2} is decreased according to the amount of lung involved; the Pa_{CO_2} is usually slightly elevated or in the upper range of normal.

Treatment consists of intensifying the prophylactic procedures. The patient is kept active, encouraged to breathe deeply and cough. If atelectasis is extensive, a lubricated catheter is passed through a nostril and advanced into the trachea while the patient inspires deeply. This stimulates violent coughing and usually dislodges secretions blocking the major bronchi. Intermittent aspiration is performed through the catheter. Bronchoscopy is indicated if aeration is not improved, when there is collapse of one lung or bilateral extensive atelectasis, or when the atelectasis is secondary to aspiration of a foreign body, profound weakness, paralysis of intercostal and abdominal musculature, disorientation, coma, stupor, or hypotension. Rarely tracheostomy is required to permit repeated aspiration of secretions. It provides access to the tracheobronchial tree but decreases the effectiveness of coughing. Tracheostomy may be needed after crush injury of the chest, severe facial or cervical burns, repeated aspiration, and severe chronic pulmonary disease. High concentration of oxygen should not be given because of the danger of oxygen toxicity.

Compression atelectasis is treated by removing fluid by paracentesis, thoracentesis, draining an empyema or subphrenic abscess, relieving abdominal distention, or removing tight abdominal binders.

A bacterial culture of tracheal secretions should be obtained and appropriate antibiotics given.

Venous Thrombosis: Thrombophlebitis and Pulmonary Embolism

Prevention. Since the time of Virchow very little more has been learned about the factors he implicated in the development of blood clots in the venous system occurring after operation. He described venous intimal damage, stasis,[22] and a change in the coagulability of blood.[12] The relative importance of each is not known, and whether or not increased coagulability of blood occurs during and after operation is indefinite. Clots form during or immediately after operation most commonly in the deep veins of the calf or thigh and less often the pelvis. Common procedures to decrease venous thrombosis are:

Decrease Stasis. The legs are elevated and elastic stockings worn during and after operation. Early leg exercises and ambulation are encouraged.

Avoid Intimal Damage. Intimal damage can be prevented by avoiding pressure on the legs. In addition, the legs should not be used for infusions or medications.

Prevent Blood Coagulation. Anticoagulants have been given to inhibit clot formation in those with a high risk of embolism as in those who have had a previous embolus or who have venous disease in the legs. Small doses of heparin given subcutaneously before, during, and after operation have been shown to be effective.

Recognition. Deep vein thrombosis is often not detected clinically until a pulmonary embolism occurs. (When symptoms or signs in the legs are absent or slight, the condition has been called phlebothrombosis.) Symptoms and signs usually develop around the sixth to ninth postoperative day. They include calf pain, tenderness, swelling, venous distention, fever, and pain in the calf on dorsiflexion of the foot (Homans' sign). Early detection requires daily examination of the legs for calf tenderness or a difference in calf circumference. Thrombophlebitis is present when the clinical features in the legs are prominent. The clot may extend upward and involve the femoral and iliac veins producing massive edema of the leg (iliofemoral thrombophlebitis). If the edema and venous occlusion are massive, the arterial inflow is reduced and there may also be arterial spasm (phlegmasia cerulea dolens). Gangrene may occur.

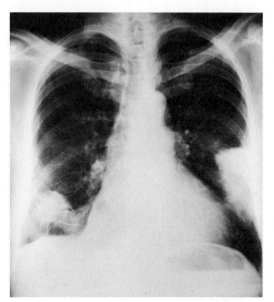

Figure 14–2. Chest x-ray showing multiple pulmonary emboli with infarcts. In the left chest is seen a somewhat triangular area of increased density with the flat portion against the chest wall and the apex toward the hilum; this is a classic example of a pulmonary infarct. There is an additional infarct in the right lower lobe that has a somewhat rounded density and appearance.

Pulmonary embolism can occur repeatedly with few symptoms or signs or can produce sudden death. This tragedy characteristically occurs on the sixth to eighth postoperative day in a patient who is walking during an otherwise uneventful convalescence. The symptoms and signs of embolism are extremely variable. A high index of suspicion is required in any patient having problems in the late postoperative period. Dyspnea is the commonest symptom. Chest pain is characteristic and may be pleuritic with cough, hemoptysis, and cyanosis. Later a friction rub may be heard. Initially the chest x-ray may be normal—later the wedge-shaped density of an infarct may be seen with a small amount of pleural fluid (Figure 14–2). A lung scan is more sensitive than a chest x-ray. When the embolus is large, an ECG may show the right heart strain pattern of cor pulmonale. There is also elevation of LDH in the blood.

Treatment. Deep thrombophlebitis with or without a pulmonary embolus should be treated by immediate administration of intravenous heparin in an initial dose of 5000 international units. A clotting time or partial thromboplastin time (PTT) is obtained before heparinization and after the second dose and then twice daily. The dose is adjusted to maintain a clotting time of about four times the normal level. Heparin is then given again every four hours subcutaneously, intramuscularly, or intravenously. The subcutaneous and intramuscular routes are inferior to the intravenous route because of the inconsistency of absorption and the frequent development of hematomas at the site of injection. The most reliable method is to run an intravenous solution continuously and give the heparin intermittently above the drip chamber.

The patient is kept in bed with the legs elevated until the signs of thrombophlebitis disappear. After several days of heparin therapy, Coumadin is also given in an initial loading dose and then in daily doses to prolong the prothrombin time two to three times the control value. After five days of Coumadin, and with a satisfactory level of anticoagulation, heparin is discontinued. Coumadin is continued for six weeks to three months. A patient with a pulmonary embolus but without evidence of thrombophlebitis is treated in the same way. If a patient has a second pulmonary embolus while adequately anticoagulated, more active measures must be taken to prevent further emboli. Since most clots come from the lower part of the body, the inferior vena cava may be ligated or partially occluded by fenestration, an external clip, or an internal umbrella or balloon so that large clots cannot pass to the lungs (Figure 14–3). On rare occasions a patient has a massive life-threatening embolus

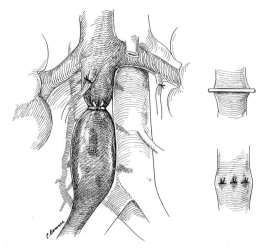

Figure 14–3. A patient who continues to have pulmonary embolism while on adequate heparin therapy may be treated by ligation of the inferior vena cava just below the renal veins or by partial occlusion of the lumen.

but survives long enough for the clot to be removed from the pulmonary artery by cardiopulmonary bypass. Deep vein thrombosis can destroy the venous valves and produce incompetence with development of the postphlebitic syndrome with chronic swelling, skin changes, and ulceration. This requires the use of elastic stockings.

Fat Embolism

The incidence of fat embolism in patients with multiple fractures may be as high as 50 percent. Clinical signs are present in about 10 percent of the critically injured. Pulmonary embolism results in hypoxia, increased respiratory rate, and tachycardia. Cerebral embolism results in confusion, irritability, and, if severe, coma with decerebrate rigidity. On examination there is generally a fever, and subcutaneous petechial hemorrhages may be seen, especially in the skin of the anterior chest and beneath the conjunctivae (Figure 14–4). Chest x-ray may show patchy consolidation giving a snowstorm appearance. Fat may be found in sputum or urine, the serum lipase may be increased, and the serum calcium decreased.

The etiology of fat embolism is not known. The older but now less popular theory was that fat in the bone marrow entered ruptured vessels at the fracture site. There may, however, be more fat in the lungs than could be derived from the bone marrow, and there is a greater amount of cholesterol in the fat in the lungs than in the bone marrow. Then, too, if the fat entered the venous system from the bone marrow, the lungs

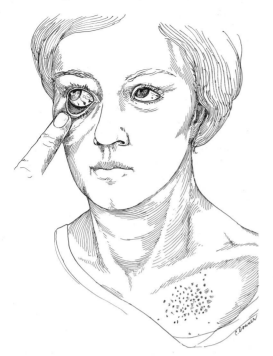

Figure 14–4. Petechial hemorrhages tend to occur on the anterior chest and beneath the subconjunctiva in fat embolism. They may be present for only several hours.

would be expected to be affected mainly, not the brain, subcutaneous tissues, and renal glomeruli. The alternate theory is that the stress of injury causes a change in the electrostatic charge on the chylomicrons and platelets in the blood, resulting in their coalescing and forming emboli which block capillaries. Increased lipase activity results in the production of free fatty acids and serotonin. The free fatty acids are irritating and result in acute inflammation. Serotonin increases capillary permeability and causes bronchospasm. There is pulmonary edema, the P_{O_2} falls, and decreased production of surfactant leads to alveolar collapse and further increases the hypoxia. Hemorrhages occur in the lungs and to a lesser extent in the subcutaneous tissues, brain, and kidneys, and result in a decrease in the hematocrit. A consumptive coagulopathy and tendency to bleed may occur if there is extensive loss of platelets.

Prophylaxis consists of the prompt immobilization of fractures and treatment of oligemic shock. Pulmonary embolism is treated by administration of oxygen. If there is marked hypoxia, endotracheal intubation may be necessary and administration of oxygen using positive end expiratory pressure (PEEP). Bronchodilators are given to overcome the bronchospasm induced by serotonin. The central venous pressure or preferably the pulmonary wedge pressure should be monitored to prevent right heart strain and congestive heart failure. Diuretics may be given to decrease the pulmonary edema. Prednisone, 50 mg every 6 hours, is given intravenously to decrease the inflammatory response. Heparin may be given for an antiserotonin effect and to prevent consumptive coagulopathy. However, the tendency of heparin to cause hemorrhage at sites of injury may contraindicate its use.

Parotitis

Acute parotitis may occur after operation and proceed quickly to suppuration. It tends to occur in aged, immunosuppressed, debilitated patients with poor oral hygiene or inadequate hydration and in those who are uremic. Atropine decreases salivary secretion and predisposes to this complication. The onset is rapid, with pain and swelling in the gland. The most common bacterial agent is the hemolytic *Staphylococcus aureus*. When the diagnosis is made, the duct of the involved gland should be massaged and smears and cultures obtained. Oral hygiene, hydration, and nutrition should be improved. Antiseptic mouth washes, cleansing of the teeth, and salivatory stimulants should be used. An antibiotic known to be effective against the staphylococcus should be given immediately while waiting for the drug sensitivity of the organism. In most instances the condition responds to this regimen. Occasionally the disease may persist and proceed to suppuration, requiring incision and drainage. This should be done before pus penetrates the capsule and invades the surrounding tissue. Radiotherapy has been advocated early in the course to decrease secretion of the gland. (See Figure 16–2, page 274.)

Pancreatitis

Acute postoperative pancreatitis occurs most commonly following surgical procedures in close proximity to the pancreas, but it may follow operations in other regions. The complication is uncommon but the mortality is high.[11] Direct surgical trauma may be important when removing a stone from the common bile duct or during gastrectomy. The diagnosis is difficult, because the symptoms and signs of pancreatitis may be overlooked in the early postoperative period and confused with changes attributable to the operation. The high mortality may be related partly to this lack of early recognition. The abdominal pain is often out of proportion to that anticipated from the procedure itself and is quickly followed by tachycardia, hyperamylasemia, prostration, tachypnea hyperpyrexia, shock, cyanosis, and death. Treatment is the same as that for acute pancreatitis (see Chapter 20).

Stress Ulcer

In 1842 Curling described acute ulceration of the stomach or duodenum following burns. Acute ulcers may develop after various types of trauma and stress including major operations[29,37] (see Chapter 18).

Abdominal Distention

Abdominal distention after operation is due to accumulation of gas and fluid in the gastrointestinal tract or blood and serous fluid in the peritoneal cavity. The colon should be emptied before operation and when indicated the stomach decompressed by a nasogastric tube. Distention and ileus can be anticipated in patients having operations on the bowel and retroperitoneal dissection for exposure of the kidney, pancreas, and aorta. In such cases a nasogastric tube should be inserted and remain until peristalsis has returned and the patient has passed flatus. Proper position and patency of the tube must be maintained. This will reduce distention, eliminate acute gastric dilatation, decrease cramps, help to protect anastomoses, and may reduce the incidence of intestinal obstruction. In operations for intestinal obstruction bowel may be decompressed on the operating table. A temporary gastrostomy is useful for prolonged decompression, particularly when ileus is predicted. Prolonged ileus is decreased by gentle handling of the bowel at operation, avoidance of intraperitoneal infection, not allowing glove powder to have contact with the bowel, and by eliminating technical errors.

Acute gastric dilatation presents with effortless vomiting of foul, dark blood-containing vomitus, usually accompanied by tachycardia, prostration, and hypotension. The patient may have insatiable thirst and little pain. The epigastrium is distended and tympanitic. A large gastric gas bubble can be demonstrated on an erect roentgenogram of the abdomen. Gastric suction should be instituted. The rapid aspiration of 2 or more liters of gas and dark, foul fluid from the stomach is sufficient to establish the diagnosis and produces immediate improvement. In most instances no organic obstructive lesion of the stomach or intestine is found. The complication can frequently accompany thoracic operations but in some cases may be caused by unsuspected cicatricial changes in the pylorus or duodenum, high intestinal obstruction from bands, hernias, and congenital

anomalies, or obstruction of the efferent stoma of a gastrojejunostomy. Hypokalemia can contribute to gastric atony.

Postoperative ileus is a common cause of postoperative abdominal distention and discomfort. It may be adynamic, where there is prolonged failure of return of normal peristalsis, or it may be mechanical. The term "ileus" is used commonly to describe the adynamic form. Differentiating the two forms may be difficult because mechanical intestinal obstruction arising immediately postoperatively is often unattended by intestinal colic. The causes of adynamic ileus are intra-abdominal infection, handling and resection of gut, hypokalemia, or reflex. The abdomen is distended and tympanitic, the patient vomits large amounts of brownish fluid, there is no peristalsis, and flatus is not passed downward. An x-ray of the abdomen which shows gas and fluid levels

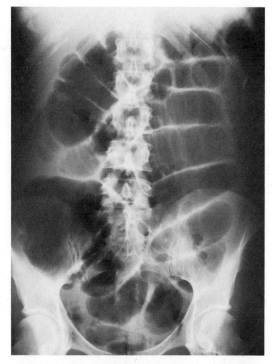

Figure 14–5. A plain film of the abdomen demonstrating adynamic or paralytic ileus, a frequent postoperative problem. Note that there is some distention of both the large and small bowel. Air is seen in the cecum on the right side around the transverse colon, in the descending colon, and in the rectal sigmoid. This x-ray film, along with the clinical picture of the patient, should clearly describe adynamic ileus. Conservative management, consisting of nasogastric suction and accurate fluid and electrolyte replacement, is indicated.

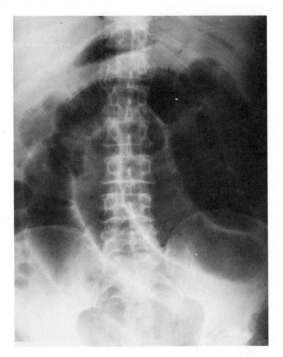

Figure 14–6. This plain abdominal x-ray provides an example of postoperative intestinal obstruction. Note small bowel distention with large loops of small bowel arranged in a somewhat circular fashion. There is a small amount of air in the stomach above, but practically no air in the large intestine. The bowel wall also seems somewhat thickened. Air fluid levels are not seen because the film was taken in the recumbent position. If, however, the film had been taken in the upright position, air fluid levels may well have been visible. This film indicates small bowel obstruction; the somewhat circular arrangement of the small intestine suggests that the bowel has been twisted. This could occur with an adhesive band or with internal herniation of the small intestine.

throughout the entire large and small bowel strongly suggests adynamic ileus rather than obstruction (Figures 14–5 and 14–6).

Treatment. Gastric dilation is treated by gastric intubation and continuous suction with fluid and electrolyte replacement. Adynamic ileus is treated by gastric suction and adequate fluid and electrolyte replacement with special attention to potassium. Antibiotics are given for peritoneal infection. Any intra-abdominal abscess is drained. Pharmacologic agents to stimulate peristalsis are usually ineffective and may be dangerous.

The differentiation between adynamic ileus and mechanical obstruction is often difficult. A prolonged trial of conservative management is required before reoperation is considered to relieve a possible obstruction. An upper gastrointestinal x-ray with a water-soluble material such as Gastrografin may be helpful in diagnosis.

Wound Disruption (Dehiscence) and Evisceration

This complication should be preventable. Contributing factors include old age, general debility, infection, abdominal distention, severe cough, steroids, and vertical incisions. The incidence is high in patients with ascites, carcinoma, hypoproteinemia, obesity, and paralytic ileus. The direct cause of wound dehiscence, however, is the manner of closure. The closure of an abdominal incision in layers with separate suture lines in the peritoneum and fascia may be inadequate in many patients. If any of the above predisposing factors is present, the incision should be closed with additional support by stay sutures of heavy nylon, dacron, or wire through the skin, subcutaneous tissue, and fascia. If there are mutiple problems as above, the wound should be closed initially as one would repair a dehiscence by heavy nonreactive sutures placed through all layers of the abdominal wall 5 to 6 cm back from the wound edges and at intervals of 2 to 3 cm. After being tied, each suture is palpated as it is tightened so the bowel is not trapped beneath the suture. The incidence of dehiscence is less with a transverse incision.

During coughing or movement a patient may feel something give way in the incision. Most commonly there is serosanguineous drainage from the wound on the fourth or fifth day. When this occurs, the wound should be inspected and palpated using sterile gloves. The absence of a healing ridge or a defect in the wound indicates a dehiscence which should be repaired. If a defect is not felt and the wound seems solid, an abdominal binder may be applied for support and the skin sutures left in for a longer period. If the defect is small, the wound may heal, but an incisional hernia will usually develop later.

Occasionally the first sign of dehiscence is the appearance of gut in the incision after removal of the skin sutures. This sudden protrusion of intestine is called evisceration.

If a dehiscence occurs with evisceration, the bowel should be covered with moist sterile towels and gloves until the patient can be taken immediately to the operating room, anesthetized, and the wound repaired. The bowel and incision are washed with saline, and the wound is repaired using heavy, all layer, through-and-through sutures. Usually with a dehiscence the wound edges are clean and debridement is not needed, but any prior sutures are removed.

Wound dehiscences closed in this way usually heal satisfactorily.

Intraperitoneal Abscesses

Pelvic. The pelvis is the most common site for an intraperitoneal abscess because it contains the appendix, fallopian tubes, and sigmoid colon, the commonest sources of intraperitoneal infection. In addition infection from extrapelvic organs may gravitate to the pelvis. The abscess may develop spontaneously or be recognized one or more weeks after operation, especially for peritonitis. Antibiotics given after operation tend to mask symptoms and often delay the diagnosis. Diarrhea and passage of mucus may be the only symptoms and pain is often absent. On rectal examination a tender mass can be palpated through the anterior rectal wall. Later the rectal wall becomes edematous, the mass becomes cystic, and the rectal interior may feel hot to the finger. The abscess lies in the pouch of Douglas and is best drained through the rectal wall. Abdominal drainage should be avoided because of the danger of contaminating the peritoneal cavity. The abdominal operation may be indicated if there is an associated bowel obstruction.

Subphrenic. There are four intraperitoneal subphrenic spaces: the right and left anterior, posterior, and one retroperitoneal behind the nonperitonealized part of the liver and extending down to the perinephric spaces. The most important clinically is the right posterior intraperitoneal space, sometimes called the subhepatic space, that drains downward into the right paracolic gutter. Perforation of an ulcer in the duodenum, rupture of the gallbladder, perforation of the hepatic flexure of the colon, or appendicitis may lead to abscess formation in this space. The left posterior intraperitoneal space, or lesser sac, may be the site of an abscess following pancreatitis or perforation of an ulcer or tumor on the posterior wall of the stomach. About one quarter of patients have infection in more than one of the subphrenic spaces. The most common predisposing cause is an operation and often an infected hematoma. The clinical picture is often obscure because most patients have been treated with antibiotics. It is well to remember the aphorism, "Pus somewhere, pus nowhere, and pus under the diaphragm." In all patients with fever, leukocytosis, and undue subcostal tenderness after operation, a subphrenic abscess must always be suspected. A swinging temperature, raised sedimentation rate, loss of appetite, shoulder tip pain, hiccough, local tenderness, and swelling may be present. Intermittent fever, leukocytosis, and an increased erythrocyte sedimentation rate may be the only findings suggesting the abscess. On x-ray the diaphragm is elevated, gas may be present below the diaphragm, the lung may be collapsed, and there may be a pleural effusion. On screening the diaphragm moves poorly or is immobile.

Treatment consists of draining the abscess and administering the appropriate antibiotics. The common subhepatic abscess is drained through the bed of the twelfth rib, obviating opening into the pleura or peritoneum. Recently it has been suggested that a lateral incision passing forward from the tip of the twelfth rib gives a better exposure. The mortality of subphrenic abscess is about 40 percent and most often results from inadequate drainage of pus.

Wound Hematoma

An accumulation of blood or serum is most likely to occur with extensive dissections, such as radical mastectomy. In such situations careful hemostasis and elimination of dead space combined with suitable drains or suction catheters will help to prevent hematomas. A collection of serum is treated by aspiration. Hematomas may require evacuation. Wound infections are discussed in Chapter 6.

Urinary Retention and Infection

It is common for patients to be unable to void in the immediate postoperative period. Local causes are diseases of the urinary tract, such an an enlarged prostate or urethral stricture, operative interference with the innervation or position of the bladder, or severe perineal pain. The most frequent cause is the inability of the patient, particularly a male, to void when lying down. This may cause overfilling of the bladder which in turn predisposes to difficulty in voiding; such a problem may be prevented by emptying the bladder before and immediately after operation.

Urinary infection may occur because the patient had bacteria in the urine before operation or because of contamination during catheterization. Proper care of an indwelling catheter requires a sterile closed drainage system to prevent ascending infection and frequent cleansing of the urethral meatus.

Urinary infection usually causes frequency, burning pain on micturition, and fever. When asymptomatic, it may be diagnosed by urinalysis. Retention of urine should be recognized early. Drugs that stimulate the parasympathetic innervation of the bladder are rarely useful and can cause cardiac arrest in patients with atherosclerosis. If the patient is unable to void after sitting or standing, catheterization should be performed using an aseptic tecnique. If the volume of urine is more than 700 ml, the catheter should be left in place and continuous drainage established for 24 to 48 hours. Repeated catheterizations and the use of an indwelling catheter for a long time may lead to infection. The infecting organism is often a gram-negative bacterium. An antibiotic should be given while cultures of the urine and antibiotic sensitivity are being determined.

Psychiatric Complications

After an operation or its complications patients may be confused and disoriented or may develop an acute psychosis. This occurs most commonly in the elderly. A previous history of mental disturbance should alert the surgeon to the possibility of a postoperative psychotic episode (see Chapter 11). Drug addiction, alcohol, and metabolic disturbances are also important.

Decubitus Ulcer

Pressure necrosis of skin and subcutaneous tissue over the sacrum, the heels, and rarely the elbows occurs more frequently in patients who are elderly, comatose, or critically ill for a prolonged period. The back and heels should be inspected daily for the development of redness over a bony prominence. The lesion can be prevented by adequate turning of the patient and weight redistribution using air mattresses and foam pads. Once the skin turns black, necrosis and liquefaction of the subcutaneous fat develop; infection frequently follows. Debridement and drainage are required. If the area is large, a skin flap from the buttock may have to be rotated later to cover the defect.

Diabetes

A patient without known diabetes may have hyperglycemia and glucosuria after operation. This is due to the neuroendocrine stimulation by the operative injury in a patient whose subclinical diabetes would otherwise be revealed by an abnormal glucose tolerance test. Ketoacidosis usually does not occur, and the condition can be treated with intravenous glucose and small doses of regular insulin. Diabetics will often have intensification of their disease or difficulty in adequate control postoperatively. Oral hypoglycemic agents should not be given, and long-acting insulin preparations are hazardous until the patient is eating a regular diet. Diabetic patients should be managed by frequent determinations of urine sugar and acetone, regular insulin according to the urine test, and a continuous infusion of 5 percent dextrose until oral intake is established. A suggested dose of insulin is 15 units for a 4 + urine sugar, 10 units for 3 +, 5 units for 2 +, and none for 1 +. Blood sugar should be measured daily. The most serious hazard after operation is hypoglycemia from too much insulin. Moderate hypoglycemia is not a problem unless an osmotic diuresis is produced, which can lead to severe dehydration.

Adrenal Insufficiency

Acute adrenal insufficiency may develop after operation in patients with impaired adrenal function. Predisposing causes are steroid therapy, tuberculosis, metastatic cancer, and previous hemorrhage into the adrenals. In many patients the etiology of the adrenal hypofunction is not known. Signs of acute adrenocortical insufficiency after operation are shock unresponsive to fluids or blood, high fever, or cyanosis. This is most likely to develop at 12 to 24 hours after operation and is not accompanied by the classic signs of Addison's disease, which are dehydration and electrolyte alterations. In some situations postoperative adrenal insufficiency may develop more slowly and may result from adrenal hemorrhage in patients given anticoagulants after operation or in patients with severe infections, particularly with burns. It may then be manifested by nonspecific symptoms of weakness and anorexia. Persistent hypoglycemia and hyponatremia suggest this possibility. (See Chapters 11 and 27.)

Gout

An acute attack of gouty arthritis may follow surgical procedures in patients who have a previous history of the disease. Rarely an initial attack of gout may be precipitated by an operation itself. This occurs especially in the joints of the foot. The diagnosis is confirmed by hyperuricemia, and treatment is with a uricosuric drug.

ORGAN FAILURE AFTER OPERATION

Any organ may fail after operation, particularly if its function was previously impaired. Failure of the cardiovascular, respiratory, and urologic systems is particularly important. The gastrointestinal or musculoskeletal systems more often fail gradually.

Serious cardiovascular complications are not common postoperatively in patients without preexisting cardiac disease unless the myocardium is subjected to a period of hypoxia or hypotension during or after operation. Cardiac complications include arrhythmias, congestive heart failure, myocardial ischemia and infarction, cardiac arrest, and decreased cardiac output.

Cardiac Arrhythmias

Patients with severe preexisting cardiac disease, particularly those who have undergone cardiac operations, may have a complex variety of arrhythmic problems. In other surgical patients supraventricular or ventricular arrhythmias may occur with no evidence of prior heart disease.

Prevention. Serious postoperative arrhythmias are not common without preexisting cardiac disease. Cardiac output should be maintained by correcting blood volume deficits to provide adequate myocardial perfusion. Full oxygenation of arterial blood should be ensured. Drugs with known arrhythmic side effects should be administered carefully with continuous monitoring of the electrocardiogram and should be discontinued if any abnormalities appear. Maintenance of normal electrolytes and particularly the serum potassium prevents ventricular irritability. This is especially important in patients treated with diuretics or digitalis.

Recognition. Monitoring the electrocardiogram in patients who may develop hypoxia or electrolyte abnormalities or who have a history of cardiac disease is essential for the early recognition of cardiac arrhythmias. Supraventricular arrhythmias are most frequent but are usually not serious. Sinus tachycardia, sinus bradycardia, atrioventricular block, wandering pacemaker, and premature atrial systoles may occur. Atrial fibrillation is not common in patients without cardiac disease except in older patients following a thoracotomy. The differentiation between some of the tachyarrhythmias may be difficult. Ventricular arrhythmias are more serious, often indicate hypoxia, commonly result from disorders of the ventricular myocardium, and lead quickly to inadequate ventricular function. These arrhythmias include complete atrioventricular block (heart block), premature ventricular contractions which may be multifocal, ventricular tachycardia, ventricular bradycardia and asystole, and ventricular fibrillation. The last two conditions, if not corrected immediately, are fatal.

Treatment. Most of the supraventricular arrhythmias appear during anesthesia or in the postanesthetic period. The cause should be determined as rapidly as possible. Since cardiac arrhythmias may occur from hypoxia, increased ventilation and improved oxygenation should be undertaken. If the blood pressure is low, it must be brought up to safe levels by appropriate measures including fluid replacement, elevation of the legs, and occasionally vasopressors. If these simple steps are not effective, drug therapy may be indicated. Atropine is useful in sinus bradycardia, while isoproterenol is useful for atrioventricular block and conditions associated with slowing of the ventricular rate. Lidocaine, in an intravenous infusion of 0.5 percent, decreases myocardial irritability manifested by ventricular tachycardia or runs of premature ventricular contractions and should be given before the arrhythmias lead to ventricular fibrillation. Rapidly acting digitalis preparations are valuable in sinus or atrial tachycardia associated with congestive failure and for atrial flutter or fibrillation with a rapid ventricular response. Electrolyte abnormalities should be recognized and corrected promptly. Patients receiving diuretics and those with digitalis toxicity may require potassium. Oxygen supplementation in the inspired air should always be used in conjunction with the pharmacologic therapy of arrhythmias. These pharmacologic agents are extremely potent and should be given with caution and careful observation. The main indication for treatment of supraventricular arrhythmias is the danger of congestive heart failure with bradycardia or of low cardiac output and cardiogenic shock in tachycardias with a rapid ventricular response which does not allow time for diastolic filling of the heart.

Congestive Failure; Pulmonary Edema

Congestive heart failure, occurring after operations other than cardiac procedures, is infrequent and usually results from problems in managing a patient with preexisting cardiac disease.

Prevention. Precipitating factors may be hypoxia, circulatory overload, or inadequate digitalization. Careful fluid balance should be maintained in patients who have known cardiac disease or are elderly. An increase in body weight suggests the possibility of circulatory overload. A patient with borderline cardiac function or congestive heart failure should be given digitalis before and after operation. If excessive fluids have been administered, digitalis and diuretics may help prevent congestive heart failure.

Recognition. Congestive heart failure may develop rapidly within a few hours or slowly over several days. If the right ventricle fails the patient may develop distended neck veins, hepatosplenomegaly, and peripheral edema. However, the usual picture is one of biventricular enlargement with elevation of the central venous pressure, crepitations and fine moist rales over the lung bases, and pulmonary venous congestion on chest roentgenograms with a butterfly distribution of increased density around both hilar regions. Rapidly developing failure may be fulminating and manifested as acute pulmonary edema with frothy pink sputum, severe dyspnea, tachypnea, orthopnea, and cyanosis.

A more common hazard is interstitial pulmonary edema from excessive dextrose and water or saline after operation. Some patients are unable to excrete this load because of the increased secretion of antidiuretic hormone and aldosterone. Much of the fluid may be in the lung in the walls of the alveoli where it interferes with oxygenation but may not produce rales or an increase in the central venous pressure. This problem may be recognized only by the presence of hypoxia.

Treatment. In addition to removing the precipitating cause, treating congestive failure includes restriction of fluid intake, diuretics, parenteral digitalis and occasionally other inotropic agents, positive pressure breathing in fulminant pulmonary edema (with positive end expiratory pressure if necessary), and reduction of venous return by tourniquets or a phlebotomy. Digitalization should be carried out with a rapidly acting preparation such as ouabain with subsequent change to a longer acting preparation such as digoxin for maintenance therapy.

Myocardial Ischemia and Infarction

A previous infarction determined from the history or electrocardiogram increases the operative risk.[1] The patient may develop hypotension, ventricular arrhythmias, myocardial failure, or another myocardial infarction after operation. Patients with a history of angina pectoris are particularly susceptible to postoperative infarction. Moreover, patients with no history of cardiac disease and with a normal electrocardiogram may also develop infarction during or after operation. For this reason a preoperative electrocardiogram should be obtained in every patient over 40 who has a general anesthetic.

Prevention. The incidence of myocardial infarction may be decreased by minimizing anxiety and pain, by avoiding deep anesthesia, hypoventilation, and hypotension, and by maintaining hydration. Oxygenation should be carefully maintained with P_{O_2} in the the range that will ensure full saturation of hemoglobin. Hypotension can usually be reversed by a mild vasopressor while the cause is being sought.

Recognition. Any patient with a history of angina pectoris or previous infarction should have continuous electrocardiographic monitoring in the surgical intensive care unit after operation. Electrocardiographic changes indicative of myocardial ischemia, such as S-T segment and T-wave changes, should be recognized promptly and investigated. A 12-lead electrocardiogram should be taken if there is any suspicion of ischemia or infarction. The electrocardiogram is usually diagnostic for this condition. Lactic dehydrogenase with its heat-stable and heat-labile components, serum glutamic oxaloacetic transaminase, and creatine phosphokinase elevations may indicate myocardial infarction and necrosis. However, these enzymes may be elevated postoperatively without myocardial infarction because of injury to skeletal muscle by the incision and exposure, and this must be taken into consideration when interpreting enzyme levels.

Treatment. This consists of observing the principles outlined under prevention and the use of antiarrhythmic and specific cardiac drugs if indicated. If infarction leads to decreased cardiac output, this should be treated in the conventional way, which usually includes the use of catecholamines and digitalis. The immediate value of circulatory-assist devices in refractory cardiogenic shock is well established, but the long-term results are unsatisfactory. Emergency myocardial revascularization procedures in these instances are currently under evaluation.

Cardiac Arrest

Sudden cessation of cardiac action can occur in any of three forms:

1. Asystole with a flaccid heart without electrical activity.

2. Profound cardiovascular collapse where the heart's electrical activity is coordinated but poor without any significant degree of mechanical contraction.

3. Ventricular fibrillation.

Many factors can lead to cardiac arrest after operation. The most common causes are hypoxia and/or hypercapnia, electrolyte imbalance, hypotension, and operative cardiac procedures. Electrolyte imbalance, particularly hypokalemia, can potentiate the effect of hypoxia or hypercapnia in increasing myocardial irritability.

Prevention. Cardiac arrest should be preventable by early recognition and treatment of hypoxia, hypovolemia, and serious electrolyte abnormalities. The onset of ventricular irritability or bradycardia should immediately indicate a search for these factors and discontinuation of pharmacologic agents that increase irritability.

Recognition. Successful treatment depends on immediate recognition.[19] A delay of only a few minutes results in irreversible damage to the central nervous system. Continuous monitoring of the electrocardiogram in the intensive care unit undoubtedly helps in recognizing sudden cardiac arrest or arrhythmias that lead to an arrest. In patients undergoing complicated cardiac operations or those at high risk for other reasons, continuous monitoring of the arterial pressure by an indwelling arterial cannula is helpful.

Treatment. Following sudden cessation of cardiac action, aerobic metabolism may continue for a few minutes until oxygen is depleted. Anaerobic metabolism then follows and rapidly produces metabolic acidosis. Tissue damage and cell death occur within 4 to 6 minutes in tissues most sensitive to lack of oxygen such as the central nervous system. Very quickly after heart action stops, ventilation stops. The initial purpose of treatment is to provide oxygen to the brain and heart. This requires mechanical ventilation to supply oxygen to the lungs and circulatory assistance to distribute this oxygenated blood. These measures allow time to apply definitive electrical and pharmacologic therapy which may then reinstitute spontaneous cardiac and respiratory activity.

Immediate ventilation is provided by mouth-to-mouth breathing or a face mask and manual ventilator. As soon as a trained persion is available, endotracheal intubation and positive pressure breathing with 100 percent oxygen are instituted. Simultaneously closed chest or external cardiac massage is begun.[13,18] The heart is compressed between the lower sternum and the vertebral column at 60 to 80 times a minute. This provides a cardiac output that is adequate to maintain the viability of the central nervous system for a few hours. Occasionally under conditions of hypoxia or hypercapnia, asystolic cardiac arrest may occur as a reflex reaction to vagal stimulation during procedures such as suctioning of the trachea. The arrest may be reversed by giving a blow to the precordium if a vasovagal reflex is the suspected cause. However, cardiac compression and pulmonary ventilation are commenced immediately if the situation does not correct itself spontaneously within seconds. The effectiveness of cardiac massage is determined by palpation of the femoral vessels by another observer. With each compression an impulse should be felt in the groin.

After initial resuscitative measures have been applied, the exact nature of the cardiac arrest should be determined and an electrocardiographic diagnosis made. If there is a delay in obtaining an electrocardiographic recording and an electrical defibrillator is available, external defibrillation is attempted, since ventricular fibrillation accounts for the majority of arrests and electrical defibrillation is the only specific therapy.

In cases of asystole or inefficient coordinated contractions that do not respond immediately to cardiac massage and ventilation, epinephrine, 0.5 mg intravenously every 3 to 5 minutes, is the drug of choice. It increases ventricular excitability, stimulates cardiac contraction, causes peripheral vasoconstriction, and directs blood to more vital centers. The rapidly developing anaerobic metabolism and metabolic acidosis alter the response of the heart and other organs to catecholamines, and thus the blood pH must be corrected by the administration of sodium bicarbonate at 10-minute intervals. After resumption of spontaneous cardiac activity, arterial blood pressure may remain low due to peripheral vasodilatation, and a vasopressor such as levarterenol in an intravenous drip may be required to break this vicious cycle. If ventricular fibrillation exists, correction of the blood pH is mandatory to maintain spontaneous activity following defibrillation. Epinephrine and calcium must be avoided in the patient with ventricular fibrillation because they may increase the refractoriness of fibrillation to electrical countershock. If there is evidence of a continuing ventricular arrhythmia, a lidocaine drip may be required to sustain effective spontaneous cardiac activity. After cardiac resuscitation the precipitating factors should be identified and corrected.

Decrease in Cardiac Output

Although a decrease in cardiac output in a postoperative patient is most commonly due to a reduction in circulating blood volume, it can also result from primary myocardial disease. Examples are acute myocardial infarction, coronary artery disease, and hypoxia developing in a patient with prior ventricular dysfunction.

Renal Failure

Decreased urine production after operation or injury results from release of antidiuretic hormone, aldosterone secretion, and sequestration of blood and extracellular fluid in the injured region. Causes of postoperative oliguria are:

1. Decreased renal blood flow due to an inadequate vascular volume, decreased cardiac output, or hypotension (prerenal failure).

2. An increased secretion of antidiuretic hormone and/or aldosterone.

3. Acute renal parenchymal failure.

4. Obstruction to urine flow due to injury to the ureters, prostatic obstruction, or a blocked catheter (postrenal failure).

Prevention. The best way to prevent acute renal failure is to maintain a normal circulation and urinary output. Acute tubular necrosis is the commonest cause and is probably produced by a combination of events of which diminished blood flow to the kidney plays a major role. As renal blood flow decreases, redistribution occurs resulting in decreased flow to the outer cortex with relatively greater deep cortical and medullary flow. In addition, hemoglobin from red cell hemolysis or myoglobin from crush or muscle injury may precipitate in the tubules to form casts, which obstruct flow and further decrease glomerular filtration rate. In a normal individual hypotension alone may not produce acute renal failure, but in patients with extensive atherosclerosis decreased renal blood flow may set the tendency to hypotension and renal problems. Thus acute renal failure occurs most commonly in elderly patients and in others with extensive atherosclerosis, abdominal aortic aneurysms, hypertension, severe injuries, dehydration, or hemolysis. Decrease in renal blood flow is avoided by maintaining a normal blood pressure and cardiac output. Urine output must be adequate not only for surveillance of renal function but also to prevent formation of casts. An adequate diuresis may help to prevent renal failure.

A catheter should be inserted in the bladder to monitor urinary output in patients with impaired renal function, with circulatory instability during a prolonged operation, or with a major injury. A urinary output in excess of 25 to 30 ml per hour should be maintained by intravenous fluids. An osmotic diuretic such as mannitol or furosemide may be given.

Early administration of an osmotic diuretic or a potent natriuretic may reverse the oliguria of acute tubular necrosis.[20,31] Kjellstrand[17] and Shalhoub and associates[28] found that if oliguria is corrected at an early stage, renal function may return to normal or nearly normal; if the oliguria is reversed at an intermediate stage, oliguric acute renal failure may be converted to high output renal failure. A large dose of furosemide, 100 mg intravenously plus 25 gm of mannitol intravenously, may be given at the first indication of a consistently low urinary output postoperatively, provided that there is no apparent mechanical cause and hydration is adequate. If a sustained increase in urinary output occurs, an intravenous infusion of 100 mg of furosemide and 500 ml of 20 percent mannitol is given over 24 hours to maintain the urinary volume.

Recognition. When the output of urine decreases below 25 ml per hour, steps should be taken to determine the reason. If the circulation and blood pressure are normal and the central venous pressure is not high, 2000 ml of saline may be given as a rapid infusion. A high urine osmolality, a urine specific gravity greater than 1.020, and a urine–serum creatinine ratio

greater than 20 also suggest the need for more fluid. A small amount of mannitol may also be given, but fluid overload and pulmonary edema should be avoided. Diuresis should be maintained if urine flow increases. If urine output remains at 5 to 10 ml per hour or less, furosemide, 50 to 100 mg, should be given intravenously. After operation sodium in the urine is low, 10 to 20 mEq/liter or less. When there is renal parenchymal failure, sodium cannot be retained or concentrated. The urine sodium increases to 50 to 60 mEq/liter or higher in the small amount of urine produced. The urine osmolality therefore approaches that of the plasma. The urine–serum creatinine ratio, normally greater than 20:1, is decreased. Diagnosis is often difficult, especially during the first 6 to 12 hours of developing renal failure. Postoperative blood loss and hypovolemia must be excluded, and a normal blood pressure must be maintained. Mechanical reasons must be excluded such as an occluded or malpositioned catheter and obstruction due to division or ligation of ureters during pelvic and retroperitoneal operations. With mechanical obstruction no urine is produced, whereas with renal failure there is generally a small amount of urine.

Treatment. Renal failure demands close control of hydration, serum potassium, and the products of protein metabolism.[23] This may be particularly difficult after operation, because there is increased breakdown of proteins, potassium is being mobilized rapidly from cells into the extracellular fluid, and the patient has often been made hypervolemic by attempts to prevent renal failure by volume expansion. Acute renal failure after injury or operation is potentially reversible. Recovery, however, may not occur until 12 to 14 days.

Volume Control. The patient is given sufficient water to replace insensible water loss minus the water produced by metabolism. An average volume for an adult is 500 ml per 24 hours and should be given as 10 percent dextrose and water. To this is added the volume of urine produced and other losses, such as from a nasogastric tube. Daily weights are necessary. The postoperative patient in renal failure and without oral intake should lose 0.2 to 0.5 kg per day if normal hydration is maintained. With recovery the first urine is dilute. Increasing volumes of water are then required as the urine flow increases and edema is eliminated. Sodium will also have to be given and perhaps potassium if losses are large.

Electrolyte Control. Sodium is not given unless there is severe hyponatremia or continuing loss of sodium. The major threat is hyperkalemia that may develop rapidly. No potassium is given. The plasma potassium and ECG are initially recorded twice daily. A serum potassium approaching 6 mEq/liter is rapidly but transiently reduced by giving glucose and insulin intravenously. More permanent control is obtained by ion-exchange resins such as Kayexalate given orally or by enema.

Catabolism and Protein Breakdown. Calories should be given as glucose to inhibit gluconeogenesis. If the gastrointestinal tract is functional, sugar and fat without protein should be given as sweetened butterballs or hard candy. A volume of 500 ml 10 percent dextrose solution intravenously is generally adequate for an adult. Recently intravenous hyperalimentation with amino acids has been advocated to decrease protein catabolism, and this shows some promise. BUN and creatinine levels may rise rapidly in the postoperative patient.

With these conservative measures the patient may be supported until renal function returns. However, dialysis is often necessary. The indications for dialysis are:

1. The presence of a fluid overload.
2. Hyperkalemia.
3. Uremia with altered mental state.

Peritoneal dialysis is satisfactory in the postoperative patient but may not be possible after insertion of an aortic graft because of adhesions and the risk of infection. Hemodialysis is then required.

High-Output Renal Failure. Usually acute renal failure produces severe oliguria or anuria. However, if the renal damage results in a moderate rather than a severe decrease in glomerular filtration rate, there may be a reasonable volume of urine but its composition may tend toward that of plasma.[33] This is similar to the diuretic phase of recovery from acute tubular necrosis. The output of urine may be 2 to 3 liters per day with a high sodium and low urine–plasma creatinine ratio. The BUN and creatinine levels in the blood rise and a creatinine plateau is usually reached after 7 to 10 days. Kidney function gradually returns and dialysis is rarely necessary.

Ventilatory Failure

Abnormalities of ventilation are common causes of mortality and morbidity after major operations. Predisposing factors are acute and chronic respiratory infections, chronic chest disease, smoking, obesity, bed rest, excessive narcosis, incisional pain, abdominal distention, and a diminished ability to cough. Atelectasis, pulmonary infection, silent aspiration, fat, and thromboembolism may occur and lead to ventilatory failure.

Prevention. Lung function should be evaluated before operation in patients suspected of having pulmonary disease. Preoperative preparation includes cessation of smoking, bronchodilator drugs, antibiotics, inhalation of humidified gases, postural drainage, and chest physiotherapy.

In the recovery room the pattern of ventilation should be carefully evaluated, deep breathing and coughing should be instituted, and humidified oxygen administered. Administration of 100 percent oxygen for 5 to 10 minutes at the termination of the anesthetic decreases the possibility of hypoxia.[21] If there is any question about the patient's ability to ventilate or oxygenate effectively, the endotracheal tube should be left in place and assisted ventilation continued for a few hours.

Other factors that may contribute to pulmonary insufficiency[24] are microemboli from multiple blood transfusions, fat embolism, the effects on the lungs of prolonged circulatory failure, resuscitative fluids, neurogenic factors, vasoactive agents released in the circulation, oxygen toxicity, intravascular coagulation, and sepsis.[3,5] Infection and peritonitis should be promptly identified and treated because of the high mortality associated with respiratory failure in patients with peritonitis.[30] Decreased serum albumen and excess body water should be corrected to decrease interstitial edema.

Recognition. Three forms of ventilatory failure occur:

Hypoventilation. Not enough air is exchanged so that alveolar ventilation is reduced and CO_2 is not eliminated. The patient with hypoventilation has respiratory acidosis and possibly hypoxia as shown by an elevated arterial CO_2 tension, reduced arterial pH, and low or normal arterial P_{O_2}. The patient may be obtunded and have an increased blood pressure and slow pulse. Hypoventilation may occur from the prolonged effects of the anesthetic, pain, analgesics, restrictive dressings, fatigue, or chronic lung disease.

Hyperventilation Leading to Fatigue. The stimulus for increased ventilation may be hypoxia, sepsis, hypotension, increased temperature, or apprehension. The patient may be anxious and have rapid, shallow, and labored respiration. Arterial P_{O_2} may be low normal and P_{CO_2} decreased. If rapid shallow ventilation continues, atelectasis and hypoxia occur. This problem must be recognized and treated before fatigue sets in.

Pulmonary Abnormalities That Alter Ventilation. In the postoperative period the factors previously mentioned may produce alveolar collapse, thickening or edema of alveolar septa, and changes in the pulmonary vasculature. The changes in pulmonary physiology include:

1. Reduction in vital capacity.
2. Pulmonary arteriovenous shunting of blood through nonaerated lung.
3. Limitations of diffusion of gases across the alveolar wall.
4. Uneven distribution of ventilation and perfusion.
5. Decreased compliance.
6. Increased dead space.

The signs of ventilatory failure are dyspnea, cyanosis, rapid shallow breathing, altered breath sounds, and mental confusion. Chest x-ray may be normal or show patchy atelectasis or more severe changes. Other, more decisive, investigations include arterial blood gas tensions, measurement of tidal volume, vital capacity, and minute volume of ventilation, and measurement of shunting by alveolar-arterial P_{O_2} gradient while breathing 100 percent oxygen (AaD_{O_2}).

Treatment. Hypoventilation requires immediate mechanical ventilatory assistance through an endotracheal tube. Hyperventilation and fatigue are treated by assisting ventilation before the condition becomes irreversible. Pulmonary function is improved by giving humidified gas with high oxygen concentration by face mask or tent. Diuretics and albumen are given when indicated. When these measures are not effective, assisted ventilation should be used.

A cuffed tracheal tube, preferably inserted through the nasopharynx, provides assisted respiration for five to six days. An elective tracheostomy is established if assisted respiration is required for a longer time. A volume-cycled ventilator provides the pressure during each breath that delivers the required volume. The best unit is a volume-limited respirator with a variable inspiratory flow rate. Minute volume of the ventilator is adjusted to provide a normal arterial P_{CO_2}. Forty percent humidified oxygen is first given in the inspired air and the concentration of oxygen adjusted to maintain an arterial P_{O_2} (Pa_{O_2}) at or above 80 to 90 mm Hg. It is important not to administer an oxygen concentration greater than 60 percent for more than 24 hours through an endotracheal tube unless hypoxia persists. Administration of 100 percent oxygen to an adult at 6 liters per minute through a face mask will deliver a 40 percent concentration of oxygen. Higher concentrations breathed for more than 24 hours result in hyaline membrane changes in the lungs and pulmonary congestion. Humidification of the gases is important to prevent drying of the airway. If the patient is agitated and breathes out of phase with the machine, a period of hyperventilation and sedation should be tried. If this is un-

successful, it may be necessary to paralyze the patient with intravenous muscle relaxants until he is brought into phase with the respirator. Frequent deep breaths or sighs should be administered to patients on the ventilator to prevent atelectasis, and blood gases should be measured every 6 to 12 hours to determine the adequacy of ventilation. Tracheobronchial suction with strict aseptic technique should be carried out at least hourly.

With prolonged need for assisted ventilation, various problems can arise that will jeopardize survival. Inspissation of tracheobronchial secretions and encrustations can build up around the tracheostomy tube and obstruct the airway. The tube should be changed frequently and high humidification should be maintained. Damage to the tracheal wall from the cuff on the endotracheal or tracheostomy tube may lead to tracheal stenosis or erosion of vessels such as the brachiocephalic artery. A soft balloon which is deflated for 5 to 10 minutes every hour is helpful in decreasing this complication.

As soon as pulmonary function has improved, the patient should be weaned from the ventilator. If tidal volume is less than 5 cc/kg, the patient needs to be maintained on the ventilator. Weaning should be done initially by using very short periods without the ventilator but with a T-connector to the tracheal tube which delivers 60 to 80 percent oxygen. The electrocardiogram is monitored and breath sounds are observed. The patient is encouraged to breathe slowly and deeply, and the periods off the ventilator are gradually prolonged until continuous ventilation can be maintained without assistance. This may require several days. With assisted ventilation for 24 hours or less, however, weaning can often be abrupt. The tracheostomy should be maintained until ventilation is adequate, cough is good, and reflexes that prevent aspiration are normal.

CITED REFERENCES

1. Arkins, R.; Smessaert, A. A.; and Hicks, R. G.: Mortality and morbidity in surgical patients with coronary artery disease. *JAMA*, **190**:485–88, 1964.
2. Baue, A. E.: Recent developments in the study and treatment of shock. *Surg. Gynecol. Obstet.*, **127**:849–78, 1968.
3. Baue, A. E.: Ventilatory failure in the surgical patient after operation or injury. In Ballinger, W. F., and Drapanas, T. (eds): *The Practice of Surgery: A Current Review.* C. V. Mosby Co., St. Louis, 1972.
4. Bendixen, H. H.; Egbert, L. D.; Hedley-Whyte, J.; Laver, M. B.; and Pontoppidan, H.: *Respiratory Care.* C. V. Mosby Co., St. Louis, 1965.
5. Clowes, G. H. A., Jr.; Farrington, G. H.; Zuschneid, W.; Cossette, G. R.; and Saravis, C.: Circulating factors in the etiology of pulmonary insufficiency and right heart failure accompanying severe sepsis (Peritonitis). *Ann. Surg.*, **171**:663–78, 1970.

6. Collins, J. A., and Ballinger, W. F.: The surgical intensive care unit. *Surgery*, 66:614–19, 1969.
7. Dudrick, S. J.; Long, J. M.; Steiger, E.; Rhoads, J. E.: Intravenous hyperalimentation. *Med. Clin. North Am.*, 54:577–89, 1970.
8. Dudrick, S. J.; Wilmore, D. W.; Vars, H. W.; and Rhoads, J. E.: Long term total parenteral nutrition with growth, development, and positive nitrogen balance. *Surgery*, 64:134–42, 1968.
9. Dudrick, S. J.; Wilmore, D. W.; Vars, H. M.; and Rhoads, J. E.: Can intravenous feeding as the sole means of nutrition support growth in the adult? An affirmative answer. *Ann. Surg.*, 169:974–84, 1969.
10. Howard, J. M., and Jordan, G. L. (eds): *Surgical Diseases of the Pancreas.* J. B. Lippincott, Philadelphia, 1960.
11. Hume, M.: The relationship of "hypercoagulability" to thrombosis. *Monographs in the Surgical Sciences*, 2:133–58, 1965.
12. Jude, J. R., and Elan, J. O.: *Fundamentals of Cardiopulmonary Resuscitation.* F. A. Davis Co., Philadelphia, 1965.
13. Kakkar, V. V., and Nicolaides, A. N.: Low doses of heparin in prevention of deep-vein thrombosis. *Lancet*, 2 (Sept. 25): 669–71, 1971.
14. Keeri-Szanto, M., and Heaman, S.: Postoperative demand analgesia. *Surg. Gynecol. Obstet.*, 132:647–51, 1972.
15. Kinney, J. M.; Egdahl, R. H.; and Zuidema, G. D. (eds): *Manual of Preoperative and Postoperative Care.* W. B. Saunders Co., Philadelphia, 1971.
16. Kinney, J. M.: The recovery room and intensive care unit. In Randall, H. T. (ed): *Manual of Preoperative and Postoperative Care*, 2nd ed., W. B. Saunders Co., Philadelphia, 1967.
17. Kjellstrand, C. M.: Ethacrynic acid in acute renal failure. *Am. Soc. Nephrol.*, November, 1968, p. 31 (abstract).
18. Kouwenhoven, W. B.; Jude, J. R.; and Knickerbocker, G. G.: Closed-chest cardiac massage. *JAMA*, 173:1064–67, 1960.
19. Lemire, J. G., and Johnson, A. L.: Is cardiac resuscitation worthwhile? A decade of experience. *N. Engl. J. Med.*, 286:970–72, 1972.
20. Maher, J. F., and Schreiner, G. E.: Studies on ethacrynic acid in patients with refractory edema. *Ann. Intern. Med.*, 62:15–29, 1965.
21. Marshall, B. E., and Millar, R. A.: Some factors influencing postoperative hypoxaemia. *Anaesthesia*, 20:408–28, 1965.
22. McLachlin, A. D.; McLachlin, J. A.; Jory, T. A.; Rawling, E. G.: Venous stasis in the lower extremities. *Ann. Surg.*, 152:678–85, 1960.
23. Merrill, J. P.: Acute renal failure. In artz, C. P., and Hardy, J. D. (eds): *Complications in Surgery and Their Management*, 2nd ed. W. B. Saunders Co., Philadelphia, 1967.
24. Moore, F. D.; Lyons, J. H., Jr.; Pierce, E. C., Jr.; Morgan, A. P. Jr.; Drinker, P. A.; MacArthur, J. D.; and Dammin, G. J.: *Post-Traumatic Pulmonary Insufficiency.* W. B. Saunders Co., Philadelphia, 1969.
25. Moore, F. D.: Volume and tonicity in body water. *Surg. Gynecol. Obstet.*, 114:276–92, 1962.
26. Moyer, C. A.: Nonoperative surgical care. In Rhoads, J. E.; Allen, J. G.; Harkins, H. N.; and Moyer, C. A. (eds): *Surgery Principles and Practice.* J. B. Lippincott Co., Philadelphia, 1970.
27. Ruth, H. S.; Haugen, F. P.; and Grove, D. D.: Anesthesia Study Commission: findings of eleven years activity. *JAMA*, 135:881–84, 1947.
28. Shalhoub, R. J.; Velasquez, M. T.; and Antoniou, L. D.: Reversal of surgical oliguric states by furosemide or ethacrynic acid. *Am. Soc. Nephrol.*, November, 1968, p. 60 (abstract).
29. Silen, W.: Stress ulcers. *Viewpoints on Digestive Diseases*, Vol. 3, No. 5, 1971.
30. Skillman, J. J.; Bushnell, L. S.; and Hedley-Whyte, J.: Peritonitis and respiratory failure after abdominal operations. *Ann. Surg.*, 170:122–27, 1969.
31. Smith, P. H.: Prevention of acute renal failure in surgical practice. *Br. J. Surg.*, 54:109–13, 1967.
32. Stephens, R. V., and Randall, H. T.: Use of a concentrated, balanced, liquid elemental diet for nutritional management of catabolic states. *Ann. Surg.*, 170:642–67, 1969.
33. Vertel, R. M., and Knockel, J. P.: Nonoliguric acute renal failure, *JAMA*, 200:598–602, 1967.
34. Vogel, C. M.; Kingsbury, R. J.; and Baue, A. E.: Intravenous hyperalimentation. A review of 2½ years experience. *Arch. Surg.*, 105:414–19, 1972.
35. Vogel, C.; Corwin, T. R.; and Baue, A. E.: Intravenous hyperalimentation in the treatment of inflammatory diseases of the bowel. *Arch. Surg.*, 108:460–67, 1974.
36. Zikria, B. A.; Spencer, J. L.; Michailoff, T.; Broell, J. R.; and Kinney, J. M.: Breathing patterns in preoperative, postoperative and critically ill patients. *Surg. Forum*, 12:40–41, 1971.
37. Zubiran, J. M.; Kark, A. E.; Montalbetti, A. J.; Morel, C. J. L.; and Dragstedt, L. R.: Peptic ulcer and the adrenal stress syndrome. *Arch. Surg.*, 65:809–15, 1952.

SUGGESTIONS FOR FURTHER READING

Baue, A. E.: Recent developments in the study and treatment of shock. *Surg. Gynecol. Obstet.*, 127:849–78, 1968.

An extensive review of shock which causes pathophysiology and various aspects of treatments. Recommended reading for intensive review of the problems of circulatory failure.

Baue, A. E.: Ventilatory failure in the surgical patient after operation or injury. In Ballinger, W. F., and Drapanas, T. (eds): *The Practice of Surgery: A Current Review.* C. V. Mosby Co., 1972.

This is an extensive review of problems of ventilatory failure in surgical patients and provides detailed information about diagnosis and support of such problems.

Bendixen, H. H.; Egbert, L. D.; Hedley-Whyte, J.; Laver, M. B.; and Pontoppidan, H.: *Respiratory Care.* C. V. Mosby Co., 1965.

A good solid treatise on respiratory care in surgical patients.

Kinney, J. M.; Egdahl, R. H.; and Zuidema, G. D. (eds): *Manual of Preoperative and Postoperative Care.* W. B. Saunders Co., Philadelphia. 1971.

This volume provides concise information about many aspects of preoperative and postoperative care of surgical patients and should be available to all surgeons.

Merrill, J. P.: Acute renal failure. In Artz, C. P., and Hardy, J. D. (eds): *Complications in Surgery and Their Management*, 2nd ed. W. B. Saunders Co., Philadelphia, 1967.

A concise consideration and review of the problems of renal failure in surgical patients.

Chapter 15

BURNS

George P. Reading

CHAPTER OUTLINE

Anatomy and Functions of the Skin
  Functions of the Skin
Types of Burns
  Thermal Burns
  Electrical Burns
  Chemical and Radiation Burns
Depth and Area of Burns
Pathophysiology of the Burn
  Fluid Loss
  Cardiovascular System
  Respiratory System
  Gastrointestinal System
  Lymphoreticular System
  Metabolism
  Renal System
  Infection

Management of Burns
  Resuscitation
    Respiratory System
    Intravenous Fluids
    Monitoring
    Drugs
    Initial Care of the Burn Wound
  Intermediate Care
    Topical Treatment
    Nutrition
    Debridement and Skin Grafting
  Rehabilitation
    Contractures
    Aesthetic Problems
    Psychological Considerations
Prevention of Burns

This chapter is included in the section on Total Care of the Surgical Patient to emphasize the widespread effects of burns. The initial resuscitation after a severe burn presents one of the most serious problems in fluid replacement. In the patient with an extensive burn and sepsis there is a greater hypercatabolic state than in any other surgical condition. Often severe sepsis and serious complications involve the pulmonary, renal, and cardiovascular systems as well as special problems with skin grafting, prevention of deformity, and prolonged rehabilitation.

ANATOMY AND FUNCTIONS OF THE SKIN

The skin consists of epidermis and dermis (see Plate I; Chapters 25 and 33). The stratum germinativam is irregular as it goes over the papillary convolutions of the dermis and is reflected down into the glands of the skin and into the hair follicles. It is from these deep reflections of the basal cell layer that the epidermis is reconstituted after partial-thickness destruction of the skin. The dermis is composed of fibrous tissue, collagen, and elastic tissue and contains the blood vessels, lymphatics, nerves, hair follicles, and the erector pili muscles. This is the tough layer responsible for the strength of the skin and much of the protection it provides. The subcutaneous tissue below the dermis is comprised largely of fat with interspaced blood vessels, nerves, and lymphatics. In some regions, such as the scalp and in the bearded portion of the face in males, the hair follicles penetrate deeply into the superficial layers of the subcutaneous tissue.

Functions of the Skin

1. The skin protects the body from invasion by pathogenic organisms
2. The skin, especially the stratum corneum, acts as a barrier separating the dry external environment from the moist internal environment.
3. It regulates heat loss through its blood vessels and secretion of sweat.
4. It protects the underlying tissues from injury.
5. It glides and stretches over joints and facilitates movement. Scarring results in loss of skin elasticity, reduced movement, and eventually

produces contractures when situated on the flexor aspect of joints.

6. It is important cosmetically. This is especially important in burns of the face and neck.

TYPES OF BURNS

Thermal Burns

The most common thermal burns follow flame or flash injuries. Flame burns are usually associated with burned clothing and destroy at least the full thickness of skin. A flash explosion more often produces a partial-thickness burn. Scalds are typically partial thickness, but if the hot fluid remains in contact for a prolonged period, a full-thickness burn occurs, for example, when an elderly patient falls into a bath of hot water and is unable to get up. Scalds are often seen in children when the contents of pots and pans are spilled. Burns caused by contact with hot objects are usually small and not full thickness, unless there are factors that keep the patient in prolonged contact with the source of heat, for example an epileptic seizure.

Electrical Burns

These are caused by low-voltage currents as in household injuries or high voltage as in some industrial accidents. Household electrical burns commonly occur in children who put electrical wires or plugs into their mouths. Saliva completes the circuit. High-tension burns are more serious. When the current is well conducted, local damage is small but damage to the central nervous and cardiovascular systems is likely to be great. When resistance is high, considerable heat is generated and tissue destruction is severe. Electrical burns are typically more extensive than is apparent on the surface, and when they involve the limbs, amputation is often required.[3]

Chemical and Radiation Burns

Chemical burns are caused by contact of caustic materials with the body and occur in industrial accidents and in personal assaults when lye is thrown at the face. These burns should be irrigated promptly with large volumes of water. Burns caused by ionizing radiation are seen in industrial or laboratory accidents. They are now seldom seen after therapy for malignant disease. Excessive exposure to ultraviolet rays in sunlight usually causes only superficial burns.

DEPTH AND AREA OF BURNS

A first-degree burn, for example sunburn, affects only the epidermis and causes pain and redness but no blistering (Figure 15–1). The burn heals in two to three days.

In a second-degree or dermal burn all the epidermis and some of the dermis are destroyed. The skin is blistered and sensitive to pinprick. Intermediate dermal burns should be distinguished from deep dermal burns. In an intermediate dermal burn there remain alive islets of the basal layer of epidermal cells from which the epidermis can be reconstituted. In a deep dermal burn few of these cells remain. Therefore considerable time may be required for reepithelization.

The epidermis and dermis are entirely destroyed in a full-thickness or third-degree burn. Except for small burns skin grafting is necessary.

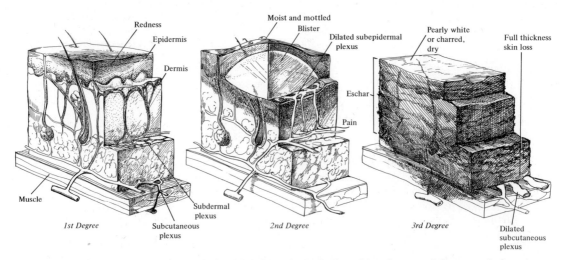

Figure 15–1. A burn may be first degree and involve only the epidermis, second degree and also include superficial dermis, or third degree with loss of the whole thickness of the skin.

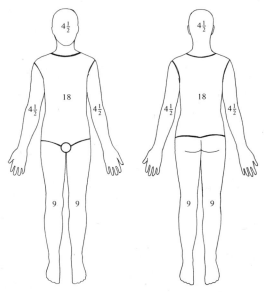

Figure 15–2. The rule of nines is used to calculate the area of a burn.

Infection can change the depth of a burn from partial to full thickness, especially when the burn is deep dermal. Burns rarely extend beyond the subcutaneous fat to the fascia or muscle or bone.

The percentage of total body surface burned is estimated using the rule of nines (Figure 15–2).[6] In an adult each upper extremity is 9 percent of the total body surface, each lower extremity 18 percent, the head and neck 9 percent, anterior trunk 18 percent, posterior trunk 18 percent, and the perineum the remaining 1 percent. In children the head is relatively larger and the lower extremity is smaller (see Chapter 35).

PATHOPHYSIOLOGY OF THE BURN

A large burn is one of the most severe injuries that an individual can sustain. Survival and morbidity are related to the depth of the burn, the percentage of the body surface involved, and age of the patient. Patients under 18 months have a relatively poor prognosis and those over 30 years have an increasingly poor prognosis with age. Other injuries, particularly respiratory injuries, such as inhalation of smoke, and systemic diseases, such as arteriosclerosis, diabetes, and alcoholism, adversely affect the prognosis.

Fluid Loss

Immediately after a 10 to 20 percent burn there is a rapid loss of fluid and, unless this deficit is treated, shock ensues. Injury to the small vessels results in increased permeability and loss of protein-rich fluid from the surface. The rate of evaporation is 10 to 15 times as great from a burn as through the intact skin.[8] Recent studies show that sequestration of fluid in the burned tissues is more important than external loss. Injured cells are unable to maintain the normal gradient of sodium of 5 mEq per liter in the cell to 140 mEq per liter in the interstitial fluid. Sodium therefore enters the cell and causes cellular edema. The breakdown of large protein molecules into smaller molecules increases the oncotic pressure and water retention. This sequestration of fluid is best seen in patients with burns of the head and neck. The hematocrit initially rises due to the loss of large volumes of fluid from the intravascular space and later falls. The initial hemoconcentration results in increased viscosity and poor perfusion of injured tissues. Whole blood is generally not required in the immediate period after a burn.

Cardiovascular System

In experimental burns the cardiac output decreases markedly even before fluid loss from the intravascular space. The decrease can be prevented by digitalization and infusion of large volumes of fluids prior to the burning, but not by either alone. A myocardial toxin has been demonstrated in the circulation 24 hours following production of an experimental burn.

Initially there is thrombocytopenia and a short blood clotting time, and later a decrease in prothrombin results in a prolonged clotting time.

A number of factors are responsible for the anemia commonly seen in burned patients. In large deep burns up to 5 percent of the erythrocytes are immediately destroyed. The life-span of the erythrocytes is decreased from the normal of 120 days. An important factor is hemolysis due to infection. Severe anemia frequently occurs about one week after a large burn.

Respiratory System

Pulmonary lesions and complications are frequent in burn patients. Thermal burns occur only in the mouth, nose, and oral pharynx. Only steam can produce a thermal burn of the lower respiratory tract. Inhalation of nitrous oxide, sulfuric acid, carbon monoxide, or hydrocyanic acid produced by the burning of paint, wood, and other materials causes necrosis of the alveolar membrane, edema, and infection.

Gastrointestinal System

A major burn causes ileus of the gastrointestinal tract. The patients are thirsty and readily develop acute gastric dilatation if allowed to drink a large amount of fluid. This can result in decreased respiratory efficiency, vomiting, and aspiration.

A "Curling's ulcer," occurring most often at 7 to 10 days, may cause an upper gastrointestinal hemorrhage. These ulcers may be in the stomach and/or duodenum and may be single or multiple. There may be epigastric pain and tenderness, but frequently there are no associated symptoms. Most patients respond to conservative treatment of nasogastric suction, antacids, and antispasmodics. Operation may occasionally be required and most often consists of partial or rarely total gastrectomy (see Chapter 18). The pathogenesis of "Curling's ulcer" is not known, but contributory factors are increase in histamine, adrenal cortex stimulation, impaired blood flow, and poor nutrition to the cells lining the stomach and duodenum.

Lymphoreticular System

The patient with extensive burns suffers a marked decrease in the cell-mediated immune response and a lesser impairment of the humoral response.[1] This may predispose to infection, especially by organisms that are not normally pathogenic, such as Candida albicans. During this period patients have prolonged "take" of skin allografts. A positive nitrogen balance maintained by intravenous hyperalimentation, and elemental diets may prevent this decrease in the immune response.

Metabolism

Severely burned patients have a markedly increased metabolic rate which may be as much as four to eight times the basal rate. The cause is not clear.[7] Factors include the loss of fluids through the burned skin and the cooling effect that evaporation of this fluid, 580 calories per liter, has on the organism. Efforts to combat this heat loss include increasing the environmental temperature and humidity and applying wet dressings. Patients with severe burns are unable to take by mouth the 4000 to 6000 calories and 100 gm of protein per day necessary to prevent severe catabolism of endogeneous proteins. Intravenous hyperalimentation and elemental diets are therefore of great value (Chapter 11).

Renal System

Renal failure may occur in the severely burned patient from circulatory changes associated with oligemia or from the effects of deep burns on erythrocytes and myoglobin. In oligemic shock there is a marked decrease in renal blood flow from intense stimulation of the sympathetic nervous system and activation of several humoral systems. Hemoglobin and myoglobin leak through the capillary of the renal tubules and are deposited as casts in the distal renal tubules. The lesions may be an upper or lower nephron nephrosis or a combination.

Infection

Infection is a major problem in the care of extensive burns because the normal barrier function of the skin is lost. In addition, protein-rich dead tissue is an ideal medium for the growth of organisms. Bacteria tend to grow in this hypoxic zone protected from drying by eschar and not in contact with the vasculature of the uninjured tissues. Bacteria multiply rapidly (e.g., Pseudomonas aeruginosa may reach 10^7 bacteria per gram of tissue), may enter the circulation, and produce septicemia. Systemic antibiotics have not been successful in controlling local infection because of the decrease in vascularity and rapid development of resistant strains of bacteria.[10] Topical bacterial agents are useful. An important principle in the treatment of deep burns is rapid removal of dead tissues.

Elaborate techniques have been developed to prevent extraneous infections, including "Life Island Techniques" and laminar air flow. Disadvantages in using isolation techniques are that treatments are more difficult, observation is impaired, and the most frequent source of infection is bacteria that normally inhabit the respiratory system, the deep glands of the skin, and, most important, the gastrointestinal tract.

MANAGEMENT OF BURNS

Management consists of resuscitation in the first two to three days, an intermediate period from resuscitation until the wound is closed, and finally rehabilitation.

Resuscitation

Respiratory System. Prime consideration should be given to maintenance of the airway and to care of related injuries which may have occurred at the time of burning and which may be more life-threatening in the immediate period than the burn. The airway may be obstructed by edema at or above the larynx immediately or up to eight hours after receiving a burn of the neck or pharynx. Intubation can usually be performed through the nose or mouth, and only rarely is tracheostomy necessary. If it is necessary to establish a tracheostomy through burned tissues, the site becomes infected and leads to infection entering the lower respiratory tract and mediastinum. If the patient is burned in an enclosed space, the nasal vibrissae are singed off. In a mucosal burn of the upper airway the likelihood of pulmonary damage is great. Undue restlessness may be a manifestation of hypoxia. Blood gases should be monitored, secretions gently removed, and the inspired gases humidified. Steroids are given if there is bronchospasm. Positive end-pressure respiration (PEEP) may be necessary. Systemic antibiotics should be withheld until the organisms and sensitivities are known.

Intravenous Fluids. In severe burns, over 10 percent body surface in children and elderly patients and 15 percent in adults, large volumes of fluid are lost from the extracellular compartment. Therefore large amounts of intravenous fluids are required. There are several regimes for fluid therapy based on body weight and percentage of body surface burned.

The Brooke formula recommends that 1.5 ml crystalloid solution (usually Ringer's lactate) per kilogram of body weight and 0.5 ml colloid solution (plasma, albumin, or dextran) per kilogram of body weight be given during the first 24 hours for each percent of body surface burn. In addition, dextrose and water, 2000 ml, are given to replace basal losses. One half of the total volume is administered during the first eight hours and also during the second day.

A ratio of one to one, colloid to crystalloid, is used with another regime. Yet another treatment consists of omitting colloids during the first 24 hours because they leak rapidly out of the intravascular compartment and may be of no value. A hypertonic salt solution may be given because there is a deficit of sodium ion in the extracellular fluid, and it is desirable not to overload the intravascular compartment with water. This regime is advocated particularly in elderly burn patients and in those with cardiopulmonary disease. Dextran has been used as the principal fluid for resuscitation to decrease the viscosity of the intravascular fluid and improve the microcirculation to burned, but not completely devitalized tissues. No matter what regime is used, it is essential to monitor the patient carefully and adjust the fluid to be given from hour to hour.

In large deep burns destruction of erythrocytes and muscle may produce hemoglobin and myoglobin that may be precipitated in the kidney tubules. A low volume of dark or syrupy urine is produced. Osmotic diuretics should be given.

Monitoring. Pulse, blood pressure, and respiratory rate are recorded every half hour. The cerebral status is carefully noted. Central venous pressure determinations are useful to detect changes which may suggest overloading or cardiac failure. A urinary catheter is inserted, and the urinary volume and specific gravity are measured hourly. In adults the rate of fluid administration is adjusted to keep the urine flow at about 40 ml per hour. A common error is to give too much fluid and produce pulmonary edema. This is most likely to occur during the second to fifth days following the burn when the sequestered fluid is being reabsorbed and in children under 18 months of age and in elderly patients.

Blood is taken on admission for "baseline values" of electrolytes and renal and liver function studies. Serial hematocrit determinations reveal the degree of intravascular dehydration. Advocates of colloid therapy increase the rate of the colloid administration if the hematocrit continues to rise. Arterial and mixed venous blood gas determinations and cardiac output determinations by dye dilution methods are helpful, particularly in those with respiratory injury or concomitant cardiopulmonary disease.

Drugs. Analgesic and sedative drugs are given intravenously as needed. It is important not to confuse the vital signs by oversedation. Early after a *deep* burn there is little pain unless the burn is handled roughly. Reassurance and calm management by all personnel may do more to calm an agitated patient than large doses of analgesics.

Patients with large burns are routinely digitalized to combat the inevitable decrease in cardiac output. It is critical to obtain a history regarding any previous drugs, and this is particularly true in older patients who may be on cardiac glycosides. Inotropic agents, such as isoproterenol, are given when indicated.

Booster doses of tetanus toxoid are given to previously immunized patients and human immune globulin (Hypertet) to those who have not been immunized.

Antibiotics are usually withheld until culture and sensitivity reports are available because of the high incidence of superinfection with resistant organisms when wide-spectrum antibiotics are used. Penicillin may be given to protect against infection by beta-hemolytic streptococci which may be rapidly invasive in the early postburn period.

Initial Care of the Burn Wound. The burn wound is cleaned with bland soap and sterile water or saline; easily removed, obviously necrotic tissues are cut away and topical treatment started. Cold applications relieve the pain of superficial burns. The patient may be placed in a water bath (Hubbard tank) for the initial cleansing.

Intermediate Care

Closing the burn wound must be foremost in treatment. Early closure prevents sepsis, inanition, and joint contractures.

Topical Treatment. Burns of the face and perineum are best treated by exposure. Exposure treatment results in a dry eschar, under which bacteria grow less readily than in the warm, moist environment under a dressing. However, a large amount of fluid evaporates from an apparently dry eschar and infection may occur beneath it. Topical antibacterial agents, such as silver nitrate, mafenide (Sulfamylon), and and silver sulfadiazine, have now superceded dressing and exposure techniques in most centers. The upper and lower extremities can be immobilized by incorporating splints of plaster, aluminum, or plastic in the dressings.

Silver Nitrate. Silver nitrate, 0.5 percent, may be applied as a solution or cream. Many layers of coarse mesh gauze saturated with silver nitrate are also applied to the wound and covered with an impervious sheet. The high humidity at the burn wound decreases water evaporation. The dressings must be changed frequently because the concentration of silver nitrate is critical. Silver nitrate is not bactericidal at less than 0.3 percent and is injurious to the tissues at greater than 1 percent.

Disadvantages of the silver nitrate dressings include:

1. The solution is hypotonic, and as a result large amounts of sodium, potassium, and other ions are lost through the burn wound.

2. Frequent wetting and changing of the dressing are necessary.

3. Silver nitrate stains materials and personnel.

4. Treatment must be started promptly after burning because silver nitrate cannot penetrate a dry eschar.

5. The eschar separates slowly because of the absence of proteolytic enzymes from bacterial contamination of the subeschar space.

Silver nitrate cream, 0.5 percent, may be used in a similar way to mafenide. It has the advantages of not causing pain on local application and rarely causes local sensitivity reactions.

Mafenide (Sulfamylon). Mafenide is a sulfa drug that is not inactivated by purulent discharge nor by para-aminobenzoic acid. Applied locally as a 10 percent cream, it is active against a wide spectrum of bacteria both in vitro and in vivo but is destroyed when absorbed into the blood stream. The drug can permeate the eschar and destroy underlying bacteria. The incidence of septicemia has been reduced as has the mortality rate in burns of less than 50 percent of the body surface.

Disadvantages are:

1. Metabolic acidosis may occur because the drug is a carbonic anhydrase inhibitor in the kidney tubules. The increased acid load results in a compensatory increase in respiration. This is usually tolerated well except in cases of respiratory injury or associated lung disease.

2. Pain occurs on initial application of the drug but may subside after three or four days.

3. Local sensitivity develops in 10 to 20 percent of patients after two to three weeks.

4. The rate of healing of granulating wounds may be decreased by mafenide.

Silver Sulfadiazine (Silvadene). Silver sulfadiazine, used as a 1 percent cream, combines the advantages of silver nitrate and sulfa drugs.[9] These advantages are that it controls infection and it does not cause pain. In addition, there is no excessive loss of electrolytes, no inhibition of carbonic anhydrase, and local hypersensitivity is uncommon. Some strains of bacteria have recently become resistant to the drug.

Nutrition. A hypermetabolic state occurs after a burn. A patient with an infected 50 percent burn requires about 10,000 calories per day to maintain a positive nitrogen balance and maintain body weight. Caloric and protein loss can be decreased by local application of heat (32°C, 90°F) and wet dressings. Intravenous hyperalimentation and elemental diets by mouth or feeding tubes have increased survival after severe burning.

Debridement and Skin Grafting. Closure of full-thickness skin loss requires removal of dead tissue. Prior to the use of the newer topical anti-infective agents, purulent infection usually occurred beneath the eschar in the second or third weeks, resulting in an easily removable eschar. With the new topical agents the eschar is considerably more difficult to remove. Removal is done at the bedside, in a bath, or in the operating room without destroying viable deep dermal tissues or producing pain or significant bleeding. Small full-thickness burns, less than 10 percent of body surface, may be excised at the level of the deep fascia and the defect closed by a graft. When possible, dead tissue should be removed within four weeks. Removal after this time results in infection, inanition, and often failure of skin grafts to "take." When the dead tissue has been removed, the full-thickness burn granulates rapidly and should be promptly covered. With extensive burns autografting may be dangerous because the donor sites are similar to second-degree burns. In massive burns autograft donor areas may be used up before all the granulations are covered.

Allografts. Allografts, obtained from cadavers within six hours of death, are useful to provide temporary closure. The grafts are taken, using sterile technique, from the lower extremities, buttocks, and lower trunk, and stored at 4°C in balanced salt solution with 10 percent plasma and an antibiotic. Significant viability is maintained even after four weeks.[5]

The time of allograft rejection depends on the immunologic competence of the host and the difference in the histocompatibility genes between the donor and the recipient. Burn patients may have so depressed an immune response that grafts "take" for six to eight weeks. Allografts are usually applied in series. Each crop is removed after three to four days, at the time of "take" or vascularization. Another allograft or an autograft may then be applied. The bacterial count in granulation tissue is markedly reduced in the first 24 hours after applying an allograft, xenograft, or nonviable graft. The count remains reduced if the graft adheres firmly but increases if the graft fails. If the allograft "takes" at three to four days, an autograft will "take" in the same region.

Xenografts. Pigskin xenografts remain viable for up to four weeks and are as successful as allografts. Grafts have been freeze-dried, using agents that prevent crystallization, and stored at −50°C for several years. Both fresh and frozen pigskin grafts are now commercially available.[4]

Autografting. The definitive cover for full-thickness burn wounds is the autograft. The grafts are cut with a motor dermatome with thicknesses between 10 to 20 × 1/1000 of an inch and are applied to the prepared recipient sites. The most convenient donor sites are the thighs and lower abdomen. Almost any site, however, may be used, including uneven regions that have to be ballooned out by injection of fluids subcutaneously to achieve a smooth surface, for example over the ribs. In massive burns donor sites may be reused after healing in two to four weeks if the grafts are cut very thin.

Small slits may be cut in a staggered fashion in an autograft to increase the area covered by the graft and to permit drainage of serous fluid or blood from beneath the graft (mesh grafting). When sutured in position, the graft appears as a net (Figure 15–3). The open areas heal by migration of epithelium within two to three weeks. The main disadvantage is that the network pattern can always be seen in the graft.

Rehabilitation

The rehabilitation phase of the treatment of burns may be said to start after the burn wound is completely closed. However, of course, the treatment of contractures and psychological problems must be carried out through the entire management. They are discussed here for convenience.

Contractures. Contractures are frequent when a burn occurs over a joint. Important deformities are flexion contractures at the hips, elbows, knees, axillae, and especially the hands and anterior neck.

Joints are splinted in position to prevent the deformity. This includes holding the knees, elbows, wrists, and interphalangeal joints in extension. The metacarpophalangeal joints are placed in flexion, while the thumb is placed in abduction and opposition. Exercises are performed regularly during the period of intermediate care and wound closure. Traction applied to skeletal pins is useful, especially with circumferential burns of the upper and lower

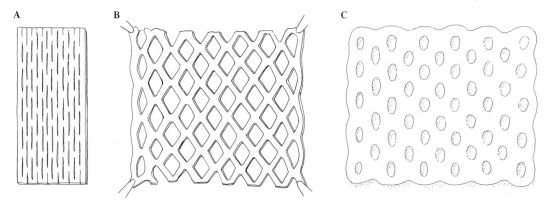

A   B   C

Figure 15–3. Mechanical devices have been produced to make a mesh graft. *A.* Multiple small incisions are placed in a patch of skin. *B.* The edges are sutured under tension, giving it a diamond-shaped pattern. *C.* Healing occurs, leaving multiple clear oval patches.

extremities, and to prevent contracture of the neck by placing a pin in the mandible. The most important preventive measure, however, is prompt closure of the burn wound. At most sites this can be achieved by early debridement and prompt application of autografts.

Established contractures are treated by stretching, dynamic splinting, traction, or by removing scar tissue and applying autografts. Z-plasties and flaps are often used (see Chapter 33). It is advisable to wait for maturation of scars, particularly in children, because considerable stretching of the tissues can occur. Too much time, however, must not be allowed to pass or contractures may become more difficult to correct, especially in the hand and anterior neck.

Aesthetic Problems. Burns on the face that are deeper than partial thickness may result in severe disfigurement due to contracture of scars and distortion of the normal features. Eyebrows, ears, and the margins of the nose are often lost. The reconstruction of these defects is extremely difficult and may be carried out using full- and split-thickness and composite grafts and local and distant flaps. Hypertrophic scars are particularly common on the face and neck and may flatten significantly over a period of months and years. Elastic compression may hasten flattening of these scars.

Psychological Considerations. The psychological impact of a severe burn is great on the patient and his family.[2] In the immediate postburn period the patient may be principally concerned with survival, but later he is more worried about permanent disability and disfigurement. Members of the family, particularly parents of burned children, may need special counseling to overcome feelings of guilt. Early involvement in occupational therapy and rehabilitative counseling is of great value.

PREVENTION OF BURNS

Many burns are caused by the ignition of clothing, for example by space heaters used in cold weather where central heating is not available. Safety regulations for space heaters are now being prepared. The American Burn Association is testing the flammability of clothing worn by burn victims, and this has led to federal regulations to ensure that clothing will not ignite easily.

Heat and smoke alarm systems should be present in all businesses and homes. Fire drills should be carried out in private businesses and housing as well as in public buildings. Smoking in bed is particularly dangerous, especially when associated with alcohol ingestion. Many burns are the result of lighting bonfires with flammable liquids and oil-soaked clothing catching fire in automobile repair areas. Abandoned cars with gasoline in the tank present a special hazard to children. Electrical wiring breakdown is a frequent cause of house fires, especially in older homes.

CITED REFERENCES

1. Alexander, J., and Fisher, M. W.: Vaccination for *Pseudomonas aeruginosa. Am. J. Surg.*, **120**:512, 1970.
2. Andreasen, N. J. C.; Worres, A. S.; and Hartford, C. E.: Incidence of long-term psychiatric complications in severely burned adults. *Ann Surg.*, **174**:785–93, 1971.
3. Baxter, R.: Present concepts in the management of major electrical injury. *Surg. Clin. North Am.*, **50**: 1401–18, 1970.
4. Bondoc, C. C., and Burke, J. F.: Clinical experience with viable frozen human skin and a frozen skin bank. *Ann. Surg.*, **174**:371–82, 1971.
5. DiVincenti, F. C.; Pruitt, B. A.; and Rechler, J. M.: Inhalation injuries. *J. Trauma*, **11**:109–17, 1971.
6. Hutcher, N., and Haynes, B. W.: The Evans formula revisited. *J. Trauma*, **12**:453–58, 1972.
7. Kukrol, J. C., and Shoemaker, W. C.: The metabolic sequelae of burn trauma. *Surg. Clin. North Am.*, **50**:1211–16, 1970.
8. Lamke, L. O., and Liljedahl, S. O.: Evaporative water loss from burns, grafts and donor sites. *Scand. J. Plast. Reconstr. Surg.*, **5**:17–22, 1971.
9. Sanford, W.; Rappole, B. W.; and Fox, C. L., Jr.: Clinical experience with silver sulfa diazine, a new topical agent for control of pseudomonas infections in burns. *J. Trauma*, **9**:377–88, 1969.
10. Waisbren, A.: Antibiotics in the treatment of burns. *Surg. Clin. North Am.*, **50**:1311–23, 1970.

SUGGESTIONS FOR FURTHER READING

Artz, C. P., and Moncreif, J. A.: *Treatment of Burns.* W. B. Saunders Co., Philadelphia, 1969.
This is a comprehensive text on the treatment of burns by well-known authorities.
Polk, H. C., and Stone, N. H.: *Contemporary Burn Management.* Little, Brown and Company, Boston, 1971.
Newer concepts in burn management are presented. A series of chapters are included describing the new and controversial methods of treatment.
Stone, N. H.: *Profiles of Burn Management.* Industrial Medicine Publishing Co., Inc., Miami, 1969.
The practical management of the burn patient is presented with little emphasis on the pathophysiology.

SURGICAL ANATOMY

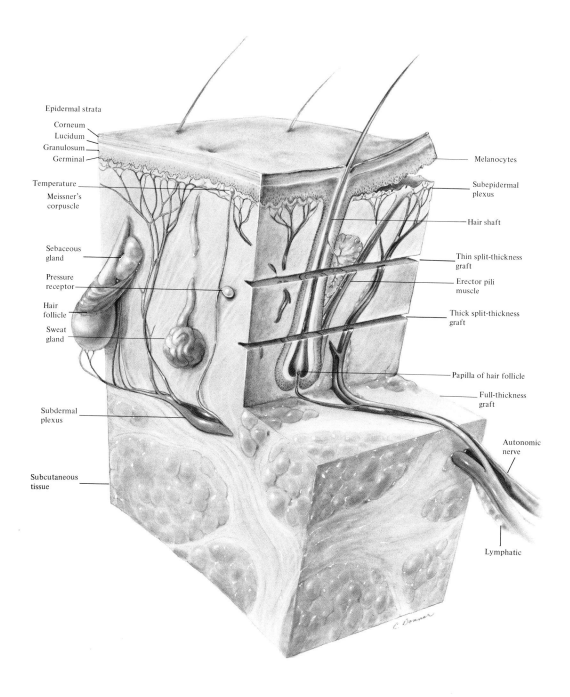

Epidermal strata

Corneum
Lucidum
Granulosum
Germinal

Melanocytes

Temperature

Subepidermal
plexus

Meissner's
corpuscle

Hair shaft

Sebaceous
gland

Thin split-thickness
graft

Pressure
receptor

Erector pili
muscle

Hair
follicle

Thick split-thickness
graft

Sweat
gland

Papilla of hair follicle

Full-thickness
graft

Subdermal
plexus

Autonomic
nerve

Subcutaneous
tissue

Lymphatic

Plate I. Skin.

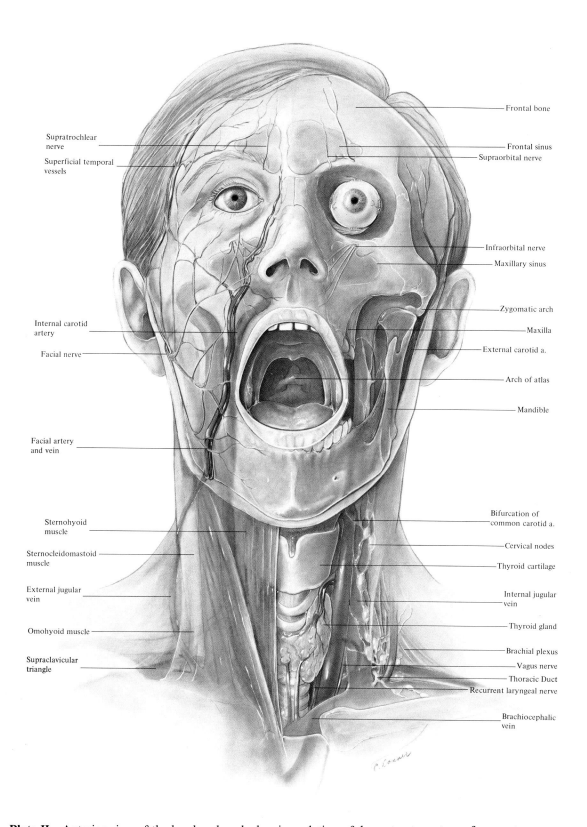

Supratrochlear nerve

Superficial temporal vessels

Internal carotid artery

Facial nerve

Facial artery and vein

Sternohyoid muscle

Sternocleidomastoid muscle

External jugular vein

Omohyoid muscle

Supraclavicular triangle

Frontal bone

Frontal sinus

Supraorbital nerve

Infraorbital nerve

Maxillary sinus

Zygomatic arch

Maxilla

External carotid a.

Arch of atlas

Mandible

Bifurcation of common carotid a.

Cervical nodes

Thyroid cartilage

Internal jugular vein

Thyroid gland

Brachial plexus

Vagus nerve

Thoracic Duct

Recurrent laryngeal nerve

Brachiocephalic vein

Plate II. Anterior view of the head and neck showing relation of deep structures to surface anatomy.

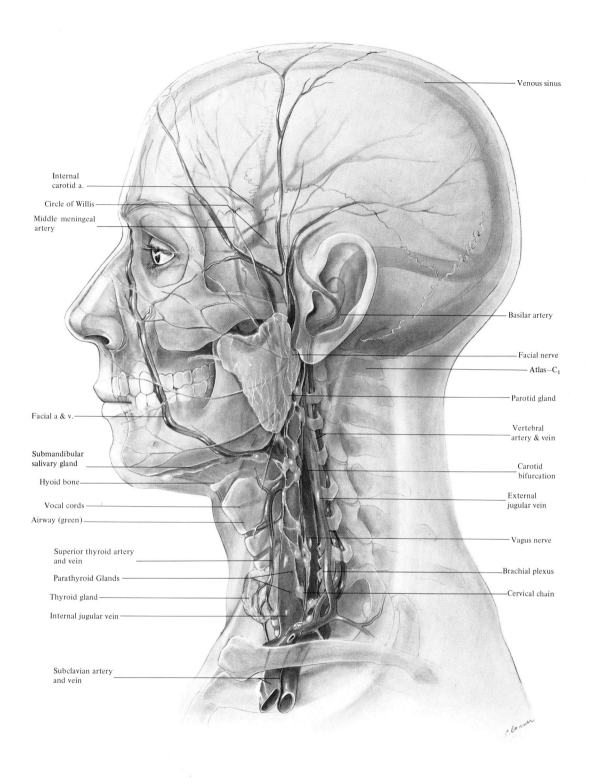

Internal carotid a.

Circle of Willis

Middle meningeal artery

Facial a & v.

Submandibular salivary gland

Hyoid bone

Vocal cords

Airway (green)

Superior thyroid artery and vein

Parathyroid Glands

Thyroid gland

Internal jugular vein

Subclavian artery and vein

Venous sinus

Basilar artery

Facial nerve

Atlas—C$_1$

Parotid gland

Vertebral artery & vein

Carotid bifurcation

External jugular vein

Vagus nerve

Brachial plexus

Cervical chain

Plate III. Lateral view of the head and neck.

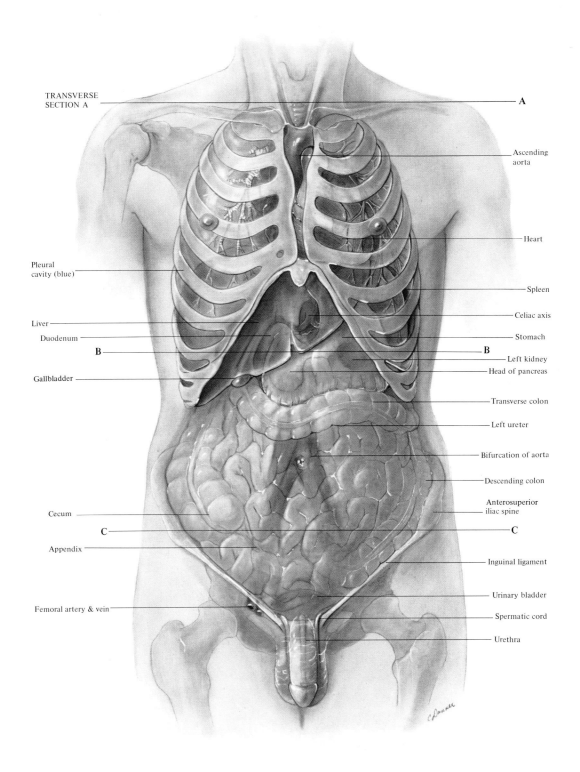

TRANSVERSE
SECTION A ———————————————————————————————————— A

Ascending
aorta

Heart

Pleural
cavity (blue)

Spleen

Celiac axis

Liver

Stomach

Duodenum

B ——— B

Left kidney

Head of pancreas

Gallbladder

Transverse colon

Left ureter

Bifurcation of aorta

Descending colon

Anterosuperior
iliac spine

Cecum

C ——— C

Appendix

Inguinal ligament

Urinary bladder

Femoral artery & vein

Spermatic cord

Urethra

Plate IV. Contents of the thoracic and abdominal cavities.

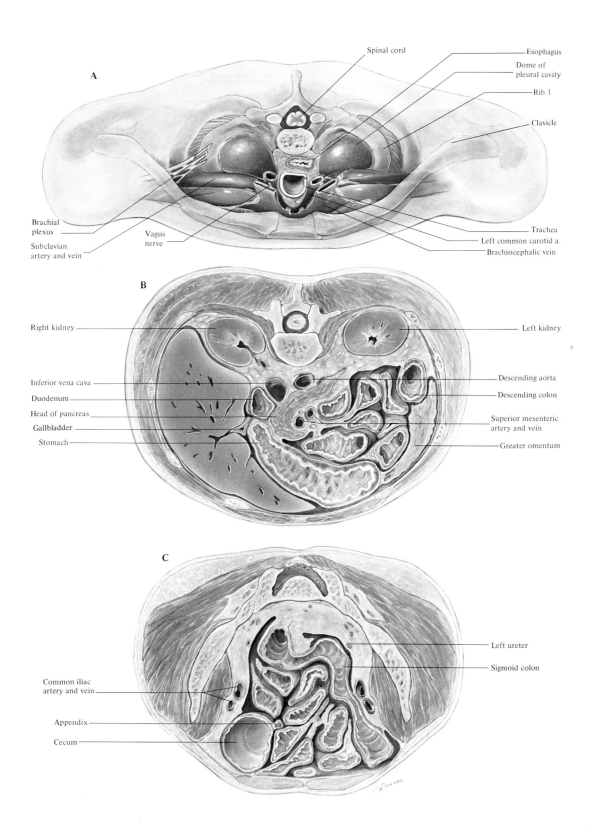

A

Spinal cord

Esophagus

Dome of
pleural cavity

Rib 1

Clavicle

Brachial
plexus

Vagus
nerve

Subclavian
artery and vein

Trachea

Left common carotid a.

Brachiocephalic vein

B

Right kidney

Left kidney

Inferior vena cava

Duodenum

Head of pancreas

Gallbladder

Stomach

Descending aorta

Descending colon

Superior mesenteric
artery and vein

Greater omentum

C

Left ureter

Sigmoid colon

Common iliac
artery and vein

Appendix

Cecum

Plate V. Transverse sections of the pleural and peritoneal cavities.

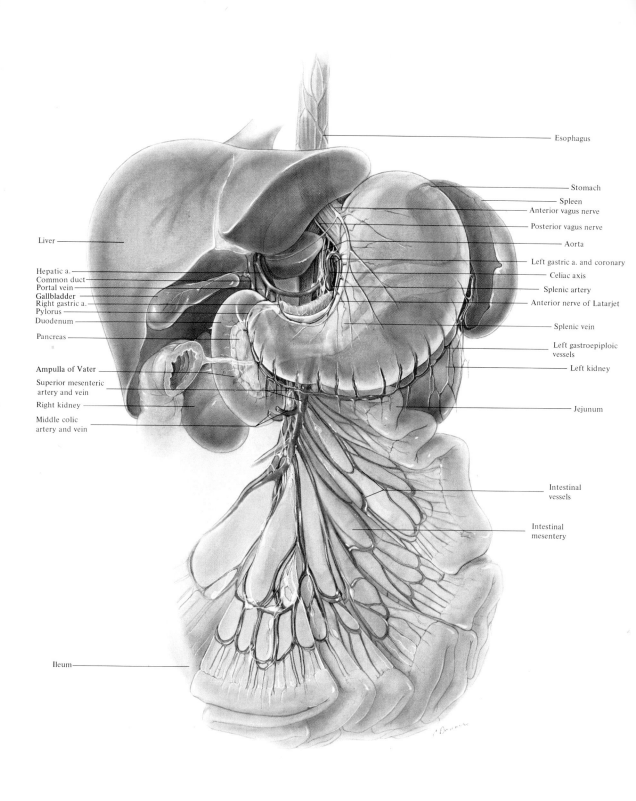

Esophagus

Stomach

Spleen

Anterior vagus nerve

Posterior vagus nerve

Aorta

Left gastric a. and coronary

Celiac axis

Splenic artery

Anterior nerve of Latarjet

Splenic vein

Left gastroepiploic vessels

Left kidney

Jejunum

Intestinal vessels

Intestinal mesentery

Liver

Hepatic a.
Common duct
Portal vein
Gallbladder
Right gastric a.
Pylorus
Duodenum

Pancreas

Ampulla of Vater

Superior mesenteric artery and vein

Right kidney

Middle colic artery and vein

Ileum

Plate VI. Stomach, duodenum, pancreas, liver, gallbladder, spleen, and small bowel.

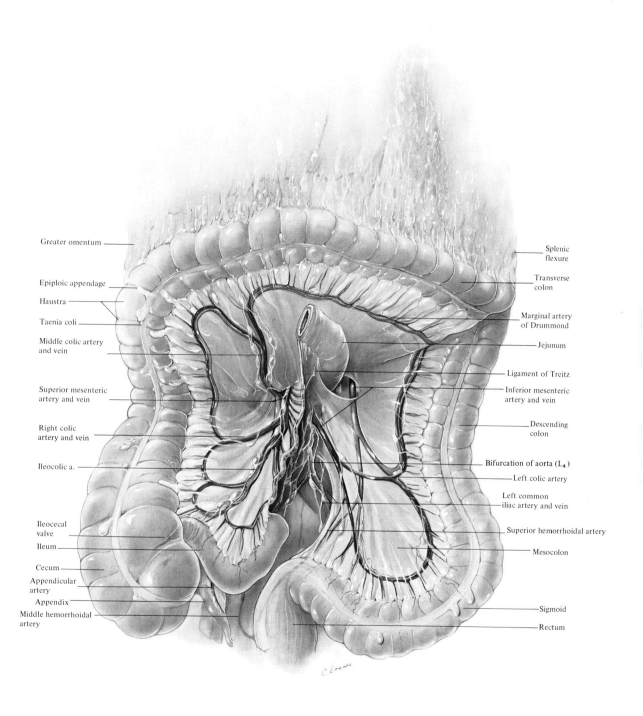

Greater omentum

Epiploic appendage

Haustra

Taenia coli

Middle colic artery
and vein

Superior mesenteric
artery and vein

Right colic
artery and vein

Ileocolic a.

Ileocecal
valve

Ileum

Cecum

Appendicular
artery

Appendix

Middle hemorrhoidal
artery

Splenic
flexure

Transverse
colon

Marginal artery
of Drummond

Jejunum

Ligament of Treitz

Inferior mesenteric
artery and vein

Descending
colon

Bifurcation of aorta (L₄)

Left colic artery

Left common
iliac artery and vein

Superior hemorrhoidal artery

Mesocolon

Sigmoid

Rectum

Plate VII. Blood supply of the colon.

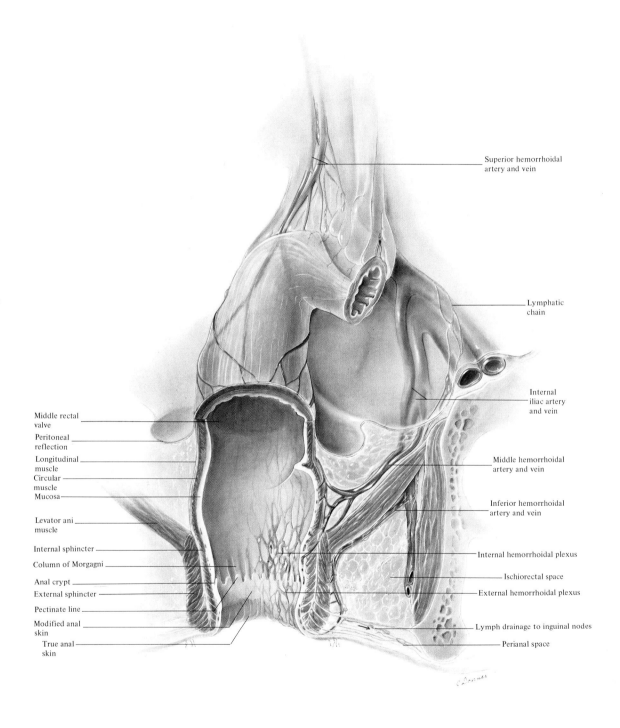

Superior hemorrhoidal
artery and vein

Lymphatic
chain

Internal
iliac artery
and vein

Middle hemorrhoidal
artery and vein

Inferior hemorrhoidal
artery and vein

Internal hemorrhoidal plexus

Ischiorectal space

External hemorrhoidal plexus

Lymph drainage to inguinal nodes

Perianal space

Middle rectal
valve

Peritoneal
reflection

Longitudinal
muscle

Circular
muscle

Mucosa

Levator ani
muscle

Internal sphincter

Column of Morgagni

Anal crypt

External sphincter

Pectinate line

Modified anal
skin

True anal
skin

Plate VIII. Pelvis, rectum, and anus.

UNIT III
PRINCIPLES OF GENERAL SURGERY

Chapter 16

HEAD AND NECK

Harold W. Bales

CHAPTER OUTLINE

Inflammatory Diseases
  Tonsillitis and Adenoiditis
  Peritonsillar Abscess
  Croup
  Cervical Adenitis
  Sialadenitis
Trauma
Neoplastic Diseases
  Leukoplakia
  Lip
  Tongue
    Treatment
    Results

Carcinoma of the Floor of the Mouth
Carcinoma of the Buccal Mucosa
Palate
Tonsil
Posterior Third of Tongue
Nasopharynx
Larynx
  Treatment
Salivary Gland Tumors
  Treatment
  Results
Mandible

The "head and neck" is a convenient anatomic unit for consideration of the biology and treatment of infections, injuries, and malignancies of this region. Congenital anomalies are discussed in Chapters 27 and 33. It does not include the brain and special sense organs but is mainly concerned with the upper respiratory and digestive tracts (see Plates II and III).

INFLAMMATORY DISEASES

The oropharynx and nasopharynx are major portals of entry for microorganisms and have a well-established defense against infection, Waldeyer's ring, consisting of the adenoids and the pharyngeal and lingual tonsils. A secondary barrier to infection is the cervical lymph nodes. Bacteria are usually destroyed, but they may persist and produce an acute or chronic inflammatory disease.

Tonsillitis and Adenoiditis

Infection in the tonsils and adenoids may lead to infection in the middle ear or elsewhere in the body. Enlarged adenoids may obstruct the eustachian tube. Their removal should then be considered.

Peritonsillar Abscess

Proliferation of pyogenic organisms within the tonsillar fossa may lead to abscess formation. The patient becomes toxic and may develop airway obstruction. Treatment is drainage of the abscess under general anesthesia with an endotracheal tube in place and administration of antibiotics. Elective tonsillectomy should be done after six to eight weeks.

Croup

Acute laryngoepiglottitis, most frequently caused by *Hemophilus influenzae*, may produce acute obstruction of the airway with cyanosis and extension of the neck. Immediate tracheostomy may be lifesaving.

Cervical Adenitis

Acute and chronic infections in the cervical nodes are frequent. A primary site for the infection in the skin, mouth, or upper respiratory tract should be looked for. A "button collar" abscess may form and require drainage (see Chapter 6). Chronically inflamed nodes may resemble lymphoma. Tuberculous cervical adenitis or scrofula is now uncommon. Nodes that do

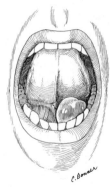

Figure 16–1. A ranula is a translucent cystic lesion of the floor of the mouth due to minor salivary gland obstruction.

not respond to antituberculous drugs should be excised.

Sialadenitis

The ducts of the major salivary glands may be obstructed by calculi or viscid saliva, as in Mikulicz's disease. The high content of mucus in the submandibular secretion may account for the higher incidence of calculi in the sub-mandibular than the parotid glands. Obstruction of the minor glands may result in the

formation of a large clear cyst, a ranula, in the floor of the mouth (Figure 16–1).

A calculus in the submandibular or parotid duct may be felt within the mouth. Pressure on the enlarged salivary gland may result in the discharge of pus from the orifice of the duct. Calculi are usually visible on plain x-ray because of their high calcium content. A radiopaque dye may be injected into the parotid duct to outline the duct pattern and show the level of obstruction (sialography). Acute suppurative parotitis, most often the result of infection by *Staphylococcus aureus*, is a serious complication in critically ill patients (Figure 16–2) (see Chapter 14).

Chronic sialadenitis without calculi is treated by sialogogues, good oral hygiene, and anti-biotics. Calculi in the major ducts should be removed through the mouth. For recurrent severe infections excision of the gland may be necessary. Abscesses may require incision, and occasionally a salivary fistula may occur.

TRAUMA

Immediate management of face and neck injuries consists of maintenance of the airway, control of hemorrhage, and protection of the spinal cord (see Chapters 33 and 34).

Common causes of airway obstruction are

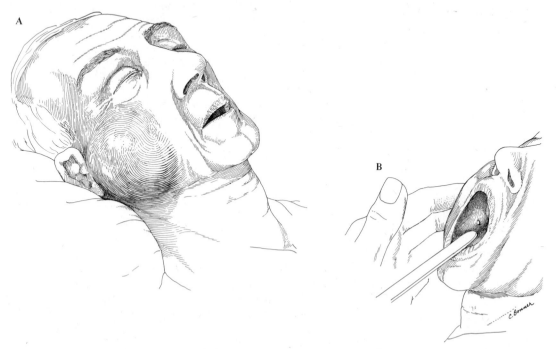

Figure 16–2. *A.* In acute parotitis, there are marked swelling and tenderness of the entire gland. *B.* Pus can often be expressed from Stensen's duct.

mandibular fractures with retrusion of the tongue, fractures of the larynx or trachea, intraoral hemorrhage, and aspiration of gastric contents. Immediate insertion of an endotracheal tube and tracheobronchial suction are essential. Emergency tracheostomy is rarely indicated and is hazardous in the presence of a cervical hematoma.

Intraoral bleeding can usually be controlled by packing around an indwelling endotracheal tube. Tears in major cervical vessels can be controlled temporarily by external pressure. All penetrating neck wounds must be explored in the operating room. A thoracotomy may be necessary to control bleeding. Fractures of the cervical spine with potential cord injury are treated by maintaining the neck in extension and distraction from the time of injury.

NEOPLASTIC DISEASES

Cancers of the skin and subcutaneous tissues of the face, head, and neck are discussed in Chapter 25. The therapeutic challenge of tumors of the head and neck is great because treatment often produces considerable impairment of function and appearance, and in addition there is often controversy over the best form of treatment. Head and neck tumors account for about 5 percent of all malignancies. Most are epithelial in origin, increase in incidence with age, and are four times commoner in men than in women. Associated etiologic factors are tobacco, alcohol, syphilis, and chronic irritation, such as dental trauma.[6,9] The incidence of second primary cancers is high.

Presenting symptoms are often minimal so that the diagnosis may be made late. For example, a carcinoma in the pyriform fossa generally presents with cervical metastases.

Exfoliative cytology is useful as a screening procedure in those at high risk, as in patients with certain types of leukoplakia. Toluidine blue supravital staining is helpful in identifying a carcinoma, in selecting a biopsy site, and in estimating the extent of the disease.

Tissue diagnosis is mandatory before therapy is planned, except in patients with enlarged cervical nodes thought to contain tumors and in those with parotid masses. The biopsy specimen should cross the tumor edge to include normal and malignant tissue. Specimens of anterior oral lesions may be obtained under local anesthesia using a cup biopsy forceps or a biopsy punch. Biopsies of more posterior lesions, including hypopharynx and larynx, usually require more extensive anesthesia and should be combined with direct laryngoscopy. A negative biopsy report of tissue from a clinically suspicious lesion must not be accepted as definitive. Further biopsies must be obtained and the patient carefully observed.

Radiographic studies are helpful in delineating the primary tumor. They include plain films of the neck using soft tissue technique, barium swallow, both standard and cine, tomography of sinuses and larynx, and contrast studies of the larynx.

Staging of tumors is helpful in selecting treatment, assessing prognosis, and identifying groups of comparable lesions for study. The most widely accepted system in international use for staging head and neck lesions is the TNM classification (Table 16–1). This system describes size and extent of the primary, nodal involvement, and metastases.

Leukoplakia

Leukoplakia is a common condition that is important because of the tendency of certain types to become malignant. Leukoplakia (Figure 16–3) is a clinical term used to describe a "white plaque" on the mucosal surface of the mouth, pharynx, esophagus, and the respiratory and genitourinary systems. It is considered to arise in response to chronic irritation, usually chemical. Tobacco, alcohol, malfitting dentures, and poor oral hygiene are the most frequent causes in the mouth.

About 50 percent of oral squamous cell carcinomas develop in a patch of leukoplakia. The earliest lesion is a white, milky film, nonpalpable patch that frequently regresses when the irritant is withdrawn. With progression the patch becomes white-smooth, white-irregular, cauliflower, carcinoma in situ, and eventually an invasive carcinoma. Those that persist or progress should be biopsied. The presence of keratosis or hyperkeratosis indicates careful followup. If there is dyskeratosis with loss of normal stratification of the layers of cells and variation in density and size of the nuclei, the region should be excised. Liquid

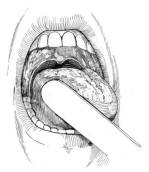

Figure 16–3. Leukoplakia of the tongue is most often seen in heavy smokers.

nitrogen cryotherapy is effective in treating larger areas.

The differential diagnosis includes chronic candidiasis, lichen planus, chronic atrophic mucositis, and superficial squamous cell carcinoma.

Lip

Carcinoma of the lip accounts for 15 percent of all head and neck malignancies. It generally occurs in the lower lip, is 20 times more common in men than women, seldom occurs under 40 years, and is rare in Negroes. In the upper lip the incidence is almost the same in males as in females. Prolonged exposure to light in outdoor workers, as in fishermen and farmers, is the most common cause. Others are chronic irritation from dental trauma and irritation by a pipe stem. The majority are squamous cell carcinomas of different grades of differentiation. Less frequent are basal cell carcinoma and malignant melanoma. The benign diseases generally differentiated readily from those that are malignant are hemangioma, lymphangioma, salivary gland tumors, hyperkeratoses, and fissures.

The squamous cell carcinoma may develop slowly from a precursor, such as leukoplakia,

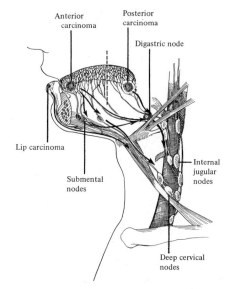

Figure 16–4. Carcinomas of the tongue tend to spread by the lymphatics. Anterior lesions spread by the submental and digastric routes, while posterior tumors primarily use the digastric pathway to the internal jugular nodes.

Table 16–1. STAGING OF PRIMARY HEAD AND NECK LESIONS

	T1	T2	T3	T4
Anterior two thirds of tongue	Less than 3 cm	3–5 cm with possible minimal extension to floor of mouth or deep muscle infiltration	5 cm to half tongue with possible limited extension of mouth	More than half tongue or massive extension to floor of mouth with involvement of mandible
Buccal mucosa	Less than 3 cm	3–5 cm with minimal extension to adjacent muscle, gingiva, faucial pillars	Greater than 5 cm with limited extension to adjacent structures	Massive
Gums	Less than 3 cm	3–5 cm with minimal extension to floor of mouth or buccal mucosa. No bone involvement	Greater than 5 cm or pressure bone defect	Massive infiltration of (moth-eaten) bone
Floor of mouth	Less than 2 cm	2–4 cm with minimal extension (up to 2 cm thick)	Greater than 4 cm or fixed to periosteum. More than 2 cm thick but still limited invasion of root of tongue	Massive invasion of root of tongue or bone
Palatine arch and oropharynx	Less than 3 cm	3–5 cm with minimal extension to adjacent structures	Greater than 5 cm with limited extension to adjacent structures	Massive

N0: No node
N1: Single node, 2 cm
N2: Large movable node or multiple unilateral nodes

N3: Fixed large unilateral node or bilateral nodes
M: Distant metastases when first seen

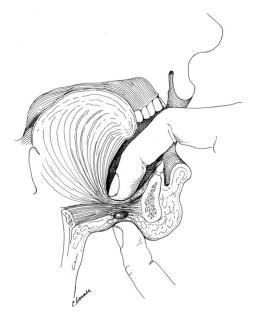

Figure 16–5. In bidigital examination, the tissue to be examined is fixed by the external finger and palpated by one placed in the mouth.

keratotic plaque, or a fissure, or arise in normal mucosa. The lesion may present as an area of induration, a firm nodule, an exophytic mass, or an ulcer. Muscle is invaded late and cervical node involvement is unusual except in advanced lesions. Spread is to the submental and submandibular nodes and then to the jugular chain (Figure 16–4).

The lip is palpated to determine the gross extent of the lesion and bidigital examination is performed of the anterior floor of the mouth to feel for enlargement of the submental nodes (Figure 16–5). Tissue diagnosis is essential. The biopsy can be performed as a simple office procedure under nerve block anesthesia.

The choice of treatment is most often based on the cosmetic result. Lesions involving a commissure and broad exophytic tumors are usually best treated by radiotherapy. More central lesions of up to one-third of the lip respond well to wedge excision and direct closure (Figure 16–6). A concomitant lip shave, removal of the exposed vermillion, is performed if the tumor is arising in a patch of leukoplakia (Figure 16–7). In such patients the cure rate rate drops to about 50 percent.[4]

Because of the low incidence of involvement of the regional nodes neck dissection is not performed until the nodes become palpable. The open ulcer, which is the most common presentation, may produce an inflammatory lymphadenopathy. The response of the nodes to antibiotic therapy should be determined before deciding on neck dissection. It is only necessary to remove the submental and submandibular nodes along with the deep fascia and the submandibular salivary gland. This is performed bilaterally if the tumor is near the midline.

Prognosis is excellent in those with cancer of the lower lip, with a five-year survival exceeding 90 percent. It is not as good in those with cancer of the upper lip because of the greater tendency to spread to the deep cervical nodes. It may then be advisable to perform a block dissection of the neck for palpable nodes when the carcinoma is in the upper lip and especially if the tumor is anaplastic.

Tongue

The anterior two thirds of the tongue is considered a separate entity from the posterior one third, which is part of the oropharynx. Most carcinomas in the anterior two thirds are squamous and occur most often on the free border at the junction of the heavily papillated mucosa of the dorsum with the smooth mucosa of the undersurface. The incidence is high in males, especially in those with excessive use of tobacco and alcohol.[10] Leukoplakia is a common precursor and less often Plummer-Vinson syndrome, Bowen's disease, or lichen planus. A carcinoma should be differentiated from leukoplakia, or chronic ulcer, syphilitic glossitis, hemangioma, salivary tumor, and rarely a sarcoma.

Figure 16–6. A carcinoma of the lower lip can be removed by excising a wedge of tissue. Closure in layers provides an excellent functional and cosmetic result.

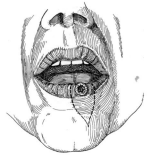

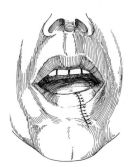

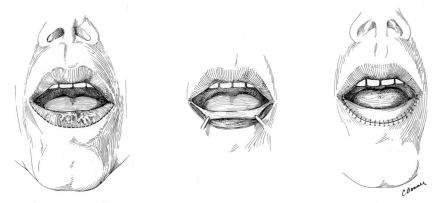

Figure 16–7. In a lip shave operation the entire vermillion tissue of the lower lip is excised down to muscle. This is commonly done for diffuse leukoplakia. Resurfacing is accomplished by advancing to the cutaneous junction.

Early symptoms are a lump or a painful ulcer often with the pain referred to the ear along the lingual and auriculotemporal nerves. Later there is impaired mobility of the tongue, hemorrhage, excessive salivation, fetor, and marked edema. Grossly the tumor may present as an ulcer, an exophytic growth, or as deeply infiltrating tumor with minimal ulceration. The rich blood and lymph flow and its mobility probably explain the early development of cervical node metastases. About 40 percent of tongue lesions have already spread to regional nodes when the patient is first seen. Spread occurs in the substance of the tongue toward the median raphe, to the digastric nodes, and then to the jugular chain (Figure 16–4). Distant metastases, particularly to lung and liver, usually occur late.

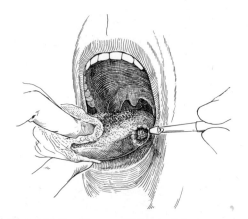

Figure 16–8. For punch biopsy of the tongue, a lingual nerve block gives adequate anesthesia. Infiltration should be avoided. Cautery using silver nitrate may be necessary to obtain hemostasis.

Microscopic diagnosis is established by a punch (Figure 16–8), incisional, or, if the lesion is small, an excisional biopsy. The biopsy specimen should cross the tumor edge to include normal and malignant tissues. A specimen is not taken from a node because of possible contamination of the extranodal tissues with cancer cells.

Treatment. The primary tumor is most often treated by radiotherapy and clinically involved nodes by neck dissection. A tumor dose of 6500 rads is generally given in five weeks by teletherapy using cobalt 60 or electrons. If there is incomplete tumor regression, additional treatment can be given using radium needles or radon seeds. Hemiglossectomy is performed if the tumor fails to regress completely, complicates syphilitic glossitis, or recurs locally. Total glossectomy is indicated when the tumor crosses the midline. Part of the mandible may have to be resected if the tumor involves bone.

Views differ on the management of the cervical nodes.[5] Most often the patients are regularly reviewed and the nodes removed by block dissection if clinically they are considered to contain metastases (Figure 16–9). Some advocate prophylactic block dissection because occult metastases are found in about 40 percent.[1]

Palliative treatment is indicated if it is not possible to remove the primary tumor completely or if cervical metastases have spread beyond the capsule of the nodes. Good palliation can often be obtained by radiotherapy. Methotrexate has been used by intravenous injection and by infusion (see Chapter 7) and has produced useful palliation.[7]

Results. The five-year survival is 50 to 60 percent in the absence of nodal metastases. Their presence reduces survival to about 20 percent.

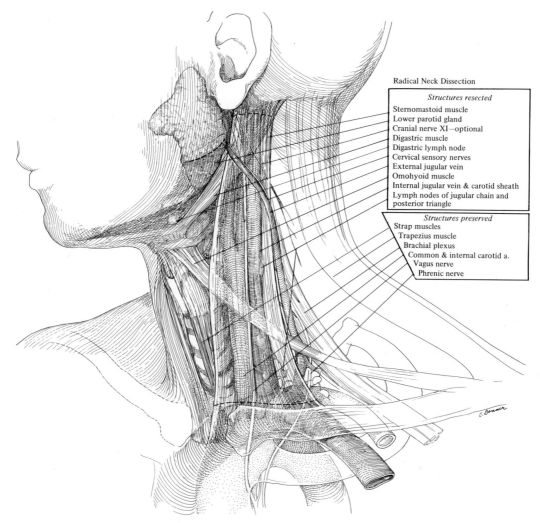

Radical Neck Dissection

Structures resected
Sternomastoid muscle
Lower parotid gland
Cranial nerve XI—optional
Digastric muscle
Digastric lymph node
Cervical sensory nerves
External jugular vein
Omohyoid muscle
Internal jugular vein & carotid sheath
Lymph nodes of jugular chain and
posterior triangle

Structures preserved
Strap muscles
Trapezius muscle
Brachial plexus
Common & internal carotid a.
Vagus nerve
Phrenic nerve

Figure 16–9. The radical neck dissection is designed to remove the principal lymphatic pathways of tumor spread, an en bloc procedure.

Carcinoma of the Floor of the Mouth

The incidence and behavior of carcinoma of the floor of the mouth are similar to those of the anterior two thirds of the tongue. A special complication is its tendency to involve the mandible at an early stage (Figure 16–10). The primary tumor can be treated by radiotherapy unless there is radiologic evidence of bone involvement. There is little likelihood of bone necrosis when megavoltage radiotherapy is used. The floor of the mouth is excised along with portions of the mandible and often with part of the tongue if bone is involved or there is local recurrence after radiotherapy.[3] When the mandible is resected, an immediate reconstruction with a prosthesis or bone graft is generally performed. If the mandible can be preserved, a

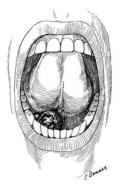

Figure 16–10. A carcinoma of the floor of the mouth tends to encroach upon the gingiva and the undersurface of the tongue.

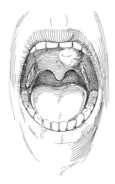

Figure 16–11. A squamous cell carcinoma of the mucosa presents as an ulcer, while a tumor of the minor salivary gland, such as a benign mixed salivary tumor, tends to have an intact overlying mucosa.

flap is necessary to cover the defect in the soft tissue.

Carcinoma of the Buccal Mucosa

The etiology and behavior of carcinoma of the buccal mucosa resemble those of carcinoma of the anterior two thirds of the tongue. The primary tumor can be effectively treated by radiotherapy. When operation is indicated because of incomplete response after radiotherapy or local recurrence, it is often necessary to remove full thickness of the cheek. A major reconstruction of the cheek is then needed using a pedicle flap.

Palate

The prognosis is much worse with carcinoma of the soft than the hard palate because of the marked tendency for metastases to develop bilaterally in the deep cervical nodes. It is important to exclude carcinoma of the antrum from primary carcinoma of the hard palate and salivary gland tumors (Figures 16–11). Carcinoma of the hard palate is most often treated by radiotherapy and operation performed if the bone is involved or there is incomplete remission following radiotherapy. Carcinoma of the soft palate is generally treated by radiotherapy to both the primary and the cervical nodes.

Tonsil

Cancer of the tonsil may be squamous cell (85 percent), lymphoepithelioma (5 percent), or a lymphosarcoma (10 percent). The so-called lymphoepithelioma is probably an anaplastic carcinoma with marked mononuclear cell infiltration. The patients most often present with unilateral pain, constant or only on swallowing. The tumor may be exophytic or more often infiltrating. Treatment is radiotherapy to the neck and cervical nodes. The prognosis is particularly bad because of early bilateral node involvement.

Posterior Third of Tongue

This tumor differs from carcinoma of the anterior two thirds in that diagnosis tends to be late, the tumor is generally anaplastic, and there are few five-year survivors because early metastases tend to occur to the deep cervical nodes. Treatment is radiotherapy to the primary tumor and cervical nodes.

Nasopharynx

Carcinoma of the nasopharynx is rare in Caucasians and common in the Chinese. The tumor is commoner in males than females and not infrequently occurs in young people around 20 years. The patient often presents with enlarged cervical nodes and no symptoms from the primary tumor. The patient may present with the petrosphenoidal syndrome consisting of supra- and infraorbital pain, paralysis of the sixth nerve, and invasion of the bones on x-ray. Others may have nasal obstruction and epistaxis. Treatment is radiotherapy to the primary tumor and cervical nodes. The prognosis is remarkably good in spite of about two thirds having invasion of the sphenoid at the time of

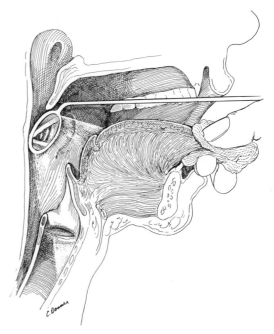

Figure 16–12. During indirect laryngoscopy, the tongue is drawn forward. A strong point light is directed at the angled mirror to illuminate the cords and reflect their image.

diagnosis. The five-year survival is about 25 percent in all patients and 50 percent in those without nodal involvement.

Larynx

Sex distribution and etiologic factors are similar to those for carcinoma of the tongue and floor of the mouth. Hoarseness is the most common presenting symptom followed by cough. In those with extrinsic laryngeal lesions involving the pyriform sinus there is pain on swallowing referred to the ear through the ninth and tenth cranial nerves.

Examination includes a thorough inspection using a bright light and a laryngeal mirror and bimanual palpation. For indirect laryngoscopy a light source and a laryngeal mirror are all that is required (Figures 16–12 and 16–13). *Any person with hoarseness persistent for two weeks must have a direct laryngoscopy.* Direct laryngoscopy requires local and topical anesthesia and is most helpful when suspicious areas have already been identified. A biopsy is necessary to establish the diagnosis and the extent of the tumor. Radiographic studies, including plain films of the neck using soft tissue technique and tomography, may help to delineate the primary tumor.

Laryngeal lesions metastasize late due to the low blood supply of the cords and the presence of surrounding cartilage. Metastases develop in the digastric node and later in the jugular chain (Figure 16–14). Diagnosis is by indirect laryngoscopy followed by direct laryngoscopy and biopsy. Tomograms and laryngograms help in defining the extent of the disease.

Treatment. Radiotherapy provides a high

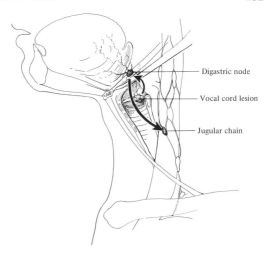

Figure 16–14. Carcinoma of the larynx spreads by the lymphatic pathway to the digastric node, then to the jugular chain.

cure rate, and there is excellent preservation of the voice when the carcinoma is confined to one mobile cord. The effectiveness of radiotherapy is sharply reduced when the tumor invades muscle or cartilage. Fixed cords and involvement of the commissure signify involvement of cartilage.

Total laryngectomy and ipsilateral neck dissection are indicated in those with advanced lesions. Methods of speech rehabilitation include "esophageal speech" (regurgitation of ingested air) and the use of mechanical vibrators held against the floor of the mouth. Both methods create intraoral air turbulence which may then be formed into speech by the tongue, teeth, and lips.

Partial laryngectomy or "conservation laryngectomy" preserves much of the speaking voice and gives good cure rates.[8] Selection of patient and procedure is critical.

Cure rates are high for intrinsic laryngeal lesions with an 80 percent five-year survival. Extrinsic lesions are more difficult to manage and have a cure rate of about 40 percent.

Salivary Gland Tumors

The bulk of salivary glandular tissue is in the parotid and the submandibular glands. It is also found throughout the submucosa of the mouth as small islands with tiny ducts. Salivary gland tumors may occur in the mouth, palate, and pharyngeal wall. The incidence is higher in the parotid than the submandibular gland because of its size. The etiology is unknown. Parotid tumors are relatively uncommon, have no sex predilection, and may occur at any age. In children parotid tumors are more likely to be

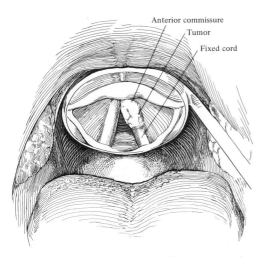

Figure 16–13. Carcinoma of the larynx involving the anterior commissure causes impaired movement of the cords.

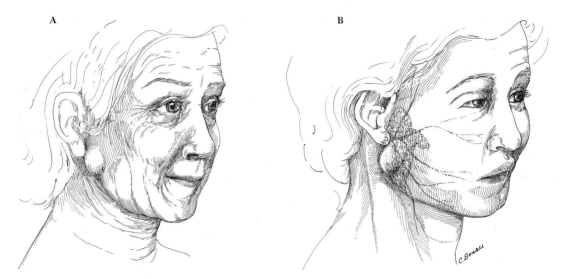

Figure 16–15. *A.* A mixed parotid tumor rarely produces weakness of the facial nerve. *B.* A carcinoma of the parotid tends to cause paralysis of the facial nerve.

malignant than in adults. About 75 percent of parotid tumors are benign, and of these two thirds are mixed parotid tumors or pleomorphic adenomas. The remainder include papillary cystadenoma lymphomatosum (Warthin's tumor), oxyphiladenoma, lymphoepithelial cyst, hemangioma, lipoma, and Mickulicz's disease. The second most frequent benign tumor is Warthin's tumor. It occurs much more commonly in males and is bilateral in about 10 percent. In Mickulicz's disease there is dense infiltration of generally a single parotid gland with mononuclear cells. It is most likely an autoimmune disease. The mixed tumor is the only benign tumor with potential to become malignant.

The group of malignant tumors is diverse. Those with moderately aggressive characteristics include mucoepidermoid, adenoid cystic, and acinic cell carcinomas. Squamous cell carcinomas and sarcomas are very aggressive.

Benign tumors usually present as asymptomatic masses (Table 16–2). Malignant tumors grow more rapidly, are usually hard, and may cause pain and paralysis in the distribution of the facial nerve (Figure 16–15). In fact pain or paralysis associated with a parotid gland mass almost always indicates a malignancy. These tumors invade the adjacent structures including skin and the pterygoid space, spread along perineural lymphatics, metastasize to the cervical nodes, and occasionally to the lungs.

The history and the physical characteristics may indicate the diagnosis. Sialography, outlining the ductal system by introducing radiopaque material into Stensen's or Wharton's

duct, may be helpful in differentiating tumors from chronic sialadenitis and sialectasis. A preoperative biopsy is generally not carried out because of the risk of seeding the skin and subcutaneous tissue with cancer cells and of injuring the facial nerve. The diagnosis may be established from a frozen section obtained at operation.

Treatment. All mobile tumors should be excised because the majority of parotid masses are malignant or have a malignant potential. The only ones that usually respond well to radiotherapy are lymphomas.

Care must be taken to preserve the facial nerve and its branches during excision of a benign tumor. The nerve emerges from the stylomastoid foramen and enters the substance of the gland where it splits into two divisions intimately related to the isthmus of the gland and then into five major branches.

Table 16–2. CHARACTERISTICS OF PAROTID TUMORS

	BENIGN	MALIGNANT
Growth	Slow, steady	Rapid
Pain	Absent	Occasionally present
Facial palsy	Absent	Diagnostic if present
Tenderness	Rare	Frequent
Consistency	Cystic to rubbery	Stony hard
Attachment	Mobile	Fixed
Trismus	None	May be present
Nodes	None	May be present

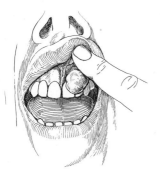

Figure 16–16. An epulis is a benign gingival lesion with intact overlying mucosa.

The nerve may be excised when removing a malignant tumor. The patient must be advised prior to operation of the risk of damage to the facial nerve. If the nerve is anatomically intact, recovery is good within up to one year. Autogenous nerve grafts using a portion of the great auricular nerve as a donor may be inserted when tumors involving the facial nerve are resected.

Results. With the current practice of precise facial nerve dissection the recurrence rate of mixed tumors is less than 5 percent. Recurrence of the other benign tumors is rare. The less aggressive malignant lesions have a cure rate of 60 to 75 percent. The outlook for the more aggressive lesions is not so good. Sarcomas have a cure rate of less than 5 percent.

Submaxillary tumors are treated in a similar manner to those of the parotid. The likelihood of a submaxillary tumor being malignant is greater than one in the parotid.

Mandible

The mandible is complex bone containing marrow, enamel organs, and gingiva. Each of these tissues can give rise to neoplasm.

Cancers of the gingiva are similar in etiology and behavior to the other squamous carcinomas of the oral cavity. They are slow to involve the regional nodes but rapidly invade the mandible.

Table 16–3. MANDIBULAR TUMORS ACCORDING TO TISSUE ORIGIN

1. Osseous
   a. Osteosarcoma
   b. Giant cell tumor
      1) Giant cell reparative granuloma (not a true tumor)
   c. Fibro-osteoma
   d. Osteochondroma
2. Ectodermal (enamel organ, etc.)
   a. Ameloblastoma (adamantinoma)
   b. Enameloma
3. Marrow
   a. Ewing's sarcoma
   b. Plasma cell, myeloma, and plasmacytoma

This is an important factor in planning treatment since radiotherapy cannot be relied on to destroy all tumor cells in bone and may cause bone necrosis. Benign gingival lesions are usually not ulcerated. A relatively common tumor is the epulis (Figure 16–16).

Bony tumors of the mandible usually present as painless masses, with the exception of an osteosarcoma which tends to produce severe pain. Pathologic fractures often occur in new and recurrent lesions. Bone lesions have specific distinguishing radiographic features which help in diagnosis. However, as with other head and neck tumors, tissue diagnosis is essential before therapy is undertaken. Tumors are typed by tissue of origin (Table 16–3) and have specific characteristics (Table 16–4).

Treatment is based on tissue type and predicted behavior. Giant cell tumors, although benign, have a high recurrence rate if excision is not adequate. Treatment is excision with preservation of the continuity of the mandible. Supplemental bone as a free graft may be necessary for structural support.

Osteosarcoma metastasizes by the blood stream and not by lymphatics.[2] A wide resection including a generous margin of bone is the preferred treatment. There is a five-year survival

Table 16–4. CHARACTERISTICS OF MANDIBULAR TUMORS

	DIRECT INVASION OR EROSION	LYMPHATIC METASTASES	DISTANT METASTASES
Fibro-osteoma (benign)	Yes	No	No
Giant cell tumor (benign)	Yes	No	No
Osteosarcoma (malignant)	Yes	No	Yes
Ameloblastoma (low-grade malignant)	Yes	Rare	No
Ewing's sarcoma (highly malignant)	Yes	No	Yes

of about 25 percent. Failure is usually due to pulmonary metastases.

An ameloblastoma arises from the enamel organ and is of low-grade malignancy. It tends to invade and destroy bone and infrequently metastasizes to the regional nodes and the lung. Early resection of the involved bone with adequate margins produces a high cure rate. Mandibular integrity should be restored at the time of resection by insertion of an autogenous bone graft. Treatment by curettage is inadequate and is generally followed by local recurrence with spread along the mandibular canal. An ameloblastoma occurs less often in the maxilla than in the mandible and occasionally is seen in the tibia.

Ewing's sarcoma is multifocal in nature and not amenable to surgical excision. Individual lesions are radiosensitive but the cure rate is low.

CITED REFERENCES

1. Beahrs, O. H.; Gossel, J. D.; and Hollinshead, W. H.: Technic and surgical anatomy of radical neck dissection. *Am. J. Surg.*, **90**:490–516, 1955.
2. Bennett, J. E.; Tignor, S. P.; and Shafer, W. G.: Osteogenic sarcoma of the facial bones. *Am. J. Surg.*, **116**:538–41, 1968.
3. Fayos, J. V.: Management of squamous cell carcinoma of the floor of the mouth. *Am. J. Surg.*, **123**: 706–11, 1972.
4. Jesse, R. H.: Extensive cancer of the lip. Surgical therapy. *Arch. Surg.*, **94**:509–15, 1967.
5. Jesse, R. H., and Fletcher, G. H.: Metastases in cervical lymph nodes from oropharyngeal carcinoma: Treatment and results. *Am. J. Roentgenol. Radium Ther. Nucl. Med.* **90**:990, 1963.
6. Keller, A. Z.: Cirrhosis of the liver, alcoholism and heavy smoking associated with cancer of the mouth and pharynx. *Cancer*, **20**:1015–22, 1967.
7. Kramer, S.: Combined chemotherapy and radiation therapy in the management of regional cancer. In Brodsky, I., and Kahn, S. B.: *Cancer Chemotherapy.* Grune & Stratton, New York, pp. 319–30, 1967.
8. Ogura, J. H.; Saltztein, S. L.; and Spjut, H. J.: Experiences with conservative surgery in laryngeal and pharyngeal carcinoma. *Laryngoscope*, **71**:258–76, 1961.
9. Sandler, H. D.: A retrospective study of head and neck cancer control program. *Cancer*, **25**:1153–61, 1970.
10. Wynder, E. L.; Bross, I. J.; and Feldman, R. M.: A study of etiological factors in cancer of the mouth. *Cancer*, **10**:1300–23, 1957.

SUGGESTIONS FOR FURTHER READING

Ackerman, L. V., and del Regato, J. A.: *Cancer: Diagnosis, Treatment and Prognosis*, 4th ed. C. V. Mosby, St. Louis, 1970.
Good for correlation with pathology.
Anderson, R., and Byars, L. T.: *Surgery of the Parotid Gland.* C. V. Mosby, St. Louis, 1965.
Detailed consideration of surgical diseases of the parotid.
Grabb, W. C., and Smith, J. W. (eds.): *Plastic Surgery: A Concise Guide to Clinical Practice.* Chapters 13 and 15. Little, Brown and Company, Boston, 1968.
Excellent basic presentation of reconstructive principles and techniques.
MacComb, W. S., and Fletcher, G. H.: *Cancer of the Head and Neck.* Williams & Wilkins, Baltimore, 1967.
Good reference for treatment and results for all head and neck tumors.

Chapter 17

ESOPHAGUS

John A. McCredie and *Gerard P. Burns*

CHAPTER OUTLINE

Basic Surgery
  Esophageal Symptoms
    Esophageal Pain
    Heartburn
  Investigation of Esophageal Disease
    Radiologic Studies
    Endoscopy
    Cytology
    Esophageal Manometry
  Foreign Bodies
  Trauma
  Corrosive Esophagitis
  Reflux Esophagitis
  Pathology
    Mechanism of Normal Continence
    Mechanism of Acid Reflux
    Symptoms and Complications
  Management
    Nonoperative

    Surgical
  Diverticulum
    Pharyngoesophageal Diverticulum
    Epiphrenic Diverticulum
  Achalasia
    Diagnosis
    Management
  Tumors
    Benign
    Malignant: Carcinoma
      Etiologic Factors
      Pathophysiology
      Clinical Features
    Management
      Excision
      Radiotherapy
      Combined Surgery and Radiotherapy
      Palliation

BASIC SURGERY

The function of the esophagus is to convey food from the pharynx to the stomach (see Plate IV). No absorption takes place. It is lined by squamous epithelium and contains a few mucus-secreting cells. The muscle of the esophagus consists in the upper one third of striated muscle, in the lower third of smooth muscle, and in the middle third of a mixture of both. Sphincteric mechanisms at the upper end prevent regurgitation of food into the air passages and at the lower end protect against reflux of acid and pepsin from the stomach. The upper sphincter is well defined anatomically as the cricopharyngeus muscle, whereas the sphincter at the lower end is not demonstrable anatomically but is physiologically measurable.

Esophageal Symptoms

The symptoms of esophageal disease are dysphagia, pain, and heartburn. *Dysphagia*, or difficulty in swallowing, may occur at the initiation of the swallowing act as a result of a neuromuscular disorder affecting the pharynx or cricopharyngeus, supplied by the ninth and tenth cranial nerves. It may occur in the middle of swallowing, usually 2 to 5 seconds after ingestion has taken place, and is then usually related to disease of the body of the esophagus, such as tumor, stricture, or spasm. Finally the dysphagia may occur late and indicates disease of the lower third or the cardioesophageal junction. The patient complains that the food appears to stick in the esophagus and usually localizes accurately the region of hold up. For example, if the lesion is in the upper third of the esophagus, the patient points to the suprasternal region or manubrium. In most lesions of the lower esophagus and cardia discomfort or pain is referred to the xiphoid region, but in some, symptoms are referred to the suprasternal region when the disease is in the lower third. For most organic conditions dysphagia is experienced initially for solid food and later for liquids. In achalasia dysphagia is frequently present for both liquids and solids even from the beginning, reflecting the disordered motility in the body of the esophagus combined with failure of the lower sphincter to relax properly.

Esophageal Pain.   Esophageal pain, which is usually burning or squeezing in character, may be felt anywhere from the suprasternal notch to the epigastrium, may be localized or diffuse and occasionally radiate to the back or into the jaw. If the pain is squeezing or crushing and retrosternal, it may be difficult to distinguish from the pain of angina pectoris. A useful distinction between esophageal and cardiac pain may sometimes be made by the Bernstein acid perfusion test.

Heartburn.   Heartburn is a common symptom of lower esophageal disease but is poorly defined both by patients and physicians. It usually refers to a diffuse burning sensation felt in the retrosternal area, anywhere from the xiphoid region to the neck, that may be accompanied by a feeling of hot water or a bitter taste in the back of the throat. Antacids provide relief. Many patients experience heartburn only after ingesting specific foods or drugs, for example, onions, aspirin, or spicy food.

INVESTIGATION OF ESOPHAGEAL DISEASE

The diagnosis of esophageal disease relies more on the clinical history than on physical examination and to a much larger extent on special investigations. General examination may show wasting as a result of dysphagia or signs of a systemic disease such as scleroderma. Examination of the neck may reveal subcutaneous emphysema in cases of esophageal rupture, involvement of cervical lymph nodes in patients with carcinoma, and rarely a palpable swelling in cases of Zenker's diverticulum. Abdominal examination may show hepatosplenomegaly in patients with esophageal varices, or metastatic disease in those with advanced cardioesophageal neoplasms. Ausculation over the lower sternum during swallowing permits timing of the arrival of the peristaltic wave at the stomach. A delay of more than 8 seconds indicates interference with peristalsis.

Radiologic Studies

The esophagus is studied by having the patient swallow a barium mixture. The act of swallowing is observed and recorded on films for later review. The stomach must always be examined at the same time. Abdominal pressure is applied in patients with symptoms of gastroesophageal reflux. In patients with suspected motor disorders cinefluoroscopy is extremely valuable in providing a dynamic record of esophageal motility.

Endoscopy.   The recent development of the flexible fiberesophagoscope has made endoscopic examination of the esophagus much more tolerable for the patient. Sedation with barbiturates or diazepam and a local anesthetic spray or gargle facilitate the procedure. The entire esophagus can be visualized easily unless there is a severe obstruction. Bougies or dilators cannot be passed through the fiberesophagoscope, but forceps can be passed to obtain biopsies of suspicious lesions. For dilatation of a stricture or larger biopsies the rigid esophagoscope must be used. Although this can be done under sedation most patients tolerate the procedure better under general anesthesia. During esophagoscopy distances are measured from the level of the incisor teeth. The cardioesophageal junction is located at 40 cm but varies with the patient's height.

Cytology.   Esophageal cytology is of considerable value in diagnosing carcinoma of the esophagus.[8] There are various methods for collecting cell samples during endoscopy. A suspicious area may be irrigated and the fluid collected. A brush may be applied to obtain cells, or a small piece of gelfoam attached to a bougie rubbed over the suspicious area. The gelfoam is then removed, fixed, sectioned, and stained. A positive diagnosis can be made in 85 to 95 percent of patients with carcinoma, and false positives are almost unknown.

Esophageal Manometry.   Information regarding esophageal motor activity can be obtained by using three open-tipped catheters introduced into the esophagus through the mouth or nasopharynx and attached to pressure transducers which are then connected to a recorder.[6] The tips of the catheters are placed 5 cm apart so that the esophageal pressure at three separate points can be recorded simultaneously. The catheters are usually infused slowly with saline, placed in the stomach, and gradually withdrawn through the lower sphincter into the body of the esophagus. Considerable information can be obtained about the pressure and position of the lower sphincter and the contractions of the body of the esophagus. In the normal act of swallowing a wave of pressure travels down the esophagus, and each swallow is accompanied by relaxation of the lower sphincter. This is an example of true peristaltic activity. Manometry is useful in diagnosing achalasia of the cardia, where the typical findings are a normal or raised pressure in the lower sphincter that fails to decrease on swallowing and the presence of uncoordinated movements in the body of the esophagus. Pressure studies are also used in diagnosing scleroderma and have been employed to investigate patients with hiatal hernia to determine the position of the lower sphincter.

Motility studies have shown that muscular contractions normally occur after the initiation of swallowing or when gastric contents reflux into the lower esophagus. In both circumstances a pressure wave develops in the upper esophagus and moves down to the stomach at a rate of about 3 cm per second. Waves starting at the upper end are primary contractions, and those that develop in the region of the aortic arch are secondary contractions. The tertiary type of contraction is abnormal, being characterized by irregular, uncoordinated muscular activity, and may give rise to a very irregular, sawtoothed appearance on barium swallow. Tertiary contractions are seen in some asymptomatic elderly patients, in some cases of reflux esophagitis, and in some cases of diffuse esophageal spasm.

FOREIGN BODIES

A large or irregular foreign body may be arrested at the level of the cricopharyngeus, or in the esophagus, especially at the lower end. Material arrested in the cricopharyngeal region can usually be removed easily through the mouth, but gentleness and dexterity are required to prevent pushing the object into the esophagus. Sharp objects, like pins, needles, or razor blades may become arrested at any point in the esophagus. Rounded objects, such as coins, which successfully pass the cricopharyngeus may be held up in the upper third where the left bronchus crosses the esophagus or at the lower end just above the cardia. A bolus of meat or other food may become impacted in the esophagus in patients with preexisting disease such as an esophageal stricture or tumor. A nonradiopaque foreign body may be outlined by a swallow of contrast material.

Sharp foreign bodies must be removed as quickly as possible because of the danger of perforation and mediastinitis. This can usually be done at esophagoscopy with gripping forceps. A food bolus at the lower end ot the esophagus may be removed or pushed into the stomach. If this is not possible, the bolus may be injected with a meat tenderizer to soften the mass and allow it to pass into the stomach. Occasionally a foreign body cannot be removed through the esophagoscope, or partial penetration of the wall may have occurred. Operative removal is then required, either through a cervical incision or a thoracotomy.

TRAUMA

Trauma to the esophagus usually occurs from instrumentation, perforation by a swallowed foreign body, or perforating injuries of the thorax. When perforation of the esophagus occurs following esophagoscopy, there has frequently been an additional procedure, either a biopsy of the esophageal wall or dilatation of a stricture by a bougie. A perforation may occur, particularly in an elderly patient with cervical spondylosis, when the rigid esophagoscope presses the esophageal wall against the spine in the region of the cricopharyngeus.

Unrecognized or untreated perforation leads to a high mortality because of the ease with which infection can travel through the relatively loose tissues of the posterior mediastinum. The condition is usually associated with severe pain in the back, a rise in temperature, tachycardia progressing to shock, and the development of subcutaneous emphysema in the neck. Injuries to the cervical esophagus are usually approached through an incision in the left side of the neck where the esophagus is more easily accessible. The perforation can be repaired directly. A perforation of the body of the esophagus is approached through a right thoracotomy incision. The perforation is sutured if possible and the mediastinum drained. Occasionally when a perforation has occured from instrumentation near a stricture or tumor, it may be advisable to resect the lesion and the perforation. If not, a fistula may develop.

CORROSIVE ESOPHAGITIS

Ingestion of a strong alkali or acid, most often the cleansing agent lye, burns the mouth and injures the esophagus. Initially there is painful dysphagia, and this may be followed by the development of a fibrous stricture. Initial treatment is intake of neutralizing fluids, antibiotics, and steroids. If a stricture forms, it is treated by repeated dilatation. Occasionally a major reconstructive procedure is necessary, substituting a piece of bowel for the stenosed segment.

REFLUX ESOPHAGITIS

Reflux esophagitis may occur with or without a hiatal hernia. A portion of the fundus of the stomach may herniate through the esophageal hiatus in the diaphragm into the lower chest and form a hiatal hernia. Two types are recognized: (1) sliding hiatal hernia (Figure 17–1), in which the gastroesophageal junction occupies a position above the hiatus in the chest and the hernial sac consists of parietal peritoneum in front and the anterior wall of the stomach behind; and (2) paraesophageal hernia (Figure 17–2), when the cardioesophageal junction remains in its normal position but a complete pouch of peritoneum extends through the hiatus into the chest and

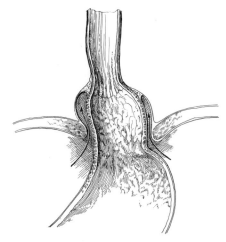

Figure 17–1. A sliding esophageal hernia showing the gastroesophageal junction situated above the hiatus.

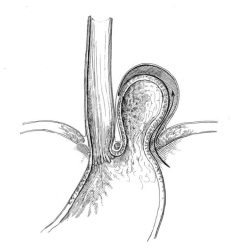

Figure 17–2. A paraesophageal hernia with the cardioesophageal junction in its normal position. Note the pouch extending through the hiatus into the chest.

usually contains a portion of the fundus of the stomach. This type is much less common, but combination of both types is frequent.

PATHOLOGY

Many hiatal hernias are discovered during radiologic examination for unrelated conditions, for example, peptic ulcer, and are asymptomatic. When symptoms occur, they depend on the type of hernia. In paraesophageal hernia symptoms are usually due to a portion of stomach either becoming incarcerated at the hiatus and produc-

ing pain, nausea, and vomiting, or pressing on the lower esophagus and causing dysphagia. Reflux esophagitis does not occur in these patients because the lower esophageal sphincter is in its normal position. In the sliding hiatal hernia reflux esophagitis is the usual cause of the symptoms. The pathology and management of reflux esophagitis can best be understood by considering the factors that normally prevent reflux.

Mechanism of Normal Continence

The exact role of the various anatomic and physiologic factors that help to maintain the gastric contents in the stomach is not entirely understood.[1] The following factors are involved: (1) contraction of the lower esophageal sphincter; (2) the effect of intra-abdominal pressure on the abdominal portion of the esophagus above the sphincter; (3) the angle of His, which refers to the acute junction between esophagus and stomach; (4) muscular contraction of the right crus of the diaphragm; (5) support of the phreno-esophageal ligament; and (6) humoral factors, including the hormone gastrin, which exerts a tonic effect on the lower esophageal sphincter. Thus when the gastroesophageal junction becomes stretched and displaced from its normal position below the diaphragm into the chest, the lower esophageal sphincter is placed at a functional and anatomic disadvantage. It is no longer exposed to the positive intra-abdominal pressure, the angle of His is straightened out, the gastric fundus no longer compresses the lower esophagus, and the anatomic sling effect of the right crus and the phrenoesophageal ligament is lost. Reflux of acid and pepsin can now occur into the lower esophagus and over prolonged periods can produce irritation and esophagitis. Severe reflux can result in peptic ulceration and stricture.

Mechanism of Acid Reflux

It should be emphasized that the radiologic demonstration of a hiatal hernia is frequently made in the absence of symptoms. Radiologic studies in which attempts were made to demonstrate a hernia in asymptomatic individuals with the use of abdominal pressure have revealed a hiatal hernia in as many as 30 percent of the normal population. Less commonly reflux of barium into the esophagus can be demonstrated in asymptomatic individuals who do not have a hiatal hernia.

The cardinal symptom of reflux esophagitis is heartburn. Of great importance is that a patient may have symptoms of reflux esophagitis in the absence of a hiatal hernia.[4] The lower esopha-

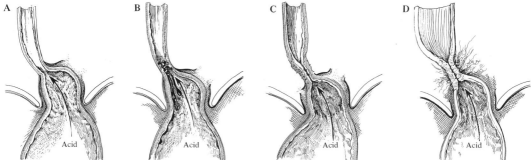

Figure 17–3. Effects of esophageal reflux on the lower esophagus. *A*. There is granular erythema of the mucosa. *B*. There is now ulceration with bleeding. *C*. Early fibrosis is present in the submucosa. *D*. There is fibrosis of the entire esophageal wall.

geal sphincter is then incompetent although located below the diaphragm. This occurs in about two thirds of normal pregnancies, becomes worse as abdominal distention increases, and then improves in the ninth month when the fetal head moves into the pelvis. In obese patients reflux symptoms may disappear after adequate weight reduction. These factors indicate that raised intra-abdominal pressure is an important factor in promoting acid reflux.

Symptoms and Complications The symptoms of esophageal reflux are aggravated by stooping, bending, or lying flat. Their severity does not correlate well with the size of the hernia. A small hernia may give rise to marked symptoms and complications, and a large hernia may be asymptomatic. Massive bleeding is rare, but chronic blood loss leading to iron deficiency anemia is frequent. When esophagitis is present, the patient often develops dysphagia initially from spasm and later from stricture formation (Figure 17–3). Inhalation of gastric contents may produce pulmonary complications. There is no correlation between the severity of symptoms and the degree of esophagitis seen at esophagoscopy. Some patients with relatively mild symptoms develop a severe stricture. For this reason esophagoscopy is essential in patients with symptomatic hernias to determine the degree of esophagitis.

A second group of symptoms may result from the mechanical effect of the hernia. Pressure on the mediastinum may produce chest pain, on the esophagus dysphagia, and on the diaphragm hiccough. Epigastric discomfort may occur from slow emptying of the gastric pouch. Occasionally the gastric fundus or a portion of colon may become incarcerated or strangulated. When a large paraesophageal hernia contains more than half the stomach, surgical repair should be considered to prevent obstruction even if symptoms are mild.

MANAGEMENT

Nonoperative

The majority of hiatal hernias are asymptomatic and do not require treatment. A significant improvement in symptoms and even their complete disappearance can be achieved by conservative means. These include reducing body weight, avoiding positions that aggravate symptoms, elevating the head of the bed, and using alkalis and regular small meals. Anticholinergic drugs are better avoided as they may delay gastric emptying and potentiate reflux. Because of the poor correlation between the severity of symptoms and the degree of esophagitis, esophagoscopy should be performed to select for operation those with moderate or severe esophagitis.

Surgical

Operation is indicated for patients who fail to respond to conservative management or who have developed severe esophagitis, stricture, or an ulcer in the gastric pouch or esophagus. A number of operations are available. In one procedure the lower esophagus is mobilized, the sac is brought down below the diaphragm, and sutures placed in the crura, posterior or anterior to the esophagus to narrow the orifice. The phrenoesophageal ligament may be sutured to the diaphragm,[1] forming a narrowed posterior crural buttress and a sling of functioning diaphragm. Recently the simpler procedure of fundoplication has been gaining in popularity[3] (Figure 17–4). In this operation the lower abdominal esophagus is mobilized and the upper ends of the lesser and gastrosplenic omentums are divided, freeing the fundus of the stomach. The fundus is then rotated posteriorly and sutured anteriorly to form a cuff around the lower esophagus. When the intragastric pressure rises, pressure in the cuff increases and presses

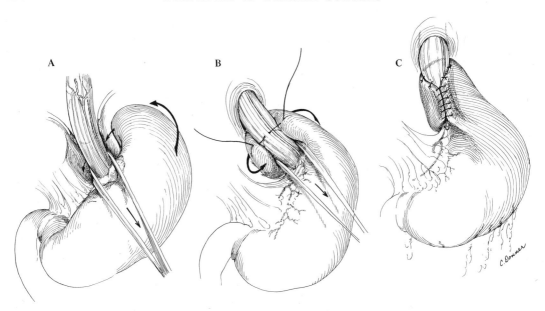

Figure 17–4.   *A*. The first steps in fundoplication for reflux esophagitis are to divide the upper part of the lesser omentum and the gastrosplenic omentum and then the gastrophrenic ligament. A tape is passed around the lower esophagus. *B*. The fundus of the stomach is then delivered posteriorly and to the right to meet the upper part of the lesser curvature. *C*. Nonabsorbable sutures are inserted so that the fundus forms a cuff around the lower esophagus.

on the lower esophagus, preventing regurgitation. Occasionally a "bloat syndrome" occurs because the patient is unable to regurgitate swallowed air. Operation relieves symptoms in 80 to 90 percent of patients. In some patients postoperative reflux may still be demonstrable even when symptoms have been completely relieved.

In patients with moderate or severe esophagitis, vagotomy and pyloroplasty may be done in addition to the hernia repair to reduce acid secretion. Vagotomy is also indicated if there is coexisting duodenal ulcer or an early esophageal stricture.

Esophageal stricture is a serious complication of reflux esophagitis. In the early stages there is fibrosis in the submucosa, but later it involves all layers of the esophagus. Early strictures are treated by graduated dilatation with bougies and when an adequate lumen has been obtained, the hernia is repaired. When the degree of esophageal shortening does not permit reduction of the hernia, a gastroplasty may be used to convert part of the fundus into a new abdominal esophagus. The gut is then enclosed snugly in the margins of the right crus (Collis). Alternatively the stricture may be incised and widened (esophagoplasty) by suturing the serosal aspect of the fundus into the defect and wrapping the rest of the fundus around the esophagoplasty (Thal). This procedure is followed by migration of

epithelial cells from the esophagus to line the serosal surface exposed to the lumen.

A number of patients with severe intractable strictures require excision and interposition of a

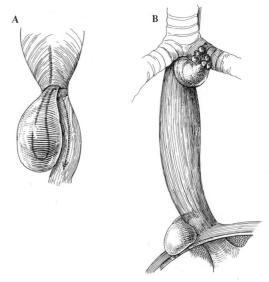

Figure 17–5.   *A*. A pharyngoesophageal diverticulum projects posteriorly above the cricopharyngeus muscle. *B*. A midesophageal diverticulum is most often a pulsion diverticulum situated just below the carina of the trachea.

portion of transverse or descending colon, or occasionally small bowel. It is essential to combine an interposition operation with an acid-reducing procedure, such as vagotomy. The vagi are always divided as an incidental procedure during esophagectomy.

DIVERTICULUM

A diverticulum or blind pouch may develop either in a juxtasphincteric position or in the midesophagus at the level of the carina (Figure 17–5). Midesophageal diverticula have previously been regarded as due to traction from inflamed lymph nodes but are probably pulsion diverticula resulting from disordered motor function of the body of the esophagus. Their location is determined probably by a congenital tracheoesophageal attachment at the bifurcation of the trachea. The diverticula are usually small, found incidentally, and rarely require treatment.

Juxtasphincteric diverticula are true pulsion diverticula that arise just above a sphincter as a protrusion of esophageal mucosa through the muscle wall and consist almost entirely of the mucosal coat. Sometimes a diverticulum arising above the upper sphincter protrudes posteriorly through the dehiscence between the transverse fibers of the cricopharyngeus and the oblique fibers of the inferior pharyngeal constrictor. This is known as a pharyngoesophageal or Zenker's diverticulum. A diverticulum located just above the lower sphincter is termed epiphrenic.

Pharyngoesophageal Diverticulum

As the diverticulum grows it extends posteriorly, then downward to the left, and may enter the mediastinum. The esophagus is displaced forward so that food or instruments tend to enter the sac, making esophagoscopy or bougienage hazardous. The patients are usually elderly and complain of dysphagia or cough with recurrent chest infections from inhaling the contents of the sac. The diverticulum may be felt as a soft mass on the left side of the neck anterior to the sternomastoid, and occasionally it may become inflamed. Rarely a carcinoma may develop. To emphasize the basic underlying motor disturbance, it has been stated that dysphagia is the cause rather than the symptom of Zenker's diverticulum. There are conflicting reports on the nature of this disturbance. It may be that the cricopharyngeus is hypertensive and fails to relax on swallowing or that relaxation does occur but is not synchronously coordinated with pharyngeal contraction so that high pressures are momentarily generated above the sphincter.

A pharyngoesophageal diverticulum may be excised through an incision in the left side of the neck. Alternatively the diverticulum may be sutured high in the neck so that it empties downward and food is unable to enter it (diverticulopexy). At the same time the fibers of the cricopharyngeus are divided (myotomy). This treatment is probably adequate, excision being reserved for large diverticula.

Epiphrenic Diverticulum

The epiphrenic diverticulum is uncommon. It develops just above the lower esophageal sphincter and usually is associated with hiatal hernia, achalasia, diffuse esophageal spasm, or a hypertensive lower sphincter. It is therefore important to study the function of the gastroesophageal sphincter by cinefluoroscopy and manometry. Many patients require a lower esophageal myotomy in addition to excision of the diverticulum. Excision as a sole procedure is frequently followed by leakage from the suture line.

ACHALASIA

Achalasia is a disease of the entire esophagus in which the lower sphincter fails to relax during swallowing and the body of the esophagus shows an elevated resting pressure, absence of true peristaltic waves, and a series of pressure peaks occurring simultaneously at different levels.[2] It is more accurate than cardiospasm because there is no increase in resting pressure in the sphincter. True propulsive movement is absent and swallowing depends largely on gravity. The basic abnormality is in the myenteric nerve plexus, and there is an excessive response to cholinergic drugs such as Mecholyl. This illustrates Cannon's law that a denervated end organ is increasingly sensitive to the normally liberated chemotransmitter substance, such as acetylcholine or its analogues. The increased contraction in response to Mecholyl has led to its use in diagnosis. As the nerve supply is primarily through the vagus, it might be expected that other abnormalities of vagal innervation might be present. It has been shown that insulin hypoglycemia in patients with achalasia often fails to elicit a gastric secretory response.

The symptoms of achalasia are dysphagia, pain, regurgitation, and weight loss. Some patients present with unusual features, such as mediastinal tumor on chest x-ray, pyrexia of unknown origin, pulmonary symptoms, or hiccough. Dysphagia is usually worse on taking liquids than solids, the reverse to an organic stricture. Patients are often aware of food being held up and experience relief as it moves on. Regurgitation may occur during eating or afterward, and may occur during sleep. The regurgitated food does not have the sour taste of gastric contents. Carcinoma may develop even after successful surgical treatment.

Diagnosis

The diagnosis is confirmed by barium swallow, cinefluoroscopy, esophagoscopy, and manometry. On x-ray there is conical narrowing at the gastroesophageal junction, and later the esophagus becomes greatly dilated, tortuous, and even sigmoid in shape. On plain x-ray an air fluid level may be visible in the chest, and as the fluid in the esophagus acts as a trap, the gastric air bubble is frequently absent. The muscular activity of the esophagus is greatly increased on giving Mecholyl subcutaneously. Manometry confirms typical muscle abnormality. Esophagoscopy often shows much retained fluid and food, but the instrument can be passed easily through the lower sphincter.

Management

Muscle relaxants and antispasmodics are of little benefit. Dilatation with mercury-laden bougies provides some degree of palliation and may be useful in frail subjects. Of more lasting benefit is forceful dilatation with a pneumatic bag passed to the level of the sphincter. If this fails, then operation should be undertaken. The recommended procedure is a Heller myotomy through the chest or abdomen, in which all the muscle fibers are divided down to the mucosa for

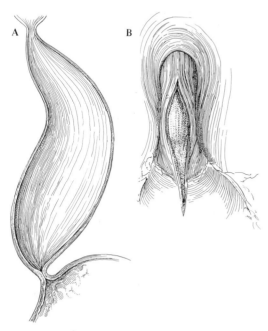

Figure 17–6. A Heller's operation for achalasia of the esophagus. The muscularis is divided longitudinally to expose the mucosa.

5 cm up the esophagus and 2 cm on to the stomach (Figure 17–6). It is advisable to dissect the muscle off the mucosa for a short distance to allow the mucosa to bulge freely. Seventy-five to 80 percent of patients experience complete relief of symptoms. Unsatisfactory results occur unless special steps are taken to repair the hiatus to prevent reflux. The esophagus does not return to normal size after operation, and follow-up must continue to detect recurrence, reflux, or carcinoma.

TUMORS

Benign

The commonest benign tumor of the esophagus is the leiomyoma. It occurs most frequently in the lower one third, is well circumscribed, rarely encapsulated, and varies in size. It may be intramural, intraluminal and pedunculated, or extramural and presenting as a mediastinal mass. Mucosal ulceration is uncommon, and bleeding is therefore usually absent. Half the lesions are asymptomatic and found incidentally. The remainder present with dysphagia or regurgitation when they have reached a critical size. On plain x-ray a tumor may be seen in the posterior mediastinum in the line of the esophagus, and sometimes it is calcified. The barium swallow may show an intraluminal filling defect, and on profile view there may be an acute angle between the tumor and the esophageal wall. Esophagoscopy may disclose a smooth mass with intact epithelium. The operative treatment is very satisfactory, as the lesion can usually be enucleated without incising the mucosa, and the defect in the muscle layers easily sutured.

Malignant: Carcinoma

Etiologic Factors.   The incidence of cancer of the esophagus is low in the United States, England, and Sweden, but high in Japan, Puerto Rico, Jamaica, and certain parts of Africa. These differences have not been explained, although it has been suggested that dietary factors such as nitrosamines may be responsible. These substances, which can be used experimentally to induce esophageal carcinoma, are found in certain plants in molybdenum-deficient soils in parts of Africa where the tumor is common.

Cancer of the esophagus tends to occur in men after the age of 50, especially in those who are edentulous, have poor teeth, are heavy smokers, are alcoholics, and in those who have had another cancer of the mouth or pharynx. Predisposing conditions include the Plummer-Vinson syndrome, achalasia, and tylosis, a hereditary disorder characterized by abnormal thickening of the palms and soles.

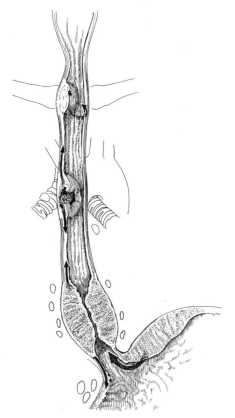

Figure 17–7. Esophageal carcinoma usually occurs at the levels of the clavicle, the carina, and, most commonly, the lower third. Such a lesion can spread through the submucosal layer around the circumference or longitudinally in either direction. The gastroesophageal junction does not act as an efficient barrier against this spread.

Pathophysiology. Carcinoma of the esophagus usually develops in the hypopharynx or postcricoid region, in the midesophagus at the level of the aortic arch, or just above the esophagogastric junction (Figure 17–7). Most tumors are squamous cell, although adenocarcinoma may be found near the cardia, probably arising from gastric epithelium, or less commonly higher in the esophagus where it can arise in isolated islands of columnar epithelium.

The tumor arises in mucosa but soon spreads along the submucosa and through the wall of the adventitia. Spread then readily occurs to the loose areolar mediastinal tissue because of the absence of a serosa and to the adjacent lymph nodes. The nodes communicate below with the left gastric and hepatic nodes and above with the paratracheal and cervical nodes. Symptoms of dysphagia usually do not occur until at least half the circumference is involved and initially do not reflect intraluminal obstruction but probably uncoordinated motor activity.

Clinical Features. The onset of dysphagia in anyone over age 45, especially in a male, should raise the suspicion of esophageal cancer. The main symptom of dysphagia frequently develops insidiously. At first meat and bread are swallowed with difficulty and later liquids and finally saliva. Acute esophageal obstruction may develop if a bolus of food becomes impacted above the tumor. Increasing weight loss is common. Pain is a late symptom, usually indicating mediastinal involvement. The barium swallow shows a persistent filling defect or stricture with gradual narrowing of the lumen and usually no dilatation of the esophagus. A soft tissue mass may be visible. At esophagoscopy the tumor can be seen and biopsed, mobility can be assessed, and washings obtained from the lumen for cytology. In midesophageal lesions bronchoscopy is useful to exclude widening of the carina, suggesting mediastinal node involvement and tracheoesophageal fistula.

The main diseases in the differential diagnosis are stricture from reflux esophagitis or corrosive esophagitis, achalasia, pressure on the esophagus by metastatic nodes, and benign tumors, especially a leiomyoma. Crohn's disease has been reported in the esophagus.

Management

The patient with esophageal cancer is generally elderly, frail, malnourished, often with pulmonary complications. Considerable preoperative preparation, including hyperalimentation, is often needed.

Excision. Excision is the commonest attempted curative treatment for carcinomas below the aortic arch. The tumor is removed as a block with at least 5 cm of normal esophagus proximal to tumor, and reconstruction achieved usually by esophagogastrostomy[9] (Figure 17–8). The operative mortality is around 20 to 30 percent, and the chances of surviving five years are less than 10 percent. Total esophagectomy may be done in patients with carcinomas high in the thorax or in the lower cervical esophagus. Reconstruction may be accomplished using a colon bypass tunneled subcutaneously or in the posterior mediastinum. Lesions of the hypopharynx can be treated by extensive resection of larynx, pharynx, thyroid, and cervical esophagus and insertion of a colon bypass.

Radiotherapy. Radiotherapy may be used to attempt cure for carcinoma situated above the aortic arch.[7] Only occasionally is it necessary to establish a gastroscopy.

Combined Surgery and Radiotherapy. Preoperative radiotherapy has been used to reduce

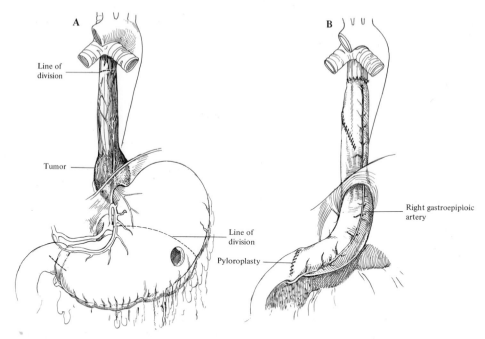

Line of
division

Tumor

Line of
division

Pyloroplasty

Right gastroepiploic
artery

Figure 17–8. *A.* The amount of esophagus and stomach removed in carcinoma of the esophagus is shown. *B.* Reconstruction is performed by anastomosing the esophagus to the remnant of the stomach. A pyloroplasty is performed to provide gastric drainage because bilateral vagotomy is performed during the procedure.

the size of the tumor and to diminish the incidence of tumor cells in the adventitia and in the edges of the resected specimen.[5] Either a short course of radiotherapy is given, 2000 to 3000 rads for about one week, followed by operation, or 5000 to 6000 rads in four to five weeks followed by operation in two weeks. The rationale of these approaches is to destroy carcinoma tumor cells in the lesion and surrounding tissues and to prevent local recurrence after excision, which is the main cause of death. The preliminary results of both methods show an increase in the five-year survival to 25 percent.

Palliation. The attempted curative treatments, even if they do not cure, provide palliation for the distressing symptoms of dysphagia and regurgitation. Good palliation is achieved by excision of the lesion, and radiotherapy will in many patients cause the stricture to open up. When the stricture does not open after radiotherapy or if excision is unsuitable, a permanent intraluminal plastic tube may be inserted through the tumor and fixed in the stomach at gastrotomy (Celestin, Mousseau-Barbin) (Figure 17–9). An alternative is to dilate the stricture with a bougie, pass a string into the stomach, and carry out intermittent bougienage over the string to permit swallowing. Most tumors are necrotic in

the center and respond to dilatation. Feeding gastrostomy provides no palliation of dysphagia and should not be done unless it is part of an overall plan for more radical treatment of the tumor.

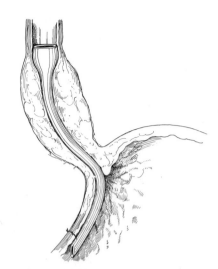

Figure 17–9. A tube may be inserted through the stricture produced by an advanced carcinoma of the esophagus. This procedure provides better palliation than a gastrostomy.

CITED REFERENCES

1. Allison, P. R.: Reflux esophagitis, sliding hiatus hernia and the anatomy of repair. *Surg. Gynecol. Obstet.*, **92**:419–31, 1951.
2. Ellis, F. H.; Code, C. F.; and Olsen, A. M.: Long esophagomyotomy for diffuse spasm of the esophagus and hypertensive gastroesophageal sphincter. *Surgery*, **48**:155–69, 1960.
3. Ellis, F. H.; Garabedian, M.; and Gregg, J. A.: Fundoplication for gastroesophageal reflux. A comparison of preoperative and early postoperative manometric findings. *Chest*, **62**:142–45, 1972.
4. Hiebert, C. A., and Belsey, R.: Incompetency of the gastric cardia without radiologic evidence of hiatal hernia. *J. Thorac. Cardiovasc. Surg.*, **42**:352–62, 1961.
5. Nakayama, K.: Preoperative irradiation in the treatment of patients with carcinoma of the oesophagus and of some other sites. *Clin. Radiol.*, **15**:232–41, 1964.
6. Olsen, A. M., and Creamer, B.: Studies of oesophageal motility, with special reference to the differential diagnosis of diffuse spasm and achalasia (cardiospasm). *Thorax.* **12**:279–89, 1957.
7. Pearson, J. G.: The value of radiotherapy in the management of squamous oesophageal cancer. *Br. J. Surg.*, **58**:794–98, 1971.
8. Prolla, J. C.; Taebel, D. W.; and Kirsner, J. B.: Current status of exfoliative cytology in diagnoses of malignant neoplasm of the esophagus. *Surg. Gynecol. Obstet.*, **121**:743–52, 1965.
9. Wilkins, E. W., and Skinner, D. B.: Surgery of the esophagus. *N. Eng. J. Med.*, **278**:824–28, 1968.

SUGGESTIONS FOR FURTHER READING

Esophagus. In: *Year Book of Surgery.* Year Book Medical Publishers, Inc., Chicago, pp. 326–42, 1974.
Abstracts of a number of articles on reflux esophagitis. Of particular interest is Denis P. Burkitt's article on the relation of constipation due to a low roughage diet on the etiology of reflux esophagitis.
Parker, E. F., and Gregorie, H. B., Jr.: Carcinoma of the esophagus. In: *Current Problems in Surgery.* Year Book Medical Publishers, Inc., Chicago, April 1967.
A comprehensive review of all aspects of carcinoma of the esophagus.
Stout, A. P., and Lattes, R.: *Tumors of the Esophagus.* Washington, D.C., Armed Forces Institute of Pathology, Fascicle 20, 1957.
An extremely well-illustrated description of the gross and microscopic findings in esophageal tumors.

Chapter 18

STOMACH AND DUODENUM

John A. McCredie

CHAPTER OUTLINE

Anatomy and Histology of the Stomach
  Blood Supply
  Lymphatic Supply
  Nerve Supply
    Sympathetic Nerve Supply
Function of the Stomach
  Mucus Barrier
  Peptic Digestion
  Secretion of Hydrochloric Acid
  Control of Gastric Acid Secretion
    Cephalic Phase
    Gastric Phase
    Intestinal Phase
Gastric Emptying
Peptic Ulcer
  Treatment
    Conservative Management
    Operative Management
  Rationale for Surgery of Peptic Ulcer
    Disease
Postoperative Complications
  Malabsorption
  Steatorrhea
  Anemia
  Osteomalacia
  Dumping Syndrome
    Treatment
  Late Hypoglycemia Symptoms
Acute Upper Gastrointestinal Bleeding
  Management
    Conservative Management

  Operative Management
  Operations
Perforated Peptic Ulcer
  Treatment
Pyloric Stenosis
Mallory-Weiss Syndrome
Injuries of the Stomach and Duodenum
Carcinoma of the Stomach
  Pathology
  Clinical Presentation
    "Silent" Presentation
    Obstruction
  Investigation
    Radiology
    Gastroscopy
    Other Investigations
  Differential Diagnosis
    Benign Ulcer
    Gastric Polyp
    Leiomyosarcoma
    Lymphoma
  Treatment
    Attempted Curative
    Palliative
Duodenum
  Peptic Ulcer
  Tumors
  Diverticulum
  Duodenal Obstruction by Superior Mesen-
    teric Artery

ANATOMY AND HISTOLOGY OF THE STOMACH

The stomach consists of the fundus, body, and antrum (see Plates IV and VI). The gastric mucosa is thrown up into a series of longitudinal folds which run roughly parallel to the greater curvature. The folds are most prominent on the greater curvature, small along the lesser curvature, and almost obliterated in the distended stomach. In patients with large outputs of gastric acid the rugal folds are large and extend high up into the fundus, while in patients with a low acid output the rugal folds are much less prominent. In achlorhydria and complete gastric atrophy the folds are absent, and the mucosa has a bald appearance.

The fundus of the stomach serves mainly as a reservoir and also secretes mucosa. It is lined by gastric pits consisting almost entirely of pale-staining, mucus-secreting cells of uniform appearance. Similar cells are seen elsewhere in the stomach. At the bottom of the gastric pits the cells are flatter and contain more mitotic figures, indicating that cell reproduction is occurring in the depths of the pits and that the cells migrate upward toward the surface epithelium. The cells of the fundus, in common with those of the tongue and esophagus, have a relatively slow turnover time of five days. However, in the body of the stomach and the antrum, the epithelial cells migrate to the surface more rapidly, taking only one day for the whole cycle. The rapid rate of turnover of mucosal cells, particularly in the body and antrum and in the small bowel, reflects the rapid rate of cell division in these tissues and makes them extremely vulnerable to cytotoxic agents.

The body of the stomach, in addition to the mucus-secreting cells, has complex branching glands which contain parietal (oxyntic) cells producing acid and peptic (chief) cells which produce pepsin. The parietal cells are large, devoid of granules, and stain bright with eosin, whereas the peptic cells are small, found only in the body of the stomach, and contain pepsinogen granules. These granules disappear from the cells on vagal stimulation.

The pyloric antrum is lined with mucus-secreting cells that produce an alkaline secretion containing intrinsic factor. In addition, the antrum secretes the hormone gastrin into the blood stream which stimulates secretion of acid by the parietal cells.

Blood Supply

The stomach has a rich blood supply from branches of the celiac axis. The left gastric artery descends along the lesser curvature and is the main blood supply to the stomach. Its terminal branches anastomose with the right gastric artery, a branch of the gastroduodenal artery. The right part of the greater curvature has the right gastroepiploic artery, a terminal branch of the duodenal artery, and the left aspect is supplied by the left gastroepiploic artery, a branch of the splenic artery. The top of the greater curvature and the fundus of the stomach are supplied by the short gastric branches of the splenic artery. Veins are closely related to the arteries.

Lymphatic Supply

There is a rich lymphatic drainage from the stomach to nodes along the greater and lesser curvatures. The main drainage of the lesser curvature is to nodes along the left gastric artery and then to the celiac nodes at the origin of the celiac arterial axis. There is a small lymphatic drainage of the lower part of the lesser curvature to nodes along the right gastric artery to nodes behind the pylorus, related to the gastroduodenal artery and hence to the celiac nodes. The right half of the greater curvature lymphatic drainage is to the nodes along the right gastroepiploic nodes and to those around the gastroduodenal artery. The upper half of the stomach and the fundus drain into nodes along the left gastroepiploic nodes, then in the gastrosplenic and gastrophrenic omentum to nodes at the hilum of the spleen, and then to nodes along the upper margin of the pancreas to the celiac nodes.

Nerve Supply

The parasympathetic nerve supply to the stomach, small bowel, and proximal colon as far as the middle third of the transverse colon is mediated through the vagus nerves. The two vagal trunks accompany the esophagus through the diaphragm, one lying anteriorly and arising mainly from the left vagus and the other lying posteriorly and arising predominantly from the right vagus. The anterior nerve divides into two branches soon after it passes through the diaphragm; the anterior gastric branch supplies the anterior aspect of the stomach down to the pyloric antrum, and the hepatic branch passes to the liver and gallbladder in the lesser omentum and also supplies a branch to the pyloric antrum (the nerve of Latarjet). The posterior nerve lies behind and to the right of the esophagus and also divides into two branches supplying the posterior part of the stomach (and pyloric antrum) and the celiac plexus for subsequent distribution to the other abdominal viscera. Total or truncal vagotomy aims at dividing both nerve trunks and any accessory trunks at the esophageal hiatus (Figure 18–1). Selective vagotomy, on the other hand, aims at dividing only the anterior and posterior branches which supply the stomach, preserving the hepatic branch of the left vagus and the celiac branch of the right vagus. Of all the nerve fibers comprising the vagal trunks, about 90 percent are afferent or sensory and the remainder are efferent. A more recent development has been the preservation of the nerves to the pyloric antrum, the nerves of Latarjet. These nerves supply the muscle of the pyloric antrum and if left intact enable the stomach to empty much better after division of the nerves to the acid-secreting cells. At present it also appears to make a gastric drainage procedure unnecessary.[14] This operation has been termed "highly selective vagotomy." Complete truncal vagotomy has the most important effect of causing a marked fall in gastric acid output and therefore is of considerable benefit in the management of duodenal ulcer. However, in addition, it denervates the gastric muscle, which results in a decrease in gastric tone and

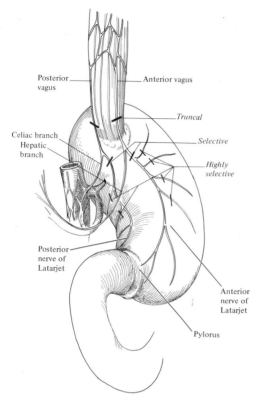

Figure 18–1. With truncal vagotomy both vagi are divided. In a selective vagotomy branches to the liver and gallbladder and to the celiac ganglion are preserved. With a highly selective vagotomy the branches to the pylorus are also preserved.

delayed gastric emptying that may last for weeks or months. Hence gastric vagotomy alone leads frequently to the undesirable side effect of gastric stasis with a feeling of gastric distention, flatulence, and perhaps vomiting. For this reason the truncal vagotomy is always accompanied by a gastric drainage procedure, which in the past was usually a gastroenterostomy but more recently pyloroplasty.

Sympathetic Nerve Supply. The efferent sympathetic fibers to the stomach arise from the sixth to ninth thoracic segments of the cord. The preganglionic fibers travel in the splanchnic nerves to their cell stations in the celiac ganglia. The postganglionic fibers follow the blood vessels to the stomach.

The vagi and the sympathetic nerves carry afferent or sensory fibers from the stomach. Pain impulses are thought to travel in the sympathetic nerves because the pain of a recurrent ulcer may persist after complete vagotomy, whereas patients who have had bilateral sympathectomy may perforate a peptic ulcer and not have pain.

FUNCTION OF THE STOMACH

The stomach acts as a reservoir for food and initiates digestion. The capacity to act as a reservoir depends on its size and also on its rate of emptying.

Mucus Barrier

In man gastric mucosa is covered by a 1.0- to 1.5-mm layer of mucus which protects the underlying mucosa from peptic digestion. The protection is physical and chemical. The mucus forms a semipermeable barrier which retains alkaline secretion in contact with epithelial cells. In addition, 100 ml of mucus can neutralize 40 ml of decinormal acid. Gastric mucus consists of a mixture of visible and dissolved mucus. Visible mucus is a thick, semiopaque material probably produced by the surface epithelial cells, whereas dissolved mucus is a viscid clear material in which visible mucus is suspended and secreted by the mucous cells at the necks of the crypts.

Peptic Digestion

Protein digestion is initiated in the stomach by hydrolysis of proteins to peptones and by combined action of pepsin and acid. It is completed in the small intestine by pancreatic enzymes which hydrolyze peptones to polypeptides and amino acids. Peptic digestion occurs only in an acid medium, which is maximal at pH 2 and stops at pH levels above 5. The vagus controls pepsin secretion. Gastric juice rich in pepsin is obtained by sham feeding, meat meals, insulin hypoglycemia, or administration of acetylcholine. The secretion of pepsin bears a close relationship to acid output, demonstrating their interdependence during peptic digestion.

Secretion of Hydrochloric Acid

The secretion of hydrochloric acid depends upon the presence of oxygen, and for each molecule of hydrochloric acid formed, a molecule of bicarbonate enters the blood stream. Acid secretion can be inhibited by a number of metabolic inhibitors, such as azide and 2:4 dinitrophenol, indicating that energy may be derived by aerobic glycolysis of various substrates, such as glucose, lactate, pyruvate, fructose, and acetoacetate, with the generation of high-energy phosphate bonds. Oxidation of these substrates liberates both electrons and energy which are capable of transferring the hydrogen ion from the cell to the gastric juice against a concentration gradient. An hydroxyl ion (OH^-) is formed for each hydrogen ion (H^+) secreted, and the interior of the cell becomes dangerously alkaline. Rapid neutralization of this pH change is accomplished with carbonic

A   B

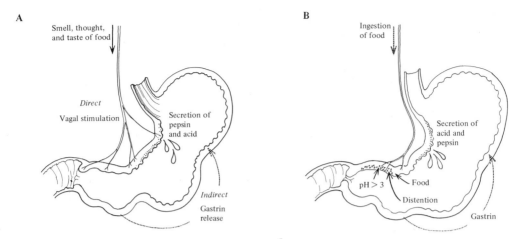

Figure 18–2. *A.* Vagal stimulation is responsible for cephalic stimulation of gastric secretion. *B.* The entry of food into the pyloric antrum initiates the gastric phase of gastric secretion.

acid catalyzed within the parietal cells by carbonic anhydrase. The hydroxyl ions formed are quickly replaced by an equal number of bicarbonate ions, which are discharged from the cells into the venous plasma, accounting for the more alkaline pH of gastric venous blood as compared with gastric arterial blood. This also explains the postprandial alkaline tide in the urine and a compensatory rise in the alveolar P_{CO_2}. Chloride is transported across the parietal cells by an active energy-consuming process or chloride pump that is coupled, ion for ion, with the pumping of hydrogen and the removal of bicarbonate from the cell.

Control of Gastric Acid Secretion

Acid secretion is controlled by (1) extrinsic nerves, (2) intrinsic nerves, and (3) humoral substances. Basal secretion is the acid output which persists after a 12-hour fast and is probably due to persisting vagal activity. It can be abolished by vagotomy or antrectomy. Patients with duodenal ulcer usually have a high basal secretion.

Cephalic Phase. This is the secretion that occurs in response to the thought, sight, or smell of food (Figure 18–2, *A*). This type of secretion comes on within about five minutes of the psychogenic stimulus and is rich in both acid and pepsin. It is abolished entirely by vagotomy.[3]

Gastric Phase. The gastric phase of secretion occurs shortly after food enters the stomach and persists for three to four hours (Figure 18–2, *B*). This is a highly acid juice, containing less pepsin than that secreted in the cephalic phase. The main stimulus for the gastric phase is the contact of food with the pyloric antrum, particularly meat products, alcohol, caffeine, and physical distention of the antrum. This phase is mediated

largely through the release of the antral hormone gastrin,[12] is abolished by antrectomy, and is considerably reduced by vagotomy. It is fairly well established that vagal innervation to the antrum makes it more responsive to the stimulus of secretagogues in the food, and that the liberated gastrin is more effective on the parietal cells in the presence of intact vagal innervation.[8]

Intestinal Phase. The intestinal phase of gastric acid secretion is less important than the other two phases in man. It is mediated through a humoral agent liberated from the small bowel, and it persists after vagotomy (Figure 18–3). The effects of the duodenal secretions on the digestion of fats, carbohydrates, and proteins are discussed in Chapters 19, 20, and 21.

GASTRIC EMPTYING

The walls of the fasting stomach are normally in contact except for the fundus, where they are separated by the gastric air bubble. Slight peristaltic activity is present in the fasting stomach, where it is possible to record small pressure rises about three times per minute as peristaltic waves are passed on to the pylorus. Every few hours bursts of more forceful and painful contractions occur called hunger contractions. When food is ingested, the gastric musculature relaxes allowing the stomach to distend and digestion to be initiated. Later movements recommence, initially to allow mixing and then to allow emptying as the pylorus relaxes. The pylorus, unlike the cardia, does not remain in a state of sustained contraction at rest but only remains closed for a few seconds after each burst of a wave from the antrum reaches it, relaxing between peristaltic waves. The pylorus therefore is not a true sphincter but serves as an

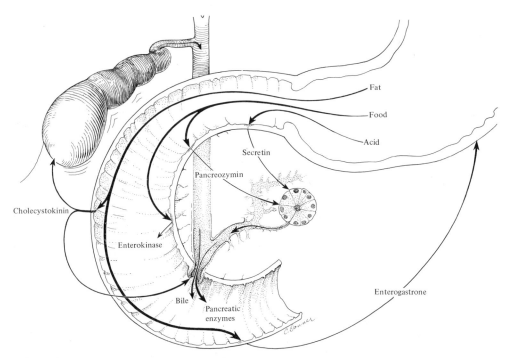

Figure 18–3. Gastric secretion is inhibited in the third or intestinal phase. The exact role of enterogastrone, duodenal secretions, and reflux of bicarbonate into the antrum is discussed in Chapter 21 (see page 356).

anatomic narrowing to prevent larger food particles from leaving the stomach. The main function of the pylorus seems to be to prevent regurgitation of duodenal contents back into the stomach during the few seconds after the peristaltic wave has passed through.

The rate of gastric emptying is proportional to the volume of the gastric content and depends upon the character of the meal and nervous factors. Large meals leave the stomach more rapidly than small meals, and large lumps of food are held back by the pylorus and delay emptying. Cold liquids leave the stomach more rapidly than hot liquids. Fatty foods, hypertonic or acid foods inhibit gastric motility and emptying. The latter effect is not abolished by vagotomy and is thought to be mediated by the release of the hormone enterogastrone which reduces gastric motility. The rate of gastric emptying can be determined by a barium meal, by aspiration of the stomach after fasting, or by aspiration two hours after giving 750 ml saline.

PEPTIC ULCER

A peptic ulcer may develop in the lower esophagus, stomach, duodenum, at the site of a gastrojejunostomy, or adjacent to a Meckel's

diverticulum (Figure 18–4). It may be associated with chronic liver or lung disease, chronic pancreatitis, Zollinger-Ellison syndrome, or hyperparathyroidism. The incidence is high in alcoholics, in those who take large amounts of

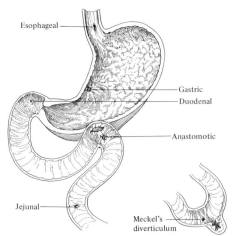

Figure 18–4. A peptic ulcer may develop in the esophagus, stomach, duodenum, at the site of a gastrojejunostomy, in the jejunum, or in or close to a Meckel's diverticulum containing gastric mucosa.

acetylsalicylic acid, phenylbutazone, and possibly prednisone.

The symptom is epigastric discomfort that is often described as burning. Pain tends to be related to eating and is frequently a hunger pain. It is relieved by food, milk, and antacids and aggravated by alcohol, smoking, spices, coffee, and often fried foods. Pain often wakens the patient at night. Remissions of several months are common, and the exacerbations last one to three weeks.

The diagnosis of chronic duodenal ulcer is most often established by barium meal. The ulcer may be visualized or its position may be recognized by persistence of barium in the ulcer. With time there is scarring and often diverticular formation if the ulcer is in its common position, the duodenal cap. Occasionally the ulcer is post-bulbar, in the second part of the duodenum. Chronic gastric ulcers are most often in the upper two thirds of the lesser curvature. Typically they are deep and penetrating and do not have rolled edges. The diagnosis, however, is frequently wrong; therefore gastroscopy and biopsy are indicated to establish it. The introduction of the flexible fiberoptic gastroscope and duodenoscope has led to visualization of the ulcer in most patients.

The 12-hour overnight secretion may be collected through a tube placed in the antrum. Normally about 20 mEq hydrochloric acid is secreted. With a chronic duodenal ulcer about 60 mEq is secreted and in a Zollinger-Ellison syndrome greater than 100 mEq. With a chronic gastric ulcer there is often a decrease in secretion of hydrochloric acid.

The pentagastrin test gives more accurate information about secretion of hydrochloric acid. Residual juice is removed from the fasting stomach and pentagastrin (6 μg/kg) is injected subcutaneously. Gastric juice is aspirated every 15 minutes for one hour. The Hollander insulin test is used to test for the completeness of vagotomy, most often in the patient who has developed an ulcer after vagotomy and pyloroplasty. A tube is placed in the fasting stomach and basal acid secretions obtained at four 15-minute intervals. Insulin, 20 units, is injected intravenously and gastric secretions aspirated every 15 minutes for two hours. The blood sugar level should be at least 35 mg/100 ml. Vagal fibers are intact if the acid secretion is increased by more than 20 mEq or by 10 mEq/liter if the basal sample had a zero concentration.

Treatment

Conservative Management. Conservative management of uncomplicated chronic peptic ulcer consists of eating six to eight times per day.[9]

The buffering action of food is important and not its content. Antacids, especially calcium carbonate, give symptomatic relief but augment gastrin release. Acetylsalicylic acid, alcohol, tea, coffee, spices, and other substances that increase gastric secretion should be avoided. Tranquilizers may be of value to decrease anxiety. Recently there has been interest in the use of carbenoxolone sodium to promote gastric ulcer healing. During acute exacerbations it may be necessary to confine the patient to bed and intensify the conservative management.

Operative Management. Operation is indicated for chronic gastric or duodenal ulcer when conservative management fails, as shown by intractability of symptoms and especially pain in the back from posterior penetration. Complications requiring operative treatment are perforation, bleeding unresponsive to conservative management, fibrotic obstruction, and any possibility of malignancy.

Rationale for Surgery of Peptic Ulcer Disease

A peptic ulcer results from the action of the enzyme pepsin on the mucosa of the alimentary tract. For pepsin to act there must be an acid environment. Peptic ulceration can occur as a result of excessive and prolonged secretion of pepsin and acid, as is probably the case in patients with duodenal ulcer disease, or it may be due to a decreased resistance of the mucosa to the action of acid and pepsin. The majority of duodenal ulcer patients have therefore excessive acid and pepsin secretion, whereas those with gastric ulcer have a normal or low-acid pepsin secretion. In gastric ulcer, since nothing can be done surgically to improve mucosal resistance, it is necessary to reduce the gastric secretion to very low levels or to combine this with removal of the ulcer-bearing region. Gastric ulcers can be cured in a high percentage of cases by a distal 40 to 50 percent gastrectomy, removing the antrum and taking the line of resection high on the lesser curve (Figure 18–5). More recently, a gastric ulcer has been treated by vagotomy and drainage without removal of the ulcer. Although this works in the majority of patients, some continue to have ulcer symptoms and a small number have a carcinoma in the ulcer. In those with an ulcer high on the lesser curve a four-quadrant biopsy should be taken to exclude the presence of a carcinoma, and the patient should be treated by vagotomy and pyloroplasty.

With duodenal ulcer simply excision is inadequate and recurrence generally follows. Surgical therapy is directed at reducing acid-pepsin secretion to a low level (Figure 18–6). This can be achieved by a high subtotal gastrectomy removing 60 to 70 percent of the stomach, by

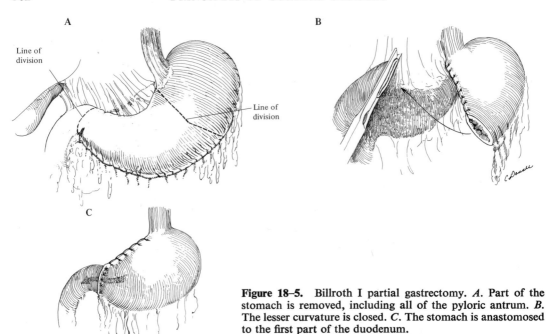

Figure 18–5. Billroth I partial gastrectomy. *A.* Part of the stomach is removed, including all of the pyloric antrum. *B.* The lesser curvature is closed. *C.* The stomach is anastomosed to the first part of the duodenum.

vagotomy and drainage, or by vagotomy and antrectomy. There is still no consensus as to the most suitable procedure.[5,6] On the one extreme, a total gastrectomy would invariably cure duodenal ulcer but would lead to a considerable mortality and morbidity. Simple gastroenterostomy, at the other extreme, has a very low morbidity, but the chance of curing the duodenal ulcer is only 50 percent. The chance of curing a duodenal ulcer by subtotal gastrectomy is 95 to 97 percent, but the mortality is 2 to 3 percent. Vagotomy combined with pyloroplasty or gastroenterostomy cures the ulcer in 90 to 95 percent of cases with a mortality of less than 1 percent[4] (Figure 18–7). Vagotomy and antrectomy occupy an intermediate position with a mortality of 1.5 to 2 percent and a cure rate of about 98 percent.[13] There is considerable interest in a number of clinical trials on the use of selective and highly selective vagotomy in the treatment of duodenal ulcer, and preliminary results show that these procedures are as effective as truncal vagotomy and have less morbidity.[10]

POSTOPERATIVE COMPLICATIONS

The physiologic side effects of gastrectomy vary from mild to severe. The alterations are greater after total than partial gastrectomy and are more marked when the gastric remnant is anastomosed to the jejunum than to the duodenum. Females are more susceptible to certain postgastrectomy symptoms than males.

The factors leading to the side effects are loss of hydrochloric acid and intrinsic factor and rapid emptying into the small intestine. Some of the nutritional defects, such as weight loss and vitamin deficiencies, may be aggravated by inadequate food intake. Also some of the postcibal symptoms such as bilious vomiting or dumping may cause the patient to decrease his food intake.

Malabsorption

Inability to put on weight occurs almost invariably after total gastrectomy and in one third to one half of patients after partial gastrectomy. The failure to gain weight is the result of diminished food intake due to postcibal symptoms, rapid gastric emptying, hypermotility of the intestine, decreased secretion of bile and pancreatic juice, poor mixing of food and secretions, decreased transmit time through the intestine reducing the time available for absorption, and bacterial contamination of the upper jejunum.

Steatorrhea

Chemical steatorrhea (fecal fat greater than 7 gm per 24 hours) occurs in 60 percent of patients after partial gastrectomy and in almost all patients after total gastrectomy. It is more frequent after a gastrojejunal than a gastroduodenal anastomosis. The concentration of bile and pancreatic enzymes is diminished following gastrectomy. The decrease in pancreatic secretion may be due to diminished stimulation from

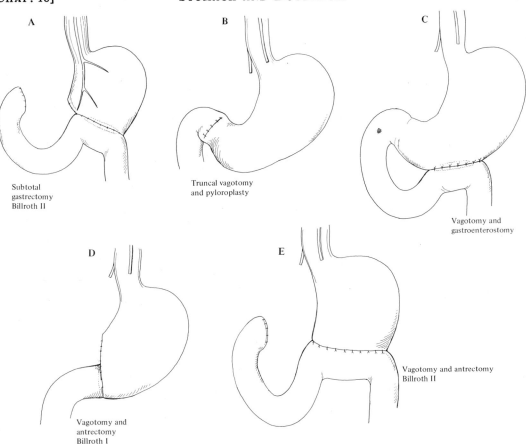

Figure 18–6.   The operations that may be performed for a duodenal ulcer. *A.* Subtotal gastrectomy with removal of all the pyloric antrum and anastomosis of the stomach to the jejunum (Billroth II procedure). *B.* Truncal or selective vagotomy with pyloroplasty or highly selective vagotomy without pyloroplasty. *C.* Vagotomy and gastrojejunostomy. *D.* Vagotomy and antrectomy with Billroth I procedure. *E.* Vagotomy and antrectomy with Billroth II reconstitution.

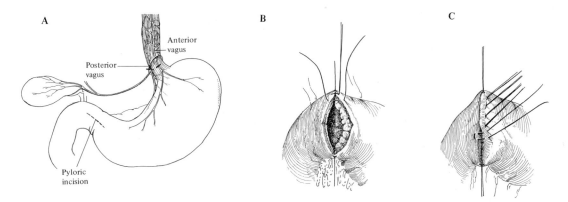

Figure 18–7.   In the operation of truncal vagotomy and pyloroplasty, (*A*) both vagi are divided below the diaphragm and a longitudinal incision may be made from the antrum, through the pylorus, and into the first part of the duodenum; (*B*) the pylorotomy incision is closed transversely; and (*C*) a second layer completes the pyloroplasty.

the gastric remnant and also from loss of duodenal stimulation when a gastrojejunal anastomosis has been made. Poor mixing of food with a diminished quantity of bile and pancreatic juice results in delay of fat hydrolysis so that a more distal level of bowel is reached before absorption can take place. Increased bacteria in the upper small bowel after gastrectomy may play a part in producing steatorrhea. Bacteria may interfere with the intraluminal phase of fat digestion, may metabolize some of the products of digestion, or may deconjugate the bile salts, which are then less effective as emulsifying agents.

Anemia

Iron deficiency anemia is less common than steatorrhea. About 30 percent of men and a greater number of women are anemic after partial gastrectomy. The rapid passage of food along the gut, bypass of the duodenum, and decrease in gastric acid are responsible for the malabsorption of iron.

After total gastrectomy vitamin B_{12} deficiency develops after three to four years. A megaloblastic anemia occurs after partial gastrectomy in about 1 percent, but subchemical deficiency, with a serum B_{12} level less than 200 μg per 100 ml, occurs in about 12 percent. Intestinal bacteria may also interfere with B_{12} absorption by metabolizing the vitamin.

Osteomalacia

Osteomalacia occasionally occurs some years after partial gastrectomy for duodenal ulcer. There are steatorrhea and failure of absorption of fat-soluble vitamin D. About 15 percent of patients after partial gastrectomy have some biochemical tendency to osteomalacia with elevation of the serum alkaline phosphatase.

Dumping Syndrome

Dumping occurs 10 to 20 minutes after eating and lasts for up to 60 minutes. The symptoms consist of dizziness, sweating, weakness, and drowsiness and may be accompanied by a feeling of epigastric distention and bilious vomiting. Physical, circulatory, nervous, or biochemical changes in the blood may be responsible. The physical factors may be related to rapid emptying of the stomach and the rapid movement of food through the small and large bowel. The circulatory changes consist of a 5 to 15 percent decrease in plasma volume, an increase in splanchnic and peripheral circulation, and perhaps shunting of blood away from the cerebrum and the heart. The reduced plasma volume appears to be due to the entry of hypertonic food into the upper jejunum and the sudden withdrawal of extracellular fluid into the bowel. Autonomic nervous stimulation may produce hypermotility of the bowel, hyperemia of the splanchnic bed, and decrease in blood flow to the brain and heart. The biochemical changes in the blood that have been implicated are both hypoglycemia and hyperglycemia. The plasma insulin levels, however, fail to support the concept that a slow insulin response may cause the symptoms. Hypermotility of the small bowel causes release of serotonin into the blood stream and may contribute to the symptoms.

Treatment. The patient should not eat hypertonic foods such as sugar, should lie down following a meal, and take small meals often separate from fluids. Atropine or hexamethonium may be given to decrease intestinal hypermotility and adrenergic blockers to antagonize the sympathetic overactivity. More recently serotonin antagonists have been used.

Dumping tends to be most severe immediately after an operation and tends to subside spontaneously within about six months. In those with persistent symptoms surgery may be indicated. Converting a gastrojejunal to a gastroduodenal anastomosis or interposing a loop of jejunum to increase the capacity of the gastric remnant may give relief.

Late Hypoglycemia Symptoms

In some patients a feeling of faintness, dizziness, and sweating occurs one to two hours after eating. It is almost always associated with a level of blood sugar below 50 mg per 100 ml. The mechanism is thought to be excessive insulin secretion after the rapid absorption of carbohydrate from the upper jejunum. These symptoms usually respond to additional sugar.

ACUTE UPPER GASTROINTESTINAL BLEEDING

Upper gastrointestinal bleeding may present with hematemesis and melena or melena alone.

The causes of upper gastrointestinal bleeding are (Figures 18–8, 18–9, and 18–10):

1. Peptic ulcer. The ulcer may be in the lower esophagus, stomach, or duodenum or at the site of a gastroenterostomy. The ulcer may be chronic and penetrate the muscularis mucosa. Alcohol, acetylsalicylic acid, prednisone, or phenylbutazone may precipitate the bleeding.

2. Stress ulcer. Patients who have undergone stress as from a burn, major operation, or multiple injuries may develop an acute hemorrhage. It is frequently encountered in intensive care departments in patients who have undergone neurosurgical operations and who have been hypoxic.[11]

3. Esophageal varices. Patients with portal

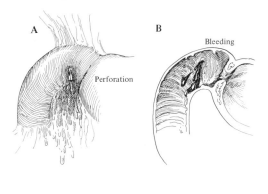

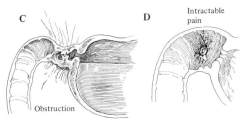

Figure 18–8. The indications for operation for duodenal ulcer are (*A*) perforation, (*B*) bleeding, (*C*) obstruction, and (*D*) intractable pain, often associated with penetration into the pancreas.

hypertension may bleed acutely from varices in the lower esophagus or cardia of the stomach. The blood tends to be plum red, profuse, and bleeding is generally not accompanied by pain.

4. Superficial gastritis. An atrophic or hypertrophic gastritis may lead to profuse bleeding. In the hypertrophic form there is often a history of alcohol consumption. The major factor in hemorrhage from gastritis is aspirin, not alcohol.

5. Mallory-Weiss syndrome. An acute bout of vomiting may tear the mucosa adjacent to the hiatus.

6. Tumors. The mucosa over a leiomyoma or leiomyosarcoma tends to ulcerate and may give rise to a brisk hemorrhage. Carcinomas of the stomach cause chronic blood loss and anemia but rarely present as a massive upper gastrointestinal hemorrhage.

7. Other causes. Reflux esophagitis may lead to chronic blood loss but rarely causes an acute hemorrhage. Other causes are foreign bodies, such as razor blades, and hemorrhagic diatheses.

Management

Conservative Management. 1. The history and physical examination are often helpful in determining the amount and the cause of the hemorrhage.

2. A gastric tube should be inserted to determine if the bleeding is from the upper gastrointestinal tract. A source of bleeding below the duodenojejunal junction is unlikely to give rise to blood in the gastric aspirate. It may be advisable initially to insert a large gastric tube, such as an Ewald tube, to remove blood clot. The subsequent course of the bleeding can be followed by aspirate through a small tube. Opinions differ on the value of gastric irrigation with cold saline. A Sengstaken–Blakemore tube may be inserted in the patient with suspected esophageal varices to control bleeding or to help establish the diagnosis.

Intravenous electrolytes, colloids, and blood are given to maintain a normal blood volume with monitoring of the general condition, pulse, blood pressure, central venous pressure, urinary output, hemoglobin, and hematocrit. An attempt should be made to maintain the hemoglobin at 10 to 11 gm per 100 ml.

Gastroscopy should be performed following initial resuscitation to visualize the cause and site of the bleed. Diazepam, 10 mg, is injected intravenously and lidocaine sprayed in the throat. A flexible fiberoptic endoscope can then be inserted. The presence of fresh or altered blood

Figure 18–9. Causes of acute upper gastrointestinal bleeding include the following: peptic ulcer complicating reflux esophagitis; varices; gastric or duodenal ulcer; acute gastritis, often associated with intake of aspirin, alcohol, prednisone, or phenylbutazone; a foreign body; the Mallory-Weiss syndrome; or a tumor, which may be polyp, leiomyoma, leiomyosarcoma, or ulcerating carcinoma. About 40 percent are due to peptic ulcer, 30 percent to acute gastritis, 10 percent to varices, and 5 percent to the Mallory-Weiss syndrome.

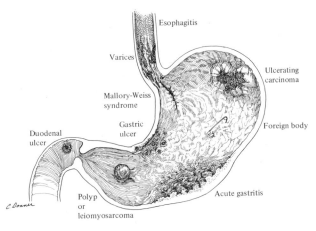

A

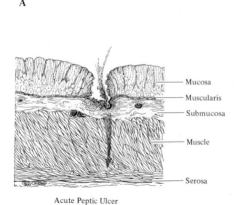

Acute Peptic Ulcer

B

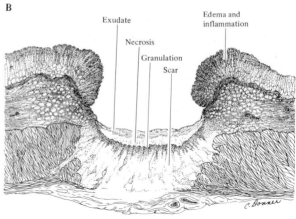

Chronic Peptic Ulcer

C

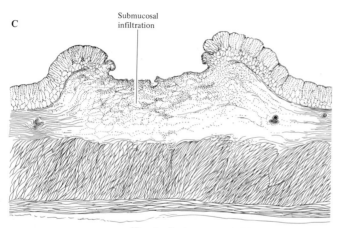

Ulcerating Carcinoma

Figure 18–10. The three main types of gastric ulceration. *A.* A superficial gastric erosion or stress ulcer that penetrates to the muscularis mucosa. This ulcer can be complicated by perforation. *B.* A chronic peptic ulcer that tends to penetrate the muscle layers. An acute erosion or chronic peptic ulcer may give rise to acute upper gastrointestinal bleeding. *C.* A carcinoma that tends to have raised edges from submucosal spread of the tumor and may infiltrate but not completely replace the muscle. It is an uncommon cause of acute upper gastrointestinal bleeding.

in the stomach is noted and whether the lesion is an erosion, ulcer, neoplasm, or angioma. It is of greater value to know if multiple lesions are present.

An upper gastrointestinal x-ray may be performed but is less accurate than endoscopy. Clot in the stomach often makes visualization of an ulcer difficult, and erosions cannot be seen on x-ray.

Selective angiography of the celiac axis or superior mesenteric artery may reveal the bleeding site and demonstrate whether the lesion is a hemangioma or tumor. Generally angiography is of less value in the diagnosis of upper gastrointestinal than of lower gastrointestinal bleeding.

Operative Treatment. Patients who are likely to continue to bleed should be identified early and operated on as soon as an optimum general condition is obtained (Figure 18–11). However, it should be appreciated that only about 20 percent of patients with upper intestinal bleeding from a peptic ulcer require surgery.

An absolute indication is a massive hemorrhage that does not respond to transfusion. This is uncommon and usually indicates that the gastroduodenal or left gastric arteries have been eroded. Occasionally an ulcer perforates, giving rise to peritonitis and in addition upper gastrointestinal bleeding. A further absolute indication for operation is bleeding in a patient with pyloric stenosis. Generally pyloric stenosis is not associated with an active ulcer, but occasionally the ulcer penetrates a vessel. The fibrosis results in the vessel being unable to retract; therefore the bleeding tends to continue.

Two or more relative indications should be present for operation to be needed. The most important is age. The older the patient, the more likely is bleeding to continue because of the high incidence of atherosclerosis which prevents vessel retraction. Also the ulcer is more likely to be associated with fibrosis. The relative indication of age is arbitrarily present when the patient is over 50. Other relative indications are bleeding

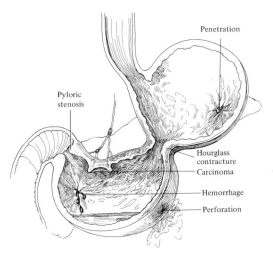

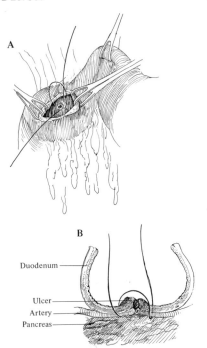

Figure 18–11. Operation is indicated for select-ed patients with bleeding from a gastric ulcer. In addition, surgery may be necessary for (1) perforation, (2) penetration producing intrac-tability of symptoms, (3) the possibility of a carcinoma, (4) obstruction in the body of the stomach producing an hourglass contracture, and (5) pyloric stenosis.

Figure 18–12. A bleeding ulcer in the posterior wall of the first part of the duodenum is treated at operation by (*A*) making a longitudinal incision in the lower stomach with extension into the duodenum, then identifying the bleeding vessel by removing a clot; and (*B*) underpin-ning each bleeding vessel. A vagotomy and pyloroplasty are then most often performed.

continuing for 24 hours while under treatment, recurrence of bleeding while under treatment, and pain radiating to the back suggesting that the ulcer is penetrating posteriorly.

Operations

Bleeding from an ulcer in the first part of the duodenum is treated by opening the stomach and duodenum through a longitudinal anterior incision through the pylorus (Figure 18–12). Clot is removed so as to identify the bleeding vessels. Each vessel is underpinned with a mattress suture. A pyloroplasty and vagotomy are then performed. Formerly treatment was by subtotal gastrectomy including the ulcer or, if it was left, bleeding vessels were underpinned. The mortality from this greater procedure is higher than for underpinning, pyloroplasty, and vagot-omy. A bleeding gastric ulcer, tumor, or heman-gioma is best treated by partial gastrectomy including the lesion. Occasionally when an ulcer is high and cannot be removed without perform-ing a total gastrectomy, the bleeding vessels may be underpinned, four-quadrant biopsies obtained to exclude a carcinoma, and a distal gastrectomy performed. In those with diffuse erosions or gastritis or the Zollinger-Ellison syndrome, treatment should be total gastrectomy.

PERFORATED PEPTIC ULCER

An ulcer on the anterior aspect of the duodenal bulb is especially liable to perforate, giving rise to local or generalized peritonitis. The patient may have a history of peptic ulcer and may have had a recent exacerbation. Frequently the patient presents with perforation without a history of peptic ulceration. The onset of the severe pain is dramatically sudden. The patient often collapses or doubles up with pain, vomits, and is pale and gray. The pain is initially epigastric but soon radiates through the whole abdomen and occasionally to the shoulders. The pain often decreases, and the color improves during the subsequent one to two hours, possibly because of exudation of fluid into the peritoneal cavity. On examination the patient lies still and breathes lightly to avoid pain from irritation of the parietal peritoneum. There are generalized abdominal tenderness and rigidity. If considerable air is in the peritoneal cavity, liver dullness may be de-creased. The serum amylase is often increased because of escape of pancreatic enzymes into the peritoneal cavity. An upright film of the abdomen generally shows air below the dia-phragm, but occasionally it is absent even with generalized peritonitis.

If the patient is not treated, the signs of para-

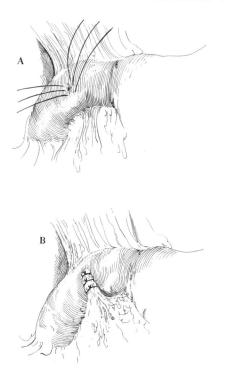

Figure 18–13. Closure of a perforation on the anterior aspect of the first part of the duodenum by (*A*) inserting interrupted sutures transversely and (*B*) tying the sutures over adjacent omentum.

lytic ileus appear after about 15 hours, namely distention, vomiting, and absence of peristalsis.

Intra-abdominal conditions that may be mistaken for perforation are acute pancreatitis, acute cholecystitis, internal strangulation, and acute appendicitis, especially in the geriatric patient. Thoracic diseases are myocardial infarction, basal pneumonia, and rupture of the esophagus, while retroperitoneal causes are acute herpes zoster and rupture of an aneurysm.

Treatment

Operation is indicated in patients with a perforated peptic ulcer. A nasogastric tube is inserted to prevent further escape of fluid into the peritoneal cavity and to prevent aspiration during induction of anesthesia. Intravenous fluids are given to correct the fluid deficit. Laparotomy is performed through an upper abdominal midline incision (Figure 18–13). The escape of gas and fluid confirms the diagnosis. The perforation is most often found on the anterior aspect of the duodenal cap. The ulcer is closed using a mattress suture or oversewn with a piece of omentum. In some centers definitive treatment of the ulcer, namely sub-

total gastrectomy or vagotomy and pyloroplasty, has been performed; however, this has not gained general acceptance. In those with a perforated carcinoma of the stomach partial gastrectomy, including the tumor, is performed. All fluid is carefully suctioned from the peritoneal cavity. Drainage is generally not established unless the perforation has lasted over 24 hours.

In some centers generalized peritonitis from perforation is treated conservatively by nasogastric suction, intravenous fluid replacement, and antibiotics. There has been little support for this treatment in North America and the United Kingdom. A perforation that has given rise to peritonitis involving the upper abdomen and even down along the right paracolic gutter to the right iliac fossa may be treated conservatively, provided the signs of peritoneal irritation do not spread to involve the whole abdomen.

The mortality is related to the duration of the perforation and the age of the patient. It is less than 2 percent in patients under 50 with less than 24 hours duration. Subsequently the mortality rises sharply.

PYLORIC STENOSIS

A chronic duodenal or antral ulcer may result in marked fibrosis with obstruction to gastric emptying. The stomach hypertrophies to overcome the obstruction but eventually distends. The patient then vomits large amounts of previously eaten food, usually every two or three days. Pain is usually absent but weight loss is generally marked. Examination may elicit upper abdominal distention and a succussion splash. The obstruction may be due to edema and may subside after several days of conservative management.

Treatment is daily insertion of a gastric tube and gastric irrigation and intravenous fluids containing a large number of calories and amino acids. A metabolic alkalosis from loss of hydrogen and potassium ions may have to be corrected. Operative treatment generally consists of partial gastrectomy, but a gastrojejunostomy may be adequate in the elderly patient. Vagotomy and pyloroplasty are not indicated because loss of parasympathetic innervation to the stomach tends to aggravate the gastric distention.

MALLORY-WEISS SYNDROME

A sudden increase in intra-abdominal pressure, as with vomiting or coughing, or of thoracic pressure, as with closed cardiac massage, may produce a mucosal tear (Figure 18–14) in the lower esophagus or cardia of the stomach.[2] The commonest cause is vomiting associated with alcoholism. The patient has trivial to severe

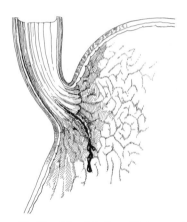

Figure 18–14. The Mallory-Weiss syndrome consists of a tear in the mucosa in the lower esophagus and upper stomach, causing upper gastrointestinal bleeding.

upper gastrointestinal bleeding without any other symptoms. The diagnosis is generally made by esophagogastroscopy. Treatment is initially conservative with insertion of a naso-gastric tube, gastric lavage, sedation, and blood and fluid replacement. Vasopressin, 20 mg, may be given intravenously to produce vasoconstriction. If bleeding continues or recurs, operation is indicated. The stomach is opened and the tear is oversewn.

INJURIES OF THE STOMACH AND DUODENUM

Injuries of the stomach and duodenum may result from penetrating wounds or closed abdominal injury, especially automobile accidents. There are frequently associated injuries to the pancreas, liver, extrahepatic biliary system, portal vein, or inferior vena cava.

Diagnosis is difficult before operation. The presence of air in the retroperitoneal tissues suggests the diagnosis. At operation there is usually a large retroperitoneal hematoma associated with crepitus and bile staining. The peritoneum is divided lateral to the second part of the duodenum and the hepatic flexure mobilized. Occasionally a single tear can be repaired by suture, but often it is advisable to suture adjacent jejunum over the defect using the serosal patch technique. Occasionally with severe duodenal injuries and tear of the head of the pancreas, especially with rupture of the pancreatic duct and common bile duct, a pancreatico-duodenectomy (Whipple resection) may be necessary.

CARCINOMA OF THE STOMACH

The incidence of carcinoma of the stomach is high in Japan, Ireland, and the Scandinavian countries, and lower in the Western world, where it is now decreasing. The incidence in the United States is 12,000 per year and is exceeded by carcinoma of the colorectum (80,000 cases), and the pancreas (16,000). The disease is commoner in men than women.

The etiology is not known but is most likely related to diet, since the incidence in Orientals born in the United States approaches that of Caucasians. Smoked fish and spices have been implicated in regions with a high incidence. The incidence is about 20 percent greater in people with blood group A, possibly because most patients have a sulfaglycoprotein in the stomach that is biochemically similar to group A substance (see Chapter 4). Patients with achlorhydria, as in pernicious anemia, atrophic gastritis, and the Paterson-Plummer-Vinson syndrome, have marked increase in carcinoma of the stomach. Benign adenomatous polyps frequently become malignant. Opinions formerly differed on the incidence of benign gastric ulcers becoming malignant, but it is now felt that the change from benign to malignant is probably extremely rare. The problem is whether the ulcer is benign or malignant to begin with.

Pathology

The tumor may be fungating, forming a polypoid mass frequently in the fundus or greater curvature, or ulcerating, especially in the lower one third of the lesser curvature (Figure 18–15). A less frequent type is the diffuse, submucous, infiltrating linitis plastica or leather-bottle stomach which tends to spread throughout the complete stomach with minimal ulceration.

Microscopically the tumors are adenocarcinomas varying from well differentiated to anaplastic. Spread tends to occur locally in the submucosal layer, especially in the lymphatics, and this may not be recognized macroscopically. The tumor penetrates the muscle in the stomach wall and eventually the serosa. A posteriorly situated tumor tends to infiltrate the pancreas. One on the anterior aspect may invade the left lobe of the liver and a lesion on the lower part of the greater curvature the transverse colon. Tumors in the fundus may spread into the lower esophagus and be mistaken for a primary carcinoma of the esophagus (Figure 17–7, page 293).

Lymphatic spread of tumors on the lesser curvature is upward to nodes along the left gastric vessels to the celiac nodes. Tumors in the lower half of the greater curvature spread to the right to nodes along the right gastroepiploic and gastroduodenal vessels and eventually to the celiac nodes. Spread from the upper half of the greater curvature is to nodes along the left

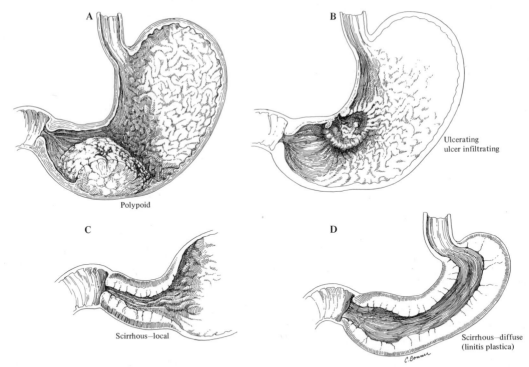

Figure 18–15.   The gross types of gastric carcinoma are (*A*) polypoid, (*B*) ulcerating, (*C*) local scirrhous infiltrating, or (*D*) diffuse submucosal infiltrating.

gastroepiploic and short gastric vessels to the hilum of the spleen and along the splenic vessels on the upper margin of the pancreas to the celiac nodes. Cancer cells in the lymphatics may reach the receptaculum chyli and thoracic duct and eventually enter the great vessels at the root of the neck. The cells may enter the jugular lymph ducts and form metastases in the left supraclavicular nodes (see Chapter 7). The nodes along the hepatic artery may contain metastases and obstruct the extrahepatic biliary ducts.

Hematogenous spread is primarily to the liver, and only occasionally are metastases seen in the lungs, brain, or bones.

When the tumor has penetrated the serous lining of the stomach, cancer cells pass freely through the peritoneal cavity and establish metastases in the great omentum, ovaries, and on the wall of the small intestine. Ascites develops as a reaction to the presence of free cells in the peritoneal cavity. Occasionally a metastasis grows deep to the umbilicus and presents as a palpable nodule.

Clinical Presentation

"Silent" Presentation.   The commonest presentation is loss of appetite of several weeks duration, epigastric discomfort, tiredness, unexplained weight loss, or anemia. Occasionally the patient notices a mass in the epigastrium or left lower neck. On routine examination a mass may be palpated in the epigastrium, umbilicus, or on rectal examination, or the patient may have ascites, jaundice, or hepatomegaly. Tumors in the fundus or the greater curvature are especially prone to a "silent" presentation.

Obstruction.   A carcinoma in the antrum is likely to cause obstruction and presents with symptoms earlier than a tumor elsewhere in the stomach. The symptoms of pyloric stenosis are vomiting generally after each meal. Patients with obstruction due to a benign ulcer have a larger stomach than occurs with a carcinoma and vomit every two to three days. The patient rapidly loses weight and develops hyponatremia, hypokalemia, and metabolic alkalosis. A tumor in the fundus may present with dysphagia and be diagnosed as a carcinoma of the esophagus.

Investigation

Radiology.   The upper gastrointestinal x-ray may suggest the presence of a carcinoma; however, the lesion may not be visualized, especially if it is situated in the fundus or along the greater curvature.[1] The position of the tumor may suggest the diagnosis. Lesions in the antrum, lower third of the lesser curvature, fundus, and along the greater curvature are most often malignant. The commonest site for a benign ulcer is the upper two thirds of the lesser curvature. The most important observation suggesting malignancy on x-ray is absence of peristalsis in the neighborhood of the tumor. This is especially demonstrable in patients with linitis plastica who may have no peristalsis in the stomach. The presence of a halo in the tumor is thought to suggest malignancy because of submucous spread at the tumor margin. Edema at the periphery of a benign ulcer may also produce this appearance. Depth and size of an ulcer are not important in suggesting the diagnosis.

Gastroscopy. Since the introduction of the flexible instrument, gastroscopy has become routine in the investigation of a gastric tumor. It visualizes lesions not seen on x-ray and allows biopsy and more accurate definition of size than on x-ray. The procedure is performed using diazepam, 10 mg intravenously.

Other Investigations. The absence of free acid in the gastric juice suggests that an ulcerating lesion is malignant. The fluid may be centrifuged and the sediment examined for cancer cells. The gastric juice has been examined for sulfoglycoprotein, a cancer-specific reversionary antigen present in the gastric secretion but not the blood of patients with carcinoma of the stomach.

Differential Diagnosis

Benign Ulcer. It was often difficult to differentiate a benign from a malignant ulcer when the diagnosis was based on history, physical findings, and radiology. With the widespread use of gastroscopy it is now possible to establish a tissue diagnosis in most patients. Views differ on the incidence of benign ulcers becoming cancers, with figures varying from 0.5 to 10 percent. The problem is more one of determining what a lesion is rather than the possibility of its becoming malignant.

Gastric Polyp. It can be difficult to differentiate a benign adenomatous polyp from a carcinoma, especially when the polyp is single. Other benign conditions that produce polyps are benign tumors such as leiomyoma, submucosa lipoma, or heterotopic pancreatic tumors. The presence of an intact mucosa suggests a benign lesion.

Leiomyosarcoma. A leiomyosarcoma may simulate a carcinoma closely, presenting as a large smooth mass that resembles a polypoid carcinoma. Frequently the mucosa becomes ulcerated and has a marked tendency to bleed often, resulting in hematemesis and melena.

Lymphoma. Hodgkin's disease, lymphosarcoma, and reticulum cell sarcoma may occur in the stomach occasionally as the only manifestation of the disease (see Chapter 24).

Treatment

The patient with carcinoma of the stomach is often anemic and has lost weight. Blood and proteins may have to be given and in addition a high-protein diet. With pyloric obstruction there are also dehydration, hyponatremia, hypochloremia, hypokalemia, and metabolic alkalosis. Several days may therefore be required to correct the electrolyte and acid-base imbalance. With complete obstruction nothing should be given by mouth and the stomach should be washed out daily. Intravenous proteins and occasionally hyperalimentation are necessary to correct a severe negative nitrogen balance.

Attempted Curative. Attempted curative treatment for carcinoma of the stomach not encroaching on the cardiac orifice consists of subtotal gastrectomy with removal of the greater and lesser omenta and the spleen.[7] The pancreas to the left of the superior mesenteric vessels is also removed if the nodes along the upper border of the pancreas are thought to contain metastases or if the tumor is penetrating posteriorly into the pancreas. The distal point of section is about 2 cm beyond the pylorus. The left lobe of liver may also be removed if the tumor directly invades the liver. A total gastrectomy is only performed if the complete stomach is involved as in linitis plastica, if the tumor has extended to

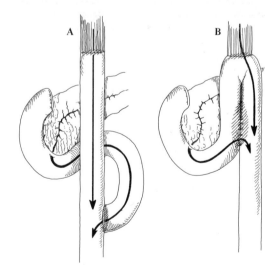

Figure 18–16. Reconstructions following total gastrectomy for diffuse infiltrating carcinoma or a carcinoma in the fundus are by (A) Roux-en-Y anastomosis or (B) anastomosing the end of the esophagus to a loop of proximal jejunum and performing an enteroanastomosis between the two limbs of the loop.

the cardiac orifice, or if it is in the fundus (Figure 18–16). A frozen section is obtained of the proximal line of section to make sure that tumor has not invaded the submucosal layer up to the point of section.

A partial gastrectomy is performed if possible, because the operative mortality is less than 5 percent and there is minimal morbidity. With total gastrectomy the operative mortality approaches 20 percent because of the high incidence of leakage at the esophageal anastomosis, possibly due to the absence of a serosa in the esophagus. In addition, there is considerable morbidity from loss of the reservoir function of the stomach, impaired absorption of iron, and loss of intrinsic factor.

The five-year survival is only about 5 percent in all patients treated for cure; it is about 25 percent in those with negative nodes.

Palliative. Partial gastrectomy is the best palliative treatment in those with liver metastases or peritoneal implants. It is questionable whether total gastrectomy should be done except in those with small metastases. In those with pyloric obstruction partial gastrectomy should be performed. A gastrojejunostomy to relieve the obstruction gives only poor palliation because the patient continues to bleed from the tumor and has marked anorexia.

Radiotherapy is disappointing in carcinoma of the stomach mainly because of the inability to deliver an adequate dose without damaging bowel. Lymphomas in the stomach are highly radiosensitive but are better treated by excision because of the possibility of producing massive tumor necrosis and perforation.

A number of primary and metastatic carcinomas of the stomach respond to 5-fluorouracil given orally or intravenously (see Chapter 7). Recently there has been increasing interest in the use of combinations of drugs, including 5-fluorouracil, cyclophosphamide, methotrexate, doxorubicin (Adriamycin), and mithramycin.

DUODENUM
Peptic Ulcer

The commonest site for a peptic ulcer is the duodenal bulb in the first part of the duodenum (see Plates IV and VI). A postbulbar ulcer may be present in the second and even the third part of the duodenum. The diagnosis may be difficult to make both radiologically and at operation when the ulcer is present at one of these uncommon sites, especially in the patient with upper gastrointestinal bleeding. The Zollinger-Ellison syndrome is especially liable to produce a peptic ulcer at these sites.

Tumors

Tumors of the duodenum are uncommon (Figure 18–17). Benign conditions are heterotopic pancreas, polyps, and leiomyomas. Malignant tumors are adenocarcinomas, lymphomas, carcinoids, and leiomyosarcomas. A primary carcinoma is difficult to differentiate from one of the pancreas, ampulla of Vater, or lower end of the common bile duct. Malignant tumors are treated for cure by pancreaticoduodenectomy and have a much better prognosis than primary carcinomas of the head of the pancreas.

Diverticulum

A diverticulum may be acquired from fibrosis associated with a peptic ulcer. Congenital diverticula are seen most often in the periampullar region and are generally asymptomatic. Occasionally they cause bleeding and produce pain but rarely do they perforate. Excision is only indicated when complications occur.

Duodenal Obstruction by Superior Mesenteric Artery

The superior mesenteric artery may obstruct the duodenum as it crosses anterior to the third part, especially in those who have had marked weight loss. The obstruction is demonstrated on x-ray. Treatment is anastomosing the dilated proximal duodenum to the proximal jejunum (duodenojejunostomy).

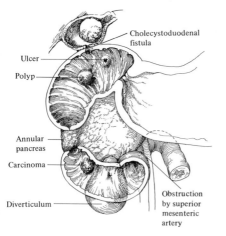

Cholecystoduodenal fistula

Ulcer

Polyp

Annular pancreas

Carcinoma

Diverticulum

Obstruction by superior mesenteric artery

Figure 18–17. Diseases of the duodenum, other than peptic ulceration, are uncommon. They consist of polyp, annular pancreas, diverticulum, cholecystoduodenal fistula, carcinoma, and obstruction by the superior mesenteric artery.

CITED REFERENCES

1. Blendis, L. M.; Beilby, J. O. W.; Wilson, J. P.; Coles, M. J.; and Hadley, G. D.: Carcinoma of the stomach: Evaluation of individual and combined diagnostic accuracy of radiology, cytology and gastrophotography. *Br. Med. J.*, 1:656–59, 1967.
2. Bruno, M. S.; Grier, W. R. N.; and Ober, W. B.: Spontaneous laceration and rupture of esophagus and stomach: Mallory-Weiss syndrome, Boerhaave syndrome, and their variants. *Arch. Intern. Med.* 112:574–83, 1963.
3. Code, C. F., and Watkinson, G.: Importance of vagal innervation in the regulatory effect of acid in the duodenum on gastric secretion of acid. *J. Physiol.* (*Lond*), 130:233–52, 1955.
4. Goligher, J. C.: Comparative results of different operations in the elective treatment of duodenal ulcer. *Br. J. Surg.*, 57:780–83, 1971.
5. Hallenbeck, G. A.: What is the best elective operation for duodenal ulcer? *Can. Med. Assoc. J.*, 103:1255–62, 1970.
6. Herrington, J. L.: Current trends in the surgical treatment of duodenal ulcer. *Surg. Gynecol. Obstet.*, 139:87–88, 1974.
7. Hoerr, S. D., and Hodgman, R. W.: Carcinoma of the stomach. *Am. J. Surg.*, 107:620–36, 1964.
8. Jordan, P. H., and Yip, B. S. S. C.: Origin of gastrin in gastric juice. *Am. J. Surg.*, 128:336–39, 1974.
9. Kettering, R. F.: Current concepts in the medical treatment of duodenal ulcer. *Surg. Clin. North Am.*, 51:835–41, 1971.
10. Kragelund, E.; Nielsen, A.; Dretler, R.; and Fischer, J.: Parietal cell vagotomy without antral drainage and selective gastric vagotomy with drainage in patients with duodenal ulcers. *Surg. Forum*, 24:365–67, 1973.
11. Menguy, R.; Gadacz, T.; and Zajtchuk, R.: The surgical management of acute gastric mucosal bleeding. *Arch. Surg.*, 99:198–208, 1969.
12. Nyhus, L. M.; Chapman, N. D.; DeVito, R. V.; and Harkins, H. N.: The control of gastrin release: An experimental study illustrating a new concept. *Gastroenterology*, 39:582–89, 1960.
13. Smithwick, R. H.; Farmer, D. S.; and Harrower, H. W.: Hemigastrectomy and truncal vagotomy in the treatment of the duodenal ulcer. *Scientific Papers*, 127:631–49, 1974.
14. Wilkinson, E. R., and Johnston, D.: Effect of truncal selective and highly selective vagotomy on gastric emptying and intestinal transit of a good barium meal in man. *Ann. Surg.*, 178:190–93, 1973.

SUGGESTIONS FOR FURTHER READING

Dragstedt, L. R.: On the cause of gastric and duodenal ulcers. *J. R. Coll. Surg. Edinb.*, 16:251–63, 1971.
Review of clinical and experimental work on the pathogenesis of peptic ulcer.

Landor, J. H.: Gastric secretory tests and their relevance to surgeons. *Surgery*, 65:523–38, 1969.
A review of the value of gastric secretory tests.

Scratcherd, T.: Gastric secretory mechanism and peptic ulcer. *Clin. Gastroenterol.* 2:259–74, 1973.
An excellent review of the physiology of gastric secretion and its relation to peptic ulcer.

Stout, A. P.: Tumors of the stomach. Armed Forces Institute of Pathology, Washington, D.C., pp. F21–9 to F21–104, 1953.
An excellent illustration account of the pathology of benign and malignant gastric tumors.

Watson, W. C.: Management of acute upper alimentary bleeding. *Can. J. Surg.*, 14:373–82, 1971.
A practical approach to the management of acute upper gastrointestinal bleeding.

Chapter 19

LIVER AND BILIARY TRACT

Bernard Langer and *Robert M. Stone*

CHAPTER OUTLINE

Introduction
Normal Structure and Function
  Gross Anatomy
  Hepatic Lobule
  Hepatic Cell
  Lymphoreticular System
  Biliary Tract
  Vasculature and Lymphatics
Common Presenting Symptoms
  Jaundice
    Pigment Production
    Transport
    Conjugation
    Canalicular Excretion
    Extrahepatic Excretion
  Pain
  Hepatomegaly
  Bleeding
  Ascites
  Hepatic Encephalopathy
  Other Clinical Signs
Diagnosis of Hepatobiliary Diseases
  History
  Physical Examination
  Laboratory Diagnosis
    Bile Pigment Abnormalities

Tests of Dye Excretion
Tests of Hepatic Cell Injury
Tests of Protein Synthesis
Tests for Obstruction
Other Tests
Radiologic Investigation
Radioisotope Scanning
Hepatic Biopsy
Diseases of the Hepatobiliary System
  Congenital Lesions
  Cholelithiasis
    Formation of Gallstones
    Symptoms
    Diagnosis
    Treatment
  Liver and Bile Duct Infections
  Injuries to the Liver and Bile Ducts
  Space-Occupying Lesions in the Liver
  Hepatic Cirrhosis and Portal Hypertension
    Pathophysiology
    Complications
    Evaluation of the Patient with Bleeding
      Varices
    Treatment
  Other Diseases of Interest to the Surgeon

INTRODUCTION

The liver is a complex organ, playing a central role in many homeostatic and metabolic functions upon which survival depends. There is a functional interdependence of the liver, the circulatory system, the hematopoietic system, and the alimentary tract. Thus the patient with primary liver disease may present with symptoms related to other organ systems, and conversely primary disease in other organs may produce manifestations of impaired hepatic function.

The liver arises embryologically from the foregut and retains a close anatomic and functional relation with the alimentary canal. The portal vein provides a direct route to the liver for substances absorbed from the gastrointestinal tract. They include nutrients, vitamins, and minerals that have been partly or wholly prepared in the gut for entry into metabolic pathways. Harmful substances are also carried to the liver where they are removed or detoxified. The biliary tract is an excretory route from the liver to the gut, through which pigments, chemicals, and drugs, or their breakdown products are eliminated. It is also the route by which bile salts, synthesized in the liver, are added to ingested food to participate in the digestion and absorption of fat before they are reabsorbed, mainly in the ileum. The portal vein and bile ducts thus provide an opportunity for recycling bile salts.

Because of its central position in the circulatory system and its relation to the alimentary tract, the liver is exposed to injurious agents such as chemicals, toxins, bacteria, and viruses. In spite of its role in removing these agents, the liver cell is particularly sensitive to injury. Damage may be dose-related and occur in any individual with high enough exposure, as in carbon tetrachloride poisoning, or it may result from a sensitivity reaction and occur only in a small number of individuals exposed, as in halothane hepatitis.

The liver compensates for its susceptibility to injury by its great functional reserve and regenerative capacity, provided that the basic architecture has been preserved. About 85 percent of the normal liver in animals can be removed, and the remainder regenerates to restore normal mass and function.[1] This may also occur in patients following diffuse hepatic necrosis. Regeneration may be restricted, however, by structural changes in the liver or by persistence of the disease process. Chronic liver disease then occurs, and treatment is directed toward minimizing further injury, supporting the impaired liver, and managing any resultant complications.

NORMAL STRUCTURE AND FUNCTION

Gross Anatomy

The liver, like the lung and kidney, has a segmental architecture that is not apparent on viewing its external surface. Classically anatomists have described the liver as being divided

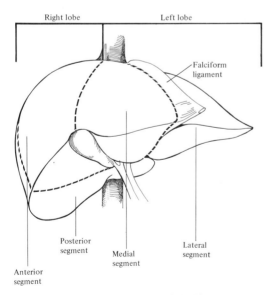

Right lobe

Left lobe

Falciform ligament

Posterior segment

Medial segment

Lateral segment

Anterior segment

Figure 19–1. The segments of the liver as seen from the external surface.

into a large right lobe and a small left lobe, separated by the falciform ligament. Careful studies of its vascular supply, however, have led to a different concept of hepatic structure[2,3] (Figure 19–1). The liver is composed of two lobes, a right and left lobe, divided by a plane extending from the gallbladder fossa anteriorly to the inferior vena cava posteriorly (see Plates IV and VI). Each of the main lobes is subdivided into two major segments. The left lobe is divided into medial and lateral segments by the falciform ligament and the right lobe into an anterior and posterior segment. The major bile ducts, branches of the hepatic artery, and portal vein enter the liver from below, travel together, and are segmentally distributed. The hepatic veins, however, leave the liver from above and are intersegmental in distribution (Figures 19–2 and 19–3).

The normal liver, 1200 to 1500 gm, is soft, located in the upper abdomen, and is largely shaped by the surrounding structures, especially the diaphragm. It is suspended from the diaphragm by reflections of peritoneum called the triangular ligaments on the right and left sides, the coronary ligament, and by the falciform ligament in the midline. The inferior vena cava is partially buried in its posterior surface.

Hepatic Lobule

Branches of the bile duct, hepatic artery, portal vein, and lymphatics enter the liver at the porta hepatis and continue together in successive divisions. The smallest divisions are surrounded by connective tissue forming portal triads on microscopic section (Figure 19–4). The end branches of the hepatic veins are separate and have been called central veins. Studies by Rappaport and others[11] suggest that the functional unit of the liver is centered about the portal triad. The branches of the hepatic vein are at the periphery of this unit and are better called terminal hepatic veins. Hepatocytes are exposed to blood as it flows from the portal triads, through sinusoids toward terminal hepatic veins. The metabolic functions of the hepatic cells depend on whether they are close to the portal triads where oxygen tension is high, or near the terminal hepatic veins where oxygen tension is low. Certain types of damage to hepatocytes are first seen close to the periphery of the lobule in this low-oxygen tension zone.

Hepatic Cell

The hepatocyte is the most important metabolic cell in the body. In addition to synthesizing proteins and detoxifying endogenous and exogenous substances, it provides materials for metabolic processes elsewhere in the body. It

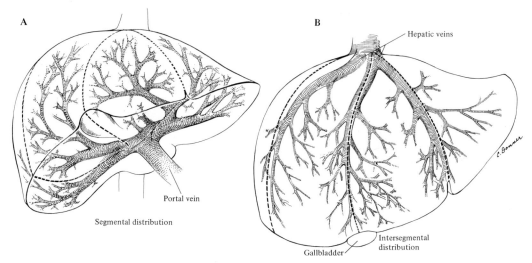

A

B

Hepatic veins

Portal vein

Segmental distribution

Gallbladder

Intersegmental
distribution

Figure 19–2.   *A.* The portal veins are within the segments of the liver. The hepatic veins have an intersegmental distribution. *B.* The segments of the liver.

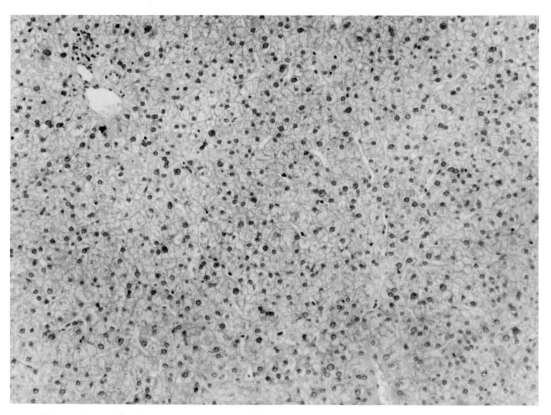

Figure 19–3.   Histologic section of normal human liver. A portal tract can be seen in the upper left corner and a central (terminal hepatic) vein on the lower right. The vacuolated appearance of the hepatocytes is due to their glycogen content. (Hematoxylin and eosin stain × 120.) (Courtesy of Dr. M. J. Phillips.)

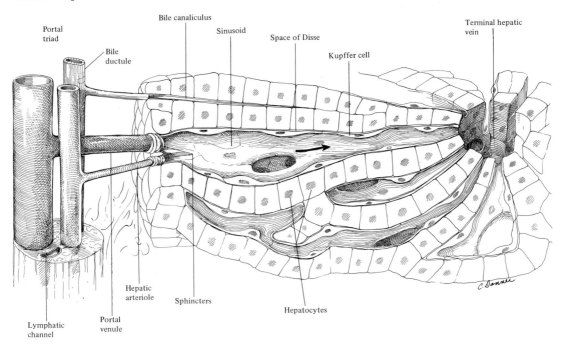

Figure 19–4. The portal triad is centrally placed and the hepatic vein in the periphery.

responds to changing requirements by converting food absorbed from the gastrointestinal tract into either readily available substrates or stored energy. The hepatic cell is ideally suited for this, having a large surface exposed to blood and a large amount of endoplasmic reticulum where these metabolic processes take place (Figure 19–5).

Lymphoreticular System

Kupffer cells, lining the hepatic sinusoids, phagocytose particulate matter and bacteria from the blood. These cells proliferate in response to systemic infection in the same way that lymphoreticular hyperplasia occurs in other regions. Other lymphoreticular cells within the liver participate in hematopoiesis in the fetus and may perform this function in later life when the bone marrow has been chronically damaged or replaced.

Biliary Tract

It is through the biliary tract (Figure 19–6) that the liver exercises its major function of excretion and contributes to intestinal absorption. Hepatic bile is formed largely by active transport from the hepatocyte into the bile canaliculus. An increase in synthesis or feeding of bile salts increases the bile flow. Secretin increases biliary flow and in particular stimulates secretion of electrolytes and bicarbonate. The cuboidal epithelial cells of the bile ducts

change the composition of bile. In the fasting state there is minimal concentration of bile as the result of absorption of electrolytes and water. On stimulation with secretin the opposite occurs, and water and electrolytes, especially bicarbonate, are added to the hepatic bile. The resting tone in the sphincter of Oddi diverts bile into the gallbladder, where water and electrolytes are absorbed and the bile is concentrated about tenfold. With ingestion of fat, cholecystokinin is released from the duodenal mucosa, causing the muscular wall of the gallbladder to contract and the sphincter of Oddi to relax (Figure 18–3, page 300). Ingestion of fat also increases the flow of hepatic bile. Bile then flows into the gut to aid in the digestion and absorption of fat. When a bile duct is obstructed, bile secretion continues until the intraductal pressure rises to about 35 cm of water. Secretion then ceases, and bile pigments and salts begin to be absorbed through ductular epithelium. If obstruction is complete, the duct system may become filled with a clear mucoid fluid that has been called "white bile."

Vasculature and Lymphatics

Total hepatic blood flow in the adult is about 1000 to 1200 ml per minute.[6] The hepatic artery contributes 30 percent and portal vein approximately 70 percent. Blood in the portal vein has a lower P_{O_2} and also differs from arterial blood in that it contains substances absorbed from the

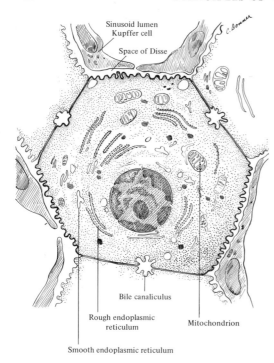

Figure 19–5. The hepatocyte is a biologically active cell.

gastrointestinal tract. The portal vein drains the alimentary canal from the esophagogastric junction to the middle of the rectum as well as the spleen and pancreas.

The hepatic artery arises from the celiac axis. Abnormalities of its origin and distribution are common and are important to the surgeon.[9] The right hepatic artery arises in part or in whole

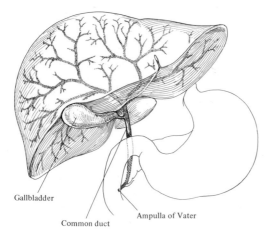

Figure 19–6. The biliary system consists of small right and left hepatic ducts, common hepatic duct, cystic duct, gallbladder, and common bile duct.

from the superior mesenteric artery in approximately 16 percent of cases, the left hepatic artery in part or in whole from the left gastric in 25 percent, and the common hepatic artery from the superior mesenteric artery in 2.5 percent. Pressure in the hepatic arterial system is the same as in the systemic circulation, while that in the portal vein is 7 to 10 mm Hg.

The few lymphatics in the liver are located along the bile ducts and in the capsule of Glisson. The hepatic lobule has no lymphatics. The interval between the hepatic sinusoid and hepatocytes, known as the space of Disse, is a plasma space and may represent a source of lymph appearing at the hilum of the liver (Figure 19–4).

COMMON PRESENTING SYMPTOMS

Jaundice

Jaundice is the visible staining of tissues by bile pigments. These pigments are normally present in blood and tissues but are not visible until blood levels reach about 3.0 mg percent. They are formed mainly from the breakdown of hemoglobin of senescent erythrocytes in the spleen and bone marrow, and to a small extent from intracellular cytochromes and catalases.[13] An abnormality at any of the five steps in the handling of bile pigments may lead to jaundice (Figure 19–7).

Pigment Production. This may be increased as a result of hemolysis in patients with congenital or acquired hemolytic anemias, with incompatible blood transfusion, with large hematomas or extravasations of blood, and with septicemia. Transfusion of large volumes of old bank blood results in breakdown of a large number of erythrocytes and the formation of unconjugated bilirubin. Patients who have had a valve prosthesis inserted may have damage to the erythrocytes with production of jaundice. Some drugs such as phenacetin must result in excess hemolysis. In addition, any severe catabolic state in which there is release of intracellular enzymes may increase the pigment load. The serum bilirubin rarely exceeds 5.0 mg percent as a result of increased hemolysis because of the capacity in the normal liver to handle the increased amount of pigment.

Transport. Bilirubin is bound to albumin in plasma and then delivered to the hepatocyte. An active transport mechanism is required for the uptake of the pigment by the hepatocyte, and this is impaired in some patients with viral hepatitis and in Gilbert's disease.

Conjugation. Bilirubin is conjugated with glucuronic acid by the enzyme glucuronyl trans-

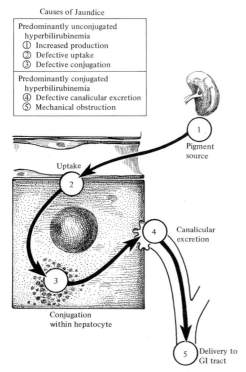

Causes of Jaundice

Predominantly unconjugated
hyperbilirubinemia
① Increased production
② Defective uptake
③ Defective conjugation

Predominantly conjugated
hyperbilirubinemia
④ Defective canalicular excretion
⑤ Mechanical obstruction

Figure 19–7. Jaundice can result from impairment in handling of bile pigments at five different stages.

ferase in the microsomes of the rough and smooth endoplasmic reticulum of the hepatocyte. This enzyme is deficient in neonates and accounts for the physiologic jaundice of the newborn. An inherited persistent deficiency of glucuronyl transferase is the cause of the Crigler-Najar syndrome.

Canalicular Excretion. Conjugated bilirubin is excreted by active transport into the bile canaliculus. There is less capacity to handle increased loads at this than at any of the other steps. Canalicular excretion is impaired in patients with sensitivity to drugs such as chlorpromazine and in the Dubin-Johnson syndrome.

Extrahepatic Excretion. The bile pigments pass through the biliary tract to the intestine, with or without storage in the gallbladder. Mechanical obstruction of the extrahepatic ducts is one of the commonest causes of jaundice.

Bilirubin is not changed in the small intestine but is converted by bacterial action in the colon to biliverdin and urobilinogen (stercobilinogen). Some water-soluble urobilinogen is absorbed into the circulation and excreted again in the bile. Trace amounts of urobilinogen are also normally excreted by the kidney. If hepatic excretion is impaired as a result of hepato-

cellular injury or obstruction to bile flow, the blood level and urinary excretion of urobilinogen increases. With complete obstruction or diversion of bile flow, bile pigment does not enter the gut, urobilinogen is not formed, and therefore none is absorbed from the intestine or excreted in the urine.

Normally only a small amount of conjugated bilirubin is found in the blood and urine. The conjugated form is less tightly bound to protein than unconjugated bilirubin so that in conjugated hyperbilirubinemia bile appears in the urine, whereas in unconjugated hyperbilirubinemia it does not. Conditions that either increase the amount of pigment or interfere with the steps up to and including conjugation increase the unconjugated pigment, whereas diseases interfering with the pathway beyond that point increase the conjugated bilirubin. A mixed picture is often found when disease processes interfere with more than one step. In addition the poor sensitivity of the standard laboratory tests may fail to clearly distinguish between conjugated and unconjugated bilirubin.

Pain

Pain is a common symptom in hepatobiliary disease. It occurs as a result of either biliary tract obstruction, inflammation, or acute stretching of the liver capsule (Figure 19–8).

Biliary tract obstruction produces either tonic contraction or acute distention of the biliary tract or gallbladder. This causes a severe, poorly localized visceral pain referred to the midepigastrium, with or without extension to the right upper quadrant and radiation into the back. The severity and quality of this pain are more helpful in diagnosis than localization. It usually starts gradually, taking 10 to 20 minutes to reach its peak, and then remains steady for up to several hours. Although called biliary colic it is not a crampy type of pain. It is unrelieved by change in position and often accompanied by retching and vomiting. The severity varies from a vague sense of discomfort to severe disabling pain requiring an analgesic.

Acute stretching of the liver capsule produces a diffuse right upper quadrant pain varying from vague discomfort to severe steady localized pain that is aggravated by movement. The liver is usually enlarged and the lower border is tender. Pain may also be produced by percussion over the right lower chest. This type of pain is seen in acute hepatic enlargements associated with congestive heart failure, hepatic vein thrombosis, and acute bile duct obstruction. It also occurs in diffuse inflammatory processes with edema, such as hepatitis.

Localized inflammatory processes produce

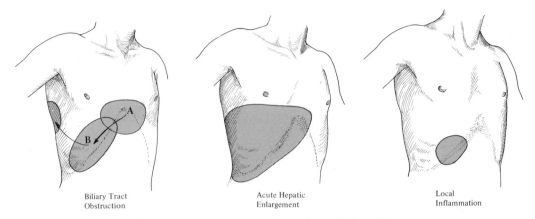

Biliary Tract
Obstruction

Acute Hepatic
Enlargement

Local
Inflammation

Figure 19–8. Localization of pain in hepatobiliary diseases.

pain due to irritation of the parietal peritoneum, as in acute cholecystitis. Local signs may also result from intrahepatic causes such as abscess or hemorrhage into a tumor. Pain is well localized and accompanied by signs of parietal peritoneal irritation. When the disease process is not directly in contact with the abdominal wall, the signs are less apparent, for example in a deep-seated liver abscess. Irritation of the diaphragm by a local process may produce pain referred to the shoulder mediated through the phrenic nerve.

Hepatomegaly

A normal liver is often palpable during deep inspiration in a thin patient. Suspected enlargement of the liver must be confirmed by outlining the upper border by percussion. The normal liver measures about 15 cm in the midclavicular line. X-rays of the chest and liver scan may also be useful in evaluating liver size.

A variety of diseases may produce diffuse hepatic enlargement. Accumulation of intracellular material such as fat in alcoholic liver disease and glycogen in von Gierke's disease may markedly increase liver size. Increases in intracellular fluid may occur in diffuse inflammatory process like viral hepatitis, or in hepatic outflow obstruction, in which distention of sinusoids is an additional factor. Hepatic enlargement also occurs in biliary tract obstruction where dilatation of bile ducts, accumulation of inflammatory cells, and deposition of connective tissue contribute to the increase in size. Diffuse infiltrative processes such as lymphoma may produce hepatomegaly, as will myeloid metaplasia in patients with bone marrow failure. Space-occupying lesions, such as cysts or tumors, may produce either localized or diffuse hepatic enlargement, depending on their position and whether they are single or multiple. Finally, the liver's great ability to regenerate after injury may give rise to an apparent localized hepatic enlargement of part of the liver in response to injury or removal of another part.

The small liver denotes absolute loss of hepatic parenchyma and indicates a poor prognosis. It may occur in acute hepatic necrosis from viral or toxic types of hepatitis. In chronic liver disease a small liver indicates that the fibrotic process is advanced, hepatic function is marginal, and there is no potential for significant regeneration.

Bleeding

Bleeding from the gastrointestinal tract may occur with liver disease as a result of impaired synthesis of coagulation factors or from gastroesophageal varices, or a combination.[15] The coagulation factors produced in the liver that require vitamin K for synthesis are factors II (prothrombin), VII, IX (Christmas factor), and X (Stuart factor). Those that do not require vitamin K include factors I (fibrinogen) and V (proaccelerin). Severe hepatocellular injury may impair synthesis of all these factors and produce bleeding. Fresh blood, fresh frozen plasma, or concentrates are used for treatment. Bleeding may also occur in chronic obstruction of the bile ducts. In this situation deficiency of bile salts in the gut results in impaired absorption of fat-soluble vitamin K and insufficient synthesis of the K-dependent factors. Treatment consists of parenteral administration of vitamin K.

An increase in plasminogen activators released from the damaged liver increases fibrinolytic activity and may also cause bleeding. Decreased hepatic inactivation of accelerator factors and increased intravascular clotting may be difficult to distinguish from fibrinolysis, especially if massive transfusion has been given. Epsilon aminocaproic acid is useful in the treatment of increased fibrinolysis. The patient with disseminated intravascular coagulation, however, should receive heparin (see Chapter 11).

Ascites

Fluid in the peritoneal cavity represents an imbalance between the rate of fluid formation and its reabsorption by the peritoneum. The mechanisms involved are increased portal pressure, decreased plasma oncotic pressure, and systemic retention of sodium. Increased portal pressure results in increased lymphatic flow and the leaking of fluid from visceral surfaces. When intrahepatic pressure is increased, as in cirrhosis, the surface of the liver leaks fluid high in protein. The ability to retain fluid in the vascular space is impaired when plasma oncotic pressure is reduced. In patients with advanced liver disease albumin synthesis is decreased and plasma albumin concentration is low. The associated increase in plasma globulin does not compensate osmotically, since globulin molecules are considerably larger than albumin. These patients tend to retain salt and water due to an increase in aldosterone secretion. It has been suggested that fluid sequestration in the splanchnic region causes systemic hypovolemia, and that this acts as a stimulus to aldosterone

secretion. Normally aldosterone is metabolized in the liver. Impaired liver function would therefore also tend to increase the amount in the blood. Other studies point to a primary salt- and water-retaining mechanism mediated by some substance released from the injured liver. Patients with liver disease may have a moderate amount of ascites for a long time with little ill effect. When ascites is severe, they may have associated peripheral edema and symptoms such as abdominal discomfort, shortness of breath, and umbilical hernia. Treatment is administration of protein, diuretics, and salt restriction.

Hepatic Encephalopathy

This refers to a neurologic syndrome seen in patients with impaired hepatic function in whom portal blood bypasses the liver. Symptoms vary from minor disturbances of cerebral function, such as memory impairment, personality change, disturbed sleep rhythm, and slowed mentation, through degrees of drowsiness and confusion to deep coma. In the intermediate stages there may be a coarse flapping tremor of the outstretched hands, cerebellar or peripheral neurologic signs, and a pungent sweet odor to the breath (fetor hepaticus).

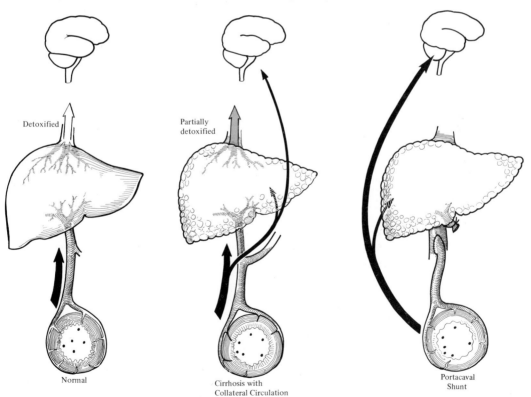

Detoxified

Partially detoxified

Normal

Cirrhosis with
Collateral Circulation

Portacaval
Shunt

Figure 19–9. Portacaval encephalopathy may develop in those with cirrhosis and well-developed collateral circulation or in cirrhotics who have blood diverted from the liver by operation.

Symptoms are increased by protein and blood in the gut and result from the effect on brain cells of protein breakdown products normally detoxified by the liver (Figure 19–9). Ammonia has received most attention, but it is likely that other substances such as volatile amines and short-chain fatty acids are more important.

Other Clinical Signs

Chronic liver disease, particularly cirrhosis, may be asymptomatic for a long time. Some patients with liver disease have only malaise, anorexia, and a low-grade fever. Splenomegaly is one of the secondary signs in portal hypertension and is due to passive congestion of the spleen. There may be an accompanying thrombocytopenia and leukopenia. Pruritus occurs most often in patients with impaired bile excretion and is thought to be related to bile acid accumulation in the skin. It is not specific for biliary tract obstruction but may be seen in intrahepatic cholestasis or even in primary hepatocellular disorders.

DIAGNOSIS OF HEPATOBILIARY DISEASES

History

A careful history may be important in elucidating the diagnosis. Patients with primary liver disease may present with symptoms that seem unrelated to hepatic function such as fatigue, weight loss, anorexia, pruritus, and easy bruising. Careful inquiries should be made regarding exposure to hepatotoxins and contact with jaundiced patients. Individuals with gallstones may present nonspecific symptoms such as belching and vague upper abdominal distress. The relation of symptoms to foods that stimulate the release of cholecystokinin may help to establish the diagnosis. In the jaundiced patient the presence of pain and chills and the color of stools and urine are significant.

Physical Examination

A number of extra-abdominal physical findings are associated with hepatic function disorders. Jaundice is the most common. The skin should also be examined for spider angiomata and the telltale scratch marks of pruritus. Other peripheral findings include muscle wasting, gynecomastia, and testicular atrophy. The size and consistency of the liver should be determined. In acute inflammation of the gallbladder tenderness is produced during deep inspiration while the examining hand is pressed below the lower border of the liver (Murphy's sign). The enlarged, inflamed gallbladder may sometimes be outlined by gentle palpation when abdominal guarding is not too pronounced. A palpable but nontender gallbladder, however, in a patient with painless jaundice usually means common duct obstruction by tumor either in the pancreas or common bile duct (Courvoisier's law). When a stone in the common bile duct is the cause of the jaundice, the patient usually has pain, and the thick-walled gallbladder is unable to distend and become palpable. Many question the value of this law.

Ascites occurs more frequently in chronic than acute parenchymal liver disease and is a bad prognostic sign. The most reliable way to detect ascites is by the demonstration of shifting dullness. In many forms of chronic liver disease splenomegaly is also found.

Laboratory Diagnosis

Bile Pigment Abnormalities. The normal plasma bilirubin level is less than 1.0 mg percent, most of which is unconjugated and called "indirect-reacting" bilirubin. When the serum bilirubin is elevated, serial determinations of conjugated and unconjugated fractions may help determine the abnormal step in pigment handling. The presence of excessive urobilinogen in the urine is an early sign of hepatic cell injury or excretory obstruction. With complete obstruction urobilinogen disappears from the urine, since its precursor bilirubin can no longer reach the gut.

Tests of Dye Excretion. Sulfobromophthalein (Bromsulphalein, BSP) and indocyanine green (ICG) are organic dyes excreted by the hepatocyte in a manner similar to bilirubin. Their excretion is diminished when hepatic blood flow is decreased or when there is hepatic cell injury or excretory obstruction. In the absence of jaundice the amount of BSP retained in the plasma 45 minutes after its intravenous injection is a good screening test for abnormal hepatic function. Normally less than 5 percent is retained in the serum. More sensitive tests include establishing clearance curves after a bolus of either dye is injected, and the application of the Fick principle to measure total hepatic blood flow following continuous infusion of ICG.

Tests of Hepatic Cell Injury. The most commonly used test for hepatocellular injury is measurement of the enzyme serum glutamic oxaloacetic transaminase (SGOT). The normal serum level does not exceed 40 units. This enzyme is present in high concentration in hepatocytes but is also found in cardiac and voluntary muscle cells. It takes part in the transfer of an amino group from glutamic acid to oxaloacetic acid. Very high levels of SGOT, greater than 300 units, are only seen in patients with hepatocellular disease, including necrosis and acute extrahepatic bile duct obstruction. Other enzymes that have been associated with cellular injury include serum glutamic pyruvic transaminase and leucine aminopeptidases.

Tests of Protein Synthesis. Serum albumin is produced only in the liver and in the absence of abnormal losses is a good indication of the liver's ability to synthesize protein. The normal value should exceed 4 gm per 100 ml of serum. The globulin fraction of the plasma proteins is synthesized in lymphoreticular tissues throughout the body and is usually not influenced by hepatic dysfunction. In certain forms of hepatic disease, however, especially those associated with some immunologic abnormality, the globulin level may be increased above normal. The albumin-globulin ratio, normally about 1.7:1.0, may fall below 1.0. The one-stage prothrombin time is a useful screening test for clotting defects in liver disease and is abnormal if there is a deficiency not only of prothrombin but also of factors V, VII, X, and fibrinogen. If the coagulation defect is due to bile duct obstruction alone, it will be rapidly corrected by the parenteral administration of vitamin K.

Tests for Obstruction. In obstruction of the bile ducts the bilirubin is usually elevated, particularly the conjugated fraction. Pigment studies, however, may not clearly distinguish between intrahepatic and extrahepatic cholestasis. The enzyme alkaline phosphatase is increased in the blood of patients with extrahepatic biliary tract obstruction. It should be remembered, however, that there are other sources of raised plasma alkaline phosphatase, such as bone, ileum, placenta, and leukocytes. The source can be determined from the isoenzymes. The elevation seen in obstruction of the hepatic ducts is not due to failure of the enzyme to be excreted but to increased synthesis by epithelial cells lining the obstructed ducts. Thus partial obstruction of small ducts, such as by infiltrating tumor, may produce elevations in the plasma level without any other abnormal biochemical finding. The enzyme 5′-nucleotidase is elevated in the same circumstances as the alkaline phosphatase but is more specific for liver diseases.

Other Tests. The hepatitis-associated antigen (HAA or Australia antigen) is found in the serum of patients with serum hepatitis and is probably a fragment of the virus. It is also present in contaminated blood and blood products, but is absent from the feces. It produces serum or type B hepatitis, has a long incubation period of 50 to 180 days, occurs at any age, and is now frequently seen in drug addicts who administer their drugs by injection often using the same needle. In addition, the disease can be transmitted in transfused blood or orally. The antigen can be seen under the electron microscope and can be checked for using immulogic tests. Routine screening of blood and its derivatives for the antigen may reduce the risk of transmitting serum hepatitis.

In type A or infectious hepatitis, the Australia antigen is absent, the incubation period is 15 to 45 days, it tends to occur in epidemics in young people, and it can be spread by fecal contamination or in blood.

Alpha fetoprotein has been found in the serum of about 40 percent of Caucasians and in 80 percent of Negroes with primary malignant hepatoma (see Chapter 7). It has also been identified in 25 percent of patients with malignant teratomas and is therefore not specific for hepatic tumors. Antimitochondrial and anti-smooth-muscle antibodies have been identified in patients with immunologic diseases of the liver, such as primary biliary cirrhosis.

The serum lactic dehydrogenase (LDH) is helpful in diagnosing hepatocellular necrosis. The subfractions I and II are elevated with muscle necrosis, III with tumor necrosis, and IV and V with liver necrosis.

Serum cholesterol tends to be elevated in obstructive biliary tract disease, especially primary biliary cirrhosis. The increase is not due

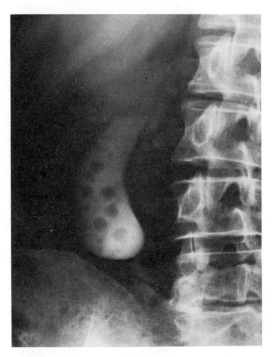

Figure 19–10. Oral cholecystogram showing radiolucent stones in the gallbladder.

to failure of excretion but to increased synthesis following interruption in the enterohepatic circulation of bile salts.

Radiologic Investigation

Oral cholecystography is the simplest and most frequently used test to determine gallbladder function and the presence of stones. The contrast material iopanoic acid (Telepaque) is absorbed from the gastrointestinal tract and excreted like bilirubin by the liver. It appears in low concentration in hepatic bile and is concentrated in the gallbladder in 8 to 16 hours (Figure 19–10). Films are taken at this time and after administration of a fatty meal to stimulate contraction of the gallbladder. If the gallbladder is not seen, another dose is given. Failure to outline the gallbladder with this technique usually indicates a diseased organ. Other causes of nonvisualization include hepatocellular disease, jaundice, gastric or intestinal obstruction, and failure to take or absorb the tablets.

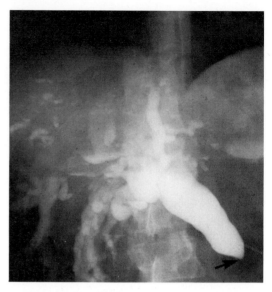

Figure 19–12. Percutaneous transhepatic cholangiogram showing low common bile duct obstruction (→) by a tumor at the ampulla of Vater. Note the gross dilatation of the common duct and its intrahepatic branches. (Courtesy of Dr. R. F. Colapinto.)

Intravenous cholangiography involves injection of a radiopaque dye (Iodipamide) which appears in high concentration in hepatic bile and outlines the duct system as well as the gallbladder (Figure 19–11). It is useful in demonstrating abnormalities of the extrahepatic bile ducts. If the gallbladder fails to fill when the common duct is normal, this indicates gallbladder disease. Deaths have occurred from intravenous cholangiography from hypersensitivity to iodine.

Operative cholangiography may be done at the time of cholecystectomy to ensure that the extrahepatic ducts do not contain stones. A fine polyethylene tube is inserted into the common bile ducts through the cystic duct and radiographs obtained after injection of a radiopaque dye.

Dye can also be injected into the intrahepatic bile ducts by percutaneous transhepatic cholangiography. This is useful when indirect methods have failed, for example, in the patient with jaundice and suspected extrahepatic duct obstruction. In major duct obstruction the proximal biliary tree becomes dilated and readily accessible to a flexible needle passed through the skin into the substance of the liver and thence into one of the dilated ducts (Figure 19–12). This procedure may produce bleeding or leakage of bile from the liver and should therefore be reserved for patients in whom laparotomy can if necessary be carried out immediately.

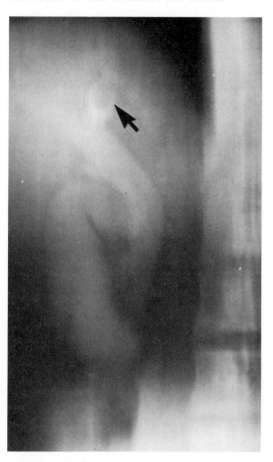

Figure 19–11. Intravenous cholangiogram showing a radiolucent stone (→) in the left hepatic duct.

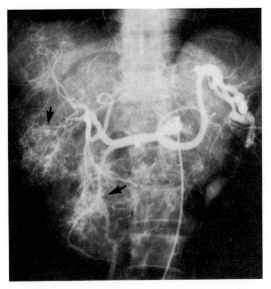

Figure 19–13. Hepatic arteriogram in the patient with a primary hepatoma. Arrows indicate large tumor masses and prominent abnormal vascular pattern. (Courtesy of Dr. R. F. Colapinto.)

Endoscopic retrograde cannulation of the papilla of Vater has recently provided another useful route for injecting radiopaque dye into the biliary and pancreatic ducts. X-rays showing ductal anatomy can be obtained with little risk, and this may provide an early definitive diagnosis in the patient with jaundice of obscure origin.

Selective hepatic arteriography is done by passing an arterial catheter percutaneously from the femoral artery in the groin into the celiac axis and its branches. Sequential films are taken after injection of radiopaque material. This procedure is useful in localizing solitary lesions of the liver and in differentiating hepatic tumors from cysts. Because the anatomic arrangement of hepatic arterial supply varies, arteriography is also indicated before any operative procedure that might require major hepatic resection (Figures 19–13 and 19–14).

Radioisotope Scanning

Liver scans help diagnose space-occupying lesions of the liver and determine liver size. ^{131}I rose bengal is taken up by hepatocytes and excreted in bile. ^{198}Au colloidal gold and ^{99m}Tc technecium sulfur colloid particles are phagocytosed by the Kupffer cells of both liver and spleen. The isotope ^{99m}Tc is currently in widest use because it has a short half-life of six hours and low energy.

These isotopes are all injected intravenously and are gamma emitters. The scanning device may be either an automated collimator or a gamma camera. The normal liver presents a uniform pattern of activity (Figure 19–15). Intra- or parahepatic lesions compressing the liver appear as filling defects on the scan (Figure 19–16) and must be at least 2 cm to be detected. Diffuse diseases such as cirrhosis produce a mottled appearance (Figure 19–17). The hepatic scan is a useful screening test, but arteriography often permits a more precise diagnosis.

Recently there has been interest in the use of ^{99m}Tc-labeled pyridoxilidine glutamate to visualize the gallbladder. There is no risk of a reaction to iodine, the result is available within minutes, and it can be used in the patient who is vomiting or jaundiced.

Hepatic Biopsy

Hepatic biopsy is the most accurate diagnostic test in liver disease. The biopsy may be obtained by percutaneous puncture using a Menghini[7] or Vimm-Silverman needle, or at laparotomy by resecting a small wedge of liver.

DISEASES OF THE HEPATOBILIARY SYSTEM

Congenital Lesions

Biliary atresia is a rare condition in which there is deficiency of part or more often all of the biliary ducts. Jaundice and hepatomegaly are

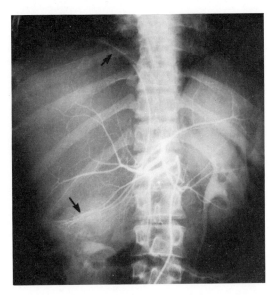

Figure 19–14. Hepatic arteriogram in a patient with a single huge hydatid cyst in the right lobe. Arrows indicate stretched-out hepatic arterial branches around the periphery of the avascular cyst. (Courtesy of Dr. R. F. Colapinto.)

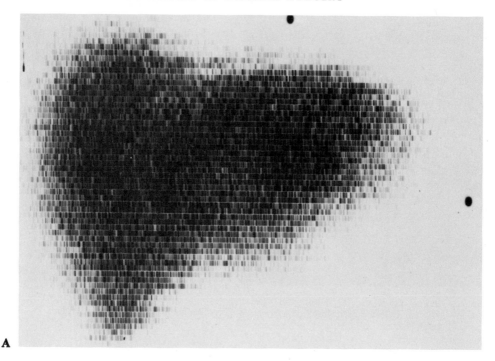

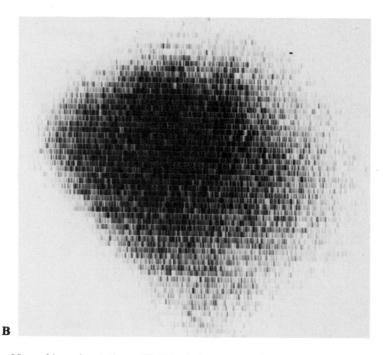

Figure 19–15. Normal hepatic scintiscan (^{99m}Tc). *A.* Anteroposterior scan. Note that the spleen picks up very little isotope. *B.* Right lateral scan. (Courtesy of Dr. D. E. Wood.)

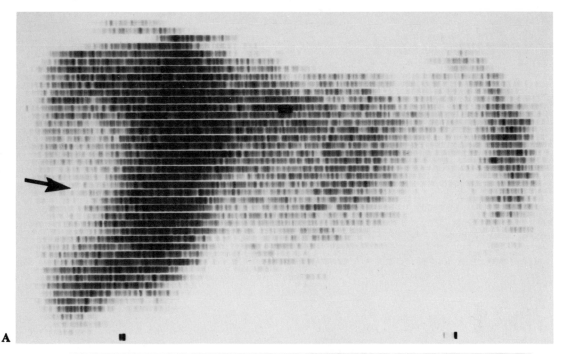

A

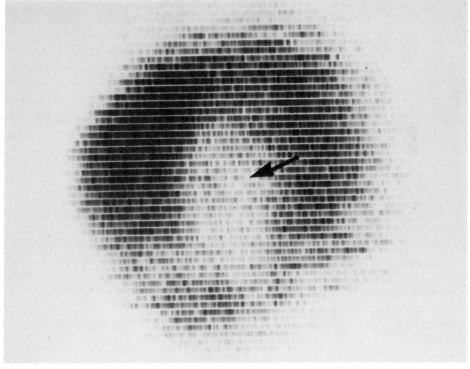

B

Figure 19–16.　Hepatic scintiscan (^{99m}Tc) showing a large "cold" area in the right lobe caused by an amebic abscess. *A.* Anteroposterior scan. *B.* Right lateral scan. (Courtesy of Dr. D. E. Wood.)

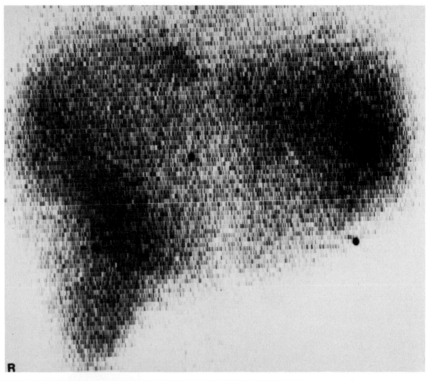

A R

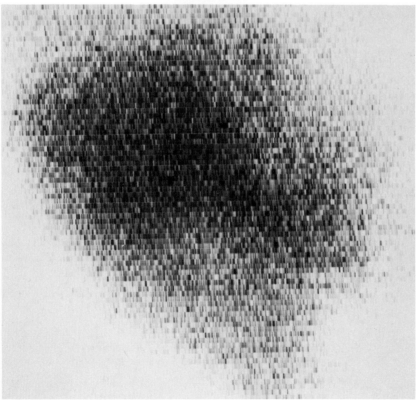

B

Figure 19–17.
Hepatic scintiscan (^{99m}Tc) in a patient with cirrhosis and portal hypertension. *A*. Anteroposterior scan. *B*. Right lateral scan. Note the patchy decrease in uptake of isotope in the liver and the marked increase in uptake in the spleen, as well as the enlargement of the spleen. (Courtesy of Dr. D. E. Wood.)

present soon after birth, and jaundice progresses inexorably until death, usually within a year. In a few cases there is atresia of only a portion of the extrahepatic biliary system, and this can be treated by anastomosing the biliary tract to bowel.

Choledochal cyst is a congenital cystic deformity of the common bile duct, presenting with jaundice from obstruction of the duct and upper abdominal pain. Symptoms usually begin in the first 10 years of life. The cyst may be decompressed by anastomosis of its wall to adjacent duodenum or jejunum.

Cholelithiasis

Formation of Gallstones. The most common type of gallstone is the cholesterol stone. Cholesterol is not water soluble but becomes soluble in bile as a result of the action of bile salts and phospholipids, which form micelles in which cholesterol particles are dissolved. In the normal individual cholesterol remains in solution in bile throughout the physiologic ranges of concentration. Cholesterol may come out of solution as a result of:

1. Supersaturation with cholesterol. This occurs when the solubilizing effect of bile salts and phospholipids is exceeded by the amount of cholesterol. It can be demonstrated in vitro, but the in vivo evidence that increased cholesterol loading is a factor is still circumstantial.

2. Decreased solubilizing efficiency of bile. Small[14] has studied bile from normal individuals and patients with gallstones and correlated the occurrence of stones with changes in the bile salt-phospholipid-cholesterol ratio. This concept of abnormal bile that predisposes to stone formation ("lithogenic" bile) is further supported by studies of inbred Indian populations, where all members have abnormal bile and virtually all develop gallstones. This also lends some support to the clinical observation of a familial tendency to gallstone formation.

3. Infection. This is not a major primary etiologic factor in stone formation except in certain parts of the world, such as China, where parasitic infestation, particularly that caused by *Clinorchis sinensis*, may result in chronic biliary tract disease with multiple stones.

4. Biliary obstruction. Biliary stasis permits the growth of bacteria which deconjugate bilirubin glucuronate to insoluble calcium bilirubinate. This precipitated material forms

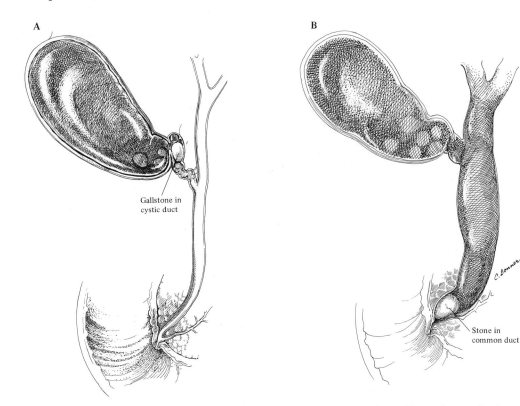

A

Gallstone in cystic duct

B

Stone in common duct

Figure 19–18.   *A.* A stone in the cystic duct is resulting in acute cholecystitis. *B.* A stone in the common bile duct is causing jaundice.

characteristic soft brown stones which may occur in the gallbladder, in the common bile duct above strictures, and are also occasionally seen in the bile duct in the absence of stricture or associated gallbladder stones.

Cholesterol stones are formed by precipitation of cholesterol crystals in the gallbladder. These coalesce with cellular debris and mucus to form concretions. Varying amounts of bile pigment and calcium carbonate may be incorporated to produce "mixed stones." In patients with chronic hemolytic anemias the bile pigment load is high, and almost pure pigment stones may develop.

Symptoms. Gallstones may be present for years without producing symptoms. Symptoms usually develop as a result of mechanical obstruction by a stone in the cystic duct or Hartmann's pouch (Figure 19–18, *A*). Tonic contraction of the gallbladder gives rise to biliary colic. If obstruction persists, edema of the gallbladder wall and chemical irritation may occur and produce acute cholecystitis, manifested by local pain, tenderness, fever, and leukocytosis. The attack may resolve or may become complicated by bacterial infection of the gallbladder. This also may subside spontaneously, but occasionally it progresses to perforation and either localized abscess or generalized peritonitis. Carcinoma of the gallbladder as a result of chronic irritation by calculi is a rare complication.

Stones may pass from the gallbladder into the common bile duct and then through the ampulla into the duodenum. The stone may obstruct the common duct (Figure 19–18, *B*), producing jaundice which is often intermittent. In 10 to 15 percent of patients with bile duct obstruction from stone, pain is not a prominent feature. With more prolonged obstruction of the common bile duct by stone, secondary infection (cholangitis) may occur and may be associated with transient episodes of high fever. This may progress to persistent high swinging temperature and toxemia due to the development of pus in the bile ducts and associated septicemia. This condition is known as suppurative cholangitis and is a surgical emergency requiring decompression of the biliary tree.[4]

Pancreatitis may complicate gallstones with or without stones in the common bile duct. About 40 percent of cases of acute pancreatitis are in fact associated with biliary calculi, and surgical removal of the gallbladder and associated stones usually prevents recurrence of this type of pancreatitis. A single large stone occasionally erodes through the wall of the gallbladder into the duodenum, passes down the small bowel, and occludes the terminal ileum, producing acute intestinal obstruction known as gallstone ileus.

Diagnosis. The history and physical examination are often sufficient to make a diagnosis of cholecystitis, but confirmation should be obtained by x-ray. Stones are seen on plain radiographs in less than 10 percent of patients. Oral cholecystography with or without intravenous cholangiography confirms the diagnosis in most of the remaining patients. Biochemical tests, especially alkaline phosphatase and conjugated bilirubin in the blood, are elevated in those with obstruction of the main extrahepatic bile ducts.

Treatment. There is controversy about the treatment of the patient who has gallstones but no symptoms.[8] Because of the likelihood of complications, cholecystectomy is usually recommended, provided that the patient is in good general health (Figure 19–19). Symptom-producing gallstones are best treated by cholecystectomy.

There are currently several clinical trials in progress in which oral feeding of chenodeoxycholic acid is being used to change bile composition to a more normal pattern. The preliminary reports suggest that dissolution of some gallstone may occur; however, this is experimental and is being used only in patients with asymptomatic gallstones or retained common bile duct stones. The long-term effects of bile salt feeding have not yet been determined.

Opinion is divided regarding the advisability of operation during an attack of acute cholecystitis. The conservative approach is based on the knowledge that most attacks settle spontaneously. Operation can then be done electively, generally after about three months, when the inflammatory process has resolved. Conservative treatment consists of giving nothing by mouth, intravenous fluids, and antibiotics. The patient is carefully observed and is operated on only if toxicity increases and there are signs of increasing peritoneal irritation. The operation consists of cholecystostomy performed through a small subcostal incision. The gallbladder is then removed after about three months.

There is increasing support for treatment of acute cholecystitis by cholecystectomy during the acute attack.[17] Those who advise immediate operation do so because the attacks do not always settle, perforation and peritonitis may occur, and the operation is not more hazardous providing patients are properly selected. The total period of hospitalization is shorter than if the patient is treated conservatively and then readmitted for cholecystectomy. The criteria for operation during an acute attack are: Diagnosis is definite, the patient's general condition is

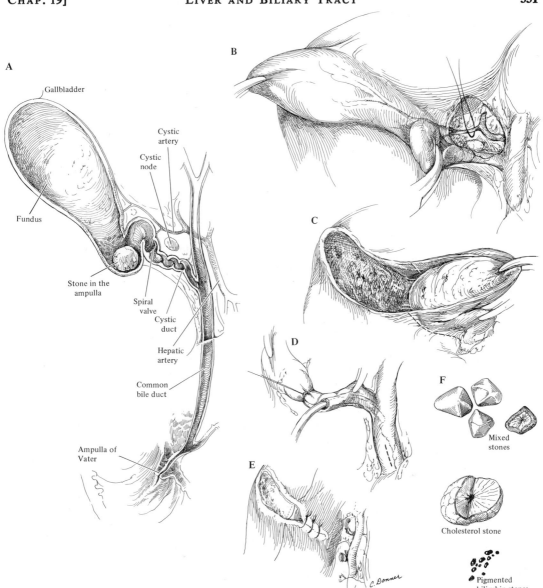

Figure 19–19. Technique of cholescystectomy. *A.* A right subcostal, transverse, or right para-median incision is generally used. After laparotomy, traction is applied to Hartmann's pouch using sponge forceps and the cystic duct is identified. The triangle defined by the cystic duct, common hepatic duct, and cystic vessels, and containing the cystic lymph node, is dissected out. *B.* The cystic artery is divided. *C.* The peritoneum is incised on the gallbladder at 1 cm from the liver and the gallbladder is mobilized from the liver. *D.* A catheter is inserted in the cystic duct and delivered into the common bile duct if an operative cholangiogram is to be performed. The cystic duct is ligated flush with the common bile duct, and the gallbladder is removed. If exploration of the common bile duct is indicated, a longitudinal incision is made in the anterior wall of the duct. *E.* The gallbladder bed in the liver is then reperitonealized. *F.* The gallstones may be mixed, cholesterol, or contain bilirubin.

good, the patient is not overweight, and the operation is performed within 48 hours of the onset of the attack.

An operative cholangiogram is particularly useful to demonstrate stones in the bile ducts. These are removed through an incision in the anterior wall of the common bile duct after removal of the gallbladder. The common bile

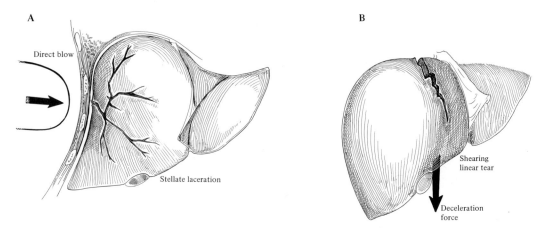

Figure 19–20. *A.* A direct blow may result in a stellate laceration or intrahepatic hematoma. *B.* Sudden deceleration results in a shearing force that tends to produce a linear tear.

duct may be anastomosed to the duodenum (choledochoduodenostomy) in patients with many stones in the extrahepatic ducts or with previous operation for stones. Antibiotics may be used to treat either bacterial cholecystitis or cholangitis, but such treatment is an adjuvant rather than an alternative to surgical therapy. Gallstone ileus is treated by operative removal of the obstructing stone. The stone is moved up into normal bowel and removed through a vertical incision in the gut. The gallbladder is usually removed after about three months.

Liver and Bile Duct Infections

Organisms may reach the liver and biliary tract either through the systemic or portal circulation. Protozoal and helminthic infections, as well as certain bacteria and viruses, enter through the portal route. Bacterial infection in the biliary tract rarely occurs in the absence of obstruction from stone, stricture, or tumor. It is characterized by high fever and biochemical signs of obstruction and may be associated with septicemic shock. Treatment is surgical decompression of the biliary tree and antibiotic therapy.

A pyogenic hepatic abscess is secondary to infection in the abdominal cavity and in other parts of the body, but in one half of reported cases a primary site cannot be found. Pyogenic hepatic abscess requires drainage and antibiotic therapy. Amebic hepatitis and abscess are always associated with intestinal amebiasis, although symptoms of the intestinal disease may be mild. Amebic abscess may be managed by aspiration and systemic antiamebic therapy and usually requires open drainage only if aspiration fails or if secondary pyogenic infection occurs.

Hydatid disease due to *Echinococcus granu-*

losus is the commonest helminthic infection of the liver in North America. It is endemic in a few areas and is frequently found in immigrant populations from the Mediterranean region. The symptoms of hydatid cyst in the liver are pain, fever, palpable mass, and jaundice, alone or in combination. The cysts can rarely be excised but are satisfactorily managed by evacuation of the contents with or without external drainage.

Viral infection may affect the liver alone, as in viral hepatitis, or may involve the liver as part of a systemic infection, as in infectious mononucleosis. Viral hepatitis is important in surgical practice because its symptoms may mimic surgical conditions. In the anicteric phase hepatic tenderness and pain may be confused

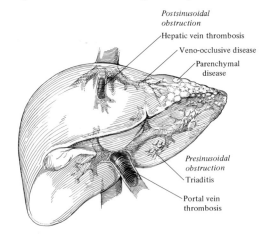

Figure 19–21. Obstructive conditions of the liver. In presinusoidal portal hypertension the portal pressure is elevated and the sinusoidal pressure is normal, while in postsinusoidal portal hypertension both pressures are elevated.

with inflammation of the gallbladder. In the subacute or chronic stage, particularly if the hepatitis is predominantly cholestatic, the differentiation from obstructive jaundice may be difficult. Viral hepatitis may occur as a complication of operation if blood or blood products contaminated with serum hepatitis virus are used.

Injuries to the Liver and Bile Ducts

The lower ribs protect the liver from injury. Closed injuries may produce hepatic lacerations either by direct force, in which case there is usually evidence of rib injury, or by sudden deceleration, as in a fall from a height when there may be no local signs of trauma (Figure 19–20). Penetrating wounds vary in severity depending on the nature of the wounding agent, its shape, and its velocity. Hemorrhage, biliary fistula, and infection are complications of hepatic injuries. Early operative treatment to stop bleeding, remove devitalized tissue, and establish adequate drainage has improved survival.

Bile duct injury due to external trauma is rare. The usual mechanism of injury is accidental damage at the time of operation on the gallbladder, common bile duct, or stomach and duodenum. Injury results in biliary fistula and bile duct stricture with resulting jaundice and infection and is treated with surgical reconstruction.

Space-Occupying Lesions in the Liver

Slowly enlarging lesions in the liver may reach great size before impairing hepatic function because of this organ's great reserves. There are no specific clinical means for differentiating hepatic tumor from cysts. Among the biochemical tests of hepatic function the alkaline phosphatase is often abnormal in the early stages. It may be elevated proportionally higher than the bilirubin or other enzymes in the case of infiltrating lesions. A radioactive scintiscan usually shows such lesions, and angiography may help distinguish between avascular cystic lesions and vascular tumors (Figures 19–13 and 19–14).

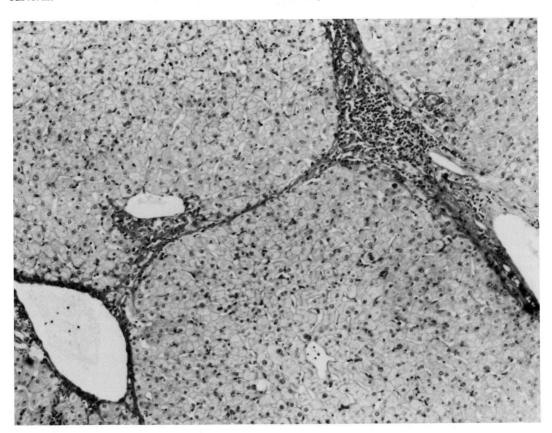

Figure 19–22.   Section of liver from a patient with advanced macronodular cirrhosis. Note the nodular character of the parenchyma. The septa are of variable thickness and contain large veins. (Hematoxylin and eosin stain × 120.) (Courtesy of Dr. M. J. Phillips.)

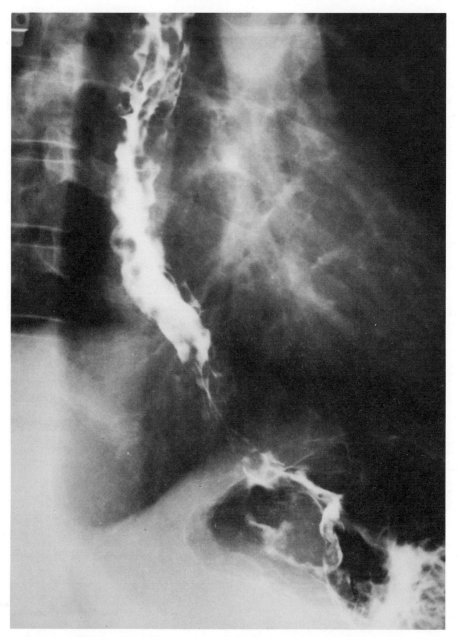

Figure 19–23. Barium examination of the esophagus showing extensive esophageal varices. (Courtesy of Dr. R. F. Colapinto.)

The commonest malignant lesion of the liver is metastatic carcinoma from the gastrointestinal tract. Primary hepatic malignancies are less common and are most likely to occur in patients with cirrhosis. Carcinoma of the gallbladder is an uncommon tumor that tends to infiltrate the liver. Cholangiocarcinoma may present as an hepatic tumor when it arises in the intrahepatic bile ducts, or as a cause of jaundice when it arises in the extrahepatic biliary tree. It may be mistaken for a benign bile duct stricture or sclerosing cholangitis. Benign lesions may be removed by local or segmental resection. Cysts may be excised when technically easy; otherwise evacuation of the contents and drainage usually suffice. Excision of hepatic lesions is technically possible[2] but may be difficult and requires an accurate knowledge of segmental anatomy.

Malignant lesions are not often curable by excision. A carcinoma of the gallbladder may be treated by cholecystectomy and segmental removal of the adjacent liver or right lobectomy. Bile duct tumors can occasionally be resected but are more often treated by palliative methods in an attempt to maintain biliary tract drainage.

Hepatic Cirrhosis and Portal Hypertension

Pathophysiology. Portal pressure is determined by the blood flow and resistance. Normally there is little resistance and the portal pressure is between 7 and 10 mm of mercury. This pressure may be measured directly through a catheter in the portal vein introduced either through a tributary at the time of operation or through the reopened umbilical vein. The portal pressure may also be estimated by measuring intrasplenic pressure through a percutaneous needle. Intrahepatic or "sinusoidal" pressure is normally the same as portal vein pressure and may be measured by percutaneous puncture of

the liver itself or the hepatic vein wedged pressure via a catheter introduced through the vena cava.

In rare instances portal hypertension may be due to increased portal inflow, as in patients with arteriovenous fistula. The majority, however, result from increased resistance in the liver. Portal hypertension can thus be classified according to the site of the lesion (Figure 19–21). When the obstruction to flow is in the portal vein or its tributaries, the portal and splenic pressures are elevated, but the hepatic wedged and intrahepatic pressure is normal. This type of obstruction is said to be "presinusoidal." When the obstruction to flow is in the main hepatic vein or its tributaries, portal and intrahepatic pressures are equally elevated. The block in this situation is said to be "postsinusoidal." The commonest condition causing portal hypertension is hepatic cirrhosis in which there is collapse of hepatic lobules, formation of diffuse fibrosis, and areas of nodular regeneration

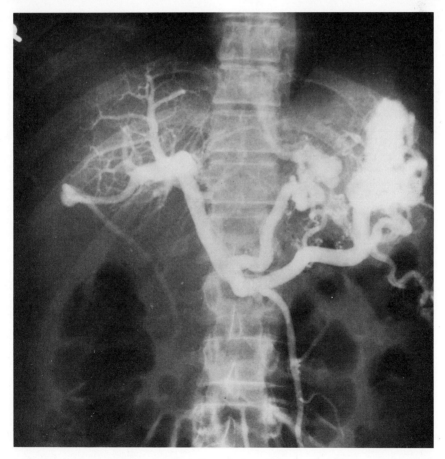

Figure 19–24. Splenoportogram showing large bolus of dye in the spleen, patent splenic and portal veins, and collateral flow through the inferior mesenteric vein and a large coronary vein. (Courtesy of Dr. R. F. Colapinto.)

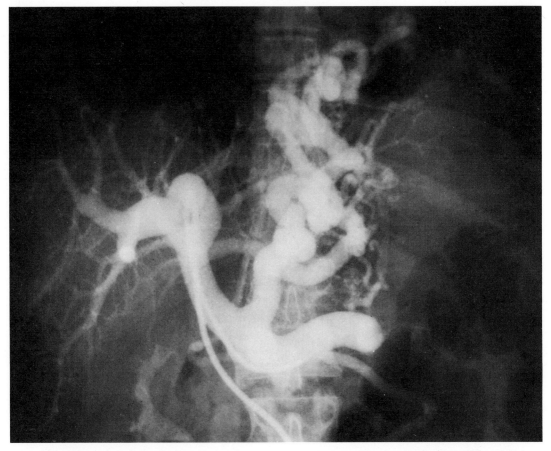

Figure 19-25.   Umbilical portogram. The catheter has been introduced through the obliterated umbilical vein into the portal vein. Note the huge coronary vein leading into dilated, tortuous, gastroesophageal varices.

(Figure 19–22). Most patients with cirrhosis have a "postsinusoidal" block.

Portal hypertension in cirrhotics is associated with a decrease in portal venous flow through the liver and the development of portasystemic shunts. The sites for the collateral flow are the submucosal gastroesophageal veins, the inferior mesenteric vein, and retroperitoneal, splenic, and paraumbilical veins.

Complications.   The major complications possible in cirrhotics with portal hypertension are bleeding from varices, hepatic encephalopathy, and ascites. Bleeding from varices is sudden, painless, and profuse. There may be other manifestations of liver disease. The immediate mortality of bleeding varices is high and the likelihood of rebleeding is frequent. Ascites usually indicates advanced liver disease or a sudden deterioration in a formerly stable, cirrhotic liver.

Evaluation of the Patient with Bleeding Varices. The clinical diagnosis of bleeding from varices

must be confirmed, and other causes of upper gastrointestinal bleeding must be excluded, such as peptic ulcer and acute gastritis. The incidence of peptic ulcer is high in cirrhotics probably because of poor nutrition, venous congestion in the bowel, and a high blood level of histamine because of impaired breakdown of the hormone by the liver. The most useful techniques to determine the cause of bleeding are barium examination of the upper gastrointestinal tract (Figure 19–23) and esophagogastroscopy. The accuracy of these examinations varies with the skill of the examiner, but each alone is approximately 75 percent accurate and together they are 90 percent accurate.

The suitability for operation and potential for survival are more closely related to the functional capacity of the liver than to the severity of the hemorrhage. It is therefore important to determine liver function accurately before operation. A liver biopsy is also useful, especially in the alcoholic patient, in evaluating liver function.

Hemodynamic abnormalities are investigated because they influence the choice of surgical treatment. Splenoportography allows measurement of portal pressure and visualization of the varices (Figure 19–24). The main complication following insertion of a needle into the spleen is a tear that may require splenectomy. This procedure should not be performed in the jaundiced or ascitic patient, when the prothrombin time is prolonged or the platelet count is low. For more accurate assessment an umbilical vein may be catheterized, and transhepatic catheterization or wedged hepatic vein pressures may be performed (Figure 19–25). These studies are useful to determine the degree of portal hypertension, the alteration in flow patterns, and the changes that may be expected after operation.

Treatment. Several major problems may co-exist in the patient with bleeding varices, including coagulation disorders, respiratory insufficiency, and in some cases renal decompensation. Treatment aims to correct the metabolic and hemodynamic abnormalities, to prevent organ failure, and to stop bleeding. Blood and fluid replacement are required to maintain circulating volume and adequate hepatic blood flow. Adequate oxygenation and ventilatory function are essential. Normal plasma glucose levels are maintained by infusing glucose. Hepatic encephalopathy is treated by colonic irrigation and oral neomycin to reduce bacterial flora in the colon. Protein is not given orally, and blood is removed from the gut using a Levin tube and enemas. Coagulation defects are treated by parenteral vitamin K, which may partially correct low prothrombin levels, and by fresh blood. Platelet transfusions are rarely required.

Bleeding from varices may stop spontaneously but in most treatment is essential. Intravenous Pitressin may be given to produce transient splanchnic vasoconstriction and decrease portal flow and pressure. Although it successfully stops bleeding in a high percentage of patients, bleeding often recurs. Pitressin may produce myocardial ischemia in patients with preexisting cardiac disease. Tamponade of varices using the Sengstaken-Blakemore tube or one of its modifications also temporarily controls bleeding (Figure 19–26). Careful continuous supervision is essential, because the balloon may be dislodged and cause acute respiratory obstruction.

Emergency operation should be considered in patients who do not stop bleeding after conservative management. The decision to operate depends on the patient's general condition and liver function. In patients with advanced hepatic failure the high mortality precludes operation. Transesophageal ligation of varices effectively

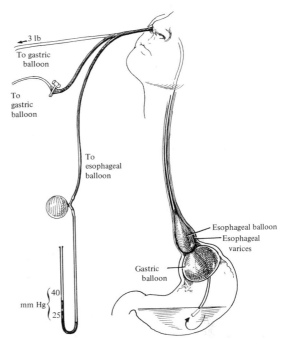

Figure 19–26. The Sengstaken-Blakemore tube is inserted to control bleeding from esophageal varices.

controls bleeding, but rebleeding is frequent. An emergency portosystemic decompression is preferred because it controls bleeding and is rarely followed by recurrence.[10]

Operation is also advisable in patients who have stopped bleeding and have reasonably good liver function. A portosystemic decompression is generally the best procedure because of the high risk of recurrence of bleeding. The common shunts are the end-to-side portacaval anastomosis and end-to-side splenorenal anastomosis[5] (Figure 19–27). The diversion of significant amounts of portal venous flow from the liver may be a factor responsible for postshunt encephalopathy and hepatic failure. There is considerable interest in modifying these operations to preserve hepatic blood flow while allowing decompression of the gastroesophageal veins. The Warren distal splenorenal shunt[16] preserves superior mesenteric flow to the liver but allows variceal decompression through the short gastric and splenic veins, and may prove to be superior to the standard procedures. Prophylactic shunt procedures in cirrhotics with known varices, who have not bled are not indicated.[12]

Other Diseases of Interest to the Surgeon

Postoperative jaundice is not a specific disease but may be seen after a variety of operations or as a result of major injury or illness. The main

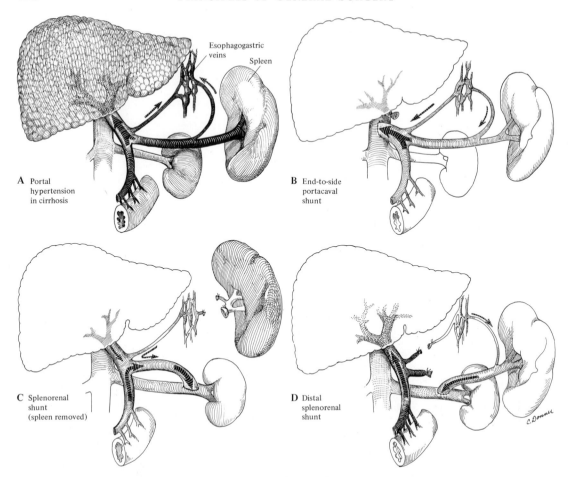

Figure 19–27. Decompression operations performed for portal hypertension. *A.* In portal hypertension from cirrhosis, the flow is reversed in the coronary and short gastric veins. *B.* With an end-to-side portacaval shunt, there is a normal direction of flow in the coronary and esophageal veins but portal blood flow to the liver is eliminated. *C.* A splenorenal shunt decreases pressure in the portal system and often causes reversal of flow of portal blood to the liver. *D.* With a Warren shunt, there is decompression of esophageal varices but maintenance of a high pressure in the superior mesenteric vein and continued portal inflow to the liver.

factors which may contribute to the hyperbilirubinemia include:

1. An increased pigment load from transfused old stored blood, blood extravasated into the tissues, and increased catabolism of cells containing heme pigments.

2. Impaired liver handling of pigment due to transient hypoxia or decreased hepatic blood flow.

3. Impaired renal excretion of conjugated bilirubin.

Other specific causes of postoperative jaundice are incompatible blood transfusion, bile duct obstruction, and hepatic artery ligation. Halothane hepatitis is a rare condition caused by hypersensitivity to the anesthetic halothane (see Chapter 12, page 227).

Alcoholic liver disease varies from fatty infiltration of the liver to advanced cirrhosis. During intensive exposure to alcohol acute alcoholic hepatitis, characterized by fever, leukocytosis, hepatomegaly, and jaundice, occurs. Liver failure may occur associated with an increase in portal pressure and bleeding.

Clinical hepatic transplantation has been carried out in several centers since the first attempt in the early 1960s. Unlike renal transplantation, however, this operation is not yet a practical clinical reality. There have been a few long-term survivors, but the problems of temporary support for the patient with the failing liver are yet to be overcome. The most suitable patients at present are those with chronic incurable, nonmalignant liver disease, where one has sufficient time to find a suitable donor.

CITED REFERENCES

1. Bucher, N. L. R.: Experimental aspects of hepatic regeneration. *N. Engl. J. Med.*, **277**:686–96, 738–46, 1967.
2. Fortner, J. G.; Beattie, E. J.; Shin, M. H.; Howland, W. S.; Watson, R. D.; Gaston, J. P.; and Benna, R. S.: Surgery in liver tumors. *Current Problems in Surgery.* Yearbook Medical Publishers, Chicago, June 1972.
3. Healey, John E., Jr.: Clinical anatomic aspects of radical hepatic surgery. *J. Intern. Coll. Surg.*, **22**:542–49, 1954.
4. Hinchey, E. J.: Acute obstructive suppurative cholangitis. *Am. J. Surg.*, **117**:62–68, 1969.
5. Jackson, F. C.; Perrin, E. B.; Felix, W. R.; and Smith, A. G.: A clinical investigation of the portocaval shunt. *Ann. Surg.*, **174**:672–701, 1971.
6. Leevy, C. M.: Clinical Aspects of the hepatic circulation. *Gastroenterology*, **48**:790–804, 1965.
7. Lidner, H.: Limitations and dangers in percutaneous liver biopsies with the Menghini needle. Proc. Third World Cong. *Gastroenterology*, **3**:373–75, 1966.
8. McSherry, C. K., and Glenn, F.: Surgical aspects of biliary tract disease. *Am. J. Med.*, **51**:651–58, 1971.
9. Michels, N. A.: The hepatic cystic and retroduodenal arteries and their relation to the biliary ducts. *Ann. Surg.*, **133**:503–24, 1951.
10. Orloff, M. J.: Emergency portocaval shunt: a comparative study of shunt, varix ligation and nonsurgical treatment of bleeding esophageal varices in unselected patients with cirrhosis. *Ann. Surg.*, **166**:456–74, 1967.
11. Rappaport, A. A.: Anatomic considerations. In Schiff, Leon (ed.): *Diseases of the Liver.* J. B. Lippincott Co., Phil. pp. 1–49, 1969.
12. Resnick, R. H.; Chalmers, T. C.; Ishihara, A. M.; Garcean, A. J.; Callow, A. D.; Schimmel, E. M.; O'Hara, E. T.; and Boston Interhospital Liver Group: A controlled study of the prophylactic portocaval shunt. *Ann. Intern. Med.*, **70**:675–88, 1969.
13. Schmid, Rudi: Bilirubin metabolism in man. *N. Engl. J. Med.*, **287**:703–709, 1972.
14. Small, Donald M.: Gallstones. *N. Engl. J. Med.*, **279**:588–93, 1968.
15. Walls, W. D., and Losowsky, M. S.: The hemostatic defect of liver disease. *Gastroenterology*, **60**:108–19, 1971.
16. Warren, W. D.; Zeppa, R.; and Fomon, J. J.: Selective trans-splenic decompression of esophagogastric varices by distal splenorenal shunt. *Ann. Surg.*, **166**:437–55, 1967.
17. Welch, C. E.: Cholecystectomy for acute cholecystitis. *Surgery*, **49**:284–88, 1961.

SUGGESTIONS FOR FURTHER READING

Child, C. G.: The liver and portal hypertension. In: *Major Problems in Clinical Surgery.* Vol. I. W. B. Saunders Co., Philadelphia, 1964.

This is a classic monograph which describes the development of surgery for portal hypertension, details the evaluation of patients, pathophysiology of collateral circulation, ascites, and coma. Operations available and unsolved problems are discussed.

Madding, G. F., and Kennedy, P. A.: Trauma of the liver. In: *Major Problems in Clinical Surgery.* Vol. III. W. B. Saunders Co., Philadelphia, 1971.

This is an excellent review of the surgical anatomy of the liver and approaches to hepatic resection. Hepatic injuries are discussed based largely on wartime experience but applicable to the civilian injuries now seen with increasing frequency.

Sherlock, Sheila: *Diseases of the Liver and Biliary System.* Blackwell Scientific Publications, Oxford, 1965.

This is a very complete, easily readable textbook of hepatology compiled by a master clinician and investigator and based on a wealth of clinical experience.

Chapter 20

PANCREAS

James Kyle

CHAPTER OUTLINE

Exocrine Pancreas
  Development
  Anatomy
  Physiology
    Control
  Clinical Features of Diseases of the
    Exocrine Pancreas
    Pain
    Jaundice
    Loss of Weight
  Pancreatic Investigations
    Biochemical Tests
    Secretory Tests

Radiology of the Pancreas
Diseases of the Pancreas
  Congenital
  Trauma
  Acute Pancreatitis
  Chronic Pancreatitis and Pancreatic
    Lithiasis
  Carcinoma of the Pancreas
  Endocrine-Secreting Tumors of the
    Pancreas
    Islet Cell Tumors
    Zollinger-Ellison Syndrome

EXOCRINE PANCREAS

Lying obliquely across the upper part of the retroperitoneum, partially masked by the costal margin and stomach, the pancreas is one of the least accessible structures within the abdomen. In a world of ever-increasing violence these structures do not protect the pancreas from trauma. Injuries of the pancreas are therefore increasingly common in penetrating wounds of the upper abdomen and in automobile accidents. Acute pancreatitis may present as one of the most dramatic abdominal surgical emergencies. The onset and progression of pancreatic neoplasms may be as insidious and even more sinister than carcinoma of the stomach.

Development

The pancreas develops in two parts from the duodenal loop between the fourth and seventh weeks of intrauterine life. Most of the pancreas—part of the head, the neck, body, and tail—is formed from a diverticulum that arises from the dorsal aspect of the duodenal loop. A ventral diverticulum, closely related to the early bile duct, forms the remainder of the head. The duodenal loop rotates to the right and posteriorly, and the two parts of the pancreas then fuse. Abnormal rotation gives rise to annular pancreas.

Initially the main duct is derived from the dorsal diverticulum, but later the ventral duct becomes the main pancreatic duct of Wirsung. The right portion of the dorsal duct usually persists as the accessory pancreatic duct of Santorini and drains the upper part of the head of the pancreas. It may or may not communicate with the main duct.

Anatomy

The pancreas is an elongated, cream-colored, compound, racemose gland (see Plates IV and VI). Its lobules are normally soft and somewhat loosely arranged, and there is no proper fibrous capsule. Flattened anteroposteriorly, the head of the gland fills the concavity of the duodenal loop. It is joined to the body by the neck, behind which passes the superior mesenteric vein to join the splenic vein and form the portal vein. The body of the pancreas passes upward and to the left at an angle of 30° to 40°, ending as the tail, which is usually in contact with the hilum of the spleen.

Behind the right upper part of the head of the pancreas lies the common bile duct which passes downward in a groove on or almost surrounded by the pancreas to join the main pancreatic duct at the ampulla of Vater. The common opening into the duodenum, or papilla, is on the medial wall at the distal end of the second part of the duodenum. The accessory duct enters the duodenum about 2 cm beyond the pylorus and may be damaged when the duodenum is mobilized during gastrectomy. The unyielding lumbar spine lies behind the neck and adjacent body, with the inferior vena cava to the right and the aorta on the left. The left kidney lies posterior to the body. The uncinate process of the pancreas is a leftward extension of the lower part of the head which passes for a short distance behind the superior mesenteric vessels.

The principal anterior relation is the stomach, which, with the lesser peritoneal sac, covers most of the body and tail of the pancreas. The hepatic flexure of the colon overlies the head with only loose areolar tissue intervening. Loops of jejunum may be in contact with the lower edge of the head and body.

The arterial supply is derived from the gastroduodenal, superior mesenteric, and splenic arteries. The anterior and posterior branches of the superior pancreaticoduodenal artery pass down in the sulci between the head and the

medial border of the duodenum to anastomose with corresponding branches from the superior mesenteric artery. Variations in the arterial branches of the celiac axis are common.

Surgically the venous drainage of the pancreas is more important and troublesome than the arterial supply. Resectability of a neoplasm is often determined by the presence or absence of invasion of the superior mesenteric or portal vein. Several short, friable tributaries usually enter the right side and front of the mesenteric vein in the region of the uncinate process and lower part of the neck. The splenic vein lies below the splenic artery and is overlapped by the body and tail from which it receives numerous fine tributaries.

At the upper border of the pancreas and surrounding the arterial celiac axis lie the celiac ganglia and autonomic nerve plexus. A chain of lymph nodes extends from the celiac axis along the upper border of the pancreas to the splenic hilum.

Microscopically the pancreas resembles the salivary glands, with which it has a pathologic relationship. The exocrine unit is the acinus, lined by secreting columnar cells. Often an inner

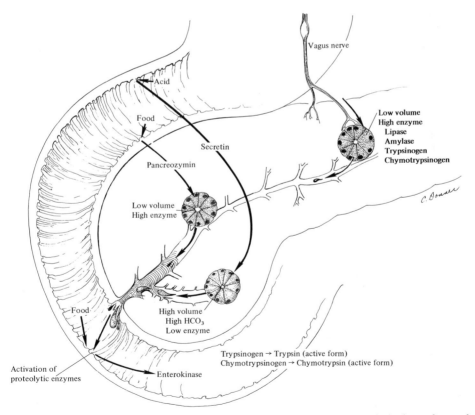

Figure 20-1.   The duodenum and pancreas secrete enzymes involved in carbohydrate, fat, and protein digestion.

darkly staining zone is seen in these cells, probably due to the presence of secretory granules. Fine ductules, lined by flattened cells, connect the acini to the main duct system. Between the acini in places lie clusters of insulin-secreting endocrine cells, the islets of Langerhans.

Physiology

The pancreas is a very active exocrine gland, secreting 1000 to 1500 ml of pancreatic juice every 24 hours. It contains enzymes essential for digestion of foodstuffs and a large amount of bicarbonate, pH 8.4, for neutralizing gastric acid that enters the duodenum. The acinar cells have a high rate of protein synthesis. Injected, tagged amino acids appear within a minute or two in the zymogen in the acinar cells.

Three main groups of enzymes are secreted. Amylase acts on ingested carbohydrate, hydrolyzing polysaccharides into maltose (Figure 20–1). Lipase splits neutral fat into fatty acids and glycerol. This process is facilitated by the presence of bile salts, which help emulsification and increase the solubility of freed fatty acids. The third group of enzymes is concerned with the digestion of proteins. Both trypsin, a powerful enzyme, and chymotrypsin are released from the cells as inactive precursors. Enterokinase in the duodenum assists in their activation. These proteolytic enzymes, along with carboxypeptidase, break down polypeptides into amino acids and small peptides that can be absorbed in the small intestine. Ribonuclease and deoxyribonuclease, which split nucleic acid, are also secreted by the pancreas.

Control. The pancreas has hormonal and nervous control systems. Hormonal regulation is the more important, but there is a close interrelationship between the two and with ingested food products, bile salts, and other gastrointestinal hormones, such as gastrin. All the possible interactions have not yet been fully established.

Stimulation of the vagus nerve (parasympathetic) in experimental animals produces a moderate flow of viscid pancreatic juice, rich in enzymes. Atropine blocks this action. In man stomachlike phases of pancreatic secretion have been described (e.g., psychic, gastric, and intestinal). They are probably the result of variations in the output of hydrochloric acid by the stomach before and during a meal. There may also be some direct stimulation of pancreatic cells by parasympathetic postganglionic nerve fibers. Highly selective vagotomy, which preserves the nerve supply to the gastric antrum and pancreas, allows a good flow of pancreatic enzymes to be obtained in response to hypoglycemia. The effect of insulin on the exocrine function of the pancreas is probably mediated by the vagus nerve.

The principal hormones regulating pancreatic secretion are secretin and pancreozymin, which is possibly identical with cholecystokinin (CCK-PZ) produced in the duodenum and jejunum. When injected intravenously secretin stimulates the flow of a large volume of alkaline pancreatic juice with a low enzyme content. The presence of acid in the duodenum and jejunum appears to be the chief factor in the liberation of secretin, but fat and to a lesser extent proteoses are also effective. However, in man it is doubtful if the luminal pH in the distal duodenum or proximal jejunum is ever sufficiently low to permit significant amounts of secretin to be released. The precise role of secretin in human physiology is less certain today than it was 70 years ago.

Breakdown products of protein and fat are responsbile for the liberation of pancreozymin, the protein products being more active. There is controversy about how effective acid in the upper intestinal tract may be in the release of CCK-PZ. Pancreozymin has an action on the pancreas similar to that produced by excitation of the parasympathetic nerves, namely an enzyme-rich juice. Atropine does not prevent this action.

Experimentally gastrin, some prostaglandins, and vasoactive peptide can stimulate secretion from the pancreas, while in certain circumstances calcitonin and glucagon may have some inhibitory effect. Other inhibitory mechanisms may exist. In disease states there may be imbalance between the complex hormonal and neural control systems. For example, in duodenal ulceration the bicarbonate pancreatic response to duodenal acidification may be deranged.

Clinical Features of Diseases of the Exocrine Pancreas

The three main clinical features of pancreatic disease are pain, jaundice, and weight loss. Frequently they coexist, especially in the chronic diseases of the pancreas.

Pain. Although within the abdomen the pancreas is completely outside the peritoneal cavity so that the classic features of peritoneal irritation are not present unless that membrane is breached. Pancreatic pain may be visceral and referred to the lower thoracic and upper lumbar regions (Figure 20–2). Immediately cephalad of the pancreas is the solar plexus, a complex network of autonomic nerves and ganglia, from which the pancreas receives fibers. A punch on this network results in collapse and nausea. The upper retroperitoneum is generously supplied with laminated pacinian corpuscles, which will

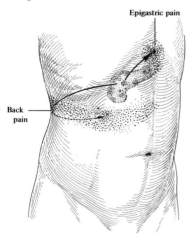

Epigastric pain

Back
pain

Figure 20–2. Pancreatic pain may be referred to the epigastrium and to the back, including the left costovertebral region.

generate afferent impulses when stimulated. The posterior parietes are frequently involved in inflammatory and neoplastic processes; their sensory nerves pass to the spinal cord through the posterior nerve roots. The diaphragm is supplied by the somatic phrenic nerve from the third, fourth, and fifth cervical segments of the cord.

There are therefore plenty of afferent nerve pathways from the pancreas, but it is not clear how the pain sensation is generated. Some fine nerve fibers are probably especially designed to transmit pain, but in many instances pain results from abnormal and excessive stimulation of an end-receptor or nerve which normally serves some other function, such as stretch or pressure. Thus distention of a duct results in pain, and the pressure quickly built up in the retroperitoneum by an effusion produces the same sensation. It is possible that digestive enzymes, kinins, histamine, and potassium ions can directly cause pain. Peristalsis does not seem to be important in the pancreas. Colic, however, can occur if the bile duct or intestine is involved. Infiltration of somatic nerves in the posterior abdominal wall, as by extension of a tumor, gives well-localized pain. Visceral pain sensation transmitted by autonomic pathways is less accurately localized.

The pain of acute pancreatitis comes on rapidly. In about 40 percent of patients it starts in the right hypochondrium, moves within an hour to the epigastrium, and later spreads to the left hypochondrium. This right-to-left progression of steady severe pain suggests that the first inflammatory reaction is in the gallbladder, that the head of the pancreas is soon involved, and that the swelling occludes the main duct and results in the pancreatitis involving the body

and tail. In many patients the pain is confined to the epigastrium. The pain rarely extends below the umbilicus but is often present in the upper lumbar region. In severe cases diaphragmatic irritation results in shoulder tip pain.

Occasionally there is an associated acute cholecystitis with right upper abdominal pain, going through to the right scapular region and right shoulder, and accompanied by fever. There is generally little pyrexia or evidence of bacterial infection in the first few days of acute pancreatitis. In severe pancreatitis enzyme-rich fluid may eventually enter the peritoneum and produce the pain of generalized peritonitis. Pain is absent in 5 percent of acute pancreatitis, especially if it occurs early after an operation.

Morphine and alcohol may cause spasm of the sphincter of Oddi. The increase in pressure inside the duct of Wirsung could cause further pain and increase the enzymatic disruption. Consequently morphine preparations are avoided in the treatment of acute pancreatitis. Although the precise action of Demerol on the sphincter is uncertain, it generally gives relief. Antispasmodics, such as propantheline, can ease the pain but only in large doses. Intravenous glucagon reduces pancreatic secretion and may relax spasm but should only be administered with care in patients with a low circulating insulin level.

Cancer of the ampullary region and of the head is painless in about one third of patients; in the remainder the pain is mild and felt deep in the epigastrium and the back. Cancer of the body of the pancreas is usually not diagnosed until the tumor is large and has infiltrated backward to involve the somatic nerves of the posterior abdominal wall. The pain is severe, unrelenting, boring in character, and located in midback. It is aggravated by lying flat and decreased by bending forward. The patient may sit for hours in a chair bent forward, or if in bed he sits leaning across a bedtable or clasping his drawn-up knees (Figure 20–3). Interruption of nerve pathways by phenol injection or operative intervention is frequently necessary.

Jaundice. Pancreatic disease can cause obstructive jaundice, with retention of bile pigments and bile salts in the circulation. Although the pigments cause the obvious yellowish discoloration of the tissues, the bile salt retention is more damaging.

Overt jaundice is uncommon in the first 24 hours of an attack of acute pancreatitis. It could be the result of pressure of a turgid, inflamed gallbladder or a swollen head of pancreas on the common bile duct. Rarely is it due to the presence of a stone impacted at the ampulla. A mild jaundice is often present on the

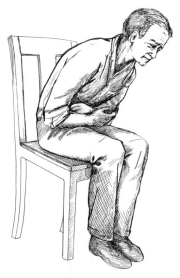

Figure 20–3. Patient with severe pancreatic pain often obtains relief by a characteristic bending-forward.

second or third day and usually disappears in 48 hours. It is probably due to edema of the head of the pancreas. If jaundice persists and deepens, then a stone is probably present in the common bile duct and operation is necessary. Jaundice first appearing after four or five days suggests that an abscess or pseudocyst is developing and compressing the lower end of the bile duct.

A small number of patients with acute pancreatitis go on to develop recurrent attacks and have an associated biliary tract disease. Fortunately later attacks are less severe than the first one, with pain less intense and jaundice less noticeable.

Intermittent and unpredictable short attacks of jaundice are a feature of chronic pancreatitis. It is doubtful if the absence of bile salts from the intestine contributes much to the steatorrhea usually present. A stricture may be present at the papilla or multiple strictures in the pancreatic duct. A sphincteroplasty stops the icteric attacks and often improves the pancreatitis but will be of no value when the multiple strictures are within the pancreas.

Jaundice is the first symptom in most patients with carcinoma at the ampulla of Vater. Its intensity may fluctuate slightly, but the serum bilirubin gradually rises to high levels. Neoplasms of the head also give rise to icterus at an early stage, which increases steadily until the patient is a greenish or mahogany color. The feces are clay colored and the urine dark amber. The gallbladder is palpable in only 50 percent of cases, showing the inaccuracy of Courvoisier's law. Jaundice is rarely caused by metastases in the hilar nodes from a primary carcinoma in the pancreas, pressing on the extrahepatic bile ducts.

Most patients with deep jaundice have severe pruritus. The exact mechanism of this disordered pain sensation is not clear, but bile salts deposited in the deep layers of the skin may play a part. The patient's greenish-brown nails may be highly polished from constant scratching. Cholestyramine in large doses may give some relief. Testosterone was formerly used, but it may produce cholestasis and this is undesirable in an icteric patient. A biliary bypass operation dramatically relieves pruritus often before the serum bile pigments or salts fall significantly.

Loss of Weight. Weight loss may be the result of inadequate intake, excessive loss, or increased catabolism.

In acute pancreatitis nausea and vomiting prevent food intake. Since food intake stimulates pancreatic secretions and increases the pain, the patient soon stops eating. In severe pancreatitis edema and swelling in the mucosa of the gastric antrum and adjacent duodenum produce nausea and loss of appetite. With chronic lesions there is sometimes mechanical distortion of the gastrointestinal tract. The presence of a peptic ulcer or portal hypertension from thrombosis of the portal vein contributes to the patient's inability to take food.

Severe impairment of lipase secretion results in steatorrhea and loss of calories. The pale bulky stool has an oily appearance and an offensive smell and tends to float on top of water. Not only is a rich source of calories lost, but the fat-soluble vitamins, A, D, E, and K, are not properly absorbed as a result of bile and pancreatic obstruction. The blood prothrombin time is prolonged. Absorption of calcium and magnesium is impaired, so that the bones become osteoporotic. Hypomagnesemia may interfere with the action of parathormone. Some patients with chronic pancreatitis develop brown discoloration on extensor skin.

Weight loss may be the first sign that a diabetic patient has developed a carcinoma. With cancer at the ampulla of Vater some blood is occasionally shed into the duodenum. When mixed with a steatorrheic stool, this blood may rarely give a silver or aluminium color to the stool.

In acute pancreatitis the proteolytic enzymes that escape among the pancreatic cells and into the retroperitoneum cause extensive tissue destruction. Repair results in a large nitrogen deficit. The complications of acute pancreatitis, especially abscess and fistula, further impair nutrition. Patients lose protein into pleural and pericardial effusions, and 5 to 10 percent bleed from the stomach or duodenum at some time in the protracted course of their illness.

The presence of ascites from peritoneal metastases results in loss of protein, water, and electrolytes.

Intravenous alimentation is advisable when there has been considerable weight loss, especially in those with fistulae. Supplementary vitamins may be needed and intramuscular injections of vitamin K if operation is contemplated.

In acute pancreatitis the blood glucagon level may rise initially and then fall later; the insulin level is reduced. In more chronic states the diabetes tends to be "brittle" or difficult to control. With insufficient insulin in chronic pancreatitis, lipids may not be cleared properly from the blood after a meal.

Pancreatic Investigations

In addition to determining the general state of patients with suspected exocrine pancreatic disease, and performing tests of pancreatic function, it is important to fully investigate the liver, gallbladder, and extrahepatic biliary system and the function of the islets of Langerhans. The investigations may be classified as biochemical, secretory, radiologic, and scanning.

Biochemical Tests. Because the pancreas plays such a major part in digestion and is closely linked to the liver, a large number of pancreatic function tests are possible. None, however, is reliable enough to be valuable in diagnosis.

There are large quantities of bicarbonate, sodium, potassium, and chloride in the pancreatic juice. Serum concentrations should be checked frequently because of the substantial losses in acute pancreatitis and pancreatic fistulae. The serum calcium level falls in those with fat necrosis. Occasionally pancreatitis is associated with the hypercalcemia of hyperparathyroidism.

Amylase is formed in the liver, salivary glands, and pancreas and is cleared rapidly from the blood. Less than 25 percent appears in the urine. The normal serum amylase is 70 to 300 IU per liter. Grossly elevated serum values are found in most cases of acute pancreatitis, but in some patients the serum amylase level remains normal. Elevated levels usually fall in a few hours. The serum amylase is also increased in other acute abdominal conditions such as perforated peptic ulcer, intestinal obstruction, and rupture of aortic aneurysm.

In health the excretion of fat in the stools should not exceed 18 m mol per 24 hours (5 gm per day). The output of pancreatic enzymes has to be decreased by 90 percent before there is obvious steatorrhea. Prolonged storage of specimens before performing the fat content estimation may lead to altered values, and the test is of no value in determining the cause of the steatorrhea.

Secretory Tests. *Lundh Test.* The concentration of pancreatic enzymes in the duodenum, after stimulation by a standard meal, is determined by the Lundh test.[2] The fasting patient is intubated with a radiopaque tube, the tip of which is weighted with a small mercury bag. The tube is placed in the duodenum using x-ray control. The patient drinks 300 ml of a solution containing water, 40 gm glucose, 18 gm corn oil, and 15 gm of the protein preparation Casilan. The duodenal contents are then aspirated every 30 minutes for two hours. The specimens are stored at $-30°C$ until enzymatic estimations are performed.

Abnormally low enzyme outputs are found in 90 percent of patients with chronic pancreatitis, and the results are abnormal in 80 percent of patients with carcinoma of the pancreas. When jaundice is due to obstruction within the bile ducts, the Lundh test is nearly always normal.

Secretin-Pancreozymin Stimulation Test. The enzyme and bicarbonate outputs of the pancreas are determined after infusions of secretin and CCK-PZ.[6] An opaque tube is placed in the duodenum of the fasting patient and gastric juice aspirated through nasogastric tube. An intravenous infusion is then given for 50 minutes, consisting of 0.15 M of sodium chloride containing secretin at a dose of 1.0 clinical unit per kilogram body weight each hour and CCK-PZ at 1.0 Ivy unit per kilogram each hour. The bicarbonate, amylase, and trypsin contents of the aspirate are then measured. The bicarbonate concentration is variable and not very helpful. Enzyme output after stimulation in normal subjects shows a skew distribution, so that interpretation can be difficult. Before a low output is ascribed to pancreatic insufficiency, the potency of the hormones must be checked.

Radiology of the Pancreas. A straight radiograph of the abdomen may show calcification in the pancreas or pancreatic lithiasis. Oblique views and tomograms may be needed to determine the exact position of the calcified material. Soft x-rays may reveal a soft tissue mass or displacement of adjacent structures, such as the stomach and kidney. A straight radiograph of the chest is advisable to exclude a primary bronchogenic neoplasm. In pancreatitis there may be a pleural effusion and fixity of the diaphragm.

Examination of adjacent viscera sometimes provides indirect evidence of pancreatic pathology. Upper GI series may show displacement, indentation of the stomach, or widening of the duodenal loop. Oblique views show if the retrogastric prevertebral space is increased in depth. A thickened lobule of pancreatic tissue behind the proximal duodenum can simulate a duodenal ulcer deformity.

Hypotonic Duodenography. Hypotonic duodenography is the best procedure to demonstrate the pancreatic duct papilla. An antispasmodic is injected to render the duodenum hypotonic during a double-contrast barium examination. An intravenous pyelogram will reveal distortion or displacement of the kidneys.

Selective Angiography. The blood supply to the pancreas can be demonstrated by catheterizing the celiac and/or superior mesenteric arteries. Minute doses of vasoactive drugs may be injected to vary the blood flow. In chronic pancreatitis there is a marked decrease in vascularity. The common carcinoma of the head of the pancreas is scirrhous, causing irregularity, infiltration, and narrowing of the arteries rather than an increase in blood flow.

Retrograde Pancreatography. It is now possible to cannulate the papilla using a fiberoptic duodenoscope[5] and to visualize the pancreatic duct after injecting a contrast medium. Pancreatic juice can be aspirated and examined for carcinoma cells after stimulation with secretin and CCK-PZ.

Pancreatic Scanning. Scintigraphic scanning is the only direct method of "viewing" the pancreas.[4] The pancreas takes up injected ^{75}Se-selenomethionine to form protein. However, the liver also takes up the radioactive compound, and its bulk may render interpretation difficult. At the end of the conventional selenium scan [198]Au colloidal gold can be injected to delineate the liver. A second scan can then be "subtracted" from the first to provide a clearer picture of the pancreas.

Uptake is reduced in pancreatitis. A neoplasm 3 cm or more in diameter may be seen as a filling defect but more often results in a diffuse reduced uptake. In skilled hands the accuracy of the investigation approaches 70 percent. False negatives are less than 5 percent, but false positives, poor uptake with a normal pancreas, vary from 10 to 30 percent.[1] Old age, diabetes mellitus, cirrhosis, and truncal vagotomy all reduce uptake.

Ultrasonic Scanning. This is only valuable in the diagnosis of pseudopancreatic cysts.

Finally it must be stressed that none of the pancreatic tests are specific or 100 percent accurate. In many patients laparotomy is necessary to establish the diagnosis.

DISEASES OF THE PANCREAS

Congenital

Annular pancreas is a very uncommon lesion, seen slightly more often in males at any time from birth to middle life. It is the result of abnormal early development, probably from duplication of the ventral duodenal bud or its rotation to the right. The duodenum is encircled by a ring of pancreatic tissue of variable thickness at the level of the ampulla. There may be duodenal stenosis with dilatation of the proximal duodenum. In adults there may be stasis ulceration in the stomach.

Vomiting is the principal symptom, but upper abdominal fullness and pain may be the presenting symptoms. Rarely there is jaundice or pancreatitis. A uniform constriction of the second part of the duodenum seen on contrast radiography or, in an adult, duodenoscopy suggests the diagnosis.

Duodenojejunostomy is the safest operative treatment. Sometimes the annulus is attenuated on the left anterior aspect of the duodenum and can be divided here, the divided ends being carefully ligated with nonabsorbable sutures.

Heterotopic pancreatic tissue may be found in the wall of the stomach, bile ducts, jejunum, and Meckel's diverticulum. Often it is a chance finding, but it can become ulcerated and bleed, precipitate an intussusception, or be mistaken for a carcinoma.

Trauma

The pancreas is damaged in only 2 to 3 percent of all abdominal injuries. In the United States two thirds are the result of penetrating abdominal wounds, mostly stabbing and shooting, while nonpenetrating blunt injuries are more common in Europe. Automobile accidents commonly cause nonpenetrating injuries.

An isolated injury to the pancreas is uncommon. Violence applied to the front of the abdomen from the right may disrupt the liver, avulse the common bile duct, tear the duodenum, split the colon, and damage the major blood vessels. If the injuring force is from the left, the spleen is likely to be ruptured, and the colon and left kidney may also be involved. A blow from in front may split part of the neck or body of the pancreas, or if more violent it will completely transect the gland by compressing it against the lumbar vertebrae; sometimes the upper jejunum or its mesentery is also damaged.

The serum amylase is nearly always raised in pancreatic injuries. An isolated closed lesion of the pancreas can readily be missed because of the organ's position outside the peritoneal cavity. A four-quadrant peritoneal tap and peritoneal

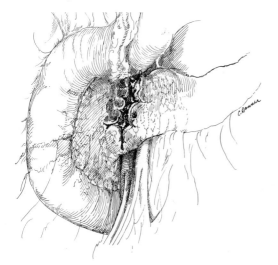

Figure 20–4. Traumatic rupture of the pancreas at the junction of the head and body is treated by resection of the pancreas to the left of the mesenteric vessels.

lavage may show no abnormality. Radiographs do not help. Repeated examination is essential. Deep epigastric tenderness may slowly increase. When in doubt it is better to perform a laparotomy, with thorough exploration of the gland, including mobilization of the duodenum and spleen and division of the gastrocolic omentum. Some cases are only diagnosed after a day or two when a mass appears. Other untreated cases progress to develop a pseudopancreatic cyst in two to six weeks.

A tear in the duodenum is a frequent and serious concomitant injury and raises the mortality to 50 percent. If it is suspected, a Gastrografin examination of the duodenum should be performed. With pancreatic injuries a large quantity of fluid and blood is lost into the retroperitoneum. Hepatic, splenic, and vascular injuries add further to the blood loss. Large volumes of intravenous fluids are therefore required and operation as soon as possible.

At operation a ruptured spleen, liver, or a torn major vessel is first dealt with. To expose the head, the peritoneum lateral to the second part of the duodenum is divided. A simple tear on the surface of the pancreas is sutured with shallow, nonabsorbable sutures. If the pancreas is transected, the left half and spleen are removed (Figure 20–4). The main pancreatic duct is transfixed and the torn pancreas oversewn with interrupted sutures. The region must always be drained, preferably with two flank drains of the sump-suction type. The skin around the drains is protected with aluminum paste. Possible wound

dehiscence should be anticipated by inserting strong tension stitches and leaving them for two weeks.

Considerable ingenuity is required when the duodenum is also torn. Occasionally it is possible to excise the edges of a small tear and close the defect in two layers. A larger defect is best covered by an adjacent loop of jejunum sutured over the defect. Alternately a vagotomy and gastojejunostomy may be performed and a Foley catheter inserted into the defect forming a duodenostomy. A pancreaticoduodenectomy may be indicated if the head of the pancreas is extensively damaged or if there is avulsion of the main pancreatic duct and common bile duct or damage to the portal vein.[3]

A fistula may follow any pancreatic injury. Most fistulae close spontaneously in a few weeks. During this time stimulation of the pancreas should be kept to a minimum and nutrition maintained by intravenous alimentation or jejunostomy feeding.

If a pseudopancreatic cyst forms in or near the lesser sac, it is drained by anastomosing it through and to the posterior wall of the stomach.

Acute Pancreatitis

Acute pancreatitis is a serious abdominal emergency with an incidence of about 7 cases per 100,000 population each year. In many patients the etiology is obscure. Trauma, mumps, corticosteroids, and neoplasm each account for 1 to 2 percent of cases. An increased pressure within the duct system is important as seen in pancreatitis following afferent loop obstruction, annular pancreas, or injudicious attempts at retrograde pancreatography. Reflux of free and especially of infected bile acids up the duct of Wirsung is toxic to the pancreas (Figure 20-5). Lysolecithin, which has a lytic action on pancreatic cells, may be formed from bile lecithin. Enzyme inhibitors within the pancreas may cease to function. Alcohol may qualitatively alter bile through its action on the liver. Alcoholism seems to be more important in America and Australia than it is in Europe. In Scotland alcohol poses major problems in psychiatric illness and liver damage, but it plays a minor role in acute pancreatitis. Many of the pancreatitic victims are abstemious old ladies who have never touched a drop of whiskey in their lives, or so they say.

Biliary tract disease is present in 50 percent of cases, but its exact role is uncertain. In most cases the disease is in the gallbladder and only rarely in the common duct. Removal of a gallbladder containing stones appears to lessen the risk of recurrent pancreatitis. The "blocked common passage" theory is rarely the cause. If the passage was obstructed by a calculus, stenosis, or pro-

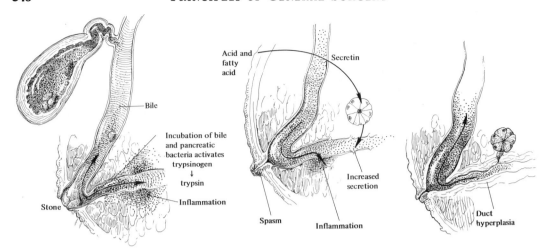

Figure 20–5. Pancreatitis is sometimes due to obstruction by a stone impacted at the ampulla of Vater and probably more often from spasm of the sphincter of Oddi. The commonest cause is multiple narrow segments in the main pancreatic duct. The sequence of events leading to pancreatitis is triggered by pressure and stasis of bile and pancreatic secretions, as pictured.

longed spasm of the sphincter of Oddi, there should be deepening jaundice. Instead jaundice is frequently absent in acute pancreatitis and when present tends to be mild and transient.

The pathologic changes result from the liberation of pancreatic enzymes, especially the proteolytic enzymes, into the substance of the gland. The first change occurs in the tissue immediately deep to the acinar cells, possibly caused by phospholipase A leaking out. All grades of severity are encountered. If mild, there may only be edema. If more severe, there is erosion of small vessels by elastase resulting in hemorrhagic pancreatitis. The most severe form causes death of pancreatic tissue. There is a considerable outpouring of fluid into the retroperitoneum and often into the peritoneal cavity. When the chemical inflammation is widespread and severe, both endocrine and exocrine secretions cease. Released lipase causes fat necrosis in the abdomen and even in the soft tissues in the limbs. An alternative explanation for the fat necrosis is that the lowered serum insulin level causes activation of intracellular lipases, particularly in the fat cells of the great omentum. Methemalbumin is sometimes formed, while kinins and other protein products may be liberated into the circulation.

Pain is usually agonizing, but the abdominal findings may be unremarkable, with only deep tenderness and guarding in the epigastrium. There is a tendency to retch, and vomiting is common. Shock varies and may be profound. In part it is due to the passage of fluid from the intravascular compartment into the retroperitoneal tissues and in part to the action of kinins

and unknown peptides. The hematocrit is high and the central venous and arterial pressures low. Glycosuria may be present. Bluish staining may occur in the loins or umbilicus after a few days in those with hemorrhagic pancreatitis.

The diagnosis is made by suspecting pancreatitis in those with sudden severe upper abdominal pain and by then checking the serum amylase. The level may be 4 to 10 times normal but usually only stays elevated for 6 to 24 hours. In 10 percent of patients the serum amylase remains within the normal range throughout the illness. There is nearly always a leukocytosis, and its persistence after a few days strongly suggests that a complication such as an abscess or pseudocyst is developing. When calcium is being used to form soaps in areas of fat necrosis, the serum calcium will fall below the normal level of 9 to 9.5 mg per 100 ml or 2.3 to 2.7 m mol per liter. A straight x-ray may show ileus in the duodenojejunal region or hepatic flexure when these structures lie in contact with the inflamed pancreas. Operation can mostly be avoided, but if there is doubt about the diagnosis laparotomy should be performed.

The complications of acute pancreatitis are tetany when there is extensive fat necrosis and decrease in the serum calcium to about 7 mg per 100 ml, abscess formation in the pancreas, retroperitoneal, or subphrenic spaces, cyst formation within the pancreas, or a pseudocyst from collection of fluid in the lesser sac, rarely diabetes mellitus, and calcification and fibrosis with recurrent attacks (Figure 20–6).

Treatment consists of nasogastric suction to

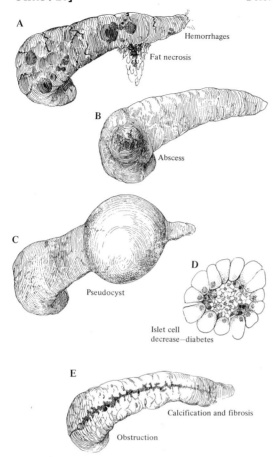

A — Hemorrhages, Fat necrosis

B — Abscess

C — Pseudocyst

D — Islet cell decrease—diabetes

E — Calcification and fibrosis, Obstruction

Figure 20–6. Complications of acute pancreatitis are (*A*) tetany following extensive fat necrosis, (*B*) abscess formation, (*C*) formation of a pseudocyst, (*D*) diabetes mellitus, and (*E*) recurrent pancreatitis from fibrosis and multiple obstructions within the pancreatic ducts.

prevent vomiting and to reduce stimulation of the pancreas, rapid infusion of adequate volumes of saline and colloids to restore the circulation, and watching for complications such as obstructive jaundice or abscess formation which require surgery. It is doubtful if antispasmodics or antibiotics are of much value. There is controversy about the use of the kallikrein inhibitor aprotinin. Kallikrein helps form the kinin bradykinin, which affects the circulation. Given prophylactically aprotinin prevents experimental pancreatitis in animals; however, in humans the disease is well established before treatment is started. Survival has improved because of better fluid replacement, and this has resulted in late complications being seen more frequently, such as abscess in the mediastinum, fat necrosis in the pelvis (causing late obstructive signs), and pseudocysts.

Chronic Pancreatitis and Pancreatic Lithiasis

Chronic pancreatitis is commoner in the United States, France, and South Africa than it is in Britain and Scandinavia and is much less frequent than acute pancreatitis, although the incidence may be increasing. Alcohol combined with a low protein intake is an important contributory factor. Heredity, hyperlipidemia, and hyperparathyroidism are occasionally important. Many patients have scattered calcification or multiple stones in the dilated pancreatic ducts. A small percentage eventually develop a carcinoma.

The main symptoms are recurrent upper abdominal pain, loss of appetite, and loss of weight. There is pancreatic steatorrhea, and calcium and fat-soluble vitamins are lost. The patient often becomes wasted physically and warped mentally. One third of the patients have mild, intermittent attacks of jaundice. Drug addiction can become a problem, diabetes mellitus may appear, and hematemesis sometimes occurs.

A normal Lundh test or pancreatic scan virtually eliminates chronic pancreatitis as a cause of malabsorption. The secretin-pancreozymin test is helpful in establishing the diagnosis and in assessing the response to treatment. The immunoglobulins IgA and IgG may be increased.

The first aim of treatment is to relieve pain. Analgesics are given, and any biliary abnormality is corrected. If symptoms persist, splanchnic blocks or splanchnicectomy may be tried. Nutrition is improved by giving pancreatic extract, provided the enzymes in the preparation are protected from destruction by acid-pepsin in the patient's stomach. Alcohol is forbidden and a low-fat, high-protein diet given.

With calculi and duct strictures it may be necessary to drain the pancreas to the left, into a Roux-en-Y loop of jejunum after opening the duct and removing the stones (Figure 20–7). When the pancreas is almost replaced by large calculi, Child's operation is recommended. Ninety percent of the diseased gland, along with the spleen, is removed, only a thin crescent of tissue being left in the concavity of the duodenum.

Tumors of the pancreas may arise from the exocrine cells, nonbeta cells giving rise to the Zollinger-Ellison syndrome or beta cells producing insulinomas.

Carcinoma of the Pancreas

The common type of cancer of the pancreas is an adenocarcinoma of the ductal or acinar cells. About 65 percent occur in the head of the gland, 20 percent in the body and tail, and 15 percent

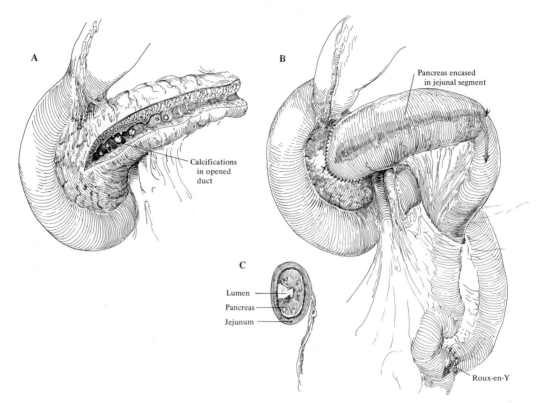

Figure 20–7. Recurrent pancreatitis associated with multiple strictures in the pancreatic duct may be treated by (*A*) laying the main duct open and (*B*) ensheathing the pancreas with jejunum; the proximal jejunum is attached to the jejunum below the anastomosis. *C* shows the completed operation.

in the ampullary region. It is still uncertain which tissue gives rise to cancer of the ampulla. True cancers of the duodenal mucosa do occur but are very rare. The ampullary lesion may arise from the lining of the terminal bile duct or from adjacent acinar cells.

Spread is mostly by direct extension to adjacent structures and in particular to the great vessels and liver. There is also lymphatic spread to nodes close to the celiac axis, bile duct, and along the upper border of the pancreas. Occasionally the patient presents with an enlarged node in the left supraclavicular triangle.

It is commonly stated that carcinoma of the pancreas is more frequent in diabetes. However, many of the patients have late-onset, unstable diabetes with jaundice developing a few months after the diabetic state was detected. In many it seems probable that the diabetes was in fact secondary to an established but still silent carcinoma. Other predisposing causes are cigarette smoking and polyposis coli. It is interesting that the incidence is high in the Polynesian race and in American female Indians.

Males develop cancer of the pancreas more often than females with a peak at 55 to 65 years. Pain is the presenting symptom with lesions in the body and tail as described above. Later generally it becomes the most distressing feature for a tumor in any position. Ampullary lesions present with jaundice, but on questioning, some patients admit to earlier vague epigastric discomfort or fullness. As jaundice deepens, pruritus becomes troublesome. Anorexia, lassitude, apathy, and weight loss may be apparent early on. A peripheral transient thrombophlebitis migrans sometimes appears, as in chronic pancreatitis.

To diagnose cancer of the pancreas early, the clinician must always be suspicious about its presence in patients with seemingly minor epigastric symptoms. A barium examination shows enlargement of the duodenal loop only when a large tumor is present in the head. A projecting ampullary lesion shows a "reversed 3" appearance, and the diagnosis can be confirmed by duodenoscopy. Cytologic studies may be helpful. A pancreatic scan may show a "cold spot" or a poorly functioning gland because there is often pancreatitis in the obstructed part of the gland. Even at laparotomy the diagnosis can be difficult. A small stone in the lower bile duct surrounded by a hard area of pancreatitis closely simulates a neoplasm of the head. Even biopsy is not entirely safe and reliable. The specimen may only show pancreatitis, while if the incision is made deeply to try to reach the neoplasm, a pancreatic fistula may follow.

Treatment is operative. Unfortunately the majority are not suitable for radical extiration of the neoplasm. When resection is impossible, a biliary short-circuit is established, usually by anastomosing the common bile duct to the first part of the duodenum, the stomach, or to a Roux-en-Y loop of jejunum. A gastroenterostomy may be added routinely or only if the duodenum is obstructed. Survival averages about nine months. In many cases this can be extended by combined therapy with 5-fluorouracil and megavoltage radiotherapy.

Cancers of the body and tail are seldom seen at an early stage. If such a tumor is found, it is treated by excising the left half of the pancreas and the spleen. Cancers at the ampulla of Vater, which are still localized, are removed by pancreaticoduodenectomy (Whipple's operation) (Figure 20–8). The distal two thirds of the stomach, lower common bile duct, head of pancreas, all the duodenum, and proximal few centimeters of jejunum are resected en bloc, dividing the pancreas at its neck. Radical resection should probably not be attempted in carcinoma of the head of the pancreas because the prognosis is bad. Experience at the Cleveland Clinic and in Copenhagen has shown that the expectation of life with carcinoma of the head of the pancreas is less after radical surgery than after a simple biliary bypass. In spite of this some surgeons are still tempted to remove a small neoplasm in the head, fearing if left it will eventually cause intractable pain which is difficult to control.

Endocrine-Secreting Tumors of the Pancreas

Islet Cell Tumors. Insulin-secreting beta cells of the pancreas may form a benign (75 percent) or malignant (25 percent) tumor of the pancreas, and in about 15 percent the tumors are multiple. Hyperplasia is only found occasionally in children.

Whipple's triad is still valuable in establishing the diagnosis:

1. Fainting attacks brought on by fasting or exercise.
2. Fasting blood sugar below 50 mg per 100 ml.

3. Symptoms relieved by oral or intravenous sugar.

A decrease in blood sugar causes release of epinephrine and glucagon. If the decrease is rapid, the sudden release of epinephrine causes weakness, sweating, and tachycardia. Because the brain requires glucose for its nutrition, many patients will present with neurologic abnormalities such as headache, mental and visual disturbances, convulsions, and coma. Symptoms may be of weeks' or years' duration. Many patients overeat to prevent symptoms and become obese. It is important to exclude other causes of hypoglycemia, such as the poorly understood idiopathic hypoglycemia of children that generally resolves spontaneously, alimentary, and hepatic hypoglycemia. Often definite diagnosis can be established by determining the blood insulin, permitting the investigator to avoid using the potentially dangerous tests such as starvation or administration of tolbutamide.

Treatment. Treatment is operative removal of the tumor. The pancreas is carefully examined for a tumor and the involved portion removed either by excising the pancreas to the left of the mesenteric vessels or the head along with the duodenum, preserving the tail. If a tumor is not found, the stomach, duodenum, and small intestine are examined for an aberrant tumor. If none is found, the pancreas to the left of the mesenteric vessels is generally removed. If symptoms persist and other causes of hypoglycemia have definitely been excluded, it may then be necessary subsequently to remove the remainder of the pancreas.

In those with metastases streptozotocin may be given to destroy the beta cells or diazoxide to prevent release of insulin from the islet cells.

Zollinger-Ellison Syndrome. In 1955 Zollinger and Ellison described the triad:

1. Fulminating and often complicated peptic ulceration in the duodenum and stomach and often in atypical locations such as the third part of the duodenum and jejunum.
2. Gastric hypersecretion with overnight secretion often exceeding 2 liters of fluid containing 200 mEq of free acid.
3. Nonbeta cell tumor of the pancreas.

Patients often present with a long history of peptic ulcer that responds poorly to both medical and surgical treatment. About one third have diarrhea, and this may be present with gastric hypersecretion but no ulceration.

About 60 percent are malignant and metastasize mainly to the regional nodes and the liver. About 20 percent of the nonbeta cell tumors are multiple within the pancreas and duodenum. Endocrine diseases are present in about 20 percent, such as pituitary disorders, hyperparathyroidism,

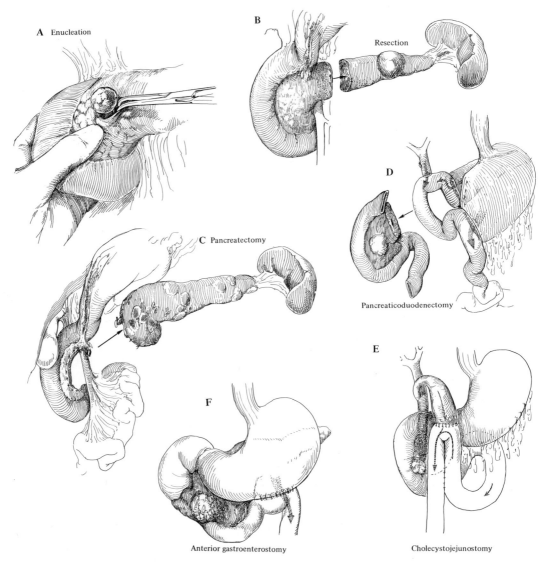

Figure 20–8.   Operations for adenocarcinomas of the pancreas. *A.* The diagnosis is confirmed microscopically by locally excising part or all of the tumor (enucleation) or taking a needle biopsy. *B.* That part of the pancreas to the left of the mesenteric vessels may be removed. *C.* A 90 percent pancreatectomy may be performed leaving a small cuff adjacent to the second part of the duodenum. *D.* A pancreaticoduodenectomy may be performed with preservation of the pancreas to the left of the mesenteric vessels. All the pancreas may be removed. *E.* For a nonresectable tumor, palliation may be obtained by anastomosing the gallbladder to the stomach, duodenum, or jejunum, as shown. *F.* A bypass procedure is often undertaken for gastric decompression by establishing a gastrojejunostomy.

Cushing's disease, and beta cell tumors of the pancreas.

The tumors secrete gastrin, and this is responsible for the gastric hypersecretion. An elevation in serum gastrin to above 1200 picograms is pathognomonic. The histamine stimulation test is negative because acid is already being secreted at maximum capacity.

Treatment. Patients should be treated by total gastrectomy rather than by excision of the tumor. Tumor resection is often followed by persistence of symptoms, because many of the tumors are malignant and have already metastasized and the tumors are often multiple. Regression of metastases has occurred in a number of patients after total gastrectomy.

A syndrome has also been described in patients with nonbeta cell tumor of the pancreas, consisting of intractable watery diarrhea, hypokalemia, and achlorhydria (WDHA syndrome). These tumors may be secreting glucagon or other substances rather than gastrin.

CITED REFERENCES

1. Bachrach, W. H.; Birsner, J. W.; Izenstark, J. L.; and Smith, V. L.: Pancreatic scanning: A review. *Gastroenterology*, **63**:890–910, 1972.
2. James, O.: The Lundh test. *Gut*, **14**:582–91, 1973.
3. Northrup, W. F.: Pancreatic trauma: A review. *Surgery*, **71**:27–43, 1972.
4. Spencer, A. M.; Patel, M. P.; Smits, B. J.; and Williams, J. D. F.: Pancreatic scanning as a diagnostic tool in the district general hospital. *Br. Med. J.*, **4**:153–56, 1974.
5. Takagi, K.; Ikeda, S.; and Nagagawa, Y.: Retrograde pancreatography and cholangiography by fiber duodenoscopy. *Gastroenterology*, **59**:445–52, 1970.
6. Wormsley, K. G.: The response to an infusion of combination of secretin and pancreozymin in health and disease. *Scand. J. Gastroenterol.*, **4**:623–32, 1969.

SUGGESTIONS FOR FURTHER READING

Beck, I. T., and Sinclair, D. G. (eds.): *The Exocrine Pancreas*. Churchill Press, London.
General coverage. The Proceedings of a Symposium held at Kingston, Canada, in June 1969.
Carey, L. C. (ed.): *The Pancreas*. C. V. Mosby Co., St Louis, 1973.
Deals with both endocrine and exocrine function in health and disease. Transplantation, diabetes mellitus, and pediatric conditions also covered.
Howat, H. T. (ed.): The exocrine pancreas. *Clinics in Gastroenterology*. Vol. 1. W. B. Saunders Co., Philadelphia, 1972.
Clinical. The first half of the book deals with investigations of exocrine pancreas and the second half with pancreatitis and cancer.

Chapter 21

JEJUNUM AND ILEUM

Alvin L. Watne

CHAPTER OUTLINE

Applied Surgical Anatomy
Physiology
   Motor Activity
   Digestion
   Absorption
Clinical Features
Special Investigations
   Tests of Absorptive Function
   Intestinal Intubation
   Radiologic Investigation
Specific Diseases
   Meckel's Diverticulum

Intestinal Short Circuit for Obesity and
   Hypercholesterolemia
Transposition of Small Bowel
Intestinal Fistula
Short-Bowel Syndrome
Blind-Loop Syndrome
Vascular Insufficiency
Injuries to Small Intestine
Tumors
Crohn's Disease
Radiation Enteritis
Specific Infections

APPLIED SURGICAL ANATOMY

The small bowel consists of duodenum, jejunum, and ileum (see Plates IV and VI). The duodenum is discussed along with the stomach because of the number of diseases common to both. The jejunum and ileum are both developed from the midgut. Both are suspended from the posterior abdominal wall by a mesentery running from the left of the second lumbar vertebra to the right sacroiliac joint. The beginning and end of the mesentery are short, making the bowel more fixed at the beginning of the jejunum and the end of the ileum. The jejunum and ileum measure about 250 cm, with the upper two thirds consisting of jejunum and the remainder of ileum.

The superior mesenteric artery and vein supply the small bowel. This artery arises from the aorta at the first lumbar vertebra and passes posterior to the pancreas and anterior to the third portion of the duodenum. Branches form interlocking arcades and give rise to many intestinal branches. Gangrene of the entire small bowel and proximal colon occurs if the flow is interrupted at the origin of the superior mesenteric artery. The veins accompanying each branch of the artery join, eventually forming the superior mesenteric vein that joins the splenic vein at the upper edge of the pancreas to form the portal vein. The lymphatics commence as lacteals in the villi of the intestinal mucosa. They drain into nodes in the mesentery and then to the para-aortic nodes and the cisterna chyli. Chylomicrons composed of long-chain fatty acids absorbed from the small intestinal lumen give the characteristic milky appearance of intestinal lymph.

Parasympathetic fibers from the posterior vagus pass through the celiac ganglion and form a mesenteric plexus that supplies the small intestine. The vagus nerve transmits both efferent and afferent impulses. The efferent cell station is in the plexus of Auerbach between the circular and longitudinal muscles and in the plexus of Meissner in the submucosa. The sympathetic fibers pass to the small intestine from the greater and lesser splanchnic nerves, the celiac ganglion, and superior mesenteric plexus. The efferent fibers synapse in the abdominal ganglia.

The mucosal surfaces of the jejunum and ileum have circular folds, valvulae conniventes, extending about two thirds around the wall which can be seen on x-ray. The mucosal absorption surface is greatly increased by microscopic villi lined by absorptive columnar cells and goblet or mucus-secreting cells (Figure 21–1). The columnar cells have microvilli that further increase the area for absorption. It now appears that the microvilli have micromicrovilli termed

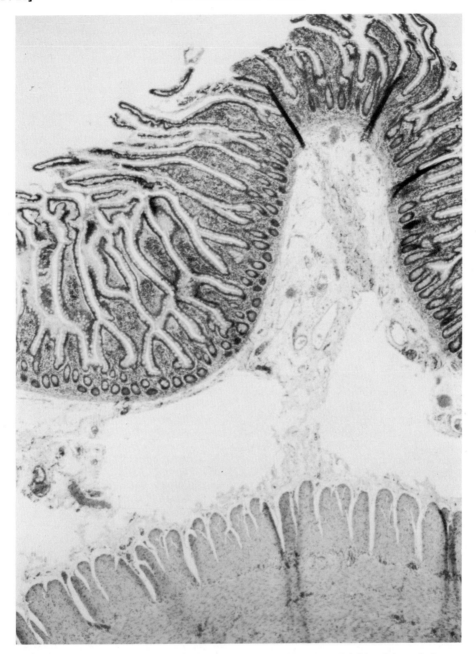

Figure 21–1. Photomicrograph of the jejunum showing the mucosal folds of the valvulae conniventes, intestinal villi, and the crypts of Lieberkuhn lined by goblet and columnar cells. (Hematoxylin and eosin stain × 75.)

the glycocalyx. The crypts of Lieberkuhn lie between the villi and are the source of new columnar cells that are formed in their depths, migrate toward the tips of the villi, and are extruded into the bowel lumen within 48 to 96 hours. The crypts of Lieberkuhn also contain Paneth cells and serotonin-secreting argentaffin cells. Each villus contains a central lacteal, an arteriole, and a venule.[1]

PHYSIOLOGY
Motor Activity

The function of the small intestine is transport and digestion of food, and absorption of water, electrolytes, and nutrients. Motor activity occurs both as segmental contractions that serve to mix the chyme and as propulsive movements that propel the contents along the length of the bowel. A duodenal pacemaker may exert some control. Absorption is aided by contraction of the muscularis mucosa that results in alternate shortening and lengthening of the intestinal villi. The chyme normally traverses the small bowel in about four hours. The circular muscle at the ileocecal valve contracts to delay the evacuation of the small bowel and enhances digestion and absorption. The valve also prevents reflux of the cecal contents into the ileum.

Digestion

During the transit of the chyme through the small intestine proteins, carbohydrates, and fats are broken down into simpler compounds that can be absorbed through the intestinal mucosa. When the chyme leaves the stomach, the proteins are in the form of polypeptides, starch digestion is incomplete, and fat digestion has scarcely begun. Hormones secreted by the duodenum stimulate the secretion of fluids and enzymes by the pancreas and small intestine, cause flow of bile into the duodenum, and inhibit further gastric secretion. Secretin triggers the secretion of water and bicarbonates by the pancreas and small intestine. Pancreozymin stimulates the secretion of pancreatic enzymes. Cholecystokinin causes contraction of the gallbladder and efflux of bile, enterogastrone inhibits gastric secretion signaling an end of the gastric phase of digestion, and enterokinin stimulates secretion of enzymes by the small intestine (Figure 18–3, page 300].

The pancreatic proteolytic enzyme trypsinogen is activated to trypsin by a duodenal enzyme, enterokinase. The pancreatic secretions also contain chymotrypsin that breaks down the proteins to long peptide chains, amylase that breaks down carbohydrates to disaccharides, and lipase that initiates the breakdown of fats to triglycerides. The digestion of polypeptides to amino acids is completed in the small intestine. The monosaccharides glucose, fructose, and galactose are formed from the disaccharides. The fatty acids and monoglycerides remain soluble by forming micelles with the conjugated bile salts. The micelles are water soluble and 3 to 10 millimicrons in diameter. The lipid portion of the micelle is able to pass into the brush border of the mucosal cells and thus be absorbed. The free bile salts pass down the small bowel to be absorbed in the terminal ileum (Figure 20–1, page 341).

Absorption

Solutes and fluids are absorbed by passive and active diffusion mainly in the small intestine. Passive diffusion is passage of a molecule across a membrane from a region of high to low concentration. Certain water-soluble substances of low molecular weight and fat-soluble compounds, such as drugs, are absorbed by passive diffusion through intestinal pores 3 to 4 Å in diameter. The water-soluble vitamins, nicotinamide, pyridoxine, inositol, ascorbic acid, choline, para-aminobenzoic acid, biotin, pantothenic acid, riboflavin, thiamine, and folic acid, can be absorbed by passive diffusion. The rate of diffusion depends upon the concentration gradient across the intestinal epithelium. Passive diffusion therefore occurs mainly high in the small bowel.

Active transport is absorption of a substance across a membrane against an electrical and/or chemical gradient and requires energy. Active transport mechanisms have been demonstrated for glucose, fructose, sodium, potassium, chloride, iron, calcium, amino acids, fatty acids, pyrimidines, bile salts, cholesterol, vitamin B_{12}, and folic acid. Proteins are absorbed almost completely as amino acids and sugars as monosaccharides.

The absorption of fat begins when the monoglycerides and fatty acids in the micelles are passively taken into the brush border of the mucosal cells. The monoglycerides and fatty acids are reesterified to form triglycerides in the apical microvesicles. The triglycerides are coated with cholesterol and then an envelope of phospholipids and protein in the Golgi apparatus to form chylomicrons. These are discharged into the intracellular spaces and enter the lymphatics and the thoracic duct. Glycerol, short-chain fatty acids, and medium-chain triglycerides may bypass these final steps and enter the portal venous system.

Water and electrolytes may pass in both directions between the intestine and the blood. The evidence for or against active and passive transport of water is controversial. Electrolyte transport is an active process, probably involving the mitochondria. The intestinal absorption of calcium depends on the presence of vitamin D and parathormone. Iron absorption depends on the body needs. Ferric iron must be reduced by hydrochloric acid or bile to the ferrous form for absorption to occur. The ferrous iron is then oxidized in the mucosal cell to the ferric form, which then combines with the protein apoferritin. Vitamin B_{12} in the diet becomes bound to the intrinsic factor in gastric fluid and then in the presence of calcium ions enters the mucosal cells. The fat-soluble vitamins, A,

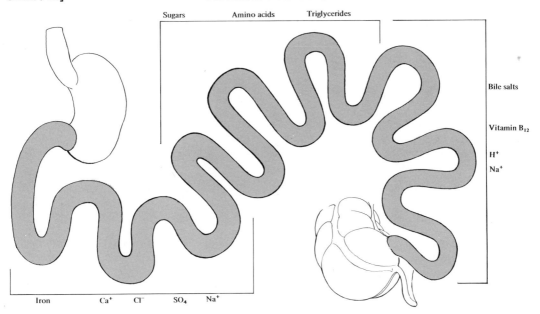

Figure 21–2. The levels at which absorption of products takes place in the small intestine.

D, E, and K, are absorbed in the same way as lipids.

Carbohydrate, protein, and fats are absorbed throughout the small intestine but mainly in the jejunum (Figure 21–2). The low pH in the upper small bowel favors the absorption of iron in this region. The bile salts, vitamin B_{12}, and gastrointestinal secretions are electively absorbed in the distal ileum.

CLINICAL FEATURES

Symptoms arise in small bowel disease as a result of obstruction, perforation, bleeding, or malabsorption. Obstruction is associated with recurrent attacks of pain or colic. Colic is a spasmodic pain that reaches a climax of intensity followed by relaxation and recurs at intervals of two to three minutes. The pain is referred to the center of the abdomen. Perforation of the small bowel gives rise to generalized abdominal pain, muscle guarding, and rigidity unless the perforation is sealed off and localized. Bleeding from the small bowel is likely to produce blood in the stool, usually appearing as melena unless the bleeding is massive, in which case red blood is passed. Less commonly, bleeding presents as hematemesis, especially if the lesion is in the upper small bowel. Occasionally, chronic iron deficiency anemia results from recurrent blood loss from the small bowel, but this is less often seen than with lesions in the stomach and colon. Malabsorption presents a variable clinical picture depending on the specific nutrient whose deficiency becomes most marked. Fat mal-

absorption results in bulky and offensive stools containing an increased proportion of fat, and generalized evidence of malnutrition. Failure to absorb vitamin B_{12} as a result of bacterial colonization of intestinal blind loops or diverticula results in a macrocytic anemia. Protein malabsorption results in hypoproteinemia, edema, and general debility.

Diarrhea may result from more rapid transit through the small bowel in such conditions as jejunocolic fistula, Crohn's disease, and after massive bowel resection.

SPECIAL INVESTIGATIONS

The small bowel is investigated by measuring absorptive function and by intubation and radiologic techniques.

Tests of Absorptive Function

Fat absorption can be measured by collecting the feces excreted in three days and estimating the average daily output of fat. Normally this is less than 6 gm per day in the adult, and levels higher than this indicate steatorrhea. No special diet is required for this test. Attempts have been made to separate the steatorrhea of pancreatic disease from other types of steatorrhea on the basis that the percentage of split fat in the stool is decreased in the absence of pancreatic enzymes. This distinction has not been of much practical value. A simple screening test for fat malabsorption is the measurement of the serum carotene. The carotenes are converted after ingestion into fat-soluble vitamin A, mainly in the wall of the small bowel. The normal serum carotene is 70 to 290 μg per 100 ml. Low values are found in steatorrhea, liver disease, and conditions of deficient carotene intake. Several radioisotopic tests for fat absorption have been devised. For example ^{131}I triolein has been given orally and the amount excreted in the stool or its level in the blood determined. These methods are subject to considerable variations and none has become popular.

Carbohydrate absorption can be measured using the D-xylose excretion test. After an overnight fast the patient empties his bladder and takes an oral dose of 25 gm of D-xylose in 250 ml of water. Urine is collected for the subsequent five hours, and a blood sample is taken two hours after the test begins. In the normal individual between 4 and 7 gm of xylose is excreted in the urine over the five-hour period, and the serum xylose at two hours is greater than 30 mg per 100 ml. The test is a measure of both the absorption of xylose and its renal clearance and so must be carefully interpreted. The oral glucose tolerance test may also be used and shows a flattened curve when intestinal absorption is impaired.

The serum cholesterol is frequently low in the presence of steatorrhea but is also decreased in abetalipoproteinemia. Disaccharide absorption can be measured by giving a 50-gm dose of either lactose, sucrose, or maltose and measuring the serum glucose levels. Deficiency of the enzyme lactase with lactose intolerance is particularly common in American blacks.

Protein absorption involves estimating amino acid absorption and metabolism and is not used as a practical clinical test. Occasionally it is important to determine the rate of protein loss from the gastrointestinal tract. This can be done using an intravenous injection of a large-labeled, proteinlike molecule such as ^{131}I polyvinylpyrrolidone (PVP) followed by stool collection for four consecutive days. Normally less than 1.5 percent is excreted in the stool, but in some patients with protein-losing enteropathy up to 30 percent of the activity may appear in the stools. Similar tests can be carried out using ^{51}Cr-labeled albumin.

Vitamin B_{12} absorption is valuable in a number of small bowel disorders. As a screening test the serum vitamin B_{12} level may be estimated, the normal value being between 100 and 720 ng per ml. This value is low when absorption of vitamin B_{12} is interfered with in the small bowel. It is also low in pernicious anemia. A more sophisticated measurement of B_{12} absorption is the Schilling test, which is usually carried out in two parts. The patient is given a dose of radioactive vitamin B_{12}, 0.5 to 1.0 μCi orally in 50 ml of water, followed by an intramuscular flushing dose of 1000 μg of nonradioactive vitamin B_{12}, given to saturate the body. The body handles both forms of the vitamin B_{12} similarly; the excess is excreted in the urine and collected over the next 24 hours. The second part of the test is carried out at least three days after the first part. The radioactive vitamin B_{12} is again given by mouth together with a capsule of 50 ml of intrinsic factor followed by the intramuscular flushing dose of nonradioactive B_{12}. Urine is collected for 24 hours and assessed for radioactivity. In the first part of the Schilling test, there is normally an excretion of between 7 and 30 percent of the dose in the first 24 hours. A low value indicates either absence of intrinsic factor or defective B_{12} absorption. During the second part of the test when the intrinsic factor is administered, B_{12} absorption is increased in pernicious anemia. Low urinary excretion of B_{12} also occurs in the blind loop syndromes and in jejunal diverticulosis. A failure of excretion to increase after administration of intrinsic factor suggests that the small bowel is diseased. Bacterial contamination of the small bowel can be confirmed by giving the patient a five-day course of tetracycline, 2 gm daily, which will inhibit bacterial contamination in the gut. If the Schilling test is repeated after five or six days without intrinsic factor, a normal result is obtained.

Excessive bacterial growth in the small intestine usually results in bacterial breakdown of dietary tryptophan to indole, which is absorbed and excreted as indoxyl sulfate or indican in the urine. The normal urinary output of indican is 48 mg per 24 hours, and values above 80 mg are abnormal. In some patients with stagnant loop syndrome the output reaches 500 mg, especially when there is a predominance of indole-producing organisms such as *Escherichia*, *Bacteroides*, and certain *Klebsiella*.

Intestinal Intubation

In some patients it is useful to measure the bacterial flora directly by intubating the small bowel and obtaining a sample using a double-lumen polyvinyl tube or with a special sampling capsule such as a Shiner capsule. A small bowel mucosal biopsy can be obtained using a suction biopsy capsule attached to a thin tube and positioned radiologically.

Radiologic Investigation

The radiologist can often detect small bowel pathology on the follow-through series after ingestion of a barium meal. A dilated portion may indicate subacute bowel obstruction. Thickening of the intestinal folds may suggest celiac disease. A fixed noncontracting loop occurs in Crohn's disease. An internal fistula or diverticulosis may be seen. The best radiologic studies of the small bowel are achieved by intubating the duodenum and injecting small amounts of dilute barium so that the whole small bowel can be outlined without filling the stomach. The terminal portion of the small bowel and the ileocecal valve can often be visualized best on the barium enema. Celiac or superior mesenteric arteriograms are of value in determining the source of gastrointestinal bleeding and sometimes reveal small bowel tumors with abnormal vasculature.

Disaccharide intolerance can be shown by giving a mixture of barium and the appropriate disaccharide, for example lactose. In patients with lactose deficiency the barium mixture is rapidly diluted in the small bowel, the bowel dilates, and there are vigorous intestinal contractions.

SPECIFIC DISEASES

Meckel's Diverticulum

The diverticulum is the result of incomplete closure of the omphalomesenteric duct during the fifth to seventh weeks of gestation. It contains all the components of the intestinal wall and is therefore a true diverticulum. The diverticulum is located on the antimesenteric border of the ileum, within 50 cm from the ileocecal valve, and varies in size from 1 to 11 cm. Males outnumber females three to one. The incidence is 0.3 to 3.0 percent, and occasionally the condition is familial. Heterotopic tissue occurs in one

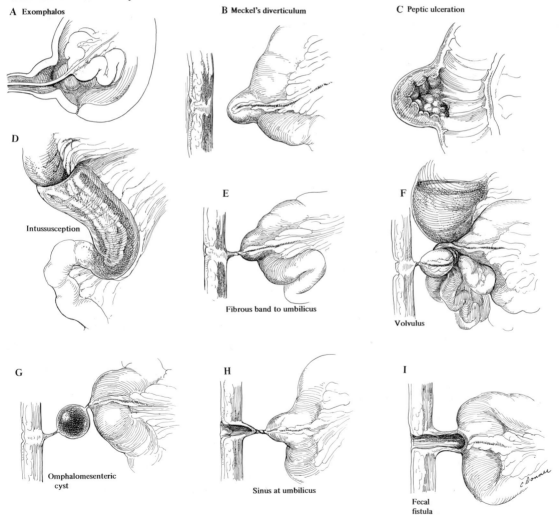

Figure 21–3. *A*. Embryologic origin of Meckel's diverticulum. *B*. Meckel's diverticulum. *C–I*. Complications of Meckel's diverticulum.

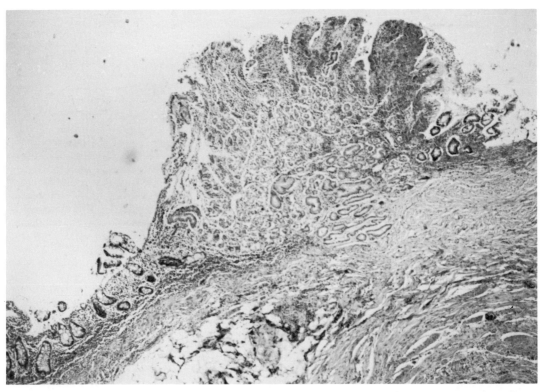

Figure 21–4. Photomicrograph of ulcerated Meckel's diverticulum. At left is normal ileal mucosa; at center is inflammatory edge of ulcer with ectopic gastric mucosa. (Hematoxylin and eosin stain × 75.)

third of Meckel's diverticula and may be gastric, duodenal, jejunal, pancreatic, or colonic. A number of anatomic derangements may occur with a Meckel's diverticulum, depending on the degree of closure of the omphalomesenteric duct (Figure 21–3). Ectopic gastric mucosa may produce free acid and peptic ulceration in the adjacent bowel or in the diverticulum (Figure 21–4). Hemorrhage is the most common complication necessitating surgery and occurs most frequently in children. Rarely the ulcer may perforate, giving peritonitis. A segmental resection of the diverticulum and adjacent bowel should be performed to remove any ectopic mucosa along with the diverticulum and ulcer. The diverticulum may become inverted and form the apex of an intussusception producing intestinal obstruction. Mechanical obstruction of the small intestine may occur in patients who have a fibrous band extending from the diverticulum to the umbilicus. Acute obstructive diverticulitis rarely, if ever, occurs, because the opening to the diverticulum is large.

A Meckel's diverticulum encountered as an incidental finding at laparotomy should generally be excised. A segmental resection should be done including the adjacent ileum and continuity established by end-to-end anastomosis.[2,3] Atresia and stenosis of the intestine are discussed in Chapter 35.

Intestinal Short Circuit for Obesity and Hypercholesterolemia

The term *morbid* obesity has been used to describe the massive obesity (two or three times the ideal weight) that persists for five or more years and resists treatment. Initially jejunocolic anastomosis was performed but was found to be unsuccessful. Many patients developed severe diarrhea with water and electrolyte depletion, nutritional deficiencies, and liver failure. The integrity of the ileocecal valve was then preserved by anastomosing the jejunum at 35 cm from the ligament of Treitz to the terminal ileum 10 cm above the ileocecal valve. Complications were less frequent. However, there are conflicting views on the value of the procedure. Many patients have serious psychologic problems that are not cured by surgery.

A distal ileal bypass has been recommended for hypercholesterolemia, since cholesterol is absorbed exclusively in the small intestine and predominantly in the distal half. The level of blood cholesterol can be effectively lowered by the bypass. The betalipoprotein blood level is also lowered, while the alphalipoprotein level remains unchanged.[4]

Recently there has been interest in the operation of gastric bypass for obesity.

Transposition of Small Bowel

The small intestine can be used for a number of substitution operations because of its availability, length, good blood supply, inherent transport mechanisms, and distensibility.

In urologic surgery a segment of ileum has been used as a conduit between the ureter and the skin following total removal of the urinary bladder (see Chapter 32, page 583). The ileum can be used to compensate for loss of a major portion of the bladder (ileocystoplasty) or to replace a segment of the ureter. A segment of jejunum has been utilized in reconstruction after resection of the esophagus. Jejunal segments have been used to form a reservoir after total gastrectomy. Jejunal isoperistaltic loops have been utilized to convert a gastrojejunostomy to a gastroduodenostomy for correction of the dumping syndrome. Antiperistaltic segments have also been used to correct rapid emptying of the stomach or small bowel.

Intestinal Fistula

A small intestinal fistula is a major catastrophe. The mortality depends upon the level of the fistula; it is 20 percent for an ileal fistula and 40 percent for one in the jejunum. An intestinal fistula may develop after drainage of an abscess complicating appendicitis, diverticulitis, Crohn's disease, carcinoma, or trauma. Seventy percent of small bowel fistulas arise as a complication of a surgical procedure, often for intestinal obstruction and often in patients who have been treated by radiotherapy. Technical excellence in intestinal anastomoses and care in avoiding incidental damage to the small bowel during surgery will prevent most of these complications.

Treatment involves local control and care of the fistula, fluid and electrolyte replacement, correction of the nutritional deficit, and surgical correction if necessary.[5] Most intestinal fistulae will heal spontaneously unless there is residual malignant disease, poor blood supply, distal intestinal obstruction, a foreign body, or chronic granulomatous disease. Small bowel secretions are rich in enzymes and cause autodigestion of the abdominal wall. The skin must be protected by inserting a soft suction catheter in the proximal limb of the fistula, applying a protective material such as aluminum or karaya powder, or

collecting the secretions in a disposable bag sealed to the margins of the fistula. The fluid and electrolyte loss depends on the level and size of the fistula. Water, sodium, and potassium deficits must be carefully assessed from the history, clinical signs, urinary and fistular outputs, and the blood electrolyte levels. Accurate replacement of deficits and anticipated losses is essential. All the secretions in the small intestine are rich in base. Patients therefore tend to develop a metabolic acidosis requiring intravenous sodium bicarbonate. The loss of proteins in the secretions and inability to digest them causes a negative nitrogen balance. The resulting gluconeogenesis produces marked muscle wasting, a low serum albumin, and poor wound healing. These nutritional deficits frequently lead to death.

It is therefore essential to maintain an adequate protein intake and to produce a positive nitrogen balance. The patient with a small fistula may be given protein by mouth, supplemented by intravenous albumin or amino acids. All patients with more than a small fistula should be treated by hyperalimentation or elemental diets (see Chapter 14, page 244). A positive nitrogen balance can be attained and with it the likelihood of spontaneous healing of the fistula. Blood should be given to patients with a low hemoglobin, since proteins are first used to form hemoglobin. Antibiotics are given as indicated. Surgical treatment may be required for a large fistula that persists in spite of good supportive management. Establishment of a bypass to the fistula is the most frequently used procedure. Local closure is rarely successful. Resection of the fistula and adjacent bowel with continuity reestablished by an end-to-end anastomosis can be extremely difficult because of the presence of inflammatory adhesions.

Short-Bowel Syndrome

Resection of the small intestine results in a loss of absorptive efficiency. Patients can maintain good nutrition after resection of 50 percent of the small intestine but lose weight and develop nutritional deficiencies after resection of a greater amount. A minimum of 30 to 40 cm of small intestine is necessary to maintain life. Extensive resection may be required for Crohn's disease, trauma, gangrene secondary to arterial or venous occlusion, congenital defects, and hernias complicated by massive gangrene.

The absorptive deficit after extensive resection of the small intestine is not well understood. There is marked decrease in fat absorption, but amino acid and carbohydrate absorption are less affected. Severe electrolyte losses are often present. Hypokalemia and hypocalcemia can reach lethal levels, and magnesium deficiency and hypophosphatemia also occur.[6]

A number of patients with only a few centimeters of small intestine have been successfully treated by repeated intravenous hyperalimentation.

Blind-Loop Syndrome

A surgically constructed blind loop following a side-to-side anastomosis sometimes results in a megaloblastic or macrocytic anemia, crampy abdominal pain, fatigue, nausea, distention, episodic diarrhea, and failure to gain weight. Steatorrhea may also occur. Occasionally a similar picture results from partial intestinal obstruction. The symptoms are due in part to growth of anaerobic bacteria in the intestinal segment with impaired absorption of fats resulting from deconjugation and dehydroxylation of bile salts.[7]

The macrocytic anemia comes from impaired absorption of vitamin B_{12}. The serum B_{12} level is decreased, and the Schilling test shows a low urinary excretion. There is often impaired xylose absorption and a low serum albumin. The anemia is treated by giving liver extract, folic acid, or vitamin B_{12}. Oral broad-spectrum antibiotics correct the megaloblastic anemia and restore the Schilling test to normal. Definitive treatment is excision of the blind loop or correction of the partial intestinal obstruction.

Vascular Insufficiency

The commonest causes of acute occlusion of the superior mesenteric artery are embolism or thrombosis. In a number of patients the reason for the occlusion is not known. The superior mesenteric artery is particularly prone to obstruction by embolism because of its large size, the high rate of blood flow, and its direction parallel with the abdominal aorta. The embolus may be formed in the heart on a diseased valve or arise from a mural thrombus following cardiac infarction, or it may form on an atheromatous plaque in the aorta. The embolus lodges at a point of vessel narrowing, either secondary to arteriosclerosis or the origin of a major branch such as the middle colic artery. A secondary thrombus is formed and propagates distally and proximally. Reflex spasm of the vessel occurs. The infarcted bowel is initially blanched secondary to the vasospasm, peristalsis of the bowel disappears, and the bowel wall after four to six hours becomes cyanotic and congested.

Thrombosis of the superior mesenteric artery occurs in patients with arteriosclerotic vessel narrowing. A history of intestinal angina may be obtained. Periarteritis nodosa may cause thrombosis of branches of the superior mesenteric artery and small segments of infarcted bowel.

The common denominator for all nonocclusive infarction of the small bowel is a decreased blood flow through the mesenteric vascular bed. This can arise from congestive heart failure, diabetic coma, infection, hypovolemia, or the injudicious use of vasoconstrictors to treat hypovolemic shock.

Intestinal angina describes a syndrome of general abdominal pain aggravated by eating and results from insufficient blood supply to the bowel. There is also weight loss because of decreased intake of food and malabsorption of fat and protein. Several major vessels must be arteriosclerotic for symptoms to appear. The diagnosis is made by the history and the demonstration of occlusive vascular disease by selective mesenteric angiography.[8]

Thrombosis of the superior mesenteric vein is now a rare cause of mesenteric vascular obstruction. It may result from hypercoagulable states associated with carcinomatosis and polycythemia, local stasis in the superior mesenteric vein due to hepatic cirrhosis, injury to the vein following trauma, intra-abdominal sepsis, or radiotherapy. The clinical picture of venous thrombosis is less acute than that following arterial occlusion.

Until recently the only treatment for mesenteric vascular insufficiency was resection of the infarcted bowel. The loss of bowel was frequently so extensive that the patient died. With the development of modern vascular surgery embolectomy can be performed successfully, or a stenosed segment of the mesenteric artery can be bypassed.

Injuries to Small Intestine

Injuries to the small intestine may arise from penetrating wounds of the abdomen through the abdominal wall, diaphragm, or perineum, or from blunt abdominal trauma (Figure 21-5). A hole may be produced in the bowel, the lumen may be completely transected, or the blood vessels may be torn. There may also be a mesenteric hematoma and edema (Figure 21-6). It has been traditional to explore all deep penetrating wounds of the abdomen. Recently in centers with great experience in the care of these patients, patients have been treated conservatively and only operated on if there were signs of bleeding or peritonitis. Blunt abdominal injuries are treated conservatively and only operated on when there is bleeding or peritonitis. Symptoms may be obscured by multiple injuries to the head, chest, and multiple fractures. Pain, tenderness, abdominal guarding, paralytic ileus, leukocytosis all point toward some visceral injury and,

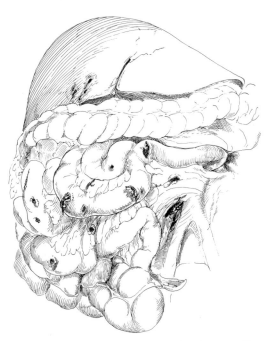

Figure 21–5. Penetrating wounds of the small intestine can involve many overlapping loops as well as the liver and blood vessels.

if the question remains, the surgeon may be obligated to explore the abdomen and examine all the viscera. An upright film of the abdomen and abdominal tap are indicated in patients treated conservatively for abdominal injuries (see Chapter 9). Trauma to the small intestine frequently occurs near the region of fixation, the ligament of Treitz, and the distal ileum and results from compression of the bowel against the vertebral column. Injury to the blood vessels may result in ischemic gangrene of the small intestine. A hole in the small bowel is repaired in two layers with the suture line at right angles to the lumen. Resection is only performed if there are multiple holes in a segment of the bowel or if damage to the blood supply has resulted in gangrene.

Tumors

Benign tumors outnumber malignant tumors of the small intestine in autopsy series. The commonest are leiomyomas, lipomas, and hemangiomas. They are often asymptomatic but may cause recurrent subacute or acute intestinal obstruction often associated with intussusception. Occasionally they give rise to chronic or massive bleeding.

Heterotopic islets of pancreatic, gastric, and duodenal mucosa in the small intestine may present as tumors. True adenomatous polyps of

the small intestine may be single or multiple and may be associated with adenomatosis of the entire gastrointestinal tract.

The Peutz-Jeghers syndrome consists of multiple polyps of the gastrointestinal tract, associated with melanin spots on the oral mucosa, lips, palms, and soles. The syndrome was first described by Peutz in 1921 and re-emphasized by Jeghers in 1949. The syndrome occurs equally in males and females and is transmitted as a mendelian dominant trait. The intestinal polyps are hamartomas and do not become malignant. The patient presents with intussusception, bleeding, or diarrhea. The portion of bowel giving rise to symptoms should be resected or individual polyps removed by enterotomy. Removal of all the involved intestine may result in the short-bowel syndrome. Bleeding may arise from hemangiomatosis associated with Osler-Weber-Rendu syndrome.

The malignant tumors, carcinomas, sarcomas, and carcinoid tumors occur in a ratio of 3:2:1. Adenocarcinoma is the most frequent malignant tumor of the small intestine (Figure 21–7). The usual clinical presentation is intestinal obstruction. Resection of the tumor and lymph node drainage is the treatment of choice.

Sarcomas are more common in the ileum than

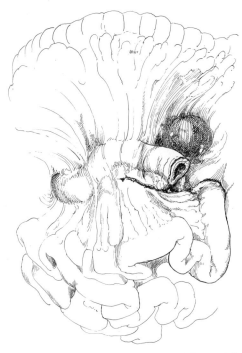

Figure 21–6. Landing on the feet after a fall may result in the complete tearing of the jejunum just below the ligament of Treitz. There can be associated tear of the mesentery or hematoma in the transverse mesocolon.

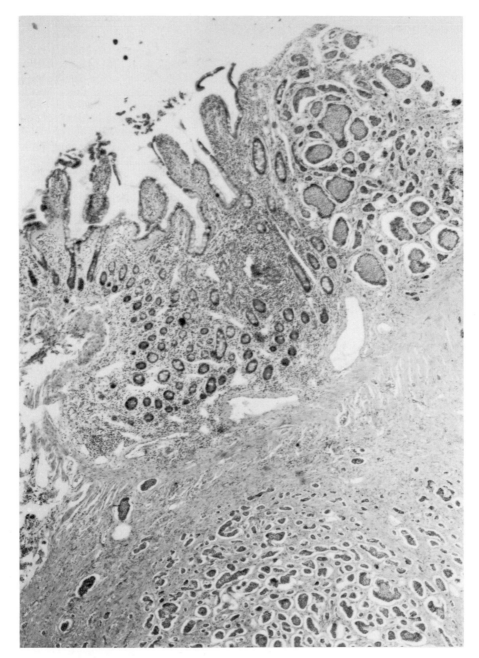

Figure 21–7. Photomicrograph of adenocarcinoma of the ileum. At left is normal ileal mucosa and junction with adenocarcinoma. Carcinoma cells are seen invading the muscularis at lower edge of micrograph. (Hematoxylin and eosin stain × 75.)

in the jejunum. They may grow external to the bowel lumen, producing an abdominal mass with or without signs of obstruction. Lympho-sarcomas are the most frequent, followed by leiomyosarcomas.[9] When the sarcoma is located in one segment of the bowel, resection is in-

dicated. Radiotherapy is effective in lymphomas. The five-year survival rate is 20 percent for adenocarcinomas, 60 percent for lymphosarcomas, and 60 percent for leiomyosarcomas.[10]

The serotonin-secreting carcinoid tumors arise from Kultschitzky cells in the crypts of

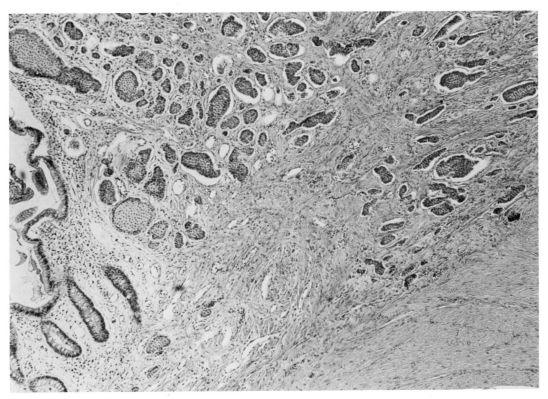

Figure 21–8.   Photomicrograph of carcinoid of the ileum. At left is normal ileal mucosa, leading into nests of large regular carcinoid tumor cells that invade the submucosa and the muscularis. (Hematoxylin and eosin stain × 75.)

Lieberkuhn. The name erroneously suggests that the tumors are benign. They can occur at any location from the cardiac end of the stomach to the anus. About 50 percent are found in the appendix, 25 percent in the ileum, and 15 percent in the rectum. They are occasionally found in the bronchus. The primary tumors remain small and do not exceed 3 cm in diameter even with gross metastases in the mesenteric nodes and liver. The tumors are yellow and rarely ulcerated. The differentiation of benign from malignant tumors is difficult on microscopic examination (Figure 21–8). Those in the appendix are almost invariably benign, while one third of those in the small intestine develop metastases. Removal of the appendix is adequate treatment if the tumor is confined to the appendix, has not invaded the mesoappendix or lymph nodes, and does not extend to the point of resection. When the tumor is in the small intestine, the segment of bowel should be excised along with the regional nodes. If the lesion is in the terminal ileum, a right hemicolectomy is done with resection of the involved small bowel. The five-year survival for malignant

carcinoids of the small intestine is about 50 percent.

The carcinoid syndrome consists of transient red-purple flushing of the trunk and face associated with diarrhea and occasionally with asthma, and sometimes collapse. Chronic manifestations of the syndrome are tachycardia, edema, pellagroid skin lesions, and valvular disease of the right heart. Subendothelial fibrosis of the pulmonary or tricuspid valves leads to cardiac decompensation.

The symptoms of the carcinoid syndrome may be due to secretion of serotonin (5-hydroxytryptamine) by the tumor and its metastases. Recently it has been shown that the pathogenesis of the symptoms is more complex. Normally only a small amount of the essential amino acid tryptophan is converted to 5-hydroxytryptophan and then 5-hydroxytryptamine. In the patient with metastases more than half the dietary intake of tryptophan is metabolized by the carcinoid tissue. This diversion of the amino acid combined with diarrhea results in a negative nitrogen balance and the symptoms of niacin deficiency. The liver metastases secrete a large amount of serotonin in the blood returning to the right heart. The lungs contain a large amount of monoamine oxidase that removes two thirds of the serotonin. The cardiac lesions are therefore right-sided. The urinary output of 5-hydroxyindoleacetic acid is increased 100 to 150 times. The diagnosis is established by demonstrating a high level of 5-hydroxyindoleacetic acid in the urine. Bananas and some medications can also produce an increase. However, a number of findings are difficult to explain. The serotonin content of tumors varies greatly, injection of serotonin does not always produce the syndrome, and the administration of serotonin antagonists or agents to block production of serotonin has not been effective in treating the syndrome. It is most likely that a number of biologically active peptides such as bradykinin and kallikrein are also involved in the syndrome.

Patients with the carcinoid syndrome should be treated by excising as much of the tumor as possible. This may involve removal of regional nodes and partial hepatectomy. Temporary relief of symptoms occurs, provided that an adequate amount of serotonin-secreting tumor is removed. Treatment by radiotherapy or chemotherapy is of no value.[11]

Crohn's Disease

In 1932 Crohn described the granulomatous bowel disease that he called regional ileitis. The disease may develop in any part of the gastrointestinal tract from the esophagus to the anus and also in the skin. A more satisfactory name is Crohn's disease.

The disease begins as a granulomatous lymphangitis in the mesentery and regional nodes and produces edema in the bowel wall leading to fibrosis, narrowing, and sometimes obstruction of the lumen. The mucosa becomes ulcerated and all coats are involved. Perforation may occur with abscess formation or development of a fistula between the bowel and other viscera or skin.

Crohn's disease occurs mainly in young adults but may arise at any age. The incidence is increasing in the colon in older patients. One half have the onset at below 20 years, and frequently the terminal ileum is involved. The onset may be acute and resemble appendicitis, or the patient may present with weight loss and crampy abdominal pain. The first symptom may be foul-smelling diarrhea with passage of mucus, pus, or blood. The granulomatous reaction may produce a palpable mass and result in intestinal obstruction. Many patients have an anal fistula, fissure, or anorectal abscess. Grossly there is a rubbery thickening of one or more accurately defined segments of bowel associated with an increase in mesenteric fat. The thickened mesentery contains enlarged regional lymph nodes. The involvement of sharply defined segments of bowel interspersed with normal "skip" regions is characteristic. Microscopically the main feature is that the inflammation and fibrosis involve all the layers of the intestine and the regional nodes. The mononuclear cell infiltration, fibrosis, and giant cell formation resemble chronic tuberculosis. There is, however, no caseation and tubercle bacilli are not present.

The etiology of Crohn's disease is unknown. The mononuclear cell infiltration, occasional response to immunosuppressive drugs, and spontaneous regression of involved segments suggest that this may be an autoimmune disease. It has also been suggested that Crohn's disease and ulcerative colitis are variants of the same disease. Ulcerative colitis predominantly affects the mucosa, while Crohn's disease affects all layers of the bowel and the regional nodes.

The diagnosis of Crohn's disease can be confirmed by barium x-ray study. The small bowel is hyperirritable, there is coarsening of the mucosa, thickening of bowel wall, and the classic string sign may be present (Figure 21–9).

Conservative management is indicated in uncomplicated Crohn's disease. If the diagnosis is made at laparotomy for suspected acute appendicitis, the involved bowel should not be removed. If the cecum is not diseased, the appendix should be removed, and in addition a mesenteric node should be removed for microscopic examination. Subsequently most patients do not have further symptoms.

Patients with diarrhea should be given a bland, milk-free, low-residue diet, antispasmodics, and antidiarrheal medications. The use of azathioprine is under investigation. Steroids may be given, especially during the acute inflammatory stage. The response to these drugs is generally less than in patients with ulcerative colitis.

Operation is indicated in patients with Crohn's disease because conservative management has failed or local or systemic complications have developed (Figure 21–10). Urgent indications are acute intestinal obstruction, perforation, massive bleeding, and acute toxic megacolon. Elective indications are chronic intestinal obstruction, abdominal mass, fistula, perianal sepsis, and the development of cancer. Cancer of the colon occurs in about 3 percent of patients with Crohn's disease in the colon of 10 years' duration. It is also increased in the small intestine in those with Crohn's disease there. There is a marked tendency for fistula formation internally into the bladder, another loop of bowel, or the vagina, externally to the skin usually following an operation, or into the perineum.

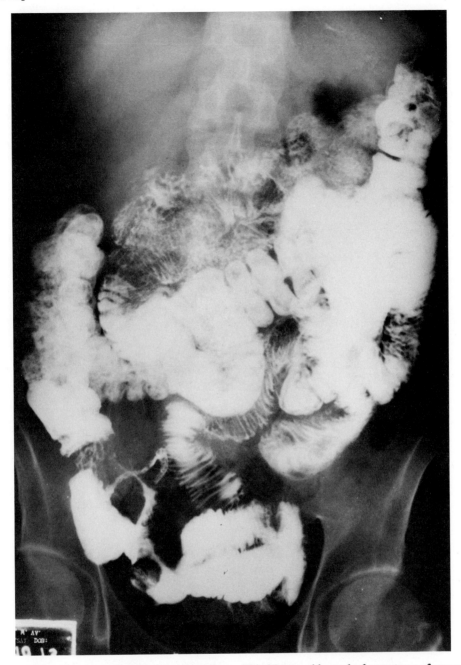

Figure 21–9.   Crohn's disease of the distal ileum. This 37-year-old man had symptoms of crampy abdominal pain, tenderness, and vomiting for two days. The small bowel x-ray study shows a partially obstructed small intestine with a thickened wall and narrowed lumen of the distal ileum, the classic string sign. The patient responded to conservative treatment. (Courtesy of Drs. C. Mendoza and T. Mehta.)

Perineal abscess may antedate diagnosis of Crohn's disease by several years. Occasionally the fistula enters the psoas producing a psoas abscess. Patients who are malnourished, as for example, with fistula, often require intravenous hyperalimentation or elemental diets before operation. Patients who have steatorrhea with Crohn's disease of the ileum have impaired

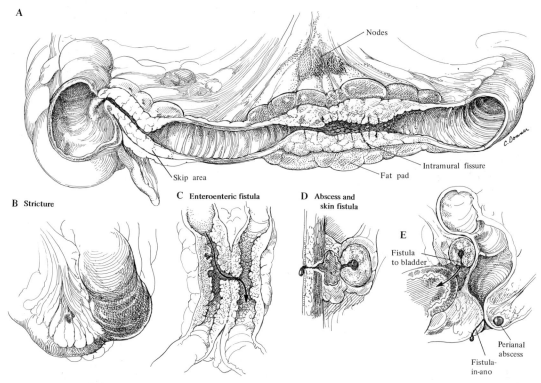

A

Nodes

Skip area

Intramural fissure

Fat pad

B Stricture

C Enteroenteric fistula

D Abscess and skin fistula

E

Fistula to bladder

Perianal abscess

Fistula-in-ano

Figure 21–10. Crohn's disease of the small intestine and its complications.

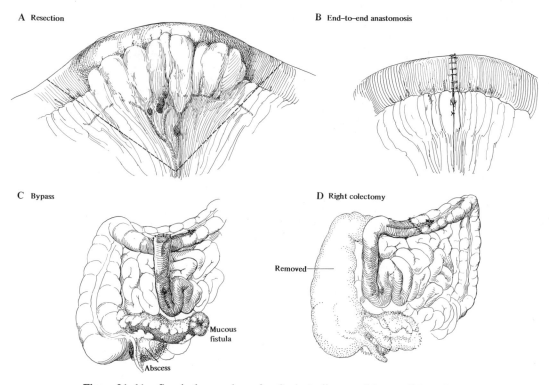

A Resection

B End–to–end anastomosis

C Bypass

Mucous fistula

Abscess

D Right colectomy

Removed

Figure 21–11. Surgical procedures for Crohn's disease of the small intestine.

metabolism of the bile salts and an increase in cholelithiasis. Hyperphosphatemia and oxalemia increase the incidence of urinary calculi. Systemic complications are similar to those in patients with ulcerative colitis and include arthritis, ankylosing spondylitis, iritis, hepatitis, and skin lesions. The treatment of choice is excision of the diseased bowel and its mesentery (Figure 21–11). Occasionally a bypass is performed because of the patient's general condition, the presence of extensive disease, or a large inflammatory mass.[12]

Operative treatment in those with disease of the colon is resecting involved bowel or establishing a bypass. Occasionally total colectomy and ileostomy are necessary when all the colon is involved. In addition, abdominoperineal resection of the rectum may be required. Sky-blue lymphangiography at operation aids in determining the level for bowel resection. The dye spreads readily through the mesenteric lymphatics in uninvolved bowel but remains localized when early disease is present. The disease may recur after operation and one third of patients need a second operation.[13] Care must be taken to avoid resecting too much bowel and creating a short-bowel syndrome. The 20-year survival is about 76 percent in Crohn's disease and about 60 percent in ulcerative colitis.

Radiation Enteritis

Radiotherapy, especially when given in high dosage to patients with gynecologic cancer or carcinoma of the bladder, may produce acute or chronic changes in the small intestine.[14] The terminal ileum is most frequently involved. In the acute stage the wall of the bowel becomes acutely inflamed and edematous, and there is damage to the mucosal cells and ulceration. Symptoms are crampy abdominal pain, diarrhea, melena, marked dehydration, and loss of electrolytes. After about 12 weeks the wall of the bowel becomes thickened and fibrotic, and the mucosa is atrophied and ulcerated. Microscopically there is marked narrowing of the blood vessels from endarteritis and perivascular fibrosis. The patient may develop acute or chronic intestinal obstruction with or without bleeding. During the acute phase the patient should be treated conservatively. When fibrosis has caused obstruction, the involved bowel should be excised. Care should be taken to resect adequate intestine so that the anastomosis is performed using normal bowel. Leakage at the suture line and fistula formation are common postoperative complications.

Specific Infections

Salmonella and typhoid organisms affect mainly the small intestine. Occasionally perforation or severe bleeding occurs and requires operative treatment. Staphylococcal or pseudomembranous enterocolitis may occur in patients treated with antibiotics. The antibiotic-resistant staphylococci replace the normal intestinal flora, and the patient becomes toxic, has severe diarrhea, and may die. Treatment is intravenous fluids and electrolytes, antidiarrhea medications, and antibiotics to which *Staphylococcus aureus* is sensitive.

Collagen diseases such as lupus erythematosus, rheumatoid arthritis, polyarteritis nodosa, and Wegener's granulomatosis can give rise to small bowel ulceration and perforation.

CITED REFERENCES

1. Aubrey, D. A.: Meckel's diverticulum. A review of sixty-six emergency Meckel's diverticulectomies. *Arch. Surg.*, **100**:144–46, 1970.
2. Bank, S.; Markes, I. N.; and Novis, B.: Progress in small bowel physiology and disease. *S. Afr. Med. J.*, **45**:1141–44, 1971.
3. Conn, J. H.; Chavaz, C. M.; and Fain, W. R.: The short bowel syndrome. *Ann. Surg.*, **175**:803–14, 1972.
4. DeCosse, J. J.; Rhodes, R. S.; Wentz, W. B.; Reagan, J. W.; Dworken, H. J.; and Holden, W. D.: The natural history and management of radiation induced injury of the gastrointestinal tract. *Ann. Surg.* **170**:369–84, 1969.
5. DeDombal, F. T.; Burton, I.; and Goligher, J. S.: The early and late results of surgical treatment for Crohn's disease. *Br. J. Surg.*, **58**:805–16, 1971.
6. Eade, M. N.; Cooke, W. T.; and Williams, J. A.: Clinical and hematologic features of Crohn's disease. *Surg. Gynecol. Obstet.*, **72**:643–46, 1972.
7. Goldstein, F.: Mechanisms of malabsorption and malnutrition in the blind loop syndrome. *Gastroenterology*, **61**:780–84, 1971.
8. Hancock, R. J.: An 11-year review of primary tumors of the small bowel including the duodenum. *Can. Med. Assoc. J.*, **103**:1177–79, 1970.
9. McIhath, D. C., and Hinnekens, P. H.: Primary tumors of the small intestine. *Surg. Clin. North Am.*, **47**:909–14, 1967.
10. Roback, S. A., and Nicoloff, D. M.: High output enterocutaneous fistulas of the small bowel. An analysis of fifty-five cases. *Am. J. Surg.*, **123**:317–22, 1972.
11. Scott, H. W.: Metabolic surgery for hyperlipidemia and atherosclerosis. *Am. J. Surg.*, **123**:3–12, 1972.
12. Weinstein, E. C.; Cain, J. C.; and Remine, W. H.: Meckel's diverticulum: 55 years of clinical and surgical experience. *JAMA*, **182**:251–53, 1962.
13. Williams, L. F. J.: Vascular insufficiency of the intestines. *Gastroenterology*, **61**:757–77, 1971.
14. Wilson, H.; Cheek, R. C.; Sherman, R. T.; and Storer, E. H.: Carcinoid tumors. *Curr. Prob. Surg.*, Nov. 1970, pp. 1–51.

SUGGESTIONS FOR FURTHER READING

Armstrong, W. McD., and Nunn, A. S., Jr.: *Intestinal Transport of Electrolytes, Amino Acids and Sugars.* Charles C Thomas, Springfield, Ill., 1972.

This sophisticated book presents the detailed knowledge of intestinal cellular activity in the absoption of various substances across the cell membrane. It is a continuation of the information contained within a standard physiology textbook.

Boley, S. J.; Swartz, S. S.; and Williams, L. F., Jr.: *Vascular Disorders of the Intestine*. Appleton-Century-Crofts Education Division, Meredith Corporation, New York, 1971.

There is a complete discussion of vascular disorders of the gastrointestinal tract including pathophysiology, radiology, and experimental investigations.

Colcock, B. P., and Braasch, J. W.: *Surgery of the Small Intestine in the Adult*. W. B. Saunders Co., Philadelphia 1968.

This book describes the surgical aspects of diseases of the small intestine. It has an excellent bibliography of the major contributions to surgery of the small intestine.

Kyle, J.: *Crohn's Disease*. Appleton-Century-Crofts Educational Division, Meredith Corporation, New York, 1972.

This excellent book summarizes our present knowledge of Crohn's disease, pathophysiology, its diagnostic and clinical features, and the medical and surgical treatment.

Chapter 22

COLON, APPENDIX, RECTUM, AND ANUS

Alexander Doolas, Richard G. Caldwell, David L. Roseman, and
Frederic A. de Peyster

CHAPTER OUTLINE

COLON
Anatomy
  Embryology
  Histology
  Blood and Lymphatic Supply
  Innervation
    Parasympathetic
    Sympathetic
    Extrinsic Afferent System
Physiology
Trauma
  Diagnosis
  Treatment
Inflammatory Diseases
  Amebiasis
  Tuberculosis
  Pseudomembranous and Staphylococcal
    Enterocolitis
  Nonspecific Inflammatory Diseases
    Ulcerative Colitis
    Granulomatous Colitis
  Diverticular Disease
    Pathology
    Clinical Picture
    Conservative Treatment
    Surgical Treatment
Cancer of the Colon
  Etiology
  Pathology
  Clinical Presentation
  Diagnosis
  Treatment
    Colonic Preparation for Operation
    Chemotherapy
    Local Radiotherapy
    Results of Treatment
Ischemic Disease of the Colon
  Clinical Picture
  Transient Ischemic Colitis
  Ischemic Strictures
Volvulus of the Colon
  Diagnosis
  Treatment

Acquired Megacolon
  Clinical Presentation
  Treatment
Radiation Injury
Hematochezia
  Diagnosis
  Treatment
Colostomy
  Care of Colostomy
APPENDIX
Anatomy
Acute Appendicitis
  Clinical Picture
  Physical Findings
  Laboratory Findings
  Differential Diagnosis
    Gastroenteritis
    Acute Mesenteric Adenitis
    Primary Peritonitis
    Crohn's Disease
    Meckel's Diverticulum
    Acute Diverticulitis
    Tumors of the Gut
    Acute Cholecystitis
    Perforation of Peptic Ulcer
    Gynecologic Conditions
    Genitourinary Conditions
  Management
  Special Types of Acute Appendicitis
    During Infancy
    During Pregnancy
    Geriatric Patient
Other Diseases of the Appendix
  Carcinoma
  Carcinoid
  Mucocele
  Diverticulitis
RECTUM
Anatomy
Physiology
Inflammatory Diseases
  Amebic Proctitis
  Ulcerative Proctitis

Trauma
Neoplasms
    Polyps
        Adenomatous Polyps
        Villous Adenomas
        Juvenile Polyps
    Carcinoid
    Carcinoma of the Rectum
    Clinical Presentation
    Diagnosis
    Treatment
        Attempted Curative Treatment
        Palliative Treatment
ANUS
Anatomy
    Anoderm
    Musculature
    Vasculature
    Lymphatics
    Innervation
Physiology
History
    Bowel Habits
    Presence of Blood

Pain
Other Symptoms
Physical Examination
    Proctoscopy, Colonoscopy
Diseases of the Anus
    Congenital Diseases
    Injuries to the Anus
    Fissure
    Stricture
    Cryptitis
    Abscesses
    Fistula
    Pruritus Ani
    Anal Incontinence
    Hemorrhoids
        Diagnosis
        Treatment
    Anorectal Prolapse
        Treatment
    Anal Neoplasms
        Treatment
    Pilonidal Cysts and Sinuses
    Presacral Retrorectal Tumors and Cysts

COLON

ANATOMY

The colon begins at the ileocecal valve, ends at the rectum, and is 1.5 meters long (see Plate IV). The following characteristics distinguish it from the small intestine.

1. The colon is twice the diameter of the small bowel except for the descending colon, where the diameter is approximately the same.

2. The external longitudinal muscle of the colon is arranged in three longitudinal bands (taeniae) 1 cm wide. The taeniae are shorter than the colon, thus allowing the bowel to balloon between them, forming sacculations or haustrae. They converge at the base of the appendix.

3. The plicae semilunares are transverse muscular and mucosal bands that separate the haustrae. On plain abdominal films of the small bowel the valvulae conniventes encircle the entire bowel.

4. The appendices epiploicae are fatty, teardropped appendages located along the two anterior taeniae of the colon.

Embryology

The portion of colon proximal to the midtransverse colon is derived from the midgut. Its vascular and nerve supply and its absorptive function therefore are similar to that of the small intestine. The distal colon arises from the hindgut (Figure 35–3, page 633).

Histology

The colon wall consists of five layers: mucosa, muscularis mucosa, submucosa, muscularis, and serosa.

1. The mucosa is a relatively flat layer containing the glands of Lieberkuhn, which are lined by goblet cells in their depth and by striated columnar cells toward the surface. The goblet cells secrete mucus, which lubricates, protects, and neutralizes acid bacterial breakdown products. Mucus is visible in the stool only in pathologic states, such as infectious diarrhea, ulcerative colitis, carcinoma, and villous adenoma. Loss of great quantities of mucus may lead to electrolyte imbalance.

2. The muscularis mucosa is a thin, smooth, muscular layer that separates the mucosa from the submucosa.

3. The submucosa is a dense layer of connective tissue that conveys blood vessels, nerves, and lymphatics.

4. The muscularis consists of an inner circular layer and the taeniae.

5. The serosa is composed of a thin layer of mesothelial cells and is absent in the retroperitoneal portions of the colon.

Blood and Lymphatic Supply

The colon derives its blood supply from the superior and inferior mesenteric arteries (see Plate VII). The former supplies the transverse colon through the middle colic artery, then the right colon by the right colic artery, and finally the ileum and cecum through the ileocolic artery. The inferior mesenteric artery supplies the left colon through the left colic artery, then the sigmoid colon by three or four sigmoidal arteries, and finally the rectum by the superior hemorrhoidal artery. The colic arteries divide to form an anastomotic arcade, the marginal artery of Drummond, located 0.5 to 1.0 cm from the colonic wall. This arcade carries sufficient blood supply to allow the sacrifice of the inferior mesenteric or right colic arteries as is routinely done in abdominal aortic resections and colonic interpositions between the cervical esophagus and the stomach. On rare occasions sacrifice of the main arteries to the colon has led to colonic ischemia and infarction, probably due to arteriosclerotic occlusion of collateral vessels. The point of bifurcation of the lowest sigmoidal artery and the superior hemorrhoidal artery, the critical point of Sudeck, has been thought to be a weak anastomotic link. In practice, ischemia of the rectosigmoid is extremely rare after this intercommunication has been ligated because of the presence of numerous intramural collateral vessels.[11]

The venous drainage of the right colon is to the superior mesenteric vein. The inferior mesenteric vein drains the left half of the colon and joins the splenic vein.

The lymphatic drainage of the colon is to the cisterna chyli. Valves prevent retrograde flow. Lymph nodes are located along the marginal artery, the vascular arcades, and the main colic vessels. Due to the abundant lymphatic collaterals, skip metastases occasionally occur in patients with carcinoma of the colon. Retrograde lymph node involvement is infrequent because of the valves unless there is proximal lymphatic obstruction.

Innervation

The colon is controlled by extrinsic and intrinsic nervous systems. The extrinsic nervous system modifies the automatic action of the intrinsic system. It consists of parasympathetic and sympathetic fibers of the autonomic nervous system.

Parasympathetic. The right colon is innervated by the vagus nerve, and the left colon by the second, third, and fourth pelvic splanchnic nerves (nervi erigentes).

Sympathetic. These fibers emanate from T_9 through L_2 levels and supply preganglionic fibers coursing through the white rami communicantes to the sympathetic chain and then to the various mesenteric ganglia and plexi. Both systems synapse in the intrinsic enteric plexi to give postganglionic fibers that terminate in the intestinal glands, vessels, and muscle. The parasympathetic system stimulates colonic motility and mucous secretions and inhibits sphincter contraction. The sympathetic system has the opposite effect.

Extrinsic Afferent System. The colon perceives stimuli of distention and stretching but not cutting, piercing, or burning. Sensory impulses travel through the pelvic splanchnics, the lumbar and thoracic sympathetics, or the vagus nerve, depending on the segment of bowel stimulated, and synapse with fibers coursing to other segments of the cord, hypothalamus, thalamus, or cortex.

The intrinsic nervous system is composed of multiple ganglionic cells forming Auerbach's plexus, located between the two muscular coats of the bowel, and Meissner's plexus, located in the submucosa. Absence of the intrinsic system results in loss of bowel motility in that segment as seen in congenital megacolon. Deprivation of the extrinsic system has little effect on bowel motility. The extrinsic mechanism therefore is not as essential to colonic function but renders a degree of voluntary control and coordination of bowel activity, especially during defecation.

PHYSIOLOGY

The colon reduces the bulk of the intestinal chyme by fluid resorption, stores fecal material in the descending and sigmoid colon, and expels feces through the act of defecation.

1. Absorption. The colon reduces 500 ml of intestinal chyme to 135 gm of feces through active salt and passive water absorption (Figure 22–1). A variety of segmental, churning, nonpropulsive contractions mix the fecal material to facilitate absorption.

2. Storage. The feces are slowly advanced to the sigmoid colon, where they are stored. If defecation does not occur, the sigmoid accommodates the feces.

3. Defecation. The act of defecation is initiated by a mass peristaltic wave, with peak pressures of 100 mm Hg beginning in the transverse colon and moving distally. This wave is initiated by a large meal, smoking, drinking coffee, or other stimuli to which the individual has conditioned himself. As the feces enter the rectum, the resulting distention causes a further

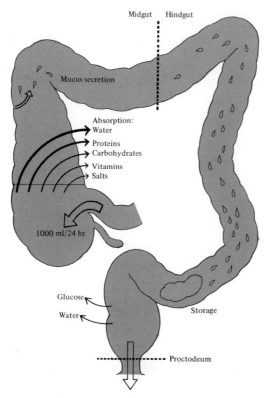

Figure 22–1. Colonic function. The function of the right colon is mainly absorptive and that of the left is transport, lubrication, and storage of feces.

reflex contraction of the colon. Simultaneously flexion of the abdominal musculature, the Valsalva maneuver, and the relaxation of the anal sphincter result in defecation.

TRAUMA

Blunt trauma does not frequently result in colonic injury because the colon is protected by the ribs and pelvic bones. Penetrating trauma to the abdomen results in colonic injuries in 20 percent of patients. Management of colonic injuries is difficult and is associated with frequent infections and anastomotic leaks due to the semisolid state of the stool, the high bacterial count, and the absence of an enveloping external longitudinal muscle. Injuries to other organs are found in 50 percent of patients with colonic injuries due to blunt trauma.[21] Car accidents are the most frequent cause of blunt trauma, followed by sports and industrial injuries.[21] The mechanism of injury is not through an increase of intraluminal pressure, as was once thought, but by compression and shearing of the colon between the external force and the vertebral column. The injury varies from hematoma of the bowel wall or its mesentery to complete transection of these structures. Transection of the mesentery may result in colonic necrosis or in a chronic ischemia with subsequent stenosis and obstruction.

Penetrating injuries result from shootings and stabbings. All segments of the colon are involved equally in penetrating injuries, whereas in blunt trauma the transverse colon is most frequently injured. Penetrating injuries in civilian life are less serious than those in war and may be handled differently.[17] Most civilian gunshot injuries are inflicted with low-velocity weapons (below 1700 ft/sec). War wounds are caused by high-velocity projectiles and inflict serious damage.

Explosive injuries of the colon are usually the result of practical jokes, when compressed air as is used in construction and sandblasting is blasted into the perineum. The colon suddenly distends and ruptures most often in the cecum. Blast injuries usually occur in underwater explosions. The energy is transmitted to the hollow viscera and causes intramural hemorrhage and colonic tears.

Ingested foreign bodies, such as pins, chicken bones, or fish bones, may occasionally lead to colonic perforation. Vigorous proctoscopy or cautery above the peritoneal reflection can perforate the sigmoid colon.

Diagnosis

Since tremendous forces are required to produce colonic injury in blunt trauma, 50 percent of the patients have other serious injuries. A preoperative diagnosis of the colonic injury is rarely made. The patient usually has signs of peritonitis, free air on decubitus abdominal films, or may be explored for intra-abdominal bleeding.

Treatment

The management of colonic injuries depends on the patient's condition, the associated pathology, the extent of colonic injury, and fecal contamination.

Small hematomas of the colonic wall or mesentery may be left alone if they are not expanding. Ligatures control bleeding from large mesenteric tears. A large hematoma may cause thrombosis of vessels. The viability of the colon should therefore be determined by the presence of pulsation, peristalsis, pink color, and bleeding when the serosa is incised. Nonviable gut should be exteriorized over a glass rod or resected and the ends brought out as colostomies. A primary anastomosis is rarely indicated (Figure 23–4, page 413).

Small tears of the right colon resulting from

blunt trauma not exceeding 5 to 6 cm may be debrided, closed primarily, and drained. Larger tears should be exteriorized. Tears in fixed portions of the left colon should be oversewn, drained, and the gut defunctioned by a proximal colostomy. Penetrating injuries of the right colon may be closed. Those on the left do better if exteriorized or defunctioned with a colostomy. Wounds from high-velocity missiles are extensive and should not be closed. A primary anastomosis or closure site of a colonic perforation should not be exteriorized. These suture lines often leak because they require contact with serosa for proper healing. To aid healing omentum may be gently wrapped around the suture line.

Broad-spectrum antibiotics should be given to patients with fecal contamination of the peritoneal cavity. The abdominal cavity should be irrigated with copious amounts of saline-containing antibiotics.[3] Neomycin and kanamycin can cause respiratory depression and should be used sparingly in the irrigating solution.

The mortality depends on the number of associated injuries and is as high as 75 percent when several organs are involved. The overall mortality rate of civilian colonic injuries is 15 percent, whereas in World War II it was about 50 percent.

INFLAMMATORY DISEASES

Amebiasis

Surgical intervention is occasionally necessary for perforation or massive bleeding. Occasionally colectomy is erroneously performed when an ameboma is mistaken for a carcinoma.

Tuberculosis

Tuberculosis involvement of the colon affects young adults, most frequently females. Two types have been noted: the primary (hypertrophic) type, usually found in the absence of pulmonary involvement, and the ulcerative type, usually associated with pulmonary tuberculosis.

Pseudomembranous and Staphylococcal Enterocolitis

The etiology of pseudomembranous entercolitis is not clear, although about half of the cases reported have been associated with staphylococci in the stools. Septic shock, ileus, chemical poisoning, drug sensitivity, and intravascular coagulation are some etiologic factors that have been considered. Frequently the onset is a few days after operation, especially when antibiotics have been used. Broad-spectrum antibiotics may diminish the growth of sensitive bacteria, while the growth of resistant bacteria, such as staphylococci and *Proteus*, is uninhibited. The staphylo-

cocci release an antitoxin that is probably responsible for the severe symptoms. The ileum is most often involved, while the colon is involved a fourth of the time. The mucosa is erythematous, edematous, and friable and may be covered by a yellow, gray, proteinaceous membrane. With progression of the disease the submucosa becomes inflamed.

The patient develops fever, cerebral symptoms, a severe watery diarrhea, abdominal distention, and hypovolemic shock usually a few days after operation. When ileus is present, there is no diarrhea, but the colon distends with large volumes of exudative fluid.

The diagnosis may be made by stool culture and proctoscopy, but above all by having a high degree of suspicion. Proctoscopy reveals an edematous mucosa and sometimes a pseudomembrane.

Therapy consists of fluid replacement, anticholinergic drugs, and discontinuation of broad-spectrum antibiotics or intestinal antiseptics. Steroids may be useful. Parenteral hyperalimentation may be necessary to maintain nutrition. Specific antibiotics against staphylococci, such as vancomycin or intravenous oxacillin, are of value. The incidence of the disease can be reduced by careful use of antibiotics.

Nonspecific Inflammatory Diseases

Ulcerative Colitis. Ulcerative colitis is a diffuse inflammatory disease of the colon of unknown etiology. The incidence is difficult to

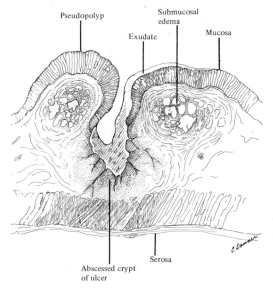

Figure 22–2. The inflammatory changes in ulcerative colitis are confined to the mucosa and submucosa. A pseudopolyp and crypt abscess are present.

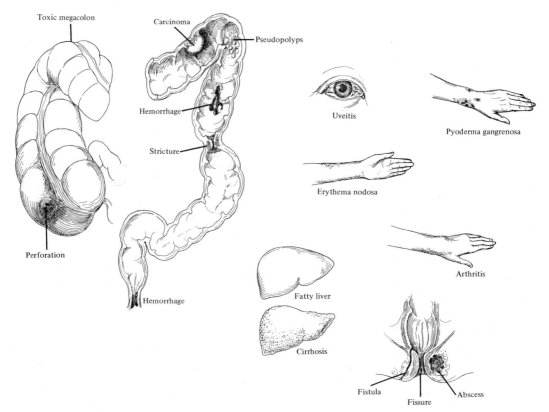

Figure 22–3. The complications of ulcerative colitis may be confined to the colon or they may be systemic.

ascertain because mild cases are often not recorded. Most patients are 20 to 40 years, but the disease can occur at any age. It is more frequent in females than males. Suggested causes are psychiatric disturbances, allergies, endotoxins, lack of protective mucosal substances, infections, collagen pathology, and autoimmune disease.

Pathology. Inflammation occurs initially in the mucosa and progresses to microabscess formation in the crypts and ulceration (Figure 22–2). The submucosa then becomes inflamed and undermined. The muscularis is seldom involved but becomes edematous. In acute fulminating toxic megacolon the muscularis is penetrated and perforation may occur.[16] With chronic and repeated bouts of inflammation, granulation tissue is formed in the mucosa producing pseudopolyps. The muscularis is eventually replaced by fibrous tissue and the colon contracts in length and width and loses its haustral markings.

Clinical Picture. The patient with mild ulcerative colitis has frequent, semiformed stools; with a severe attack he has watery diarrhea and passes mucus, blood, and pus. Blood is passed more frequently in ulcerative colitis than in Crohn's disease. There are cramping abdominal pain, tenesmus, abdominal tenderness, and fever. In the severe fulminating type the temperature rises, the colon becomes dilated sometimes to the point of rupture, and the abdomen is silent and tender.

Three fifths of patients with ulcerative colitis have a relapsing form that persists for one to three months. One third have symptoms lasting for six months or longer.

Complications. Ulcerative colitis exhibits systemic and colonic complications (Figure 22–3).

The acute intestinal complications are perforation, abscess, massive hemorrhage, and toxic megacolon. The patient who develops toxic megacolon has severe diarrhea, becomes toxic, has severe abdominal pain and distention, and develops abdominal tenderness with guarding. On x-ray there is marked distention of the colon, involving mostly the transverse colon. This is a particularly serious complication and if not promptly treated by operation is followed by perforation and a mortality of about 20 percent. It may also occur in patients with Crohn's disease and pseudomembranous colitis. Chronic complications are the development of pseudopolyps, stricture, perianal abscesses, fistulae, and cancer. Perianal complications are more frequent in Crohn's disease than ulcerative colitis. A stricture seen on barium enema should be carefully investigated to exclude the presence of a cancer. The incidence of cancer depends on the duration and extent of the disease. When confined to the rectum and sigmoid colon the incidence is not great but has been reported as high as 40 percent in those who have had diffuse disease for more than 25 years.[7] Others have found that it occurs in about 3 percent in the first 10 years and in 20 percent by 20 years. The cancers are often multiple and have a marked tendency to metastasize early, so that the survival is about half that in patients with cancer of the colon without ulcerative colitis.

Systemic complications are inanition, arthritis, hepatitis, erythema nodosum, dermatitis gangrenosum, stomatitis, arteritis, iridocyclitis,

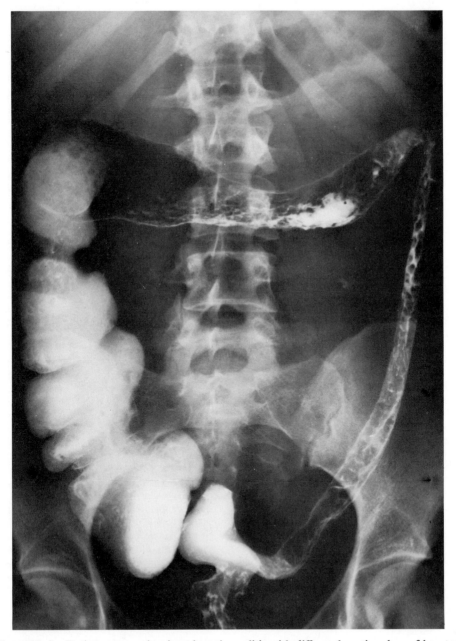

Figure 22–4. Barium enema showing ulcerative colitis with diffuse ulceration, loss of haustration, shortening of the colon, and presence of pseudopolyps.

myocardial degeneration, and anemia due to blood loss and bone marrow suppression.

Diagnosis. The history and physical findings are most important in making the diagnosis. The mucosal changes can be seen in the majority of cases on proctoscopy, and biopsy confirms the diagnosis. In the early stage the mucosa is red, granular, and friable. In the severe form there is a purulent discharge, ulceration, a fibrinous pseudomembrane, and even pseudo-polyps. Multiple ulcers are seen on barium enema (Figure 22–4). Later pseudopolyps, loss of haustrae, and shortening of the colon may be seen and occasionally a carcinoma. The differential diagnosis is with other diseases producing diarrhea, such as Crohn's disease, ischemic colitis, amebiasis, tuberculosis, and carcinoma.

Treatment.   CONSERVATIVE.   Although ulcerative colitis cannot be cured, relief can be obtained by conservative management in 70 to 80 percent of patients.

1. The intestinal tract is rested in the acute and relapsing forms of the disease. Nothing is given by mouth.

2. Hydration and nutrition are maintained by intravenous infusion. In the patient with a severe attack or with profound inanition, hyper-alimentation may be necessary.

3. Anticholinergic drugs are given to relieve cramps. Care must be taken to avoid inducing ileus by giving excessive antispasmodics and producing toxic megacolon.

4. Chemotherapy. Systemic antibiotics are given in acute ulcerative colitis since there is bacterial invasion of the mucosa and submucosa. Broad-spectrum antibiotics, such as ampicillin, cephalothin, gentamicin, in combination with Lincocin, are recommended. Azulfidine is a nonabsorbable diazocompound of salicylic acid and sulfapyridine which has more favorable effects on ulcerative colitis than the other sulfa preparations. The dose varies from 0.5 mg orally four times a day to three tablets six times a day, and is reduced as the patient improves.

5. Steroids have been credited with a favorable effect in all phases of the disease except in the late fibrotic stage. They reduce the inflammatory response and the hypersensitivity reaction which may be involved in ulcerative colitis.[13] Steroids are contraindicated in patients with perforation of the colon and in those with toxic megacolon.

When remission has been obtained, the diet should be high in protein and calories, but low in residue, spices, and irritating ingredients.

Tranquilizers and psychotherapy play an important role in patient care.

SURGICAL.   Eventually, 20 percent of patients require operation for ulcerative colitis.[5] The emergency indications are toxic fulminating megacolon, perforation, and bleeding.

Total abdominal colectomy is required for patients with massive bleeding or toxic megacolon. The rectum should be examined through a proctoscope to ascertain that it is not bleeding. An abdominoperineal resection of the rectum may be required if bleeding continues. The rectum is removed later when the patient is in optimal condition.

Turnbull recommends exploration, ileostomy, and multiple colostomies for toxic megacolon rather than colectomy. This avoids breakdown of sealed-off areas of perforation and has resulted in a low mortality.[18] Colectomy is performed later when the infection subsides.

Elective colectomy is indicated in patients with chronic disease not controlled by conservative management and in patients who exhibit the sequelae of chronic disease, such as pseudopolyps, fibrosis, strictures, cancer, chronic inanition, blood loss, and systemic complications, such as arthritis, skin lesions, and hepatitis. Total proctocolectomy and removal of the rectum are usually performed at the same time. It is important to dissect as close to the rectum as possible to avoid damaging the nervi erigentes, which control sexual and urinary functions. Impotence is uncommon.

The rectum is free of disease in less than 20 percent of patients, yet only 5 percent requiring operation live symptom-free with an ileoproctostomy.[1] This procedure may be considered in young patients who do not have disease in the rectum and have not had a family.

RESULTS.   Younger patients have more severe disease and 30 percent require operation with a mortality rate of 20 percent, while patients over 60 require operation less frequently. The 20-year survival is about 60 percent in patients with ulcerative colitis not treated by resection and about 75 percent in those with Crohn's disease. The main complication causing death in ulcerative colitis is the development of a carcinoma.

CARE OF ILEOSTOMY.   Ileostomies are established after a total colectomy for such diseases as ulcerative colitis, familial polyposis, or rare collagen disease of the colon. Two types of ileostomy bags are available: the disposable plastic or cellophane bag with an adhesive back in which a stoma is created by cutting it to the desired size, and the permanent bag, also made of rubber or plastic pouch, and a faceplate to which a skin cement or a karaya gum ring can be applied to fit snugly around the stoma (Figure 22–5). The karaya gum ring can be applied over inflamed and ulcerated skin. Ileal contents

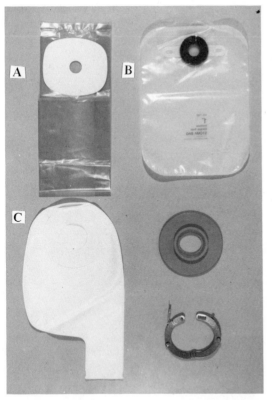

Figure 22–5. Ileostomy. *A.* Disposable plastic bag with gum. *B.* Permanent bag with karaya seal. *C.* Permanent bag with separate faceplate.

should not come in contact with the skin since this will cause erosion.

Immediately after operation a temporary appliance is placed snugly around the stoma. After the ileostomy is mature, a permanent plastic bag and faceplate may be reapplied with a special skin cement or with a karaya gum ring. The faceplate and the bag may remain on the skin for up to two or three days, at which time they should be changed, the skin washed clean, and the bag reapplied. Even the so-called permanent bag is discarded every few months because of discoloration and odor.

Complications of Ileostomy. Complications of ileostomies are recurrence of the primary disease such as Crohn's disease, stricture of the skin due to recurrent irritation and ulceration, ulceration of the skin, bowel obstruction. peristomal abscess, and prolapse.

The ileostomy contents are usually watery, have the consistency and coloring of apple jelly, and are not fecal smelling. When the contents become watery, more abundant, and foul smelling, an obstruction near the stoma should be suspected. Ulcerations of the skin can be prevented by a snugly fitting faceplate. If the more complicated faceplate, which requires skin gum, cannot be used, a karaya gum ring may be utilized. Finger dilatation of the stoma prevents skin stricture.

Granulomatous Colitis. Crohn's disease affects most often the right colon but may affect any segment, multiple segments, or the entire colon and may occur at the anastomotic site after a right hemicolectomy for Crohn's disease. Grossly and microscopically all coats of the bowel, the mesentery, and lymph nodes are involved. The mucosa has a cobblestone-like surface with intervening normal mucosa. There are ulceration and a deep fissure penetrating deeply into the muscle (Figure 22–6). There is an increase in cancer of the colon in patients with Crohn's disease of the colon, the incidence being about 3 percent after ten years. Conservative management is similar to that for Crohn's disease in the small intestine (see page 366). Operation is indicated in patients who do not respond to conservative management and in those who develop complications such as obstruction, perforation, abscess, fistula, or rarely severe bleeding. Treatment is most often resection of the involved bowel or occasionally establishment of a bypass. Total colectomy and ileostomy may be required in those with diffuse colonic disease. If the rectum is involved, an abdominoperineal resection is also performed.

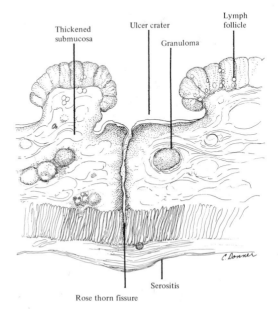

Figure 22–6. A superficial ulcer, thickened submucosa, and a deep-penetrating, rose thorn fissure are seen in a patient with Crohn's disease. All layers are involved, including the serosa.

Diverticular Disease

Diverticula are teardrop-shaped outpouchings of serosa and mucosa, most frequently found in the sigmoid and left colon, but which may occur throughout the entire large bowel. They are seen more often in males than in females, and their incidence increases with age, so that by the age of 70 they are found in 40 percent of the population.[20] Solitary diverticula of the right colon are congenital, occur in young individuals, possess all layers of colonic wall, and may develop the same complications as do the acquired or false diverticula.

The etiology of diverticula is not clear. They may be the result of an increase in intraluminal pressure and uncoordinated peristaltic activity. This theory is supported by the finding of hypertrophic, thickened colonic musculature in patients with diverticulitis and by relief of symptoms after stripping the taeniae coli.[15] Constipation produced by low bulk in the diet of the Western world may lead to diverticula. African vegetarian tribes do not develop diverticulosis. Perhaps another cause of diverticula is loss of elastic tissue, as seen with the increased incidence of hernias, diverticulosis, and varicose veins with aging. The association of diverticulosis, hiatus hernia, and cholelithiasis is called "Saint's" triad. The anatomy of the colon favors the formation of diverticula since there is no enveloping external longitudinal muscle layer. Diverticula occur next to the antimesenteric taeniae, adjacent to the penetrating blood vessels. The rectum, which has a complete external longitudinal muscle layer, does not develop diverticula.

Pathology.   The prediverticular stage can be seen on x-ray as a fine serrated border in the

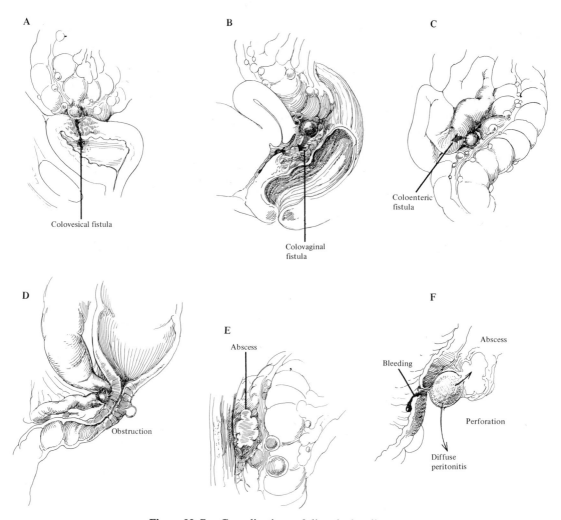

Figure 22–7.   Complications of diverticular disease.

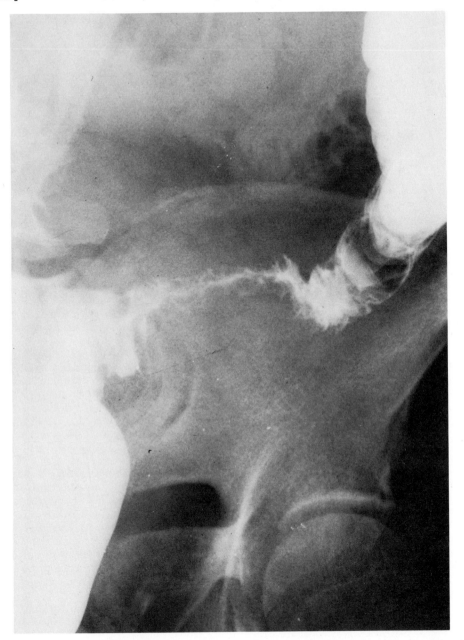

Figure 22–8. Barium enema showing diverticular disease of the sigmoid colon with marked constriction of the lumen. The stricture is long and has tapering edges, unlike an annular carcinoma.

sigmoid colon. The fully developed diverticulum is rounded and flask-shaped and may contain a fecolith. When the fecolith erodes the diverticular wall, serous fluid escapes and bacteria proliferate, causing a localized cellulitis and edema which occlude the stoma of adjacent diverticula. This process forms phlegmon or perforates the diverticula. Diverticular disease

may have the following complications (Figure 22–7):

1. Obstruction. Obstruction is caused by the progressive fibrosis and stricture of the bowel wall. It is also found in acute diverticulitis, when edema and spasm are severe, or when an abscess compresses the lumen from without (Figure 22–8).

2. Perforation. When a diverticulum perforates, local or generalized peritonitis occurs. Generalized peritonitis is infrequent and usually results from perforation of a single diverticulum without preceding symptoms. Localized perforation with abscess occurs when the infection is walled off by surrounding viscera and omentum. The abscess may slowly regress or may enlarge and rupture, causing peritonitis. It may perforate into adjacent organs, such as the bladder, small bowel, uterus, or abdominal wall, producing a fistula.

3. Fistula. A fistula may develop between the colon and the bladder, vagina, small intestine, or the skin. The cutaneous variety is seen most often after draining an abscess adjacent to the diseased bowel. In many patients an abscess communicating with a diverticulum perforates into the other organ and forms a fistula.

4. Bleeding. About 5 percent of patients with diverticulitis require operation for massive bleeding.[8] The bleeding is usually associated with a low-grade inflammation of the neck of the diverticulum, often without other symptoms. Massive bleeding often occurs from the right colon.

Clinical Picture. Diverticulosis is an anatomic description and not a symptom complex. Diverticulitis occurs in 20 percent of the people with diverticulosis. In phlegmonous nonperforated diverticulitis the patient may have constipation due to spasm and also intermittent diarrhea. There are fever, malaise, anorexia, and left lower quadrant pain, and red blood may be passed. If perforation occurs with a widespread peritonitis, the patient has severe abdominal pain, vomits, and becomes extremely ill. There are fever and leukocytosis, tenderness, rebound, free air under the diaphragm, distention, and vomiting. If a walled-off abscess develops, there are spiking fever, localized abdominal tenderness, constipation, and distention. The patient may present with a pelvirectal or isochiorectal abscess. A colovesical fistula most often presents as acute or chronic cystitis and occasionally with pneumaturia or fecaluria. A fistula to the small intestine causes severe diarrhea. Not infrequently a fistula is diagnosed at operation.

Conservative Treatment. The patient with diverticulosis should eat a high-residue diet consisting of whole-grain cereals, bran muffins, whole-wheat bread, raw and cooked vegetables and fruits, and keep the stools hydrated by drinking extra water and taking a stool softener. He should avoid too many starchy and concentrated foods such as potatoes, rice, macaroni, spaghetti, rich pastries, candies, rich desserts, and bananas. When diverticulitis occurs, the patient should be placed on bed rest, given broad-spectrum antibiotics intravenously, and kept fasting, except for oral stool softeners and nonabsorbable stool sterilizers such as Sulfasuxidine. Intravenous fluids are infused to maintain hydration, and nasogastric suction may be necessary if there is ileus or a small bowel obstruction.

Surgical Treatment. *Elective.* Most patients with diverticulitis respond to conservative treatment. About 20 percent require operation because of repeated attacks or development of complications. Since the mortality of patients requiring operation for complications is about 10 percent and hospitalization is long, it is preferable to operate on high-risk patients electively before they develop complications. Mortality is then less than 1 percent, and the hospital stay is about two weeks.[8] Indications for elective resection are:

1. One attack of diverticulitis in a patient with many diverticula who is under 55 years of age.

2. Two or more attacks of diverticulitis.

3. A fixed narrowing of the colon due to chronic diverticulitis on barium enema.

4. Presence of a fistula.

5. A mass associated with diverticulitis.

Before a resection and primary anastomosis can be safely accomplished, there must be absence of infection or tension, the vascular supply must be excellent, and the colon empty of feces. If the diverticula are limited to the sigmoid area, resection and anastomosis give good results. Patients with more diffuse diverticulosis may need a left colectomy.

Immediate Operation. The indications for immediate operation in diverticular disease of the colon are massive hemorrhage, general peritonitis, abscess, and acute intestinal obstruction. Massive hemorrhage from the colon is most often due to diverticular disease. Localizing the source of bleeding may be difficult, especially in those with diffuse diverticular disease involving the right and left colon. Barium enema, sigmoidoscopy, and angiography help, but a number of patients come to operation without the source being known. These patients should be treated by total colectomy with establishment of an ileostomy and the distal colon brought to the surface as a mucous fistula. Subsequently an ileorectal anastomosis is performed. When bleeding is from the sigmoid colon, the bowel is removed and a colostomy and mucous fistula established. It would be hazardous to resect the colon containing the diverticula and establish continuity with an end-to-end anastomosis in the patient who does not have an adequately prepared bowel. In the patient with general peritonitis treatment has usually consisted of evacuation of pus from the peritoneal cavity, drainage, insertion of kanamycin, and establishment of a transverse colostomy. The involved colon is then resected after about three to six months and continuity reestablished using an end-to-end anastomosis. The colostomy is then resected and continuity reestablished after about three weeks.

Many patients continue to have infection adjacent to the involved bowel, possibly because of feces contained in the bowel distal to the colostomy. Therefore a trial dissection may be attempted at the site of leakage, and if the bowel can readily be mobilized resection is performed, an end-type left iliac colostomy established, and the rectal stump brought out as a mucous fistula in the midline. Occasionally it is possible to mobilize the bowel sufficiently to perform an exteriorization resection (Mickulicz procedure), but more often mobilization is not adequate, in which case the rectal stump can be closed (Hartmann's procedure) and the proximal bowel brought to the surface as an end-type iliac colostomy. Continuity can later be reestablished by anastomosing the two ends of bowel. This two-stage procedure is now increasingly being used for diverticulitis with peritonitis or with an abscess. When a fistula is present and in acute intestinal obstruction, the three-stage resection is generally performed.

CANCER OF THE COLON

The colon and rectum are the most frequent sites of cancer, with the exception of the skin. Females predominate slightly in the incidence of colonic cancer, whereas males have more rectal cancer. About 70 percent of cancer of the large bowel occurs in the rectosigmoid. The rest is distributed equally throughout the remaining colon, with a higher incidence in the cecum. The most frequent age is 50 to 80 years but it occurs at all ages.

Etiology

The cause of colonic cancer is not known. There is a slight increase in relatives of patients with colonic cancer, excluding those with multiple polyposis, but a definite genetic relation has not been established. There is no relation with the blood groups, diverticulitis, or infectious disease of the colon. There is a high incidence in patients with ulcerative colitis. A low-residue diet, such as that in the United States, promotes constipation and allows possible dietary carcinogens to remain in contact with the colonic mucosa for long periods of time.[6]

The possibility that colonic cancer arises in previously benign adenomatous polyps has been extensively explored, but no definite conclusions have been reached. Morson believes that at least one half of colonic carcinomas have arisen

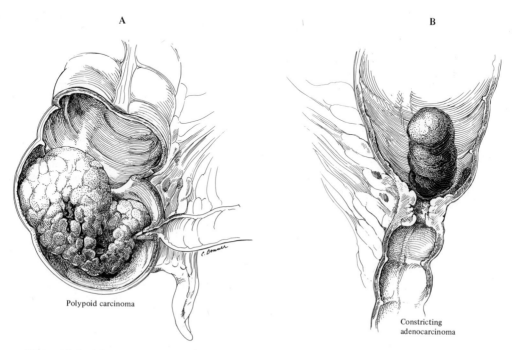

A

B

Polypoid carcinoma

Constricting
adenocarcinoma

Figure 22–9. Gross appearance of colorectal carcinomas. *A.* Large polypoid tumor. *B.* Annular scirrhous causing intestinal obstruction. Less frequently an ulcer is found.

in a previously benign polyp. This raises the question whether the other half of the carcinomas arise de novo from the colonic mucosa.[12] Almost all patients with polyposis coli develop cancer of the colon by age 40.

Pathology

Although other malignant tumors, such as leiomyosarcomas, fibrosarcomas, lymphomas, and carcinoid tumors, can be found in the colon, approximately 98 percent of cancers of the colon are columnar cell adenocarcinomas. The histologic grading of the carcinoma is pertinent in that the higher the grading, the more frequent the lymph node metastasis. Another method of defining the extent of tumor growth is through a modification of Dukes' classification. In stage A the muscle is not involved, in stage B the muscle is infiltrated, in stage C the regional nodes are involved, and in stage D there are distant metastases.

There are three gross types of colonic carcinoma (Figure 22–9):

1. The polypoid or proliferative type is found usually in the right colon or the rectum, is bulky and cauliflower-like. It rarely causes obstruction because the rectum and right colon have wide lumens; however, they often ulcerate and bleed. A variant is the mucoid or colloid adenocarcinoma. This is a soft gelatinous tumor, composed mostly of mucus-secreting cells, which grows slowly.

2. The annular is a hard, small, encircling tumor with little proliferation and much fibrosis that tends to obstruct the lumen. On barium enema it resembles a napkin ring or apple core.

3. The ulcerating carcinoma has a raised edge, a necrotic center and often bleeds.

Colonic cancer spreads along the length of the bowel wall through the layers of the bowel wall, through venous channels to the liver, lungs, etc., transperitoneally to contiguous organs, and intraluminally (see Chapter 7, pages 143–47).

Clinical Presentation

The symptoms and signs of colonic cancer depend on the location of the tumor and its gross type.

Cancer in the right colon is often asymptomatic or may produce anemia, weight loss, or discomfort in the right abdomen. It may present with a palpable mass with few or no gastrointestinal symptoms. The anemia is probably the result of blood loss and suppression of the bone marrow. The bleeding is not massive and often presents as melena.

Carcinomas in the left colon most often present with intermittent constipation alternating with diarrhea. With obstruction there are abdominal distention, colicky lower abdominal pain, and audible borborygmi. The change in bowel habit results from sloughing of the tumor or the accumulation of bowel material overcoming the obstruction and allowing feces to pass.

Large bulky tumors ulcerate, become infected, and are palpable. Smaller encircling tumors produce change in bowel habits and obstruct. Colonic obstruction is particularly dangerous in patients who have a competent ileocecal valve, since the ileal contents continue to enter the colon. This results in a great dilatation of the colon and particularly the cecum. This distention causes vascular embarrassment to the cecal wall, stercoral ulceration, and perforation. Occasionally cancers of the colon perforate and form sinuses or fistulae.

Diagnosis

On barium enema the proliferative tumors are seen as persistent spherical filling defects. The annular carcinomas often cause obstruction and are visualized as short, napkin ring-like defects with sharp shoulders (Figure 22–10). Carcinomas in the right colon are liable to be missed because of the large diameter of the gut. Occult blood determination of the stool is valuable in diagnosing ulcerating and bleeding lesions. The differential diagnosis includes diverticulitis, granulomas, benign tumors, extraluminal tumors, and inflammatory diseases of the colon.

Treatment

Attempted curative treatment is operative removal of the tumor and its lymphatics. The no-touch technique of dissection is the ideal method.[19] To minimize anastomotic recurrence the bowel is tied with tapes proximal and distal to the tumor. The vascular pedicle and mesentery of the colon are transected, and then the colon containing the tumor is mobilized and resected. In case of perforation the tumor may be resected with exteriorization of both ends of the colon. In obstruction a proximal colostomy is the safest procedure, with plans for a later resection. When adjacent tissues are involved in the cancer, these may also be excised en bloc, with the expectation of curing some patients.

Colonic cancers should be removed even in the presence of metastases because they grow, become infected, ulcerate and bleed, or perforate. A proximal colostomy with no plans for later resection or local radiotherapy is rarely indicated except in the extremely debilitated, obstructed patient.

Colonic Preparation for Operation. The most important factors in preventing suture line breakdown and infection are a clean empty

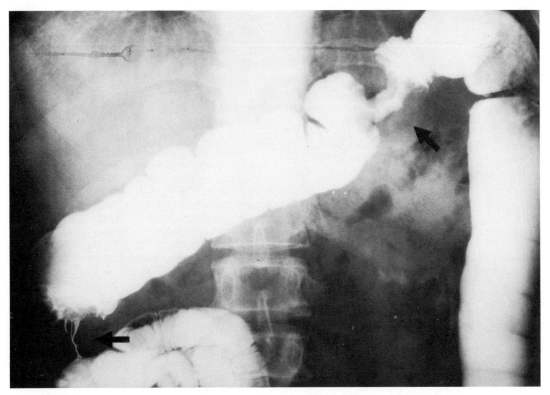

Figure 22–10.   Barium enema showing synchronous "napkin ring" carcinoma of the ascending and transverse colon causing intestinal obstruction. The strictures are short and have well-marked "shoulders." The incidence of synchronous lesions is about 5 to 8 percent.

bowel and proper operative technique. An empty bowel is obtained by placing the patient on a low-residue diet three days prior to operation, full liquids on the second day, and clear liquids on the final day. Cathartics, 45 ml of phosphosoda or 60 ml of castor oil, are given on each of the two days prior to the operation. Saline enemas are given each of the three evenings. In the geriatric or partially obstructed patient a slower preparation is undertaken to prevent fatigue, abdominal pain, and dehydration.

The use of antibiotics to reduce the bacterial flora in the colon is controversial, since they may increase enterocolitis and suture line recurrence.[10] A 36-hour preparation with neomycin and Sulfathaladine or neomycin and erythromycin is effective.

Chemotherapy.   In patients with metastases or recurrent tumors oral or intravenous 5-fluorouracil can produce useful palliation.[2] The oral use of 5-FU, 500 mg twice weekly or 10 to 15 mg per kilogram intravenously, produced objective tumor regression in 25 percent of patients with carcinoma of the gut. 5-FU has also been placed within the lumen of the gut and in the peritoneal cavity, but its value has not been established in controlled clinical trials.

Local Radiotherapy.   Local radiotherapy is seldom useful in carcinoma of the colon because of the difficulty in localizing treatment and avoiding the highly radiosensitive small intestine.

Results of Treatment.   The five-year survival of patients with carcinoma of the colon treated surgically is about 56 percent.[9] Survival is 90, 80, and 30 percent in patients with grades A, B, and C, Dukes' classification. Turnbull, in a noncontrolled trial, stated that survival was doubled in those with stage C tumors when he used a "no-touch" technique. Stage D patients have only a 15 percent five-year survival.

ISCHEMIC DISEASE OF THE COLON

The blood supply to the colon is abundant, and under normal circumstances branches may be divided without hazard—for example, the inferior mesenteric artery may be ligated during resection of the abdominal aorta, and the right colic artery when the right colon is used for substitution of the esophagus. When collaterals are occluded by arteriosclerosis, or periarteritis nodosa, interruption of a major vessel by operative ligation, trauma, embolus, or thrombosis may result in ischemia or necrosis of the bowel. Patients with low cardiac output and hypotension are especially prone to develop arterial thrombosis. Ischemic disease may be the result of arterial thrombosis or embolism, venous thrombosis, small vessel disease, or a low-flow state, as in those with congestive heart failure. Ischemic colitis is frequent in patients with rheumatoid arthritis and other collagen diseases and is now recognized to be a complication of immunosuppressive therapy after kidney transplantation. An angiogram is therefore often normal. The left colon is the commonest site of ischemic disease.

The patient may develop gangrenous colitis, a stricture, or transient ischemic colitis. The mucosa is injured first, since it is supplied by the terminal arterioles. The severity of the damage depends on the duration of the ischemia and the number of vessels occluded. When the damage is mild, there is mucosal edema or necrosis; a severe injury results in complete bowel infarction. An intermediate injury with necrosis extending into the muscle results in fibrosis and stricture, but not complete infarction.

Clinical Picture

The patient, usually elderly, develops abdominal pain, which may be slight or severe and may be gradual or sudden in onset. An embolus produces acute pain, whereas a thrombosis, as in a patient with congestive heart failure, causes gradual onset of pain. The patient may vomit, have dark bloody diarrhea, hypotension, fever, ileus, and abdominal tenderness with guarding or rigidity. If the rectosigmoid is involved, proctoscopic examination reveals a dusky, edematous, bleeding mucosa.

Laparotomy is often performed with the provisional diagnosis of perforated viscus or peritonitis. The bowel is dark and edematous, and if a major vessel is occluded, the mesentery is dusky and pulseless. When there is only distal occlusion or there has been a low-flow state, normal arterial pulsations are present.

Treatment is administration of broad-spectrum antibiotics, such as kanamycin and gentamicin, and specific antibiotics such as Lincocin for the anaerobes. Adequate intravenous fluids are essential to maintain the peripheral microcirculation and prevent spread of the thrombosis. Low-molecular-weight dextran may be given to prevent sludging of the platelets. Sympatholytic agents may be given to relieve spasm and steroids to combat septic shock. Resection of the colon with proximal colostomy and distal mucous fistula is the safest procedure. Frequently the small bowel is also involved. The underlying cause of the occlusion is treated to prevent progression of the ischemia. Congestive heart failure and arrhythmias are reversed. An embolus present in a major vessel is removed if the bowel is viable.

Transient Ischemic Colitis

About one half of patients with ischemic disease have complete spontaneous recovery, and only about 5 percent of all patients have a recurrence. The symptoms are less severe than those of infarction. They are mild abdominal pain, bloody diarrhea, and few abnormal abdominal findings. A barium enema reveals "thumbprinting" of the edematous mucosa and is best seen in the splenic flexure and transverse colon (Figure 22–11). If ischemia does not progress, the edema settles in about one week.

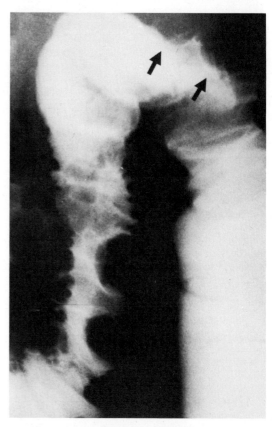

Figure 22–11. Barium enema showing acute ischemic colitis maximal in the region of the splenic flexure. There is well-marked "thumbprinting" from edema of the mucosa (arrows). Haustral markings of the transverse colon mimic "thumbprinting" in this x-ray.

Ischemic Strictures

A delayed stricture may occur when ischemia has not caused infarction but has resulted in fibrosis of the submucosa and muscularis. There is an acute onset; the patient then improves after a few days and develops obstructive symptoms months later. Persistence of bleeding for more than one month suggests that a stricture may occur. The development of "funneling" in a stricture near the splenic flexure is characteristic. The differential diagnosis is Crohn's disease, ulcerative colitis, and carcinoma. Treatment is resection of the stricture and reanastomosis.

VOLVULUS OF THE COLON

Volvulus of the colon is second to carcinoma as a cause of colonic obstruction. In the Western world where diets are low in residue it is infrequent, whereas in regions where diets are high in residue and the colon is heavy with feces, it is more frequent. The predisposing cause in about 20 percent is a long mesentery to the sigmoid colon or cecum associated with a narrow base. In patients with volvulus of the cecum the rotation is clockwise toward the left upper quadrant and involves the ileum and ascending colon. In those with volvulus of the sigmoid the upper limb rotates over the inferior limb one, two, or three times. A ball valve effect results in intestinal contents entering the partially closed loop faster than they are evacuated. This causes further distention, obstruction of the bowel, venostasis, and finally the arterial flow is impeded, resulting in gangrene and peritonitis.

Volvulus may be acute or subacute. Previous attacks are frequent. The acute form occurs in younger individuals, is characterized by intense pain, tenesmus, bloody diarrhea, vomiting, tenderness, vascular collapse, and rapid progression to gangrene often without much abdominal distention. The subacute form occurs in older individuals, is more insidious in onset, and is characterized by constipation and great abdominal distention, but little tenderness, pain, or vomiting.

Diagnosis

Abdominal x-rays show a greatly distended loop of colon in the right or left upper quadrant, depending on whether the sigmoid or cecum is involved. With a sigmoid volvulus there may be two fluid levels, one in each limb of the gut, whereas there is only one fluid level with a cecal volvulus. A barium enema shows the obstruction at the base of the sigmoid. In cecal volvulus there may be distended small bowel loops to the right of the distended cecum, and the right lower quadrant may be empty to palpation. The ileocecal valve may occasionally be seen in the distended cecum.

Treatment

A rectal tube is passed through a proctoscope, preferably with the patient in the knee-elbow position in volvulus of the sigmoid colon. This often produces relief as a great gush of fluid and air escapes. The tube should be left in place for 48 hours because recurrence is frequent. If the volvulus persists or there is strangulation, operation is indicated. The distended loop is aspirated with a trocar to prevent tearing before it is untwisted. A gangrenous colon is exteriorized or resected and no attempt made at anastomosis. The mortality is high when gangrene is present but is low with a simple volvulus.

ACQUIRED MEGACOLON

Acquired megacolon may be organic or functional. The organic megacolon results from chronic stenosis of the left colon, rectum, or anus due to a previous injury, ischemia, cancer, chronic infection, or radiotherapy. Rarer causes are avitaminosis B and Chagas' disease, which result in degeneration of the muscularis. Functional megacolon may begin in infancy, as the infant withholds its bowel movements for secondary gains. It also occurs in elderly patients, usually in nursing homes and mental institutions. These individuals eat very little, exercise little, and often do not respond to the defecatory urge.

Clinical Presentation

Patients with organic megacolon may have rectal tenderness due to an anal fissure, fistula, or hemorrhoids. There are also abdominal distention, perhaps a palpable colon, and often no other symptoms. In extreme cases dyspnea and loss of appetite are present. In the patient with functional megacolon there is stool in the ampulla of the rectum, and on barium enema the entire colon is dilated to the anus.

Treatment

The treatment of functional megacolon in young individuals is directed toward correcting their psychological problem. In older patients confined to the nursing home treatment consists of uplifting their mood, more activity, a diet high in bulk, such as fluids, fruits, and vegetables, and administering bowel stimulants and stool softeners. In megacolon due to localized organic stricture a local resection is the treatment of choice, usually preceded by a decompressing colostomy.

RADIATION INJURY

Local radiotherapy may cause an early acute inflammatory reaction in the colon with severe diarrhea. Later the blood supply may be decreased as a result of perivascular fibrosis and endarteritis. The patient may develop an ulcer with characteristic telangiectasia in the surrounding mucosa. Since the most common reason for irradiating the abdominal contents is carcinoma of the uterus, cervix, or bladder, the rectosigmoid colon is the most frequent site of large bowel involvement. The patient develops proctitis with pain, diarrhea, and bleeding, and later stenosis or fistula. A previous operation causes adhesions that fix the bowel in one region and predispose to irradiation injury.

Obstruction is treated by resecting the involved segment of gut and anastomosis. When a complete obstruction or perforation exists, a preliminary defunctioning colostomy is necessary.

HEMATOCHEZIA

Massive bleeding per rectum is a difficult diagnostic therapeutic problem. The blood may originate anywhere from the esophagus to the rectum.

The most frequent causes of hematochezia in the colon are diverticulosis, ulcerative colitis, infectious diseases of the colon, and less frequently cancer, polyposis, and Crohn's disease.

Diagnosis

Proctoscopy should be performed while the patient is bleeding. Abundant irrigation with saline permits observation of the rectal mucosa. Colonoscopy is usually unsatisfactory when the patient is bleeding. A barium enema may show diverticulosis, ulcerative colitis, polyps, or a tumor. Occasionally bleeding from diverticula ceases after a barium enema, presumably due to inspissation of barium against the bleeding source. Arteriography, with selective mesenteric arterial injections, should be performed after the barium has been evacuated with enemas. A bleeding point may be found with a flow rate of as little as 0.5 ml per minute.

Treatment

Operation is indicated if the patient continues to bleed after administration of four units of blood. In the absence of a diagnosis the gut is carefully examined for a cause of the bleeding. If a reason is not found, total colectomy with anastomosis of the ileum to the rectum is the safest procedure. The advantages are that a source of bleeding is not missed and there is no contamination as occurs after making multiple colotomies for examining the lumen with a proctoscope.

A left colectomy has been performed presuming that the source of bleeding is diverticula in the left colon. Unfortunately the source of bleeding is the right colon in about one half of the patients. A transverse colostomy is not indicated because it fails to treat the source of bleeding. Atraumatic clamps have been applied to segments of the colon to find the portion of the gut that fills with blood. The source of bleeding is rarely found.

COLOSTOMY

A temporary colostomy is created to defunction the distal colon in patients with perforation, obstruction, or a low anastomosis. The colostomy is usually established in the transverse colon since this segment is easily exteriorized. It may occasionally be established using the descending colon or cecum (cecostomy). A permanent colostomy is established after abdominoperineal excision of the rectum.

The simplest colostomy is the loop colostomy. The colon is brought out over a rod to keep the gut above the skin level. The colon is opened usually after several days. It is not necessary to suture the gut to the skin because the two tissues adhere within one to two days, and in three to six weeks the mucosa and skin firmly unite as the colostomy matures. The gut should be completely transected if complete diversion of feces is desired. The proximal end is established as an end colostomy and the distal as a mucous fistula.

The early complications of a colostomy are retraction of the gut below the skin and necrosis of the colon. Later complications are small bowel obstruction due to herniation through an abdominal aperture, prolapse of the colostomy, stricture of the skin around the colostomy, or a pericolostomy abscess.

Care of Colostomy

In the patient with a right colostomy the stool is semisolid and escapes continuously. A one-piece plastic disposable bag, with a ring that fits snugly around the stoma, is required at all times. A colostomy in the descending colon usually produces solid stool, and the time of evacuation is known by the patient. These patients often use no bag at all and often have one bowel movement every one or two days. Irrigation with 500 ml of water in the morning causes a massive peristalsis and evacuates the colon. Irrigations may be discontinued after the rhythm of the colon has been established. To prevent skin retraction and narrowing of the colostomy, finger dilatation may be performed daily for the first few months.

APPENDIX

The appendix, often referred to as a vestigial organ, is by no means innocuous, for it is one of the commonest causes of the "acute abdomen." Morbidity and mortality have decreased due to careful adherence to surgical principles and the availability of antibiotics. However, long-term morbidity still occurs from sepsis and adhesions.

The specific function of the appendix is not known. There is a large amount of lymphoid tissue in the appendix up to the age of about 30, and then it decreases with age until none is present in the geriatric patient.

ANATOMY

The vermiform appendix averages 8 cm in length. Its base is at the posteromedial aspect of the cecum where the taeniae coli merge to form the outer longitudinal muscle layer of the appendix. The tip of the organ is freely mobile and may occupy a number of positions. The commonest positions are retrocecal and pelvic; less frequent are retroileal, anterioleal, retroperitoneal, right subcostal, and left lower abdomen.

Microscopically the layers of the appendix are similar to those in the cecum: serosal covering, two muscular layers—longitudinal and circular, a tunica propria containing numerous lymphoid follicles, and a mucosa containing the mucus-secreting glands of Aschoff. The blood supply is derived from the appendicular artery, which is the end branch of the ileocolic and the superior mesenteric arteries. The arteries are accompanied by the venous and lymph channels and lie in the free margin of the mesoappendix.

ACUTE APPENDICITIS

Acute appendicitis is rare in African Negroes who take a high-roughage diet and have frequent bowel movements. Its incidence in Negroes in the States is the same as in Caucasians. The cause is therefore most often dietetic and rarely genetic. A low-residue diet predisposes to stagnation of bowel content in the lumen of the appendix, absorption of water, and formation of inspissated fecal material. Calcium-rich mucus is deposited with the formation of a hard mass, a fecolith, that readily obstructs the lumen and results in acute appendicitis. Acute appendicitis is uncommon below the age of 3 years, increases until puberty, and then decreases with age. The sex incidence is about equal

In about 70 percent of patients the cause is obstruction of the appendiceal lumen. In the lumen the usual cause is a fecolith and less commonly a foreign body or worms. Hyperplasia of submucosal lymphoid follicles, fibrosis from previous attacks of appendicitis, and benign or malignant tumors are causes within the wall. Extraluminal causes are congenital bands or acquired adhesions. The obstruction from hypertrophy of the lymphoid follicles may occur in patients with generalized systemic infections such as acute respiratory infection, measles, and mononucleosis. Acute appendicitis may occur without obstruction. It is sometimes called "catarrhal" appendicitis and most likely results from viral infection.

Experimentally produced obstruction of the lumen of the appendix results in inflammatory changes similar to those seen in acute appendicitis.[11] The increasing pressure within the lumen from mucus secretion and inflammation impairs the venous and arterial blood supply and is followed by ulceration, invasion of the wall by bacteria from the lumen, vascular thrombosis, gangrene, and perforation. The escape of fecal and purulent fluid into the peritoneal cavity results in peritonitis. The infections, most of which are mixed, are aerobic and anaerobic organisms in symbiosis. The most frequently found aerobic bacteria are *Escherichia coli* and *Streptococcus faecalis*.[1]

An acute attack of appendicitis may not progress to perforation but resolve and predispose to further attacks. Occasionally the infecting organism is of low virulence, and if the obstruction persists, an empyema may be formed. Rarely obstruction occurs without infection with formation of a mucocele.

Clinical Picture

The earliest symptom of appendicitis is abdominal pain usually felt in the periumbilical region and less commonly in the right lower quadrant or epigastrium. The pain is ill defined and steady, with superimposed intermittent colicky spasms. Localization generally occurs within 12 hours in the right lower abdomen. The exact location of the pain depends upon the position of the appendix. It is low in the right side when the appendix is in the pelvis, in the flank when the appendix is retrocecal, and even in the right subcostal region when the cecum is high. The initial pain is visceral, the result of powerful muscle contraction to overcome the obstruction in the lumen, and is referred to the midgut pain distribution in the umbilical region. The pain felt at the site of the appendix is somatic and is the result of irritation of the parietal peritoneum. Nausea and vomiting occur in about 75 percent of patients and commence usually after onset of the pain. Anorexia is even more frequent and generally precedes the pain. Diarrhea may occur when the appendix is pelvic or retroileal in position. Frequency of micturition when the appendix is in the pelvic or retrocecal position may also occur. On rupture the pain becomes more severe and diffuse. The patient often gives a history of similar mild attacks that settled spontaneously.

Physical Findings

Common signs are furring of the tongue and halitosis. The temperature may be elevated by about 1° C but is frequently normal. The pulse rate may be increased or normal. Reproducible tenderness in the right lower abdomen is the most reliable sign in the diagnosis of acute appendicitis. The point of maximal tenderness is most often at the junction of the outer and middle thirds of a line drawn from the umbilicus to the anterosuperior iliac spine (McBurney's point). Tenderness may be elicited in the right lower abdomen when the pain is entirely visceral and felt in the periumbilical region. Muscle guarding occurs when there is tenderness in the right lower abdomen and is the result of involuntary contraction of the muscles on deep palpation. Rigidity occurs when the inflammatory process has extended to the parietal peritoneum.

Rebound tenderness signifies irritation of the parietal peritoneum. Care must be taken in interpreting this sign, especially in children, because of the high incidence of false positives. A mass may be palpated in the right iliac fossa. The bowel sounds are not useful in the diagnosis of acute appendicitis, because they may be absent with a normal appendix and occasionally hyperactive in the patient with peritonitis. Rectal examination is essential as there are tenderness and often a tender mass when the appendix is acutely inflamed and lying in the pelvis.

On rupture abdominal pain increases and is more constant, the pulse and temperature increase, and there is increasing abdominal rigidity.

Laboratory Findings

The total leukocyte count is usually elevated, but the degree of leukocytosis does not correlate well with the extent of the inflammatory process. The differential count shows a relative increase in polymorphonuclear leukocytes, and the number of young forms is usually increased.

Protein, pus cells, and a few erythrocytes may be found in the urine when the appendix is in contact with the right ureter. Bacteria are not found.

X-rays are of little value. The small bowel may be dilated and contain fluid levels adjacent to an acutely inflamed appendix. A fecolith may be seen on x-ray of the abdomen and on rare occasions a gas-filled cylinder distal to the fecolith.

Differential Diagnosis

The diagnosis of acute appendicitis with or without peritonitis is often difficult to make because of the large number of conditions that mimic the disease. It is often necessary to make the decision to operate with only the diagnosis of an acute surgical abdomen. It is good surgical practice to operate and find that the diagnosis is correct in 80 to 90 percent of patients. An accuracy below 80 percent suggests that too many laparotomies are being performed, while that above 90 percent suggests that conservative management is practiced in too many patients.

Gastroenteritis. In the patient with gastroenteritis vomiting and diarrhea are generally more marked than in acute appendicitis, the pain is more diffuse, and the findings on abdominal examination are minimal. With appendicitis these symptoms are most likely to occur when the appendix is retroileal.

Acute Mesenteric Adenitis. It is difficult to determine the incidence of acute mesenteric adenitis.[8] The lymph nodes in the mesentery vary in size with age and are large, especially at puberty. They may at operation be mistakenly considered to be inflamed. The condition does not occur after 30 years and affects both sexes equally. The infecting organism or virus enters the mesenteric nodes from the gut or less often the blood. Often there is a history of a recent respiratory infection. The acute inflammatory reaction causes constant severe abdominal pain, often with nausea and vomiting, and generally a higher fever and leukocytosis than in the patient with acute appendicitis. The most striking feature is the paucity of abdominal signs in a patient with severe symptoms and a high temperature. Frequently the only finding is tenderness without guarding or rigidity below and to the right of the umbilicus. Shifting tenderness may be elicited when the patient is examined on his side. The patient should be treated conservatively if the diagnosis is definite. Acute mesenteric adenitis can mimic acute appendicitis so closely that laparotomy is often necessary. A regional node should not be removed because the diagnosis is based on gross findings and is not necessarily confirmed on microscopic examination of the node. Also complications may occur from removal of the node. The appendix should be removed because it might be the portal of infection for the adenitis, it might be abnormal although not grossly inflamed, and removal will prevent a subsequent attack of appendicitis.

Primary Peritonitis. Peritonitis may develop suddenly, especially in malnourished girls around six years. The child develops acute lower abdominal pain, becomes toxic, vomits, and often has frequency of micturition. On examination there are diffuse lower abdominal tenderness and rigidity and tenderness on rectal examination. The infecting organism is most often the pneumococcus and is thought to ascend from the vagina and reach the peritoneal cavity along the fallopian tubes. Primary peritonitis may occur in boys and is probably hematogenous. The condition simulates acute appendicitis so closely that operation is necessary to establish the diagnosis. The appendix should be removed and pus evacuated from the peritoneal cavity; drainage is not necessary. The child should be treated with antibiotics. Complications are uncommon.

Crohn's Disease. The patient with Crohn's disease may develop acute abdominal pain and vomiting with tenderness in the right lower abdomen. At operation the sharply demarcated inflammatory process involving all the wall of the gut, the presence of "skip" lesions, the large edematous regional lymph nodes, and the palisading of the mesenteric fat about the ileum confirm the diagnosis. The involved gut should not be resected. An enlarged node and the appendix should be removed for microscopic examination. The appendix should not be removed if the cecum is inflamed at the base of the appendix because of the danger of producing a fecal fistula (see Chapter 21, page 366).

Meckel's Diverticulum. A peptic ulcer associated with a Meckel's diverticulum may result in right lower abdominal pain and vomiting. There may be a history of passing blood.

Acute intestinal obstruction may occur from intussusception of the diverticulum, or bowel may be obstructed by a band passing from the diverticulum to the umbilicus (Figure 21–3, page 359).

Acute Diverticulitis. A true diverticulum of the colon, generally in the right colon, may become acutely inflamed and present as acute appendicitis. Acquired diverticulosis may occur in any part of the colon but is more often on the left side. Acute diverticulitis may present as acute appendicitis, especially when the diverticulum is in the right colon, but also when the sigmoid colon is involved.

Tumors of the Gut. Tumors in the small intestine often intussuscept and result in abdominal pain, vomiting, and abdominal tenderness. A carcinoma of the cecum may perforate and produce local or general perito-

nitis. A carcinoma of the sigmoid colon causing intestinal obstruction results in distention of the cecum and may produce stercoral ulceration with or without perforation. The local tenderness in the right abdomen may lead to the diagnosis of acute appendicitis.

Acute Cholecystitis. The patient with acute cholecystitis may have nausea and vomiting, right subcostal pain, and no radiation of pain to the back. The condition closely simulates acute appendicitis in the patient with a high cecum or an appendix lying in the subcostal region.

Perforation of Peptic Ulcer. After perforation of a gastric or duodenal ulcer, gastric and duodenal content tends to collect in the right posterior intraperitoneal subphrenic space and to pass down the right paracolic gutter to the right iliac fossa. The rigidity in the right iliac fossa may lead to the wrong diagnosis of acute appendicitis, especially in elderly patients.

Gynecologic Conditions. Gynecologic diseases, such as acute salpingitis, hemorrhage into or torsion of an ovarian cyst, or ectopic pregnancy, are the most frequent reasons for a wrong diagnosis of acute appendicitis.

Mittelschmerz. Ovulation may result in considerable bleeding into the peritoneal cavity. The patient develops sudden severe constant pain in the lower abdomen at about 14 days after the last period. There is no toxicity, the tongue is clean, there is usually no fever or leukocytosis, but there is marked tenderness often with rigidity across the lower abdomen. The condition should be treated conservatively.

Acute Salpingitis. Acute salpingitis occurs most often following pregnancy or a menstrual period and is usually bilateral.[6] There are severe constant lower abdominal pain and often frequency of micturition. Examination discloses toxemia, fever, and tenderness, often with rigidity low on both sides of the abdomen and on both sides of the pelvis on vaginal examination. The patient is treated with antibiotics.

Ectopic Pregnancy. A ruptured pregnancy causes severe colicky lower abdominal pain with shock, tenderness, and rigidity in the lower abdomen. On vaginal examination the uterus is enlarged, a mass may be felt, and there is extreme tenderness on moving the cervix uteri. There is usually a history of a delayed period. The patient should be treated by operation.

Ovarian Cyst Torsion or Hemorrhage. Torsion or hemorrhage into an ovarian cyst may give rise to severe lower abdominal pain associated with tenderness and rigidity. The enlarged tender cyst may be felt on vaginal examination. Laparotomy is indicated.

Genitourinary Conditions. A ureteral calculus, pyelonephritis, a congenitally low kidney,

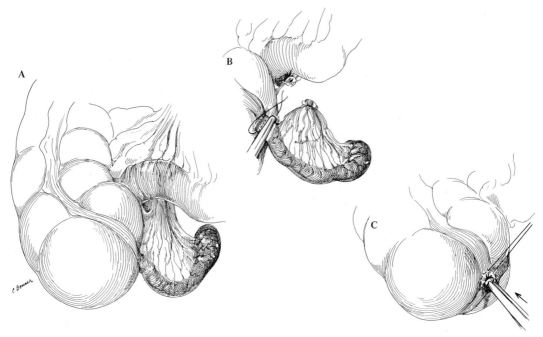

Figure 22–12.   Steps in appendectomy. *A.* The appendix is exposed through a right grid iron incision (McBurney). *B.* The mesentery of the appendix is divided and the base of the appendix ligated. *C.* The appendix is removed and the stump invaginated by a purse string suture in the cecum.

torsion of the testis, or epididymitis may simulate appendicitis.

Management

The acute inflamed appendix should be removed as soon as possible (Figure 22–12). With generalized peritonitis early operation is indicated as soon as the patient's general condition has been improved maximally. The operative mortality is now less than 5 percent as compared with 50 percent about 50 years ago. Intravenous fluids and antibiotics are given and continuous gastric suction established. At operation the appendix can almost invariably be removed. A careful search is made for a fecolith that may have escaped from the ruptured appendix. Pus is aspirated from the peritoneal cavity. Opinions differ on the value of irrigating the cavity with isotonic saline or antibiotics. Formerly the abdomen was drained and the appendix rarely removed. Now it is appreciated that removal of the infecting organ and pus is important for prompt recovery.

If the patient has an abscess in the right lower abdomen, the pus should be evacuated, drainage established, and no attempt made to remove the appendix. It is generally safer not to remove the appendix when draining the abscess because it is often incorporated in the wall of the abscess, and

its removal might result in bleeding or development of a fecal fistula. Interval appendectomy is performed after about three months.

Opinions differ on managing a patient with a mass in the right lower abdomen that is the result of edema in the tissues around the organ and in the omentum. If operation is performed, the appendix can usually be removed, often along with adherent omentum. Alternatively the patient may be treated conservatively and the appendix removed after about three months. Conservative management of generalized peritonitis with or without abscess formation is rarely indicated (Ochsner treatment).

Special Types of Acute Appendicitis

During Infancy. Acute appendicitis is uncommon during the first three years.[5] It is often misdiagnosed with the result that most children have peritonitis at operation. It is more serious than in older children, possibly because the greater omentum is not fully developed and localization of infection is impaired. An adequate history is not obtainable, the signs are mistaken, especially for those of gastroenteritis, and the pathologic process proceeds rapidly, leading to general peritonitis. The infant should be treated by operation.

During Pregnancy. The diagnosis of acute appendicitis is difficult to make during pregnancy because the position of the organ is altered by the large uterus.[9] The condition may simulate acute cholecystitis, acute pancreatitis, onset of labor, torsion of an ovarian cyst, or pyelonephritis. General peritonitis is often present when the diagnosis is made. The mother is prepared for operation as rapidly as possible. Progesterone may be given to inhibit uterine contraction and appendectomy performed with minimal handling of the uterus. Unfortunately labor often occurs after operation and infant mortality is high. Toxemia is profound in the mother with peritonitis because of the large blood supply in the uterus and surrounding tissues. Maternal mortality is greatest when acute appendicitis occurs in the third trimester (Figure 11–6, page 217).

Geriatric Patient. Acute appendicitis is uncommon in the aged because the organ atrophies and the lumen is often obliterated.[10] The initial pain in the periumbilical region followed by pain in the right lower abdomen is often missing, because the poor musculature in the obstructed appendix is unable to contract powerfully and produce pain. The patient therefore often feels anorexic for one or two days and may have vague abdominal discomfort. Sudden severe generalized abdominal pain occurs when the appendix perforates. The condition is readily mistaken for perforation of a peptic ulcer, perforation of carcinoma of the colon or stomach, or perforated diverticulitis. Laparatomy should be performed.

OTHER DISEASES OF THE APPENDIX

Carcinoma

Carcinoma of the appendix is rare and has been reported in less than 0.1 percent of appendectomies.[4] Right hemicolectomy should be performed.

Carcinoid

Carcinoid of the appendix is generally an incidental finding at the time of laparotomy for some unrelated condition, but occasionally it causes acute appendicitis.[2] The tumor is generally located at the distal end of the appendix and is small, well localized, submucosal, and yellow-brown in color (Figure 22–13). Microscopically the tumors are identical with those in the small intestine, but they rarely invade the muscle or metastasize. Removal of the appendix and mesentery is all that is required. A wedge of

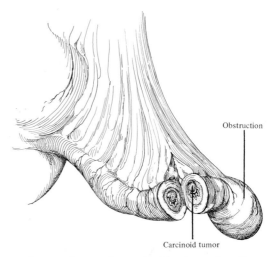

Figure 22–13. A carcinoid obstructing the appendix and causing acute appendicitis. Appendectomy is adequate treatment.

cecal wall may be removed if the tumor is at the base of the appendix.

Mucocele

Benign mucocele of the appendix is the result of obstruction of the lumen by a stricture and accumulation of mucus.[7] This condition has been reported in approximately 0.2 percent of appendectomies and is most prevalent in the fifth to sixth decade of life. Appendectomy is all that is required. Care should be taken not to rupture the mucocele and possibly lead to the development of pseudomyxoma peritonei. This is an unusual condition affecting the parietal and visceral peritoneum in which widespread accumulation of gelatinous material becomes distributed throughout the peritoneal cavity following rupture of a mucocele of the appendix. Less commonly it occurs as a complication of a pseudomucinous cystadenoma of the ovary, and the mucous cells may be implanted on the peritoneum and continue to secrete mucus. If pseudomyxoma peritonei is found at operation, the appendix is removed and pseudomyxomatous material evacuated from the peritoneal cavity.

Diverticulitis

Diverticulitis of the appendix presents in similar manner to acute appendicitis.[3] There is a marked tendency for perforation because the wall of the diverticulum does not contain a muscular coat. Treatment is removal of the appendix.

RECTUM

ANATOMY

The rectum, derived from the distal hindgut, is 10 to 12 cm in length, begins at the level of the third sacral vertebra, and lies in the hollow of the sacrum (see Plate VIII). The curvature of the rectum and the acute flexion at the rectosigmoid junction act as valves that help to support the weight of the stool. The caliber in the upper rectum is the same as that of the sigmoid colon; in the lower rectum it is dilated to form the ampulla. There are three valves of Houston, which are mucosa-covered fibrous indentations of the wall, two on the right and one on the left; these valves are thought to support the weight of the stool. The relationship of the peritoneum to the rectum is important. Posteriorly the entire rectum is uncovered, while anteriorly and laterally the cul de sac of Douglas extends for a variable distance. The peritoneal reflection terminates at about 7 cm from the anus in the male and 5 cm in the female. The wall of the rectum has the same layers as the remainder of the colon. The longitudinal muscle layer is continuous around the circumference of the rectum and does not form taeniae as in the colon.

The main arterial blood supply is the superior hemorrhoidal artery and the terminal branches of the inferior mesenteric artery. The superior hemorrhoidal veins drain into the inferior mesenteric vein. The paired middle hemorrhoidal branches of the hypogastric vessels and the inferior hemorrhoidal branches of the pudendal artery and vein supply the lower rectum. The middle hemorrhoidal artery and vein are surrounded by a condensation of fibrous tissue called the rectal stalks, structures which are significant anatomic landmarks in some rectal operations.

The rectum is supplied by sympathetic and parasympathetic nerves from the inferior mesenteric and hypogastric plexuses. The upper rectal lymphatics drain into the superior hemorrhoidal nodes and from these to the inferior mesenteric nodes. The ampulla drains laterally to nodes on the pelvic diaphragm.

PHYSIOLOGY

The rectum stores stool and absorbs water and electrolytes. Mucus is secreted to facilitate passage of stool. The main function of the rectum is participation in the complex act of defecation (see pages 373, 374).

INFLAMMATORY DISEASES

The rectum may become inflamed from within or without (see page 375). Extrinsic infections (pararectal abscesses) are discussed on page 402. Intrinsic inflammation of the rectum (proctitis) is caused by a number of agents.

Amebic Proctitis

Amebic proctitis may exist independently or may accompany a more widespread colonic or extracolonic infection. Rectal involvement results in diarrhea. The definitive diagnosis depends on laboratory documentation of *Entamoeba histolytica*, although proctoscopic visualization of the characteristic punched-out ulcers is highly suspicious. Laboratory demonstration of the organism may be difficult even when multiple warm stools are examined. Empiric treatment with diiodohydroxyquin (Diodoquin) will often stop diarrhea even if amebae are not demonstrated and is recommended if a specific cause for the diarrhea is not found.

Ulcerative Proctitis

Ulcerative colitis usually starts in the rectum and is diagnosed by proctoscopic examination (see page 378).

Other causes of proctitis are schistosomiasis, tuberculosis, ischemia, radiation, and venereal diseases including gonorrhea, syphilis, chancroid, and lymphogranuloma venereum. The last mentioned is one of the most common causes of benign rectal stricture, especially in women.

TRAUMA

The wide variety of foreign bodies which have found their way into the rectum staggers the imagination, and their removal may severely tax the surgeon's ingenuity.

Injuries to the rectum are considered with those to the colon (see pages 374, 375).

NEOPLASMS

Polyps

The term polyp refers to a lesion that originates in the wall of the bowel and protrudes into the lumen. Polyps with pedicles are pedunculated, while those that have no pedicle are sessile. The term polyp does not imply particular histology; in fact there is a wide variety of lesions that are polypoid.

A polyp may be diagnosed during a proctoscopic examination or on a barium enema. Those seen through the proctoscope can usually be removed or biopsied through the proctoscope. Those seen on barium enema present a special difficulty since the transabdominal removal of

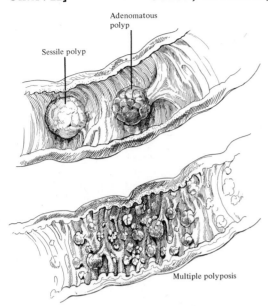

Adenomatous
polyp

Sessile polyp

Multiple polyposis

Figure 22–14. Pedunculated polyps possess a definite stalk, while sessile polyps are directly attached to the bowel wall. Patients with multiple polyposis have innumerable polyps scattered throughout the colon and rectum.

such polyps carries a significant (more than 1 percent) mortality and a significant risk of morbidity, such as wound infection. Several considerations aid the decision as to whether or not surgical removal of the polyp is indicated:

1. The risk that a polypoid lesion is malignant increases with the size of the lesion. Only about 1 percent of polyps 1 cm in diameter or less are malignant. The risk of removal at laparotomy nearly equals the likelihood of malignancy. Polypoid lesions 3 cm in diameter are almost invariably malignant.[1]

2. Polyps with a definite pedicle metastasize infrequently. Such a polyp in a poor-risk patient should be observed by repeated examinations.

3. The entire colon can be visualized using a flexible colonoscope. The histology of questionable colon lesions can therefore be determined preoperatively. In addition, it is sometimes possible to remove a polyp, especially if it is pedunculated, using the colonoscope.

Adenomatous Polyps. Adenomatous polyps arise from mucosal glands and consist of a connective tissue stroma covered with hyperplastic, uniform glandular epithelium (Figure 22–14). They are rarely found in patients under 20 unless the patient has familial polyposis. About one third of adults in North America have polyps; in 8 percent the polyps are greater than

0.5 cm in diameter, and in 4 percent they are greater than 1 cm.[2] It was once thought that adenomatous polyps were invariably premalignant; it now appears that they seldom undergo malignant change. Adenomatous polyps are evenly distributed throughout the colon, approximately 30 percent being within reach of the proctoscope.

Most adenomatous polyps are asymptomatic. The most common symptom is passage of bright red blood, generally on the surface of the stool. Some polyps intussuscept and cause cramplike pain. Large rectal polyps can cause tenesmus.

There are several syndromes in which patients have innumerable adenomatous polyps in the colon and rectum. Familial polyposis is transmitted as an autosomal dominant and must be treated by total colectomy if carcinoma of the colon is to be prevented, since unoperated patients invariably develop carcinoma by the age of 40. Other syndromes are the Gardner syndrome (colonic polyposis with osteomata, fibromata, and sebaceous cysts),[3] the Turcot syndrome (colonic polyposis and brain tumor),[4] the Oldfield syndrome (colonic polyposis and sebaceous cysts),[5] and the Cronkhite syndrome (gastrointestinal polyposis, alopecia, pigmentation, and atrophy of the fingernails and toenails).[6]

In patients with the Peutz-Jeghers syndrome (see Chapter 21, page 363) the polyps are not adenomatous polyps but rather hamartomas and are not premalignant.

Villous Adenomas. Villous adenomas are important because about one third contain invasive adenocarcinomas. They have a papillary mucosa that gives them a characteristic velvety appearance, are mostly sessile, and are often more than 5 cm in diameter. In contrast to adenomatous polyps, villous adenomas are not evenly distributed throughout the colon; about 90 percent are found in the rectum and distal sigmoid colon. They are generally asymptomatic until large, at which time they present with symptoms similar to a polypoid carcinoma. A rare but interesting presentation is diarrhea with loss of a large volume of potassium-rich mucus resulting in hypokalemia and weakness.[7] Lesions causing these symptoms are large and located in the rectum or low sigmoid colon.

Villous polyps are soft and readily missed on rectal examination. On barium enema they appear as proliferative masses generally in the rectum or sigmoid colon (Figure 22–15). The velvety appearance at proctoscopy is pathognomonic. Ulceration and induration suggest malignancy. Biopsy and microscopic confirmation of diagnosis are essential. Small lesions

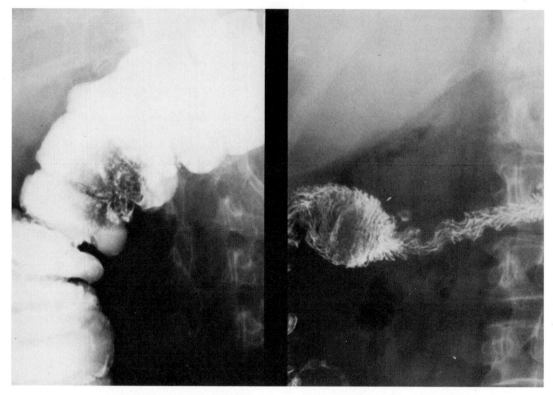

Figure 22–15. A villous adenoma is present in the hepatic portion of the transverse colon seen in barium enema and evacuation x-rays.

can be removed completely through the proctoscope, while larger lesions should be excised or biopsied at several sites. If invasive cancer is found, the lesion is treated as an adenocarcinoma. If the polyp is benign, the treatment of choice is complete excision. The resected lesion is then examined using multiple microscopic sections.

Juvenile Polyps. Juvenile polyps, more properly known as retention polyps, are smooth, pedunculated lesions that contain gross and microscopic cysts and have a normal colonic mucosa. They are often ulcerated and are therefore inflamed and contain granulation tissue. They are the most common type of colon polyp in patients below 21 years. The majority are asymptomatic. Symptoms are rectal bleeding and intussusception. They never become malignant but should be excised if they are producing symptoms.[8]

Carcinoid

About 1 percent of rectal tumors are carcinoids. They may be benign or malignant, the distinction not always being apparent microscopically. They are firm, smooth, yellowish tumors covered by intact mucosa. Ulceration suggests malignancy. They differ from carcinoids at other sites in that they do not take up a silver stain (see Chapter 21, page 363). Rectal carcinoids have rarely produced the carcinoid syndrome.

Treatment is based mainly on the size of the tumor. Carcinoids less than 1 cm are rarely malignant, while half of those 1 to 2 cm and nearly all greater than 2 cm are malignant. Lesions less than 2 cm and without muscle invasion should be excised locally. Large lesions and those with muscle invasion should be treated as an adenocarcinoma. Prognosis is poor in those with malignant lesions.[9]

Carcinoma of the Rectum

Carcinoma of the rectum is increasing in North America and is now the most frequent site of carcinoma of the colon.

Clinical Presentation

The clinical presentation varies with the level of the tumor (Figure 22–16). Those in the upper third of the rectum are most frequently annular scirrhous carcinomas that cause intestinal obstruction. The symptoms are distention, colicky lower abdominal pain, borborygmi, and

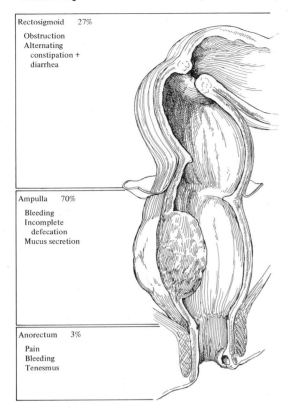

Rectosigmoid   27%

  Obstruction
  Alternating
    constipation +
    diarrhea

Ampulla   70%

  Bleeding
  Incomplete
    defecation
  Mucus secretion

Anorectum   3%

  Pain
  Bleeding
  Tenesmus

Figure 22–16. The gross appearance of recto-sigmoid carcinomas varies with the anatomic level and influences the symptoms with which they present. The figures indicate the percentage of rectosigmoid tumor occurrences at the various levels.

flatulence. There is increasing constipation often alternating with diarrhea. Passage of blood and mucus is uncommon. Growths in the middle third or ampulla of the rectum are usually large tumors. The patient generally passes red blood and often mucus and has a feeling of incomplete defecation. The symptoms from growths in the lower one third of the rectum resemble those of carcinoma of the anal canal. The tumor is usually an annular scirrhous tumor with an ulcer, which causes painful, difficult defecation. The stools may be narrow and are often covered with blood.

The patient with carcinoma of the rectum often presents with hemorrhoids. The venous distention may be the result of obstruction of the superior hemorrhoidal veins by the tumor. The patient may mistake the symptoms of the carcinoma for those of the hemorrhoids.

Diagnosis

Most rectal carcinomas can be felt on digital examination. All are within reach and can be biopsied using a proctoscope. The amount of local spread should be accurately determined. Fixation to the sacrum, invasion of the prostate or bladder, and extension into the vagina or uterus influence treatment. In those with advanced tumor a "rectal shelf" may be felt, the result of diffuse spread within the pelvis. The patient is examined for ascites, liver enlargement, jaundice, and an enlarged left supraclavicular lymph node.

A carcinoma of the rectum should be differentiated from a benign polyp, extension of carcinoma from a neighboring organ such as the bladder, prostate, vagina, uterus, or the anal canal, Crohn's disease, diverticulitis, carcinoid or chronic inflammatory diseases such as amebiasis, lymphogranuloma venereum, or actinomycosis.

Treatment

In spite of the accessibility of the rectum to digital and proctoscopic examination, the diagnosis of rectal cancer is often delayed. One quarter of patients are incurable at the time of diagnosis.

Attempted Curative Treatment. Attempted curative treatment is surgical. The amount of tissue removed depends upon the site of the tumor in the rectum (Figure 22–17). Those above the peritoneal reflection can usually be removed with the regional lymphatic drainage and continuity of the bowel reestablished by an end-to-end anastomosis (anterior resection). Carcinomas at a lower level require an abdominoperineal resection of the rectum and formation of a permanent left iliac colostomy (Figure 22–18). The prognosis is related to the microscopic findings in the operative specimen (Dukes' classification) (see page 385).

The five-year survival is about 50 percent for all patients treated for cure. Survival is about 90 percent in patients with grade A lesions and none in those with grade D.[10]

A short course of radiotherapy has been given before operation in an attempt to decrease local recurrence and increase survival. Preliminary results suggest that survival is increased in those who have metastases in the regional nodes, but further confirmation is needed before preoperative radiotherapy is generally accepted. The use of prophylactic postoperative radiotherapy has been advocated in patients with nodal metastases and in those with tumors in the lower one third of the rectum. Adjunctive chemotherapy has not proven to be of value in patients with rectal carcinoma.

Palliative Treatment. Best palliation is obtained by removal of the "operable" primary tumor even in the presence of distant metastases.

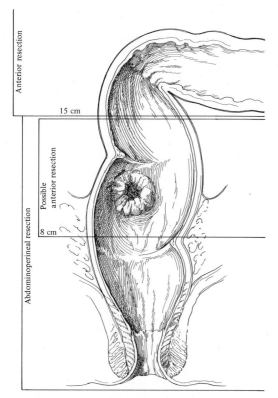

Anterior resection

15 cm

Possible anterior resection

8 cm

Abdominoperineal resection

Figure 22–17. The rectum can generally be preserved when the cancer is more than 12 cm above the anal verge, but it usually must be removed (by abdominal-perineal resection) when the tumor is less than 6 cm from the verge. The choice of procedures for tumors between 6 and 12 cm is based on such factors as the patient's age, size of tumor, and technical considerations.

If the primary tumor is left, the patient becomes anemic and toxic and develops abscesses and pain in the pelvis and perineum. A locally advanced tumor is best treated by local radiotherapy. It may occasionally be necessary to establish a colostomy in the patient with intestinal obstruction and a nonresectable

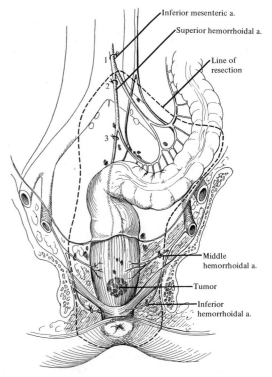

Inferior mesenteric a.

Superior hemorrhoidal a.

Line of resection

Middle hemorrhoidal a.

Tumor

Inferior hemorrhoidal a.

Figure 22–18. Curative resection of rectal cancer requires the removal of all tissue encompassed by the dashed line.

tumor. Local radiotherapy can then be given after operation to the primary tumor. The surgeon marks the region with hemoclips to facilitate subsequent radiotherapy.

Chemotherapy with intravenous 3-fluorouracil causes objective response in 25 percent of patients with metastatic colon cancer, and those that respond live an average of 19 months, compared with seven and a half months in untreated controls.[11] In addition, many nonresponders have subjective improvement, especially relief of sacral root pain. The oral use of 5-FU is of value in patients with carcinoma of the rectum (see page 385).

ANUS

ANATOMY

The anal canal, 2 cm to 3.5 cm, has an external slitlike orifice and has walls held contiguous by annular compression of the sphincter muscles (see Plate VIII). It is derived chiefly from the invaginated ectoderm (proctodeum). The proximal portion, occasionally designated as the terminal rectal segment, is formed by the union of the urorectal septum anteriorly with the fused anal tubercles. Evidence of the embryonic proctodeal membrane is the serrated pectinate line. Persistence of this membrane forms one type of imperforate anus. The mucus-containing anal sinuses or crypts of Morgagni when compressed by stool exude mucus and aid in evacuation. The four to eight anal glands that communicate with the crypts probably do not have any secretory function. They may play a role, however, in the pathogenesis of perianal infection.

Anoderm

The wall of the upper part of the anus immediately proximal to the dentate line consists of a series of vertical folds of mucous membrane, the columns of Morgagni, which are connected distally at the pectinate line by a common anal valve. The epithelial lining immediately above the valves is cuboidal, giving way to columnar more proximally. Distal to the pectinate line the anal canal is lined with modified skin firmly adherent to the underlying structures and devoid of mucus-secreting glands.

Musculature

The muscles of the anal canal are the external and internal sphincters and the levator ani complex. The external sphincter is an elliptical, muscular cylinder of voluntary muscle that surrounds the anal orifice. The distal part is fixed to the subcutaneous tissues and anal verge, and proximally it is continuous with the puborectalis and pubococcygeus muscles. The internal sphincter, an involuntary muscle, is the terminal portion of the circular muscular coat of the rectum and ends about 1 to 1.5 cm proximal to the anal orifice. The levator ani complex consists of two broad muscles that arise from the inner surface of the pelvis, unite medially, and are inserted into the anococcygeal raphe, the coccyx, and into an aponeurosis which is attached to the sacrococcygeal ligament. The levator complex forms the pelvic diaphragm and supports the abdominal viscera. The puborectalis and pubococcygei components constrict the anal canal, support the sphincters, and are involved in defecation.

Vasculature

The anorectal blood supply consists of three principal arteries with accompanying veins that supply the lower rectum and anus (see Plate VIII). The superior hemorrhoidal artery is the terminal branch of the inferior mesenteric. The paired middle hemorrhoidal branches arise from the internal iliac vessels, while the external hemorrhoidal arteries are terminal branches of the pudendal vessels that stem from the internal iliacs. Venous drainage into the portal system is by way of the superior hemorrhoidal veins and into the systemic circulation by the middle and inferior hemorrhoidal branches of the internal iliac veins. The veins surrounding the lower rectum and anus form a dense intercommunicating network.

Lymphatics

The lymphatic network of the anus is intramural and extramural. The intramural network is similar throughout the intestine and consists of an intercommunicating network lying in the submucous and subserous layers of the bowel wall. Drainage superiorly accompanies the superior hemorrhoidal vessels to the para-aortic nodes. Lymphatics also pass through the retrorectal lymph nodes and along the plexus of the perianal skin to the inguinal nodes.

Innervation

The motor nerves of the internal sphincter (involuntary) are from the sympathetic and parasympathetic (inhibitory to sphincter) pathway via the pudendal plexus. The plexus consists of nerve fibers from the anterior divisions of the second, third, and fourth sacral nerves. The voluntary external sphincter is bilaterally innervated by the inferior branch of the internal pudendal and perineal branch of fourth sacral nerves. A high degree of discrimination is achieved by the anorectal sensory nerve fibers. Voluntary selective sphincter action results in the ability to distinguish between the gaseous, liquid, and solid state of intraluminal contents.

PHYSIOLOGY

The anus and lower rectum control evacuation of the intestinal tract. The anal sphincter muscle is surpassed by none as a protector of man's dignity, yet it is so ready to come to his relief. The act of defecation is complex. Stretch receptors in the lower rectal mucosa respond to distention and generate impulses that pass via the dorsal root ganglia to the cord and are then relayed:

1. To the cerebral cortex which is responsible for voluntary closure of the glottis and diaphragmatic fixation.

2. To the ventral horn cells to promote relaxation of the anal sphincters and contraction of the abdominal and perineal muscles.

3. To the pelvic autonomic nerves stimulating the rectum to expel its contents by a peristaltic-type action. The urge to defecate may be controlled by voluntary contractions of the sphincter muscles which force the rectum to respond by adaptive relaxation.

HISTORY

Bowel Habits

Important points in the history are changes in bowel function, the nature and consistency of the stool, regularity of movement, pain, itching, and the presence of blood, pus, or mucus. There is great variation in the regularity of movements.

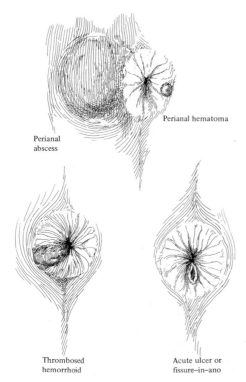

Perianal hematoma

Perianal abscess

Thrombosed hemorrhoid

Acute ulcer or fissure-in-ano

Figure 22–19. Severe anal pain is most often caused by perianal abscess, perianal hematoma, thrombosed internal hemorrhoid, or an acute anal fissure.

One individual may be regular with three movements daily, another may normally have one to three movements per week. Movements are also influenced by disease, diet, cathartics, temperature, chemicals, pathogenic microorganisms, humidity, food allergies, and anxiety.

Presence of Blood

Blood arising in the anal canal is red and coats the surface of the movement, or it may collect in the rectum and be passed independent of a bowel movement. Blood may be observed on the tissue, in the bowel, or on the outside of or mixed in the stool.

Pain

Sharp, lancinating pain on defecation is most commonly due to stretching the anoderm in the patient with a fissure or tear in the anus. Localized, constant, throbbing pain is frequently associated with thrombosed hemorrhoids or a pararectal abscess. The common causes of perianal pain are anal fissure, thrombosed hemorrhoids, perianal hematoma, and perianal abscess (Figure 22–19).

Other Symptoms

Perianal discharge may indicate a fistula, hidradenitis suppurativa, or a pilonidal sinus. A history of chronic constipation with tenesmus leads to protrusion of mucosa or bowel. An estimate of the degree of anal eversion or rectal prolapse can often be made from the history. Anal pruritus or itching is a frequent symptom.

PHYSICAL EXAMINATION

Examination is generally performed with the patient in the left lateral position. Anorectal protrusion or prolapse is best demonstrated with the patient straining in the squatting position.

A tap water or phosphosoda enema is advisable before an anorectal examination except in those who have just evacuated their bowel or in those with colitis in whom cultures are desirable.

Inspection is done with the buttocks abducted, noting abnormal openings, ulcers, swellings, warts, pigmentation, discharge, inflammation, or external hemorrhoidal tags. Digital examination is routinely performed except in patients with severe sphincter spasm and pain. The skin of the anal verge is gently retracted to reveal a fissure or ulcer which is usually in the midline posteriorly. Regions of induration and tenderness are sought. The sphincter tone is noted. The prostate and seminal vesicles are palpated in the male (Figure 22–20). The rectovaginal septum may be readily palpated by bimanual technique.

Internal hemorrhoids, hypertrophic papillae, abnormal openings, and anorectal neoplasms can be seen through an anoscope.

Proctoscopy, Colonoscopy

Examination with a standard, rigid, 25-cm proctoscope can be performed with the patient in different positions (Figure 22–21). Abnormal mucosal pigmentation (cascara), loss of light reflex of the mucosa denoting early inflammation, ulcerations, bleeding sources, polyps, or submucosal excrescenses should be sought. Flexible colonoscopy provides vision of the colonic mucosa from the sigmoid colon to the cecum. Tumor biopsy and excisions of small polyps may also be performed without anesthesia. Exudates for cultures and smears should be taken if indicated. Friability of the mucosa denoting inflammation is readily determined by gently scraping the end of the instrument over the mucosal surface, producing petechial hemorrhages. The degree of tumor fixation can also be judged by manipulating the bowel wall with the end of the scope without anesthesia.

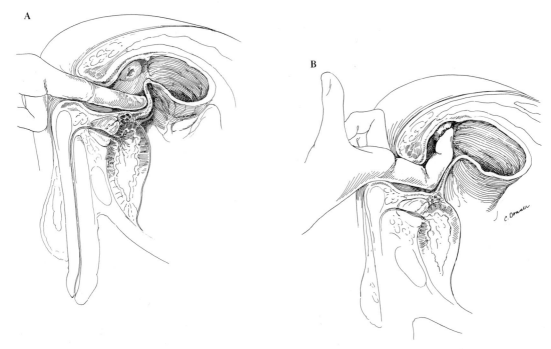

Figure 22–20. Rectal examination in the male. *A*. The prostate, bladder base, seminal vesicles, and rectovesical pouch are palpated anteriorly. *B*. On palpating posteriorly the coccyx and curvature of the sacrum can be felt. Shown is an ulcerating carcinoma in the posterior wall of the rectum.

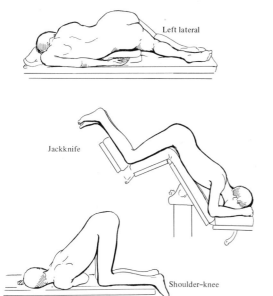

Figure 22–21. Sigmoidoscopy can be performed with the patient in the left lateral, jackknife, and shoulder-knee positions. Under general anesthesia the Trendelenburg-lithotomy position is generally used.

A punch biopsy should be taken from the base of rectal lesions (Figure 22–22). In contrast, biopsies from the anus or anal margin may require infiltration anesthesia.

Electromyography records muscle response to an electrical stimulus and aids in defining the location and integrity of the anal sphincter.

DISEASES OF THE ANUS
Congenital Diseases
See Chapter 35.

Injuries to the Anus

Common results of anal trauma requiring medical attention are anal ulcers, fissures, or iatrogenic strictures following operation for hemorrhoids, fistula, or prolapse. Occasionally the anal sphincter is damaged from third-degree tears of the perineum at childbirth, often resulting in a fistula, stricture, and incontinence.

Fissure

The commonest localized inflammatory lesion is an ulcer or fissure. It is a slitlike lesion occurring in the midline posteriorly in 80 percent of patients, more frequent in women than men

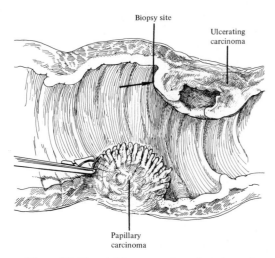

Biopsy site

Ulcerating carcinoma

Papillary carcinoma

Figure 22–22. A biopsy can be taken through the sigmoidoscope. Several biopsies should be taken, including one from the junction of the normal mucosa with the lesion.

and uncommonly in the aged. The anoderm in the posterior midline is fixed to the underlying structures and is subject to direct pressure from the passage of hard, dry stool. Pain is the cardinal feature. If the ulcer is not painful, the diagnosis may be cancer, syphilis, chancroid, donovanosis (granuloma inguinale), or tuberculosis. These ulcers are often located laterally on the anoderm. The pain of the nonspecific anal ulcer is lancinating on defecation and disappears a varying time after the movement. As sphincter spasm recurs, an intense burning anal discomfort returns. A few drops of blood are often seen in the toilet bowl, on the tissue, or on the surface of the stool. The dread of pain on defecation often results in stool suppression and constipation.

The diagnosis is based on the history and by observing the ulcer by gently separating the anal margins. An inflamed sentinel pile (Brodie) may mark the distal ulcer site. Pain caused by dilating the anal sphincter precludes diagnostic instrumentation during the acute phase and should be deferred for a short time until healing has occurred or be performed under local anesthesia.

Most ulcers respond to conservative management. The stools should be kept soft, a low-residue diet given, and fluid intake increased. Pain from anal spasm is relieved by hot compresses and sitz baths. The local application of an anesthetic or astringent ointment is of little value. Operation should be performed if the ulcer persists for more than six weeks in a patient on strict conservative management.

Surgical treatment consists of excising the ulcer, dilating the sphincter, and dividing the superficial fibers of the anal sphincter in the posterior lateral quadrant. This may be done under local or general anesthesia. Histologic examination of the excised ulcer elements is essential.

Stricture

Anal strictures or stenoses may follow operations for hemorrhoids, fistula, or prolapse. Senile anal stenosis, however, occurs without operation and is the result of fibrosis of the muscularis submucosae in patients who habitually take cathartics. Instrumental anal dilatation provides only temporary relief and causes painful fissuring. Surgical treatment consists in Z-plasty rotation of skin flaps or interposing the underlying mucosa, drawing it into the midline at the point of superficial sphincterotomy. Specific inflammatory stenoses from granuloma inguinale or chronic lymphogranuloma venereum and late syphilis may occur low in the anorectum. The diagnosis[2] is based on microscopic examination of the tissue from the anus and regional nodes and examination of smears for the specific organisms (Donovan bodies,[9] *Treponema pallidum*,[10] and the tubercle bacillus). Definitive skin sensitivity tests are essential (Frei, tuberculin, and serologic tests for syphilis). In addition to the surgical treatment of the stricture, specific systemic chemotherapy is employed. Severe strictures of the lower rectum occasionally require colostomy.

Cryptitis

Cryptitis, an entity not universally recognized, refers to nonspecific inflammation of one or more anal crypts of Morgagni associated with hypertrophy of the adjacent papilla. If the inflammatory process extends into the anal ducts, rupture occurs into the ischiorectal fat with abscess and often later a fistula. The chief symptom is pruritus. Cryptitis responds to warm compresses, sitz baths, low-residue diet, stool softeners, oral Sulfasuxidine, and topical corticosteroid creams or suppositories. Surgical treatment for indolent cases consists in "unroofing" the pathologic crypts and excising the associated hypertrophied papillae.

Abscesses

Abscesses are classified according to their relation to the anal canal, levator muscles, and ischiorectal fossa (Figure 22–23). Inflammation within the bowel (Crohn's disease, colitis, etc.), perforation by a foreign body, and inflammatory diseases from the prostate, pelvis, and perineum may also produce abscesses. General symptoms are malaise and anorexia with local tenderness,

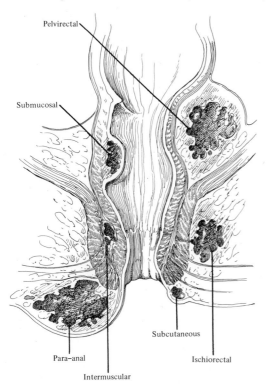

Pelvirectal

Submucosal

Para-anal

Intermuscular

Subcutaneous

Ischiorectal

Figure 22–23. The most frequent abscesses in the anal region are the para-anal and ischiorectal abscesses.

swelling, and erythema if the abscess lies superficial to the levator muscles. Supralevator abscesses (pelvirectal) produce a dull throbbing pain without external localizing signs. The pain of a perirectal abscess is aggravated by defecation and sitting. Occasionally urinary retention occurs through reflex stimulation of the pelvic plexus.

An ischiorectal abscess lies in the ischiorectal space bounded medially by the musculature of the anus and the levator ani and laterally by the ischial tuberosity. It lies deep to a layer of deep fascia that forms the floor of the ischiorectal space. Infection may reach the space following cryptitis, from downward extension of a pelvirectal abscess, from a penetrating injury of the buttock, or from hematogenous spread. Local signs are fullness and tenderness between the anus and ischial tuberosity. If treatment is delayed, the abscess tends to rupture into the anal canal or spread behind the anus to the opposite ischiorectal space. Downward extension tends to be late because the deep fascia prevents spread. The patient is given intravenous antibiotics and is operated on as soon as possible. A cruciate incision is made over the space and the edges excised. The deep fascia is incised, and

the space is thoroughly drained. The operative site is allowed to heal by secondary intention. Late or inadequate surgical treatment is frequently followed by a fistula. A pelvirectal abscess is drained through the ischiorectal fossa (Figure 22–24).

Fistula

An anorectal fistula refers to a pathologic tract between the lumen of the bowel and the skin of the perineum. Fistulas may be (1) simple, having an internal and external opening with an interconnecting tract; (2) complex, consisting of several branching tracts; or (3) horseshoe, characterized by two external openings symmetrically placed on either side of the anus and entering the rectum through a common internal opening, usually posterior. The diagnosis is based on the presence of a chronic intermittent perineal discharge. Often there is a history of a previous abscess and/or an anorectal operation. Palpation reveals an indurated tract directed to the anorectum from the external stoma frequently associated with a previous operative scar. Probing the external opening usually does not demonstrate a continuous tract, nor is the internal opening found in all patients. The presence of a sentinel pile in the same quadrant as the external opening of the fistula shows that a crypt is involved.

Treatment consists of excising the tract. If the tract passes deep to the superficial and through fibers of the deep sphincter, incontinence is prevented by staged excisions using the Seton suture technique.

Pruritus Ani

Pruritus ani is an anogenital neurodermatitis characterized by localized itching with lichenification and moisture of the anal skinfolds. The cause is idiopathic in 50 percent of patients. Allergies, infections, intertrigo, eczema, parasites, and seborrhea account for 20 percent, and systemic diseases such as lymphoma, diabetes, and hepatic disorders for 10 percent, while organic disease of the anorectum (fissures, hemorrhoids, cryptitis, fistulae) for the remainder. Many patients with anogenital pruritus have a strong psychological overlay or are prone to anxiety neuroses.

Definition of the exciting agent is based on a careful history to eliminate dermatologic, systemic, and psychological causes. General and anorectal examination and laboratory tests are performed to exclude systemic diseases. Perineal excoriations, edema, and moisture of the perianal skinfolds are characteristic.

The treatment of pruritus ani from psychological, dermatologic, and systemic disease is

A   B

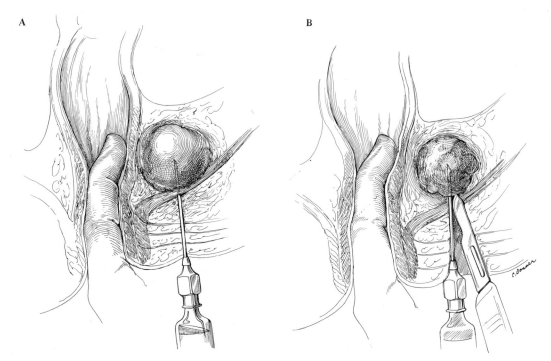

Figure 22–24. *A*. A pelvirectal abscess is localized by inserting a wide-bore needle and aspirating pus. *B*. The abscess cavity is then opened and the pus evacuated. The opening is enlarged and a wide excision of the ischiorectal fossa performed so that the region heals by secondary intention.

medical. Idiopathic, anogenital neurodermatitis is managed by sedatives or tranquilizers, cool compresses, sitz baths, and topical corticosteroids. Sanitary toilet habits should be stressed with particular emphasis on keeping the anal verge and perineal tissues dry by the use of a cotton wafer.

The surgical correction of coexisting hemorrhoids, fissures, cryptitis, papillitis, and fistulae is often curative. Surgical treatment of idiopathic chronic pruritus ani is less successful and includes such procedures as "cloverleaf" excisions centered about the anus, and the subcutaneous injection of absolute ethyl alcohol by multiple puncture techniques or tattooing with mercury sulfide.[16] Unfortunately there is no one successful treatment for refractory anogenital pruritus.

Anal Incontinence

Incontinence of the anal sphincter or loss of voluntary sphincter control is commonly associated with iatrogenic trauma, occasionally in the aged, or secondary to severe and spontaneous degenerative disease of the spinal cord or central nervous system. Conservative treatment consists of diet and bowel regulation and active and passive muscular contraction to improve sphincter tone. Complete division of the sphincter

muscle laterally causes some degree of incontinence and may be averted by a staged technique (Seton suture). Immediate or delayed repair by direct apposition of the divided muscle can be accomplished by primary suture or the Bunnell pull-out wire technique.[4] In the aged, with incontinence due to atony, sphincter reefing procedures[5] or fascial slings[15] may control incontinence. The gracilis transplant procedure[13] is reserved for younger patients with marked incontinence from either certain congenital or acquired causes. Colostomy may be required, especially in those with disease in the spinal cord or central nervous system.

Hemorrhoids

Hemorrhoids are varicose dilatations of one or more of the veins of the inferior or superior hemorrhoidal plexi, or both.

Varicosities of the superior hemorrhoidal plexus which lie proximal to the dentate line are internal hemorrhoids. Varicosities of the inferior hemorrhoidal network of veins, situated distally and covered with modified anal skin, are external hemorrhoids. Multiple intercommunicating vessels join the two plexi (Figure 22–25). When one or more of the communicating veins are dilated together with varicosities of the superior and inferior hemorrhoidal plexus,

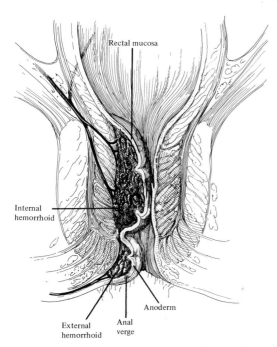

Rectal mucosa

Internal
hemorrhoid

Anoderm

External
hemorrhoid

Anal
verge

Figure 22–25. Internal hemorrhoids are situated above the pectinate line and covered by mucous membrane. External hemorrhoids are at the anal verge and covered partially by skin.

mixed hemorrhoids result. Thrombus formation is more common in the external rather than the internal hemorrhoidal plexus. Rupture of a vessel results in a painful, tender perivascular hematoma which should be distinguished from a perianal abscess or fissure in ano. Stretching of the perivascular supporting tissue produced by tenesmus or straining on defecation promotes hemorrhoidal protrusion or prolapse. Hemorrhoids prolapsing through the external sphincter are compressed, impeding the blood supply, and tend to ulcerate and strangulate.

Contributing factors to hemorrhoid formation are man's upright position, heredity, and occupations requiring muscular straining, such as for athletes and laborers. Exciting causes are constipation, cardiac failure, portal hypertension, chronic cough, pregnancy, and infections.

Diagnosis. The diagnosis is based on a history of protrusion and often painless bleeding on the tissue, the stool, and in the bowl. Only complicated hemorrhoids are painful, i.e., when they are ulcerated, thrombosed, infected, or strangulated. Inspection, digital examination, and anoproctoscopy are performed with the patient in the squatting, Sims', shoulder-knee, or lithotomy position. Proctoscopy should always be performed to eliminate other causes of rectal bleeding, except when the pain of hemor-

rhoidal complications render instrumentation intolerable.

Treatment. Prophylactic therapy consists of a high-roughage diet to promote regular soft stool. In the patient with hemorrhoids the use of mineral oil or stool softeners and the inclusion or two cooked fruits and vegetables in the diet cannot be overemphasized to promote soft movements. Five to eight glasses of water a day are also desirable. Nuts, seeds, popcorn, and corn on the cob should be excluded. The application of 1 percent silver nitrate to the ulcerated areas may promote healing, and astringent or emolient suppositories also offer some aid. Warm compresses may be applied with the patient in the recumbent position for thrombosed, superficially ulcerated, or bleeding hemorrhoids. Immediate excision of an acute thrombosed hemorrhoid brings rapid relief.

Surgical treatment consists of injection,[17] ligation,[3] or excision of the hemorrhoids. Injection and ligation are indicated only for uncomplicated internal hemorrhoids. The most satisfactory treatment is total excision that can be performed by various techniques under local, regional, or general anesthesia (Figure 22–26). Postoperative management includes hot compresses, sitz baths, analgesics, stool softeners, and a diet to induce normal movements. Postoperative anal dilatations are not required.

A perianal hematoma is treated by evacuation of the clot using local anesthesia (Figure 22–27).

Anorectal Prolapse

Anorectal prolapse is a condition in which one or more layers of the rectum protrude through the anal ring.

The prolapse may include only the mucosa and be incomplete or involve all layers of the bowel wall and be complete (Figures 22–28 and 22–29). The complete form is usually associated with a peritoneal sac. Significant predisposing causes are tenesmus, attenuation, and degeneration from aging or multiple pregnancies. Rectal prolapse is encountered in all ages from infancy to senescence. Prolapse must be distinguished from rectosigmoid intussusception, procidentia, anal eversion, and prolapsed hemorrhoids.

Treatment.   *Indications.*   Conservative measures of reducing the prolapse and keeping it reduced by support are usually adequate in infancy and early childhood. Operation is usually not indicated. By contrast, surgical repair is usually required in adults and may be accomplished by a perineal, transabdominal, or combined approach.

Procedures. Generally the perineal repair is reserved for aged and debilitated patients, employing cerclage with a Thiersch silver wire,[7]

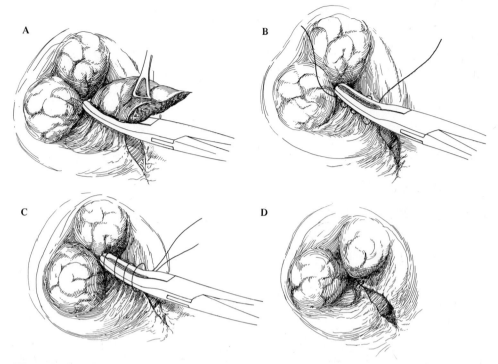

Figure 22–26. Steps in the excision of a hemorrhoid. The left lateral and right posterior and right anterior primary hemorrhoids are excised in order.

the Rehn-Delorme[8] or Altemeier[1] procedures. Transabdominal coloproctopexy (Ripstein)[14] (Figure 22–29) or anterior resection[18] has yielded excellent results in good-risk patients. The combined perineal-abdominal procedure[6] also provides excellent results.

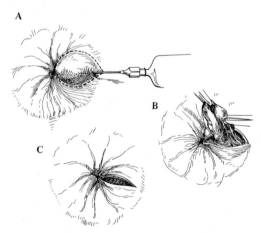

Figure 22–27. *A.* The skin underlying a perianal hematoma is infiltrated with local anesthetic. *B.* An incision is made and the blood clot evacuated. *C.* The region is left open.

Anal Neoplasms

Benign neoplasms are papillomas and hypertrophied papillae associated with infection or cryptitis. They are best treated by excision. Condylomata acuminatum, warty growths of viral origin of the anus and perineum, are controlled by podophyllum in 20 percent collodion, tincture of benzoin, fulguration, or excision.

Malignant tumors of the anus are keratinizing, epidermoid, or squamous cell carcinomas and nonkeratinizing tumors, including basal cell, Bowen's disease, Paget's extramammary disease, cloacogenic cancer, and melanoma. Anal cancer accounts for about 2 percent of all malignancies of the colon and anorectum. It occurs equally between the sexes and is less frequent in the black race. The commonest manifestations in order of frequency are bleeding, pain, and tenesmus. About one third of the patients have associated benign conditions of the anorectum such as hemorrhoids and fistulae which may mask the primary malignancy.

All chronic anorectal or perianal ulcerating lesions and long-standing fistulae should arouse suspicion of associated cancer and be excised or biopsied to establish a definite diagnosis. Particular attention should be directed to the inguinal lymph nodes.

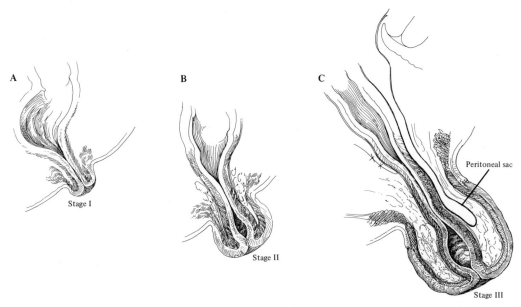

Figure 22–28. *A.* In stage I prolapse of the rectal mucosa has descended below the anal verge. *B.* In stage II the whole wall of the rectum is included. *C.* In stage III there is, in addition, prolapse of the peritoneum on the anterior wall of the rectum.

Treatment. Noninvasive epidermoid lesions, such as Paget's, Bowen's disease, and basal cell cancer, can be treated by irradiation or local excision, particularly if the lesion is located distal to the dentate line.[11,12] Abdominoperineal excision of the anorectum is indicated for infiltrating anal epidermoid carcinoma because of the neoplasm's tridirectional pathways of spread. The adjunctive use of preoperative irradiation therapy combined with operation is currently being evaluated. The five-year survival is about 50 percent in patients treated by abdominoperineal resection for epidermoid cancer of the anus who do not have metastases in the inguinal nodes. There are few survivors when the nodes contain metastases.

Pilonidal Cysts and Sinuses

A pilonidal cyst occurs in the midline of the sacrococcygeal region. Some are congenital and arise from a persistent remnant of the neurenteric canal. The majority are trichogranulomas and result from penetration of a hair into the subcutaneous tissues. They also occur at the umbilicus, axillae, face, finger webs of barbers, soles of the feet, anteriorly in the perineum, and in the scar of an amputation stump. They are four times commoner in men than women, uncommon in Negroes, and occur most often in those who are dark and hirsute. A midline sinus is present over the sacrum or coccyx and often has hairs projecting from the orifice. They may present with a painless discharging sinus but

more often with recurrent abscesses that can be extremely painful. The condition should be distinguished from anal fistulas, hidradenitis suppurativa, and simple subcutaneous abscess formation.

Treatment by excision and primary closure is followed by a recurrence rate of about 25 percent. Marsupialization, removing the roof of the sinus and any associated tracts and suturing the skin to the remaining deep portion of the cyst, has a recurrence rate of about 1 percent. A depilating dose of local radiotherapy was given to prevent recurrence but is now omitted because of the possibility of developing a squamous cell carcinoma in the irradiated skin.

Noninfected midline sinuses may be successfully treated by various surgical techniques employing en bloc excision with partial or no closure. Healing occurs by secondary intention.

Presacral Retrorectal Tumors and Cysts

Presacral dermoids or epidermal cysts are congenital benign neoplasms situated between the posterior wall of the rectum and coccyx. Uncomplicated cysts are usually asymptomatic and detected only on routine rectal examination. The enlarging cyst produces rectal pressure and mild pelvic discomfort. Spontaneous rupture secondary to infection leads to chronic sinus formation and/or recurrent abscesses of the postanal skin.

Extrarectal surgical excision is the treatment of choice performed through a subcoccygeal

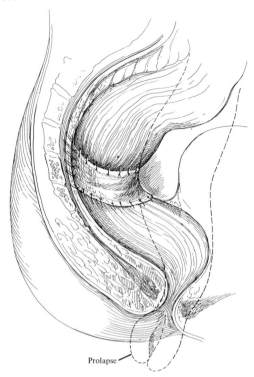

Prolapse

Figure 22–29. A complete prolapse of the rectum may be repaired by an abdominal approach, by placing a synthetic fiber mesh around the rectum and anchoring it to the tissues attached to the sacrum. The subsequent fibrotic reaction prevents descent of the rectum and recurrence of the prolapse.

approach. Removal of the coccyx, often not required, provides wider exposure. Primary closure is performed in the absence of infection. In infection an effort should be made to remove the pyogenic cyst wall. The wound then should be allowed to heal by secondary intention. Sacrococcygeal teratomas, derived from all germinal layers, are rare congenital neoplasms occurring principally in the female with malignant change reported in from 9 to 20 percent. Surgical excision is the treatment of choice.

CITED REFERENCES

COLON

1. Aylett, S. O.: Three hundred cases of diffuse ulcerative colitis treated by total colectomy and ileorectal anastomosis. *Br. Med. J.*, 1:1001–1005, 1966.
2. Brennan, M. J.; Talley, R. W.; San Diego, E. L., *et al.*: Critical analysis of 594 cancer patients treated with 5-fluorouracil. In Plattner, P. A. (ed.) *Proc. Int. Symp. Chemotherapy Cancer.* Elsevier, New York, pp. 118–50, 1964.
3. Brockenbrough, E. C., and Moylan, J. A.: Treatment of contaminated surgical wounds with topical antibiotics: Double-blind study of 240 patients. *Am. Surg.*, 35:789–92, 1969.
4. Brooke, B. N.: Management of ileostomy, including its complications. *Lancet*, 2:103–104, 1952.
5. Brooks, J. R., and Veith, F. J.: The timing and choice of surgery for ulcerative colitis: The influence of corticosteroids. *JAMA*, 194:115–18, 1965.
6. Burkitt, D. P.: Epidemiology of cancer of the colon and rectum. *Cancer*, 28:3–13, 1971.
7. De Dombal, F. T.; Watts, J. M.; Watkinson, G.; and Goligher, J. C.: Local complications of ulcerative colitis: Stricture, pseudopolyposis and carcinoma of the colon and rectum. *Br. Med. J.*, 1:1442–47, 1966.
8. Doolas, A.; Economou, S.; and Gilchrist, R. K.: Prophylactic surgery for diverticular disease of the colon. *Contemp. Surg.*, 1:62–66, 1972.
9. First National. Conference on Cancer of the Colon and Rectum. *Cancer*, 28:1–3, 1971.
10. Herter, F. P., and Slonetz, C. A., Jr.: Preoperative intestinal preparation in relation to the subsequent development of cancer at the suture line. *Surg. Gynecol. Obstet.*, 127:49–56, 1968.
11. McGowan, J. R.: Collateral circulation in the sigmoid colon. *Arch. Surg.*, 71:531–37, 1955.
12. Morson, B. C., and Bussey, H. J. R.: Predisposing causes of intestinal cancer. *Curr. Probl. Surg.*, Feb. 1970.
13. Nugent, F. W.: Medical management of inflammatory disease of the colon. *Surg. Clin. North Am.*, 51:807–13, 1971.
14. Prohaska, J. V.; Govostis, N. S.; and Taubenhaus, M.: Postoperative pseudomembranous enterocolitis successful treatment with corticotropin (ACTH) *JAMA*, 154:320–23, 1954.
15. Ransom, J. H. C.; Lawrence, L. R.; and Localio, S. A.: Colomyostomy: A new approach to surgery for colonic diverticular disease. *Am. J. Surg.*, 123:185–91, 1972.
16. Roth, J. L. A.; Valdez Dapena, A.; Stein, G. N.; and Bockus, H. L.: Toxic megacolon in ulcerative colitis. *Gastroenterology*, 37:239–55, 1959.
17. Tucker, J. W., and Fey, W. D.: The management of perforating injuries of the colon and rectum in civilian practice. *Surgery*, 35:213–20, 1954.
18. Turnbull, R. B.; Hawk, W. A.; and Weakley, F. L.: Surgical treatment of toxic megacolon. *Am. J. Surg.*, 122:325–31, 1971.
19. Turnbull, R. B.; Kyle, K.; Watson, F. R.; and Spratt, J.: Cancer of the colon: The influence of the no-touch isolation technic on survival rates. *Ann. Surg.*, 166:420–27, 1967.
20. Welch, C. E.; Allen, A. W.; and Donalson, G. E.: An appraisal of resection of the colon for diverticulitis of the sigmoid. *Ann. Surg.*, 138:332–43, 1953.
21. Williams, R. D., and Yurko, A. A.: Controversial aspects of diagnosis and management of blunt trauma. *Am. J. Surg.*, 111:477–82, 1966.

APPENDIX

1. Altemeier, W.: The pathogenicity of the bacteria of appendicitis peritonitis. *Surgery*, 11:374–84, 1942.
2. Crowder, B. L., II; Judd, R. S.; and Dockerty, M. G.: Gastrointestinal carcinoids and the carcinoid syndrome: Clinical characteristics and therapy. *Surg. Clin. North Am.*, 47:915–27, 1967.
3. Deschênes, L., *et al.*: Diverticulitis of the appendix: Report of sixty-one cases. *Am. J. Surg.*, 121:706–709, 1971.
4. Edmondson, H. T., and Hobb, M. L.: Primary adenocarcinoma of the appendix. *Am. Surg.*, 33:717–32, 1967.
5. Fields, I. A., and Cole, M. M.: Acute appendicitis in infants thirty-six months of age or younger: Ten-year survey at the Los Angeles County Hospital. *Am. J. Surg.*, 113:269–78, 1967.

6. Girardet, L., and Enquist, I. F.: Differential diagnosis between appendicitis and acute pelvic inflammatory disease. *Surg. Gynecol. Obstet.*, **116**:212–16, 1963.

7. Hughes, J.: Mucocele of the appendix with pseudomyxoma peritonei: A benign or malignant disease. *Ann. Surg.*, **165**:73–76, 1967.

8. McDonald, J. C.: Nonspecific mesenteric lymphadenitis. *Surg. Gynecol. Obstet.*, **116**:409, 1963.

9. Thomford, N. R.; Patti, R. W.; and Teteris, N. J.: Appendectomy during pregnancy. *Surg. Gynecol. Obstet.*, **129**:489–92, 1969.

10. Thorbjarnarson, B.: Acute appendicitis in patients over the age of sixty. *Surg. Gynecol. Obstet.*, **125**:1277–80, 1967.

11. Wangensteen, O., and Dennis, C.: Obstructive origin of appendicitis in man. *Ann. Surg.*, **110**:629–47, 1939.

RECTUM

1. Spratt, J. S., Jr.; Ackerman, L. V.; and Moyer, C. A.: Relationship of polyps of the colon to colonic cancer. *Ann. Surg.*, **148**:682–98, 1958.

2. Arminski, T. C., and McLean, D. W.: Incidence and distribution of adenomatous polyps of the colon and rectum based on 1,000 autopsy examinations. *Dis. Colon Rectum*, **7**:249–61, 1964.

3. Gardner, E. J., and Richards, R. C.: Multiple cutaneous and subcutaneous lesions occurring simultaneously with hereditary polyposis and osteomatosis. *Am. J. Hum. Genet.*, **5**:139–47, 1953.

4. Turcot, J.; Deprés, M. P.; and St. Pierre, F.: Malignant tumors of central nervous system associated with familial polyposis of colon. *Dis. Colon Rectum*, **2**:465–68, 1959.

5. Oldfield, M. C.: The association of familial polyposis of the colon with multiple sebaceous cysts. *Br. J. Surg.*, **41**:534–41, 1954.

6. Cronkhite. L. W., Jr., and Canada, W. J.: Generalized gastrointestinal polyposis. An unusual syndrome of polyposis, pigmentation, alopecia and onychotrophia. *N. Engl. J. Med.*, **252**:1011–15, 1955.

7. Lee, R. O., *et al.*: Villous tumors of the rectum associated with severe fluid and electrolyte disturbance. *Br. J. Surg.*, **57**:197–201, 1970.

8. Holgersen, L. O.; Miller, R. E.; and Zintel, H. A.: Juvenile polyps of the colon. *Surgery*, **69**:288–93, 1971.

9. Wilson, H.; Cheek, R. C.; Sherman, R. T.; and Storer, E. H.: Carcinoid tumors. *Curr. Probl. Surg.*, Nov. 1970, pp. 37–40

10. Bussey, H. J. R.: The long-term results of surgical treatment of cancer of the rectum. *Proc. R. Soc. Med.*, **56**:494–96, 1963.

11. Moertel, C. G., and Reitemeier, R. J.: Effect of 5-fluorouracil therapy on survival. In Moertel, C. G., and Reitemeier, R. J. (eds.): *Advanced Gastrointestinal Cancer*. Harper & Row, New York, pp. 129–34, 1969.

ANUS

1. Altemeier, W. A.; Culbertson, W. R.; and Alexander, J. W.: One-stage perineal repair of rectal prolapse. *Arch. Surg.*, **89**:6–16, 1964.

2. American Public Health Association: *Diagnostic Procedures for Virus and Rickettsial Diseases*, 4th Ed. New York, N.Y., pp. 869–903, 1969.

3. Barron J.: Office ligation treatment of hemorrhoids. *Am. J. Surg.*, **105**:563–70, 1963.

4. Birnbaum, W. D.: A method of repair for a common type of traumatic incontinence of the anal sphincter. *Surg. Gynecol. Obstet.*, **87**:716–18, 1948.

5. Blaisdell, P. C.: Repair of the incontinent sphincter ani. *Am. J. Surg.*, **79**:174–83, 1950.

6. Dunphy, J. E.; Botsford, T. W.; and Savlov, E.: Surgical treatment of procidentia of the rectum: an evaluation of combined abdominal and perineal repair. *Am. J. Surg.*, **86**:605–12, 1953.

7. Gabriel, W. B.: The Thiersch operation for rectal prolapse. *Dis. Colon Rectum*, **7**:383–85, 1964.

8. Preston, F. W. (ed.): *General Surgery, Gastrointestinal Tract VI: 11N*. Harper & Row, Hagerstown, Md., pp. 69–72, 1972.

9. Frankel, Sam, *et al.* (eds): *Gradwohl's Clinical Laboratory Methods and Diagnosis*. Vol. II. 7th ed. C. V. Mosby Company, S. Louis, Mo., pp. 1287–89, 1970.

10. *Ibid.*, pp. 1366–72.

11. Holm, W. H., and Jackman, R. J.: Ano-rectal squamous cell carcinoma, conservative or radical treatment? *JAMA*, **188**:241–44, 1964.

12. Kuehn, P. G., *et al.*: Epidermoid carcinoma of the perianal skin and anal canal. *N. Engl. J. Med.*, **270**:614–17, 1964.

13. Pickrell, K. L.; Broadbent, T. R.; Masters, F. W.; and Metzger, J. T.: Construction of a rectal sphincter and restoration of anal continence by transplanting the gracilis muscle. *Ann. Surg.*, **135**:853–62, 1952.

14. Ripstein, C. B., and Lanter, B.: Etiology and surgical therapy of massive prolapse of the rectum. *Ann. Surg.*, **157**:259–64, 1963.

15. Stone, H. B., and McLanahan, S.: Results with fascia plastic operation for anal incontinence. *Ann. Surg.*, **114**:73–77, 1941.

16. Turell, R.: Treatment of intractable anal pruritus. In Turell, R. (ed.): *Diseases of the Colon and Anorectum*, 2nd ed. Vol. II. W. B. Saunders Co., Philadelphia, pp. 1007–28, 1969.

17. Terrell, R. V., and Chewning, C. C.: The present status of injection treatment of internal hemorrhoids. *Am. J. Surg.*, **79**:44–48, 1950.

18. Theuerkauf, F. J., Jr.; Beahrs, O. H.; and Hill, J. R.: Rectal prolapse, causation and surgical treatment. *Ann. Surg.*, **171**:819–53, 1970.

SUGGESTIONS FOR FURTHER READING

COLON

Bockus, H. L.: *Gastroenterology, The Small Intestine, Absorption and Nutrition, The Colon, Peritoneum, Mesentery and Omentum*, 2nd ed. W. B. Saunders, Philadelphia, **2**:595–1087, 1964.
A most complete textbook of gastroenterology, interestingly written, and presenting both surgical and medical views. Many useful references.

Burdette, W. J.: *Carcinoma of the Colon and Antecedent Epithelium*. Charles C Thomas, Springfield, Ill., 1970.
A very thorough yet concise book about colon cancer. The sections on epidemiology, antigenicity, and cellular physiology are excellent.

Goligher, J. C.; DeDombal, F. T.; Watts, J. M.; and Watkinson, G.: *Ulcerative Colitis*. Ballière, Tindall and Cassell, London, 1968.
All about ulcerative colitis in one compact volume.

Perry, J. F.: Blunt and penetrating abdominal injuries. *Curr. Probl. Surg.*, May, 1970.
A complete monograph of abdominal trauma. Describes diagnostic methods, complications and treatment of specific injuries. Many good references.

Turell, Robert (ed.): *Diseases of the Colon and Anorectum*, 2nd ed. 2 vols. W. B. Saunders, Philadelphia, 1969.
A very complete set discussing colonic and anorectal problems mainly from the surgical viewpoint. Surgical procedures are described as in a surgical atlas.

APPENDIX

Hawk, J. C., Jr.; Backer, W. F.; and Lehman, E. P.: Acute appendicitis. III. An analysis of one thousand and three cases. *Ann. Surg.*, **132**:729, 1950.
Review of clinical experience with modern treatment of appendicitis.
Reynolds, J. T.: Appendicitis: Basic consideration of choice of therapy. *Surg. Clin. North Am.*, **42**:128–45 1944.
Good review of the pathogenesis of appendicitis.

RECTUM

Burdette, Walter J. (ed.): *Carcinoma of the Colon and Antecedent Epithelium.* Charles C Thomas, Springfield, Ill., 1970.
An excellent summary of the current knowledge with good coverage of clinical as well as experimental colon and rectal cancer.

Davenport, Horace W. (ed.): *Physiology of the Digestive Tract*, 3rd ed. Year Book Medical Publishers, Inc., Chicago, 1971.
Concise, clear coverage of gastrointestinal physiology.
Turell, Robert (ed.): *Diseases of the Colon and Anorectum*, 2nd ed. 2 vols. W. B. Saunders, Philadelphia, 1969.
The most thorough single reference.

ANUS

Morson, Basil C. (ed.): *Diseases of the Colon, Rectum and Anus—Tutorials in Post Graduate Medicine. Vol. I.* Appleton-Century-Crofts, New York, 1969.
An excellent British compendium directed to graduate students who desire an introductory knowledge of anorectal diseases.
Turell, Robert (ed.): *Diseases of the Colon and Anorectum*, 2nd ed. 2 vols. W. B. Saunders Co., Philadelphia, 1969.
The most informative text by multiple contributors.

Chapter 23

INTESTINAL OBSTRUCTION AND HERNIA

Richard W. Williams

CHAPTER OUTLINE

Intestinal Obstruction
  Etiology
    Mechanical
    Nonmechanical
    Patient's Age
  Pathophysiology
    Secretion
    Absorption
    Distention
    Peristalsis
    Mucosal Cell Turnover
  Clinical Management
    History and Physical Examination
    Laboratory Procedures
    Roentgenography
  Treatment
    Antibiotics
    Operation
  Specific Bowel Obstructions
    Neonatal Obstructions
    Intussusception

    Foreign Bodies
    Gallstone Ileus
    Fecal Impaction
    Neoplasms
    Volvulus
    Crohn's Disease
    Diverticular Disease of the Colon
    Adhesions
    Ischemic Enteritis and Colitis
    Paralytic Ileus
Hernia
  External Hernias
    Indirect Inguinal
    Direct Inguinal
    Femoral
    Umbilical
    Epigastric
    Incisional
  Internal Hernias
  Diaphragmatic Hernias
    Hiatal

INTESTINAL OBSTRUCTION

Intestinal obstruction may result from mechanical or nonmechanical causes and may be simple or strangulated depending on the state of the blood supply. There are approximately 8000 deaths per year in the United States from bowel obstruction, the mortality varying from 5 to 20 percent. Mortality has decreased over the past 50 years as a result of nasogastric and intestinal intubation, better management of fluid and electrolyte losses, administration of antibiotics, and better surgical and anesthetic techniques. However, it remains high when there is delay in treatment, coexisting malignancy, or congenital abnormality.

Etiology

Obstruction may be acute, subacute, or chronic.

Mechanical. Mechanical causes of bowel obstruction include

With Occlusion of Lumen

Intraluminal	Polypoid tumor
	Gallstone
	Foreign body
	Fecal impaction
Intramural	Stenosing tumor
	Crohn's disease
	Diverticulitis
	Intussusception
	Atresia or stenosis
Extraluminal	Adhesion
	Hernia
	Volvulus
	Annular pancreas

Without Occlusion of Lumen

	Ischemic enteritis
	Colitis

411

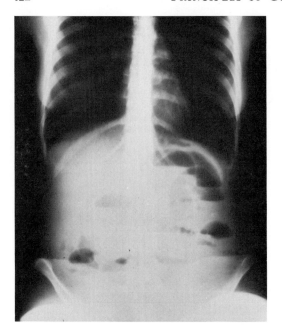

Figure 23-1. In acute small bowel obstruction there are multiple fluid levels in the upright position.

Nonmechanical. Paralytic ileus is a nonmechanical cause of intestinal obstruction.

Patient's Age. The most likely cause of bowel obstruction depends on the patient's age. In the newborn congenital abnormalities predominate. In the adult intra-abdominal adhesions, usually from a previous operation, are the most frequent cause. After 40 years there is an increasing incidence of carcinoma, especially of the colon.[4] At any age a hernia predisposes to intestinal obstruction.

Pathophysiology

The functions of the bowel are secretion, digestion, absorption, motility, and excretion. It is necessary to understand how these processes are affected by obstruction.

Secretion. Oral and intestinal secretions continue and even increase during bowel obstruction and are an important factor in the production of distention. In obstruction of the small intestine fluid is lost in large quantities into the lumen and by emesis. The consequences of the large loss of fluid and electrolytes are decreased extracellular volume and hypovolemic shock. With simple colonic obstruction there is often no vomiting.

Absorption. Normally most of the secretions into the upper gastrointestinal tract are reabsorbed in the ileum. With obstruction of the small intestine much of the fluid may not reach the absorptive region and is therefore vomited or remains in the lumen. The higher the obstruction, the greater the loss of fluid and electrolytes.

Distention. Gaseous distention is the result of air swallowing (aerophagia), gas production by bacteria, and diffusion of gas from the blood into the lumen. Air swallowing is the major source. Intraluminal pressure is normally about 2 to 4 mm Hg and increases to 20 to 30 mm Hg during peristalsis. The pressure increases with obstruction and causes venous and eventually arterial occlusion. With large bowel obstruction there is marked distention of the colon and especially of the cecum. On the other hand, acute jejunal obstruction presents with minimal distention. If the ileocecal sphincter remains closed, there is a closed loop obstruction, which if not rapidly treated will perforate. Secondary effects of abdominal distention are elevation of the diaphragm with impairment of pulmonary function and decreased venous return from the lower extremities. The decreased venous return results in accumulation of fluid in the legs and its loss from the circulation. Later ileus may occur as a result of the prolonged distention, accumulation of fluid in the wall, and hypokalemia.

Peristalsis. Intestinal motility increases in an attempt to overcome the obstruction, and there may be reverse peristalsis. The pain from

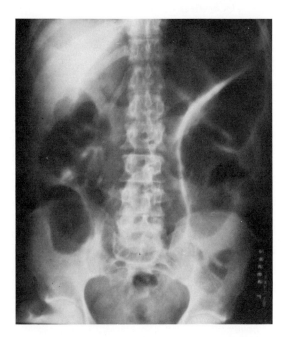

Figure 23-2. In acute volvulus of the sigmoid colon a markedly distended loop is seen arising from the pelvis.

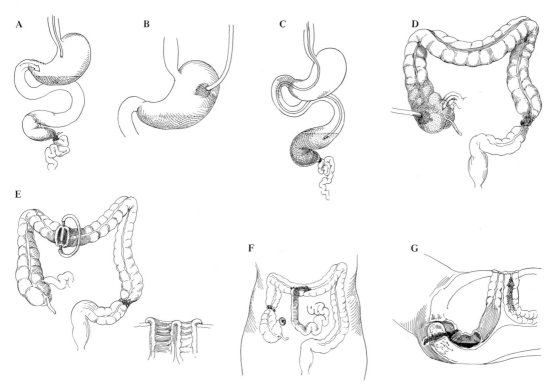

Figure 23–3.   Methods of gastrointestinal decompression. *A*. Nasogastric tube. *B*. Gastrostomy. *C*. Motor tube. *D*. Cecostomy. *E*. Transverse colostomy. *F*. Ileotranverse anastomosis and mucous fistula. *G*. Left iliac double-barrelled colostomy.

the increased peristalsis is more severe with small bowel than colon obstruction because the muscle layer is much thicker in the small than in the large intestine.

Mucosal Cell Turnover. The mucosal cell

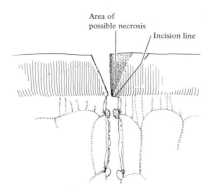

Figure 23–4. Gangrenous bowel has been resected and a V-shaped segment of mesentery excised. The line of section is in healthy bowel beyond the area of necrosis, at an angle that affords a good blood supply.

turnover is markedly decreased as a result of edema and impairment of the blood supply. Bacteria and toxins within the lumen can then readily enter the wall, blood stream, and peritoneal cavity. Perforation and peritonitis may occur.

Clinical Management

History and Physical Examination. Information is sought about the type, severity, and duration of pain, emesis, and the time of the last bowel movement or passage of flatus. The patient is asked about previous abdominal operations and gastrointestinal symptoms. On physical examination attention is directed first to the patient's general condition for evidence of dehydration, oligemic shock, and the cardiopulmonary status. The abdomen is examined for previous incisions, distention, visible peristalsis, and loops of bowel, tenderness, masses, and the state of the bowel sounds. The groin is carefully examined for hernia, especially in the obese female when a small femoral hernia may readily be overlooked. The rectum must be checked for stool, blood, or an

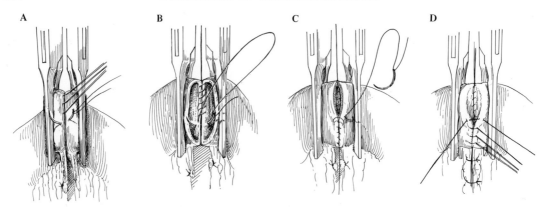

Figure 23–5. Technique of end-to-end anastomosis. *A.* The posterior row of interrupted nonabsorbable seromuscular sutures is being inserted. *B.* The all-coat continuous layer of catgut sutures is placed in the posterior wall of the anastomosis. *C.* The all-coat catgut layer is continued anteriorly. *D.* The anterior interrupted layer of nonabsorbable sutures is completed.

obstructing mass. Vaginal examination may further help in abdominal evaluation. With small bowel obstruction there is severe colicky, poorly localized, midabdominal pain with vomiting. The amount of distention increases as the level of obstruction approaches the ileocecal valve, and there may still be bowel movements. With simple colonic obstruction there may not have been a bowel movement for many days; there is marked distention, and pain is often not severe and is poorly localized to the lower midabdomen. Often there is no emesis.

Strangulation of the bowel is a serious complication that markedly increases mortality. Signs of strangulation are deterioration in the patient's general condition, fever over 38° C, and tachycardia. With the onset of strangulation the intermittent crampy pain of simple obstruction becomes more severe and more constant. On abdominal examination there is increasing tenderness with guarding and rigidity and signs of involvement of the parietal peritoneum in the inflammatory process.

Laboratory Procedures. The hematocrit, BUN, and electrolytes help in the initial assessment of the fluid and electrolyte status. There may be considerable hemoconcentration from loss of fluids and electrolytes, and the electrolytes may therefore be normal or even increased in the presence of marked electrolyte depletion. There is usually little change in acid-base balance because emesis results in loss of hydrogen ion from the stomach and base from the intestinal secretions. Leukocytosis is present when strangulation occurs. The total white cell count must be interpreted in relation to hemoconcentration.

Roentgenography. An upright or lateral decubitus x-ray of the abdomen is the most important investigation in acute intestinal obstruction. Positive findings include free air under the diaphragm, indicating perforation, gaseous distention, air-fluid levels, and edematous loops of bowel (Figure 23–1). The radiologic and typical findings may be pathognomonic as in gallstone ileus or a volvulus (Figure 23–2). A barium enema indicates the site of a large bowel obstruction.

Small bowel obstruction is diagnosed on x-ray by the presence of valvulae conniventes in the distended loops and the absence of cecal distention. In colonic obstruction haustrae can be seen in the distended colon, and small bowel may also be distended. Mechanical obstruction usually presents a small number of loops that are distended, while in paralytic ileus numerous loops including both the large and small bowel are involved and air is often seen in the rectum.

Treatment

Intravenous fluids are given to restore extracellular losses.[3] Operation may be postponed for

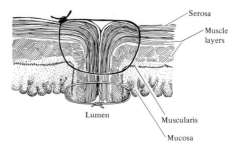

Figure 23–6. The completed anastomosis shows the deep all-coat continuous layer of catgut sutures and the outer interrupted seromuscular sutures.

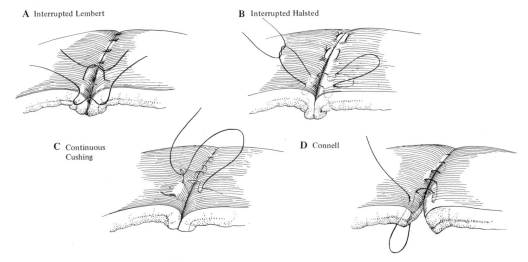

A Interrupted Lembert

B Interrupted Halsted

C Continuous
   Cushing

D Connell

Figure 23–7.   A number of different stitches can be used for the anastomosis. *A.* A simple end-on seromuscular suture can be used. *B.* The Halsted stitch is a horizontal seromuscular mattress stitch. *C.* A Cushing stitch is similar to the Halsted but continuous. *D.* A Connell suture resembles the Cushing except that it penetrates all layers of the bowel.

several hours while intravenous solutions are given. If there is evidence of strangulation, resuscitation should be as rapid as possible, and in addition to fluids and electrolytes, plasma, albumin, or blood may be required. Central venous pressure monitoring, especially in older patients and those with preexisting cardiac disease, is essential when large volumes of intravenous fluids are required. A catheter passed into the bladder is necessary to accurately measure urine output.

A nasogastric tube is passed to relieve distention by removal of fluid and gas (Figure 23–3). In certain circumstances it may be possible to pass a longer tube, such as a Cantor or Miller-Abbott tube, into the small intestine to the level of the obstruction. These tubes are 2 to 3 meters long and have a balloon on the distal end. When filled, the balloon acts as a bolus and is propelled along by peristalsis. It is best to use fluoroscopy to direct the tube through the pylorus so that it may pass freely through the small intestine. However, retrograde peristalsis often makes passage of the tube impossible. With the tube in the small bowel it may be necessary to pass a nasogastric tube into the stomach for proximal decompression. These tubes should only be used in limited circumstances, such as recurrent bowel obstruction from adhesions, in postoperative bowel obstruction, and in extremely ill patients. They are of no value in paralytic obstruction.

A number of patients with acute intestinal obstruction are kept under observation and only operated on if the obstruction does not resolve spontaneously or if there are signs of impaired blood supply to the bowel. Acute obstruction is frequent about two weeks after laparotomy, is usually due to fibrinous adhesions, and generally settles on conservative management. Adhesions may cause acute obstruction at any time after laparotomy. A trial period of conservative management is justifiable provided that the patient is examined frequently. Generally patients with acute intestinal obstruction who have not had a previous operation should be treated surgically.

Antibiotics. Antibiotics are given intravenously before operation in those with strangulated bowel or peritonitis. They are not indicated in simple obstruction.

Operation.   Operation is directed to relieve the obstruction by division of adhesions, reduction and repair of a hernia, and resection or bypass of an obstructing lesion.

In those with strangulated bowel special measures prevent contamination of the peritoneal cavity by the bowel content. Packs are inserted into the peritoneal cavity, and suction and intestinal clamps prevent escape of intestinal contents and facilitate their prompt removal. The obstruction is relieved and the bowel resected if it is gangrenous. Often the viability of the bowel is in doubt. Moist warm packs are then placed around it for at least 10 minutes. The changes in the appearance of the bowel are often dramatic. A segment which was congested, dark, and without peristalsis frequently becomes pink, develops pulsations in the vessels of the mesentery, becomes bright and shiny

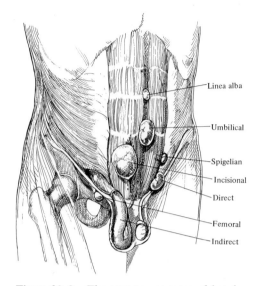

Linea alba

Umbilical

Spigelian

Incisional

Direct

Femoral

Indirect

Figure 23–8. The commonest external hernias are the inguinal (direct and indirect), femoral, umbilical, and incisional. A hernia through the linea alba above the umbilicus (epigastric hernia) is less frequent. A hernia at the lateral border of the rectus muscle (spigelian hernia) is uncommon.

on its serosal surface, and transmits contraction waves. Decompression of the intestine with reduction of intraluminal pressure to normal often dramatically improves the blood supply. If these changes fail to occur, the bowel has undergone necrosis and the segment must be removed (Figures 23–4 to 23–7).

Strangulation of the omentum is treated by excision.

Specific Bowel Obstructions

Neonatal Obstructions. The cause of intestinal obstruction in the neonate is often suggested by the age. Esophageal atresia, duodenal atresia, and volvulus neonatorum present at or within a few days of birth, while pyloric stenosis occurs most often at about three weeks (see Chapter 35).

Intussusception. Intussusception is invagination of one part of the intestine into another. It occurs most commonly in infants and may result from lymphoid hyperplasia (see Chapter 35). In older children and adults a neoplasm is usually present at the apex of the intussusception.[8] The patient presents with acute or recurrent bowel obstruction, often with the passage of blood per rectum.

Foreign Bodies. Foreign bodies are a common cause of intestinal obstruction in patients institutionalized for mental retardation and psychiatric diseases. The most frequent is the phytobezoar from eating hair. Ascaris worm infestation may lead to small bowel obstruction.

Gallstone Ileus. Gallstone ileus accounts for only 1 to 2 percent of all mechanical obstructions (see Chapter 19). However, in patients over 65, gallstones are responsible for 20 percent of small bowel obstructions. The death rate is five to ten times higher than for other types of intestinal obstruction because the diagnosis is often made late.[1,6]

There is often a recent history of acute abdominal pain, nausea, emesis, and elevation of temperature indicating acute cholecystitis. A single large stone ulcerates through the gallbladder wall into the duodenum and passes through the intestines where it often impacts about 6 cm from the ileocecal valve. A flat film of the abdomen may, in addition to showing signs of acute obstruction, reveal a stone in the right lower quadrant and gas in the biliary tract indicating the presence of the cholecystoduodenal fistula.

Fecal Impaction. This is a common cause of acute left colonic obstruction, especially in elderly patients and the mentally retarded. It may also occur in those who do not have all the barium removed after an upper gastrointestinal series or barium enema. The hard fecal mass can often be broken up digitally by a finger in the rectum and the colon evacuated by enemata. Rarely is it necessary to operate and remove the feces by colotomy.

Neoplasms. Neoplasms of the small intestine are a rare cause of obstruction (see Chapter 21). Benign lesions are usually found incidentally at laparotomy while malignant tumors more commonly cause symptoms. Polypoid tumors may cause intussusception. A malignant neoplasm is the most common cause of large bowel obstruction (see Chapter 22). Treatment is directed to relief of acute obstruction and removal of the tumor.

Volvulus. Volvulus is a twisting of the bowel, including its blood supply. There are both a closed loop obstruction with marked distention of the rotated segment and mechanical obstruction of the proximal bowel. The early onset of strangulation makes this a particularly dangerous form of obstruction. It occurs most commonly in the sigmoid colon but is also found in the stomach, small intestine, and cecum. Volvulus of the colon is the result of excessive mobility of the colon associated with a high-roughage diet (see Chapter 22). Volvulus of the stomach occurs in hypermobile stomachs that are associated with paraesophageal hernias (see Chapter 16). Midgut volvulus occurs in the neonate because of a defect in the mesenteric fixation associated with malrotation of the gut

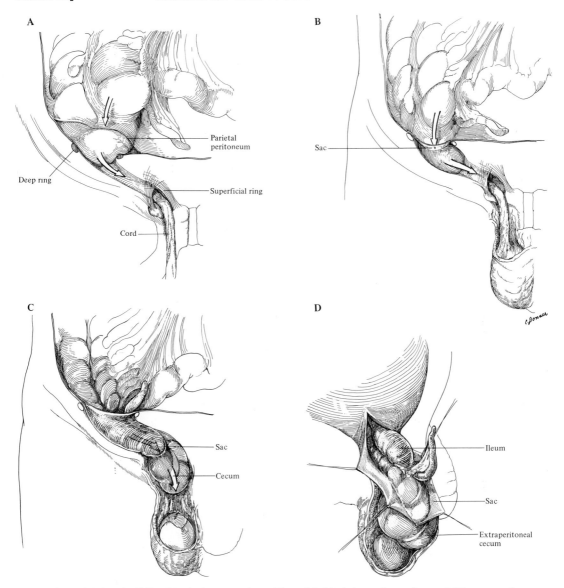

Figure 23–9.   A sliding hernia is protrusion of bowel behind the peritoneal sac. *A*. The cecum is commencing its descent to the groin in an extraperitoneal position. *B*. The bowel has passed through the internal ring with the peritoneal sac following its descent. *C*. The cecum has entered the scrotum uncovered by peritoneum and could readily be mistaken for a hernial sac at operation. *D*. Bowel has now descended into the true hernial sac anterior to the sliding hernia.

and failure of the cecum to descend (see Chapter 35). The mesentery consists of a narrow pedicle around which the intestine rotates, usually in a clockwise direction. The syndrome occurs mainly in infancy and rarely in adults. Epigastric distention, pain, and bile emesis are the common features. Strangulation is common and early operation is indicated.

Crohn's Disease.   Crohn's disease may cause intestinal obstruction at any level from the duodenum to the rectum (see Chapter 21). The obstruction may be due to edema, intramural fibrosis, adhesions, or abscess formation. At operation the involved segment is either by-passed or resected.

Diverticular Disease of the Colon.   Diverticulitis of the sigmoid colon may present as a large bowel obstruction (see Chapter 22). There may be a previous history of intermittent attacks of pain in the left lower quadrant and

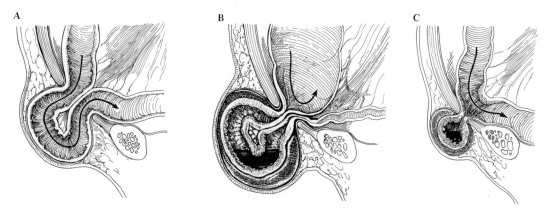

A   B   C

Figure 23–10. *A.* Small intestine is in the hernial sac, but the lumen is not obstructed and the blood supply to the bowel is normal. *B.* The hernia is now irreducible, its lumen is obstructed, and the blood supply to the bowel has been cut off. There is blood-stained fluid in the hernial sac, the wall is dark and thickened, and there is blood in the lumen. There is acute intestinal obstruction with marked distention of the proximal bowel. *C.* The wall of the bowel is strangulated, but the lumen of the bowel is not obstructed (Richter's hernia).

fever. On examination the abdomen is distended with a palpable tender mass in the left lower quadrant. Occasionally the site of obstruction is a loop of small bowel adherent to the inflamed colon. A diverting proximal colostomy relieves the obstruction, but primary resection of the involved colon is gaining in popularity.

Adhesions. About two thirds of small bowel obstructions are due to adhesions, whereas large bowel obstruction secondary to adhesions is uncommon. Predisposing factors are peritonitis, pelvic procedures, extensive dissections, talc or starch glove powder, and multiple operations. Occasionally adhesions may be present with no known predisposing cause.

The diagnosis of acute obstruction secondary to adhesions is made on the basis of history of previous operations or intra-abdominal infection. Conservative treatment is indicated, and operation is performed if the obstruction persists or there are signs of impaired blood supply to the bowel. Surgical treatment is directed to dividing the adhesive bands causing the obstruction. The essential part of the procedure is to define the region where there is a junction between dilated and collapsed bowel. If the bowel is markedly dilated, a needle attached to suction may be inserted for decompression.

Ischemic Enteritis and Colitis. Obstruction to the blood supply or a low-flow state may cause intestinal obstruction without mechanical obstruction of the lumen (see Chapter 22). The superior mesenteric artery may obstruct the third part of the duodenum in normal individuals and more often in those who are malnourished and confined to bed. The patient has

intermittent attacks of epigastric pain and often vomiting. On barium x-ray there is obstruction at the middle of the third part of the duodenum. Conservative treatment is tube decompression, antispasmodics, intravenous fluids, and elevation of the foot of the bed. Duodenojejunostomy is the best operative procedure.[2,7]

Paralytic Ileus. Paralytic or adynamic ileus occurs from lack of intestinal motility (see Chapter 14). The common causes are peritonitis, bowel resection, and retroperitoneal hemorrhage.

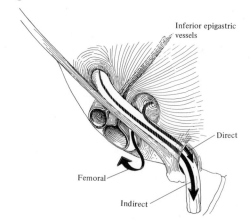

Figure 23–11. The paths of hernias. An indirect hernia passes with the cord through the internal ring and tends to descend into the scrotum. The direct hernia arises medial to the epigastric vessels and has less tendency to enter the scrotum than the indirect inguinal hernia. A femoral hernia lies below and lateral to the pubic tubercle and produces a lateral and upward impulse on coughing.

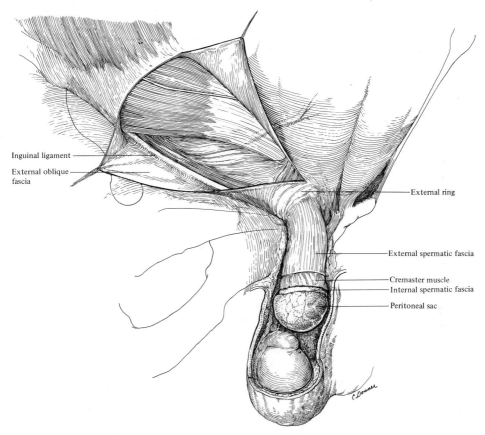

Inguinal ligament

External oblique fascia

External ring

External spermatic fascia

Cremaster muscle
Internal spermatic fascia
Peritoneal sac

Figure 23–12.   The anatomy of an indirect inguinal hernia is shown. Note the order of the layers as they enter the scrotum.

HERNIA

A hernia is an abnormal protrusion of the contents of a cavity through its wall at the site of a congenital defect or of weak fibrous and muscular tissues. Abdominal hernias are external or internal and may be reducible or irreducible. The hernia may be irreducible because of adhesions or because of the presence of obstructed bowel. When bowel obstruction is complicated by vascular impairment, strangulation is said to have occurred. The incidence of external abdominal hernias is indirect inguinal 60 percent, direct inguinal 15 percent, umbilical and incisional, each 9 percent, while femoral and epigastric hernias each occur in only about 3 percent (Figure 23–8).

Congenital defects account for most indirect inguinal hernias, the umbilical hernia in the infant, and certain types of diaphragmatic hernia. Some may present with respiratory distress as a neonatal emergency, such as exomphalos or diaphragmatic hernia. An irreducible hernia may result from adhesions between the sac and its contents, especially with

an umbilical hernia. A hernia may also be irreducible because it is a sliding hernia (Figure 23–9). A portion of bowel, usually the cecum or sigmoid colon, has descended in an extra-peritoneal position and forms the posterior wall of the inguinal hernial sac. Obstruction occurs when a segment of small bowel descends into the sac and is unable to return to the peritoneal cavity due to the presence of a constricting ring at the neck of the sac. Strangulation occurs as progressive swelling interferes with the venous return and later the arterial inflow. The bowel, omentum, or rarely the ovary may become strangulated. When part of the circumference is strangulated but the lumen is not obstructed, the clinical features of acute intestinal obstruction are absent (Figure 23–10). The diagnosis may not be made until peritonitis has developed.

External Hernias

Indirect Inguinal.   An indirect inguinal hernia lies in the inguinal canal, its neck lateral to the inferior epigastric vessels. With enlargement it

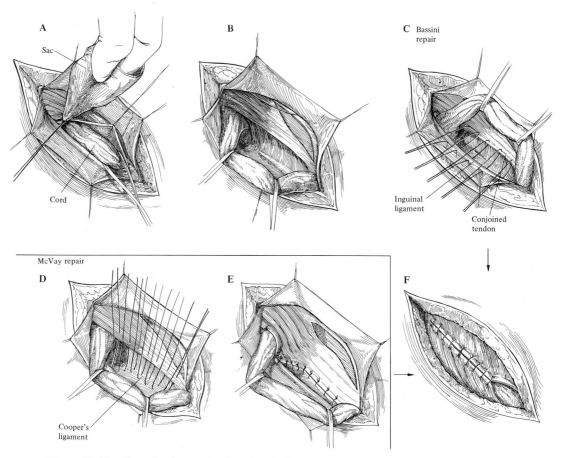

Figure 23–13. Steps in the repair of an inguinal hernia. *A.* In the Bassini repair the external oblique aponeurosa is divided and the indirect hernial sac removed. *B.* The conjoined tendon and inguinal ligament are exposed. A relaxing incision can be made to allow the conjoined tendon to reach the inguinal ligament. *C.* The posterior wall of the canal is reinforced with interrupted sutures placed between the conjoined tendon and fascia transversalis and the inguinal ligament. Frequently the conjoined tendon is not present. Sutures are then inserted through the lower muscular margins of the internal oblique and transversus abdominis muscles. *D.* In the McVay repair the fascia transversalis is divided and the sutures placed between the conjoined tendon and fascia transversalis and Cooper's ligament on the ileopectineal line. *E.* The most lateral sutures approximate and then include the inguinal ligament. *F.* With both repairs the external oblique is closed anterior to the cord.

passes above and medial to the pubic tubercle into the scrotum (Figures 23–11 and 23–12). Most are probably the result of failure of the processus vaginalis to close and may be present at birth or develop later spontaneously or after a sudden stress (see Chapter 35). They are commoner in males than females and present most often in childhood or early adult life.

The patient may present with a bulge in the groin that may or may not be painful. On coughing the hernia tends to descend into the scrotum and can be kept reduced by pressing over the internal inguinal ring midway between the anterior superior iliac spine and the pubic tubercle.

The indirect inguinal hernia has to be differentiated from a direct inguinal hernia, femoral hernia, scrotal swellings, such as hydrocele and varicocele, enlarged inguinal nodes, and a varix of the long saphenous vein.

A truss can maintain reduction of an indirect inguinal hernia but is only for those in whom operation is contraindicated. Operative repair in the infant consists of removal of the sac; in the child and young adult the internal ring is also tightened, and in the adult the posterior wall of the inguinal canal needs to be reinforced (Figure 23–13). In elderly men with large inguinoscrotal hernias orchiectomy may be indicated because the operation can be per-

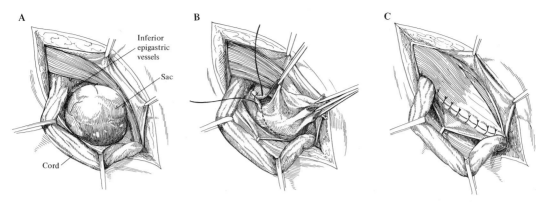

Figure 23–14. *A*. A direct inguinal hernia is seen in the posterior wall of the inguinal canal. *B*. The sac is excised or may be left in position. *C*. Repair is performed suturing the conjoined tendon to the inguinal ligament. Medially, sutures are inserted through the anterior rectus sheath, and, laterally, they are placed in the lower margins of the internal oblique and transversus abdominis muscles.

formed more rapidly and the inguinal canal can be completely closed, as in the female. The presence of a sliding hernia must always be suspected in those with large, especially irreducible hernias. The overall recurrence rate should be less than 1 percent.

Direct Inguinal. A direct inguinal hernia is situated medial to the deep epigastric vessels and is due to acquired weakness in the posterior wall of the inguinal canal. It occurs in older patients, is rare in females, seldom obstructs, and rarely descends into the scrotum. On examination the rupture projects forward on coughing, usually reduced spontaneously on lying down, and is not kept reduced on coughing when the pressure is applied over the internal ring. A careful history and physical examination must be performed to rule out important causes of increased abdominal pressure, such as obstruction of the colon, retention of urine from prostatic disease, and ascites. In some centers sigmoidoscopy is performed in patients over 40 years.[5]

Intestinal obstruction is a less frequent complication of a direct than an indirect hernia. A portion of the bladder frequently descends on the medial wall of the hernia, and a sliding hernia is not uncommon. At operation it is important to reinforce the weak posterior wall of the inguinal canal (Figure 23–14). Removal of the sac is not important.

Femoral. A femoral hernia occurs where the deep lymphatics ascend from the thigh. The hernia presents as a mass below and lateral to the pubic tubercle and lies medial to the femoral vein in the femoral canal (Figure 23–15). Femoral hernia is more frequent in woman than men; however, inguinal hernia is more frequent in women than a femoral hernia. There is a marked tendency for a femoral hernia to become strangulated because of the sharp boundaries to the femoral canal formed by the lacunar ligament medially, the inguinal ligament anteriorly, and Cooper's ligament posteriorly. A femoral hernia often presents as a Richter's hernia. It may then present as general peritonitis of unknown origin if the hernia is not palpable in an obese patient. An enlarged inguinal lymph node or a varix at the termination of the long saphenous vein is particularly

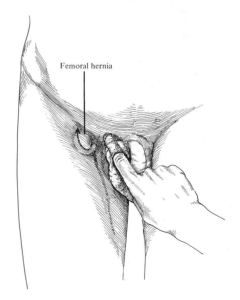

Figure 23–15. The femoral hernia lies below and lateral to the pubic tubercle. Its path curves upward.

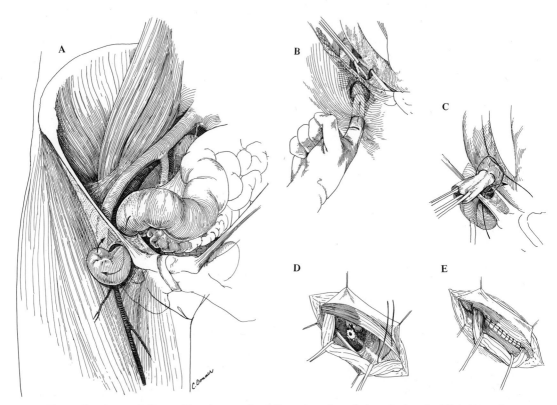

Figure 23–16. *A*. A femoral hernia must be delivered up from below the inguinal ligament after division of the external oblique and fascia transversalis in the posterior wall of the inguinal canal. *B*. The sac is being delivered above the inguinal ligament. *C*. The hernial sac is transfixed and excised. *D*. Repair is performed, suturing the inguinal ligament to the fascia on the ileopectineal line. *E*. Repair of the posterior wall of the canal has been completed, suturing the conjoint tendon to Cooper's ligament on the ileopectineal line.

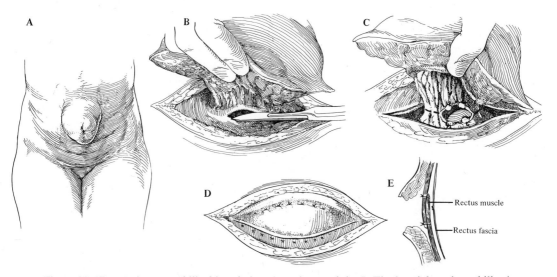

Figure 23–17. *A*. A paraumbilical hernia is present in an adult. *B*. The hernial sac is mobilized. *C*. The neck of the sac is incised, and the hernia, including the umbilicus, is removed. *D*. A two-layer overlap repair is performed using nonabsorbable sutures. *E*. This is a side view of the repair.

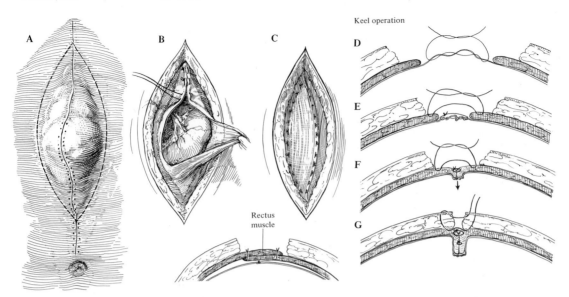

Figure 23–18. Steps *A*, *B*, and *C* show excision and repair of an incisional hernia. *D*, *E*, *F*, and *G* show details of placing the sutures in the Keel operation. In this operation the peritoneal cavity is not opened and the sac is not excised. The sac is invaginated into the abdomen, followed by the muscles and fascia at the margins of the defect.

liable to be mistaken for a femoral hernia (Figure 31–12, page 559). A truss is of no value because the inguinal region moves on walking. Operation consists of dividing the external oblique and the fascia transversalis in the posterior wall of the inguinal canal (Figure 23–16). The hernial sac is then excised. Repair is performed by suturing the internal oblique and transversus abdominis to Cooper's ligament along the ileopectineal line.

Umbilical. A true umbilical hernia occurs through the defect created by the umbilical vessels. It is an extremely common hernia and usually disappears spontaneously by two years. Intestinal obstruction is a rare complication. The local application of pads to keep the hernia reduced is of no value. The occasional hernia that persists should be operated on after three to four years. Surgical repair is closure of the fascial defect with preservation of the umbilicus.

An umbilical hernia in an adult is really a paraumbilical hernia through the linea alba above or below the umbilicus. It tends to occur after 40 years and is often associated with obesity. Extraperitoneal fat herniates through the linea alba at the site of penetration of a blood vessel and is followed by a peritoneal sac. As the hernia enlarges there is a marked tendency for the peritoneum lining the sac to atrophy. Intestine or omentum then adheres to the wall, and the hernia frequently becomes irreducible or partly reducible. Because of the adhesions intestinal obstruction is frequent. Abdominal

hernias in the adult should therefore be treated by operation (Figure 23–17). Redundant fat is removed generally along with the umbilicus and the hernial sac excised. Care is taken in mobilizing gut from the wall of the sac to avoid opening into bowel. Repair is performed by overlapping the upper and lower portions of the rectus sheath in a "vest over pants" manner using a double layer of sutures. Occasionally the defect is so large that a sheet of prosthetic material has to be inserted.

Epigastric. The epigastric or linea alba hernia occurs through a defect in the midline of the epigastrium. The sac is small and most often contains the omentum. The pain and discomfort caused by the small hernia may be confused with peptic ulcer disease. Treatment is operative repair.

Incisional. The factors predisposing to incisional hernia are wound infection, increased intra-abdominal pressure from paralytic ileus, ascites, and coughing, poor surgical technique, and constitutional factors such as hypoproteinemia, old age, and the use of steroids. There is a marked tendency for the wall of the sac to become atrophied; therefore adhesions are frequent between the sac and the omentum or intestine. Strangulation is liable to occur, especially in those with a sharp, well-defined margin to the defect. Incisional hernias should be treated by operation except in those with a diffuse bulge, as for example after a renal incision when there is often a defect extending from the costal margin to the iliac crest (Figure 23–18).

Internal Hernias

Internal hernias are an uncommon cause of intestinal obstruction or peritonitis. Congenital hernias may be present at the root of the mesentery of the sigmoid colon, at the ileocecal valve, and around the ligament of Treitz. A hole in the mesentery may allow bowel to pass through. Herniation of the intestines through the foramen of Winslow into the lesser sac is rare. The patient with an internal hernia generally presents with acute intestinal obstruction or general peritonitis. Treatment is operative relief of the obstruction and closure of the hernial defect.

Diaphragmatic Hernias

Hiatal. Sliding hiatal and paraesophageal hernias are common and are discussed elsewhere (see Chapter 18). Traumatic rupture of the diaphragm is frequently the result of closed and penetrating upper abdominal injury (see Chapter 9). Hernia through the foramen of Bochdalek, a congenital defect in the posterolateral portion of the diaphragm, may present as acute respiratory distress in the neonate (see Chapter 35). The foramen of Morgagni, located anteriorly in the parasternal region, is a rare congenital cause of diaphragmatic hernia.

CITED REFERENCES

1. Anderson, R. E.; Woodward, N.; Diffenbough, W. G.; and Strohl, E. L.: Gallstone obstruction of the intestine. *Surg. Gynecol. Obstet.*, **125**:540–48, 1967.
2. Barner, H. B., and Sherman, C. D., Jr.: Vascular compression of the duodenum. *Surg. Gynecol. Obstet.*, **117**:1–16, 1963.
3. Billig, D. M., and Jordan, P. H., Jr.: Hemodynamic abnormalities secondary to extracellular fluid depletion in intestinal obstruction. *Surg. Gynecol. Obstet.*, **127**:1274–82, 1969.
4. Floyd, C. E., and Coh, I., Jr.: Obstruction in cancer of the colon. *Ann. Surg.*, **165**:721–31, 1967.
5. Patton, J. J., and Benfield, J. R.: Evaluation of routine barium enema and proctosigmoidoscopy before hernia repair. *Rev. Surg.*, **27**:145, 1970.
6. Safoei-Shirozi, S.; Zike, W. L.; and Printen, K. J.: Spontaneous enterobiliary fistulas. *Surg. Gynecol. Obstet.*, **137**:769–72, 1973.
7. Strong, E. K.: Mechanics of arteriomesenteric duodenal obstruction and direct surgical attack upon etiology. *Ann. Surg.*, **148**:725–30, 1958.
8. Stubenbord, W. T., and Thorbjarnasson, B.: Intussusception in adults. *Ann. Surg.*, **172**:306–10, 1970.

SUGGESTIONS FOR
FURTHER READING

Nyhus, L. M., and Harkins, H. N.: *Hernia*. J. B. Lippincott, Philadelphia, 1964.
Describes techniques of hernia repair.
Wagensteen, O. H.: *Intestinal Obstructions*, 3rd ed. Charles C Thomas, Springfield, Ill., 1955.
Although this book needs to be updated, it is a classical review of the subject of intestinal obstruction.
Zimmerman, L. M. (ed.): Symposium on surgery of hernia. *Clin. Surg. North Am.*, **51**:1247–1421. W. B. Saunders Co., Philadelphia, 1971.
All aspects of surgical management of hernias are discussed.

Chapter 24

LYMPHORETICULAR SYSTEM

William R. Jewell and *Loren J. Humphrey*

CHAPTER OUTLINE

Lymphatic System
  Anatomy
  Physiology
  Clinical Lymph Node Enlargement
    Clinical Evaluation
    Lymphangiography
    Treatment
  Lymphedema
  Lymphomas
    Classification
    Stages
    Clinical Evaluation
    Treatment
Spleen
  Anatomy
  Physiology
  Indications for Splenectomy

Trauma
Hypersplenism
Primary Hypersplenism
  Congenital Hemolytic Anemia
  Primary Splenic Neutropenia
  Acquired Hemolytic Anemia
  Primary Idiopathic Thrombocytopenia
Secondary Hypersplenism
Other Conditions
Splenectomy
Thymus
Anatomy
Physiology
Thymic Tumors
Myasthenia Gravis
Transplantation
Thymectomy

The lymphoreticular system includes the five secondary immunologic organs, the lymph nodes, spleen, Kupffer cells in the liver, bone marrow, and the lymphoid tissues in the alimentary tract (see Chapter 4). Their primary functions are defense against foreign organisms and materials and removal of dead cells. They contain B-cell lymphocytes that give rise to plasma cells and are responsible for the humoral immune response, T-cells that are responsible for cellular immunity, and large mononuclear phagocytic cells that take up foreign materials and effete erythrocytes.

LYMPHATIC SYSTEM

The lymphatic system is a complex system of ducts and nodes that provides an interface between the blood vascular circulation and tissue fluid (Figure 24–1). Of its many functions, the roles played in infections and the spread of malignant tumors are of particular importance to the surgeon.

Anatomy

The functional unit of the lymphatic system is the lymph node with its afferent and efferent ducts (see Chapter 4 and Figure 24–2). Lymph from the afferent ducts enters a reticular reservoir, the subcapsular sinus, and then passes slowly through cortical internodal and then the medullary sinuses and leaves in efferent lymphatics. Numerous capillaries and post-capillary venules, mainly in the nonfollicular regions of the cortex and the primary follicles, provide an important blood-lymph interface. Most germinal centers and each medullary cord possess a central blood vessel. Lymphatics tend to have a similar distribution to blood vessels. They are absent in the central nervous system and cartilage.

Physiology

Lymph is formed by the filtering of fluid from vascular capillaries and postcapillary venules into the interstitial space. Plasma electrolytes and other small molecules pass readily through

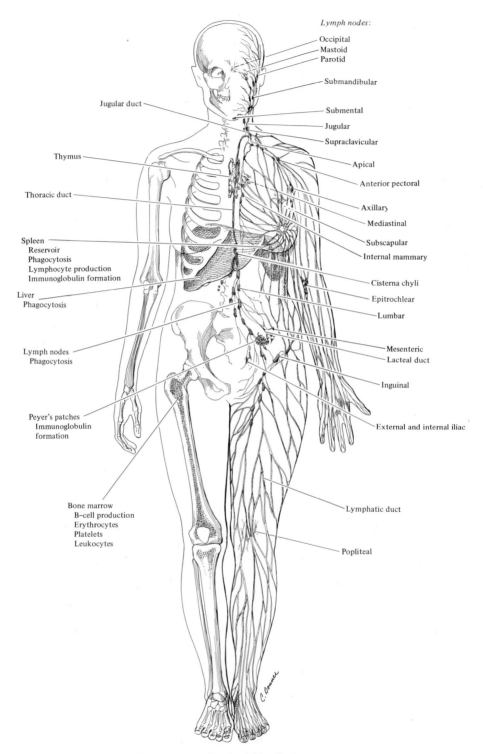

Figure 24–1.   The lymphoreticular system.

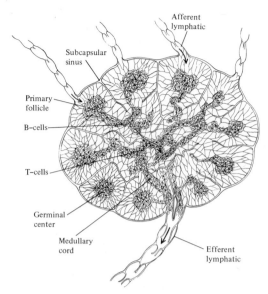

Figure 24–2. Although T-cells and B-cells are not produced by the lymph nodes, they are found there. B-cells are located in primary follicles and medullary cords and T-cells in the deep cortical zone. The flow of lymph is indicated by the arrows.

intercellular pores in the vascular endothelium and maintain concentrations in the extracellular spaces almost identical to plasma. Larger molecules, for example albumin, leave the blood vessels at a slower rate. Therefore the concentration of albumin in the interstitial fluid is about one fourth that in plasma, and the larger globulin molecules are present in even smaller quantities. Since the product of cations and anions is the same on both sides of the semipermeable vascular membrane, the concentration of the anions, HCO_3^- and Cl^-, is lower and that of the cations, Na^+, K^+, Ca^{++}, and Mg^{++}, is slightly higher within the blood vessels than in the interstitial fluid (Donnan and Gibbs law, see Chapter 3). The interstitial fluids pass readily through the large openings in the walls of the lymphatics. Lymph therefore has nearly identical concentrations of electrolytes and proteins as interstitial fluid. The lymphatics in the small intestine play an important role in the transmission of the products of fat digestion to the vascular system. The chylomicrons they contain after a fatty meal result in the lacteals having a whitish-yellow color (lacteals—see Chapter 21). Lymph is moved through the lymphatic channels to the lymph nodes by interstitial tissue pressure generated by muscle contraction and by pressure transmitted from the vascular system. The lymph may pass through several sets of nodes or may

bypass nodes entirely. The lymphatic channels enlarge progressively to end in two or more major ducts to enter the great veins at the root of the neck. Lymph from the right upper extremity and right side of the head and neck enters the right subclavian vein via the right lymphatic duct. All other lymph enters the left subclavian vein through the thoracic duct. Lymph can also enter small blood vessels through numerous intercommunications between lymphatics and small blood vessels. The volume of lymph entering the vascular system per day is approximately equal to the plasma volume.

With movement through the node foreign materials and bacteria are removed by fixed macrophages in the cortex and the medulla. The regional nodes play an important role in the immune response, particularly with its initiation (see Chapter 4). Foreign antigens are carried in the lymph to the nodes and sensitize specific lymphocytes. Long-lived thymus-dependent ("T") lymphocytes that have been sensitized in the tissues enter the nodes from the lymphatics. The sensitized lymphocytes transform in the nodes, giving rise to lymphoblasts with cytotoxic potentiality. The T-cells are responsible for cell-mediated immunity. Examples are the delayed hypersensitivity reaction to tubercle bacillus, dinitrochlorobenzene, chronic rejection of a tissue homograft, and the cell-mediated resistance to cancer. The T-cells produce humoral mediators that help activate specific lymphocytes produced in the bone marrow. These B-cells transform in the nodes and produce plasma cells and more B-cells. There is initially rapid production by the plasma cells of IgM (19S, M.W. 900,000), followed by slower but more prolonged production of IgG (7S, M.W. 150,000). After the initial or primary response a population of committed lymphocytes with "memory" for the particular antigen remains. Should the lymphoid complex again be exposed to the same antigen, a faster and more pronounced secondary antibody response follows due to the presence of many "memory" cells. It is likely that antigen processing by sinusoidal cells and their reaction against the antigen are important steps in both cellular and humoral immunity. Individual lymph nodes contain both T- and B-cells and can therefore produce both cellular and humoral responses. Immunologic memory does not remain in one node but is soon present in distant parts of the lymphoreticular system.

Clinical Lymph Node Enlargement

Clinical Evaluation. A carefully taken history and physical examination will often provide the diagnosis in patients with enlarged lymph nodes. Laboratory and x-ray studies should be carefully selected for each patient.

In those with no obvious tumor or infection a distal focus of infection or tumor may provide the reason for nodal enlargement. It is often difficult to differentiate enlargement due to chronic infection from neoplastic enlargement. An important differentiating point is pain. An infected node is usually painful and tender, whereas nodes containing metastatic carcinoma or a lymphoma are usually not. Generally it is wise to remove suspicious nodes if after completing relevant investigations the reason for enlargement is not obvious. Location of an enlarged node is often significant. For example, a patient with an enlarged node in the supraclavicular triangle should be fully investigated for a source of metastatic carcinoma or lymphoma, as chronic infection is uncommon in this site. A single enlarged node in the midneck may contain metastases from thyroid carcinoma or squamous cell carcinoma in the head and neck area. Infection occurs more frequently in upper cervical than lower cervical nodes. An infection in a tooth socket, tonsil, nasopharynx, or nasal sinus is a common cause of enlargement of a single or multiple nodes in the upper neck. Tuberculosis in the neck most often presents with enlargement of a node just behind the angle of the jaw. Lymphoma should always be considered whenever solitary or multiple nodal enlargement occurs in any location in the neck. Carcinomas in the mouth, pharynx, and larynx may produce metastases in cervical nodes at any level (Figure 16–4, page 276). Enlargement of single or multiple axillary nodes may be the result of infection originating in the forearm, arm, or especially the fingers. Epitrochlear nodal enlargement is rare. In women occult carcinoma of the breast must be excluded. The assessment of enlarged inguinal nodes is difficult because they are often palpable in normal people. The portal for infection or source of metastatic disease may be in the anal region, perineum, or legs. A small or nonpigmented melanoma may not be clinically recognized but may produce metastases in inguinal nodes.

Hodgkin's disease often presents as multiple discrete nodes, which are nontender and rubbery in consistency. As the disease progresses, the nodes become firmer and matted to one another. In patients with lymphosarcoma the nodes can become extremely large, although they tend to remain soft, and ulceration may occur. The nodes tend to become adherent, hard, and calcified in tuberculosis. In the subacute phase they develop central necrosis and may produce an abscess (see Chapter 6).

Lymphangiography. Lymphangiography is useful in investigating patients with lymphomas due to the presence of large, foamy cells which often replace the entire node. Its use to determine the presence of metastases in nodes from carcinomas and malignant melanomas has been disappointing, because of the high incidence of false negative and positive results. Small deposits of malignant cells, which are common, are often too small to be seen, and hyperplastic nodes are not only enlarged but may have filling defects suggesting tumor involvement. However, lymphangiography can at times be useful in demonstrating nodal involvement above the level of planned resection, for example metastases in the para-aortic nodes in a patient with a malignant melanoma in the leg. When possible involvement exists beyond the extent of planned resection, a biopsy should be performed. Lymphangiography should never be relied upon to exclude the feasibility of radical lymphadenectomy. Another use of lymphangiography is to demonstrate the completeness of a radical lymphadenectomy. As the dye remains in the nodes for several weeks, an x-ray taken at the time of operation reveals any residual lymph nodes. Also, chlorophyll injected with the radiopaque material makes the nodes readily visible by the surgeon.

The technique of lymphangiography is simple but requires considerable skill and patience. The vessels are so small in the hand that its use is confined to the lower extremity. Methylene blue dye is injected subcutaneously into a digital web interspace in the foot, an incision is made, a lymphatic is chosen, and a small polyethylene catheter is inserted into the vessel. Radiopaque dye is slowly injected with a mechanical pump, and serial x-rays of the node-bearing areas are taken for 48 hours or longer.

Complications of lymphangiography are infection of the incision or the dorsum of the foot, iodine hypersensitivity, and pulmonary embolism from the oily dye.

Treatment. *Drainage.* Acutely inflamed lymph nodes are treated by antibiotics and operative drainage when pus is present (see Chapter 6).

Node Biopsy. An enlarged node should be excised for histologic examination when the reason for enlargement is not clear. When adenopathy occurs secondary to a known distal infection, biopsy is not necessary, providing the nodes decrease in size as the infection subsides. At times, particularly with cervical node enlargement, it is difficult to be certain whether or not an infection is the cause of the adenopathy. For example, some patients present with a vague history of a sore throat or a low-grade dental infection of long duration associated with enlargement of a node. A broad-spectrum antibiotic should be given for three weeks. If significant regression does not occur, the node should be removed. Generally, excisional biopsy is favored to minimize wound contamination and to give the pathologist an adequate amount of tissue for examination. Incisional biopsy or needle biopsy may be used when the node is found in the deeper structures (Figure 7-7, page 147).

Radical Lymphadenectomy. Nodes considered clinically to contain metastases should be excised, provided that there are no distant metastases and the primary tumor can be completely removed at the same operation or has previously been successfully treated by operation or radiotherapy. Views differ on the prophylactic excision of regional nodes (see Chapter 7, page 149). Generally, the authors recommend the routine removal of regional nodes in breast carcinoma and for melanoma of an extremity.

Lymphedema

Lymphedema is the accumulation of excessive lymph in the interstitial space. The causes are congenital deficiencies of the lymphatic system or acquired lymphatic obstruction.

Congenital lymphedema may involve one or both lower extremities and is the result of an absence or a decrease in functional lymphatic vessels. The swelling may occur at birth or in later life and is more common in females than males. Conservative management consists of diuretics, wrapping the leg with elastic bandages, elevation, and treating recurrent lymphangitis and cellulitis with antibiotics.

Secondary lymphedema is due to obstruction of the lymphatic flow following removal of nodes, treatment by radiotherapy, or extensive involvement by tumor or filarial infection. The edema should be treated vigorously, as early as possible. If allowed to persist, intractable edema occurs with fibrosis and impaired nutrition of the skin.

Intractable lymphedema can be treated surgically.[7,8] The results, however, are disappointing. The procedures include bridging normal and involved tissues with omental or skin flaps, creating subcutaneous tunnels and radically excising the edematous tissues and skin grafting. Since lymphedema rarely involves subfascial tissues, attempts have been made to drain the superficial edematous tissues into the deep lymphatic system. Early results with this approach have been encouraging.

Lymphangiosarcoma may develop in a limb with persistent lymphedema. This is seen most often in the postmastectomy patient with arm edema. Small, single or multiple, red-purple, flat lesions develop in the skin and subcutaneous tissues. Excisional biopsy confirms the diagnosis. Treatment is amputation of the limb because the disease spreads rapidly through the lymphatics.

Lymphomas

Major advances in the management of patients with lymphomas are the recognition that many patients with Hodgkin's disease can be cured using extended field radiotherapy and that treatment using combination chemotherapy in patients with advanced lymphomas can greatly increase survival. The role of the surgeon has changed. There is no place for radical excision of nodes. The surgeon is required to remove a node to establish the diagnosis, and he often performs laparotomy to define the extent of spread of the disease.

Classification. The lymphomas are classified as Hodgkin's disease that occurs in about 50 percent of the patients, lymphosarcoma, and reticulum cell sarcoma. Hodgkin's disease occurs most frequently at 20 to 40 years. Microscopically the disease is described as lymphocyte predominant, nodular sclerotic, mixed cellular, or lymphocyte depleted. The prognosis is best when there are few Reed-Sternberg cells, considerable fibroblasts and lymphocytes, and the pattern is nodular and not diffuse. Lymphosarcoma has two peaks, one in boys and the other for both sexes around 60 years. Reticulum cell sarcoma also occurs most often at about 60 years, and the cell type may be histiocytic or undifferentiated mesenchymal. The nonHodgkin's lymphomas may also be nodular or diffuse. The term histiocytic sarcoma is preferred by some to reticulum cell sarcoma.

Stages. Patients with Hodgkin's disease are staged according to the extent of spread.

Stage I. Disease is present in one node or one anatomic group of lymph nodes.

Stage II. Disease is present in two separate groups of nodes on one side of the diaphragm.

Stage III. Disease is present in nodes on both sides of the diaphragm but limited to involvement of the lymph nodes, spleen, and Waldeyer's ring.

Stage IV. The lymphoma has spread to extranodal tissues such as the bone marrow, liver, lungs, intestine, kidneys, or skin.

The letter A added to the stage means that the patient has no systemic symptoms. When fever, pruritus, night sweats, and greater than 10 percent body weight loss in three months has occurred, the letter B is added. The presence of anemia does not justify use of B.

Initially all patients with a lymphoma confined to tissues or organs other than lymph nodes were placed in stage IV. However, it became apparent that prognosis was good after excision of the extranodal tissues followed by radiotherapy, as for example a lesion in the gastrointestinal tract. These lesions are therefore staged as Ie (extranodal). When the regional nodes are also involved, the patient is in IIe.

Clinical Evaluation. A history is taken inquiring about weight loss, fatigue, itching, and sweating. On physical examination special attention is paid to all lymphoreticular tissue such as the spleen, liver, lymph nodes, and Waldeyer's ring in the pharynx. The erythrocyte sedimentation rate is determined because it is a useful indicator of the activity of the disease. A complete blood examination is made with careful study of the differential smear for lymphoma cells. Other investigations include bone marrow biopsy, chest x-ray, skeletal x-ray and bone scan, liver function studies and liver scan, intravenous pyelogram, upper gastrointestinal series with follow-through, and lower limb lymphangiography. At laparotomy the extent of lymphomatous involvement of the abdominal nodes, liver, and spleen is determined. A wedge of liver tissue is removed, and two needle biopsies are taken of deep liver tissue. Nodes thought on lymphangiography to contain disease are removed. A number of para-aortic nodes and those at the hilum of the spleen are routinely removed. The site of nodes excised is marked with hemoclips for subsequent localization. The spleen is removed, and hemoclips are placed to mark the splenic vessels. Splenectomy, in addition to providing more accurate staging information, reduces the amount of radiation that has to be given, particularly to the left kidney, lower left lung field, and intestine. A biopsy of iliac crest bone is taken for microscopic examination of the marrow. In females of childbearing age the ovaries are sutured together in the midline. The inverted Y field for radiotherapy can then be used. The results of laparotomy in Hodgkin's disease have shown that there is a 50 percent error in nonsurgical staging,[4,6] Laparotomy is not indicated in patients in stage IV. Laparotomy is primarily indicated to determine whether spleen and/or liver are involved and to substantiate the findings on lymphangiography and venography.

Treatment. Patients in stages I to IIIA are best treated by radical extended field radiotherapy. A mantle technique is used above the diaphragm with extensions upward to include both sides of the neck. In the abdomen an inverted Y-shaped pattern of radiation is given with a spur to the left to treat nodes in the splenic pedicle. It is unclear at present whether all patients should receive total nodal therapy. Patients in stage IV are best treated by chemotherapy, and this probably also applies to patients with stage IIB and IIIB disease.

Staging of Hodgkin's disease helps in determining prognosis. Stage I and II patients have a five-year survival of 85 to 95 percent. In stage IIIA survival is about 60 percent. About 85 percent of stage IIIB and IV patients treated with combination chemotherapy go into remission and many remain disease-free for more than five years.

The principles of management of patients with Hodgkin's disease can largely be applied to those with nonHodgkin's lymphomas. For example, the patient with a reticulum cell sarcoma confined to the stomach is in stage I. When the regional nodes are involved, the stage is II. Disease in the para-aortic nodes would result in stage III and in the lungs in stage IV.

SPLEEN

Anatomy

The spleen develops from several mesenchymal swellings in the dorsal mesogastrium. With growth the masses coalesce and project from the left side of the dorsal mesogastrium. The mesogastrium ventral to the spleen forms the gastrosplenic omentum and that posteriorly the lienorenal ligament. Accessory spleens are present in about 15 percent and result from persistent independent splenic masses.

The spleen contains the largest amount of lymphoid tissue in the lymphoreticular system. It is situated deep in the left upper quadrant of the abdomen and is protected by the ninth to the eleventh ribs (see Plate VI). The parietal convex surface rests on the diaphragm posteriorly. The visceral portion is in contact with stomach, left kidney, and colon. The splenic artery and vein run along the upper border of the body and tail of the pancreas. A palpable spleen is enlarged and can occasionally be distinguished from other left upper quadrant masses by the presence of a notch on its anterior border. An enlarged spleen may be recognized on an upper gastrointestinal x-ray by displacement of the stomach. The size can also be determined by a radioactive scan using ^{51}Cr-tagged autologous erythrocytes or ^{99}Tc-labeled sulfur colloid particles.

Microscopically the spleen contains red and white pulp with a junctional marginal zone (Figure 24–3). The red pulp consists of cords of reticular cells and vascular sinuses. The white pulp consists of spherical nodules of lymphocytes, plasma cells, and macrophages, each nodule containing a central artery. Branches of

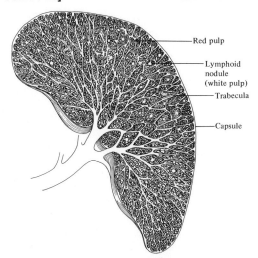

Red pulp

Lymphoid
nodule
(white pulp)

Trabecula

Capsule

Figure 24–3. The structure of the spleen consists of red and white pulp threaded with trabeculae through the whole substance.

the artery pass through the marginal zone at the junction of the two pulps and drain into the large sinusoids in the red pulp. The marginal zone is a vascular space that contains plasma cells and often foreign particles.

Physiology

The spleen stores cellular elements of the blood and under certain conditions produces them. It functions as a clearing house for antigens and damaged autologous erythrocytes, leukocytes, and platelets and produces humoral and cellular immune factors. Aged erythrocytes are sequestrated in the sinusoids. There is a large blood flow approximating 350 liters per day. In dogs the smooth muscle in the capsule and parenchymal trabeculae contracts following exercise, secretion of epinephrine, or hemorrhage leading to discharge of erythrocytes into the systemic circulation from the vascular sinuses. This probably also occurs to a lesser extent in man. The reticuloendothelial cells of the spleen are abundant and contribute to its important role in phagocytosis. The fixed macrophages in the walls of the sinusoids remove effete erythrocytes and take up circulating antigens. The reticular dendritic cells in germinal follicles trap circulating antigen. This is followed by the conversion of B-cells into IgG-forming plasma cells. The spleen is normally hematopoietic in intrauterine life. It resumes this function in the adult with myelofibrosis of the bone marrow.

Indications for Splenectomy

With expanding knowledge of hematology the indications for splenectomy have changed,

and it is important for the surgeon to know the principles of the splenic disorders that are so treated.

Trauma

The spleen is frequently ruptured after blunt trauma although it is situated deeply and protected by ribs. Direct injury by a knife, bullet, or by a retractor during operation is common. Rupture is occasionally spontaneous, especially in those with splenomegaly, e.g., chronic malaria or infectious mononucleosis. Rupture may result in immediate hemorrhage with local signs of blood in the peritoneal cavity and systemic reactions of shock. The diagnosis is often not made in patients who are comatose following a head injury, as the only signs may then be hypotension and increasing abdominal distention. The diagnosis should be considered in every patient with injury to the chest or abdomen and in the unconscious patient who is showing signs of oligemic shock following a head injury. General symptoms of decreased blood volume are dizziness and fainting when the patient is upright. Diaphoresis and lethargy, cold, damp skin, tachycardia, and change in blood pressure are signs of hypovolemia. Abdominal findings are left upper quadrant tenderness, which may be difficult to differentiate from contusion of the abdominal wall, guarding, and sometimes rigidity. Bowel sounds are decreased or absent. Abdominal distention occurs with the accumulation of blood. The white blood cell count is generally increased. Upright films of the abdomen may show displacement of the gastric air bubble to the right and fractures of the ribs. The left diaphragm may be elevated and move poorly. The blood hematocrit is initially increased but after several hours is decreased. A peritoneal tap using a catheter to irrigate the peritoneal cavity may be used to help establish the diagnosis. Laparotomy should be performed when rupture of the spleen is suspected. An upper abdominal midline incision will permit thorough inspection of the abdomen.

A delayed splenic hematoma may develop after injury to the spleen. A hematoma develops deep to the capsule of the spleen and in the adjacent tissues, the gastric splenic omentum, and lienorenal ligament. There is a history of trauma and of initial shock and on examination some tenderness and guarding in the left subcostal region. The general condition then improves. The hematoma may rupture after days or weeks into the general peritoneal cavity and may result in death. Patients should be operated on when the diagnosis of delayed splenic hematoma is made. Spleen scans should be done in patients with possible splenic damage, and selective angiography is often of value.

The spleen should be removed in all patients who have signs at laparotomy of damage to that organ. The remainder of the lymphoreticular system takes over most of the functions of the spleen.

Hypersplenism

The spleen normally participates in forming the cellular components of the blood and in removing aged and damaged cells from the circulation. Hypersplenism is excessive destruction of the cells by the spleen.[1] The condition may arbitrarily be considered primary when the spleen is responsible for the excessive removal of the cells, or it may be secondary to another disease. One or all of the cell types may be involved.

The normal life of an erythrocyte is about 120 days. The biologic half-life of ^{51}Cr-tagged erythrocytes is normally about 30 days. In patients with excessive removal of erythrocytes from the circulation the half-life is less than 25 days.

Primary Hypersplenism

Congenital Hemolytic Anemia. In congenital hemolytic anemia the erythrocytes are small and spherocytic and excessively fragile. The condition is often familial and is transmitted as a mendelian autosomal dominant. Patients may present with an enlarged spleen, a chronic anemia associated with ulceration of the legs, or they may develop crises with marked hemolysis, anemia, and jaundice. About one third develop biliary cholelithiasis. Peripheral blood and bone marrow studies show that the erythrocytes are decreased and spherocytic, the reticulocyte count is increased, and there is a hyperplastic bone marrow. The Coombs' test is negative, and splenomegaly is regularly present. Splenectomy is indicated in all patients. The operation corrects the anemia but does not affect the erythrocyte fragility or spherocytosis. Since bilirubin pigment stones are frequently present in the gallbladder and biliary tract, cholecystectomy and exploration of the bile duct are frequently necessary.

Primary Splenic Neutropenia. Patients usually present with acute or chronic infections. There are a severe neutropenia and hyperplastic bone marrow, and the spleen may or may not be enlarged. Splenectomy arrests the neutropenia. A panhematocytopenia may also occur affecting all the cellular elements in the blood.

Acquired Hemolytic Anemia. Anemia may develop as a result of overactive erythrophagocytosis by the spleen due to coating of the cell surface with antibodies (warm IgG type). The cause may be from infection or drugs or be idiopathic. There is a marked decrease in the erythrocyte count and a hyperplastic bone marrow. The Coombs' test is generally positive, indicating the presence of blocking antibody. Cortisone or ACTH should be given. Splenectomy generally helps and should be performed if the patient fails to respond to steroid therapy or relapses after treatment. There is great difficulty in cross-typing and cross-matching blood in patients with acquired hemolytic anemia.

There is also an IgM cold type of autoimmune hemolytic anemia, in which the patient has a negative Coombs' test and does not benefit from splenectomy because the erythrocyte destruction is mainly in the liver.

Primary Idiopathic Thrombocytopenia. The spleen may remove platelets excessively, producing thrombocytopenia. An antiplatelet factor is probably present in the serum that results in the platelets being removed more readily. Petechial hemorrhage, hemoptysis, or hematuria may lead one to suspect the diagnosis. The spleen is usually not palpable. The bone marrow contains many megakaryocytes. Secondary thrombocytopenia, most often drug-induced, must be excluded. Drugs that produce thrombocytopenia include organic arsenicals, quinidine, quinine, sulfonamides, oxytetracycline, chlorothiazide, hydrochlorothiazide, chlorpropamide, chloramphenicol, penicillin, meprobamate, paraaminosalicylic acid, streptomycin, phenylbutazone, antipyrine, sodium salicylate, Tridione, estrogens, and digitoxin. The thrombocytopenia in patients with lupus erthematosus must be excluded. Splenectomy is the treatment of choice in patients with chronic primary idiopathic thrombocytopenia. Steroids should initially be used in those with symptoms of short duration. Prednisone increases the platelet count and also decreases bleeding by directly acting on small blood vessels. Transfusion of blood or platelet concentrates is indicated during thrombocytopenic crises.

Secondary Hypersplenism

Increased destruction of one or more of the cellular elements in the blood may occur in congestive splenomegaly as seen complicating portal hypertension, Felty's syndrome, Gaucher's disease, xanthomatosis, leukemias, sarcoidosis, Hodgkin's disease, syphilis, and tuberculosis.

Other Conditions

Cysts of the spleen are rare and are often found at laparotomy. Hemorrhage into a cyst may result in pain.

Tumors of the spleen are uncommon and generally asymptomatic. Sarcoma, fibroma, fibrosarcoma, dermoid, hemangioma, and others are found and should be treated by splenectomy.

Splenectomy

A midline incision is favored because it is relatively avascular and can be extended readily. The organ is mobilized from its bed by incising the phrenicolienal ligament. The gastrolienal ligament is clamped, divided, and ligated to ensure hemostatic control of the short gastric vessels. The splenic artery and vein are divided and ligated, and the organ is removed. The artery should be doubly ligated. The vein should be ligated separately from the artery to prevent subsequent arteriovenous fistula. Care is taken to avoid damage to the pancreas and splenic flexure of the colon. A drain is specifically avoided unless the pancreas is injured. It is important to look for and remove accessory spleens, present in about 15 percent of patients, when performing splenectomy for hematologic diseases. Recently there has been been considerable interest in the role of splenectomy in the management of lymphomas (see page 430).

Postoperatively the erythrocytes and white blood cell count increase. Lymphocytes usually increase from a normal of 20 percent to about 50 percent. Platelets may increase within a few hours after operation to over one million per cubic millimeter. Serial counts should be done, and if the count exceeds 750,000, heparin should be given. The likelihood of venous thrombosis, however, after splenectomy has probably been overemphasized.

Most patients tolerate splenectomy without serious sequelae. However, it appears that children are more susceptible to infection, especially with diplococcus pneumonia. Some hematologists feel that this may be true of adults as well but as yet this is unproven.

THYMUS

Anatomy

The thymus is a bilobed organ, 4 × 5 × 1 cm, located in the anterior superior mediastinum anterior to the great vessels and behind the sternum. The gland extends from the fourth rib to the lower border of the thyroid gland. Blood supply is from the internal mammary vessels. Microscopically the thymus has a cortex consisting of reticular tissue and lymphocytes and a medulla containing reticular tissue and Hassall's corpuscles.

Physiology

The only known function of the thymus is production of T lymphocytes, which are responsible for cell-mediated immunity and aid in the production of certain antibody responses (see Chapter 4). The thymus is large at birth, increases in size until puberty, and then undergoes involution. Eventually fat replaces the lymphocytes.

Thymic Tumors

The commonest tumor is the "thymoma." The name derives from the difficulty in differentiating benign from malignant lesions. Patients with these tumors usually present with an asymptomatic enlargement in the anterior superior mediastinum. Thymomas should be removed surgically through a sternal splitting approach. Occasionally myasthenia gravis is associated with thymoma and may be relieved by removal of the tumor. Other lymphocyte-associated malignant diseases such as Hodgkin's disease and lymphosarcoma also occur.

Myasthenia Gravis

Since Blalock performed the first thymectomy for myasthenia gravis in 1936, surgical interest in this disease has waxed and waned considerably. Generally operation has been reserved for patients, particularly young females, who developed brittleness to drug therapy or rapid progression of disease. Recently a more aggressive surgical attitude has emerged.[5,9] Thymectomy should probably be considered for all patients except those with isolated focal (usually ocular) symptoms and mild generalized disease. The course after thymectomy in 80 percent of the patients is gradual improvement with final stabilization of disease after several months or years. The remaining 20 percent do not benefit. Relapse in patients without thymoma is rare, as is worsening of disease after operation.

The loss of T-cells seems too slow to account for the observed rate of improvement, and attrition of cells is not likely in the face of a response. There is some evidence that the thymus is the target of the autoimmune attack, and that the thymus liberates a small-molecular-weight factor which interferes with neuromuscular transmission and the structural integrity of motor end plates. It may be the regeneration of motor end plates which takes time after thymectomy to allow return of normal function.

Transplantation

There is no evidence that removal or local radiotherapy to the thymus prolongs allograft survival in humans, and therefore it has no place in human organ transplantation at present.

Thymectomy

Most surgeons prefer a sternal splitting approach. A vertical midline incision is made downward to the third interspace from a 3-cm transverse cervical incision. The sternum is split with a Lebshe knife to the same level and then transversely into both third intercostal spaces. The divided bone fragments are spread, exposing the anterior superior mediastinum. The thymus can be easily removed by hemoclipping around the periphery of the gland. If a thymoma is present, a significant section of parietal pleura may have to be removed, requiring chest tube drainage of the pleural space. Small pleural rents can be closed without a chest tube.

The sternal splitting approach should be used in all patients with suspected thymoma. However, some surgeons prefer a transcervical approach in patients with myasthenia gravis,[3] without evidence of tumor. A low thyroid-type collar incision is made. The median raphe is divided vertically and the strap muscles are spread laterally. The thymus is identified under the origins of the sternohyoid muscles and is delivered into the incision by combined sharp and blunt dissection using hemoclips to secure hemostasis. The gland is then removed. Advocates of this approach claim less postoperative discomfort than with the sternal splitting approach. Others, however, feel that the cervical approach provides inadequate exposure to guarantee consistent complete removal of the gland.

All patients should have a tracheostomy. Postoperative mechanical ventilatory assistance is routine.[2] Muscle relaxants should be avoided during surgery, and the use of anticholinesterases should be minimized for several days. Oral anticholinesterases may be started once the patient is improved to the point that accurate clinical performance can be assessed.

CITED REFERENCES

1. Dameshek, W., and Estren, S.: Hypersplenism—some preliminary observations. *Acta Med. Scand. (Suppl.),* **231**:106–19, 1948.
2. Jenkins, Leonard C.; Chang, Jone; and Saxton, George D.: Myasthenia gravis: anesthetic and surgical management of the patient undergoing thymectomy. *Can. Med. Assoc. J.,* **93**:198–203, 1965.
3. Kirschner, P. A.; Osserman, K. E.; Kark, A. F.: Studies in myasthenia gravis: transcervical total thymectomy. *JAMA,* **209**:906–10, 1969.
4. Lowenbraun, S.; Ramsey, H.; Sutherland, J.; and Serpick, A. A.: Diagnostic laparotomy and splenectomy in Hodgkin's disease. *Ann. Intern. Med.,* **72**:655–63, 1970.
5. Papatestas, A. E.; Alpert, L. I.; Osserman, K. E.; Osserman, R. S.: Kock, A. E.: Studies in myasthenia gravis: effect of thymectomy. *Am. J. Med.,* **50**:465–74, 1971.
6. Prosnitz, L. R.; Meloud, S. B.; and Kligerman, M. M.: Role of laparotomy and splenectomy in the management of Hodgkin's disease. *Cancer,* **29**:44–50, 1972.
7. Stone, Elizabeth J., and Hugo, Norman E.: Lymphedema. *Surg. Gynecol. Obstet,* **135**:625–31, 1972.
8. Thompson, N.: Surgical treatment of chronic lymphoedema of the lower limb. *Br. Med. J.,* **5319**:1566–73, 1962.
9. Zeldowicz, L. R., and Saxton, G. P.: Myasthenia gravis: comparative evaluation of medical and surgical treatment. *Can. Med. Assoc. J.,* **101**:609–14, 1969.

SUGGESTIONS FOR FURTHER READING

Alexander, J. W., and Good R. A.: *Immunobiology for Surgeons.* W. B. Saunders, Philadelphia, 1970.
This text provides an excellent survey of immune mechanisms in clear, concise terms. Particular emphasis is given to the immunology of surgical problems, e.g., transplantation and cancer.

Mathiew, A., and Kahan, B. D.: *Immunologic Aspects of Anesthetic and Surgical Practice.* Grune & Stratton, New York, 1975, pp. 1–400.
A general review of the role of immunology in clinical practice.

Williams, W. J.; Bettler, E.; Erslen, A. J.; and Rundles, W.: *Hematology.* McGraw-Hill, New York, 1972.
This text is a comprehensive review of hematology in general. The section on "Hypersplenism", pp. 511–20, written by Harry S. Jacob, is of particular value for further information concerning this topic from a hematologists' point of view.

Yoffey, J. M., and Courtice, F. C.: *Lymphatics, Lymph and Lymphomyeloid Complex.* Academic Press, New York, 1970.
This book represents a complete in-depth review of the lymphatic system with emphasis on basic anatomy and physiology.

Chapter 25

SKIN AND SOFT TISSUES

John A. McCredie and *Thomas A. Watson*

CHAPTER OUTLINE

Anatomy
Physiology
  Protection
  Absorption
  Temperature Regulation
  Circulatory Changes
  Sensory Functions
  Storage
Investigations
Preoperative Assessment and Care
The Skin as an Indicator of Systemic Diseases
Benign Diseases of the Skin
  Hemangioma
  Cysts
  Benign Hyperplastic Diseases
    Seborrheic Keratosis
    Actinic or Senile Keratosis
    Keratoacanthoma
  Warts
    Verruca Vulgaris

Verruca Plantaris
Condylomata Accuminata
Malignant Diseases of the Skin
  Basal Cell Carcinoma
  Squamous Cell Carcinoma
  Malignant Melanoma
    Clinical Examination
    Differential Diagnosis
    Prognosis
    Treatment of a Pigmented Nevus
    Treatment of Malignant Melanoma
  Other Cancers of Skin
  Lymphomas and Metastases
Tumors of the Soft Tissues
  Lipoma and Liposarcoma
  Fibroma and Fibrosarcoma
  Neuroma and Neurofibrosarcoma
  Tumors of Smooth and Voluntary Muscle
  Lymphovascular Tumors

ANATOMY

The skin consists of the ectodermal-derived epidermis connected by the rete pegs to the underlying dermis developed from mesoderm (see Plate I). The epidermis contains four layers:

Germinal Layer. The deep layer is a single row of columnar hyperchromatic cells that give rise to the cells in the superficial layers. Injury is followed by an increase in the number of mitotic figures. Single clear cells, melanocytes, are interspersed at intervals between the germinal cells and produce melanin granules that are often taken up by the basal cells.

Prickle Layer. The cells are held together by interconnected processes that produce the "prickle" appearance. In normal skin more mitoses are seen in the prickle than the basal layer.

Granular Layer. The cells contain basophilic granules of keratohyalin.

Keratin Layer. The dense horny layer, the stratum corneum, is the main protective layer of the skin and largely determines its thickness. The cells are dead and are continuously shed from the surface.

An additional lucidum or thin translucent layer is present between the granular and keratin layers in the skin of the palms and soles. The hair and nails are derived from specialized cells of the epidermis. The sweat glands in the dermis transmit their secretions through pores on the surface of the skin.

The dermis is thicker than the epidermis and consists of fibroelastic tissue containing blood vessels, lymphatics, nerves, hair follicles, sebaceous, sweat, and scent glands. The sweat or eccrine glands present on the palms, soles, head, and neck play an important role in controlling body temperature. The scent or apocrine glands in the axillae and perineum open into the hair follicles. They are long and deep and more prone to infection than the sweat glands. The sebaceous glands secrete sebum, derived from dead cells, into the most superficial part of the hair follicles. They are absent in the palms and soles. The muscles of the hair follicles, responsible for "gooseflesh," are the arrectores pilorum. The supporting stroma consists mostly of collagen secreted by fibroblasts and to a lesser extent of elastic and reticulum fibers.

PHYSIOLOGY

The skin is not only a protective covering separating the external from the internal environment but is also a dynamic organ with many functions (see below). It weighs about 15 percent of body weight and its thickness varies from 1.5 to 5 mm. The functions include protection from injury, infection and ultraviolet light, temperature control, and maintenance of homeostasis.

Protection

A thin film of emulsified, acid material derived from the cells of the stratum corneum and the secretions of the cutaneous glands lies on the surface of the skin and forms the first protective layer. Its main function is to prevent penetration of water and water-soluble substances. Lipid-soluble substances can pass through this material. The stratum corneum is thickest in regions of repeated trauma, such as the soles and palms, and forms the main protective layer against injury and entry of microorganisms. On injury cells in the stratum germinativum rapidly proliferate. The pigment melanin protects against injury by ultraviolet light.

Absorption

The ability of the skin to inhibit absorption of water-soluble products is lipid dependent, while its ability to prevent absorption of gases is water dependent. A number of toxic materials such as phenol, heavy metals, and carbon tetrachloride can penetrate normal skin. Salicylic acid, fat-soluble vitamins, and the hormones testosterone, progesterone, estrogens, and desoxycorticosterone penetrate skin readily. Hydrocortisone can be absorbed in amounts sufficient to produce a systemic effect. Substances are more readily absorbed through injured skin.

Temperature Regulation

The skin plays a major role in regulating body temperature. The metabolism of 3000 calories in 24 hours results in considerable heat, most of which is eliminated through the skin. Heat leaves the cutaneous vessels in the water that passes through the skin to be lost as insensible perspiration. The amount depends upon the blood flow. Additional heat, as produced during strenuous exercise, is lost by secretion of sweat by the small sweat or eccrine glands. Sweat secretion is mainly controlled by the autonomic nervous system. The efferent pathway is sympathetic. Acetylcholine is liberated at the nerve endings and causes stimulation, while atropine decreases sweating. Sweat is mostly water but also contains sodium chloride and potassium. Their concentrations vary with the amount of sweat secreted. The loss of heat from the surface of the skin is by convection, conduction, or evaporation of infrared rays.

Circulatory Changes

Changes in cutaneous blood flow, controlled by the autonomic nervous system and local tissue mediators, are important in maintaining the blood pressure. Epinephrine, norepinephrine, and Pituitrin cause vasoconstriction of mainly the arterioles, while acetylcholine increases blood flow. The color of the skin depends on the amount of blood in the capillaries and the temperature on the arteriolar blood flow. Arteriovenous shunts are present in the skin of the fingers; their myoepithelial elements give rise to neuroectodermal glomus tumors.

Sensory Functions

Pain sensation is registered mainly in the nonmyelinated fibers in the diffuse plexiform plexus immediately deep to the stratum germinativum. Fibers pass between the cells in the epidermis and are responsible for accurate localization of pain. Cold sensation was considered to be registered in the Krause end bulbs, temperature in the Ruffini endings, touch in Meissner's corpuscles, and pressure in the Pacinian corpuscles; however, the concept of their being specific sensory receptors is now being challenged. The density of these end organs varies in different regions of the body.

Storage

With extensive skin loss, as in burns, the patient may develop iron deficiency anemia because of the storage of large amounts of iron in the skin.

INVESTIGATIONS

Skin lesions may be erythematous, macular, papular, vesicular, or bullar. A hand lens helps in the diagnosis of many skin diseases, for example identification of the scaly pitted surface of seborrheic hyperkeratosis. Scales can be removed and help diagnose fungal infections.

Skin tests may determine the presence of allergies and the immune status. A biopsy is frequently needed to establish the diagnosis of malignant diseases, as in mycosis fungoides and scleroderma.

PREOPERATIVE ASSESSMENT AND CARE

The patient should be asked about a history of skin reactions to antiseptics, adhesive tape, and medicines. Exceedingly sensitive skin is often needlessly irritated by preoperative shaving. Satisfactory shaving can now be done with an electric razor. Excessive washing with antiseptic soaps may produce a contact dermatitis that increases the risk of infection.

In patients with dermatologic disease proper preoperative and postoperative treatment may prevent an exacerbation after operation. Prolonged use of a corticosteroid ointment causes atrophy of skin and may lead to slow wound healing. The patient should be questioned about the use of systemic corticosteroids for the treatment of a skin disease.

Previous incisions should be inspected for keloid formation. If present, the patient should be warned of recurrence. Keloid is an overgrowth of connective tissue that occurs after injury in predisposed persons, especially Negroes. It occurs most often on the face, neck, and presternal regions. The scar becomes pink, broad, and elevated and often causes a burning sensation especially when warm. The condition settles spontaneously in about six months and leaves a broad, cosmetically bad scar. Hypertrophic scar formation can be treated by intralesional corticosteroid injections and by liquid nitrogen cryotherapy. This is especially important when the scar is visible.

THE SKIN AS AN INDICATOR OF SYSTEMIC DISEASES

Endocrine dysfunction is present in most patients with hypermelanosis. In Addison's disease the brownish pigmentation is most marked in the creases of the palms and soles, the oral mucosa, and the flexures such as the axillae. Hypermelanosis may also occur in Cushing's syndrome, pheochromocytoma, or thyrotoxicosis and with malignant diseases such as Hodgkin's disease, lymphosarcoma, or lymphatic leukemia. Acanthosis nigricans is a marked pigmentation in the axillae and anogenital regions in some patients with adenocarcinoma, especially of the stomach.

A diffuse yellowish-brown pigmentation may develop in chronic renal disease (see Chapter 32). Jaundice is first recognized in the conjunctivae (see Chapter 19). Patients with malabsorption syndromes, pellagra, scurvy, and vitamin A deficiency may have localized or generalized pigmentations.

About one half of patients with hemochromatosis develop an addisonian type of pigmentation from excessive melanin deposits. The remainder have excessive hemosiderin, giving a slate-gray pigmentation, especially in the face, arms, skinfolds, and genitals.

BENIGN DISEASES OF THE SKIN

Hemangioma

Cutaneous hemangiomas are strawberry, port-wine, or cavernous. The strawberry nevus is present at birth and usually disappears by seven years. No treatment is needed other than reassuring the parents. Port-wine stains occur most often on the face and upper trunk and do not tend to regress. Lesions on the face are often best left untreated and covered with opaque cosmetic creams. Cavernous hemangiomas are usually in the subcutaneous tissues, may grow and ulcerate through the skin, and are best treated by surgical excision. A cavernous hemangioma is rarely due to an arteriovenous fistula. A sclerosing hemangioma is a subepidermal hemangioma associated with fibrosis and occurs most often in the extremities. It may be black and readily mistaken for a malignant melanoma.

Cysts

A sebaceous cyst is a unilocular cyst firmly attached to the skin and occurs most often in the head, neck, and upper torso. A punctum can often be seen where the sebaceous gland is obstructed. The cyst contains cheesy material and frequently becomes infected. It should be excised through an elliptical incision including the site of attachment to the skin. When infected the cyst may be drained, the wall avulsed, and the area left open to heal by secondary intention.

Epithelial cells misplaced in the subcutaneous tissues as a result of trauma may grow and form a unilocular epidermal-lined cyst containing keratin. Dermoid cysts are congenital but usually present clinically years after birth. They are most likely occlusive cysts and tend to occur in the midline in the scalp, face, neck, and trunk. Treatment of epithelial and dermoid cysts is surgical excision.

Ganglia are described in Chapter 33 and pilonidal cysts in Chapter 22.

Benign Hyperplastic Diseases

Hyperkeratosis means thickening of the keratin layer of the skin and occurs in senile keratoses and warts. Acanthosis is thickening of the prickle layer as in psoriasis.

Seborrheic Keratosis. This is a yellowish-brown, hyperkeratotic, greasy-surfaced, plaque-like tumor that has a characteristic "stuck-on" appearance. It occurs especially on the trunk, is often multiple, and increases in incidence with age. Occasionally the lesion is deeply pigmented and is mistaken for a malignant melanoma. It is not a premalignant lesion. Treatment is electro-desiccation and curettage or liquid nitrogen cryotherapy. Liquid nitrogen applied to the lesion results in desquamation in two weeks with little or no residual scarring.

Actinic or Senile Keratosis. This is a hard, hyperkeratotic, papular lesion that occurs on areas exposed to sunlight, the face, ears, and dorsum of hands and arms. It is induced by ultraviolet light, is premalignant, and occurs most often in fair-skinned Caucasians. Treatment is similar to that for seborrheic keratosis. Multiple actinic keratoses of the face can be treated by local application of 2 per cent 5-fluorouracil in propylene glycol. An acute inflammatory reaction occurs followed by disappearance of the lesions with usually no scarring.

Keratoacanthoma. A keratoacanthoma is a rapidly growing red papule in the center of the face that is difficult to distinguish from a squamous cell carcinoma grossly and microscopically (Figure 25–1). Eventually the lesion ulcerates, exposing a central core of keratin. Spontaneous regression usually occurs within three months. Biopsy of part or all of the lesion is necessary to confirm the diagnosis.

Warts

Verruca Vulgaris. The common wart is a virus-induced hyperplasia of the epidermal cells

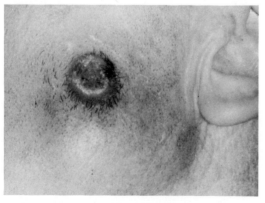

Figure 25–1. A keratoacanthoma in a 64-year-old man.

that does not extend into the dermis. Untreated, the majority disappear spontaneously without producing a scar. Surgical excision may be followed by prompt recurrence of the lesion due to the persistence of the virus in the surrounding epidermal cells. Local electrodesiccation is often successful. Persistent and recurrent lesions can be successfully treated with a single exposure of superficial x-rays.

Verruca Plantaris. A plantar wart is a common wart on the sole. The dermal-epidermal junction is pushed in to form a firm, rubbery mass which is painful on walking. The virus is acquired by walking on infected wet floors, as for example at public swimming pools. Spontaneous remission is frequent.

For diagnosis the lesion is pared with a scalpel and the cut surface moistened and studied with a magnifying lens. The plantar wart has numerous bleeding points and a sharply demarcated border separating it from the epidermis. At the deepest point there is an exquisitely tender blue spot. The lesion should be differentiated from a callus, a mosiac wart, a mosaic wart in a callus, and a foreign body granuloma.

A plantar wart may be pared until there is bleeding at the base. It is then cauterized with silver nitrate and a single drop of cantherone solution applied. The region is then covered with a small square of Blenderm tape held firmly to the foot by adhesive tape. An inflammatory reaction occurs in the wart within the following 24 hours and subsides in one to two days. The wart then gradually dries up and falls out over the succeeding two weeks. A plantar wart may be treated under anesthesia by curettage and electrodesiccation or by a single dose, 1300 to 1500 rads, of x-rays.

Condylomata Accuminata. Condylomata accuminata are papillomatous lesions on the penis, vulva, and perineum produced by the common wart virus. Small lesions that have been present for a short time may be successfully treated by application of 20 percent podophyllum resin in 70 percent alcohol. Recurrence, however, is frequent. Large lesions are treated by electrodesiccation and curettage or by liquid nitrogen cryotherapy. The liquid nitrogen is applied to the lesions without an anesthetic. Several treatments are usually necessary at 10-day intervals. Circumcision may be required in those with recurring penile lesions.

MALIGNANT DISEASES OF THE SKIN

Cancer of the skin is the most common malignant disease and accounts for 25 percent of cancers in men and 10 percent in women.[2]

About 90 percent occur on surfaces exposed to sunlight. The commonest tumors are basal cell and squamous cell carcinomas and less frequently malignant melanomas, Kaposi's sarcoma, and dermatofibrosarcomas. Lymphomas and metastases from carcinomas are common in the skin. Skin cancers, excluding malignant melanoma, have been staged clinically according to the UICC classification:

T1N0 Lesion with surface diameter less than 2 cm and depth less than 1 cm.

T2N0 The surface diameter 2 to 5 cm and depth less than 2 cm.

T3N0 Surface diameter more than 5 cm and depth greater than 2 cm and attached to bone or cartilage.

T4N0 The lesion has invaded cartilage or bone.

The nodes and distant metastases are classified as in patients with carcinoma of the breast (see Chapter 26).

Basal Cell Carcinoma

Basal cell carcinomas are the commonest malignant tumors of the skin and account for about 60 percent of skin cancers. They are often multiple, occur mainly on or adjacent to the nose, and occasionally elsewhere on the body (Figure 25–2). The lesions develop mainly after 50 years but at a younger age than squamous cell carcinomas. They are common in fair-skinned Caucasians and rare in Negroes. Ultraviolet light is important in the production of those on the face. In some patients there is an important genetic factor. The tumor is initially a firm nodule covered by stretched-out pearly epidermis containing telangiectatic vessels. Later the nodule ulcerates and penetrates deeply. The edge of the ulcer is sharply demarcated and often elevated and has a rolled or beaded appearance.

A basal cell tumor grows more slowly than a squamous cell carcinoma, reaching a diameter of 1 cm in about one year, and very rarely metastasizes to the regional nodes.

Treatment is excision or local radiotherapy. Excision is adequate if the line of excision is wide of the tumor in all directions. Basal cell tumors are extremely radiosensitive and have a local recurrence rate of less than 2 percent. Lesions around the eyelids are successfully radiated with good cosmetic results. Initial treatment is often by radiotherapy, and surgical removal is reserved for those with incomplete regression or recurrence. Complete regression may take as long as six months following radiotherapy. Surgical treatment is indicated in preference to radiotherapy in those under 40 years and when good radiotherapy is not available. Skin excessively damaged by radiotherapy produces cosmetic impairment which becomes worse with time and may develop a squamous cell carcinoma, especially when the region is exposed to sunlight. Basal cell carcinomas are also effectively treated by electrodesiccation and curettage. Moh's chemosurgical technique can be used to treat multiple lesions. Cryotherapy with liquid nitrogen is a promising form of therapy.

Regular follow-up is essential because new lesions frequently occur.

Squamous Cell Carcinoma

About 30 percent of skin cancers are squamous cell carcinomas. They occur mainly in the face, pinna, dorsum of the hands, and adjacent to orifices such as the mouth, urethra, or anus (Figure 25–3). They occur in farmers and fishermen, who are exposed to ultraviolet light, and especially in people of Celtic origin. A

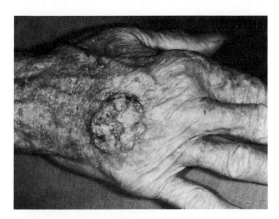

Figure 25–2. A basal cell carcinoma of the dorsum of the hand, present for five years.

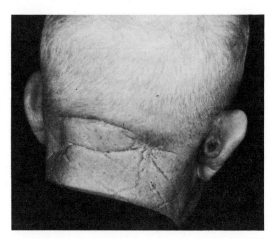

Figure 25–3. A squamous cell carcinoma in a 72-year-old farmer.

common premalignant condition is an actinic hyperkeratosis. They often arise in the scar of a burn (Marjolin's ulcer), previously irradiated skin, or at the site of chronic infection such as a fistula or chronic abscess. Other premalignant conditions are keratotic lesions secondary to the ingestion of arsenic and xeroderma pigmentosum.

The tumor commences as a firm cutaneous nodule with a hyperkeratotic surface and rapidly ulcerates. The margin of the ulcer tends to be irregular and slightly raised. Spread can occur to the regional nodes. Microscopically the cells vary from well-differentiated producing epithelial pearls to anaplastic with no attempt at keratinization. Broder has classified the degree of differentiation as grades I to IV, more than 75 percent to less than 25 percent of the cell differentiated. Other factors such as depth of penetration, size, mononuclear cell infiltration, blood and lymphatic invasion, and the presence of metastases in the regional nodes also help to determine the prognosis.

All chronic skin ulcers should be examined microscopically because a squamous cell carcinoma is frequently misdiagnosed. A small lesion may be excised or an incisional biopsy, including the edge of the ulcer, performed on a larger lesion. Treatment is wide local excision often with application of a skin graft. When the carcinoma has arisen in previously damaged skin, as in the scar of the burn, all the damaged tissues should be excised. Local radiotherapy can be used to treat a squamous cell carcinoma and is just as effective, at the same dose, as in the treatment of a basal cell carcinoma. The regional nodes are not excised prophylactically but are removed by block dissection when they are enlarged and mobile. Nodes fixed to one another or to the skin or deeper structures are treated by radiotherapy. Palliation can also often be obtained by chemotherapy. Amethopterin and bleomycin are the drugs of choice.

Malignant Melanoma

Malignant melanoma is the most dangerous type of skin cancer. The incidence is about three per 100,000 per year, and the mortality at five years is about 50 percent. It occurs most often in Caucasians and is uncommon in blacks. Before puberty melanomas are almost invariably benign, although grossly and microscopically they may appear to be malignant. The incidence increases and is greatest in the third, fourth, and fifth decades, with a median age for both sexes of about 45 years. The incidence is the same in both sexes, but the mortality is greater in males. In females malignant melanoma is more fre-

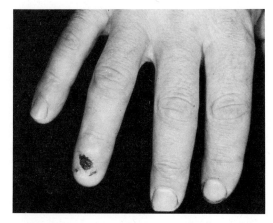

Figure 25–4. A subungual malignant melanoma that has resulted in loss of the nail.

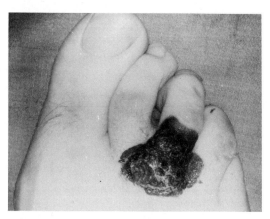

Figure 25–5. A large, deeply invasive malignant melanoma of the foot.

quent in the legs, in males in the trunk, and in blacks about 70 percent are in the soles. Distribution is almost uniform. It is higher per square centimeter only in the face and neck, probably because of exposure to ultraviolet light (Figures 25–4 and 25–5).[1] There is no evidence that injury to or incomplete removal by operation or fulguration of benign nevus precipitates malignant change.

The melanocyte-stimulating hormone (MSH) of the anterior pituitary increases melanocyte activity, while cortisone and ACTH cause a decrease. A decrease in epinephrine and norepinephrine inhibits the action of MSH.

A malignant melanoma usually develops in a pigmented nevus that has been present since birth or for many years. Most patients do not know how long the lesion has been present. A malignant melanoma develops from cells that are derived from the primitive neural crest. Cells from the neural crest migrate and give rise to melanoblasts, cells of pigmented nevi, and Schwann cells of peripheral nerves. Any of these three cells can probably give rise to a malignant melanoma. For example, the spindle cells in a blue nevus are most likely derived from Schwann cells.

Clinical Examination. A careful examination is made of the primary lesion noting its position, color, area, volume, and the presence of ulceration, a surrounding halo, and satellite lesions. Dangerous signs are darkening in color, enlargement, itching, ulceration, development of a surrounding pink halo, or satellite lesions. Occasionally the lesion is amelanotic and is particularly difficult to diagnose. Mihm et al.[4] have stated that early signs of malignant change are the development of a variegated color with shades of red, white, or blue, the presence of an irregular edge, or an irregular surface. Exact measurements and a photographic record are made. The regional nodes are recorded as clinically negative or positive. The number and size of clinically involved nodes are recorded and whether they are fixed to one another or to the skin or deep tissues. Cutaneous nodules are looked for, especially between the primary tumor and the regional nodes (in transit metastases). The skin is examined for other pigmented spots. A diffuse brown pigmentation is only seen rarely in patients with widespread metastases. The abdomen is examined for hepatic enlargement, enlarged para-aortic nodes, and ascites. The chest is examined for a pleural effusion. Neurologic examination is important because of the high incidence of cerebral metastases. Metastases are found occasionally in the breast.

Special Investigations. Pulmonary metastases may be seen on chest x-ray. A pleural effusion or broadening of the mediastinum requires further investigation to exclude metastases. An isotope bone scan should be obtained because of the high incidence of bony metastases. If the scan is positive, a skeletal survey is performed to exclude benign diseases such as Paget's disease, osteoarthritis, or a pathologic fracture. Liver and brain scans are performed because of the high incidence of metastases at these sites.

The serum alkaline phosphatase is often increased in patients with small hepatic metastases. With increasing growth of metastases the LDH, SGOT, and bilirubin increase and the serum albumin falls. Bony metastases also increase the serum alkaline phosphatase. Hypochromic anemia occurs in patients with widespread bony metastases. The diagnosis can be confirmed by percutaneous marrow biopsy in those with negative surveys.

An electroencephalogram, electrocardiogram, gastrointestinal series, and intravenous pyelogram may be performed. Lymphangiography or angiography is seldom indicated. Melanemia and melanuria only occur in patients with widespread metastases.

Differential Diagnosis. *Junctional Nevus.* Most malignant melanomas develop from junctional nevi or the junctional component in a compound nevus. Nevi on the soles, palms, and genitalia are junctional. The junctional nevus is flat or forms a plaque and is light to dark brown. The compound nevus and juvenile melanoma in children probably become junctional nevi at puberty. Microscopically the nevus is in the superficial dermis and often has processes extending into the epidermis to reach the surface, producing "skip lesions."

Intradermal Nevus. The intradermal nevus is the commonest pigmented nevus but never develops into a malignant melanoma. It is flat or nodular, light to dark brown, and may or may not have hairs. All hairy moles are intradermal nevi. It never occurs on the soles, palms, or genitalia. Microscopically it is in the dermis and has a normal overlying epidermis.

Compound Nevus. Clinically the compound nevus is identical to an intradermal nevus. About 98 percent of nevi in children are compound. Microscopically the cells are in the dermis and epidermis. The intraepidermal component may become malignant.

Juvenile Melanoma. The juvenile melanoma is a pink or red nevus occurring most often on the face of a child before puberty. The lesion appears malignant grossly and microscopically, but its course is benign. Microscopically it is a compound nevus with spindle and epithelioid cells in the deep epidermis and dermis.

Blue Nevus. The blue nevus is deeply pigmented, discrete, has a thinned-out, covering epidermis that occurs on the face, dorsum of hands, feet, and the buttock. It is entirely intradermal and rarely becomes malignant.

Hutchinson Freckle. The Hutchinson freckle is a large, flat, brownish-black nevus most often on the face. It develops most often after 50 years and can become a malignant melanoma. The malignant region forms a nodule, darkens in color, and ulcerates.

Pigmented Basal Cell Tumor. Brown or black pigment is often present in a basal cell carcinoma.

Seborrheic Keratosis. Multiple pigmented plaques often develop in elderly patients, especially on the trunk. When deeply pigmented, they can be mistaken for malignant melanoma.

Hemangioma. A black area may develop in a hemangioma, ulcerate, and simulate a malignant melanoma. The sclerosing form is particularly liable to misdiagnosis.

Prognosis. The appearance gives considerable information about prognosis. A malignant melanoma that grows horizontally has a better prognosis than one that grows vertically. The larger the surface area and volume, the worse the prognosis. Bad features are lack of pigmentation, ulceration, satellite lesions, clinically involved regional nodes, and a subungual position. The prognosis is best in women when the lesion is in the leg and when the malignant melanoma develops in a Hutchinson freckle.

The prognosis is better in patients with superficial malignant melanoma with cancer cells confined to the epidermis and superficial dermis than in those with deep malignant melanoma when the cells extend into the deep dermis and subcutaneous fat.[5] The five-year survival is about 75 percent for superficial melanoma and 25 percent for the deep type. The degree of anaplasia, hyperchromatism, number of mitoses, vascular and lymphatic invasion, and lymphoid infiltration also influence the prognosis. The most important single feature is the presence or absence of metastases in the regional nodes. There are few long-term survivors when nodes contain metastases.

Recently the importance of the depth of penetration has been emphasized by describing five levels. In level I the malignant melanoma cells are confined to the epidermis; in level II the cells are present in the narrow papillary zone that contains few fibroblasts; in level III they are deforming the reticular zone of the dermis; in level IV they have invaded the reticular zone, and in level V they have reached the subcutaneous fat. The mortality is approximately equal to the depth of penetration, measured by a micrometer, multiplied by 10.

Microscopically three lesions have been described, each with a different prognosis. In the superficial spreading malignant melanoma there are large cells in the papillary zone in contact with stratum germinativum, and cells can be seen infiltrating the epidermis in a pagetoid manner. Normal regions may be seen within the lesion. The superficial spreading melanoma is equivalent to an in-situ carcinoma, radial growth may occur for many years, and probably less than 1 percent develop distant metastases. When it becomes invasive, the prognosis is worse than when malignancy develops in a Hutchinson freckle. The lentigo maligna lesion is grossly a Hutchinson freckle. Densely pigmented cells can be seen in the papillary zone of the dermis, and the cells do not infiltrate the epidermis in a pagetoid manner.

Regions with only a few macrophages containing melanin pigment can be seen corresponding to the clear regions seen grossly in the Hutchinson freckle. The occurrence of vertical deep penetration is recognized clinically by thickening in the tissues. The origin of a malignant melanoma from a superficial spreading melanoma is differentiated from that developing in a lentigo maligna by microscopic examinination of the lesion's periphery. The third lesion, the nodular melanoma, has the worst prognosis and is malignant and infiltrating from its onset.

Treatment of a Pigmented Nevus. Any pigmented nevus that shows signs of becoming malignant should be excised and examined microscopically. An intradermal nevus is only removed for cosmetic reasons or when the diagnosis is in doubt. Compound nevi and Hutchinson freckles should be excised or regularly reviewed because the epidermal component may become malignant. All juvenile nevi should be excised because there is inadequate information on the natural history of the untreated lesion. The great problem is managing the patient with one or often many junctional nevi. Formerly excision was recommended for those on the soles, palms, deep to the nails, perioral, and in the perineum because they were thought to frequently become malignant. This is not necessary. Junctional nevi exposed to sunlight are more likely to become malignant and should be removed. All lesions that are removed must be examined microscopically.

Treatment of Malignant Melanoma. Retrospective studies on the management of patients with malignant melanoma show that up to one half have improper treatment of the primary lesion. The signs of malignant change are often ignored by the patient or physician, the primary tumor is treated by fulguration or local excision, and the specimen is not examined microscopically or the definitive excision is not adequate.

Lesions with "dangerous" signs should be excised and examined microscopically. It may be possible to make the diagnosis on frozen section, but frequently examination of multiple paraffin sections is necessary. When the diagnosis of malignant melanoma is confirmed, the lesion should be excised with a minimum of 2 cm surrounding normal skin. The superficial and deep fascias are removed, and at most sites a skin graft is applied.

There is controversy about the management of clinically uninvolved regional nodes.[6] The nodes are generally removed in continuity with the primary lesion when the tumor is close to the nodes, as for example when the melanoma is in the thigh or upper arm. About 25 percent of clinically negative nodes contain metastases. It is illogical to perform an incontinuity dissection when the primary is at a distance, for example in the lower leg or forearm, because the lymphatics freely communicate around the limb. Alternately the nodes may be observed and removed when they are thought to contain metastases. Nodal and hematogenous metastases tend to occur at the same time in patients with malignant melanoma. The findings on microscopic examination of clinically negative nodes therefore give information about prognosis. There have been no clinical trials using random controls comparing prophylactic with therapeutic removal of regional nodes.

Crile has suggested that prophylactic removal of the regional nodes is harmful. He states that the cancer cells tend to grow more readily in the limb that is often edematous after removal of the nodes and that prophylactic nodal excision impairs the host's immune response and increases metastases.

Radiotherapy. Malignant melanoma is relatively radioresistant. There is no place for prophylactic radiotherapy in the patient treated by an attempted curative operation. Useful palliation can sometimes be obtained in the patient with local recurrence of the primary tumor, in transit metastases, metastases in the regional nodes, and pain from bony metastases. Cerebral, pulmonary, and liver metastases do not respond well to radiotherapy. The isotope ^{32}P sometimes gives useful palliation in the patient with anemia and bone pain from widespread metastases in bone.

Chemotherapy. The alkylating antimetabolite phenylalanine mustard (PAM) causes regression of a number of syngeneic malignant melanomas in mice. It has been used extensively in patients by intravenous injection or by perfusion but with disappointing results. Recently there has been considerable interest in combination drug therapy using agents such as vincristine, cyclophosphamide, imidazole carboxamide, and bishydroxy urea.

Immunotherapy. There is considerable evidence of an immunologic response in patients with malignant melanoma (see Chapter 4). Cancer-specific antigens and antibodies have been demonstrated. Spontaneous regression can occur and prolonged regression followed by rapid widespread growth of metastases. Mononuclear cell infiltration is generally present in the primary tumor when it is small and disappears as the tumor grows.

Local active nonspecific immunotherapy, using dinitrochlorobenzene, BCG, or vaccination, can cause regression of skin metastases in patients with malignant melanoma.[3]

Other Cancers of Skin

Adenocarcinomas occasionally develop from sebaceous or sweat glands. They tend to grow slowly and are best treated by excision. The sweat gland tumors are very aggressive, rapidly growing, and often fatal.

Mycosis fungoides is a lymphomatous disease of the skin. There may be a skin rash followed by formation of skin plaques and ultimately cutaneous tumors and ulceration. The lesions respond well to local radiotherapy. They can also be treated by local or systemic chemotherapy.

Kaposi's sarcoma is a nodular tumor that occurs in the edematous legs mainly of Jewish and Italian men. Treatment is excision or radiotherapy.

Lymphomas and Metastases

Patients with Hodgkin's disease, reticulum cell sarcoma, and lymphosarcoma may develop nodules in the skin and subcutaneous tissues. This may be the initial presentation of the disease. Metastases are frequent in the skin and subcutaneous tissues especially in patients with carcinoma of the breast, lung, and malignant melanoma. The deposits develop in the lymphatics and lymphoid tissues in the dermis and subcutaneous fat. A single or several lesions may be treated by excision. More often, local radiotherapy, chemotherapy, and, in patients with possible hormone-dependent tumors, hormonal manipulation are the treatments of choice.

TUMORS OF THE SOFT TISSUES

Lipoma and Liposarcoma

A lipoma is a soft multilobular tumor occurring in the subcutaneous tissues and less often in deep organs and tissues, such as the gut and retroperitoneal fat. Superficial lipomas are generally attached to the skin and have a characteristic edge that "slips from the fingers like soap in a bath." Multiple lipomas may be hereditary. Benign lipomas probably never become malignant and are best treated by local excision.

The malignant liposarcoma occurs most often in the leg, buttock, and retroperitoneal fat. The tumor enlarges rapidly, infiltrates the underlying muscles, and ulcerates through the skin. It tends to recur locally after excision and metastasizes to the regional nodes and lungs only after it has been present for a number of years. Treatment is wide local excision often with application of a skin graft. Amputation of a limb is only indicated after one or more attempts at wide excision have been unsuccessful and function of the limb is markedly impaired. Some palliation can be obtained by local radiotherapy to tumors that cannot be removed. The results with chemotherapy have been disappointing. Recently it has been found that a number of liposarcomas and other soft tissue sarcomas respond to Adriamycin.

Fibroma and Fibrosarcoma

A pure fibroma is rare. A malignant fibrosarcoma is more frequent and occurs most often in the legs and often in a scar. The tumor grows slowly and has a marked tendency to recur locally after excision. Treatment is wide local excision and only rarely amputation of a limb. Lung metastases may develop after a number of years.

Neuroma and Neurofibrosarcoma

Neuromas arising from the cells of Schwann are neurilemmomas, and those from all the neural tissues are neurofibromas. The neurilemmoma tends to be small and arises from small peripheral nerves. Neurofibromas are often multiple and associated with genetically determined von Recklinghausen's syndrome, consisting of neurofibromatosis, café au lait spots, and scoliosis. Rapid growth and pain in a neurofibroma suggest development of a neurofibrosarcoma.

A neurilemmoma should be excised. A solitary neurofibroma can sometimes be removed without damage to the nerve. The patient with von Recklinghausen's disease generally has so many tumors that their removal is impossible. Those tumors that are growing rapidly, causing pain, or cosmetic impairment should be excised. A malignant neurofibrosarcoma should be excised widely.

Tumors of Smooth and Voluntary Muscle

Benign muscle tumors are uncommon in the soft tissues except in the female genital tract. A malignant rhabdomyosarcoma or leiomyosarcoma should be treated by wide local excision and rarely by amputation.

Lymphovascular Tumors

The benign cystic hygroma occurs mainly in the neck and thighs of infants. It is a multilobular cystic tumor that grows and may obstruct vital structures in the neck such as the trachea. Wide local excision is often not possible because of its position, and local recurrence is frequent. Cavernous hemangiomas are multilobular blood-filled tumors that are often present at birth and tend to grow with the child. They may contain arteriovenous communications and produce local gigantism and heart failure.

The malignant lymphangiosarcoma is uncommon but may develop in lymphedematous tissue such as a swollen arm after radical mastectomy, filariasis, or congenital lymphedema. Treatment is amputation of the limb. Most patients die rapidly from pulmonary metastases.

CITED REFERENCES

1. Block, G. E., and Hartwell, S. W.: Malignant melanoma: A study of 217 cases. Part I: Epidemiology. *Ann. Surg.*, **154**:74–87, 1961.
2. De Cholnoky, T.: Cancer of the face: A clinical and statistical study of 1062 cases. *Ann. Surg.*, **122**:88–101, 1945.
3. Klein, E.: Hypersensitivity reactions at tumor sites. *Cancer Res.*, **29**:2351–62, 1969.
4. Mihm, M. C., Jr.; Fitzpatrick, T. B.; *et al.*: Early detection of primary cutaneous malignant melanoma. *N. Engl. J. Med.*, **289**:989–96, 1973.
5. Peterson, R. F.; Hazard, J. B.; *et al.*: Superficial malignant melanoma. *Surg. Gynecol. Obstet.*, **119**:37–41, 1964.
6. Polk, H. C., and Linn, B. S.: Selective regional lymphadenectomy for melanoma: A mathematical aid to clinical judgment. *Ann. Surg.*, **174**:402–13, 1971.

SUGGESTIONS FOR FURTHER READING

Cade, Sir Stanford: Malignant melanoma. *Ann. R. Coll. Surg. Engl.*, **28**:331–66, 1961.
An excellent review by a surgeon who has had extensive experience with this disease.
Conway, H.: *Tumors of the Skin.* Charles C Thomas, Springfield, Ill., 1956.
Review of benign tumors of the skin.
Human cutaneous melanomas. In: *Seminars in Oncology.* Vol. 2. No. 2. Grune & Stratton, New York, 1975.
A multiauthor presentation of all aspects of malignant melanoma with special reference to pathology. There is a detailed presentation by W. H. Clark on the importance of depth of penetration and prognosis.
Pack, G. T.: End results in the treatment of sarcomata of the soft somatic tissues. *J. Bone Joint Surg.*, **36A**:241–63, 1954.
A comprehensive review of the subject.

Chapter 26

BREAST

John A. McCredie

CHAPTER OUTLINE

Development and Function
Anatomy
  Congenital Abnormalities
Infections of the Breast
Carcinoma of the Breast
  Methods of Spread
    Interstitial
    Lymphatic
    Hematogenous
    Intraductal
    Transserous
  Microscopic Types
  Staging
  Grading
  Clinical History
  Clinical Examination
  Other Investigations
    Cytology
    Thermography and Infrared Photography
    Mammography
    Xeroradiography

X-rays
Isotope Scans
Laboratory Tests
Screening Programs
Differential Diagnosis
  Mammary Dysplasia
  Cysts
  Fibroadenoma
  Duct Papilloma
  Fat Necrosis
  Chronic Breast Abscess
  Cystosarcoma Phylloides
Treatment
  Operations
  Radiotherapy
  Hormones
  Chemotherapy
Personal Regimen for Initial Treatment
Diseases of the Male Breast
  Carcinoma
  Gynecomastia

DEVELOPMENT AND FUNCTION

The breast, a modified sweat gland, commences as a series of thickenings in the ectoderm of the milk line that extends from the midclavicle to the center of the inguinal ligament. One in each pectoral region persists. About 20 solid cords of ectoderm extend from the plaque into the deeper tissues; they become canalized and form the main ducts and open independently at the elevated nipple. In the adult only about six ducts are patent and functional; the remainder have "blind ends."

The gland, under the influence of maternal estrogens, becomes functional at birth. It enlarges, develops acini, and produces a small amount of secretion. These changes regress after the first week. The functional changes in the breast result from the interaction of a number of ovarian and pituitary hormones. In the female the breast enlarges at puberty; the ducts pass deeper, divide, and are surrounded by periductal fibrous tissue. Lobules appear with the onset of ovulation. The breast enlarges at the end of the first week of the menstrual cycle due to proliferation of the parenchyma, increase in vasculature, and interlobular edema and is often tense and tender prior to menstruation. The changes rapidly regress with the onset of menstruation. If conception occurs, the gland enlarges, the nipple becomes more prominent, the areola darkens, and there is a marked increase in vascularity. During the menopause the breast slowly involutes, the lobules are replaced by fibrous tissue and fat, the acini disappear, and only the large lobular ducts remain.

ANATOMY

The glandular tissue consists of about 20 discrete lobules arranged radially around the nipple and lying approximately in the same plane. The periphery of the lobules extends beyond the mammary prominence. The mammary lobules extend from the second to sixth ribs and from just lateral to the sternum to the midaxillary line. A process of glandular tissue, the axillary tail of Spence, extends from the upper lateral part of the gland through the axillary fascia to lie under the lateral border of pectoralis major muscle in the third intercostal space in contact with the anterior pectoral lymph nodes. The deep fascia behind the gland covers mainly the pectoralis major muscle and on its lower lateral aspect the serratus anterior muscle. In the resting state breast size is determined by the amount of fat superficial and deep to the lobules rather than the amount of glandular tissue. Fibrous bands, the ligaments of Cooper, connect the superficial surface of the lobules to the skin, and others lie in the retromammary fat and connect the deep surface to the pectoral fascia. The nipple consists of mainly circular and longitudinal smooth muscle fibers. The surrounding areola is pigmented and also contains smooth muscle fibers.

Perforating branches of the internal mammary artery are the main blood supply of the breast. They pass through the second, third, and fourth intercostal spaces, the pectoralis major muscle, and deep fascia about 1 cm lateral to the sternum and supply about half the blood to the breast. The lateral thoracic branch of the axillary artery, lying just lateral to the pectoralis major muscle, and perforating branches of the intercostal arteries supply mainly the gland's deep and lateral aspects. The venous drainage is mainly to a subareolar plexus and then to the internal mammary, lateral thoracic, and axillary veins. Some deep veins enter the intercostal veins and may account for the high incidence of metastases in the ribs, sternum, and dorsal vertebrae. The lymphatic drainage is of particular importance in the spread of breast carcinoma (see page 447).

Microscopically each lobule is a compound alveolar gland. Several lobules drain into a single lactiferous duct. The main duct is dilated just below the skin and forms a lactiferous sinus. Small ducts with acini projecting from their walls drain into the main duct. The epithelium of the lactiferous sinus is squamous, and that of the ducts has two layers of cuboidal cells. The alveoli have an outer basement membrane, spiral myoepithelial cells, and an inner layer of low columnar glandular cells, Estrogens produce hyperplasia of the ductal epithelium during the first half of the menstrual cycle and sensitize the acinar cells to subsequent exposure to progesterone. Progesterone then induces hyperplasia of the acinar cells and increases fibrous tissue throughout the breast. During pregnancy the number of ducts and acini increase markedly. Colostrum is secreted by the glandular acinar cells at the sixth month, and milk granules are shed into the alveolar lumen just after delivery.

Congenital Abnormalities

Absence of a breast, amazia, is usually unilateral, occurs more often in men than women and may be associated with absence of the underlying pectoralis major muscle or of ribs. A small breast, micromazia, may occur on one or both sides. Supernumerary breasts, polymazia, are quite common. They are the result of persistence of portions of the milk ridge and may be present in tissues between the buttock and neck. Supernumerary nipples, polythelia, are more frequent than polymazia. Congenital inversion of the nipple may occur and may in the adult suggest the presence of carcinoma of the breast.

INFECTIONS OF THE BREAST

An acute breast abscess may occur at birth, at puberty, or, most frequently, after delivery. Mastitis, occurring at birth or puberty, may progress to abscess formation and require drainage. The common acute puerperal form occurs most often within four weeks after childbirth when infection enters a duct or lymphatic through an abrasion on the nipple. Good hygiene is therefore the best prophylaxis. The infecting organism is most frequently *Staphylococcus aureus*. Drainage of milk is impaired, and infection rapidly becomes established in the protein-rich milk. Initially it is confined to a single lobule but soon spreads to adjacent lobules. The patient is toxic, has a high temperature, and the breast becomes swollen and extremely painful. In the early stages support, antibiotics, and cessation of lactation may abort the infection. An established abscess should be drained under general anesthesia through a skin incision over the mass, or if the lower half of the breast is involved, through an inframammary skin crease incision. Fibrous septa in the abscess cavity should be carefully broken with a finger (Figure 6–5, page 134).

A chronic breast abscess may develop spontaneously or follow treatment of an acute abscess with antibiotics. It may present months or years after pregnancy. More frequently it is not a complication of pregnancy but follows obstruction to a duct. The names mammary duct ectasia, plasma cell mastitis, and comedomastitis have also been applied to this condition. The mass may not be painful or tender and is ill defined and hard. It can be attached to skin or deeper structures and cause retraction of the nipple, produce edema in the overlying skin, and enlargement of the axillary nodes. It may therefore closely simulate a carcinoma. Chronic breast infection due to actinomycosis or syphilis is rare. Tuberculosis occurs usually in patients with open pulmonary tuberculosis.

CARCINOMA OF THE BREAST

Carcinoma of the breast is the most frequent cancer in the female and is the commonest cause of death in women of 35 to 44 years. In North America the incidence is about 21 per 100,000 women per year. About 1 in 15 women develops breast carcinoma. Public education, better medical supervision, and the use of mammography have led to earlier diagnosis and better prognosis in an increasing number of patients. Surgical excision of the primary tumor and regional nodes with or without radiotherapy effectively controls local disease in the majority of patients. There is, however, no curative treatment for disseminated disease. Improved results are unlikely to be obtained from changes in treatment methods of the primary tumor but rather from earlier diagnosis of the primary and treatment of metastases.

The etiology of breast carcinoma is not known. It is frequent in North America and Western Europe and less common in Asia, Russia, and Africa. In Japan the annual incidence is about 4 per 100,000 women per year. There is a positive correlation between the unsaturated fat content of the diet and the incidence of the disease.[40] The bacterial flora in the colon differs in those on high- and low-fat diets. It has been suggested that with a high intake of unsaturated fats the bacteria produce carcinogenic estrogens from the bile salts and these are absorbed into the systemic circulation. Animal studies suggest that estrogens increase the incidence of breast carcinoma. Clinical reports, however, fail to confirm the results of the animal studies.[9]

The incidence of carcinoma of the breast is lowest in women who have the menopause induced before 35 years and in those who have had their first pregnancy before 20 years. The low incidence in those who have had many children is probably more related to the age at which they had the first pregnancy than the number of pregnancies. Breast feeding is probably not important. The incidence is greatest in those who have had carcinoma of the contralateral breast, who are nulliparous, have had miscarriages, or have their first pregnancy after 28 years. Views differ on the significance of a family history of breast carcinoma. There appears to be a greater incidence when the patient's mother had a carcinoma of the breast at less than 50 years and especially if the mother had bilateral mammary tumors. The daughter also tends to develop the disease at an early age. A history of a sister or other relatives having the disease is probably not important.

Women under 20 rarely develop carcinoma of the breast. The incidence then increases until about 45 years when it plateaus for about 10 years and then increases. The incidence at 80 is about twice that at 50.

Methods of Spread

Spread of breast carcinoma occurs within the mammary lobules, toward the overlying skin, to the deep structures on the thoracic wall, to the regional lymph nodes, and by distant metastases.

Interstitial. Carcinoma of the breast grows locally by increase in cell mass and by infiltration of the mammary lobules and eventually the fat and adjacent tissues. Prognosis is better when growth is by expansion, producing a tumor with a smooth or nodular margin; it is worse when the tumor grows by infiltration. The infiltrating tumor with its stellate margin occurs in two thirds of patients. It can often be recognized clinically and can readily be seen on mammography, on section of the gross specimen obtained at operation, and by microscopic examination of the tumor edge. Superficial spread in continuity with the primary tumor causes tethering, fixation, and ultimately ulceration of the skin. Deep spread in continuity is to the deep fascia, muscle, and eventually the thoracic wall and pleural cavity.

Lymphatic. The rich lymphatic drainage from the breast is responsible for the high incidence of metastases in the regional nodes. The lymphatics of the mammary lobules drain into periductal lymphatics that enter the large subareolar plexus (Figure 26–1). Lymphatics pass mainly to the anterior pectoral lymph nodes and to a lesser extent to the internal mammary nodes. The subepidermal and subdermal plexi over the breast drain mainly into the subareolar plexus and also communicate with similar plexi on the contralateral side. There are communications between the subdermal plexus and the lymphatics in the mammary lobules but they are important only when the large periductal lymphatics are obstructed. Similar communications exist between the lymphatics on the deep surface of the mammary lobules and the lymphatic plexus on the surface of the deep fascia covering the pectoralis major and serratus anterior muscles. Again these connections are only important when the major

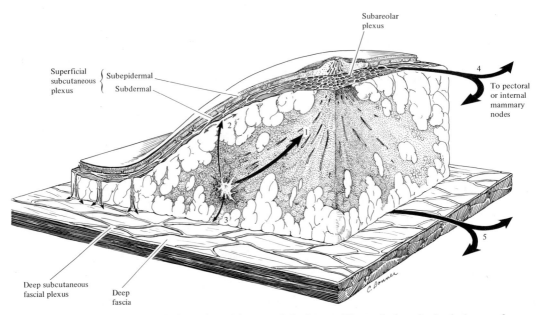

Figure 26–1. Lymphatic drainage in carcinoma of the breast. The main lymphatic drainage of the breast is to the subareolar plexus and then to the anterior pectoral or internal mammary nodes. The subepidermal and subdermal plexuses over the breast drain to the large subareolar plexus and have little connection with the mammary lobules. The plexus over the deep fascia and the cutaneous plexuses do not normally communicate with those in the mammary lobules but drain into the anterior pectoral and internal mammary nodes. In the patient with a locally advanced carcinoma there is obstruction of the lymphatic flow. Cancer cells may then spread by embolism and permeation to the cutaneous and deep fascial plexuses and then to the regional nodes. With an early carcinoma, spread tends to occur only by routes 1 and 4.

lymphatic channels within the breast are obstructed. Two thirds of the lymphatic drainage from the mammary lobules is to the anterior pectoral nodes, and most of the remainder is to the internal mammary nodes. There is probably a small amount of drainage, less than 10 percent, along the intercostal vessels to the posterior mediastinal and interpectoral nodes. There is a higher incidence of metastases in the anterior pectoral than the internal mammary nodes when a carcinoma is in the lateral quadrants of the breast (Figure 26–2). When the carcinoma is retroareolar or in a medial quadrant, metastases are more frequent in the internal mammary nodes. The anterior pectoral nodes lie deep to the axillary fascia on the second and third intercostal spaces under the lateral margin of the pectoralis major muscle. The other lower axillary nodes, the lateral axillary and posterior subscapular, at the base of the truncated conal space of the axilla, contain metastases only when the anterior pectoral nodes are largely replaced by tumor. Lymph from the anterior pectoral nodes passes in lymphatics that lie medial to the axillary vein and deep to the pectoralis minor muscle, to the

apical nodes lying on the first intercostal space, deep to pectoralis major muscle and the costo-coracoid membrane, below the clavicle and medial to the coracoid process. Efferent lymphatics from the apical nodes pass deep to the clavicle to enter the thoracic duct on the left side and the jugular duct on the right side. Lymph then enters the great veins at the base of the neck. The supraclavicular nodes drain directly into the thoracic or jugular duct.

Lymphatic drainage to the internal mammary nodes occurs through the medial ends of the anterior intercostal spaces to the nodes lying medial to the internal mammary vessels and behind the sternum. The largest nodes are in the second intercostal space. The anastomotic lymphatics between the internal mammary nodes on both sides only carry cancer cells to the contralateral internal mammary nodes and to the contralateral breast and axillary nodes when the ipsilateral nodes are largely replaced by tumor. The internal mammary nodes drain to the large lymph ducts at the root of the neck.

A small amount of lymphatic drainage also occurs from the deep fascial plexus along the

Figure 26–2. Lymphatic drainage of breast to regional lymph nodes. The lymphatic drainage from a laterally placed carcinoma goes to the anterior pectoral nodes (*1*), to the apical nodes (*2*), and then to the great veins at the root of the neck. The supraclavicular nodes may then contain metastases (*3*). There is a small amount of lymphatic drainage to the internal mammary nodes. A medially placed or retroareolar tumor drains mainly into the ipsilateral internal mammary nodes; a smaller amount is to the anterior pectoral nodes. The subscapular, lateral axillary, supraclavicular, and contralateral internal mammary and axillary nodes only receive lymph from the breast when the primary groups are extensively infiltrated with tumor.

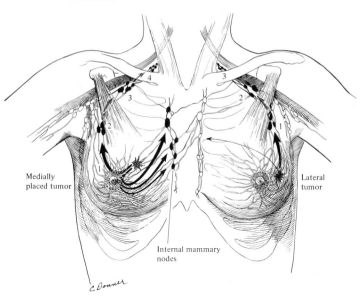

Medially placed tumor

Lateral tumor

Internal mammary nodes

C. Donner

intercostal vessels to nodes in the posterior mediastinum. This accounts for the high incidence of tumor seen at autopsy in the ipsilateral chest wall and ribs. The lymphatic communications between the deep aspect of the breast and the interpectoral nodes lying between pectoralis major and minor muscles probably only carry cancer cells in patients with advanced breast carcinoma. Lymphatic drainage from the breast was also thought to occur to the deep fascial plexus on the rectus abdominis muscle and along the falciform ligament to nodes at the porta hepatis of the liver, and anterior to the clavicle to the supraclavicular nodes. However, these routes are not important in patients with "operable" carcinoma of the breast.

Lymphatic spread is initially by embolism of single cancer cells or clumps of cells. Metastases develop first in the cortex of the node; they grow and largely replace the nodal tissues, impairing flow of lymph and permitting retrograde permeation of the afferent lymphatic to the primary tumor with a continuous cord of cancer cells. Foci of cancer cells growing in the permeated lymphatics form palpable subcutaneous nodules. Edema develops in the skin and subcutaneous tissues and can be recognized clinically and on mammography. The superficial surface of the mammary lobules is attached to the skin by fibrous bands, the ligaments of Cooper. The attachments produce dimpling of the edematous skin and a "peau d'orange" appearance. Its presence signifies that the lymphatics are extensively permeated with cancer cells and that the prognosis is bad.

Hematogenous. Cancer cells enter the systemic venous circulation by direct infiltration of capillaries or veins, through numerous communications between small lymphatics and blood vessels, or through the jugular or thoracic ducts. Some establish metastases in the lungs, while others pass through and establish metastases in the bones, liver, skin, brain, adrenal glands, and ovaries. The bones are the commonest site of distant metastases. The red marrow-containing bones close to the breast, the ribs, sternum, and thoracolumbar vertebrae have the highest incidence of bony metastases. This suggests that some of the cancer cells enter the red bone marrow through the vertebral system of veins rather than the general systemic circulation (see Chapter 7, page 146).

Intraductal. Cancer cells may grow within the lumen of the lobular ducts and, when combined with secretions, form a cheeselike material, the comedocarcinoma. Examination of the fluid from the ducts has not proven a useful routine cytologic test for the diagnosis of breast carcinoma.

Transserous. Cancer cells can spread directly from the deep fascial plexus through the intercostal spaces to the parietal pleura and cause effusion of blood-stained fluid containing cancer cells. Pleural effusion is more often the result of metastatic spread in the lungs or mediastinal nodes to the visceral or mediastinal pleura.

Metastases in the nodes at the porta hepatis, in the liver, or ovaries may infiltrate the visceral peritoneum and produce ascites.

Microscopic Types

The classification by Foote and Stewart[18] has been adopted with some modifications by the World Health Organization. This provides a detailed description of the different types of tumor based on the origin of the cancer cell and its tendency to metastasize. The cancer cell may arise from the epithelium of the nipple (Paget's disease of the nipple), the ducts (infiltrating or noninfiltrating, including the common scirrhous carcinoma), or the mammary lobules (infiltrating or noninfiltrating).

Benign tumors of the breast may be classified as:

1. Epithelial. A papilloma may be intraductal or subareolar.

2. Mixed epithelial and mesodermal. A fibroadenoma may be intra- or pericanalicular. The distinction is not important, and both types can be found in most tumors. Cystosarcoma phylloides is a giant intracanalicular fibro-adenoma.

3. Mesodermal. The tumor may be a lipoma, fibroma, or a granular cell myoblastoma. The latter tumor is now considered to be of Schwann-cell origin.

Malignant tumors of the breast may be classified as:

1. Carcinoma of mammary ducts. (a) A noninfiltrating intraductal carcinoma may be papillary, comedo (with central necrosis), or solid. (b) Infiltrating ductal carcinoma.

(i) The papillary type is responsible for about 2 percent of breast cancers. It is soft and has a good prognosis.

(ii) With productive fibrosis. Seventy to 80 percent of breast cancers are of this type. It is hard, has irregular processes, and metastasizes early.

(iii) Comedo infiltrating. This tumor has a better prognosis than the scirrhous tumor.

(iv) Medullary. The tumor is large and soft, metastasizes late, and has a good prognosis. About 2 percent of breast cancers are of this type. Microscopically the tumor is quite cellular (epithelial) and has scanty fibrous tissue infiltrated with many lymphocytes. These cells may be a manifestation of a good cell-mediated immune response.

(v) Mucinous. The mucus is produced by the duct cells, and the tumor has a good prognosis.

(vi) Paget's. There is always an associated ductal carcinoma.

2. Carcinoma of mammary lobules. (a) Noninfiltrating in situ lobular. (b) Infiltrating lobular. About 5 percent of breast carcinomas are of this type. Multiple tumors are often present in the same breast, and in 30 percent the tumors are bilateral.

3. Miscellaneous carcinomas. These include sweat gland and cutaneous tumors.

4. Sarcomas. These uncommon tumors include the malignant form of the cystosarcoma phylloides and soft tissue sarcomas.

Another classification by Ackerman[1] is of particular value to the clinician as it reflects prognosis.

Type I: Noninvasive carcinoma. This is carcinoma in situ.

Type II: Invasive carcinoma but rarely metastasizing. Examples are medullary carcinomas with lymphocytic infiltration and well-differentiated carcinomas.

Type III: Invasive carcinomas with moderate tendency to metastasize. Examples are the common scirrhous carcinomas and infiltrating intraductal carcinomas. The scirrhous carcinoma occurs in 75 percent of patients.

Type IV: Invasive carcinomas with marked tendency to metastasize. Examples are undifferentiated carcinomas and those that invade blood vessels.

Staging

A clinical classification of the extent of spread is valuable in planning treatment, making a prognosis, and comparing results between centers. The stage is determined before treatment is begun, is based on the most advanced findings on clinical and special investigation, and is not changed because of operative findings or the results of microscopic examination of the operative specimen. The Manchester system of staging has been used extensively (Figure 26–3). It is based on spread of the primary tumor toward the skin or chest wall, the state of the regional nodes, and the presence or absence of distant metastases (Figure 26–4). Patients in stages I and II are often stated to have early or operable tumors and to be suitable for "attempted curative" treatment. Those in stages III and IV are said to have advanced tumors and should be given palliative treatment. Five-year survival is approximately 85 percent in stage I, 50 percent in stage II, 30 percent in stage III, and 10 percent in stage IV. The TNM (tumor, nodes, and metastases) classification proposed by the International Union Against Cancer provides a more precise classification and is being increasingly used.[28]

T (Tumor)

T–0 A nonpalpable tumor diagnosed by mammography.

T–1 Tumor measures less than 2 cm.

T–2 Tumor measures 2 to 5 cm.

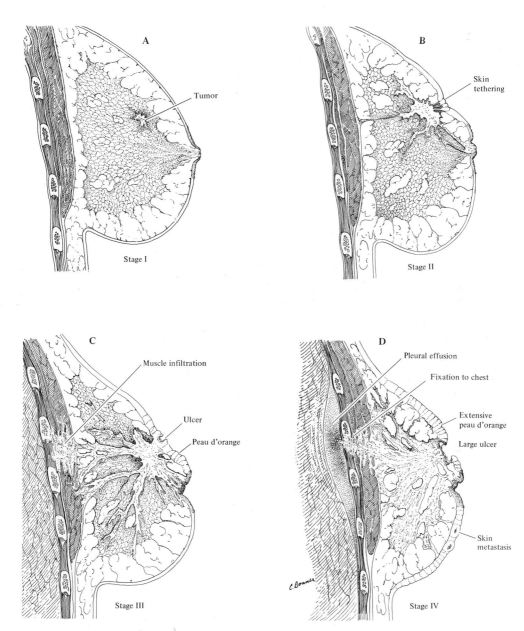

Figure 26–3. Staging of carcinoma from clinical examination of the breast. A carcinoma of the breast can be staged according to the extent of spread into the superficial or deeper tissues. *A.* In stage I the carcinoma is confined to the mammary lobules. *B.* In stage II it is tethered to the skin or deep fascia. *C.* In stage III the tumor has infiltrated the skin and may have caused ulceration, or it has invaded the lymphatics and produced edema (peau d'orange). Deep penetration may have occurred into the pectoralis major or serratus anterior muscles. *D.* In stage IV there is gross ulceration, peau d'orange over the whole breast, or multiple skin nodules. Deep extension may have occurred with fixation to the ribs and extension into the pleural cavity, producing a blood-stained effusion containing cancer cells.

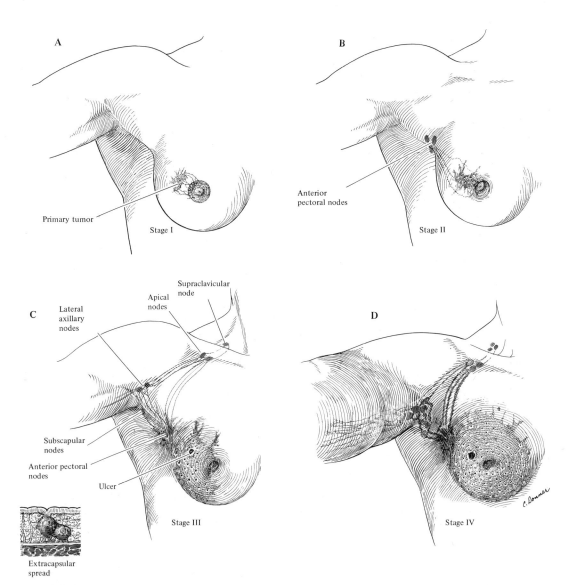

Figure 26–4. Clinical staging of patients with carcinoma of the breast. A carcinoma is staged clinically according to the most advanced sign in the breast or the regional nodes. *A.* In stage I the carcinoma is confined to the mammary lobules and the regional nodes do not clinically contain metastases. *B.* In stage II there is early extension outside the lobules with tethering to the skin or deep fascia, and the axillary nodes clinically contain metastases. *C.* In stage III there is further involvement of the skin with obvious infiltration or early ulceration, and peau d'orange may be present over the tumor. There is penetration through the deep fascia. The metastases in the axillary nodes have extended beyond the capsules. There may be metastases in an ipsilateral supraclavicular node. *D.* In stage IV the skin is grossly ulcerated, peau d'orange is present over the whole breast, or deep fixation has occurred to the ribs. A pleural effusion may be present. The axillary and supraclavicular nodes are fixed, and edema of the arm is present. The presence of distant metastases places the patient in stage IV.

T–3 Tumor measures greater than 5 cm or has extended to the skin or deep fascia.

N (*Nodes*)

N–0 The nodes do not clinically contain metastases.

N–1 {
N–1A Nodes are palpable but are thought not to contain metastases.

N–1B The nodes are thought to contain metastases.
}

N–2 The metastases in the nodes have extended beyond the capsule. The nodes are fixed to one another, to the skin, or to the deep tissues.

M (*Metastases*)

M–0 Distant metastases are not found clinically or on preoperative investigation.

M–1 Distant metastases are present.

The TNM classification can be applied to the Manchester system.

Manchester Stage	*TNM Classification*
I	T–1, N–1A, M–0
II	T–1, T–2, N–1B, M–0
III	T–3, N–2, M–0
IV	M–1

Criticisms of the TNM classification are that patients with tumors greater than a 5-cm diameter are placed in T–3 and said to be equivalent to those in stage III. They may therefore be considered for palliative and not attempted curative treatment. This places considerable importance on determining the size of the tumor. It is extremely difficult to measure accurately the size of a tumor, especially in the patient with a large breast and a deeply placed tumor. The size on mammography is generally smaller than on clinical examination and is more accurate. Unfortunately all tumors are not outlined on mammography. There is therefore no completely satisfactory means of accurately determining tumor size. Also, a number of patients with large tumors, expecially medullary carcinomas with lymphoid infiltration and infiltrating ductal papillary carcinomas, have a good prognosis and should have attemped curative treatment. It would therefore appear that giving palliative treatment to patients with tumors greater than 5 cm is incorrect. Patients placed in stage III because axillary metastases have extended beyond the capsule of the nodes have about 25 percent five-year survival, while those placed in the same stage because of local extension of the tumor have about 70 percent five-year survival. Those with locally advanced tumors and clinically negative axillary nodes are therefore better treated in an "attempted curative" manner. Their best treatment is preoperative radiotherapy followed by mastectomy.[13]

Grading

The degree of malignancy may be assessed by microscopic examination of the tumor (grading). Initially the degree of differentiation of the cancer cell was the only feature considered. Anaplastic cancer cells infiltrate and metastasize more rapidly than those that are well differentiated. A good host response, however, inhibits their growth. For example, certain groups of patients with anaplastic carcinoma who have marked infiltration of the tumor with lymphocytes, plasma cells, and large mononuclear cells have a five-year survival of about 90 percent. Grading is based on the degree of differentiation, chromatin uniformity, size of the nuclei, and the number of mitotic figures; the presence of cancer cells in lymphatics, blood vessels, and nodes; the amount of infiltration with lymphocytes, plasma, and large mononuclear cells; the size of the tumor; and the presence of a smooth or irregular margin. Grading is made after a number of microscopic sections have been examined and according to the findings in the area with the most advanced features. It is described as low, intermediate, or high, or as grades I, II, III, or IV.

A more accurate prognosis can be made when clinical staging and microscopic grading are both used than by employing one scheme.[6] Patients in stage I, grade III have a bad prognosis and about 30 percent five-year survival, while those in stage III, grade I have about 70 percent five-year survival. A bad grade in a patient who is in clinical stages I or II is the main reason for poor survival.

Clinical History

Tumors of the breast in women under 40 are most often benign and in those over 50 are most often malignant. Carcinoma of the breast, however, is often seen in women in the fourth decade and occasionally in those under 30.

About three quarters of patients give a history of finding a painless tumor while washing or on routine self-examination. Sometimes a minor injury may lead to its recognition. About 10 percent of patients have a mild discomfort or tingling sensation. The same percentage have a discharge from the nipple. A blood-stained discharge with a palpable tumor, greater than 1 cm, suggests a malignant papilloma or intraductal carcinoma. In Paget's disease there are local irritation and a blood-stained discharge from the areola or nipple. Prognosis is better when the tumor has been present for a long-time and has grown slowly; it is worse when the tumor has increased rapidly in size.

The commonest sympton suggestive of distant metastases is bone pain, especially in the ribs and thoracolumbar vertebrae. Occasionally a pathologic fracture results in acute severe pain. The patient with extensive bone metastases may have hypercalcemia with a clinical presentation suggesting brain metastases. Spread to the liver may result in right upper abdominal discomfort and if extensive, loss of weight, anorexia, and

occasionally jaundice. Deep jaundice suggests the presence of metastases in the porta hepatis obstructing the extrahepatic bile ducts. Abdominal distention may occur from ascites. Brain metastases may be the presenting symptom. Lung metastases only cause symptoms when they are advanced.

Clinical Examination

Various types of breast carcinoma may be recognized on clinical examination (Figure

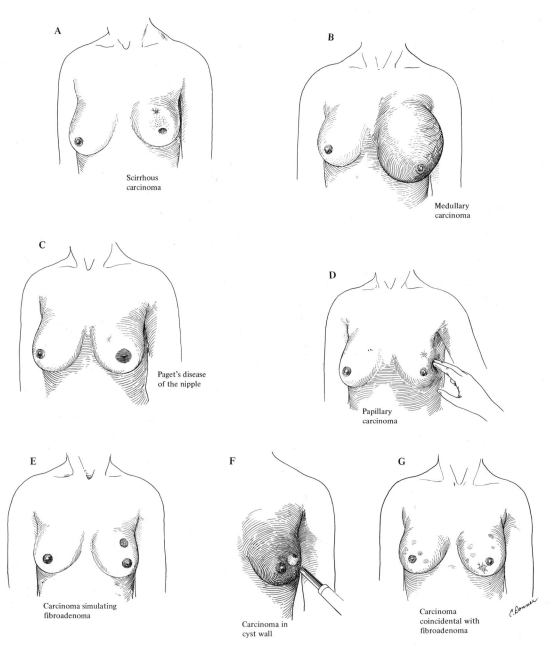

A Scirrhous carcinoma

B Medullary carcinoma

C Paget's disease of the nipple

D Papillary carcinoma

E Carcinoma simulating fibroadenoma

F Carcinoma in cyst wall

G Carcinoma coincidental with fibroadenoma

26–5). The patient is examined by inspection in the sitting position with the arms relaxed by the side and also with the arms raised (Figure 26–6, A, B). The breasts are then palpated with the flat of the fingers, with the patient upright and lying down (Figure 26–6, C, D, E, F, G). Evidence for spread to the skin and deep structures is looked for. The nodes in the axillae are then palpated, particularly the anterior pectoral group. The apical nodes, below the clavicle medial to the coracoid process, can sometimes be felt in a thin patient. Palpation of the supraclavicular region is important (Figure 26–6, H). Slight swelling in the fingers signifies that the axillary nodes are extensively infiltrated with metastases and that the prognosis is poor (Figure 26–6, I). Edema of the skin overlying the entire breast or satellite skin nodules signifies that only palliative treatment is indicated.

The correct diagnosis of carcinoma of the breast using clinical examination and mammography is now over 90 percent. Clinical assessment of axillary lymph nodes is much less accurate. About 50 percent of women without palpable nodes have metastases on microscopic examination. Those who have palpable nodes but are thought to be hyperplastic and not contain tumor (N–1A) often contain metastases, and conversely those thought to contain tumor (N–1B) are often hyperplastic. Clinical assessment of nodes as N–1A or N–1B is wrong in 25 to 40 percent of patients.

The patient is examined for distant metastases. Tenderness over bone, especially the ribs, sternum, and vertebrae suggests bony metastases. Abnormality in breath sounds suggests pleural effusion from lung metastases. Metastases in the liver may increase its size. Occasionally metastases in the pelvis producing a "rectal shelf" or ovarian enlargement can be detected on rectal or vaginal examination. Ascites may be present. A neurologic abnormality may indicate cerebral metastases. Clinical signs of Addison's disease are uncommon and suggest extensive metastases in the adrenal glands.

In the patient with breast carcinoma who has been treated for cure, the first sign of local recurrence is most often the development of one or more skin nodules at the operative site. The prognosis is bad, because distant metastases are generally found elsewhere on clinical or special investigation or they soon develop at a distance. They are therefore not a sign of local recurrence but of widespread disease. Recurrence in the axillary nodes is uncommon in those in stage I who had been treated by radical or modified radical mastectomy. It occurs in about 15 percent in stage II. Edema in the arm more than six months after the initial treatment is most likely the result of recurrent disease in the axilla.

Other Investigations

A thorough investigation is necessary, especially to help diagnose the tumor and to detect distant metastases. A cyst is translucent on illumination if it is superficial and contains clear fluid (Figure 26–6, J). Most cysts contain turbid fluid and do not transilluminate.

Cytology. Fluid from the nipple has been examined for cancer cells. Individual ducts have been cannulated and washings obtained. This has not proved a useful investigation.

Thermography and Infrared Photography. There is often an increase in emission of infrared radiation by the tissues overlying a carcinoma of the breast. The "hot spots" in the overlying skin can be recognized by applying a thermocouple to the skin or by infrared photography.[27] The increased temperature results from increased

---

Figure 26–5. Types of carcinoma of the breast. A. The scirrhous tumor is most frequent. It is hard in consistency and can usually be felt with the palm of the hand, the edge is generally irregular, and the periphery is not sharply defined. The tumor tends to spread to the skin and deep fascia and metastasizes frequently to the regional nodes and by the blood. B. The soft or medullary tumor may or may not be associated with pregnancy. It is often large and soft, has a smooth margin, and induces local hyperemia. The medullary type with lymphoid infiltration tends to remain localized. The medullary type without lymphoid infiltration or inflammatory carcinoma spreads rapidly to the skin and deep tissues, metastasizes to the regional nodes, and produces hematogenous metastases. C. The patient with Paget's disease of the breast has ulceration of the nipple and adjacent skin with partial or complete loss of the nipple, and a well-defined margin to the area of ulceration. There is always an underlying carcinoma of the breast, which may or may not be palpable. D. A papillary carcinoma often presents with passage of red blood from the nipple. The blood may be expressed by palpation of the tumor or a region in the breast. Small tumors, less than 1.0 cm, are usually benign duct papillomas; larger lesions are more likely to be malignant. E. A carcinoma of the breast may be discrete, soft, and freely mobile and simulate a fibroadenoma. F. A carcinoma may be present in the wall of a cyst. G. A patient with diffuse fibroadenosis may also have a carcinoma of the breast. The patient may present with metastases in the axillary nodes or distant metastases, and the primary tumor cannot be found clinically but may be diagnosed on mammography or xerography.

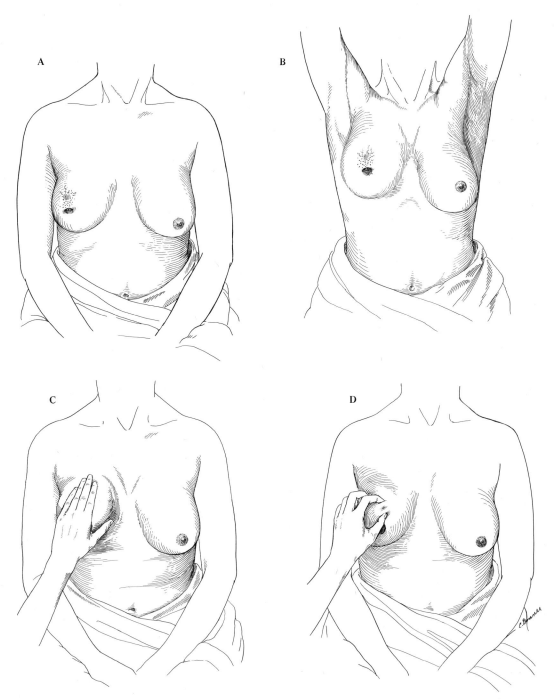

Figure 26–6. Examination of the breasts. *A.* The breasts are inspected with the patient upright. A carcinoma may produce slight asymmetry on the affected side and the nipple may be retracted. A swelling, retraction of the skin, peau d'orange, ulceration, skin nodules, and prominent veins may be visible. *B.* When the arms are raised, the asymmetry and the nipple and skin retraction are accentuated. *C.* The tumor is gently palpated with the flat of the hand and then with the fingers. Its consistency, the presence or absence of tenderness, the margin, and relation to the surrounding breast tissues are noted. The state of the remaining breast tissues is noted. *D.* Dimpling when the skin is approximated over the tumor signifies tethering. *E.* To demonstrate tethering to the deep fascia it is necessary to make the fascia over the pectoralis major muscle tense by contracting the muscle. The hand is pressed firmly against the iliac crest and the breast moved medially and laterally.

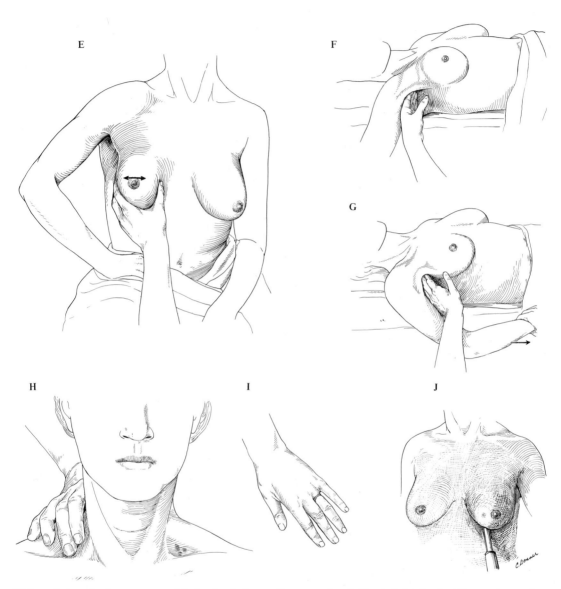

If there is impaired movement with the fascia tense, the tumor has infiltrated the fascia. The carcinoma has infiltrated the muscle if movement of the breast is impaired when the pectoral muscles are relaxed. The tumor is fixed to the ribs and intercostal muscles when no movement can be elicited. *F.* The breasts are next palpated with the patient lying supine. Examination of the axilla is more complete than in the upright position. Special attention is paid to the anterior pectoral nodes on the second and third intercostal spaces under the lateral margin of the pectoralis major muscle. *G.* The axillary nodes are most easily palpable when the arm is relaxed at the side. Nodes containing tumor are generally hard in consistency. They are recorded as not palpable, or palpable clinically but not containing metastases. If they are thought to contain tumor, they are described as single, multiple, fixed to one another, or fixed to the skin or deep tissues. *H.* The supraclavicular triangle is palpated on both sides for enlarged lymph nodes. *I.* The arm is examined for swelling. Recently developed tightness of a ring signifies extensive infiltration of the axillary nodes with metastases. *J.* The breast may be examined by transillumination for a cyst.

457

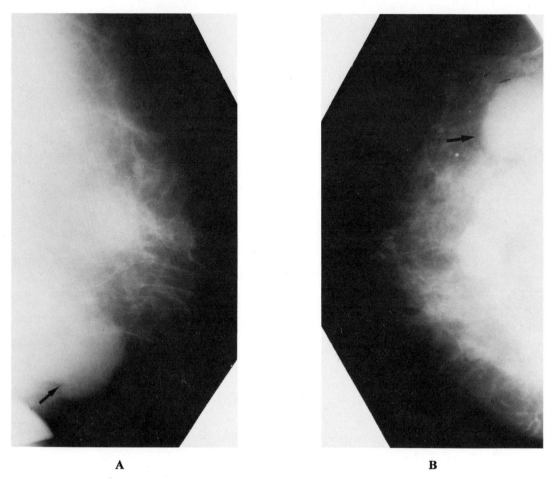

A   B

Figure 26–7. Mammography. *A.* There is a well-defined fibroadenoma with nodular margin. *B.* The breast shows diffuse mammary dysplasia with fibrosis and cyst formation.

metabolism in the tissues and not from an increase in blood flow. The test is positive in about 80 percent of patients with breast carcinoma, a similar incidence to that on mammography. The incidence of false positives is generally about 20 percent. The test is of value in women under 50, while mammography is more sensitive in older women. Burn[10] in a controlled trial comparing thermography with mammography found that the incidence of false positives, especially in patients with mammary dysplasia, was too high for the test to be of value. A chronic breast abscess may also produce hyperemia and simulate a carcinoma.

Mammography.   The soft-tissue structure of the breast can be seen on mammography[15] (Figure 26–7). The technique differs from that for routine radiography in that low-voltage, high-current x-rays and screened fine-grain photographic film are used. Fine granules or

thin lines of calcification are almost pathognomonic of breast carcinoma but are found in only about one third of patients. Suggestive signs are an ill-defined or stellate margin to the tumor or prominent blood vessels in the surrounding tissues. Thickening occurs in the overlying skin even without clinical edema. Bands tethering the skin to the tumor or skin infiltration with dimpling are readily seen. One of the most useful signs is the discrepancy between the size of a carcinoma on clinical examination and that on mammography. The tumor appears much larger on clinical examination because of the reaction induced in the surrounding tissues. Benign tumors are only slightly larger on clinical examination than on the mammogram.

Some recommend that mammography and thermography be performed at the first examination and thermography on subsequent visits. If any changes appear on thermography, then

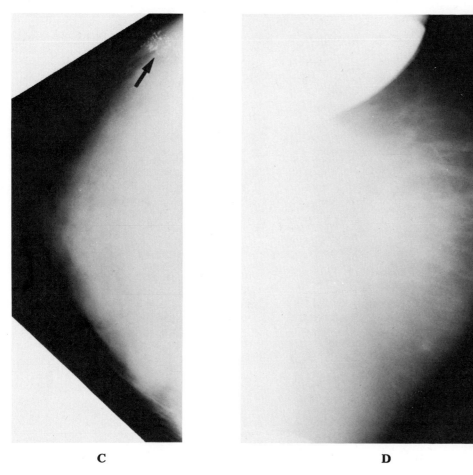

C   D

Figure 26–7 [*continued*].   Mammography. *C*. There are minute calcifications in a nonpalpable carcinoma. *D*. There is a large carcinoma, and the nipple is retracted.

mammography is done. This minimizes the amount of radiation the patient receives. Others feel that too many false positives are detected on thermography and that the investigation is of no value. Even those who are enthusiastic about its use stress that biopsy is not indicated in a woman who has a positive thermogram but has a normal mammogram and no abnormality on clinical examination. Thermography does not accurately localize a tumor, and mammography is therefore essential in those with a positive thermogram.

The indications for mammography are:

1. Mammography should be performed yearly in patients who have had breast carcinoma. The annual incidence of carcinoma of the contralateral breast is just less than 1 percent per year and remains the same each year up to 20 years.[30]

2. It is indicated in patients with breast carcinoma to exclude a synchronous carcinoma of the opposite breast.

3. The significance of a high incidence of breast carcinoma in a family is not clear. Mammography performed once and followed by repeated clinical examinations and possibly thermography is indicated in these women.

4. It is of value in the patient with nodular breasts when biopsy of an area is not indicated from clinical examination and in the patient with symptoms confined to a particular segment.

Mammography is not justified in asymptomatic women under 40 because of the small number of tumors detected, the cost, and the relatively large dose of radiation, 5 to 20 rads. Better definition of the mammary lobules is obtained by using a molybdenum rather than a tungsten anode. The technique is known as senography.

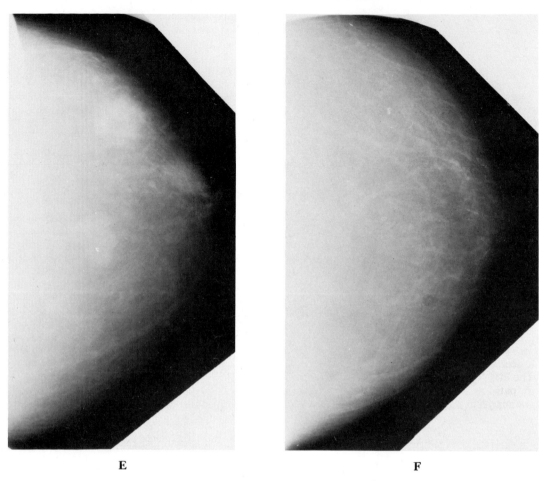

E   F

Figure 26–7 [*concluded*].   Mammography. *E.* There are two carcinomas and a fibroadenoma in the same breast. *F.* A normal breast.

Xeroradiography. Xeroradiography has a number of advantages over mammography. The dose of radiation is lower, about 5 rads; all the breast tissue can be visualized on a single plate; the axillary nodes can often be seen, and the changes in breast architecture are better defined. An electrostatic charge is placed on a selenium-coated aluminum plate. The charge is absorbed by the overlying soft tissues according to their density. The plate is then sprayed with a negatively charged blue thermoplastic powder, called toner, that adheres in amounts proportional to the residual charge. The toner image on the plate is transferred to paper by electrostatic means. Cysts, however, are not as well defined on xeroradiography as on mammography.

X-rays. The chest should always be x-rayed in patients with possible carcinoma of the breast. It is common for lung metastases to be present without any symptoms or abnormal physical signs. Intrapulmonary opacities, pleural effusion, and irregularity or broadening of the mediastinum suggest metastases. A skeletal survey should be performed in patients who have any abnormality in the isotope bone scan. A routine skeletal survey in patients thought to have the tumor confined to the breast reveals metastases in only about 2 percent. Osteolytic or occasionally osteoblastic metastases may be seen, especially in the ribs, sternum, or dorsal vertebrae.

Isotope Scans. A bone scan using isotopes should be obtained in all patients thought to have a carcinoma of the breast. When only strontium-85 was available, the investigations took several days. The scan can now be done within one hour after intravenous injection using the isotopes fluorine-18, strontium-87M, or polyvalent phosphate tagged with technecium ^{99}Tc. Galasko[19] found, using fluorine-18 scans, that 25 percent of patients being considered for attempted curative treatment had bony metastases that were not diagnosed on skeletal survey. The isotope is taken up by new bone produced adjacent to the metastases and not by the cancer cells. All patients who were positive on the isotope scan and had benign disease, about 6 percent, had the diagnosis established on the skeletal survey. The benign conditions were Paget's disease of bone, osteoarthritis, and pathologic fractures. A skeletal x-ray survey is therefore essential for patients with positive isotope scans to exclude false positives. In patients with advanced disease the scans were positive in 84 percent and in 50 percent on skeletal survey.

A liver scan may help diagnose liver metastases (see Chapter 19, page 325). A brain scan is indicated when a neurologic abnormality is found on history or physical examination.

Laboratory Tests. The serum alkaline phosphatase and blood calcium levels may be increased when there are metastases in bones. An increase in alkaline phosphatase and SGOT and a decrease in albumin suggest liver metastases. The blood sedimentation rate may be increased in patients with metastases. A normochronic anemia may be present due to extensive bony metastases. The marrow shows the characteristic picture of myeloid metaplasia. Preliminary results suggest that the ratio of androgenic to total steroids in the urine is abnormal in patients who are likely to develop carcinoma of the breast and in those with established disease.[8]

Screening Programs

There has been only one prospective trial using random controls to determine the value of screening normal women for the early detection of breast carcinoma.[38] In the Hospital Insurance Policy (H.I.P.) 31,000 women who were insurance policyholders were asked to attend for clinical examination of the breasts and mammography. A similar number wa⁻ designated but not screened. The response rate was only 65 percent, and 15 percent were lost to follow-up. More cancers were detected and survival was better in the screened patients. The detection rate was 2.8 cancers per 1000 patient years and 1.4 per 1000 patient years in the controls. At five years the mortality was 2.6 per 10,000 patient years and 4.1 per 10,000 in the controls. The main problem is whether the results of this study should be accepted and widespread screening be recommended, or whether further studies are required.

Differential Diagnosis

It is often difficult to diagnose breast carcinoma from the history and clinical examination (Figure 26–8).

Mammary Dysplasia. Many names, chronic cystic mastitis, fibroadenomatosis, and mammary dysplasia, describe the condition characterized by fibrosis, duct hyperplasia, and cyst formation (Figure 26–8, *D*). It is the commonest benign disease of the breast, is first seen in the twenties, and increases with age. The most likely cause is exaggeration of the hyperplasia-involutionary changes that occur during the menstrual cycle. During the first half of the cycle estrogens produce hyperplasia of the ductal epithelium and sensitize the acinar epithelium to subsequent exposure to progesterone. Progesterone then induces hyperplasia of the acinar epithelium and increases fibrous tissue throughout the breast. Menstruation occurs and is accompanied by involution of the epithelial and fibrotic changes. Mammary dysplasia is probably the result of a relative increase in estrogens. This is supported by the observation that symptoms and signs are most marked following an anovulatory cycle. It should be noted, however, that the results of hormonal treatment are generally disappointing. The dysplastic changes in the breast are generally mixed; however, one often predominates:

Hyperplasia. Hyperplasia of the epithelial cells in ducts and acini persists, producing papillomatosis or epitheliosis with partial or complete blockage of the ducts. Localized nodules or fibroadenomas may develop.

Cyst Formation. The ductal and acinar epithelia remain thin. Cysts are formed that are initially microscopic. They coalesce and can be recognized clinically or are seen on section of the operative specimen. Cyst may also develop as a result of hydrolysis of desquamated cells in an obstructed duct.

Fibroplasia. The fibrous tissue that increases during the latter half of the cycle may persist and become hyalinized or calcified. The fibrosis may be marked and cause distortion of the ducts, simulating a carcinoma both clinically and microscopically (sclerosing adenosis). The uniformity of the epithelial cells, lack of mitoses, and the presence of larger cysts in the periphery show that the condition is benign.

At operation dilated ducts can be seen containing greenish-yellow pseudopurulent material. A single large cyst is known as a blue-domed cyst of Bloodgood. The specimen containing many small cysts and marked fibrosis is known as Schimmelbusch's disease.

Opinions differ on the relation of mammary dysplasia to carcinoma of the breast. Willis[39] stressed the high incidence of epithelial hyperplasia associated with cystic disease in patients with breast carcinoma. He stated that noncystic lobular hyperplasia, mazoplasia, or adenosis seen in women below 30 was not premalignant. He considered that the diffuse microscopic cystic hyperplasia, often not detected clinically, was premalignant, and not the gross cystic disease obvious on clinical examination. Gallager and Martin[20] studied serial sections of the breast in patients with carcinoma in the same breast and found multiple malignant nodules in

half the specimens. In addition, epithelial hyperplasia was always present. The evidence from microscopic sections certainly suggests that the microcystic form of mammary dysplasia associated with epithelial hyperplasia is premalignant. Devitt,[14] on the other hand, found no relation between benign and malignant diseases of the breast and stated that there was no need to terrorize patients with fibrocystic disease by continual follow-up examinations.

Pain in the breast, especially before menstruation, is the most common symptom of mammary

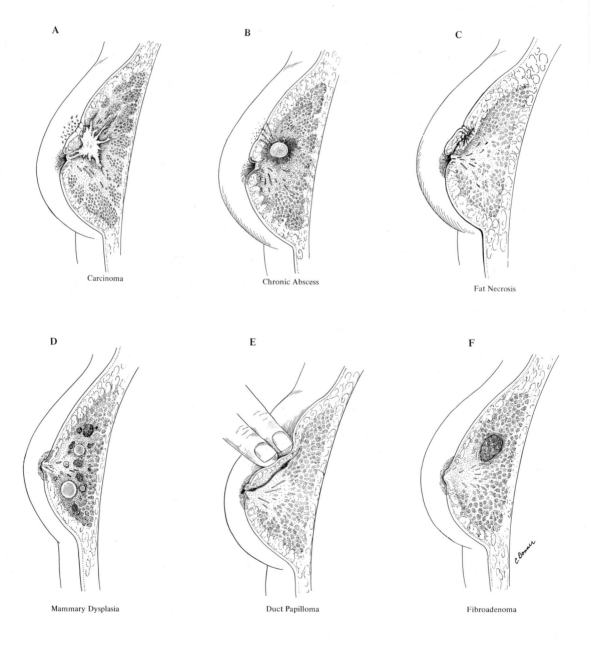

A   Carcinoma

B   Chronic Abscess

C   Fat Necrosis

D   Mammary Dysplasia

E   Duct Papilloma

F   Fibroadenoma

dysplasia. Rapid increase in size of a cyst from hemorrhage or accumulation of fluid may produce local pain and tenderness. There may be a clear, brown, semipurulent or blood-stained discharge from the nipple. There may be tender, diffuse, ill-defined thickening with accentuation of the breast lobulation in one or both breasts or in a segment of a breast. A nodule is generally less readily palpable to the palm of the hand than a carcinoma. The findings on clinical examination are most marked during the week prior to menstruation. It is useful therefore to repeat the examination during the week after menstruation.

Mammography should be performed. Any portion of the breast that shows changes suggestive of malignancy on mammography or clinical examination should be excised and examined microscopically. Excision of a segment of breast is generally all that is required. Subcutaneous mastectomy with preservation of the fat around the breast and the areola and nipple is occasionally necessary in those with persistent and incapacitating symptoms. Instruction in self-examination, six-monthly clinical examinations, and mammography when indicated are called for in patients with mammary dysplasia.

Conservative treatment is indicated when the diagnosis is definite. A firmly fitting brassiere should be worn day and night. Estrogens given at the beginning of the menstrual cycle and progesterone later or diuretics administered during the week before menstruation occasionally relieves discomfort. Relief sometimes occurs on discontinuing birth control pills.

Cysts. Cysts may occur in the breast with or without mammary dysplasia. Opinions differ on their management. Some advise that a solitary cyst in a normal breast be excised and examined microscopically. Others recommend aspiration of the cyst and examination of the fluid for cancer cells. A conservative approach with or without aspiration is indicated in patients with multiple cysts. A cyst should be excised after aspiration if fluid is not obtained, a mass remains palpable, the fluid is blood stained, the cyst rapidly recurs, or cancer or atypical cells are found on microscopic examination.

A milk-containing cyst, a galactocele, may develop close to the nipple after lactation stops. Inspissated milk and epithelial debris block and cause dilatation of usually the ampullary portion of a duct. The cyst should be excised because it may become infected or may later become fibrotic and calcified and simulate a carcinoma.

Fibroadenoma. Single or multiple fibroadenomas may occur in association with mammary dysplasia or in normal breast tissue (Figure 26–8, F). They occur most often in women at 20 to 30 years, are multiple in about 15 percent of patients, are discrete, mobile, and rubbery in consistency. They are usually not painful but may be tender on palpation. The segment of breast containing the tumor should be excised, because a fibroadenoma tends to increase in size, or the diagnosis may be wrong and the tumor indeed be a carcinoma. A fibroadenoma rarely, if ever, becomes sarcomatous.

Duct Papilloma. A blood-stained discharge from the nipple suggests a duct papilloma (Figure 26–8, E). A tumor may be palpable most often close to the areola, or its position be found by obtaining a blood-stained discharge on pressing over the involved segment of the breast. The segment should be excised and examined microscopically. Duct papillomata are often multiple and situated in the large lobular ducts. All the large ducts can be excised through a curved incision at the junction of the skin with the lower half of the areola. A cannula can

Figure 26–8. Differential diagnosis of lesions of the breast. *A.* Scirrhous carcinoma. The classic scirrhous carcinoma is shown for comparison with the other, benign conditions. The edge is stellate and there are skin and nipple retraction and peau d'orange. *B.* Chronic breast abscess. A chronic breast abscess may present months after or without pregnancy and may closely mimic a carcinoma. The tumor is hard, ill-defined, may be tethered to the overlying skin and produce edema, and cause slight retraction of the nipple. *C.* Traumatic fat necrosis. Fat necrosis may or may not follow an injury to the breast. It closely resembles a carcinoma; it is hard, irregular, and may be tethered to the skin or deep fascia and cause retraction of the nipple. *D.* Mammary dysplasia. This is the most frequent disease of the breast. The patient often complains of pain, especially premenstrual. Multiple tender nodules are usually present. The tumors are cysts, fibroadenomas, or areas with fibrosis. The condition may be widespread, including both breasts, or be confined to all or part of one breast. The axillary nodes are often enlarged and soft. There is frequently a watery or brownish discharge from the nipple. *E.* Duct papilloma. The patient most often presents with passage of red blood from the nipple. A tumor may be palpated, the region may be tender, or blood may be expressed by pressure over the site of the papilloma. Tumors less than 1 cm are generally benign. *F.* Fibroadenoma. A fibroadenoma may occur in an otherwise-normal breast or in a patient with fibroadenosis. Most occur in patients under 40 years of age and may or may not be painful. The tumor is well defined, not hard, and freely mobile.

sometimes be inserted into the duct and the papilloma excised locally. It is probably advisable to do a wider excision, however. A subcutaneous mastectomy should be considered if the condition recurs or the findings are diffuse on microscopic examination. The contralateral breast often shows similar changes. There is increasing support that duct papillomatosis is benign or malignant and that one rarely changes to the other.

Fat Necrosis. Injury to the breast may cause release of lipolytic enzymes, breakdown of fat to glycerol and fatty acids, formation of irritating calcium soaps of fatty acids, and a fibrotic reaction with infiltration of chronic inflammatory cells (Figure 26–8, *C*). More often fat necrosis does not follow an injury but occurs spontaneously in the dependent portion of a large pendulous breast, probably as the result of vascular stasis. The tumor is hard and irregular, and there may be retraction of the skin and nipple. On mammography coarse calcification is present. The tumor resembles a carinoma so closely that it should be excised and the diagnosis confirmed microscopically.

Chronic Breast Abscess. A chronic breast abscess may simulate a carcinoma as closely as fat necrosis (see page 446). The findings on physical examination and mammography suggest the presence of a carcinoma (Figure 26–8, *B*). The segment containing the lesion should be excised.

Cystosarcoma Phylloides. This is an uncommon tumor of the breast. It is a variant of a fibroadenoma, occurs most often over age 40, and is malignant in only 10 percent of patients. The term "sarcoma" describes its fleshy appearance. The tumor is large, discrete, and rubbery in consistency, and on section it contains cysts with polypoid masses of epithelial cells in the walls. The malignant form metastasizes to the lungs, bones, and soft tissues and rarely to the regional nodes. The benign and malignant forms should both be treated by simple mastectomy.

Treatment

Interest at present is in diagnosing breast carcinoma at an early stage and in thoroughly investigating patients before operation to find metastases. Women are being advised to perform self-examination after each period and to report to their doctor any change in the breasts. Those at high risk of developing the disease are advised to have regular physical examinations and mammography. The patient with carcinoma of the breast is now extensively investigated before operation for distant metastases. The woman with bony metastases, as determined by bone scan, is not treated by an attempted curative operation but is given chemotherapy or hormones.

Radical mastectomy was considered until about 1940 to be the "attempted curative" treatment of choice for patients with carcinoma of the breast; its role has since been the subject of considerable controversy.[11] The alternatives proposed have been excision of a segment of the breast, simple mastectomy, modified or radical mastectomy, and even more radical procedures. Local radiotherapy has been omitted, or given before or after operation. When one adds hormone manipulation and anticancer drugs, the present state of confusion and the difficulty in performing controlled clinical trials can be appreciated. The average survival of an untreated patient from first symptom until death is about 40 months.[5] About one third of the patients survived for five or more years. It is therefore of little value to quote survival figures at five years when comparing attempted curative treatments. Survival decreases exponentially with time, with the same fraction of surviving patients dying each year. Ten-year survival should therefore be used when studying the effect of a treatment.

The effects of handling the tumor on entry of cancer cells into the blood and lymphatic systems and the establishment of distant metastases are not clear. It is advisable therefore to examine the tumor as gently and as seldom as possible. Diagnosis should be confirmed by microscopic examination because some benign diseases, especially fat necrosis and chronic breast abscess, can simulate carcinoma. Views differ on the value of needle biopsy (see Chapter 7, page 148). The number of false positives is low, but false negatives are high and may result in delay in diagnosis. There is also the possibility that needle biopsy may increase local recurrence and distant metastases. Often several days elapse between taking the biopsy and definitive treatment when cancer cells may spread from the broken capsule of the tumor and enter blood and lymphatic vessels. A segmental excision and immediate examination of the frozen section is indicated when the tumor is small. Incisional biopsy is indicated when the tumor is large or situated in such a position that the biopsy site might be opened into during the definitive excision. The possibility of local or distant dissemination of cancer cells is slight when the definitive operation is performed on receiving the report of the frozen section. Gloves, gowns, and drapes are changed following closure of the biopsy site to avoid implanting cancer cells into the definitive operative field.

Operations. *Segmental Excision.* In patients

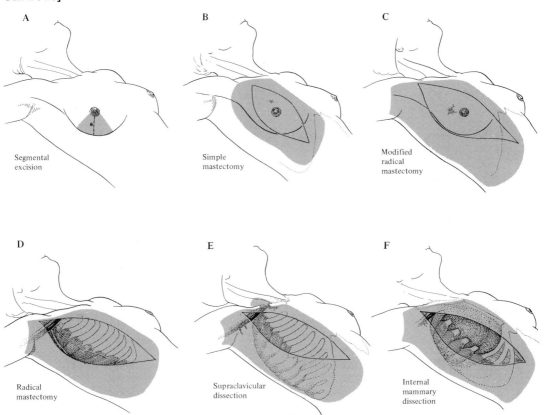

Figure 26–9. Operations in patients with carcinoma of the breast. *A.* The segment of the breast including the tumor is excised. The line of excision should be at least 3 cm wide of the tumor in all directions. *B.* Simple mastectomy requires removal of all the mammary tissues, surrounding fat, nipple, areola, and skin over the tumor. The deep fascia under the breast may or may not be removed. *C.* During modified radical mastectomy there is more extensive removal of fat and deep fascia than during simple mastectomy. The anterior pectoral, lateral axillary, and posterior subscapular nodes are removed. The pectoralis minor and the apical nodes may or may not be removed. The tissues are removed, en bloc, to produce a single specimen. *D.* During radical mastectomy the pectoralis major and minor muscles are removed to allow more complete removal of the apical nodes. *E* and *F.* Supraradical operations are not indicated because they increase morbidity and there is no evidence that they improve survival.

with stage I carcinoma of the breast the primary tumor has been removed along with a minimum of 3 cm of adjacent mammary tissues (Figure 26–9, *A*). An ellipse of overlying skin and underlying deep fascia is also removed. A minimum of one third of the breast tissue is therefore excised.[11] This has been recommended for patients with small tumors, less than 2 cm, and in those with tumors diagnosed on mammography and not palpable on clinical examination. Gallager and Martin[20] serially sectioned the complete breast in patients with carcinoma and found multiple additional carcinomas in 45 percent of the specimens. It has been stated that it is dangerous to leave breast tissue with such a high incidence of microscopic carcinomas. It is now recognized that there is about the same

incidence of nonpalpable carcinomas in the contralateral breast. Carcinoma of the breast is therefore generally a multicentric disease. At present the natural history of these small carcinomas is not known. The results of clinical trials now in progress should be available before the adequacy of segmental excision for small tumors is widely accepted.

Simple Mastectomy. Crile[11] recommended that patients with breast carcinoma be treated by simple mastectomy, and that the axillary nodes be removed only if they were felt to contain metastases on clinical examination or at operation on palpation after the axillary fascia were divided (Figure 26–9, *B*). He considered that prophylactic excision of the axillary nodes impaired the immune response of the host and increased local recurrence and distant metastases. He stated that the apical nodes should not be excised because their removal impaired lymphatic drainage and predisposed to local recurrence. The term "total" is sometimes used instead of simple mastectomy to emphasize the extent of the operation. As described in the section on anatomy, however, the mammary lobules extend beyond the mammary prominence. In addition, the axillary tail of Spence extends into the axilla. This dissection is therefore extensive and not "simple."

The term "extended simple" has been used to describe removal of the anterior pectoral nodes along with the breast. An extensive axillary dissection is not performed as in the modified radical operation.

The role of the regional nodes in the immune response to cancer is not known. Billingham and coworkers[4] showed that the regional lymph nodes were the main site of the cell-mediated immune response to an allograft placed in the subcutaneous tissues. This occurred when there were major differences in the histocompatibility genes between the two tissues, but it has not been demonstrated when there are minor differences, as with a spontaneous tumor. Adoptive immunity can be transferred shortly after transplantation, using cells from distant parts of the reticuloendothelial system, such as the spleen. A tumor has been present at least months before it is recognized clinically. The regional nodes are therefore not the only part of the central component of the immune response. Gewant and his coworkers[21] grew cancer cells in tissue culture from patients with carcinoma of the breast and found that lymphocytes from the regional nodes inhibited growth of the cancer cells when the nodes contained no or small metastases. The lymphocytes had no effect when the nodes contained large metastases. The work needs confirmation because the number of patients was small.

Baum[3] has found in the King's Cambridge trial that 70 percent of the nodes that were palpable and thought to contain tumor regressed after simple mastectomy. Some of these nodes may have been hyperplastic because of the presence of the tumor, but the trial also suggests that nodes containing small amounts of tumor may regress after simple mastectomy. In this prospective controlled trial one group is treated by simple mastectomy, and the axillary nodes are only treated by radiotherapy or excision if the nodes enlarge after operation. The other group is treated by simple mastectomy and prophylactic postoperative radiotherapy. After five years survival is the same in the two groups, but the incidence of local recurrence is higher in those treated by simple mastectomy without radiation.

Modified Radical and Radical Mastectomy. The operations are based on the assumptions that axillary nodes may contain metastases in the absence of supraclavicular, internal mammary, or hematogenous metastases; that secondary metastases may arise from microscopic foci of cancer cells in the axillary nodes as they grow to clinically recognizable tumors; and that surgical excision of the axillary nodes is superior to their treatment by radiotherapy (Figures 26-9, C and D). Radical mastectomy assures that the primary tumor and breast tissues are widely excised, that the axillary nodes are extensively removed, and that there is little chance of dividing lymphatics containing cancer cells. This is confirmed by the low incidence of recurrence at the operative site: about 1 percent in those in stage I and 15 percent in those in stage II.

Radical mastectomy, however, is a greater procedure than simple mastectomy. Most patients require blood transfusion, the operating time is at least doubled, and skin grafting is often required. Also impaired wound healing, persistent pain, decreased shoulder movement, and lymphedema may occur. A "winged scapula" occasionally occurs after division of the long thoracic nerve to the serratus anterior muscle. There have been no clinical trials, using random controls, comparing radical mastectomy with another operation in patients not treated by radiotherapy.

Modified radical mastectomy is similar to the radical operation except that the pectoralis major muscle is not excised and the pectoralis minor muscle may or may not be removed. The apical lymph nodes may or may not be removed with the anterior pectoral, lateral axillary, and subscapular nodes.[35] Their excision is probably not important, because prognosis is bad when they contain metastases. The modified radical operation is as major a procedure as radical mastectomy; however, it is followed by less impairment of arm movement, a lower incidence of edema in the arm, and less cosmetic impairment of the chest wall. When properly performed, the axillary dissection should be as complete as after radical mastectomy.

Superradical Mastectomies. Part of the sternum and the medial ends of the costal cartilages have been removed along with the ipsilateral internal mammary vessels and their medially placed nodes (Figure 26-9, E). A "monobloc" technique has been used, including these tissues as an extension of the operation of radical mastectomy.[37] The operation has been recommended in patients with carcinomas behind the areola and in the medial half of the breast, and in those with metastases in the axillary nodes. It provides excellent removal of the primary lymphatic drainage of the breast but is a greater operation and produces more cosmetic impairment than radical mastectomy. The clavicle has been divided and the tissues in the supraclavicular triangle removed in continuity or discontinuity with the internal mammary nodes.[12]

There has not been a clinical trial, using random controls, comparing the results after extended radical mastectomy with a lesser operation without radiotherapy.

Summary. Less radical operations are now being performed for carcinoma of the breast. This is based on the realization that 80 percent of those with axillary metastases will develop distant metastases within 10 years. It therefore appears most likely that nodal and hematogenous metastases occur at the same time. Also, the results of clinical trials do not show that prophylactic removal of the axillary nodes improves survival. It would therefore appear unlikely that nodal metastases rarely give rise to distant metastases while they grow from microscopic foci to clinically evident tumor.

There may be a place for segmental excision in those with early tumors. The results of clinical trials now in progress should be available before this procedure is widely accepted. There is increasing support that simple mastectomy is adequate in patients with "operable" breast carcinoma when the axillary nodes do not clinically contain metastases. It does not appear that removal of the axillary nodes influences survival. Microscopic examination of the nodes gives information about prognosis. Those with positive nodes have a poor prognosis and should be considered for chemotherapy.

Radical mastectomy gives the optimum removal of the breast and axillary nodes. The criteria for selection of patients for this procedure are now more stringent.[22] Morbidity has been decreased by leaving thicker skin flaps and excising less skin. There is considerable theoretic support for modified mastectomy with its lesser morbidity and probably similar survival. The extensions of radical operation, including removal of the internal mammary or supraclavicular nodal excision, are not indicated because of the increased morbidity and failure to show that they increase survival.

Radiotherapy. Radiotherapy is the principal treatment of patients with stages III and IV carcinoma of the breast. Its place in the earlier stages is controversial.

Preoperative Radiotherapy. There has been little interest in the administration of radiotherapy before operation to patients with breast carcinoma. However, a number of theoretic advantages exist for its preoperative rather than postoperative use. The well-oxygenated cancer cells are damaged more than after impairment of their blood supply; therefore any that are disseminated during operation or left at the operative site are less likely to establish metastases. The delay in operation gives extra time to observe for distant metastases and avoid an unnecessary operation. Modern therapy does not make the operation more difficult or impair wound healing.

Preoperative radiotherapy has been extensively used in patients with locally advanced, "borderline operable" tumors. Patients who are in stage III because of local extension of the primary tumor and who do not have clinically positive axillary nodes have a much better prognosis than those who are in stage III because they have extensive nodal metastases. They are best treated by conventional fractionated preoperative radiotherapy followed by mastectomy in about four weeks.

Prophylactic Postoperative Radiotherapy. There are conflicting views on the value of prophylactic postoperative radiotherapy in patients with carcinoma of the breast. The "maxi-therapy" school suggests that a radical operation is not really radical and should be supplemented by radiotherapy to the regional nodes that are not excised and to the chest wall in those with locally advanced tumors. The more conservative view is that radiotherapy does not improve survival, that morbidity is increased, and the immune response of the host may be damaged.

Radiotherapy is given using a fractionated "attempted curative" regime when the operative site is healed. The supraclavicular, upper axillary, and the internal mammary regions are treated. Those with locally advanced primary tumors also receive treatment to the chest wall (Figure 26–10). A total dose of 4000 to 4500 rads is most often given in 15 fractions during three weeks.

Atkins *et al.*[2] in a controlled clinical trial of 370 patients over age 50 compared local excision of the carcinoma (tylectomy) and prophylactic postoperative radiotherapy with radical mastectomy and prophylactic postoperative radiotherapy. Tylectomy consisted of removing 3 cm of the tissues around the tumor. During the first three years of the study patients in both groups were also given three intravenous doses of thio-TEPA immediately before operation and two and four days after operation. Survival at 10 years did not differ significantly between the groups. Those patients treated by tylectomy who had negative axillary nodes on clinical examination (stage I) had the same incidence of local recurrence, metastases, and survival as those

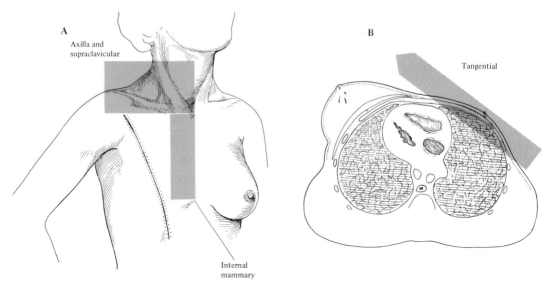

Figure 26–10.   Regions treated by radiotherapy in patients with carcinoma of the breast. *A.* Supraclavicular and upper axillary regions are irradiated. The internal mammary field extends from 2 cm lateral to the ipsilateral border of the sternum to 1 cm beyond the middle of the sternum on the opposite side and from the suprasternal notch to the xiphoid process. *B.* The chest wall is sometimes irradiated, using parallel opposed fields to minimize exposure to the lungs and heart.

treated by radical mastectomy and radiotherapy. Those with clinically positive nodes (stage II) had greater local recurrence, metastases, and poorer survival than those treated by radical mastectomy and radiotherapy. When all the patients in each group were considered together, there was no difference in survival at any time. Edema of the arm and limitation of movement were greater in those treated by radical mastectomy. The authors pointed out, however, that a number of women treated by tylectomy had "marbling" of the skin over the tumor, fibrotic breasts, and limitation of arm movement. The results suggest that patients with clinically positive axillary nodes are best treated by radical mastectomy and prophylactic postoperative radiotherapy and those with clinically negative nodes by tylectomy and radiotherapy.

Radiotherapy may be given after simple mastectomy to treat metastases in the nodes. Dahl-Iversen[12] showed that one third of patients with metastases in the axillary nodes had supraclavicular metastases. Handley[23] demonstrated that one half of patients with operable tumors had metastases in the internal mammary nodes. McWhirter[31] suggested therefore that it was illogical to remove the axillary nodes and treat the remainder by radiotherapy and that instead intensive postoperative radiotherapy should be given to all the regional nodes. He advised removal of the breast because the

primary tumor was not as effectively controlled by radiotherapy as were lymph node metastases. A wide simple mastectomy was performed without opening into the axilla, a skin graft was not applied, and the drain was brought out through the incision. Superficial palpable axillary nodes were removed through a small incision. Kaae and Johansen,[25] in a randomly controlled study including 668 patients with "operable" tumors, compared simple mastectomy and postoperative radiotherapy with superradical mastectomy and no radiotherapy. The operation consisted of radical mastectomy and removal of the supraclavicular and internal mammary lymph nodes in discontinuity. Survival at 10 years was the same in the two groups as was local recurrence, and morbidity was lower in those treated by radiotherapy. Radiotherapy therefore controlled metastases in the regional lymph nodes as effectively as operative excision.

Brinkley and Haybittle[7] found that survival at 10 years was the same in patients with stage II carcinoma of the breast treated by an extended simple mastectomy (the anterior pectoral nodes were removed if thought to contain metastases) and prophylactic postoperative radiotherapy as in those treated by radical mastectomy and prophylactic postoperative radiotherapy.

The effect of prophylactic radiotherapy on host resistance to cancer has been of particular concern. Meyer[32] found that prophylactic postoperative radiotherapy decreased the number of lymphocytes in the peripheral blood for more than two years. He suggested that lymphopenia decreased the cell-mediated host response and increased metastases. Others have confirmed the lymphopenia and have shown that the population of lymphocytes in the peripheral blood is changed by treatment.[29] The results from two clinical studies, using random controls, suggest that radiotherapy does not affect survival but may possibly increase growth of metastases. Paterson and Russell[34] found that survival of patients with breast carcinoma was the same at 10 years in those given prophylactic postoperative radiotherapy as in those treated therapeutically for local recurrence. There was a suggestion, however, that liver metastases were increased in those given prophylactic postoperative radiotherapy. The National Surgical Adjuvant Breast Project (NSABP) trial found that survival was not significantly affected by prophylactic postoperative radiotherapy.[17] The five-year survival rate was 6 percent lower, and the fraction first presenting with distant metastases was 8 percent higher in irradiated patients. Criticisms of this study were that 40 percent of 1900 patients were excluded, it was not shown that selection of patients was not biased, and the data suggested that those treated by radiotherapy had more advanced disease.

Johnstone[24] reviewed the effect of prophylactic postoperative radiotherapy in 88 patients who had negative apical axillary and internal mammary lymph nodes. Those with negative axillary nodes received radiotherapy to the supraclavicular and internal mammary fields. The results were compared with 33 patients who were not irradiated. The recurrence rate was 16 percent in those who were irradiated and 9 percent in the controls. This suggests that radiotherapy may have increased metastases.

These studies suggest that radiotherapy is as effective as operative excision in the treatment of the regional nodes. They also show that a well-done simple mastectomy followed by good radiotherapy is as effective as a radical or extended radical mastectomy. The value of prophylactic radiotherapy given after radical mastectomy is controversial. Treatment reduces recurrence in the irradiated areas but does not increase survival. The effect of radiotherapy on the immune response is still not known.

Summary of Attempted Curative Treatments. Fortunately there have been more controlled clinical trials of the treatment of breast carcinoma than of any other surgical disease. The results of attempted curative treatments show that the results at 10 years after simple mastectomy and radiotherapy are as good as after any greater treatment (Table 26–1). It should be emphasized that the simple mastectomy was carefully performed by well-trained surgeons and the standard of radiotherapy was higher than is generally available. Results are not available at 10 years of any clinical trial that did not include at least simple mastectomy and treatment by excision or radiotherapy to the axillary nodes. A number of clinical trials have recently been commenced excluding treatment to the axillary nodes. The results should be available, preferably at 10 years, before this treatment is widely accepted. The studies show that there is no indication that radical mastectomy with its associated morbidity is necessary. An extended simple or modified radical mastectomy does not significantly increase morbidity over simple mastectomy and may be preferred to simple mastectomy, especially when the standards of radiotherapy available vary so greatly.

Hormones. At the end of the last century it was known that oophorectomy sometimes caused regression of breast carcinoma and that pregnancy and the puerperium often affected the rate of cancer growth. Attempts have therefore been made to alter the hormonal environment by irradiation or removal of the ovaries; by administration of testosterone, estrogen, or progesterone; by excision or suppression, using prednisone, of the adrenals; or by irradiation or removal of the pituitary gland.

Opinions differ on whether ovarian function should be suppressed prophylactically at the time of the initial treatment for cure or whether castration should be withheld until recurrence. Nissen-Meyer[33], in a study with random controls, showed that prophylactic castration by excision or radiotherapy increased survival in postmenopausal women up to the age of 70 years and that the addition of prednisone further improved results. He also showed that local radiotherapy to the ovaries was as effective as surgical oophorectomy. Kennedy[26], in a retrospective study, found that prophylactic castration delayed clinical recognition of metastases but did not improve survival. The National Surgical Adjuvant Breast Project trial showed that prophylactic castration by operation was of no benefit in patients treated by radical mastectomy.[36] There is considerable support for not performing castration at the initial curative treatment, reserving its use until metastases develop.

The presence of estrogen receptors in the cytoplasm of cells of carcinoma of the breast suggests that the patient is likely to respond to hormonal manipulation, and their absence

Table 26–1. CLINICAL TRIALS OF ATTEMPTED CURATIVE TREATMENT OF CARCINOMA OF THE BREAST

GROUPS	AUTHORS	NO. OF PATIENTS	YEARS OF OBSERVATION	CONCLUSIONS
1. Radical mastectomy + PPR*	Paterson (1962)	709	10	Survival and local recurrence same
2. Radical mastectomy + therapeutic radiotherapy		752		Morbidity less in group 2
1. Simple mastectomy + PPR	Kaae and Johansen (1968)	331	10	Survival and local recurrence same
2. Radical mastectomy + removal internal mammary and supraclavicular nodes		335		Morbidity less in group 1
1. Radical mastectomy	Fisher et al. (1970)[17]	235	5	Survival same
2. Radical mastectomy + PPR		180		? earlier metastases in group 2
1. Stage II Extended simple mastectomy + PPR	Brinkley and Haybittle (1971)[7]	113	10	Survival same Morbidity greater in group 2
2. Stage II Radical mastectomy + PPR		91		
1. Tylectomy + PPR	Atkins et al. (1972)[2]	182	10	Survival better in group 2, if nodes positive but same if nodes negative
2. Radical mastectomy + PPR		188		More local recurrence in group 1

* PPR: Prophylactic postoperative radiotherapy.

strongly suggests that they will not respond. Sixty to 80 percent of women have estrogen receptors, the number increasing with age, but only about 55 percent respond to endocrine therapy. However, only about 8 percent of those who are negative will respond. The absence of receptors therefore suggests that hormonal therapy should not be used and that the patient should be treated by chemotherapy.

Age determines the type of hormonal therapy to be given to patients with advanced or recurrent breast carcinoma. In women up to two years after the menopause the initial treatment should be castration by operation or radiotherapy. This may be supplemented by testosterone. Women more than five years postmenopause are unlikely to benefit from castration but often respond to estrogens. The keratinizing index from a vaginal smear was used to determine the amount of ovarian function and the time up to which castration might be of benefit. Its accuracy is now questioned. Initially it was found that about 50 percent of women had hormone-dependent tumors; however, the incidence is probably nearer 25 percent. The response rate is about 50 percent in patients who have metastases in the ovaries. A hormone-dependent tumor regresses and then invariably

recurs. The recurrence may be treated by bilateral adrenalectomy or hypophysectomy. The best response is obtained in those with metastases in bone and skin. Hormonal suppression of the adrenals by prednisone or ACTH is equally effective. Unfortunately the side effects produced by prednisone make surgical ablation generally the treatment of choice.

Postmenopausal women who do not respond to estrogens may have tumor regression when the estrogens are discontinued (estrogen withdrawal), and some may respond to androgens. Conversely premenopausal women who have not responded to testosterone occasionally have tumor regression after the administration of estrogens.

In patients with tumors that have never been or have ceased to be hormone-dependent, partial regression may be obtained using cyclophosphamide or thio-TEPA, or radioactive phosphorus.

Radiotherapy often provides good palliation in locally advanced breast carcinoma and in those with distant metastases. Metastases in bone and subcutaneous tissue respond well, while those in the liver, lungs, and brain respond poorly.

Chemotherapy. There was great interest 10

to 15 years ago in the adjunctive use of chemicals, such as nitrogen mustard, cyclophosphamide, thio-TEPA, or 5-fluorouracil, at the time of operation. The drugs were given by the topical, systemic venous, or intra-arterial routes. Thio-TEPA was found to decrease recurrence at three years in women just before the menopause who had metastases in four or more axillary nodes.[16] They were treated by radical mastectomy and given the drug intravenously at the time of operation and on the two subsequent days. Total survival was not increased. There is the possibility that thio-TEPA inhibited tumor growth by inhibiting ovarian function rather than by directly affecting the cancer cells.

More recently it has been suggested that a drug may be necessary for a prolonged time when the tumor volume is at a minimum. Women with metastases in the axillary nodes have about an 80 percent chance of developing metastases within 10 years. They may therefore benefit from courses of a drug, or combinations of drugs, one to two years after the primary tumor has been removed. The drugs currently under evaluation are L-phenylalanine mustard (L-PAM), cyclophosphamide, 5-fluorouracil, Adriamycin, and methotrexate, all of which have been shown to be effective in patients with established tumor. There has been concern that the prolonged use of combinations of drugs may decrease the immune response and increase infections and new primary cancers. These patients will therefore need to be observed for a number of years.

Chemotherapy sometimes induces partial regression and useful palliation in patients who have never responded or have ceased to respond to change in their hormonal status. The agents, however, are toxic, and the harmful effects must be balanced against a possible temporary partial regression. Cyclophosphamide (Cytoxan)

doxorubicin (Adriamycin), or 5-fluorouracil given systemically can produce useful palliation. Recently there has been considerable interest in the use of combinations of drugs such as doxorubicin, cyclophosphamide, 5-fluorouracil, methotrexate, and vincristine. Complete or partial remissions can be obtained in 50 to 80 percent of patients.

Personal Regimen for Initial Treatment

Views differ markedly on the treatment of breast carcinoma. The conflicting opinions have been discussed. It is necessary, however, to evolve a line of action from the evidence available at the present time. Table 26–2 summarizes a personal regimen for the initial treatment of patients with breast carcinoma.

Diseases of the Male Breast

Carcinoma. About 1 percent of breast carcinomas occur in the male and 25 percent in breasts that were previously hyperplastic resembling mammary dysplasia in the female. The incidence is the same as in women for patients with Klinefelter's syndrome (XXY). The tumor is hard, rapidly fixes to the skin, ulcerates, and tends to infiltrate the deep fascia and pectoralis major muscle. Radical mastectomy should be performed with removal of the pectoralis major muscle, and a skin graft is generally necessary. The prognosis is much worse than in the female. Since the tumors are often hormone-dependent, local recurrence of metastases should be treated by orchidectomy and estrogens.

Gynecomastia. In gynecomastia one or both breasts enlarge, become painful and tender, and the mammary lobules feel discoid and rubbery in consistency. When bilateral, there is usually an increase in estrogens from an exogenous source, as in the patient treated for carcinoma of the prostate, or from an endogenous source, as

Table 26–2. INITIAL TREATMENT OF CARCINOMA OF THE BREAST

STAGE	OPERATION	RADIOTHERAPY	CASTRATION AND HORMONE THERAPY	CHEMOTHERAPY
I	MRM*	—	—	—
II	MRM	—	—	—
III				
Primary tumor	MRM	+ Preoperative	—	—
Axillary nodes	None	+ To primary and nodes	—	—
IV	None	+ To primary and nodes	Castration < 2 years after menopause	—
		+ To skin and bony metastases	Estrogens > 2 years after menopause	—

* MRM: Modified radical mastectomy.

in hepatic cirrhosis and an estrogen-secreting tumor, for example in the testis. It is often seen in the male at puberty. A cause is usually not found when the condition is unilateral. Gynecomastia is not premalignant. Occasionally it is necessary to excise the breast to establish diagnosis, for cosmetic effect, or because of persistent pain and tenderness.

CITED REFERENCES

1. Ackerman, L. V., and del Regato, J. A.: *Cancer—Diagnosis, Treatment and Prognosis*, 4th ed. C. V. Mosby Company, St. Louis, pp. 837–38, 1970.
2. Atkins, H.; Hayward, J. L.; Klugman, D. J.; and Wayte, A. B.: Treatment of early breast cancer: a report after ten years of a clinical trial. *Br. Med. J.*, 2:423–29, 1972.
3. Baum, M.: Surgery and radiotherapy in breast cancer. *Semin. Oncol.*, 1:101–08, 1974.
4. Billingham, R. E.; Brent, J.; and Medawar, P. B.: Quantitative studies on tissue transplantation immunity: origin, strength, and duration of activity and adoptively acquired immunity. *Proc. R. Soc. Lond.*, Series B. 143:58–80, 1954.
5. Bloom, H. J. G.; Richardson, W. W.; and Harries, E. J.: Natural history of untreated breast cancer (1805–1933). Comparison of untreated and treated cases according to histological grade of malignancy. *Br. Med. J.*, 4299:213–21, 1962.
6. Bloom, H. J. G.: The influence of delay on the natural history and prognosis of breast cancer. *Br. J. Cancer*, 19:228–62, 1965.
7. Brinkley, D., and Haybittle, J. L.: Treatment of stage II carcinoma of the female breast. *Lancet*, 2:1086–87, 1971.
8. Bulbrook, R. D.; Greenwood, F. C.; and Hayward, J. L.: Selection of breast cancer patients for adrenalectomy of hypophysectomy by determination of urinary 17-hydroxycorticosteroids and aetiocholanolone. *Lancet*, 1:1154–57, 1960.
9. Burch, J. C., and Byrd, B. F.: Effects of long-term administration of estrogen on the occurrence of mammary cancer in women. *Ann. Surg.* 174:414–18, 1971.
10. Burn, J. I.: Diagnostic methods in breast cancer. *Proc. R. Soc. Med.*, 64:254–56, 1971.
11. Crile, G., Jr.: Rationale of simple mastectomy without radiation for clinical stage I cancer of the breast. *Surg. Gynecol. Obstet.*, 120:975–82, 1965.
12. Dahl-Iversen, E.: An extended radical operation for carcinoma of the breast. *J. R. Coll. Surg. Edinb.*, 8:81–90, 1963.
13. Delarue, N. C.: The management of primary breast cancer. *Surg. Gynecol. Obstet.*, 118:133–52, 1964.
14. Devitt, J. E.: Fibrocystic disease of the breast is not premalignant. *Surg. Gynecol. Obstet.*, 134:803–806, 1972.
15. Egan, R. L.: Fifty-three cases of carcinoma of the breast, occult until mammography. *Am. J. Roentgenol.*, 88:1095–1101, 1962.
16. Fisher, B.; Ravdin, R. G.; Ausman, R. K.; Slack, H. N.; Moore G. E.; Noer, R. J. (and cooperating investigators): Surgical adjuvant chemotherapy in cancer of the breast: results of a decade of cooperative investigation. *Ann. Surg.*, 168:337–56, 1968.
17. Fisher, B.; Slack, N. H.; Cavanaugh, P. J.; Gardner, B.; and Ravdin, R. G.: Postoperative radiotherapy in the treatment of breast cancer: results of the NSABP clinical trial. *Ann. Surg.*, 172:711–32, 1970.
18. Foote, F. W., and Stewart, F. W.: A histologic classification of carcinoma of the breast. *Surgery*, 19:74–99, 1946.
19. Galasko, C. S. B.: The detection of skeletal metastases from carcinoma of the breast. *Surg. Gynecol. Obstet.*, 133:1019–24, 1971.
20. Gallager, H. S., and Martin, J. E.: Early phases in the development of breast cancer. *Cancer*, 24:1170–78, 1969.
21. Gewant, W. C.; Chasin, L.; Tilson, M. D.; Rutledge, C.; and Goldenberg, I. S.: Lymph node—breast carcinoma interrelations in tissue culture. *Surg. Gynecol. Obstet.*, 133:959–62, 1971.
22. Haagensen, C. D., and Cooley, E.: Radical mastectomy for mammary carcinoma. *Ann. Surg.*, 157:166–69, 1963.
23. Handley, R. S.: Symposium on early carcinoma of the breast: the early spread of breast carcinoma and its bearing on operative treatment. *Br. J. Surg.*, 51:206–208, 1964.
24. Johnstone, F. R. C.: Postoperative radiation in the treatment of carcinoma of the breast. *Am. J. Surg.*, 128:276–81, 1974.
25. Kaae, S., and Johansen, E.: Simple mastectomy plus postoperative irradiation by the method of McWhirter for mammary carcinoma. *Prog. Clin. Cancer*, 1:453–61, 1965.
26. Kennedy, B. J.; Mielke, P. W., Jr.; Fortuny, I. E.: Therapeutic castration versus prophylactic castration in breast cancer. *Surg. Gynecol. Obstet.*, 118:524–40, 1964.
27. Lawson, R. N., and Chughtai, M. S.: Breast cancer and body temperature. *Can. Med. Assoc. J.*, 88:68–70, 1963.
28. MacKay, E. N., and Sellers, A. H.: A clinical trial of TNM staging of breast cancer—Ontario 1960–62. *Int. J. Cancer*, 1:515–24, 1966.
29. McCredie, J. A.; Inch, W. R.; and Sutherland, R. M.: Effect of postoperative radiotherapy on peripheral blood lymphocytes in patients with carcinoma of the breast. *Cancer*, 29:349–56, 1972.
30. McCredie, J. A.; Inch, W. R.; and Alderson, M.: Consecutive primary carcinomas of the breast. *Cancer*, 35:1472–77, 1975.
31. McWhirter, R.: The value of simple mastectomy and radiotherapy in the treatment of cancer of the breast. *Br. J. Radiol.*, 21:599–610, 1948.
32. Meyer, K. K.: Radiation-induced lymphocyte immune deficiency: a factor in the increased visceral metastases and decreased hormonal responsiveness of breast cancer. *Arch. Surg.*, 101:114–21, 1970.
33. Nissen-Meyer, R.: Prophylactic endocrine treatment in carcinoma of the breast. *Clin. Radiol.*, 15:152–60, 1964.
34. Paterson, R., and Russell, M. H.: Clinical trials in malignant disease. Part III—breast cancer: evaluation of postoperative radiotherapy. *J. Fac. Radiol.*, 10:175–80, 1959.
35. Patey, D. H., and Dyson, W. H.: The prognosis of carcinoma of the breast in relation to the type of operation performed. *Br. J. Cancer*, 2:7–13, 1948.
36. Ravdin, R. G.; Lewison, E. F., *et al.*: Results of a clinical trial concerning the worth of prophylactic oophorectomy for breast carcinoma. *Surg. Gynecol. Obstet.*, 131:1055–64, 1970.
37. Urban, J. A.: Extended radical mastectomy for breast cancer. *Am. J. Surg.*, 106:399–404, 1963.
38. Venet, L.; Strax, P., *et al.*: Adequacies and inadequacies of breast examinations by physicians in mass screening. *Cancer*, 28:1546–51, 1971.
39. Willis, R. A. (ed.): *Pathology of Tumours*, 4th ed. Butterworth and Co., London, pp. 230–33, 1967.
40. Wynder, E. L.: Identification of women at high risk for breast cancer. *Cancer*, 24:1235–39, 1969.

SUGGESTIONS FOR FURTHER READING

Bonadonna, G.; Brusamolino, E.; et al.: Combination chemotherapy as an adjuvant treatment in operable breast cancer. N. Engl. J. Med., 294:405–10, 1976.
   The administration of three drugs prophylactically—cyclophosphamide, methotrexate, and 5-fluorouracil—decreased recurrence of tumor to about one-fifth in women with positive nodes. The effect on survival is still not known.

Fisher, B.; Carbone, P.; et al.: 1-Phenylalanine mustard (L-PAM) in the management of primary breast cancer. N. Engl. J. Med., 292:117–22, 1975.
   This is an important study in that it is the first that showed that prophylactic postoperative chemotherapy to women with positive nodes, using a single drug for a prolonged time, decreased recurrence by about 50 percent.

McCredie, J. A.: Management of the contralateral breast. In: Stoll, B. A. (ed.): Management of Breast Cancer—Early and Late. Wm. Heinemann Medical Books Ltd., London, in press.
   A review of the controversial subject of management of the remaining breast in women with carcinoma of the breast.

McDivitt, R. W.; Stewart, F. W.; and Berg, J. W.: Tumors of the breast. In: Firminger, H. I. (ed.): Atlas of Tumor Pathology. Armed Forces Institute of Pathology, Washington, D.C., pp. 9–156, 1968.
   This is an excellent description of the pathology of tumors of the breast. The figures are of outstanding quality. The classification used in the text is based on this atlas.

Report of First National Conference on Breast Cancer. Cancer, 24:1101–1378, 1969.
   A multiauthor presentation covering most aspects of the diagnosis and treatment of carcinoma of the breast.

Watson, T. A.: Cancer of the breast; The Janeway lecture. Am. J. Roentgenol., 46:547–59, 1965.
   The author is in favor of prophylactic radiotherapy after radical mastectomy.

Willis, R. A.: Epithelial tumours of the breast. In: Willis, R. A. (ed.): Pathology of Tumours. Butterworth and Co., London, pp. 208–56, 1967.
   A lucid description of the pathology of tumors of the breast.

Wittliff, J. L.: Specific receptors of the steroid hormones in breast cancer. Semin. Oncol., 1:109–18, 1974.
   A general review of the subject.

Chapter 27

THYROID, PARATHYROID, AND ADRENAL GLANDS

Robert N. Green

CHAPTER OUTLINE

Thyroid
  Development and Anatomy
  Physiology
  Laboratory Assessment of Thyroid
    Function
    Serum Thyroxine by Competitive Binding
      Assay
    Radioimmunoassay for T-3
    Radioimmunoassay for TSH
    T-3 Resin Uptake
    Kinometry
    Basal Metabolic Rate
    Radioactive Iodine Uptake
    Thyroid Stimulation Test
    Thyroid Suppression Test
    Radioactive Iodide Scanning
    Antithyroglobulin Antibodies
  Clinical Examination
  Hyperthyroidism
    Treatment of Thyrotoxicosis
    Choice of Therapy
  Hypothyroidism
  Thyroiditis
    Hashimoto's Disease
    Subacute Thyroiditis
    Reidel's Thyroiditis
    Acute Pyogenic Thyroiditis
  Nontoxic Goiter
    Solitary Thyroid Nodule
  Benign Tumors
  Malignant Tumors
    Clinical Findings and Investigations
    Pathology
    Thyroxine and Carcinoma of the Thyroid
    Radioactive Iodine

  Local Radiotherapy
Parathyroid
  Disorders of Calcium Metabolism
    Hypocalcemia
    Hypercalcemia: Primary Hyperpara-
      thyroidism
    Hypoparathyroidism
Adrenal Cortex
  Development and Anatomy
  Physiology
  Laboratory Studies
    17-Hydroxysteroids
    17-Ketosteroids
    Cortisol
    Aldosterone
  Functions of Steroid Hormones
  Adrenocortical Hypofunction
    Acute Adrenal Insufficiency
    Chronic Primary Adrenal Insufficiency
  Adrenocortical Hyperfunction (Cushing's
    Syndrome)
    Signs and Symptoms
    Laboratory Studies
    Radiologic Examination
    Treatment
  Primary Aldosteronism
  Secondary Aldosteronism
  Syndromes of Masculinization or Femini-
    zation
Adrenal Medulla
  Pheochromocytoma
    Clinical Presentation
    Investigations
    Treatment
  Neuroblastoma

THYROID

Development and Anatomy

The thyroid develops at one month of fetal life as a midline pocket in the pharyngeal floor and grows ventrally and caudally. The thyroglossal duct closes, leaving a caudal remnant (the pyramidal lobe of the thyroid) and a cephalad remnant (foramen cecum of the tongue). In its caudal growth the

474

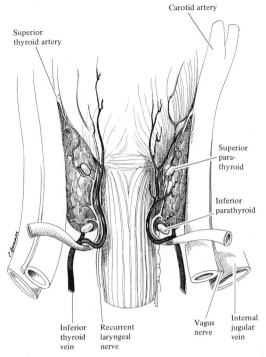

Figure 27–1. Posterior view of the thyroid showing the relations of the deep portion of the gland to the parathyroids, recurrent laryngeal nerves, and the blood vessels.

thyroid is closely associated with the third and fourth pharyngeal pouches and the ultimobronchial bodies which give rise to the parathyroid glands and the parafollicular cells. Iodinated thyroglobulin is first formed at about 11 weeks.

The thyroid is bilobed with a central isthmus and is attached to the anterolateral trachea just below the cricoid cartilage (Figure 27–1). The lateral lobes overlie the larynx and trachea and extend as high as the middle of the thyroid cartilage. The parathyroid glands are situated on the posterior aspect of the lateral lobes. The recurrent laryngeal nerves are also on the posteromedial surface of the lobes in the groove between the trachea and esophagus. The thyroid has a rich arterial supply with a flow of 5 ml each minute per gram of tissue from the superior and inferior thyroid arteries, branches of the external carotid and subclavian arteries, respectively. There are also extensive venous and lymphatic supplies. The gland is composed of indistinct lobules separated by connective tissue. The lobule contains 20 to 40 follicles, each measuring 200 to 300 microns in diameter. The spheroid follicle is lined by a single layer of cuboidal epithelial cells and contains an amber viscous fluid composed mainly of thyroglobulin (Plates II and III).

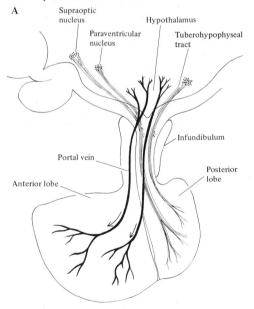

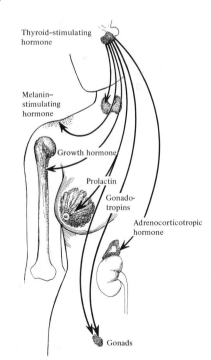

Figure 27–2. The hypophyseal portal system (*A*) closely integrates the activities of the hypophysis and pituitary glands (*B*).

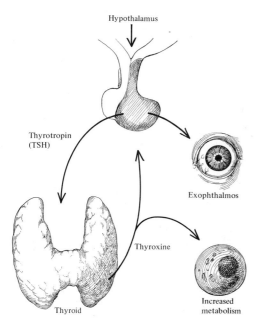

Figure 27–3. The pituitary-thyroid axis acts as a feedback control of the pituitary on thyroid function.

Physiology

The hypothalamus secretes thyrotropin-releasing hormone (TRH), a tripeptide that travels down the neural axons to the median eminence where it is released into the hypophyseal portal system that serves as the arterial supply to the pituitary (Figure 27–2, *A* and *B*). TRH triggers release of thyroid-stimulating hormone (TSH) from the pituitary. TSH then stimulates secretion of thyroid hormone (Figure 27–3). The two active hormones secreted by the thyroid are T-4 (L-thyroxine) and T-3 (triiodothyronine) (Figure 27–4). Most of the circulating T-3 is derived by peripheral deiodination of T-4.

The first step of hormone formation is trapping the large monovalent iodide anion within the basal cell. This is followed by fixation of the iodine on the tyrosine molecule by a peroxidase reaction. Large anions such as perchlorate ($ClO_4{}^-$) or thiocyanate (SCN^-) competitively interfere with trapping, while peroxidase inhibitors such as methimazole or propylthiouracil can interfere with the second step. Monoiodotyrosine (MIT) and diiodotyrosine (DIT) are the iodinated amino acids that are converted to T-3 and T-4 by coupling. T-3 and T-4 are stored in the colloid in the acini in combination with the thyroprotein thyroglobulin. When thyroglobulin is hydrolyzed in the cell, T-3 and T-4 are released into the circulation. The normal thyroid gland contains four to six-weeks' supply of hormone in the cells and colloid. The small amount of thyroid-binding globulin (TBG) in the serum binds T-4 avidly and T-3 about one tenth as strongly. Thyroid-binding prealbumin (TBPA) is present in greater quantity than TBG but binds T-4 less avidly and T-3 very weakly. Because of binding differences T-3 is more potent than T-4 and has a shorter biologic half-life (T-4 six days and T-3 one day). It is the amount of free (unbound) T-4 or T-3 that is active physiologically.

Laboratory Assessment of Thyroid Function

The clinical features of thyroid dysfunction are sometimes striking but are often subtle, requiring attention to detail in the history and physical examination. Once clinical suspicion has been aroused, proper selection of laboratory techniques should lead to a diagnosis.

Serum Thyroxine by Competitive Binding Assay. The thyroxine in the serum displaces isotopically labeled T-4 from a standard preparation of thyroid-binding globulin (TBG). The labeled T-4 is taken up on a resin and assessed for radioactivity. Three elements are allowed to associate until a dynamic equilibrium is established:

1. Standard preparation of binding protein.
2. Standard amount of radioactive hormone.
3. (a) Standard amounts of hormone (to determine standard curve) or (b) serum containing unknown amount of hormone (for assay).

Number 3 is added to 1 and 2 and results in displacement of some of 2 that is bound to the protein in 1.

Radioimmunoassay for T-3. This procedure

"T4"

$$HO - \bigcirc - O - \bigcirc - CH_2 - \underset{\underset{NH_2}{|}}{CH} - COOH$$

L-Thyroxine

"T3"

$$HO - \bigcirc - O - \bigcirc - CH_2 - \underset{\underset{NH_2}{|}}{CH} - COOH$$

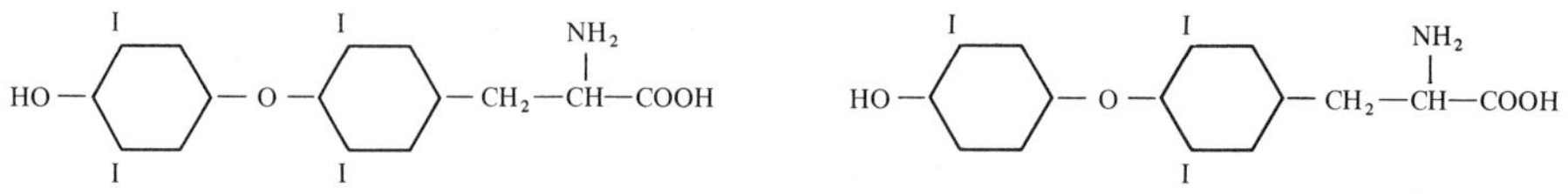

3, 5, 3'-L-Triiodothyronine

Figure 27–4. Molecular structure of thyroxine and triiodothyronine.

has only recently become available and is particularly useful in diagnosing T-3 toxicosis. In this type of hyperthyroidism the T-4 and T-3 resin uptake is normal and the T-3 is elevated.

Radioimmunoassay for TSH. The TSH in plasma is a sensitive index of primary hypothyroidism. The level is elevated as soon as physiologically inadequate levels of thyroid hormone are presented to body target tissues, including the pituitary gland.

T-3 Resin Uptake. Thyroxine is mainly bound to three proteins: (1) TBG (thyroxine-binding globulin), a small amount of circulating protein that specifically and avidly binds about 60 percent of thyroxine in the serum; (2) TBPA (thyroxine-binding prealbumin), a moderate amount of circulating protein that binds about 30 percent of serum thyroxine less specifically and less avidly than TBG; (3) serum albumin, a large circulating protein reservoir that usually binds only about 10 percent of serum thyroxine in a nonspecific manner.

The patient's serum containing his endogenous circulating proteins is incubated with a standard amount of radioactive T-3. The serum and radioactive T-3 are than filtered through a resin which absorbs all the radioactive T-3 not bound to serum protein. The magnitude of the resin uptake (expressed as percent of total T-3) is inversely proportional to the available binding sites on TBG. T-3 resin uptake is always determined along with serum T-4 measurement to adequately define abnormal T-4 measurements due to variation in endogenous binding proteins.

Kinometry. The duration of the Achilles tendon reflex jerk can be measured on electrocardiographic paper. This is characteristically slow in hypothyroidism and increased in hyperthyroidism. The test is simple, but there is considerable overlap between normal and that found in hypothyroidism or hyperthyroidism. It is not clinically useful.

Basal Metabolic Rate. Initially the only test of thyroid function was the BMR. Unfortunately it was often not "basal." The level was often increased in nonthyroidal diseases such as leukemia, lymphomas, emphysema, congestive heart failure, and perforated eardrums, and depressed in anorexia nervosa, marked obesity, and certain types of depression. The BMR is only accurate in about 50 percent of patients and is no longer used.

Radioactive Iodine Uptake. This is a measure of organ partition of the available endogenous iodide pool. A tracer dose of radioactive iodide is administered orally and is 100 percent absorbed to mix with and therefore effectively label the body pool of available iodide. Distribution occurs throughout most body tissues, including plasma and muscle. The kidney and the thyroid actively clear iodide from the body pool and compete for its removal. With a steady state of intake and loss of iodide from the body the pool of available body iodide remains stable. When the thyroid gland is functioning normally, the inorganic iodide taken up each day by the gland is about equal to the amount of organic iodide secreted by the thyroid.

Commonly the uptake in the neck is measured 24 hours after giving about 30 mCi of radioactive iodide by mouth. The normal range of 24-hour uptake varies with locality, depending upon the iodine in diet and laboratory technique.

Elevated uptakes may be found in conditions other than hyperthyroidism, such as iodide deficiency (small endogenous iodide pool), the rebound phase after subacute thyroiditis or thyroid administration, and in certain enzymatic defects within the thyroid gland.

Conversely the uptake may be suppressed in conditions other than hypothyroidism; values may be low with iodine contamination (markedly enlarged endogenous iodide pool), congestive heart failure (diminished tissue perfusion with delayed iodide delivery to organs of clearance), acute thyroiditis, antithyroid drugs, and thyroid administration.

Thyroid Stimulation Test. The thyroid stimulation test was used to differentiate primary thyroid insufficiency from secondary hypothyroidism of pituitary origin. The test has been largely replaced by the serum TSH measurement.

The baseline radioactive iodine uptake is determined. Ten units of TSH are given intramuscularly for three days, and the radioactive iodine uptake is measured again. Normally the second value is more than twice the baseline value.

Thyroid Suppression Test. The thyroid suppression test helps diagnose thyrotoxicosis. The baseline radioactive iodine uptake is determined. T-3, 75 μg, is given orally for seven days and the radioactive iodine uptake determined. Normally suppression is less than 40 percent of the baseline value. In thyrotoxicosis there is little or no suppression.

Radioactive Iodide Scanning. Radioactive iodide scanning is used to delineate functioning thyroid tissue. It helps diagnose palpable thyroid nodules and locate aberrant thyroid tissue.

Antithyroglobulin Antibodies. Antibodies are moderately to markedly elevated in 90 percent of Hashimoto's thyroiditis. Techniques used include tanned cell agglutination and complement fixation.

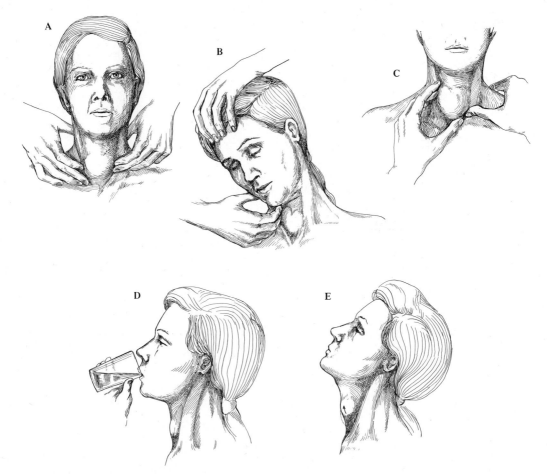

Figure 27–5.   Clinical examination. *A.* The neck is examined from behind with the neck slightly flexed. *B.* The head is bent to each side to relax the sternomastoid muscle and permit thorough palpation of the cervical nodes. *C.* A tumor is tested for mobility. *D.* The patient takes water into the mouth and holds it. *E.* When the patient swallows, the tumor can be felt to move up if it is within the thyroid.

Clinical Examination

The patient is examined for signs of hypo-thyroidism and hyperthyroidism. The neck is first visualized from in front and the patient asked to swallow (Figure 27–5).

Hyperthyroidism

Hyperthyroidism is a symptom complex resulting from excessive circulating amounts of thyroxine (T-4) or triiodothyronine (T-3), or both.

Etiologic factors in thyrotoxicosis are Graves' disease, Plummer's disease (autonomous hyper-functioning nodule), subacute thyroiditis (transient), T-4 or T-3 medication, tumor production of thyroid-stimulating material, thyroid carcinoma, and, rarely, hypersecretion of TSH by pituitary adenoma.

The symptoms of hyperthyroidism result from the direct effects of excessive thyroid hormone, increased sensitivity to catecholamines, and extrathyroidal factors.

1. Increased catecholamine effects: nervousness, palpitations, tachycardia, and tremor.

2. Hypermetabolism: increased perspiration, heat intolerance, fatigue, increased appetite, and weight loss.

3. Increased gastrointestinal activity: diarrhea

4. Myopathy: weakness and/or paralysis and dyspnea.

5. Miscellaneous: personality changes or psychosis, decreased central nervous system efficiency, menstrual irregularities, symptoms of congestive heart failure, hair loss, and eyelid retraction, lid-lag, and stare (exophthalmos).

Over 80 percent of patients have goiter,

tachycardia, weight loss, fatigue, heat intolerance, increased perspiration, and nervousness. Appetite is usually increased but may be depressed in the elderly. Muscular weakness is common, involving the legs and trunk. Fatigue may be related to the muscular weakness, to the intense increase in muscular activity over prolonged periods, or to congestive heart failure.

Treatment of Thyrotoxicosis. Therapy is directed toward controlling the production and secretion of thyroid hormone. Antithyroid agents may be given which temporarily block the synthesis or the release of thyroid hormone, or the acinar cells may be destroyed by radioiodine or removed surgically.

Antithyroid drugs commonly used are the thionamides, propylthiouracil, and methimazole, and certain monovalent anions such as perchlorate and stable iodine. Guanethidine, reserpine, and propanolol have been used to treat the clinical and hemodynamic manifestations of thyrotoxicosis. These drugs are antiadrenergic, blocking the augmented catecholamine effects.

Radioactive iodine damages the thyroid cells, suppresses thyroid hormone secretion, and damages the thyroid cell replication system with resulting gradual atrophy of the gland from failure of cell division. There is no increase in leukemia in patients with hyperthyroidism treated with ^{131}I. Advantages are ease of administration, minimal morbidity, and freedom from tetany and vocal cord paralysis. Disadvantages are delay in controlling hyperthyroidism and the high incidence of hypothyroidism. Hypothyroidism developing shortly after therapy starts is usually temporary, but that occurring after one year is usually permanent. Hypothyroidism occurs in 10 to 20 percent of patients in the first year and 2 to 3 percent per year thereafter.

Subtotal thyroidectomy is an effective form of treatment for thyrotoxicosis. A small portion of thyroid is left on each side to decrease the likelihood of damage to the recurrent laryngeal nerves and the parathyroids and to decrease the incidence of hypothyroidism. Thyroxine should be given after operation to suppress TSH production. Young adults with marked thyrotoxicosis should be treated with antithyroid drugs until they are euthyroid. They are then given iodine orally two weeks before subtotal thyroidectomy.

Choice of Therapy. Young and middle-aged adults are most often given full-dose radioiodine or low-dose radioiodine along with thionamide for about two years. Selected patients may be treated by subtotal thyroidectomy. Surgery is the treatment of choice in the pregnant female, as radioiodine is always contraindicated and high-dose thionamides, crossing the placental barrier, suppress the fetal thyroid. Children are initially treated with antithyroid drugs. A toxic adenoma is often excised by hemithyroidectomy, but some centers routinely use high doses of radioiodine.

Hypothyroidism

Hypothyroidism or myxedema occurs in 1 to 2 percent of the elderly and is seven times more frequent in women than in men. A number of patients have a familial predisposition. Some environmental factors are viral thyroiditis and severe stress. It may result from thyroid-inhibiting drugs, such as thiocynate, thiouracil, resorcinol, and cobalt, or follow administration of large doses of iodide to susceptible individuals with a defect in organic iodination. Other causes are nonsuppurative thyroiditis or chronic thyroiditis, destruction of thyroid tissue by therapeutic radioiodine or operation, and pituitary deficiency of TSH production. In most patients the cause of hypothyroidism is not known and may be on an immunologic basis.

The low level of circulating thyroxine results in a decreased rate of protein synthesis and catabolism. Often the total serum proteins are increased due to increased globulins and mucoproteins. There is also an increase in urate secretion, a decreased rate of glucose utilization, decreased cardiac output due to bradycardia and diminished stroke volume, and anemia. There may be vitamin B_{12} deficiency due to associated pernicious anemia.

Symptoms are decreased tolerance for cold, decrease in sweating, dryness of the hair and skin, hoarseness, muscle weakness, myalgias, stiffness, and cramps. General fatigue, weakness, and drowsiness, personality changes, constipation, and menorrhagia or polymenorrhea are common.

On examination the face is expressionless and placid, round, and moderately edematous (Figure 27–6). The eyelids are puffy. The nose, mouth, and tongue are thickened, the hair is fine and dry, the voice is husky and froglike. There is often deafness. The skin is swollen and does not pit; it is rough, cool, inelastic, and dry. The cardiac silhouette may be enlarged due to pericardial effusion. On neurologic examination the deep tendon reflexes reveal a normal rate of contraction and a prolonged rate of relaxation. There may be objective sensory loss, sluggish pupillary reflexes, and diplopia. Intellectual function is often impaired.

The serum cholesterol is generally elevated, and the circulating thyroid hormone is low. The earliest abnormality found by the laboratory

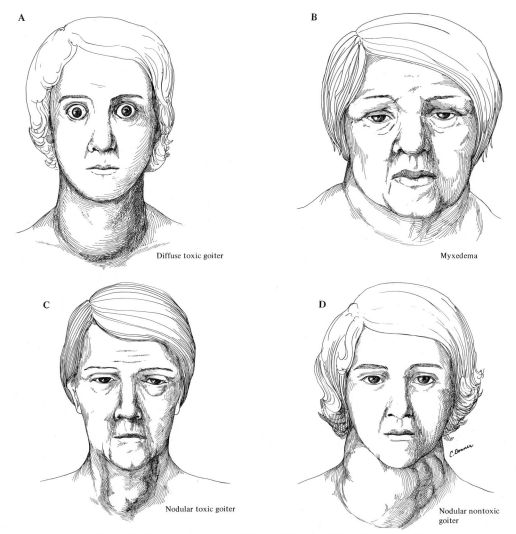

A   Diffuse toxic goiter

B   Myxedema

C   Nodular toxic goiter

D   Nodular nontoxic goiter

Figure 27–6. Facial characteristics of diseases of the thyroid gland.

is an elevation of serum TSH. Serum TSH is low in secondary hypothyroidism. Other evidence of pituitary hypofunction may be present, such as decreased urinary gonadotropins, 17-keto-steroids, and corticoids.

Treatment is administration of oral thyroid hormone. In long-standing hypothyroidism therapy is usually begun at low levels of replacement such as 0.025 mg of L-thyroxine daily. If this dose is well tolerated, it is doubled every two weeks to the usual maintenance dose of 0.2 mg daily. The prognosis with treatment is generally excellent.

Thyroiditis

Hashimoto's Disease. Hashimoto's disease or lymphocytic thyroiditis is not uncommon and occurs most often in women of 30 to 50 years. Diagnosis is made by the clinical picture of a moderately firm goiter and high serum titers of thyroid antibodies. Autoimmunity likely plays a significant role in the pathogenesis of this disease. Tissue specimens show diffuse lymphocytic infiltration, obliteration of thyroid follicles, and progressive fibrosis. There is a defect in organic binding of thyroidal iodine with an accelerated turnover of a depleted organic iodine pool. Abnormalities in hormone biosynthesis may be found in relatives of these patients.

The onset of Hashimoto's thyroiditis is usually slow and insidious but may be rapid with a tender thyroid, mimicking subacute thyroiditis. Sometimes symptoms of mild thyrotoxicosis appear during the early phase of the disease. About 20 percent of patients are hypothyroid when first seen. The goiter is generally moderate in size, firm, and smooth, and moves freely when the patient swallows. It remains unchanged or may enlarge gradually over several years.

Early thyroid function tests indicate the presence of thyroidal hyperfunction without overproduction of metabolically active hormone. ^{131}I uptake may be increased. There is glandular hypersecretion of TSH. The excessive glandular secretion is of abnormal iodoproteins. Serum T-4 level is normal. With the passing of time evidence of hyperfunction diminishes, and the ^{131}I uptake and serum T-4 approach subnormal values. Ultimately the metabolic indices and the patient's clinical state reflect inadequate hormone secretion.

The diagnosis of Hashimoto's disease is confirmed by high titers of thyroid antibodies in the serum. Since this test is at least as reliable as needle biopsy, the latter is not indicated.

Many patients require no treatment because the goiter is small. Thyroid hormone is indicated in those with hypothyroidism. Those patients with acute onset of the disease accompanied by pain and tenderness may benefit from glucocorticoids together with thyroid hormone. Occasionally surgical excision is necessary to remove a large goiter or to biopsy a suspicious region that may be malignant. There may be an increase in cancer of the thyroid and other sites in Hashimoto's disease.

Subacute Thyroiditis. This disease is probably the result of a viral infection of the thyroid gland, often following an upper respiratory illness. The disease is uncommon but is often mistaken for pharyngitis. Women are more frequently affected than men, and the maximum incidence is in the fourth and fifth decades.

In mild cases aspirin adequately controls symptoms. In more severe cases prednisone, 15 to 20 mg per day, rapidly alleviates the symptoms but does not influence the course of the underlying disease. Operation is not indicated.

Reidel's Thyroiditis. Reidel's thyroiditis is rare and is observed chiefly in middle-aged women. The etiology is unknown. It is characterized by extensive fibrosis of the thyroid gland and adjacent structures and may be associated with fibrosis elsewhere, especially in the retroperitoneal area. Thyroid hormone is given for any associated hypothyroidism, and thyroidectomy may be necessary to relieve pressure symptoms.

Acute Pyogenic Thyroiditis. Acute pyogenic thyroiditis is an uncommon disorder due to infection of the thyroid gland by pyogenic organisms. It is characterized by severe pain and tenderness in the thyroid gland with fever, dysphagia, and malaise. Treatment is with antibiotics and surgical drainage when fluctuation is present.

Nontoxic Goiter

Nontoxic goiter may be defined as any thyroid enlargement that is not associated with thyrotoxicosis or hypothyroidism and is not the result of an inflammatory or neoplastic process. Glandular hypertrophy occurs as a compensatory response to factors that impair the gland's ability to manufacture adequate quantities of the hormone. TSH secretion is hyperactive, glandular compensation is adequate, and the patient is euthyroid. This disorder differs only in degree from goitrous hypothyroidism, possibly resulting from the same etiologic factors.

Sex incidence slightly favors female over male. Iodine deficiency is now rarely a cause. Dietary goitrogens may be implicated, but generally the etiology is a defect in biosynthesis within the gland.

The patient may have noticed the enlarged gland and not have any symptoms or may present with dysphagia, local discomfort, stridor, or an unproductive cough. Thyrotoxicosis may complicate multinodular disease of long duration.

Serum T-4 and T-3 resin uptake are normal or borderline low. Radioactive iodine uptake is generally normal but may be increased as much as two or three times normal in certain enzyme defects that are causing this hormone dysgenesis. Serum TSH may be elevated and is the cause of increasing glandular size.

Treatment is directed at removing the stimulus to thyroid hyperplasia. Sufficient thyroxine is given to inhibit TSH secretion. Iodine should not be given.

A diffuse goiter of short duration generally regresses on thyroxine. Long-term multinodular nontoxic goiters often do not regress, but further enlargement is prevented.

Operation may become necessary because obstructive symptoms persist in spite of treatment with thyroxine or because of cosmetic disfigurement. Sometimes operation is indicated because malignancy is suspected in a multinodular goiter. A bilateral subtotal thyroidectomy is performed, leaving 2 to 3 gm of thyroid in each side to preserve some thyroid function and to avoid damage to the recurrent laryngeal nerves and hypoparathyroidism from removal of the parathyroids (Figure 27-7).

Solitary Thyroid Nodule. Patients frequently present with a nontoxic, mobile, solitary nodule in the thyroid. If there is no uptake of radioactive iodine by the nodule in the thyroid

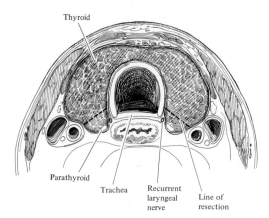

Thyroid

Parathyroid

Trachea   Recurrent
            laryngeal   Line of
            nerve   resection

Figure 27–7. The line of section of the thyroid is shown in bilateral subtotal thyroidectomy. The recurrent laryngeal nerves and parathyroids are closely related to the remnant of the thyroid.

scan, the nodule is most likely a cyst, benign adenoma, or carcinoma. A subtotal lobectomy should therefore be performed. About 10 percent of "cold" nodules will be found to be malignant. When the nodule takes up the radioactive iodine in normal or increased amounts, treatment should be administration of thyroid hormone. Many nodules will regress with this treatment. If the nodule enlarges or becomes firmer, partial lobectomy is indicated.

Ultrasound is of value in differentiating a cyst from a tumor. In those patients in whom a cyst is suspected, needle aspiration is justified. No further treatment is indicated if the fluid does not contain malignant cells on cytologic examination and if the swelling disappears completely. A nonsurgical approach is now being advocated by some surgeons for solitary cold nodules, because only about 10 percent are malignant and most of these are papillary carcinomas with an exceptionally good prognosis, especially in those below 40 years. Thyroxine is given and the tumor removed only if it fails to respond or becomes larger.

Benign Tumors

Benign adenomas of the thyroid generally present as slowly growing solitary nodules. Microscopically they consist of embryonal, fetal, follicular, papillary, or Hürthle cells. It is often difficult to differentiate benign from malignant tumors. Radioiodine uptake does not help in the diagnosis because uptake may be increased, normal, or decreased.

Treatment consists of removing the nodule with a rim of normal thyroid tissue. This usually requires a subtotal or hemithyroidectomy. About 80 percent of the excised nodules are benign.

Malignant Tumors

Cancer of the thyroid is one of the few extra-genital cancers that is more frequent in women than men and accounts for about 5000 new cases per year in the United States. About one third occur below 45 years, and below 25 years the ratio of female to male is 8:1. It is responsible for about 0.5 percent of all deaths from cancer. The ratio of deaths for males to females is 1.5:1 because of the higher incidence of more malignant microscopic types in males. The prognosis is related more to the microscopic type of tumor than to the extent of the disease.

There are a number of predisposing causes of thyroid cancer. There is a definite increase in this cancer in patients with multinodular goiters but probably not in those with endemic goiters. Some have observed a 12 percent incidence of thyroid cancer in patients with Hashimoto's disease, but others have observed no increase. A single dose of radiotherapy, 50 to 500 rad, is carcinogenic, as recorded in neonates given radiotherapy to the thymus and victims of atomic explosions. Cancer of the thyroid is not increased in patients given radioactive iodine for thyrotoxicosis. A single dose of 2000 rad is necessary to completely destroy the thyroid acinar cells. The dose for thyrotoxicosis is much greater and is therefore unlikely to be carcinogenic.

Clinical Findings and Investigations. A carcinoma of the thyroid usually presents clinically as a firm nodule in a normal gland or a multinodular goiter. A history of rapid increase in size suggests malignancy. The tumor is best felt with the examiner behind the patient and the neck flexed forward. Extension of the tumor beyond the thyroid capsule is demonstrated by impaired movement of the tumor on swallowing or extension into adjacent tissues. Another sign is hoarseness from paralysis of a recurrent laryngeal nerve. Palpable nodes, especially in the supraclavicular triangle, suggest nodal metastases. The radioactive iodine uptake is often valuable in establishing the diagnosis. Generally a carcinoma does not take up the isotope, so the tumor appears as a "cold" spot on the scan. The frequency with which thyroid tumors take up ^{131}I is follicular 75 percent, papillary 50 percent, Hürthle cell 30 percent, and anaplastic < 1 percent. Only occasionally does a carcinoma take up an increased amount of isotope. Other thyroid function tests are generally normal.

The differential diagnosis includes benign adenomas, multinodular goiter, cysts, and thyroiditis.

Pathology. The American Thyroid Association has classified carcinomas of the thyroid as papillary, follicular, medullary, and anaplastic. Prognosis is increasingly poor in the four types.

Papillary Carcinoma. This is the most common thyroid carcinoma, occurring in about 65 percent of patients. It is three times more frequent in females than males and occurs most often at 20 to 40 years.

The patient usually presents with a slowly growing discrete solitary nodule in the thyroid. Microscopically the epithelium projects as papillae into the acini, and in about 30 percent focal calcification is present. It is often difficult to differentiate a benign papillary adenoma from a papillary carcinoma. The commonest variant of the papillary carcinoma is the mixed papillary-follicular type. The tumor, however, behaves as a papillary carcinoma and not as the more malignant follicular carcinoma. The tumor is sometimes associated with marked fibrosis and grossly resembles a scirrhous carcinoma of the breast. Sometimes the carcinoma is small, the micropapillary type, and gives rise to nodal metastases in the neck; this was formerly known as a "lateral aberrant thyroid." In about 5 percent there are more than one tumor in the same lobe, and in about 1 percent the tumors are bilateral. Metastases

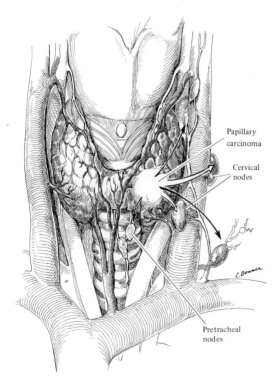

Figure 27–8. A papillary carcinoma of the thyroid tends to spread locally and to the cervical lymph nodes but not by the blood stream.

(labels on figure: Papillary carcinoma; Cervical nodes; Pretracheal nodes)

tend to occur late to the cervical nodes and only rarely to distant tissues (Figure 27–8).

Opinions differ in the treatment of papillary carcinoma of the thyroid. Some authorities advocate total thyroidectomy because tumors may be bilateral. More often a hemithyroidectomy is performed on the side containing the tumor, and the opposite side is removed only if it is believed that it contains a tumor. Nodes in the neck are generally not removed prophylactically. When a node is palpable, it was formerly the custom to remove clinically involved nodes (node picking). Most frequently a modified block dissection is performed with preservation of the sternomastoid muscle and the jugular vein.

Prognosis is extremely good for papillary carcinomas with a 10-year survival of 80 to 90 percent. This is one of the uncommon malignancies in young people that has a good prognosis. About 90 percent of thyroid cancers in children are papillary. About 85 percent have nodal metastases and 15 percent have lung metastases; yet the five-year survival is 95 percent.

Follicular Carcinoma. This tumor occurs at an older age and has a worse prognosis than papillary carcinoma. About 12 percent of all thyroid cancers are encapsulated follicular, and 8 percent are invasive follicular. The tumor usually presents as a hard mass in a normal thyroid or a multinodular goiter. It tends to infiltrate the surrounding muscles and involve the recurrent laryngeal nerve. Spread may occur to the regional nodes, but in addition there is a marked tendency for hematogenous spread to the bones and lungs.

Treatment is by hemithyroidectomy or total thyroidectomy. The regional nodes are only removed if they are clinically involved. All patients are given thyroid continuously after operation to inhibit TSH secretion. When distant metastases occur, radioactive iodine may be given to treat metastases that take up the isotope. Distant metastases may also be treated by local excision or radiotherapy. The results are disappointing with chemotherapy. The mortality is about 3 percent for the encapsulated tumor and 50 percent for the invasive follicular carcinoma.

Medullary Carcinoma. Medullary carcinoma accounts for 5 to 10 percent of thyroid cancers. The cells are in sheets and resemble those in medullary carcinoma of the breast except that the cells are better differentiated. Amyloid is frequently present. The cells are parafollicular cells derived from the ultimobranchial body and therefore originate from the neural crest. Granules consisting of calcitonin can be seen on electronmicroscopy. The blood level of calcitonin may be as high as 1000 times the normal level. About 30 percent of patients have diarrhea, and this is often severe in those with metastases. The diarrhea may be due to prostaglandins secreted by the tumor. Other hormones that are occasionally secreted are histaminase, adreno-corticotropin, and serotonin. There is a familial history in only about 5 percent of patients, and in about 70 percent the tumors are bilateral. A pheochromocytoma is present in about 5 percent. The tumor is often painful and has a marked tendency to be bilateral. Metastases are present in the cervical nodes in about 50 percent and also by the hematogenous route to bones, liver, and lungs.

Many patients, especially those with bilateral disease, have an associated pheochromocytoma. Tests for adrenal catecholamines should therefore be performed in all patients. Occasionally other endocrine disorders are also present such as hyperparathyroidism,

Treatment consists of total thyroidectomy and removal of the regional nodes if they are clinically involved. Distant metastases tend to respond poorly to thyroid suppression, radiotherapy, or radioactive iodine. Prognosis is worse than in those with follicular carcinoma. The 10-year survival is intermediate between that for follicular carcinoma (50 percent) and anaplastic carcinoma (less than 5 percent).

Anaplastic Carcinoma. Anaplastic carcinoma accounts for about 10 percent of thyroid malignancies. It tends to occur in elderly women, and there is often difficulty in differentiating the small cell type from a lymphoma. There is local pain accompanied by a marked tendency to rapidly infiltrate the tissues around the thyroid. Metastases tend to occur to the regional nodes and lungs more often than to bone. Treatment is generally by local radiotherapy. The mortality at five years is about 95 percent with an average survival of about six months.

Other Types. About 1 percent of cancers of the thyroid are squamous cell, Hürthle cell, or clear cell carcinomas.

Thyroxine and Carcinoma of the Thyroid. All patients with thyroid cancer should be given thyroxine, generally 0.3 mg of L-thyroxine daily, to inhibit production of TSH, because a number of the tumors are at least partially TSH dependent.

Radioactive Iodine. About 10 percent of the thyroid tumors take up radioactive iodine (^{131}I), and most are well-differentiated follicular carcinomas. It is usually necessary to completely remove or destroy the thyroid to obtain adequate uptake of the isotope by thyroid metastases. All patients with metastatic carcinoma should have:

1. Complete ablation of all normal thyroid tissue either surgically or with ^{131}I.

2. A high dose of ^{131}I (10 mCi) with total body scanning at 48 to 72 hours and where facilities permit counting of total body ^{131}I retention. In the absence of normal thyroid tissue a retention of > 15 percent of administered dose after 48 hours indicates iodine-concentrating tissue somewhere even if it cannot be located on a scan. It is worthwhile to administer a therapeutic dose of ^{131}I (100 to 150 mCi) if other clinical considerations allow.

Where external irradiation and ^{131}I are required, the ^{131}I should be given first, since a modest dose of irradiation may impair subsequent ^{131}I concentrating ability.

Local Radiotherapy. Thyroid tissue and the differentiated carcinomas are relatively radio-resistant. It is seldom, if ever, possible to administer curative radiation from an external source because of limitations imposed by tolerance of adjacent normal tissues (especially cervical spinal cord). Radiotherapy, 4000 to 6000 rad in four to six weeks, is given if there is residual tumor after operation or if the tumor was opened into during the resection.

PARATHYROID

There are generally four parathyroid glands, each weighing 30 to 45 mg, with the number varying from two to six. They are developed from the third and fourth branchial clefts, the superior parathyroids from the fourth and the inferior glands from the third. The superior glands are usually on the posterolateral border of the upper third of the thyroid gland. The inferior glands are usually at the lower level but may be found within the thyroid or in the anterior or posterior mediastinum. The gland contains chief cells which secrete parathyroid hormone and oxyphil cells whose function is not known.

Parathyroid hormone, parathormone, is a polypeptide with a molecular weight of about 10,000. The level of ionized calcium perfusing the parathyroid gland controls secretion. A low serum calcium results in an increase in secretion, and a high level causes inhibition. Parathormone acts mainly on the skeleton where it stimulates bone resorption, releases calcium into the extracellular fluid, and increases the serum calcium. Vitamin D is an essential cofactor, because bone resorption cannot occur when there is an extreme deficiency of the vitamin (permissive role for vitamin D). In addition, parathormone raises the serum calcium by increasing renal tubular absorption of the ion and increasing absorption of calcium from the gut.

Calcitonin is a polypeptide secreted by the parafollicular cells of the thyroid and probably also by the parathyroid and thymus. The hormone decreases plasma calcium by inhibiting bone resorption. Hypercalcemia is the main stimulus for its secretion. The importance of calcitonin in human physiology is not yet clear. Its role may be limited to emergency situations when there is calcium overloading.

Disorders of Calcium Metabolism

Hypocalcemia. Hypocalcemia may result from hypoproteinemia, parathyroid hormone deficiency, vitamin D deficiency, hyperphosphatemia, neoplastic disorders, corticosteroid excess, acute pancreatitis, and renal tubular acidosis.

Causes. Causes of hypocalcemia and hyperphosphatemia are:

1. Renal failure. The concomitant metabolic acidosis prevents the development of symptoms, such as tetany. They may, however, be precipitated by administration of bicarbonate. Correction of hyperphosphatemia by diet and administration of aluminum hydroxide gel result in an increase in serum calcium.

2. Idiopathic hypoparathyroidism. This may occur in children with Addison's disease, pernicious anemia, steatorrhea, and monilial infections, and less often with these diseases in the adult. Parathormone cannot be detected in the blood in these patients.

3. Pseudohypoparathyroidism. This is a disorder inherited as an X-linked dominant. It is characterized by hypocalcemia, phenotypic features (short stature, obesity, and mental retardation), skeletal abnormalities (short metacarpals and metatarsals, exostoses, and genu valgum), ectopic (subcutaneous) calcification. Parathormone is markedly elevated during periods of hypocalcemia and is decreased when the serum calcium is raised. End-organ refractoriness to parathormone is manifested by a lack of phosphaturia or rise in urinary cAMP after infusion of exogenous hormone. Disorders which share some of the phenotypic features of pseudohypoparathyroidism (Turner's syndrome, Gardner's syndrome, basal cell nevus syndrome, familial brachydactyly) are not associated with hypocalcemia or refractoriness to parathyroid hormone.

Hypocalcemia may occur with a normal or low serum phosphate:

1. Malabsorption syndromes. This may result from malabsorption of calcium with or without magnesium. If hypomagnesia is responsible for tetany, then the symptoms respond to replacement with magnesium but not with calcium. The cause of "magnesium-deficient hypocalcemia" may be deficient secretion of parathormone or end-organ refractoriness to the hormone. Current studies fail to support the latter hypothesis.

2. Rickets. Hypocalcemia is usually not marked in these patients.

3. Pancreatitis. Hypocalcemia is secondary to formation of calcium soaps and possibly to glucagon-mediated release of calcitonin.

4. Pregnancy.

5. Medullary carcinoma. Medullary carcinoma of the thyroid occasionally causes hypocalcemia.

Symptoms and Signs. The decreased ionized calcium results in personality changes, muscle cramps, and paresthesia which may progress to tetany with severe muscular spasms and laryngeal stridor. The patient with mild hypocalcemia may develop tetany during stress such as pregnancy and lactation. Ectopic calcification may occur in the basal ganglia and lens.

Treatment. Treatment consists of administration of vitamin D with or without supplementary calcium. The serum calcium must be followed frequently since the dose range for inadequate, adequate, and excessive therapy is narrow. Hypercalciuria and nephrocalcinosis can also complicate treatment even at low or normal concentrations of serum calcium. New preparations of vitamin D may provide safer and more efficient preparations.

Hypercalcemia: Primary Hyperparathyroidism. Hypercalcemia may be the result of excess secretion of parathormone (hyperparathyroidism) or may occur with diseases not related to the parathyroids (metastatic malignancy, blood dyscrasias such as multiple myeloma, lymphoma, and leukemia, sarcoidosis, milk-alkali syndrome, hypervitaminosis D, immobilization, hyperthyroidism, and acute adrenal insufficiency).

Primary hyperparathyroidism occurs when there is increased parathormone secretion by a parathyroid tumor or as a result of hyperplasia of the glands. Secondary hyperparathyroidism may develop in patients on dialysis or with kidney transplantation because of decreased absorption of calcium. Hyperplasia of the parathyroids occurs to compensate for calcium loss. There are often metastatic calcification, kidney calcification, and bony changes (renal osteodystrophy). Tertiary hyperparathyroidism occurs occasionally in patients with secondary hyperparathyroidism. The stimulated gland becomes autonomous.

A functioning adenoma occurs more often in women than men and most often at 30 to 60 years. Only rarely are the adenomas palpable;

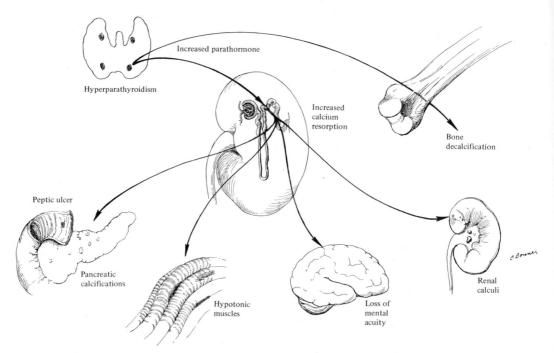

Figure 27–9. Increased secretion of parathormone affects the bones, kidneys, brain, voluntary muscles, and pancreas.

therefore most present with incidental hypercalcemia or complications of hypercalcemia. The chief cell type is the commonest, and about 5 percent of the tumors are bilateral. A carcinoma is rare. Hyperplasia may occur involving all four glands, and the cell type may be either chief cell or water-clear.

Hyperparathyroidism is often familial. It may occur as the only endocrine abnormality or be associated with the multiple endocrine adenomatosis syndrome which most often includes the pituitary, thyroid, islet cells in the pancreas, and the adrenal cortex and medulla.

Peptic ulceration is increased in patients with hyperparathyroidism, possibly from increased acid secretion. Pancreatitis is a well-recognized complication but its cause is unknown.

Clinical Presentation. The performance of a routine screening SMA-12, including the serum calcium, and investigating all patients with renal calculi have resulted in a marked increase in the diagnosis of hyperparathyroidism. The incidence of asymptomatic hypercalcemia varies from 0.1 to 1.5 percent.

GENERAL SYMPTOMS. Weakness, abdominal pain, loss of appetite, nausea, vomiting, constipation, increased frequency of micturition, and changes in mental status are nonspecific symptoms (Figure 27–9).

URINARY SYSTEM. About two thirds of patients with hyperparathyroidism present with urinary calculi and have some calcification of the kidneys (nephrocalcinosis). Most patients with hyperparathyroidism have some degree of kidney damage even without stones or renal calcification. Renal damage may result in hypertension, and this may cause heart failure and death, especially in those with a parathyroid crisis.

BONES. The occurrence of bony pain or a pathologic fracture may lead to the diagnosis being made on an x-ray. A subperiosteal absorption of bone in the phalanges, outer clavicle, and distal ulna is the most frequent early change. Later multicystic disease of bone (von Recklinghausen's disease) is pathognomonic.

PARATHYROID CRISIS. Symptoms of hyperparathyroidism may occasionally be acute in onset and consist of extreme weakness, abdominal pain, vomiting, drowsiness, and even coma. Treatment is administration of fluids, electrolytes, and diuretics (furosemide) and immediate parathyroidectomy.

Investigation. LOCALIZATION IN NECK. The tumors are small and are most often not palpable or demonstrable by x-ray. Occasionally tracheal displacement or esophageal deformity in the patient with a posterior mediastinal tumor suggests its presence.

LABORATORY STUDIES. An elevated serum

calcium is the most important test in the diagnosis of hypercalcemia. The serum phosphate is usually low but may be normal. The blood alkaline phosphatase and urine hydroxyproline concentrations are usually elevated when there is significant bone involvement. Hypercalciuria is common, an excretion exceeding intake clearly reflecting an abnormality.

SPECIAL TESTS OF PARATHYROID FUNCTION. *Corticosteroid.* The hypercalcemia of sarcoidosis, hypervitaminosis D, hypoadrenalism, as well as 50 percent of cases of malignancy respond to prednisone, 10 mg, tid, for 10 days. Primary hyperparathyroidism rarely responds to this treatment.

Phosphate Clearance. Normal subjects have a phosphate clearance of 10.8 ± 2.7 ml per minute. Values 50 percent or more above this occur in hyperparathyroidism. There are many false positives and false negatives.

Urinary Cyclic AMP. Urinary cyclic AMP is available in most clinical centers. It has been shown to be useful in establishing a diagnosis in conjunction with other procedures.

Parathormone Determination. The radioimmunoassay for PTH is the most useful procedure to establish the diagnosis of parathyroidism. The biologically active hormones produced by tumors such as of the lung, kidney, esophagus, cervix, ovary, parotid, liver, and pancreas differ antigenically from PTH. Preoperative attempts to localize abnormal parathyroid tissue using radioisotopes, angiography, or stimulation and suppression tests are often of no value.

Treatment. The primary treatment of hpyercalcemia is to control the underlying cause and provide the patient with adequate fluids. Intravenous saline is given along with potassium. Vasopressors may be used as indicated, and furosemide, 100 mg per hour, may be given intravenously. If the response is poor, phosphates and mithramycin (23 mg/kg) may be given intravenously. With renal failure unresponsive to diuretics corticosteroids and calcitonin can be used safely. Hemodialysis or peritoneal dialysis may be indicated in the patient with renal failure. Optimal management for hyperparathyroid patients with asymptomatic low-grade hypercalcemia has not been established. At the Mayo Clinic 21 of 147 patients followed for 30 months developed urinary calculi, bone disease, increasing hypercalcemia, deterioration in renal function, or psychological changes that required operative intervention. Normocalcemic hyperparathyroidism occasionally occurs; however, the value of exploring the parathyroids has not been established. In patients with symptomatic primary hyperparathyroidism neck exploration is essential. The operation is usually done without knowing whether the condition is due to a tumor or hyperplasia. A thorough dissection is performed and a tumor removed if it is found. In those with hyperplasia a frozen section is obtained of the glands, and three and one-half glands are removed. Not infrequently, all the glands or the tumor cannot be found. It is then necessary to look for parathyroid tissue in the upper mediastinum. The results of surgical treatment are excellent in those who have an adenoma removed and in those with hyperplasia who have adequate parathyroid tissue excised.

Patients with secondary hyperparathyroidism respond well if all the parathyroids are removed or a portion of a single gland is left.

Hypoparathyroidism. This may occur early after operation and recover spontaneously. Occasionally removal of parathyroid tissue has been almost complete and chronic hypothyroidism occurs (see page 479).

ADRENAL CORTEX

Development and Anatomy

The cells of the adrenal cortex arise, at four to six weeks of development, from the celomic mesoderm of the posterior abdominal wall and condense into a small cluster of acidophilic cells between the root of the mesentery and the genital ridge. At about the seventh week ectodermal neurogenic cells migrate from the neural crest to form the adrenal medulla.

The adrenal glands, each weighing about 5 gm, are flattened, caplike structures covering the superior pole of each kidney. They are richly supplied by multiple arteries that break up into sinusoids in the cortex and end in venous lacunae in the medulla. The short right adrenal vein drains directly into the inferior vena cava; the left generally enters the left renal vein. The peripheral zona glomerulosa in the cortex produces mostly mineralocorticoids, notably aldosterone. The inner layers form glucocorticoids, 17-ketosteroids, progestins, and estrogens.

Physiology

The adrenal cortex secretes three groups of hormones: the mineralocorticoids, glucocorticoids, and the sex hormones. Aldosterone is secreted by the zona glomerulosa in response to angiotensin, to an increase in potassium in the blood, and only to a slight extent to adrenocorticotropic hormones (ACTH) of the anterior pituitary. Hypovolemia stimulates production of renin, which catalyzes the generation of angiotensin, which in turn stimulates aldosterone release.

Aldosterone stimulates transport of electrolytes by epithelial cells of the sweat glands, the gastrointestinal tract, and, most important, the kidney. It conserves sodium and increases potassium loss. Aldosterone deficiency leads to sodium depletion, loss of extracellular fluid, hypovolemia, and hypotension. Excess aldosterone results in sodium retention, expansion of extracellular volume, hypokalemic alkalosis, and hypertension.

Aldosterone is extremely potent; the concentrations in clinical disorders are so low that they can only be measured with extremely sensitive radioimmunoassay techniques.

Secretion of the glucocorticoids, 11-17-hydroxycorticoids, is mainly under control of ACTH. The most important of these are cortisol and cortisone. A fall in plasma cortisol leads to an increase in ACTH secretion by the basophil cells in the anterior pituitary. An increase in cortisol inhibits ACTH secretion. Cortisol acts mainly at the hypothalamic level, causing release of a corticotropin-releasing factor (CRF). Normally the cerebral cortex inhibits CRF release. A stressful stimulus reaching the cerebral cortex releases the inhibition on the hypothalamic centers and allows large neurons to secrete CRF. ACTH activates cyclic AMP on the cell membranes of adrenocortical cells and increases the rate of conversion of cholesterol to an early steroid precursor, pregnenolone. There is a daily diurnal rhythm consisting of a low level of ACTH and cortisol during late afternoon and a peak during sleep. ACTH is rapidly destroyed by blood and tissue enzymes and has a half-life of only 5 to 10 minutes.

Testosterone, produced mainly in the testes, is the most potent androgen. In the male the small amount of testosterone produced in the adrenals equals 50 percent of that produced in the female. Female ovaries produce the remainder of circulating testosterone. Other circulating androgens, such as androstenedione and androsterone, are formed mainly in the adrenal and are much weaker androgenically. Adrenal androgen is responsible for growth of axillary hair and contributes significantly to the maintenance of adequate bone mineral mass.

Estrogens are produced mainly in the ovary but small amounts are derived from adrenal and testicular precursors.

Laboratory Studies

17-Hydroxysteroids. The plasma 17-hydroxysteroids are an estimate of circulating cortisol. Ninety percent are bound to plasma protein and 10 percent are "free." The 17-hydroxysteroids in 24-hour specimens of urine reflect the cumulative excretion of the urinary metabolites of cortisol and a few of its precursors.

17-Ketosteroids. The 17-ketosteroids in a 24-hour specimen of urine are a rough measure of the daily production of adrenal androgen.

Cortisol. The amount of cortisol in the urine reflects the amount of "free" unbound plasma 17-hydroxycorticoids (17-OH). In Cushing's syndrome there is an eightfold to tenfold increase in urinary free cortisol. The weak binding of larger quantities of circulating hormone results in an increase in glomerular filtration of cortisol.

Aldosterone. Aldosterone may be measured in a 24-hour urine specimen, mainly the conjugated tetrahydro-derivative, or may be determined in the plasma.

Functions of Steroid Hormones

The mineralocorticoids increase sodium retention and potassium excretion (see Chapter 3).

The glucocorticoids increase gluconeogenesis, resulting in hyperglycemia and breakdown of muscle proteins. They also enhance water diuresis and allow epinephrine to mobilize free fatty acids. In the blood lymphocytes and eosinophils are decreased and erythrocytes increased. The inflammatory response is inhibited. The catabolic protein-wasting effect of excess cortisol leads to muscle wasting, thinning of skin, and loss of matrix from bone. The increased acid secretion by the stomach inhibits mucus secretion. Patients with Cushing's syndrome therefore often develop a peptic ulcer. They also often have mental disturbances.

Adrenocortical Hypofunction

Adrenocortical insufficiency may be primary, as in Addison's disease, or secondary to a deficiency in pituitary ACTH.

Acute Adrenal Insufficiency. An absolute or relative lack of adrenocortical hormones results in lassitude, confusion, restlessness, vomiting, abdominal or costovertebral angle pain, and circulatory collapse. It may progress to unconsciousness and death.

Under stress the output of cortisol from the adrenal may be increased tenfold. A transient adrenocortical insufficiency may develop even in the presence of a normal gland. Causes of primary atrophy (possibly an autoimmune disease) are tuberculous destruction, hemorrhage or thrombosis, and bacterial toxins (meningococcal or streptococcal).

Since there is no rapid laboratory test of adrenocortical function, cortisol must be given, 100 mg intravenously every six hours, when a deficiency is suspected. Intravenous fluids, antibiotics, and norepinephrine may be required.

Chronic Primary Adrenal Insufficiency. Chronic primary adrenal insufficiency is generally insidious in onset, although stress may precipitate a crisis. The signs and symptoms of Addison's disease are weakness and fatigability, abnormal pigmentation, weight loss and dehydration, hypotension with small heart size, anorexia, nausea, vomiting, and diarrhea, dizziness and syncope, hypoglycemic attacks, nervousness and mental symptoms, and absence of axillary hair. Chronic adrenal insufficiency should be suspected in hypotensive patients complaining of fatigue, weight loss, gastrointestinal disturbances, and especially with pigmentation in the mouth and skin creases.

Laboratory studies that raise suspicion are unexplained anemia, low blood sugar, and a low serum sodium to potassium ratio. The ratio is normally 30 and falls toward 20 in adrenocortical insufficiency. The response to ACTH is the best test of adrenal function and can unmask potential adrenal insufficiency in the presence of a normal basal secretion.

Treatment is administration of cortisol (or other glucocorticoid) and 9-fluorohydrocortisone (mineralocorticoid). Extra cortisol is given during stress.

Secondary adrenocortical insufficiency may occur as part of panhypopituitarism or in a pluriglandular deficiency syndrome. Very rarely an isolated deficiency of corticotropin secretion occurs.

The diagnosis is suspected when there is an inadequate response to stress, such as a failure to maintain blood pressure, urine volume, blood sugar level, and general strength. Suspicion is strengthened by finding hypothyroidism, hypogonadism, a fawn-colored pigmentation, and wrinkled facial skin. The diagnosis is confirmed by the presence of diminished baseline cortisol excretion that responds to ACTH but not to the metyrapone test.

Adrenocortical Hyperfunction (Cushing's Syndrome)

Hyperplasia of the adrenal cortex or the presence of an adenoma or adenocarcinoma produces a variety of syndromes, depending on excess production of one or more of the glucocorticoids, androgens, estrogens, or mineralocorticoids. Cushing's syndrome is mainly the result of excessive cortisol. It is more frequent in women than men and occurs most often at 20 to 40 years. It may occur from chronic stress without any pathologic changes in the glands. More often it is the result of:

1. Administration of glucocorticoids.
2. Excessive pituitary ACTH with adrenocortical hyperplasia.

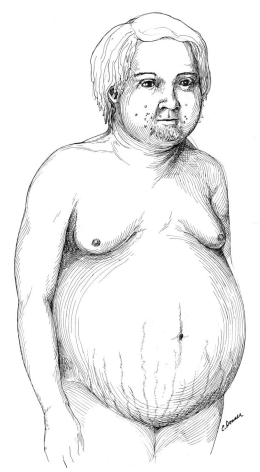

Figure 27–10. In Cushing's syndrome, there are centripetal obesity, a moonface, and abdominal striae, and there may be a buffalo hump and facial hirsutism.

3. Ectopic production of ACTH with adrenocortical hyperplasia.

4. The presence of an adrenocortical neoplasm. A tumor is present in about 25 percent of patients with Cushing's syndrome, and in about one half the tumor is malignant.

Signs and Symptoms. Excessive cortisol secretion leads to obesity with a centripetal distribution of fat (Figure 27–10). There are a characteristic moonface and often a "buffalo hump." Other signs are thinning of the skin, red cheeks, purple striae on the abdomen and thighs, easy bruising with ecchymoses, muscle wasting, osteoporosis, atherosclerosis, and hypertension. Diabetes may be overt or latent. There is frequently a metabolic alkalosis with low serum potassium and chloride.

Excessive androgens may be present and produce hirsuitism, baldness, deepening of the voice, acne, and amenorrhea. An excess of mineralocorticoids results in hypertension, hypokalemia, hypernatremia, and an increase in plasma volume.

Laboratory Studies. Laboratory findings suggestive of Cushing's syndrome are a low lymphocyte count, neutrophilia, a diabetic glucose tolerance curve, and hypokalemic, hypochloremic alkalosis.

Laboratory findings diagnostic of Cushing's syndrome include:

1. The overnight dexamethasone suppression test may be done for screening purposes. The synthetic steroid dexamethasone induces a marked decrease in ACTH secretion. Patients with Cushing's syndrome are resistant to this glucocorticoid suppression and continue to have a high output of 17-hydroxycorticosteroid. The patient is given 1 mg dexamethasone orally 2 to 3 hours after adequate sedation with barbiturate. The plasma 17-hydroxycorticoid at 8 hours should be less than 5.0 μg per 100 ml in the normal person.

2. Elevation of 24-hour urinary free cortisol is a sensitive test for excessive cortisol production.

3. Twenty-four-hour urinary 17-hydroxycorticoids is an indirect indicator of the secretory rate of cortisol and its metabolites.

Elevated baseline excretion of 17-hydroxycorticoids is suggestive of excessive cortisol production. Failure to suppress the level in the urine to 3 mg per 24 hours on the second day after administering 2 mg dexamethasone in four divided doses is diagnostic of Cushing's syndrome. If the syndrome is due to bilateral hyperplasia, suppression is noted in patients given 8 mg dexamethasone daily for two days. Suppression of urinary 17-hydroxysteroids, even with high doses of dexamethasone, is not seen when Cushing's syndrome is due to adenoma, adenocarcinoma, or ectopic ACTH production.

Radiologic Examination. When the diagnosis of Cushing's syndrome has been made by demonstrating a failure to suppress endogenous output of glucocorticoids after dexamethasone, further studies include:

1. X-ray studies of the sella turcica may show enlargement of the pituitary. This is especially liable to be present in the hyperpigmented patient.

2. Older radiographic techniques including intravenous pyelography, retroperitoneal pneumography, and arteriography are seldom helpful.

3. New methods such as adrenal scanning after giving the isotope 19-iodocholesterol or adrenal venography show promise of being discriminating. However, the former is associated with high levels of radiation exposure to the patient and the latter test with a significant incidence of adrenal infarction. The radiologic studies are an attempt to delineate anatomic abnormalities. If the clinician has decided from clinical and chemical studies that the diagnosis is definite, it is justifiable to omit these procedures because they carry significant risk to the patient.

Treatment. In adrenal hyperplasia total bilateral adrenalectomy is the therapy of choice, especially in those with rapid progression of the syndrome characterized by psychosis, marked osteoporosis, and muscle wasting or hypertension. Recent studies suggest that radiation of the pituitary and hypothalamus results in the remission of Cushing's syndrome from bilateral adrenal hyperplasia in 40 to 50 percent of cases within six months of treatment. Side effects are minimal. Cushing's syndrome from adrenal adenoma is cured by surgical removal of the adenoma. The remaining tissue will in time return to normal function. Treatment of adrenal carcinoma and most ectopic ACTH tumors (generally malignant) is palliative, using potent antimetabolic agents.

Primary Aldosteronism

Primary aldosteronism results from the autonomous hypersecretion of aldosterone. Usually primary aldosteronism is due to an aldosterone-secreting adenoma (Conn's syndrome), but occasionally it is associated with adrenal hyperplasia or with normal adrenals (idiopathic hyperaldosteronism). Excessive conservation of sodium leads to expansion of extracellular volume, elevation of the blood pressure, and suppression of renin production. In the absence of circulatory insufficiency, modest expansion of extracellular volume leads to physiologic adjustments that enable the excretory system to come into equilibrium with the sodium intake. Progressive expansion of extracellular volume is thus avoided, and overt edema is absent or only slight. These adjustments are sometimes referred to as "the escape phenomenon."

The diagnosis of primary aldosteronism begins with the recognition that a patient has hypertension. If there is hypokalemia, either persistent or intermittent, that is not the result of diarrhea, vomiting, laxatives, diuretics, or licorice, the diagnosis of primary aldosteronism must be suspected. Hypercortisolism should be ruled out. The blood level of aldosterone (under standard conditions of salt loading) and plasma renin activity (under standard conditions of sodium depletion) should be determined. The combination of abnormally high aldosterone and abnormally low plasma renin activity is pathognomonic of primary aldosteronism. Treatment consists of adrenal exploration and removal of an adenoma or removal of one and one-half glands if an adenoma is not found.

Although "normokalemic primary aldosteronism" does occur, it is rare and is likely to be included in the syndrome of essential hypertension with low or suppressed renin.

Secondary Aldosteronism

The renin-angiotensin system is the principal regulator of aldosterone secretion. The adrenal cortex responds to increased stimulation by the renin-angiotensin system by secreting aldosterone. Aldosterone promotes sodium conservation and potassium excretion. The retention

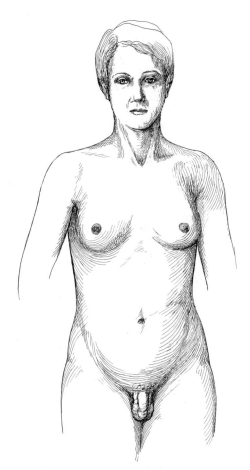

Figure 27–11. Male feminization may be produced by an adrenocortical tumor. About 85 percent are malignant.

of sodium results in expansion of extracellular volume and inhibits renin production by maintaining blood flow to the kidney. Severe dehydration, sodium depletion, hemorrhage, hypoalbuminemic states, renal arterial constriction, and sequestration of blood on the venous side of the circulation are all associated with decreased blood flow to the kidneys. This results in increased production of renin and aldosterone. Secondary aldosteronism is not a disease but rather a response of the normal adrenal to physiologic demands arising in the course of a number of diseases, such as congestive heart failure, the nephrotic syndrome, and hepatic cirrhosis.

Syndromes of Masculinization or Feminization

Excessive circulating levels of sex hormones can result in the above syndromes in the susceptible individual. Excessive androgen production can result from adrenal or ovarian tumors. Tumors of the cortex secreting excess estrogen in the male give rise to adrenal feminism (Figure 27–11), while those secreting excessive testosterone in the female give rise to adrenal virilism (Figure 27–12). Hirsutism is a relatively common syndrome in the human female, the great majority being classified as simple (idiopathic) hirsutism. A significant number of these simple hirsutes may have a very mild form of congenital adrenal hyperplasia. The classic or usual form of congenital adrenal hyperplasia occurs at birth or infancy and is manifested as masculinization, sometimes with salt wasting. The cause is a partial hormone block in the hydroxylation of cortisol (usually at position 21 or 17) with excessive production of adrenal androgens by the hypertrophied, overactive adrenals.

Rare, usually malignant, adrenal tumors produce excessive estrogens causing impotence, gynecomastia, and feminization in the male.

ADRENAL MEDULLA

The main hormones secreted by the medulla are the catecholamines epinephrine, norepinephrine, and dopamine. Control is entirely through the preganglionic autonomic nerves, the efferent cell station being cells within the medulla. There is no hormonal control of medullary function. Epinephrine functions mainly in acute stress, while norepinephrine maintains homeostasis in the resting condition. Norepinephrine acts mainly on the peripheral arterioles, where it causes vasoconstriction and a marked increase in peripheral resistance and

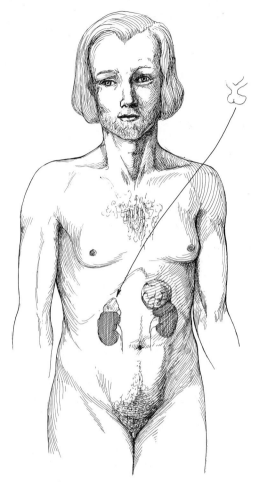

Figure 27–12. Female virilism occurs with adrenocortical tumors and is rarely seen with hyperplasia.

blood pressure. Epinephrine has an important direct effect on the heart, resulting in increased cardiac output. In addition, it increases glycolysis and produces hyperglycemia, increases the metabolic rate, and causes excitation of the central nervous system. Both hormones increase breakdown of fats and raise the serum lipids.

Pheochromocytoma

Tumors may develop in the adrenal medulla, the sympathetic nervous system, and the chromaffin tissue extending from the base of the skull to the pelvis. Those in the adrenal may secrete epinephrine or norepinephrine, while those in the extra-adrenal tissues mostly produce norepinephrine. About 10 percent of the tumors are extra-adrenal and about 40 percent are multiple or bilateral. They are more common in adults than children and are commoner in women than men. Unlike adrenocortical tumors causing Cushing's disease, pheochromocytomas may be large, and their size is not related to the amount of hormone secreted. They can be familial and are often associated with von Recklinghausen's neurofibromatosis. The incidence of malignancy is difficult to determine because the usual criteria for defining malignancy in the primary tumor do not apply. There may be the cellular criteria for malignancy along with invasion of vessels and the capsule, yet the tumors do not metastasize. The only criterion for malignancy is the development of metastases.

Clinical Presentation. The symptoms depend on the amount of hormone secreted and whether the catecholamine is mostly epinephrine or norepinephrine. Epinephrine affects mainly metabolism and norepinephrine the vascular system.

Paroxysmal Tachycardia. The elevation in blood pressure is usually intermittent, being precipitated by exertion or pressure on the tumor, but the pressure may be continuously elevated with occasional hypertensive crises. Headache, flushing, sweating, and tachycardia are the most frequent symptoms.

Hypermetabolism. The patient may develop diabetes mellitus.

A crisis may be precipitated during preoperative examination of the tumor or at the time of its removal. An unsuspected tumor may cause an increase in blood pressure during operation and result in death from heart failure, pulmonary edema, and ventricular fibrillation. Most anesthetic agents decrease systemic blood pressure, so any unexplained increase should make the anesthesiologist suspect a pheochromocytoma.

Investigations. *Pharmacologic Tests.* Histamine increases systemic blood pressure by causing release of the hormones, while phentolamine (Regitine) decreases presssure by preventing their release. These tests may be used as screening tests for pheochromocytoma but are being replaced by direct determination of epinephrine and norepinephrine in the blood and urine.

Localization. Intravenous pyelography, retroperitoneal pneumography, and arteriography may help localize the tumor. A catheter is placed in the inferior vena cava at the level of the adrenal veins and specimens obtained to directly measure the hormones in the blood.

Treatment. Great care is necessary before and during operation to prevent a hypertensive crisis. Phentolamine should be given before and up to the time the tumor is removed, while norepinephrine is generally needed after removal because there is almost invariably a profound drop in blood pressure.

Neuroblastoma

This common malignant tumor of the nervous system occurs in the adrenal medulla in about 40 percent of patients and tends to metastasize to the regional nodes, liver, lungs, and bone. This is one of the commonest sites of spontaneous regression of cancer. Occult neuroblastomas are found frequently at autopsy in children who have died from other causes, and most of these must normally regress. They are among the most antigenetic tumors that occur in man and appear to promote a strong cell-mediated immune response (see Chapter 4).

Attempted curative treatment consists of removing the adrenal, kidney, and adjacent fat. The tumors are radiosensitive, so prophylactic postoperative radiotherapy is generally given with a five-year survival in these patients of about 80 percent. Good palliation can be obtained by removing as much tumor as possible and administering postoperative radiotherapy. Those with residual primary tumor or distant metastases should receive cyclophosphamide and vincristine. The use of vitamin B_{12} to induce maturation of the tumor to a benign ganglioneuroma is rarely effective.

SUGGESTIONS FOR FURTHER READING

Diseases of the adrenal cortex—1:333–598, July 1972. Disorders of the parathyroid glands—3:171–421, July 1974. Investigations of endocrine disorders—3:423–626, November 1974. *Clin. Endocrinol. Metabol.*
Diseases of adrenal cortex and parathyroid glands are reviewed. November 1974 outlines and evaluates investigative procedures.

Endocrine disorders—56:841–1049, July 1972. Therapeutic problems; Hyperthyroidism—56:583–838, May 1972. *Med. Clin. North Am.*
Selected topics are concisely reviewed.

Endocrine surgery. *Surg. Clin. North Am.* Feb., 1969.
Selected topics in surgical aspects of endocrine disease are concisely outlined and reviewed.

Ezrin, C.; Goddin, J. O.; Volpe, R.; and Wilson, R.: *Systematic Endocrinology*. Harper & Row, New York, 1973.
Concise, palatable reading on all topics covered in this chapter.

Montgomery, D. A. D., and Welbourn, R. B.: *Clinical Endocrinology for Surgeons*. E. Arnold Publishers, London, 1963.
Excellent textbook covering the field of endocrine surgery.

Thyroid function tests. In: Stollerman, G. H. (ed.): *Advances in Internal Medicine*, Vol. 18. Year Book Medical Publishers Inc., Chicago, pp. 345–62, 1972.
Helpful, concise review of thyroid function tests.

Yearbook of Endocrinology. Year Book Medical Publishers, Chicago.
Annual collection of abstracts of the significant recent advances in endocrinology. This is a fast, easy entry into the recent literature on selected topics.

Chapter 28

HAND

George P. Reading and *John H. Schneewind*

CHAPTER OUTLINE

Applied Anatomy
Injuries to the Hand
  Assessment
  Preoperative Care
  Anesthesia
  Operation
    Tourniquet
  Postoperative Care
  Special Injuries to the Hand
    Fingertip Injuries and Finger Amputations
    Wringer or Roller Injuries
    Thermal Injuries
    Frostbite
    Grease and Paint Gun Injuries
  Common Injuries to the Digits
    Subungual Hematoma
    Dislocations and Sprains
    Metacarpophalangeal Joint of the Thumb
    Fractures of the Phalanges
    Mallet Finger
    Boutonnière Deformity
    Avulsion of Flexor Digitorum Profundus Tendon
    Foreign Bodies

Hand Infections
  Minor Infections
    Felon or Distal Pulp-Space Infection
    Paronychia
    Web-Space Infections
  Major Hand Infections
    Acute Suppurative Tenosynovitis
    Abscesses of the Deep Palmar and Thenar Spaces
Cysts of the Hand
  Ganglion
  Mucous Cyst
  Inclusion Cyst
Tumors of the Hand
  Benign
    Glomus Tumor
    Hemangioma
  Malignant
Other Surgical Conditions of the Hand
  Dupuytren's Contracture
  Nerve Compression Syndromes
    Carpal Tunnel
    Ulnar Nerve Compression
  Trigger Finger or Snapping Finger
  DeQuervain's Tenosynovitis
  Deformities Due to Rheumatoid Arthritis

APPLIED ANATOMY

A knowledge of the bony anatomy of the hand and its surface landmarks is essential to understand the more common diseases and injuries. The frequently fractured carpal scaphoid, the most radial of the proximal row of carpal bones, may be palpated through the anatomic snuffbox. Lateral radiographs of the wrist demonstrate the relationship of the lunate to the radius proximally and the capitate distally. This is the most common region for dislocation of the wrist. The distal and proximal interphalangeal joints lie beneath the flexion creases on the fingers, but the metacarpophalangeal joints are proximal to the creases at the bases of the fingers and lie at the distal palmar flexion crease (Figure 28–1).

The volar aspect of the wrist contains important tendons, vessels, and nerves and is frequently injured (Figure 28–2). The centrally placed flexor carpi radialis and palmaris longus tendons can be felt. Deep to them lies the median nerve. The palmaris longus, often used for tendon grafts, is absent in about 15 percent of patients. The radial artery lies radial to the flexor carpi radialis. On the ulnar aspect of the wrist lies the flexor carpi ulnaris tendon overlying the ulnar nerve and artery.

The palmar skin is specialized, with a thick

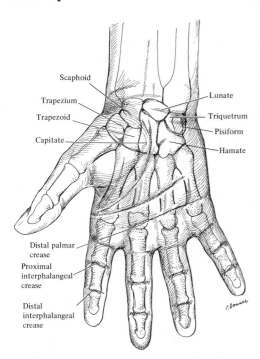

Figure 28–1. Skin creases as landmarks.

cornified epidermis and a relatively thin dermis, and is firmly attached by strong bands to the underlying palmar aponeurosis. This structure protects the long flexor tendons, nerves, and vessels in the palm. Superficial to the tendons lies the superficial volar arch formed by the junction of the radial and ulnar arteries. From the arch arise the arteries to the fingers. The digital nerves are parallel to the arteries. Deep to the tendons lie the deep volar arterial arch and deep branch of the ulnar nerve which innervates the interosseous muscles and the adductor and short flexors of the thumb. At the level of the carpal bones the transverse carpal ligament bounds anteriorly the tunnel containing the long tendons to the fingers and the median nerve. The motor branch of the median nerve to the thenar musculature leaves the median nerve just distal to the volar carpal ligament.

The skin on the dorsum of the hand is thinner, more mobile, and more easily distended than that on the palm (Figure 28–3). The long extensor tendons are fused with the extensor hood at the level of the metacarpophalangeal joints and are inserted into the proximal portion of the middle phalanx. The extensor hood is the principal insertion of the lumbrical and interosseous muscles and is inserted into the distal phalanx. The four fingers receive tendons from the extensor digitorum communis.

The index and little fingers have additional extensor tendons.

The radial aspect of the wrist is frequently injured (Figure 28–4). There are separate tendons extending to the distal phalanx and the proximal phalanx of the thumb. Between these two tendons at the level of the wrist is the anatomic snuffbox containing the carpal scaphoid and radial artery.

The sensory distribution of the three nerves to the hand is important in the diagnosis of nerve injuries. There is considerable overlap in their distribution, especially on the dorsum of the hand, so that if the radial sensory nerve to the hand is divided, the hand is numb only in a small area just distal to the anatomic snuffbox (Figure 28–5).

Congenital anomalies of the hand are described in Chapter 33.

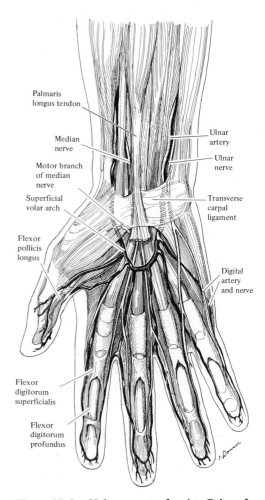

Figure 28–2. Volar aspect of wrist. Palm of hand.

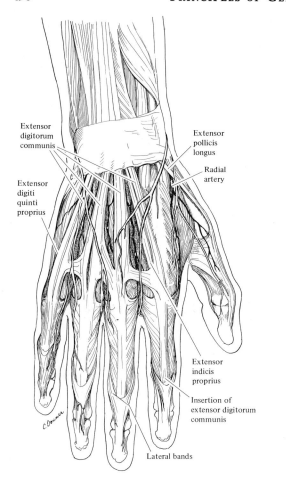

Figure 28–3. Dorsum of hand.

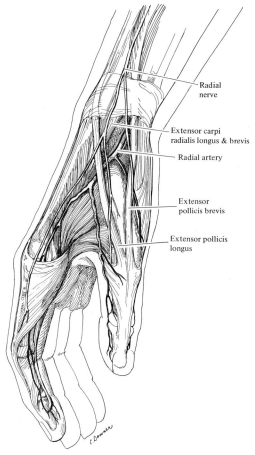

Figure 28–4. Radial aspect of wrist.

INJURIES TO THE HAND

Assessment

The patient with an apparently minor injury of the hand should not be left waiting in the busy emergency department because there is a direct relationship between the time of injury and definitive treatment and the incidence of infection.

The hand should not be placed for a long time in an antiseptic solution because this results in maceration and swelling. A severely injured hand should be initially splinted in the position of function, the bones gently aligned, a dressing applied, and radiographs taken through the dressing and splint.

A history of how, where, when, and by what agent the injury was sustained is necessary. The injury may result from a high-energy or a low-energy gunshot wound, a penetrating sharp object, or a crushing force. The degree of contamination is greater in injuries received in

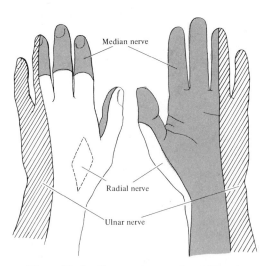

Figure 28–5. Sensory innervation of hand.

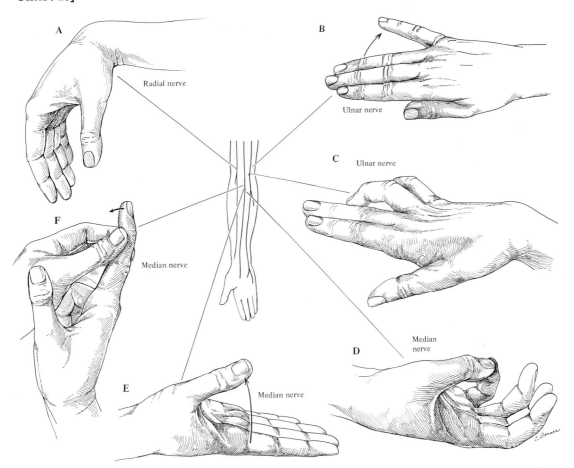

Figure 28-6. Tests of motor function of the radial, ulnar, and median nerves. *A.* Radial nerve paralysis: there is inability to dorsiflex the wrist. *B.* Ulnar nerve paralysis: paralysis of the interossei and lumbricals makes it impossible to adduct the fifth finger. *C.* Ulnar nerve paralysis: deformity consists of flexion of the interphalangeal joints of the fourth and fifth fingers and the metacarpophalangeal joints held in extension. *D.* Median nerve paralysis: opposition of the thumb is not possible. *E.* Median nerve paralysis: there is inability to elevate the thumb from the plane of the hand. *F.* Median nerve paralysis: the terminal phalanx of the index finger cannot be flexed because of paralysis of the flexor digitorum profundus.

a farmyard than in a machine shop. Animal and human bites are severely contaminated. The patient's general condition, age, and activity are also important in determining the type of treatment as well as the final result.

Associated injuries must be recognized and treated. The examiner should wear a mask and sterile gloves when examining open wounds. An assessment is made of loss of tissues, blood supply to distal parts, motor and sensory function, and bony injuries. It is imperative that the sensory function of the fingers be assessed before administering local or regional anesthesia. It is also important to check for motor function of the median, ulnar, and radial nerves (Figure 28–6).

Injuries frequently missed at the initial examination include avulsion of the long extensor tendon from its insertion on the distal phalanx, interruption of the central slip of the extensor tendon at the proximal interphalangeal joint, and injuries to the digital nerves.

Preoperative Care

A minor injury can be treated satisfactorily in the emergency department. When the injury is more serious, the hand is covered with a sterile dressing, bandaged, splinted, and not examined again until the injury is treated in the operating room. Gentle handling, immobilization, and elevation are often effective in relieving pain. Severe pain may require intravenous analgesia. Tetanus toxoid is given to immunized patients and human antitoxin to nonimmunized patients (see Chapter 6). Antibiotics are given before operation if infection is likely to occur, as in wounds with extensive destruction of tissue and severe contamination.

Anesthesia

Injection of a local anesthetic into the wound distorts the anatomy and may predispose to infection and should only be used for small superficial lacerations. Digital nerve blocks are useful in treating injuries of the fingers. A brachial plexus block produces anesthesia of the hand and forearm and permits use of a pneumatic tourniquet (see Chapter 12). General anesthesia is not used in patients who have eaten within six hours of the injury. General anesthesia is generally necessary for long procedures or if reconstruction involves the use of a distant flap.

Operation

Complicated hand injuries are treated in a bloodless field using a pneumatic tourniquet to facilitate identification of small structures. The skin is prepared as for an elective operation. The wound is irrigated with a large amount of sterile saline and protected from soap and antiseptic solutions. The order of priority for treatment is debridement to avoid infection and impairment of wound healing, skin closure to minimize scarring and preserve mobility, stabilization of bones and joints to allow accurate positioning of the structures, and repair of nerves and tendons.

The principles of wound debridement are critical in determining the outcome in hand injuries. The tissues are handled gently, and crushing instruments are not used. Small rubber drains are used as slings to retract tendons and nerves. Magnification by optical loupes helps identify small nerves and vessels. Nonviable tissue is removed by sharp excision with a knife or sharp scissors, and foreign bodies are carefully removed. Fractures are often stabilized by passing small Kirschner wires across the fracture. Continuous traction may be applied through a pin placed transversely through bone or the distal digital pulp.

If simple approximation of the skin is not adequate, free skin grafts or local or distant flaps are used. In high-energy wounds conservative debridement may be advisable, sparing important structures such as tendons, nerves, and blood vessels, and dressing the wound without any attempt at closure. The wound is reexamined in two to four days and further debridement performed if necessary. This may be repeated one or two times until closure can be accomplished without infection.

When primary wound healing is anticipated, tendons are generally repaired at the time of debridement (Figure 28–7). When the long finger flexor tendons are divided between the distal palmar crease and the proximal interphalangeal joint ("no-man's land"), late repair using a graft gives the best results. Primary repair is not advisable in this region, because the two tendons lie in a narrow fibrous tunnel, and a small amount of scar tissue results in marked decrease in movement.

Nerves should be repaired on the day of injury unless primary wound healing is doubtful. However, if the nerve is divided by a crushing injury, definitive repair should be delayed for two to three weeks when the length of injured nerve can be better assessed. Some form of magnification should be used to repair nerve

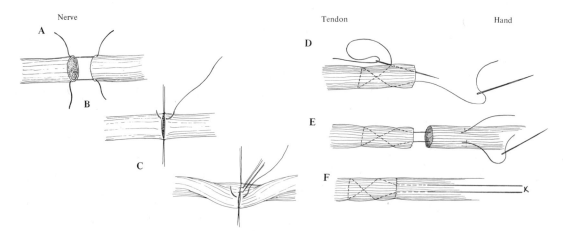

Figure 28–7. Suture of nerve and tendon.

injuries in the hand, such as four-power optical loupes or operating microscopes ranging from 4–25 power. Fine suture, 7-0 to 10-0 nylon, has been used satisfactorily. Tension at the site of nerve repair leads to an unsatisfactory result. If the defect in the nerve cannot be overcome without tension by flexing of a joint, a nerve graft should be inserted.

Formerly arteries beyond the wrist were not repaired, but recently they have been successfully sutured using microscopic techniques.

Tourniquet. A pneumatic tourniquet may be placed on the arm and kept inflated above systolic pressure for 90 minutes without ischemic damage to the hand. If a longer time is required, the tourniquet should be deflated for at least 10 minutes and then reinflated. The tourniquet is released and bleeding controlled before the wound is closed.

Postoperative Care

The hand is generally placed in the position of function with padding between the fingers. An exception is placing the wrist and fingers in flexion following repair of flexor tendons or nerves. The hand is immobilized by plaster splints placed on the volar or dorsal surface. In children a circular plaster cast extending above the elbow helps to prevent the child from interfering with the dressings. In the immediate postoperative period the most common cause of severe pain is a dressing that is too tight. The hand and forearm should be elevated using a sling when the patient is ambulatory or on pillows when the patient is in bed. Suspension from an overhead device is useful, but it is imperative that excessive circumferential pressure on any part of the limb be avoided. In general, sutures in the skin of the hand should remain in place for two weeks because healing is relatively slow. Fine, monofilament, synthetic sutures produce least reaction (see Chapter 13).

It is important to maintain movement of uninjured structures. Even a short period of immobilization may result in prolonged stiffness, especially in older individuals. After healing of the soft tissues, which may take three and a half weeks for flexor tendons and nerves, the hand is mobilized. The patient should be carefully instructed in active movements and encouraged to perform them frequently. Attendance at the department of physical therapy several times a week is useful to reinforce the instructions and encourage the patient. Passive exercises are occasionally useful. Overenthusiastic stretching, however, results in injury to healing structures, swelling, pain, and inability or unwillingness of the patient to continue active movement. Dynamic splints, made by attaching springs and rubber bands to splints, provide prolonged gentle traction and are often able to achieve a wide range of motion without excessive stretching.

Many of the complications following hand injuries are due to inadequate debridement and inappropriate closure of wounds under tension. The result is scarring, unsatisfactory rehabilitation, and often amputation.

Special Injuries to the Hand

Fingertip Injuries and Finger Amputations. These injuries are frequent and of great importance, especially those of the thumb and index finger. In general, length should be maintained, especially in the thumb. It is essential to have a healed wound with a nontender stump and, if possible, good sensation. Many different techniques have been used to cover the defects, including full-thickness skin grafts, split-thickness grafts, local flaps, and cross-finger flaps. A free graft is often used for the primary repair and more elaborate flaps applied later. Occasionally it is necessary to remove bone and shorten the finger to achieve primary closure and rapid restoration of function. This procedure is indicated in older workingmen who should not be out of work for prolonged periods for elaborate reconstructive procedures and also when the injury is to one of the ulnar three fingers. If the index or little finger requires amputation between the palm and the proximal interphalangeal joint, a midmetacarpal amputation provides a better appearance and function for fine work. However, if the patient needs a strong grip, the metacarpal head should not be removed.

Wringer or Roller Injuries. Wringer or roller injuries crush tissues often without producing a laceration. Their seriousness is therefore often underestimated. There is a shearing force that separates the skin through the dermis from the underlying tissues. A hematoma beneath the fascial envelope of the forearm may compress muscles, vessels, and nerves. If pressure is not released, necrosis, fibrosis, and contracture (Volkmann's contracture) may result with severe permanent disability. This complication can be prevented by early fasciotomy.

Thermal Injuries (see Chapter 15). Burns of the hands may be associated with extensive burns and are frequently neglected. The principles of debridement and wound closure should be applied. Isolated burns are common and require careful treatment. Electrical burns are often more severe than is initially apparent and may require repeated debridement.

Frostbite. Frostbite of the fingers is seen frequently in alcoholics, mental defectives, and people in rural settings who are exposed to cold over long periods of time. The eventual loss of tissue is usually less than that anticipated from the early appearance of the injury.

Grease and Paint Gun Injuries. Certain jobs require the use of paint and grease guns which operate at very high pressures (up to 15,000 lb/sq in.). When a small hole occurs in the tubing or other part of the system, the agent may be injected into the operator's hand and diffuse throughout large portions of it. Early after the injury the pinhole wound may appear quite innocent and be ignored. Later pain and swelling become intense. There are tissue necrosis and stiffness, loss of sensation is frequent, and amputation may be required. Treatment is early exploration, decompression, removal of the agent, and debridement.

Common Injuries to the Digits

The fingers and thumb are often exposed to injuries of relatively minor nature which if wrongly diagnosed and treated may result in significant disability. Finger injuries are the most common injuries seen in emergency departments.

Subungual Hematoma. A blow or crush injury to the fingertip may result in the collection of blood beneath the nail and sometimes fracture of the distal phalanx. X-rays should always be taken. The blood may be seen as a blue discoloration beneath the nail, and there are marked pain and tenderness. Prompt relief may be obtained by making a hole in the nail over the hematoma using a paper clip heated until it is red hot. The procedure is not painful and does not require anesthesia. However, the patient needs reassurance as he is approached with a red-hot paper clip.

Dislocations and Sprains. The finger joints are delicate and precise structures which do not tolerate trauma well. The swollen, tender joint with limitation of motion is x-rayed to rule out fractures involving articular surfaces. Anesthesia using a finger block is necessary when taking stress films to test for ligamentous tears. Complete disruption of a collateral ligament is best treated by operative repair. Sprained fingers are splinted in the position of function and active motion started in one to two weeks. The injured finger is immobilized by taping it to an adjacent finger. The uninjured finger provides lateral stability and encourages flexion-extension movement.

Metacarpophalangeal Joint of the Thumb. Injury to this joint is common after a fall on the outstretched hand. The thumb is stressed into extreme abduction. The collateral ligament on the ulnar side of the joint is strained or torn.

The entirely disrupted ligament is often displaced so that normal healing cannot occur and a chronically weak hand with a deficient pinch between the thumb and fingers results. Stress films should be taken. Operative repair is necessary if the tear is complete. Incomplete tears may be treated by splinting for four to six weeks.

Fractures of the Phalanges. The distal phalanx is the most commonly fractured bone in the body and usually heals well unless the fragments are displaced. However, if the nail bed is disrupted and not accurately reduced, severe disabling and aesthetically unpleasant deformity of the regrowing nail may ensue. Fractures of the distal phalanx with any displacement of the nail should be treated by removal of the nail and accurate approximation of the nail bed with fine sutures.

Fractures that enter the joints may result in chronically painful and stiff fingers. Accurate reduction is necessary. This may require open operation with pinning of the fractures or joints using small Kirschner wires. Markedly comminuted fractures are best treated in traction by placing a pin through the distal phalanx. The finger is then placed over a curved volar splint in the position of function. Rubber bands from outriggers provide the traction.

Mallet Finger. A force applied to the extended finger may result in rupture of the extensor tendon just proximal to its insertion on the distal phalanx or avulsion of the insertion including a small fragment of bone. The injury most often occurs when a ball strikes the finger. The patient is unable to extend the distal phalanx. A number of splints have been devised to hold the finger in extension for six weeks. An alternative treatment is to pin the joint in extension with a transarticular Kirschner wire. If a large fragment of bone is avulsed or the injury occurred two weeks or before, an open reduction and repair of the tendon is indicated. The deformity is not serious, and in certain patients the condition may be left untreated.

Boutonnière Deformity (Figure 28–8). If the central slip of the extensor apparatus is cut or ruptured at the level of the proximal interphalangeal joint, the patient may be able to extend the joint immediately after the injury. Later the lateral bands prolapse along either side of the joint and exert their force volar to the axis of the joint, resulting in flexion of the PIP joint and extension of the DIP joint. This buttonhole or boutonnière deformity occurs because the joint protrudes through the two lateral bands as through a buttonhole. If neglected, this deformity is difficult to repair

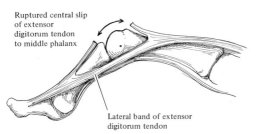

Ruptured central slip
of extensor
digitorum tendon
to middle phalanx

Lateral band of extensor
digitorum tendon

Figure 28–8. Boutonnière deformity.

because secondary joint contractures develop. The results are excellent if the extensor apparatus is repaired immediately after injury. Closed injuries may be treated with a splint which keeps the PIP joint straight and allows flexion of the distal joint and metacarpophalangeal joint. The splint must be used for five to six weeks.

Avulsion of Flexor Digitorum Profundus Tendon. This injury often occurs when the distal phalanx is flexed strongly and then extreme stress placed on the flexed fingertip. For example, a tackler catches his finger in the jersey of a football player and then falls. There is inability to flex the distal joint with pain in the palm where the end of the tendon has retracted. If treated early by surgical repair, the result is excellent, but after two weeks the contracture of the tendon, muscle, and tendon sheath militates against regaining function.

Foreign Bodies. Most foreign bodies in the hand are radiopaque on x-ray. Glass is visualized if there is an adequate lead content, as in most beer bottles. Any wound that fails to heal should be suspected of containing a foreign body. The foreign body should be removed using a tourniquet with regional or general anesthesia. Needles placed through the skin in different planes help localization on x-ray. Foreign bodies can sometimes be readily removed under local anesthesia with fluoroscopy and image intensifier.

HAND INFECTIONS

Minor hand infections are frequent but the severe types are uncommon. A minor hand infection may progress to a more serious type if treatment is inadequate. Lymphatics pass mainly from the palm and fingers to the loose tissues on the dorsum of the hand. Infections on the volar surface of the hand and fingers therefore cause considerable swelling on the dorsum.

Minor Infections

The portal of entry is most often a pinprick or laceration. Frequently, however, there is no history of injury. Most hand infections are caused by gram-positive cocci which are sensitive to penicillin or to one of the semi-synthetic penicillins that are not destroyed by penicillinase-producing bacteria. Patients with infections should be seen repeatedly to determine whether or not pus is present. Occasionally it is possible to obtain material for bacteriologic examination by injecting a small volume of sterile saline into the infected region and aspirating the fluid. The immediate recognition of cocci in a Gram stain of the specimen may aid in selecting the antibiotic. It is imperative, however, to start the antibiotic before the results of the culture are obtained. Immobilization of the hand in the position of function and with a sling is important. Failure to rest the hand may be the principal reason for persistence and spread of the infection. There is no place for the application of soaks or poultices in the care of hand infections. They produce maceration of the skin, decrease the blood supply, and increase edema and tissue necrosis.

Pus in hand infections should be drained promptly. A diamond-shaped incision made directly over the abscess evacuates the pus and ensures continued drainage. In the past the position of incisions was standardized to avoid damaging important structures. However, with the use of a tourniquet and bloodless field, the incision for drainage can be placed in any portion of the hand.

Felon or Distal Pulp-Space Infection. This is often secondary to a minor injury such as a pinprick. There are throbbing pain, inability to sleep, and a tense, tender fingertip. Pressure rapidly increases within the space because of the presence of fibrous bands which connect the skin to the ventral surface of the terminal phalanx. A felon should be drained promptly. The incision is placed directly over the most tender region as determined by gentle palpation with a blunt instrument (Figure 28–9). A direct incision over the pus avoids contamination of the

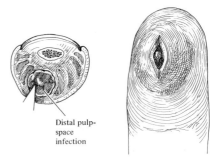

Distal pulp-
space
infection

Figure 28–9. Drainage of distal pulp-space infection.

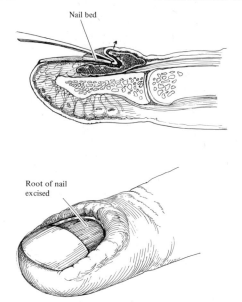

Nail bed

Root of nail
excised

Figure 28–10.   Surgical drainage of paronychia.

other spaces in the fingertip and it heals without producing a tender scar in the tactile region of the finger as had previously been feared. Inadequate drainage of a pulp-space infection may result in osteomyelitis of the terminal phalanx, acute tenosynovitis of the flexor tendon sheath, and rarely septic arthritis of the distal interphalangeal joint.

Paronychia. Infection through a ragnail may result in infection of the skinfold surrounding the dorsum of the nail (Figure 28–10). The position of the swelling and tenderness are diagnostic. Drainage is necessary when pus is present. The nail fold is elevated and if pus is present deep to the proximal nail, the proximal half of the nail is removed.

Web-Space Infection. Infection may develop in the web space as the result of a puncture injury. It is seen most frequently in heavy laborers with thick palmar skin. Infection passes deeply between the division of the bands of palmar aponeurosis going to each finger with development of a dumbbell-type abscess ("collar button") (Figure 6–6, page 135). Swelling is maximal on the dorsum of the web space with tenderness greatest on the volar aspect. Surgical drainage of both pockets is essential. Inadequate drainage may result in tenosynovitis or deep palmar space infection.

Subcutaneous abscesses on the dorsum of the hand should be treated as furuncles elsewhere.

Major Hand Infections

Acute Suppurative Tenosynovitis. This is an acute infection within the flexor tendon sheath of a finger or the thumb. The sheaths of the second, third, and fourth fingers commence at the level of the metacarpophalangeal joints. The flexor sheath of the thumb and fifth finger extends proximally to the forearm in the radial and ulnar bursae. Acute suppurative tenosynovitis usually occurs from a puncture wound which may have been forgotten. The finger is held in slight flexion, passive extension causes extreme pain, and there are fusiform diffuse swelling and tenderness over the sheath. Immediate operation is essential to drain the tendon sheath and to prevent fibrous adhesions forming between the tendons and the sheath resulting in a stiff finger. Good results have been obtained by opening the sheath distally at the level of the distal interphalangeal joint and proximally in the distal palm and irrigating the the sheath with dilute antibiotic solution.

Abscesses of the Deep Palmar and Thenar Spaces. These infections produce massive swelling of the hand and, if not promptly drained, result in marked disability.

CYSTS OF THE HAND
Ganglion

Ganglia are cysts that communicate with joints or tendon sheaths. They occur most often on the dorsum of the wrist and are attached to the wrist joint at the level of the scapholunar joint. The etiology is not clear. They may follow trauma or develop spontaneously. Recent studies show that there is a one-way communication between the joint and the ganglion. Ganglia may change in size with time, and they may be asymptomatic for many years. Treatment includes rupture, aspiration, and injection with a sclerosing agent or excision. Excision is the most reliable and is followed by a low recurrence rate. Excision is performed using regional or general anesthesia and a tourniquet. To obtain adequate removal it is necessary to excise a segment of the joint capsule or tendon sheath. Often pain and disability persist postoperatively for as long as four to five weeks. The affected joint should therefore be splinted for about one week. Ganglia also commonly arise from the radiocarpal joint and present as a swelling on the volar surface of the wrist near the radial artery. They also develop from the tendon sheaths of the fingers at the level of the proximal phalanx. Ganglia occasionally cause nerve compression syndromes.

Mucous Cyst

A mucous cyst may develop just proximal to the fingernails. These are small ganglia of the distal interphalangeal joints presenting lateral to the extensor tendons.

Inclusion Cyst

An inclusion cyst derived from epithelial elements implanted below the skin following trauma is common.

TUMORS OF THE HAND

Benign

Glomus Tumor. A glomus tumor arises from the glomus, a structure associated with heat regulation through the vasomotor system. Histologically small arteriovenous communications can be seen lined by neuromuscular cells. These tumors most commonly present as extremely painful and tender subungual masses accurately localized to the tumor. Excision relieves the intense pain dramatically.

Hemangioma. Hemangiomas are frequent in the hand. They are often congenital and may become large enough to cause disability. They are often entwined about the nerves and tendons making excision difficult.

Malignant

Squamous cell carcinoma of the skin is the most common malignant tumor of the hand. It occurs in association with excessive exposure to sunlight as in outdoor workers, with arsenical keratosis, and in those exposed to ionizing radiation. Melanomas of the hand are not common. Those that are nonpigmented or subungual are especially liable to misdiagnosis. All pigmented lesions beneath the nail should be excised. Other malignant tumors of the hand, including hemangioendotheliomas, neurofibrosarcomas, and synoviomas, are rare. Amputation may be necessary, but occasionally wide local resection of the tumor with reconstruction by skin graft or a flap is adequate.

OTHER SURGICAL CONDITIONS OF THE HAND

Dupuytren's Contracture

In Dupuytren's contracture there is increasing fibrosis of the palmar aponeurosis, most often of both hands. This results in contracture of the longitudinal fibers with the development of palpable nodules and contractures at the metacarpophalangeal joints and later the proximal interphalangeal joints. The ring finger and the little finger are usually first affected. The condition is frequently familial and usually seen in middle age. The nodularity may be present for many years without producing disability or or may progress rapidly to severe deformity. Treatment is excision of the involved fascia. Complications are delayed skin healing and injury to the digital nerves which are closely related to the fascia.

Nerve Compression Syndromes

Carpal Tunnel. The median nerve may be compressed in the carpal tunnel by any process that produces swelling of the tendons or their sheaths or by fracture or dislocation of the carpal bones. There is pain especially at night in the median nerve distribution, paresthesia, and weakness of the opponens and short abductor muscles. Exercise tends to relieve the pain. Electrical conduction studies help in the diagnosis. The most effective treatment is division of the transverse carpal ligament.

Ulnar Nerve Compression. The ulnar nerve may be injured by direct trauma at the elbow where it passes behind the medial epicondyle, or it may be stretched as a result of a growth defect secondary to injury of the distal humerus in childhood. Tension is relieved by transplanting the nerve to the anterior aspect of the elbow.

At the wrist the ulnar nerve passes adjacent to the hook of the hamate beneath the palmaris brevis muscle in a tight compartment, the canal of Guyon, where it may be injured or compressed. The compartment is opened surgically.

Trigger Finger or Snapping Finger

The long flexor tendons pass beneath a distinct margin of the fibrous digital tendon sheath (theca) at the level of the distal flexion crease (Figure 28–11). A localized swelling of the tendon may develop, perhaps secondary to trauma. The nodule snaps across the thecal

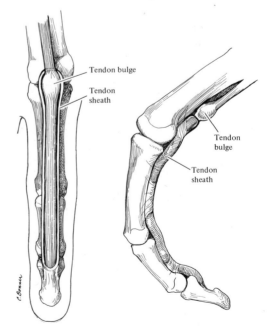

Tendon bulge

Tendon sheath

Tendon bulge

Tendon sheath

Figure 28–11. Trigger finger.

margin as the finger is flexed and may become entrapped on the palmar side with inability to extend the finger. Division of the proximal one-half centimeter of the digital theca relieves the snapping and repeated trauma to the tendon.

DeQuervain's Tenosynovitis

The flexor pollicis brevis and abductor pollicis longus tendons are held at the level of the distal radius in a firm fibrous sheath, the radial compartment of the dorsal retinaculum. Repeated rapid motion of the thumb and wrist may produce inflammation, pain, and tenderness at this site. The pain is elicited by forcibly adducting the wrist. The condition is most commonly seen in middle-aged female factory workers. If rest and injection of steroids fail to give relief, the fibrous tunnel should be opened.

Deformities Due to Rheumatoid Arthritis

Rheumatoid arthritis frequently affects the wrist, metacarpophalangeal, and proximal inter-phalangeal joints of the hand. Pain and severe deformities and disability may result with subluxations of joints and tendons. Reconstructive surgery includes synovectomy, repair and repositioning of tendons, arthrodesis, and prosthetic replacement of destroyed joints.

SUGGESTIONS FOR FURTHER READING

Boyes, Joseph H.: *Bunnell's Surgery of the Hand*, 5th ed. J. B. Lippincott, Philadelphia, 1970.
This is the latest edition of the "classic" hand textbook. One method is presented consistently. Specific topics may be difficult to find using the index.

Flynn, J. E.: *Hand Surgery*, 2nd ed. Williams & Wilkins Co., Baltimore, 1975.
Advanced comprehensive text by multiple authors each presenting his special interest. The authors do not always agree with one another.

Rank, B. K.; Wakefield, A. R.; and Hueston, J. I.: *Surgery of Repair as Applied to Hand Injuries*, 4th ed. Williams & Wilkins Co., Baltimore, 1973.
Limited to consideration of early and late repair of hand injuries from the reconstructive surgeon's point of view.

Weckesser, Elden C.: *Treatment of Hand Injuries*. Case Western Reserve University Press, Cleveland, 1974.
Practical guide to emergency and later care of hand injuries and infections.

UNIT IV
PRINCIPLES OF SPECIALTY SURGERY

Chapter 29

ORTHOPEDIC SURGERY AND FRACTURES

Eugene R. Mindell

CHAPTER OUTLINE

Normal Function
Normal Development and Structure
Principles of Diagnosis
Principles of Treatment
Congenital Abnormalities
    Upper Extremity
    Lower Extremity
        Congenital Dislocation of the Hip
        Clubfoot
        Metatarsus Varus
    Congenital Spinal Anomalies
        Spina Bifida
        Congenital Scoliosis
        Congenital Torticollis (Wryneck)
    Generalized Congenital Abnormalities
        Osteogenesis Imperfecta
        Osteopetrosis (Marble Bones or Albers-
            Schonberg Disease)
        Multiple Osteocartilaginous Exostoses
        Heritable Disorders of Connective
            Tissues
Growth Disorders
    Osteochondroses
        Legg-Perthes Disease
        Osgood-Schlatter's Disease
        Osteochondritis Dissecans
        Other Sites
    Slipped Capital Femoral Epiphysis
    Idiopathic Scoliosis
Fractures
    General Management
    Open and Closed Fractures
    Undisplaced Fractures
    Displaced Fractures
    Intra-articular Fractures
    Fractures in Children
        Birth Injuries
        Battered Children
    Complications of Fractures
        Nonunion
        Fat Embolism
    Specific Fractures
        Hand Injuries
        Colles' Fracture

Forearm Fractures
"Nursemaid's Elbow"
Radial Head Fracture
Fracture of the Olecranon
Fractures of the Humerus
Dislocation of Shoulder
Acromioclavicular Joint Separation
Spinal Fractures
Pelvic Fractures
Dislocation of the Hip
Fracture of the Femoral Neck
Intertrochanteric Fractures
Femoral Shaft
Patella
Tibial Condyles
Tibia
Ankle
Talus
Calcaneus
Metatarsals and Phalanges
Ligamentous Injuries
Meniscus Tears in the Knee
Inflammatory Disorders
    Osteomyelitis
    Pyogenic Arthritis
    Tuberculosis
    Rheumatoid Arthritis
    Ankylosing Spondylitis
Degenerative Disorders
    Degenerative Arthritis
    Degenerative Disk Disease
Bursitis and Tendonitis
    Trigger Finger
    Tennis Elbow
Foot Disorders
Metabolic Disorders
    Rickets and Osteomalacia
    Primary Hyperparathyroidism
    Osteoporosis
    Gout
    Paget's Disease
Bone Neoplasms
    Benign Tumors
        Metaphyseal Fibrous Defect

Osteoid Osteoma	Chondrosarcoma
Osteoblastoma	Ewing's Sarcoma
Osteocartilaginous Exostosis	Reticulum Cell Sarcoma
Enchondroma	Multiple Myeloma
Benign Chondroblastoma	Metastatic Carcinoma
Bone Cysts	Neuromuscular Disorders
Primary Malignant Neoplasms	Cerebral Palsy
Giant Cell Tumor	Poliomyelitis
Osteogenic Sarcoma	Stroke Patients
Paraosteal Osteogenic Sarcoma	Amputees

Musculoskeletal clinical problems are so common that all physicians must be familiar with them. This chapter will discuss in general terms the normal and abnormal functioning of the musculoskeletal system, its structure and development, and principles of diagnosis and treatment, including congenital abnormalities, growth disorders, injuries, inflammatory, degenerative, and metabolic disorders, neoplasms, and neuromuscular disorders.

NORMAL FUNCTION

The primary function of the musculoskeletal system is locomotion. Alterations in this system with age, injury, and disease produce predictable locomotor changes which may result in disability. The skeleton also protects vulnerable organs in the chest, abdomen, skull, and spine. In addition, bone has an important metabolic function, serving as a reservoir for calcium, sodium, phosphorus, and magnesium. Abnormalities in the metabolism of these minerals, especially calcium, may produce changes in bone. Approximately 99 percent of the total body calcium is present in the skeleton as calcium apatite crystals. Calcium in the circulation and tissue fluids is in equilibrium with the crystalline calcium in bone. The calcium content of bone is directly influenced by the hormones parathormone and calcitonin which maintain the serum calcium at a normal level, controlling bone resorption and formation. Bone marrow may be affected by hematologic disorders, and conversely bone disease may affect the normal functioning of the hematopoietic tissue.

NORMAL DEVELOPMENT AND STRUCTURE

The skeleton first appears at five weeks of fetal life as a cartilaginous anlage. By the seventh week a primary center of enchondral ossification begins to develop in some of the cartilaginous models of the bones. Longitudinal growth of the shaft or diaphysis occurs by proliferation of epiphyseal cartilage and its replacement by bone extending from the primary ossification center. The perichondrium around the diaphysis becomes periosteum. Bone width increases by intramembranous ossification of the deep layer of cells in the periosteum. By six months of fetal life the cortices are defined in a long bone and the medullary space is formed. Secondary ossification centers then appear at varying ages within the epiphyses.

Some epiphyses, as in the distal femur, appear before birth; others develop at a later age. The cartilage between the primary and secondary centers of ossification becomes the epiphyseal cartilage plate, while that persisting on the secondary ossification center in the joint forms the articular cartilage.

Joints appear at about the tenth fetal week as clefts between the cartilaginous bones. The surrounding mesoderm develops into the synovium and capsule.

Most of the skeleton is formed in cartilage. The clavicle and base of the skull are exceptions, being formed directly from fibrous tissue or by intramembranous ossification. When growth is complete, the epiphyseal cartilage plate disappears and the ossification centers unite. The articular cartilage is the only portion that persists of the original cartilaginous anlage.

Bone matrix is formed by the cellular activity of osteoblasts. The matrix is composed mainly of mucopolysaccharides and collagen fibrils. Calcium apatite crystals are then deposited in the osteoid with the assistance of alkaline phosphatase. The bone is maintained by osteocytes, the cells within the bone, and removed by cellular activity, usually by osteoclasts but also by osteocytes. Remodeling of bone occurs as a result of osteoclastic resorption and osteoblastic formation of new bone. The bone gradually matures into cancellous bone, as found in the medullary spaces, and also into dense cortical bone with its osteons of lamellar bone. Bone is a dynamic tissue continually reacting to mechanical and biologic stresses at any age. The greatest potential for remodeling is in the young. Mechanically bone is very strong, able to withstand considerable strain.

The ends of two articulating bones are covered by hyaline articular cartilage which provides gliding surfaces and protects the underlying subchondral bone. Synovial fluid is secreted by the synovial membrane. The capsule of thick fibrous tissue lies immediately outside and reinforces the synovial membrane. Articular hyaline cartilage contains chondrocytes and a ground substance which is rich in mucopolysaccharide. Cartilage is avascular, its cells surviving on nutrients that diffuse in from the synovial fluid. Movement of the joint aids passage of nutrients through the cartilage. Synovial fluid is secreted continuously by the synovial membrane, is present normally in all joints, tendon sheaths, and bursae, and acts as a lubricant for joint motion. It contains hyaluronic acid or mucin and most of the components of serum except for large protein molecules, such as fibrinogen.

Skeletal muscles move and support the skeleton. Their function determines their size and shape. Individual muscle cells or fibers may run the length of the muscle. The muscle cell protoplasm or sarcoplasm is surrounded by nuclei and the cell membrane or sarcolemma. The sarcoplasm is divided longitudinally into myofibrils, which in turn are divided transversely into contractile sarcomeres.

PRINCIPLES OF DIAGNOSIS

The diagnosis of musculoskeletal abnormalities usually requires a careful synthesis of information obtained from the history, physical examination, radiographic evaluation, laboratory tests, and occasionally gross and histologic examination of tissues.

The history is of great importance and will often suggest the correct diagnosis.

Pain is frequently the chief complaint, and its characteristics of onset and severity should be determined. All other symptoms are completely delineated. Past history and symptoms in other systems are also recorded.

A thorough physical examination is then conducted. For instance, the patient is observed while using the affected part. Careful inspection, palpation, and measurement are usually required. Observation of deformity, swelling, atrophy, limb length discrepancy, joint motion limitation, and joint stability are all noted and recorded. Masses are examined for size, fluctuation, tenderness, localization, warmth, and are sometimes auscultated.

Radiographs are usually obtained after the history and physical examination. Special x-ray studies may be necessary to visualize soft tissues. A radiopaque dye may be injected and radiographs obtained as in an arthrogram or myelogram or to demonstrate a draining sinus. Laboratory tests are particularly helpful in a patient with generalized disease, such as gout, or in evaluating the systemic effect of a localized disease, such as osteomyelitis.

It may be necessary eventually to obtain a sample of tissue for microscopic examination by needle, incisional, or excisional biopsy (see Chapter 7).

A definite diagnosis can usually be made after the above information has been synthesized.

PRINCIPLES OF TREATMENT

The abnormality may be self-limited, and simple observation to be certain of the diagnosis may be the only course to follow, as for example with mild injuries.

The treatments required vary greatly. They include drugs such as antibiotics for infection. Immobilization with plaster casts, braces, and splints may be necessary. Surgical procedures may be required for the best results and are applicable in a wide range of abnormalities. Radiation treatment has its role. Physical therapy may be useful, including exercise programs for strengthening muscles and improving joint function. Occupational therapy, vocational guidance, and personal counseling are often necessary to rehabilitate the patient to normal.

CONGENITAL ABNORMALITIES

Congenital anomalies of the musculoskeletal system are common and may include other organ systems. They may occur as a result of inherited or genetic defects or result from environmental influences, such as those seen following thalidomide ingestion during pregnancy.

Patients with congenital amputations should usually be provided with a prosthesis early in life to heighten the likelihood of its use.

Upper Extremity

Hypoplasia or absence of certain bones produces unique deformities which require specific treatment. For instance, congenital absence of the radius leads to an unsightly and weak "radial club hand." Treatment consists of soft tissue release and repositioning the wrist on the distal end of the ulna.

Sprengel's deformity, or congenital failure of the scapula to descend, results in limitation of shoulder movement. Treatment is rarely indicated except for cosmetic reasons.

Radial ulnar synostosis causes loss of pronation and supination of the forearm. Operative treatment is usually of no benefit.

Abnormalities of the hand, such as syndactyly or webbing, polydactyly or supernumerary digits, and hypoplasia of the thumb, must be carefully evaluated before surgery is recommended.

Lower Extremity

Congenital Dislocation of the Hip. Congenital dislocation of the hip is a common abnormality occurring in 1.5 per 1000 live births. It is bilateral in one half the cases and usually occurs in females. Careful examination of the newborn's hips should be routine and will usually reveal the dislocation. When diagnosed and promptly treated in the first three to four months of age, the child may become close to normal. Treatment at this time should be splinting in abduction. The diagnosis, however, is often not made until the child is one to two years old, and then permanent disability may result. On examination there may be decreased abduction with the hip flexed to 90 degrees, the hip may be felt to snap into and out of the acetabulum, and telescoping or sliding of the femur along the ilium can sometimes be detected. On x-ray the proximal femur is displaced laterally, there is late development of the ossification center for the femoral head, and if the child is over one year old there may be inadequate development of the acetabulum.

Treatment aims at reducing the dislocation or subluxation as early as possible and then maintaining the reduction until the acetabulum deepens and the danger of redislocation is over. In the child one to two years of age some time in traction may be advisable to stretch the tight muscles before reduction. Adductor tenotomy is then often performed and the dislocation reduced by manipulation or occasionally by operation. Care is taken to avoid placing the hip in extreme abduction, as the blood supply to the femoral head may be impaired and lead to aseptic necrosis. Closed methods are often not successful after one year of age, and open surgical reduction may be necessary. If the acetabulum is inadequate to contain the femoral head, an osteotomy or sectioning of the iliac bone above the acetabulum is often then necessary to redirect the acetabulum and provide a stable cover over the femoral head.

Many adults with degenerative arthritis of the hip are suffering from untreated or inadequately treated congenital dislocation or subluxation of the hip.

Clubfoot. Clubfoot, or talipes equinovarus, if untreated leads to severe deformity and disability. It is often bilateral and occurs more often in boys. The primary defect is in the neck of the talus, resulting in varus deformity of the heel and midfoot, equinus of the ankle, and adduction and supination of the forefoot. Treatment consists of gradual correction of the deformity by frequent manipulation and application of plaster casts over several months. Some correction is obtained at each change of the cast. This is then followed by an active dynamic splint to maintain the correction. This deformity may resist correction if there are associated joint abnormalities such as arthrogryposis multiplex congenita.

Surgery is sometimes required in clubfeet resistant to correction in casts. This usually consists of lengthening the tendo Achillis and posterior capsulotomy of the ankle.

If untreated in the older child bony correction by triple arthrodesis is indicated. Occasionally simple osteotomy of the calcaneus is used for persistent heel varus and equinus.

Metatarsus Varus. Metatarsus varus is an increasingly common foot abnormality in which the forefoot is adducted or bent inward. It can usually be corrected early in life by manipulation with cast changes.

Congenital Spinal Anomalies

Spina Bifida. Spina bifida includes varying degrees of incomplete closure of one or more neural arches, most often in the lumbosacral spine. The incidence is 2 per 1000 live births. Usually the finding is asymptomatic, being detected radiographically. Occasionally there are associated neurologic defects such as meningomyelocele. Neurologic involvement also carries varying degrees of paralysis, sensory disturbance, bladder complications, and hip dislocations. These conditions may require extensive neurologic, urologic, and orthopedic management.

Congenital Scoliosis. Congenital spinal deformities may result in scoliosis, either from fusion of vertebrae or presence of hemivertebrae. Early surgical fusion is occasionally necessary to prevent progressive deformity.

Congenital Torticollis (Wryneck). The baby's head is tilted and rotated to one side since birth due to a tight, contracted sternocleidomastoid muscle. The head is tilted toward but rotated away from the involved muscle. A swelling is noted in the sternocleidomastoid muscle soon after birth. It is soon replaced by scar tissue, which leads to contracture. The deformity often resolves spontaneously, and simple stretching is recommended during the first years of life to enhance the resolution. However, if the deformity persists after four to five years of age, permanant facial asymmetry may result. The older child therefore may need surgical division of the muscle at one or two levels. The etiology is unknown.

Generalized Congenital Abnormalities

Osteogenesis Imperfecta. Osteogenesis imperfecta is a heritable condition of increased fragility of all bones, transmitted as an autosomal dominant disorder. The severity of the disease is reflected by the age at which the first fracture occurs. The child is usually first seen because of multiple fractures, each after minimal injury. Severe deformity with marked curving of the femur and tibia may eventually occur which limits or prevents walking. On examination the children may have blue sclerae and in the advanced cases some degree of deafness. Pathologically the bone is made up of weak trabeculae and thin cortices and is seen to be very cellular. The defect may be in collagen formation, and there is no effective medical treatment. Straightening of the markedly deformed long bones can be accomplished surgically and may improve ambulation. The bones do become less fragile in adult life, as fewer fractures occur after puberty.

Osteopetrosis (Marble Bones or Albers-Schonberg Disease). Osteopetrosis is characterized by dense bones. Failure of osteoclastic resorption in the remodeling process is noted histologically. Complications are progressive aplastic anemia from bone encroachment on marrow cavity, nerve entrapment syndromes resulting in nerve deafness or blindness, and pathologic fractures. There is no treatment.

Multiple Osteocartilaginous Exostoses. Multiple osteocartilaginous exostosis, a disorder transmitted as an autosomal dominant, is characterized by multiple bony outgrowths capped by cartilage that develop from abnormally broad metaphyses of long bones.

The exostoses may cause symptoms due to pressure on soft tissues such as tendons, nerves, or vessels, or deformity due to growth disturbances. Malignant degeneration, usually into chondrosarcoma, occurs in about 1 percent of cases and should always be searched for. If asymptomatic these exostoses are best left alone. If symptoms, significant deformity, or sarcoma develops, operation is required.

Heritable Disorders of Connective Tissues. This category includes a number of syndromes, each with its own set of symptoms and signs, depending on the system and severity of involvement. Represented are such entities as osteogenesis imperfecta, Marfan's syndrome, and the mucopolysaccharidoses. The patients must be recognized, as specific treatment is available for some.

GROWTH DISORDERS

Osteochondroses

Osteochondroses include a number of clinical conditions caused by idiopathic avascular necrosis of epiphyseal centers. They are self-limiting and heal spontaneously, although permanent deformity may occur.

Specific osteochondroses include:

Legg-Perthes Disease. This disease affects the femoral head, occurs most commonly in boys of three to seven years, and is bilateral in 15 percent of cases. There is an early phase of epiphyseal necrosis which is clinically asymptomatic. The dead epiphysis is revascularized, pathologic fracture may occur in the subchondral bone, and eventually the dead bone is replaced by new bone. This may result in pain, joint effusion, and limitation of movement. Joint surface incongruity may result which could lead to degenerative joint disease in later life. The child develops a limp and pain in the hip, thigh, or knee. Examination discloses a limitation of flexion and internal rotation at the hip. Early radiographs may demonstrate only widening of the articular cartilage space as the uninvolved cartilage continues to proliferate. Later the femoral head becomes dense and deformed. Treatment consists of minimizing deforming forces on the epiphysis during the vulnerable periods of revascularization, healing, and new bone formation. Treatment, which must begin early before deformity has occurred in the femoral head, includes nonweight-bearing splinting in abduction and operation in selected cases.

Osgood-Schlatter's Disease. The tibial tubercle may undergo vascular disturbances at 12 to 15 years. Local pain, swelling, and minimal disability result with mild symptoms sometimes lasting for several years. Treatment is usually symptomatic and may include application of a plaster cylinder for several weeks. Rarely is operation indicated.

Osteochondritis Dissecans. A segment of subchondral bone may undergo avascular necrosis, separate, and act as a loose body in the joint. This abnormality is particularly common in the knee joint and less frequent in other joints such as the elbow and ankle. The treatment depends on the stage of the process. If the involved segment of subchondral bone has not been displaced and if the patient is young, healing may be expected. If the fragment is loose in the joint or in its bed, it should be removed to relieve symptoms and prevent later arthritis.

Other Sites. Osteochondrosis of secondary centers of ossification in the spine leads to permanent wedging of the vertebral bodies, a condition which is only occasionally symptomatic (Scheuerman's disease). Aseptic necrosis may occur in the second metatarsal head (Freiberg's disease). Shoe correction is often adequate treatment and operation only occasionally required. Aseptic necrosis of the carpal lunate may occur with or without an injury (Kienbock's disease). Treatment is usually symptomatic. Aseptic necrosis of the tarsal scaphoid occurs in young children and usually results in mild symptoms (Kohler's disease) Specific treatment is usually not necessary.

Slipped Capital Femoral Epiphysis

The capital femoral epiphysis may slip off the femoral neck through the substance of the epiphyseal cartilage plate, usually in boys around puberty. It is bilateral almost 25 percent of the time. In addition there may be necrosis of the femoral head and thinning of the articular cartilage. These children usually present with pain, a limp, and have limited movements at the hip. The diagnosis is often missed but must be suspected in every teenager who develops hip pain and a limp. The slipped epiphysis is seen on x-ray. The diagnosis must be made early to prevent marked deformity. The treatment in the early cases is aimed at preventing further slip by pinning the femoral head to the neck with multiple pins. The late case often requires surgical reconstruction of the upper femur.

Idiopathic Scoliosis

Idiopathic scoliosis is a condition of unknown etiology occurring usually in teenage girls at a time when trunk growth is rapid. The curvature generally does not progress after puberty. It is usually asymptomatic, but in later life the postural abnormality may cause pain. Neurologic complications are rare. The deformity may be very disfiguring, and after it has been present for several years, permanent changes develop in the bony structure, such as lateral wedging of the vertebral bodies and local arthritic change. For patients with mild scoliosis exercises and observation are all that is necessary. If, however, a young girl is seen with a mild curve and considerable additional growth is expected, marked progression of the curve may be anticipated. A specially constructed Milwaukee brace should be worn for a number of years. The brace extends down to the pelvis and may include the head. If the curve is severe but still limber, a brace or a cast may be applied followed by spinal fusion.

FRACTURES

Injuries constitute one of the world's greatest medical problems. With the increasing speed of vehicles, more leisure time, and interest in athletics, the number of injured continues to rise. In the United States 60,000 are killed annually on the highway, and there are about 3,000,000 fractures.

The first event in healing of a fracture is formation of a hematoma which clots in a few days and then becomes organized by the ingrowth of vascular fibrous tissue. After one to two days the periosteum thickens, and embryonic cells are converted to osteoblasts and lay down immature bone along the cortices and in the medullary space. Extensive stripping of soft tissues during open reduction may cause further necrosis of bone. The fragments are initially joined by fibrous tissue, which is gradually converted to bone. Immature woven bone is first formed and is gradually converted to mature bone under the influence of mechanical and perhaps electrical forces. Motion at the fracture promotes cartilage formation. Remodeling of the fracture occurs and in time, particularly in the young, the fractured bone tends to become normal.

General Management

Priority in treatment must be established. After it has been determined that the patient is breathing, or has an adequate airway, and is not bleeding, fractures and dislocations receive attention. Adequate splinting of skeletal injuries should then be carried out at the scene of the accident using formal or improvised splints. The patient may then be transported safely for definitive care.

Open and Closed Fractures

Unlike closed fractures open or compound fractures have a soft tissue wound connecting the fracture with the outside. Thus open fractures are contaminated and vulnerable to infection. All open fracture wounds must be thoroughly cleansed, debrided, and generally left open to be closed later when the danger of infection is minimal. Antibiotics may be given.

Undisplaced Fractures

Undisplaced fractures are those in which the fracture fragments have not deviated out of their normal relationship. They are usually managed by simple immobilization.

Displaced Fractures

Fracture fragments may be displaced from each other by the initial deforming forces, muscle pull, gravity, or manipulation. For treatment the distal fragments are usually aligned on the proximal by overcoming compensatory muscle pull, by manipulation, traction, or open reduction. If external manipulation is successful, the position may be maintained for the necessary time by external support, such as a plaster cast or brace. Immediate function of the injured part increases the rate of fracture healing and hastens complete rehabilitation. This may consist of early weight bearing in a plaster cast and active function of nonimmobilized regions.

Intra-articular Fractures

Intra-articular fractures may lead to incongruity of articular surfaces and predispose to later degenerative joint disease. They must be accurately reduced and securely fixed, often by open reduction and internal fixation.

Fractures in Children

Fractures in children heal more rapidly than those in adults, and nonunion is rare. The remodeling process in the child is more active and allows for better spontaneous realignment than in the adult. In addition, the child's potential for growth allows for some correction of shortening. On the other hand, if growth is disturbed in a child, permanent shortening or deformity may ensue. Epiphyseal injuries may result in growth disturbances if the vulnerable embryonic cells located near the epiphyseal side of the plate are damaged from a fracture crossing the plate or diffuse crushing of the plate. Fortunately most epiphyseal fractures occur through the provisional zone of calcification in the epiphyseal plate, and growth is not disturbed. Salter has classified epiphyseal injuries.

Birth Injuries. The trauma of delivery may produce bone and soft tissue injuries. The infant's brachial plexus may be markedly stretched, leading to varying degrees of paralysis in the upper extremity which may or may not be permanent. Treatment consists of splinting and maintaining joint mobility. When the child is older and permanent residual paralysis is present, reconstructive operation, including muscle transfers, division of tight tendons, or corrective osteotomy of the humerus may be indicated.

Fractures of the clavicle and the femur may occur during a difficult delivery but usually heal uneventfully and with simple treatment.

Battered Children. Children and infants are sometimes regularly and severely injured by someone in their home. The battered child syndrome may be recognized by fractures in different stages of repair. The main problem here is to make the diagnosis and then change the child's living environment. Laws now are in effect to encourage the reporting of cases to protect the child.

Complications of Fractures

Nonunion. Nonunion should be suspected if the patient has local pain and tenderness at the fracture site after the usual time for union has elapsed. If there is considerable movement, a pseudarthrosis with a fibrocartilaginous joint-like surface may develop. Local factors leading to nonunion are inadequate immobilization, distraction of fracture fragments by excessive traction or a wrongly applied bone plate, or infection or neoplasm in the fracture site. Poor blood supply, as in the femoral neck or talar neck, may delay but not prevent union.

The treatment of nonunion depends on the cause. If there is distraction with poor immobilization, the fragments should be placed in excellent contact and rigidly immobilized, often using a compression plate. If the position of the fragments is satisfactory, an onlay graft of autogenous cortical and cancellous bone may be applied. The grafts stimulate osteogenesis at the nonunion site and form a bony bridge which enhances internal immobilization. The sclerosed bone ends may or may not be excised.

Fat Embolism. Fat embolism may occur within the first few days after a severe injury, particularly if long bones are fractured (see Chapter 14).

Thrombophlebitis and pulmonary embolism are particularly common with fractures (see Chapter 14).

Specific Fractures

Hand Injuries. Open fractures in the hand are sometimes associated with tendon injuries, and their problems may be complicated as injured tendons adhere to underlying fractured bones (see Chapter 28).

Closed fractures of metacarpal and phalanges are common and may lead to disability unless angular and rotary displacements are corrected. Angular deformity in the phalangeal fracture must be corrected, or flexor and extensor tendon function is disturbed with resultant limited joint motion. Displaced articular fractures may require open reduction and fixation.

Metacarpal fracture may result in rotational changes which are not appreciated unless the fingernail relationships are observed as all the fingers are flexed at the same time. Closed reduction with splint or plaster fixation may be adequate, but internal fixation with insertion of intramedullary Kirschner wires is sometimes needed.

Fractures of the carpal navicular occur after a fall on the outstretched hand. The patient develops pain, swelling, and tenderness in the anatomic snuffbox. Initial x-rays may not reveal the fracture. A repeat radiograph should be taken two to three weeks after the injury when resorption of bone at the fracture line may make the fracture visible. Treatment consists of plaster immobilization until union occurs, which may take many months. Complications include nonunion and aseptic necrosis of the proximal fragment leading to disabling degenerative joint disease which may require operation for pain relief.

Colles' Fracture. A Colles' fracture is a fracture of the distal end of the radius, often along with a fracture of the styloid process of the ulna, and is usually the result of a fall on the outstretched hand. The typical silverfork deformity comes from upward and backward tilting of the distal fragment. In addition, the bone is displaced to the radial side. The fracture can usually be reduced under local anesthesia and then immobilized in a plaster cast with the wrist in slight flexion and displaced to the ulnar side. Occasionally with a comminuted fracture, a pin is placed in the metacarpals and another in the proximal radius. Both are then incorporated in a plaster cast to maintain the traction required for proper alignment of the fragments.

Forearm Fractures. Forearm fractures in children can usually be managed by closed reduction and immobilization in plaster casts. In adults nonunion and malunion may occur; therefore open reduction, internal fixation, and application of compression plates may be done to obtain the best results in the shortest time.

"Nursemaid's Elbow." Transitory radial head subluxation may occur in children of two to three years who have been lifted by one arm. Reduction is performed by supinating the forearm and then flexing and extending the elbow. Residual disability does not occur.

Radial Head Fracture. Radial head fracture with little displacement is treated symptomatically, and movement is encouraged. If fracture fragments are interfering with elbow motion, the entire radial head should be excised.

Fracture of the Olecranon. This should be considered an interruption in the triceps mechanism. Open repair is indicated if there is displacement to maintain normal extension in the elbow.

Fractures of the Humerus. *Supracondylar Fracture.* Supracondylar fracture of the humerus in children is potentially serious because of the danger of arterial injury with resultant ischemia of the forearm musculature and the later development of Volkmann's ischemic contracture. The first symptom of ischemia is severe pain. In addition there may be damage to the epiphyseal cartilage and rotational deformity which may lead to permanent elbow disability and deformity.

The fracture is reduced by traction, correction of any varus deformity, and bringing the elbow into flexion. The arm is placed in a sling, being careful not to impair circulation by tight bandaging or marked elbow flexion. Occasionally skin or skeletal pin traction is required, particularly when the circulation is embarrassed. Open operation must be performed immediately if there is any evidence of ischemia.

Supracondylar fractures in the adult are common injuries and may be followed by elbow stiffness and pain. If the articular surface is markedly disrupted, open reduction and internal fixation with early motion constitute the treatment of choice.

Humeral Shaft. Fractures of the humeral shaft can usually be treated by closed reduction, application of a plaster slab, and immobilization of the arm in a sling. Occasionally nonunion will occur if the immobilization is neglected. Another complication of this fracture is radial nerve palsy, most likely when the fracture is at the junction of the middle and distal third of the shaft. This is usually a traction injury that recovers completely. Occasionally, however, the radial nerve is divided, indicating operative repair. Since it is often difficult to differentiate between these two injuries, careful repeated clinical and EMG studies are needed.

Neck of Humerus. Fractures of the surgical neck of the humerus are common, particularly in the elderly. If the fragments are in contact, union occurs readily and treatment is early exercise designed to maintain shoulder mobility. If the fracture is comminuted and the fragments are separated, surgical reconstruction and even arthroplasty may be necessary.

Dislocation of Shoulder. Dislocations of the shoulder occur most often in the aged and generally result from a fall on the outstretched hand. Most often the head of the humerus passes through the anterior capsule and comes to lie inferiorly. Traction with the arm in slight abduction and external rotation usually effects a reduction. Alternatively the Kocher maneuver may be used. This consists of traction on the arm, adduction, and external and then internal rotation. Dislocation of the shoulder in young people is generally posterior and often followed by recurrent dislocation, but the diagnosis may be difficult to make clinically and radiographically. The history may be helpful since these injuries are prone to develop during an epileptic seizure. Special axillary views demonstrate the posteriorly located humeral head. With early recognition closed reduction is effective; later operation may be required.

Acromioclavicular Joint Separation. Separation of the acromioclavicular joint is often seen following direct falls on the superior surface of the shoulder. The injury is incomplete if only the ligaments between the acromion and the clavicle are torn. Symptomatic treatment is then only necessary. If the separation is complete with all the lateral ligaments torn, specific treatment should be considered. The extent of the separation should therefore be determined clinically and radiographically with the patient upright stressing the acromioclavicular joint by holding a weight in each hand. With a complete separation the clavicle may be held down to the acromion by pins. If untreated, the outer end of the clavicle remains prominent but symptoms are mild.

Spinal Fractures. Vertebral body fractures are potentially serious because of the possibility of injury to the spinal cord or cauda equina (see Chapter 34).

Pelvic Fractures. Fractures of the pelvis are common, often complicated by blood loss and damage to the urinary system. A great deal of blood may be lost as "concealed hemorrhage" and significantly contribute to hypovolemic shock, particularly in association with other injuries. The diagnosis of injury to the urethra and bladder must be made early, often by cystogram, and usually operation is required.

Since the pelvis is a ring, fractures occur usually in at least two places and may lead to displacement with shortening of the leg. Skeletal traction using a femoral traction pin for several weeks may then be necessary to obtain length. If the fracture involves the acetabulum, degenerative posttraumatic arthritis may follow. Occasionally open reduction and internal fixation are required for marked intra-articular displacement. If there is separation of the symphysis pubis with a displaced iliac fracture or sacroiliac dislocation, a pelvic sling or even plaster immobilization may be indicated. The result following even markedly displaced pelvic fracture is usually good unless the hip joint is incongruous.

Dislocation of the Hip. Dislocation of the hip usually follows severe indirect violence. It is most often posterior and sometimes associated with fracture of the acetabulum or femoral head. If the vascular soft tissue attachments to the femoral neck are severely damaged or if the dislocation is not reduced within 24 hours, aseptic necrosis of the femoral head occurs. This complication is usually not recognized until the necrotic head collapses under the stress of weight bearing, often months or years after the initial injury. It is then followed by disabling degenerative arthritis. The sciatic nerve may be stretched with a posterior dislocation and cause sciatic nerve palsy. Hip dislocation is treated by immediate reduction. The hip is placed in the position in which it was when the injury occurred, usually in 90° hip flexion. Traction is then applied at 90° and reduction usually occurs readily. Open reduction is generally indicated if there is a fracture dislocation or if the reduction is inexact or unstable.

Fracture of the Femoral Neck. Femoral neck fractures occur most often in elderly white women with osteoporosis and are associated with a significant morbidity and mortality. The fracture often follows a twisting injury to the upper femur. Pain, shortening, and external rotation of the limb develop, and radiographs demonstrate the femoral neck fracture with varying degrees of femoral head displacement. These fractures are prone to nonunion and aseptic necrosis of the femoral head with collapse and later degenerative arthritis because of the poor local blood supply to bone within the hip joint capsule. These fractures are best treated surgically to obtain accurate reduction, impaction of the fracture fragments, and rigid internal fixation using one or more nails or screws.

Intertrochanteric Fractures. Intertrochanteric fractures are similar to femoral neck fractures except that they occur outside the hip joint capsule where the circulation is richer and union of the fracture occurs more readily. They can be treated by skeletal traction for two to four months in bed. However, the prolonged immobilization in an elderly patient leads to a high incidence of pneumonia, thrombophlebitis, decubitus ulcers, and cerebrovascular changes, and these fractures are now more often treated by open reduction, rigid internal fixation, and early ambulation.

Femoral Shaft. Femoral shaft fractures are most common in children and young adults. Closed reduction and maintenance of reduction in traction followed by cast immobilization constitute the treatment of choice in children, usually producing excellent results. Management in adults is controversial. They may be treated by open anatomic reduction and rigid internal fixation, usually with an intramedullary nail or by skeletal traction for several weeks followed by a plaster cast or cast brace with early weight bearing. Early weight bearing in a cast or brace improves local circulation and appears to stimulate fracture healing.

Supracondylar fractures of the femur in adults can be treated by traction or plaster immobilization. If, however, the fragments are significantly displaced, they should be treated by open reduction, internal fixation with a compression blade plate, and early knee movement.

Patella. The patella is a sesamoid bone in the quadriceps mechanism. Fracture with separation leads to decrease in the power of the quadriceps. Treatment consists of wiring the patellar fragments together or repairing the quadriceps mechanism after excising one or all fragments, depending upon the severity of the injury.

Tibial Condyles. If the fragments of a tibial plateau fracture are in satisfactory position, early motion with late weight bearing is usually permitted. If the fragments are displaced, the knee is unstable, or the articular surface is markedly altered, open reduction and internal fixation are generally indicated.

Tibia. Tibial shaft fractures tend to occur in young working people and often lead to marked economic loss, as union may require many months. Most can be treated by closed reduction, walking plaster cast immobilization, and early ambulation. Some authorities prefer open reduction and fixation, but this may delay the return to unrestricted use of the limb. Complications include vascular injury, particularly with fractures high in the tibia, and dislocation of the knee. An arteriogram and arterial exploration may be necessary. Nonunion is generally treated by bone grafting with or without compression plating.

Ankle. Ankle fractures may include the malleoli and be associated with widening of the ankle mortise or dislocation of the ankle joint. Treatment is designed to restore the normal architecture of the ankle. If closed reduction is stable and the fragments are congruous, simple external plaster immobilization is adequate; otherwise open reduction and internal fixation may be required. Hopefully degenerative arthritis can be minimized by this treatment. If painful, disabling degenerative arthritis does develop years after a fracture, fusing the ankle can provide excellent pain relief with satisfactory function.

Talus. Fracture of the talus must be accurately reduced. Often closed manipulation into an equinus position is successful. Occasion-

ally the displacement of the proximal fragment is such that open reduction and internal fixation must be performed.

Fractures of the talar neck or total dislocation of the talus may be complicated by aseptic necrosis with late collapse of the talus and degenerative arthritis. Reconstructive surgery is then necessary.

Calcaneus. Fracture of the calcaneus usually results from a fall from a height and may vary from being undisplaced to severely comminuted with marked flattening and widening of the bone and marked disturbance of the subtalar joint. Closed or open reduction may be performed, but the results are about the same as after symptomatic treatment and early movement. If symptoms persist years after injury, subtalar arthrodesis can be considered for pain relief but usually is not required.

Metatarsals and Phalanges. Simple immobilization for several weeks usually produces excellent results. Fracture of toe phalanges is very common and is treated symptomatically, often by taping the injured toe to its uninjured neighbors.

LIGAMENTOUS INJURIES

Partial tears or sprains of ligaments about joints may lead to joint strain with pain, swelling, and disability. Treatment includes rest, supporting bandages, and sometimes immobilization in a plaster cast. If a complete tear of a major ligament is not recognized and treated, the patient has permanent weakness, pain, swelling, and instability. This applies particularly to the knee, ankle, and metacarpophalangeal joint of the thumb. An accurate diagnosis may be made by clinical evaluation and confirmed by stress x-rays with the injured ligament stretched. To obtain normal function operative repair may be necessary, as with knee ligament injuries in athletes. Ankle ligament injuries are usually managed by plaster immobilization, generally with satisfactory results.

MENISCUS TEARS IN THE KNEE

Rotational injuries may result in tear of one of the menisci in the knee, most often the medial meniscus. Locking, giving way, and localized pain may suggest the diagnosis. Localized tenderness over the meniscus, effusion into the joint, and muscle atrophy help in arriving at a diagnosis. The diagnosis is usually made on clinical evidence, but in doubtful cases an arthrogram or arthroscopy may be of value. Arthrotomy with excision of the torn meniscus and repair of other injured structures is generally indicated.

INFLAMMATORY DISORDERS

Osteomyelitis

Acute hematogenous osteomyelitis is a children's disease and most often secondary to staphylococcal bacteremia and less often other organisms. The infection is usually in the metaphysis of a long bone, such as the femur, tibia, or humerus, and is more frequent in boys than girls. The rich, sluggish blood flow in the metaphysis may predispose to infection at this site. If unchecked, the infection tends to spread through the diaphysis, leading to bone necrosis and formation of sequestra and subperiosteal abscess. Septicemia with pneumonia and metastatic abscesses may also occur. The epiphyseal cartilage inhibits spread to the joint, but septic arthritis can develop, especially in infants and where the capsular attachment is below the epiphyseal plate as in the hip and shoulder.

Early diagnosis and prompt treatment can lead to complete resolution without complications. The diagnosis is made on the presence of pain, bony tenderness, and fever. Needle aspiration may confirm the diagnosis, and it often provides the organism for culture and sensitivity. Radiographic changes do not appear until almost three weeks after onset of the disease. Later radiographs may demonstrate periosteal new bone, bone destruction, reactive bone formation, and in later stages bone necrosis and replacement. Bone scans are positive before there are radiographic changes and are therefore valuable in confirming the clinical diagnosis.

Osteomyelitis is treated with large doses of the appropriate antibiotics and local rest. If the treatment is begun within the first few days, the disease can be aborted. If, however, treatment is delayed or if the infection is virulent, abscesses may form that require drainage and decompression of the metaphysis. Damage to the epiphyseal cartilage may result in growth disturbance. With chronic osteomyelitis there may be wound drainage. Surgical removal of necrotic bone or sequestra and infected bone is then necessary.

Pyogenic Arthritis

Pyogenic arthritis may follow a penetrating wound, be hematogenous, or develop secondary to adjacent osteomyelitis. Newborn infants are particularly susceptible to pyogenic arthritis of the hip secondary to osteomyelitis of the femoral neck, since the femoral neck is intracapsular. The most common organism in adults is *Staphylococcus aureus*, producing severe pain, stiffness in the joint, and fever. On examination there are local tenderness and an effusion into the joint. The patient will also not permit movement of the joint due to pain.

Lysozomal enzymes released from bacteria and polymorphonuclear leukocytes may digest the articular cartilage, leading to marked permanent joint damage.

Treatment is immediate joint aspiration with or without insertion of an antibiotic into the joint cavity, immobilization of the joint in a functional position, and appropriate systemic antibiotics. Arthrotomy with joint decompression and removal of exudate may be required to prevent articular cartilage destruction, epiphyseal necrosis, and late disabling degenerative joint disease.

Tuberculosis

Bone and joint tuberculosis is usually secondary to hematogenous spread from primary disease in the lungs and less often from active disease in the genitourinary or gastrointestinal tracts or lymph nodes. The process is often indolent at first but may gradually lead to abscess formation and joint destruction. The spine is often involved as a result of spread from the urinary tract along Batson's plexus of veins. Several bones may then be compromised. Marked destruction of bone and intervertebral disks results in deformity and kyphosis. Pressure on the spinal cord may produce paraplegia, either during the acute process or from the late deformity. The hip and knee are also common sites. There tends to be bone and joint destruction leading to marked deformity. The diagnosis is usually substantiated by demonstrating the tubercle bacillus on culture.

Treatment consists of rest and administration of streptomycin, para-aminosalicylic acid, and isoniazid, usually in combination. Surgical debridement is possible in the presence of active disease. For instance, the paraplegic patient may be treated by decompression of the spinal cord and arthrodesis, using an anterior approach through the abdomen or the chest. If the joint has been destroyed, arthrodesis is still occasionally required.

Rheumatoid Arthritis

Rheumatoid arthritis is a common systemic disease of unknown etiology which affects women three times more often than men and has a peak incidence at 20 to 40 years. There is often symmetrical inflammatory polyarthritis with exacerbations and remissions, leading to progressive deformities.

The synovial membrane is inflamed, hypertrophied, and covered by granulation tissue (pannus) which interferes with nutrition and causes cartilage necrosis. The pannus then erodes subchondral bone, initially at the joint margins and then the entire joint surface, causing considerable destruction and deformity. Progressive deformities develop with contracture, joint subluxation, and dislocation. The tendon sheaths may also be involved, resulting in contracture and even tendon rupture. The hip, knee, and metacarpophalangeal joints of the feet are frequently affected, producing severe deformity and disability. Bilateral hip destruction may confine a patient to a wheelchair. Typical deformities in the hands are ulnar deviation of the fingers at the metacarpophalangeal joints and fusiform swellings of the proximal interphalangeal joints.

Rheumatoid arthritis seems to run a predetermined course in each patient. In most the disease is not severe, and only in about 10 percent does it produce permanent disability.

The treatment is aimed at relieving pain, suppressing inflammation, preventing joint deformities, and improving function. Medical treatments and anti-inflammatory drugs, such as salicylates, steroids, and gold salts, are useful. Removable splints provide local joint rest, relieve pain, and prevent deformity. Physical therapy maintains muscle strength. Operation is indicated in the disabled patient or when the disease is progressing despite medical management. Excision of the involved synovium may prevent damage to the articular cartilage and subchondral bone. It should be considered when joint involvement has been progressing for many months despite medical treatment and the patient still has fairly good articular cartilage. Excision is most appropriate in rheumatoid involvement of the knee and the metacarpophalangeal joints of the hand, wrist, and elbow. Synovectomy may permanently arrest joint destruction.

Arthroplasty is often of value in the patient with marked joint destruction and severe crippling. Total replacement of one or more joints is particularly helpful in those with disease in the hip, knee, and fingers. In general, these patients do well after operation, and spectacular rehabilitation is sometimes possible. Arthrodesis may be valuable, particularly in the hand. Tendon ruptures may be treated by tendon transfers or tendon grafts. Before surgery careful evaluation is essential over a significant period of time. The surgical procedure should be considered one episode in the treatment of a chronic disease that will require regular observation for many years.

Juvenile rheumatoid arthritis varies greatly in severity but complete recovery usually occurs. The syndrome of polyarthritis, splenomegaly, and lymphadenopathy in a child is Still's disease. Growth disturbance may complicate juvenile rheumatoid arthritis. Prolonged medical treatment is required and only rarely is operation necessary.

Ankylosing Spondylitis

Ankylosing spondylitis is a form of chronic arthritis involving the spine, sacroiliac joints, and occasionally the hips. It resembles in many ways rheumatoid arthritis but appears to be a separate entity. The patient presents with progressive stiffness and pain in the back. Ossification may eventually occur in the spine with progressive stiffness and deformity. The disease may arrest spontaneously at any point, or it may progress to flexion deformity of such severity that the patient has difficulty in raising his head to see in front. On x-ray the sacroiliac joints tend to be involved first, and their obliteration often confirms the diagnosis. Ultimately ossification occurs in the intervertebral ligaments of the whole spine. Treatment is generally symptomatic. The progressive "chin-on-chest" deformity may be secondary to a fracture of the cervical spine and should be prevented by splints or braces, and sometimes by traction. Osteotomy may occasionally be indicated.

DEGENERATIVE DISORDERS
Degenerative Arthritis

Degenerative or osteoarthritis is a joint disorder characterized by wearing away of the hyaline articular cartilage, progressive joint deformity, and often contractures and subluxation. The earliest changes in the articular cartilage are fissures, clusters of cells, and increased activity of the chondrocytes. Chemical changes in the glycosaminoglycans can be detected. Where the cartilage has worn away, the subchondral cortex thickens and subchondral cysts may form. The formation of osteocartilaginous osteophytes at the edges is apparently an attempt at repair.

Degenerative osteoarthritis occurs most often in the elderly but is sometimes secondary to injury, particularly if there is joint incongruity after an intra-articular fracture or ligamentous instability. Many joints may be involved, particularly the spine, hip, and knee.

On x-ray the diagnosis is made by the presence of articular cartilage space narrowing, sclerosis of subchondral cortices, subchondral cyst formation, and osteophytes. Joint deformity may also be seen.

Treatment of degenerative joint disease is

usually symptomatic and consists of rest and anti-inflammatory drugs given systemically and occasionally into the joint. Guidance about the advisability of changing job, athletic activities, and judicious use of rest is worthwhile. If symptoms persist, operation may be indicated. Surgical procedures include osteotomy to realign the joint and improve the mechanics, as in tibial osteotomy for bowlegs secondary to degenerative arthritis. Arthrodesis may help in a joint such as the ankle severely damaged by a fracture.

Arthroplasty effectively relieves pain and lessens disability, particularly in the hip and knee. Total hip replacement is often of great benefit. The use of total knee joint replacement for degenerative joint disease is also now being widely applied and appears to have great merit.

Degenerative Disk Disease

Pain in the lower back is one of the commonest complaints physicians have to deal with. Often the cause of the back pain cannot be definitely determined. The complaints may be due to soft tissue abnormalities such as muscle or ligamentous strain; not infrequently, however, they are due to degenerative disk disease, most often in the lower lumbar spine. The clinical picture varies markedly, with some patients having vague pains in the low back, while others have severe pain in the back with or without radiation down one or both legs. There may or may not be a history of injury, and the symptoms are usually aggravated by activity and relieved by rest. An accurate diagnosis can be established by a careful history, physical examination, and radiographic studies. The distribution of pain depends upon the nerve roots that are compressed. The low back is held rigid and is tender, and straight leg raising may elicit the pain and be restricted. Neurologic deficits should be noted. X-rays are obtained to rule out a congenital anomaly, fracture, infection, or tumor. There may be protrusion of the disk or sequestration of a fragment of the disk into the spinal canal. Treatment consists of rest and analgesics. Injection of trigger spots with a local anesthetic, the use of nerve blocks, traction, and manipulation may be helpful. After the acute pain subsides, protection in a back support is followed by exercises of the lumbar back and abdominal muscles designed to increase the patient's ability to protect his lower spine. If symptoms persist, more specific measures should be considered. If surgery is contemplated, a preliminary myelogram or discogram should be performed to localize the involved area and confirm the diagnosis. Surgical removal of the disk may then be done in carefully selected patients. A new technique still being evaluated is instillation of an enzyme, chymopapain, directly into the disk. The ground substance of the disk is changed, resulting in shrinkage and relief of pressure on the nerve roots. Occasionally spinal fusion is necessary.

Patients with disk disease whose disability is chiefly emotional do poorly following operation and should not have surgery.

Degenerative disk disease is not uncommon in the cervical spine and is often seen radiographically in asymptomatic patients. Local neck pain may be present with or without radiation into the arms. Occasionally several levels are involved in the cervical spine. The term cervical spondylosis is used when there are symptoms and signs of spinal nerve compression. Treatment is generally symptomatic, including rest, heat, occasionally a surgical collar, and intermittent head halter traction. On rare occasions operation is necessary to decompress the nerve roots and sometimes spinal fusion.

BURSITIS AND TENDONITIS

Degenerative changes may develop in tendons and bursae, most often at the shoulder. Circulatory changes occur in a tendon that has been injured or used a great deal, such as the supraspinatous tendon. An inflammatory reaction produces swelling in the tendon or overlying bursa and calcification may also develop. These patients have an acute episode of severe pain, swelling, and limitation of motion, but the acute process is generally self-limited. On x-ray a calcific deposit may or may not be noted.

Treatment consists of rest, heat, or cold, and x-ray therapy may be useful. If the contents in the distended bursa can be removed through a needle, prompt relief of symptoms results. Often breaking up the deposits of calcium with a needle under local anesthesia and injecting steroid are beneficial. In the rare patient who is unresponsive to conservative measures and whose pain is intense, incision and curetting of the calcified material may provide relief.

Not infrequently the bursitis produces intermittent symptoms for a long time and becomes chronic. Treatment is symptomatic and designed to produce pain relief and to restore or maintain a normal range of motion. Local heat, exercises, and occasional injection of steroids all are of value as is excision of a large calcific deposit.

Periarticular fibrosis is not uncommon about the shoulder and may lead to marked restriction in shoulder motion, referred to as adhesive capsulitis or "frozen shoulder." This is often seen in bedridden patients or those whose shoulders are not being used normally. They have pain and loss of glenohumeral movement and are able to elevate their arm to only 90°

through motion between the scapula and the rib cage. Treatment is directed to regaining shoulder motion by proper exercises. Complete recovery usually occurs although it may take many months. Manipulation under general anesthesia may occasionally be indicated.

Trigger Finger

Trigger finger, or stenosing tenosynovitis of one or more flexor tendons in the hand, is usually secondary to trauma or overuse. Pain and episodes of catching or locking occur in one of the fingers or the thumb. The digit is caught in the flexed position and straightens suddenly, often with difficulty. Crepitus can be felt over the involved flexor tendon sheath at the meta-carpophalangeal joint, and the patient may be able to reproduce the snapping or locking. The treatment is rest and occasionally injection of steroids directly into the tendon sheath. Opera-tion may be indicated, consisting of widely opening the tendon sheath. The same process involving the abductor pollicis tendon sheath of the thumb at the level of the wrist may produce severe pain and tenderness over the radial aspect of the wrist and is called DeQuervain's disease. The treatment is similar to that for a trigger finger (Figure 28-11, page 503).

Tennis Elbow

Epicondylitis, or tennis elbow, is a common abnormality characterized by pain and point tenderness over the lateral, or occasionally the medial, aspect of the elbow, particularly in the soft tissue attachments to the lateral epicondyle of the humerus. Symptoms usually respond to rest. Treatment is to change the patient's activities and inject steroids. Only rarely is operation indicated.

FOOT DISORDERS

Many patients have symptoms in their feet as a result of poor local mechanics because of congenital bony abnormalities, old injury, or poorly fitting shoes. These include corns, calluses, bunions, hammer toes, claw toes, claw feet, and heel spurs. These patients can usually obtain relief by wearing proper shoes, often with pads for corns and bunions and metatarsal arch supports. Occasionally specific measures in-cluding surgery are needed.

Bunions, or hallux valgus, may develop in women who wear pointed toe shoes and high heels, but occasionally the deformity is heredi-tary. Surgery does relieve the patient whose symptoms persist despite conservative treatment. Osteotomy may realign the metatarsophalangeal joint into a normal position. This is indicated

in young people who do not have arthritis of the metacarpophalangeal joint. Alternatively arthro-plasty of the metatarsal joint may be performed. The results are good, although control of the MP joint is not normal. This operation is performed in the older patient who has signifi-cant arthritic change at the joint.

Hammer toes may be treated by division of the extensor tendons or by arthrodesis of the of the proximal interphalangeal joint.

Painful heels, often seen in individuals who are on their feet a great deal, may or may not be associated with a calcaneal spur. Symptoms are usually due to a painful tender bursitis and can often be treated by relieving pressure with a pad. Occasionally steroid injection is helpful. Pain from prominent calluses under the metatar-sal heads that is not relieved by special pads or a metatarsal bar on the shoe may be successfully treated by resection of the metatarsal head.

Metatarsalgia, or pain under the metatarsal heads, is common. Proper shoe pads or a meta-tarsal bar usually relieves the pressure on the irritated plantar digital nerve and provides relief. Excision of a painful tender digital nerve neu-roma at the level of the metatarsal heads may be necessary to relieve those patients with "Morton's toe."

METABOLIC DISORDERS

Metabolic bone disease may result from abnormalities affecting the rate or quality of bone formation or bone resorption and includes defects in mineralization, such as rickets or osteomalacia, and defects in bone resorption, such as hyperparathyroidism.

Rickets and Osteomalacia

Rickets results from a lack or faulty metabo-lism of vitamin D. The decrease in calcium absorption from the gut causes inadequate mineralization of newly formed osteoid and the developing epiphyseal plate. Growth is retarded, and the epiphyseal cartilage and metaphyses are widened and irregular. Bone is weak because of the relatively large amount of osteoid compared with normally mineralized bone, and it may fracture or gradually become deformed. The skeletal and epiphyseal changes are usually reversible in children with nutritional rickets who are given vitamin D. In vitamin D-resistant rickets, which is relatively rare, the clinical findings are similar to those of nutritional rickets. However, the former patients respond only to large doses of vitamin D and always remain short in stature.

Osteomalacia, or adult rickets, may be the result of failure of calcium absorption from the gastrointestinal tract, as in steatorrhea, or it may develop in patients with renal disease. Newly formed osteoid is not mineralized because of the lack of calcium. This results in osteoporosis, fractures, and eventual deformity. Pathologic fractures in ribs and pelvis, due to infraction of bone with healing by poorly mineralized osteoid, are known as "milkman's fractures."

Renal osteodystrophy is occurring more frequently because of the large number of patients being kept alive on dialysis or by kidney transplant. Glomerular disease leads to an increase in serum phosphorus, a compensatory decrease in serum calcium, and secondary hyperparathyroidism. The changes in secondary hyperparathyroidism are similar to those in primary except that calcification occurs in small arteries, especially of the hand, metastatic calcification is noted, and brown tumors do not develop in the bones. In renal tubular disease resorption of calcium from the urine is impaired and secondary osteomalacia results.

In children with renal osteodystrophy severe skeletal deformities may occur, including knockknees and femoral neck fractures. Occasionally surgical correction is indicated. The skeletal changes improve markedly following improvement in renal function, as after kidney transplantation.

Primary Hyperparathyroidism

An increase in secretion of parathormone by the parathyroids results in hypercalcemia because of the increase in mobilization of calcium from the skeleton and a secondary fall in serum phosphorus. The alkaline phosphatase is elevated from the attempt at skeletal repair by the osteoblasts. The hypercalcemia may lead to the formation of kidney stones, which may be the chief manifestation of hyperparathyroidism. Osteitis fibrosa cystica is present when there is marked bone resorption and deposition of fibrous tissue. The osteoporosis is the result of greatly increased osteoclastic activity. Collections of fibrous tissue and osteoclasts may expand and completely destroy portions of the skeleton. They are sometimes known as "brown tumors." Subperiosteal cortical erosion may be seen radiographically, especially in the hand, upper humerus, and mandible. Bone biopsy may help establish the diagnosis; however, the changes in primary and secondary hyperparathyroidism are the same histologically.

The renal tubular failure seen in hyperparathyroidism may produce osteomalacia. It may therefore be difficult to decide which is the primary disease, because secondary hyperparathyroidism may develop from primary renal disease. The elevated serum calcium early in hyperparathyroidism is most important in establishing the diagnosis.

Primary hyperparathyroidism is treated by removing the adenoma or most of the hyperplastic glands (see Chapter 27, page 487).

Osteoporosis

Senile osteoporosis is a generalized decrease in bone tissue in which the cortices become thin and the medullary spaces wide. Although scanty, the bone is normal histologically and biochemically. The cause is unknown but may be precipitated by the menopause in women. Pathologic fractures are common, especially in the spine where they may follow minimal trauma and usually produce few symptoms. In the elderly fractures of the femoral neck and wrist may follow minor injury and can be considered pathologic. Healing occurs readily. The treatment of senile osteoporosis is unsatisfactory, but hormone, calcium, vitamin D, calcitonin, and more recently fluorides have been used. Many patients diagnosed as having senile osteoporosis probably also have some degree of osteomalacia.

Gout

Gout, a common familial error of purine metabolism occurring more often in men, is characterized by recurrent attacks of arthritis and is usually accompanied by an increase in the serum uric acid. Trauma or an illness often precipitates an acute attack. Podagra or involvement of the metacarpophalangeal joint of the great toe is the commonest presentation, but other joints may also be involved. Urate crystals deposited in the synovium and articular cartilage lead to an acute inflammatory reaction with sudden marked painful swelling and erythema around the involved joints. The diagnosis may be difficult at the time of first attack, especially when it involves the knee joint, but urate crystals in the synovial fluid are confirmatory. The disease may progress, particularly if not treated, to extensive joint destruction with tophus formation or deposit of large amounts of urate.

Colchicine, Benemid, Butazolidin, allopurinol, and phenylbutazone are all effective in treating a recent attack and preventing further attacks. Careful management is necessary to prevent hypercalciuria causing renal disease. If recognized early and treated properly, little disability or morbidity results.

Paget's Disease

Paget's disease, or osteitis deformans, is a common bone disorder characterized by progressive enlargement and deformity of one or more bones as a result of regional increase in the bone remodeling process. Radiographically the involved cortices are thickened, the trabeculae are broader than normal, and osteoporosis may be present. The distinction between normal and involved bone is usually clear. Joints are involved secondarily and only become symptomatic in the late stages. The patient may be asymptomatic, have pain, or may notice bowing of the tibia and femur, or enlargement of the skull. Osteosclerosis may produce deafness. Although the bone is thicker than normal, pathologic fractures occur, leading to progressive deformity. Microscopically there are formation and destruction of many osteones. Cement lines, from the increased osteoclastic activity, cause the "mosaic" appearance of the bone. If the resorption process is preponderant, the patient radiologically is in an osteolytic phase, while if new bone production dominates, he is in the more common osteoblastic phase and the bone is dense. The serum alkaline phosphatase is markedly elevated when the disease is active and widespread. During the active phase there is increased circulation in the involved bones, and a localized increase in temperature is noted clinically. Opening of small arteriovenous shunts explains the local warmth and the increased load on the heart, the signs and symptoms of cardiac strain. A highly malignant osteogenic sarcoma may develop in Paget's disease. Its presence is suggested by increasing pain, an enlarging mass, and the radiologic findings.

Treatment is usually symptomatic. Fractures are treated by immobilization and early ambulation. Internal fixation may be advisable to allow patients to be ambulated early to avoid prolonged bed rest which may lead to hypercalcemia and kidney stones. Calcitonin, mithramycin, and diphosphonates have been used recently, but their value has not been determined.

BONE NEOPLASMS

Primary bone tumors may be classified as benign or malignant; however, many of the benign lesions are not true neoplasms. Some benign lesions may become malignant, while others never do. Bone tumors may be classified according to the preponderant tissue they form or from which they arise, such as cartilage, bone, fibrous tissue, and marrow contents.

Management of a patient with a bone tumor includes clinical evaluation, x-ray interpretation, and examination of the gross and microscopic material. The history may indicate how long the bone lesion has been present and suggest its degree of biologic activity. The physical examination indicates the extent of the lesion and involvement of adjacent tissues. Radiographs help decide the tissues that are present and show how the host tissue has responded to the lesion.

Since the diagnosis often depends on histologic examination of the tumor, biopsy is of considerable importance. In general, open biopsy is preferred. The biopsy is taken at the periphery of the tumor and includes normal bone. Frozen section is often obtained to be certain that the procedure is adequate. Occasionally, when open surgical biopsy is contraindicated, a needle biopsy may provide the necessary tissue.

Benign Tumors

Benign bone lesions include those arising from or forming fibrous tissue, cartilage, or bone such as metaphyseal fibrous defect, osteoid osteoma, osteoblastoma, osteocartilaginous exostoses, enchondroma, benign chondroblastoma, and bone cyst.

Metaphyseal Fibrous Defect. One of the most common bone lesions is the metaphyseal fibrous defect. The lesion is located in the metaphysis, is eccentrically placed, characterized radiographically by areas of bone destruction, and almost always has a sclerotic bony margin. The x-ray appearance is quite characteristic. Most are asymptomatic and are an incidental finding on x-ray and do not need treatment. When occasionally they are large enough to lead to pathologic fracture, they may require curettage and bone grafting. Histologically they consist of benign fibrous tissue with occasional multinuclear cells and histiocytes. They are probably not true neoplasms since they tend to remodel with growth and fill in spontaneously.

Osteoid Osteoma. An osteoid osteoma is a painful tumor most often in the femur and tibia. The pain occurs even at rest and is often relieved by aspirin. Local tenderness is always present, and sometimes synovitis in an adjacent joint may produce limited joint motion. Radiographs characteristically show an area of decreased density surrounded by a zone of increased density. In the center is an area of increased density or nidus, measuring a few millimeters in diameter. Microscopically the central nidus is a network of highly mineralized new bone surrounded by a region with considerable bone formation and resorption.

Removing the tiny central nidus can effect cure. More than one nidus may be present.

Osteoblastoma. Osteoblastoma or giant osteoid osteoma is an osteolytic lesion which often develops in a vertebra. Microscopically it is similar to osteoid osteoma except that the heavily mineralized central nidus is often several centimeters in diameter. Osteoblastoma is usually cured by curettage. If the lesion recurs, wide surgical resection may be necessary.

Osteocartilaginous Exostosis. These lesions are cartilage-capped bony growths protruding most often from the metaphyseal regions of the long bones. The lesions may be solitary or multiple (hereditary multiple exostosis). Growth continues until puberty when the cartilage cap, which is presumably under the influence of growth hormone, ceases to grow. A bursa may develop over the tumor and cause pain, pressure on nerves or blood vessels, or in the hereditary multiple form interfere with epiphyseal growth.

Occasionally malignant degeneration may occur with the formation of chondrosarcoma. Treatment depends on symptoms and whether or not there is the possibility of malignancy. If removal is indicated, the entire cartilage cap must be excised to prevent recurrence.

Enchondroma. These common lesions are often present in the phalanges and metacarpals of the hand and occasionally in the long bones of the limbs. Radiologically they cause bone destruction and not infrequently they are calcified. Most patients present with a pathologic fracture or deformity. If fracture appears imminent, the lesion can be curetted and the defect packed with bone. Enchondromas in the long bones or pelvis should be strongly suspected of being chondrosarcomas.

Benign Chondroblastoma. This cartilage-forming tumor occurs in the epiphysis in children or young adults, contains multinucleated cells, and radiographically contains regions with bone destruction, bone formation, and calcification. It is generally treated by curettage and bone grafting. Occasionally recurrence may follow curettage, and in rare cases malignant degeneration may occur.

Bone Cysts. Bone cysts are common lesions of unknown etiology occurring in the metaphyses of long bones in children, especially at the proximal end of the humerus or femur. They are asymptomatic unless fractured. The fracture heals but the cyst usually persists. In time the lesion heals spontaneously, but if repeated fractures occur or if deformity has occurred or is imminent, curettage and bone grafting should be performed.

Primary Malignant Neoplasms

Malignant bone tumors are giant cell tumor, fibrosarcoma, osteogenic sarcoma, paraosteal osteogenic sarcoma, chondrosarcoma, Ewing's sarcoma, reticulum cell sarcoma, and multiple myeloma.

Giant Cell Tumor. Giant cell tumor of bone is an osteolytic lesion occurring in the epiphyseal ends of long bones usually at 20 to 40 years. Occasionally it occurs in the vertebral column or small bones and in the elderly. Histologically there are numerous multinucleated cells with intervening mononuclear cells and often areas of necrosis and hemorrhage. These tumors often extend into the subchondral cortex and rarely into a joint. Some giant cell tumors are aggressive, with local recurrence and metastasis, while others run a benign course. They should all be considered potentially malignant and be treated by resection with local reconstruction, which may involve arthrodesis and massive autogenous allograft or prosthetic replacement. Those with local recurrence and metastases can still be cured by aggressive surgical treatment, including amputation of the primary and resection of pulmonary metastases. The best chance for a cure, however, depends on the adequacy of the initial surgical treatment. Radiotherapy was used extensively but has now been shown to stimulate malignant degeneration.

Osteogenic Sarcoma. Osteogenic sarcoma is the most frequent primary malignant bone tumor after multiple myeloma. It usually occurs in children, although it may develop in adults as a complication of Paget's disease or radiotherapy. It is often present in the metaphysis of long bones but may be found elsewhere in the skeleton. Unfortunately most osteogenic sarcomas are large before they produce symptoms. Diagnosis can often be suspected from physical findings and radiographic appearance but must be confirmed microscopically. Hematogenous spread tends to occur to the lungs within two years. Treatment was formerly amputation of a limb, often by disarticulation, with a cure rate of about 20 percent. Recently chemotherapy with one or more drugs, and generally including Adriamycin and methotrexate, has been commenced immediately after operation and has markedly improved survival rates.

Paraosteal Osteogenic Sarcoma. Paraosteal osteogenic sarcoma is a bone-forming sarcoma with distinctive radiographic and histologic features that distinguish it from an osteogenic sarcoma. The former grows more slowly and has a five-year cure rate of about 50 percent following radical surgery. Occasionally resection with preservation of the limb can be performed.

Chondrosarcoma. Chondrosarcoma usually appears at a later age than osteosarcoma and tends to grow at a slower rate. The lesion is often large, especially when it is in the pelvis. On x-ray there is characteristic calcification within the tumor. Treatment is surgical resection. Amputation may be necessary when the tumor is in a limb.

Ewing's Sarcoma. Ewing's sarcoma is a

highly malignant, rapidly growing, bone-destroying neoplasm commonly situated in the bone of the trunk or limbs. Often a large soft tissue mass is present and there is anemia with a low-grade fever. Biopsy reveals sheets of round cells with areas of necrosis due to the rapid growth of the tumor. Radiotherapy causes disappearance of the soft tissue mass and marked clinical improvement. Usually there is local recurrence with metastases to other bones and the lungs, and death supervenes. Recently several drugs along with local or whole body radiotherapy have been used with marked prolongation of life and possibly cure.

Reticulum Cell Sarcoma. Reticulum cell sarcoma tends to occur in older patients than Ewing's sarcoma, has a much better prognosis, and has a somewhat similar picture microscopically. Radiographs demonstrate a mottled, irregularly destructive neoplasm. These tumors grow slowly and are very sensitive to x-ray therapy. A number of cures have been reported.

Multiple Myeloma. Multiple myeloma is a malignant neoplasm of the skeleton originating from the hematic cells of the bone marrow and found only occasionally in extraskeletal sites. The greatest incidence is at 40 to 60 years. Osteolytic lesions result which may weaken the bone enough to lead to fracture. Signs and symptoms may persist for many years before death occurs. Not infrequently a patient with myeloma is first seen because of skeletal pain, and on x-ray only osteoporosis is noted. Investigations include serum proteins, bone marrow aspiration, and occasionally direct biopsy of a lesion. Treatment includes local x-ray therapy, sometimes open reduction and internal fixation for a pathologic fracture, and chemotherapy for disseminated disease.

Metastatic Carcinoma

Carcinomas of the breast, prostate, kidney, lung, and thyroid frequently metastasize to bone. Radiographically most of the lesions are osteolytic, but those of carcinoma of the prostate and some from carcinoma of the breast are osteoblastic. Most patients present with bone pain and less often with pathologic fracture. Local radiotherapy is highly effective in relieving bone pain. Unless the patient is extremely ill, the pathologic fractures should generally be treated by open reduction and internal fixation, sometimes using methyl methacrylate as additional fixation material. Metastases from the prostate and frequently the breast are often hormone dependent and can be effectively treated by hormonal manipulation.

NEUROMUSCULAR DISORDERS

Neuromuscular disorders, such as cerebral palsy, polio, strokes, and neuropathic arthropathy, lead to symptoms that require specific orthopedic management.

Cerebral Palsy

Children and adults with cerebral palsy may have difficulty with gait and function of the upper extremity which can be improved by exercises, splints, braces, and occasionally operation. The children are generally seen by a multidisciplinary group, including pediatricians, orthopedic surgeons, physical therapists, and occupational therapists, in order for proper rehabilitation to be carried out. Splinting may be necessary to prevent joint contracture when the patient is at rest, and braces may improve gait. Surgical procedures include operations to correct joint contracture, transfer of muscles to improve function in the arm and leg, osteotomy to correct fixed abnormal deformity, and occasionally arthrodesis to stabilize a joint. It should be recognized that any procedure must have very specific limited goals of which the patient, the relatives, and the physician must be clearly aware, and that the specific surgical procedure is only one part of the overall care.

Poliomyelitis

Acute poliomyelitis is a viral infection affecting the anterior horn cells of the spinal cord and producing various degrees of motor paralysis. Most recovery occurs during the first year and little after two years. Braces may help to improve gait and function of an extremity and also support the back if the spinal muscles are involved. Surgical procedures to realign bones and joints, muscle transfers to improve function, and arthrodesis to stabilize joints should all be considered. Operation to arrest bone growth may compensate for limb shortening in a child when the lower limbs are unequally involved.

Stroke Patients

Specific measures can speed the rehabilitation of a patient disabled by a stroke. A team approach is required with care being given to the patient's medical and socioeconomic problems. Occasionally braces may improve gait and may also improve function of the upper extremity. Surgical procedures should be considered in selected patients; for example, triple arthrodesis and tendon transfer may be indicated in the young patient with a marked equinovarus deformity.

Amputees

The initial care the amputee receives plays a large role in determining how well he will be rehabilitated. Application of the artifical limb in the operating room immediately after amputation provides an excellent dressing for the stump and is a great psychological aid in recovery. Many of the artificial limbs made today are of strong lightweight materials for easier ambulation.

This broad overview of the musculoskeletal system as seen by an orthopedic surgeon should serve as an introduction for the interested physician. The advent of new techniques in diagnosis and treatment, including improved internal fixation devices, better biomaterials for joint replacement, and new methods of frac- ture treatment, indicate that much more useful information for the practicing physician will be forthcoming in the future.

SUGGESTIONS FOR FURTHER READING

Aegerter, Ernest, and Kirkpatrick, John A., Jr.: *Orthopaedic Diseases*, 3rd ed. W. B. Saunders Co., Philadelphia, 1968.

Crenschaw, A. H.: *Campbell's Operative Orthopaedics*, Vol. 2, 5th ed. C. V. Mosby Company, St. Louis, 1971.

Dahlin, David C.: *Bone Tumors, General Aspects and Data on 3987 Cases*. 2nd ed. Charles C Thomas, Springfield, Ill., 1973.

Jaffe, Henry L.: *Tumors and Tumorous Conditions of the Bone and Joints*. Lea & Febiger, Philadelphia, 1958.

Salter, Robert B.: *Textbook of Disorders and Injuries of the Musculoskeletal System*. Williams & Wilkins Co., Baltimore, 1970.

Chapter 30

CARDIOPULMONARY SURGERY

Robert E. Madden

CHAPTER OUTLINE

Introduction
The Lungs
    Embryology
    Anatomy
Investigations
    Radiography of the Chest
    Other Diagnostic Procedures
Preoperative Evaluation and Anesthesia for
        Thoracic Surgery
Pulmonary Operations
Thoracic Trauma
    Initial Management
Diseases of the Pleura
Diseases of the Trachea
Infectious Diseases of the Lung
    Bronchiectasis
    Lung Abscess
    Pulmonary Tuberculosis
    Fungal Infections
Congenital Abnormalities of the Lung:
        Bullous and Bleb Diseases
Tumors of the Lung
    Bronchial Adenoma

Bronchogenic Carcinoma
    Roentgenographic Features
    Diagnosis and Staging
    Treatment
Metastatic Tumors of the Lung
Diseases of the Mediastinum
Heart
    Embryology
    Anatomy
    Special Diagnostic Procedures
    Cardiopulmonary Bypass
    Congenital Lesions
    Acquired Heart Disease
        Mitral Stenosis
        Mitral Insufficiency
        Aortic Stenosis
        Aortic Insufficiency
        Tricuspid Disease
    Cardiac Trauma
    Coronary Artery Disease
    Pericarditis
    Pacemakers

INTRODUCTION

Intrathoracic surgery developed much later than surgery of the abdomen and the musculoskeletal system due to technical difficulties in entering the thoracic cavity and the major physiologic changes that result. Before endotracheal anesthesia, novel experimental devices, such as the Sauerbruch chamber, were tried in an attempt to overcome the natural recoil and collapse of the lungs when exposed to atmospheric pressure. The handling of battlefield penetrating chest wounds taught early surgeons the necessity of immediately sealing off the thoracic cavity. Early thoracic surgery, mainly for tuberculosis, involved collapse procedures that did not require opening the chest cavity.

Having mastered the technique of entering the chest, it was possible to resect lobes and even an entire lung, but with a high complication rate following massive ligation of structures at the hilum. Evarts and Graham among others dissected out and divided the individual structures, the arteries, veins, and bronchi, with a marked reduction in complications, such as bronchial fistula. The technique culminated in the first successful pneumonectomy for cancer in 1933.

The heart, however, remained the ultimate challenge. Souttar attempted cardiac surgery in 1927, but it was not until 1947 that Bailey and Harken, working independently, successfully operated upon the mitral valve. In 1954 Gibbon performed the first successful intracardiac or "open heart" procedure utilizing total cardiopulmonary bypass. The development of cardiac catheterization and angiography led to accurate diagnosis and operation for many congenital and acquired heart diseases. The first successful total cardiac transplant was performed by Barnard in 1969.

THE LUNGS

Embryology

The lungs develop from the ventral foregut. In the 4-mm embryo, a single tube situated caudal to the paired pharyngeal pouches bifurcates and further divisions give rise to ten segmental tubes on the right and eight on the left. Subsequent generations of branchings lead to a bushlike system of epithelial tubes that eventually become the respiratory bronchioles, alveolar ducts, and alveolar sacs. An estimated 300 million alveolar sacs are ultimately produced. The mesenchyme into which the branches project contains the developing pulmonary vasculature, lymphatics, and the cartilage and muscle of the bronchi. The respiratory epithelium is initially cuboidal and glandular and later becomes flattened in the periphery. Cells resembling macrophages and known as "great alveolar cells" appear and later produce surfactant. The enlarging primitive lungs extend into the lateral pleural cavities, and the dorsal mesentery becomes the mediastinum. The layer covering the lung condenses to form the visceral pleura.

The pulmonary arteries arise from the most caudal pair of aortic arches (Figure 30–1). They are connected to the pulmonary portion of the longitudinally dividing truncus. The left sixth arch persists as the ductus arteriosus. The pulmonary veins arise as vascular sprouts from the primitive atrium. Originally four in number, they are reduced to two main veins, right and left, by encroachment of the enlarging atrium. Peripherally the pulmonary veins fuse with the capillary vasculature of the organizing mesenchyme in the lungs.

Anatomy

The larger right lung is composed of upper, middle, and lower lobes, while the smaller left lung has upper and lower lobes. The lobes are divided into 17 segments (Table 30–1). The major (oblique) fissure divides the upper from the lower lobe on the left and the upper and middle lobes from the lower on the right. The minor (straight) fissure divides the right upper from the middle lobe. Frequently part or all of a fissure incompletely separates the lobes. On the other hand, fissures occasionally may completely separate the segments within the lobes. The trachea bifurcates at the level of the seventh dorsal vertebra into the short and sharply angulated left and the longer and straighter right main bronchi. On the right the upper lobe bronchus passes over the pulmonary artery

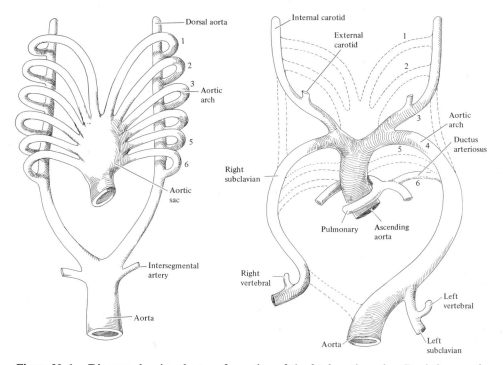

Figure 30–1. Diagram showing the transformation of the fetal aortic arches. Persisting vessels remain solid. Atrophic vessels and those that have disappeared are indicated by dashed lines.

Table 30–1. BRONCHOPULMONARY SEGMENTS

	RIGHT LUNG	LEFT LUNG
Upper lobe	Apical	Apical posterior
	Anterior	Anterior
	Posterior	Superior lingular
		Inferior lingular
Middle lobe	Lateral	
	Medial	
Lower lobe	Superior	Superior
	Medial basal	Anteromedial basal
	Anterior basal	Lateral basal
	Lateral basal	Posterior basal
	Posterior basal	

(eparterial) and the main bronchus continues as the bronchus intermedius. On the left the pulmonary artery lies beneath the main bronchus. Both upper lobe bronchi angulate sharply upward. The right middle lobe bronchus projects anteriorly, as does the lingular segmental bronchus. Both superior segmental bronchi project posteriorly. Both main bronchi then continue caudally as basilar bronchi, each giving off four segmental bronchi.

The main pulmonary artery arises to the left of the aorta and passes anterior to the left main bronchus, where it divides into the right and left pulmonary arteries. As the arteries leave the pericardial sac, they deliver a number of segmental arteries, variable in number and position. Two pulmonary veins on each side pass through the pericardium and drain into the left atrium. Peripherally the venous drainage generally follows the segmental anatomy.

The bronchial arteries provide the major blood supply to the lung parenchyma. They arise mainly from the aorta, but some also arise from the intercostal arteries, the subclavian arteries, and the innominate arteries. These nutrient arteries are closely applied to the bronchi. Venous drainage is mainly into the pulmonary veins.

Lymphatic drainage from the periphery of the lung parenchyma is to the visceral pleura and the remainder of the lung, to the nodes at the origin of the segmental and lobar bronchi, and then to the nodes in the hilum and mediastinum. Pleural drainage is to the hilar nodes. This complex of major bronchus, pulmonary artery and veins, and the lymph nodes is called the primary hilum.

The primary function of the lungs is to exchange blood gases with the environment and additionally to regulate acid-base balance, heat exchange, and fluid dissipation (see Chapter 2).

INVESTIGATIONS

Radiography of the Chest

The most frequent investigations are posteroanterior (PA) and lateral radiography of the chest taken at 72-in. tube to plate distance. The letters PA indicate that the beam enters the body posteriorly. The reverse, AP, is used chiefly in emergency radiographs taken with the patient in bed. The diverging beam causes the heart to cast a wider shadow which obliterates more of the thoracic contents. Lateral films visualize the regions behind the sternum, the posterior mediastinum, and the posterior diaphragmatic sulcus. Oblique films help to locate lung or mediastinal masses and separate them from the chest wall. Decubitus films help determine if free or loculated fluid is present and demonstrate air-fluid levels. In the apical lordotic view the patient is angled backward with the tube in front. The clavicles are thus elevated and the apices of the lung are better visualized. Films are usually taken on deep inspiration, but a pair of films will disclose excursion of the diaphragm or shift of the mediastinum. With laminography (tomography) the film and tube are moving reciprocally. This results in only one plane of the chest being in focus and helps to localize a lesion (Figure 30–2). Fluoroscopy may be used to study breathing dynamics, to localize lesions and look for chest wall and diaphragmatic movement.

In bronchography a contrast medium is introduced into the trachea and thence into the segmental bronchi. This technique is useful to determine intrabronchial disease such as tumors, bronchiectatic dilatations, or fistulae into the esophagus. Pulmonary angiography helps demonstrate vascular malformations and aneurysms and is of greatest value in showing the size and location of pulmonary emboli. It has recently been employed to estimate resectability in lung cancer. Radionuclide scanning permits gross estimation of arterial perfusion and is mostly used in suspected pulmonary embolism. Pulmonary masses, blebs, and shunts will also produce abnormal scans.

Other Diagnostic Procedures

Bronchoscopic examination can be performed under general or local anesthesia, most often using the rigid tubular bronchoscope preferably with right-angled viewing. The carina, major bronchi, and segmental bronchial orifices are inspected, and suspicious areas are biopsied. Foreign bodies can be extracted. Widening and immobility of the carina often indicate metastases in the subcarinal nodes. Saline is introduced and then aspirated to obtain fluid for cytologic

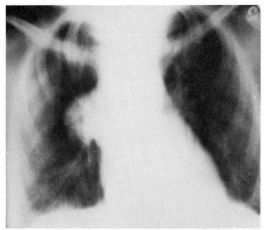

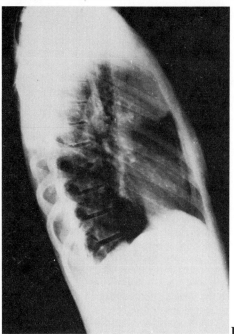

A

B

Figure 30–2.　*A*. An AP laminogram of a patient with a thymoma in the anterior mediastinum. The anterolateral ribs are in focus, and the spine is blurred. *B*. Lateral projection also shows tumor in anterosuperior mediastinum.

studies for tumor cells and for smears and cultures. Recently the flexible fiberoptic bronchoscope has been used. It can be passed more distantly into the tracheobronchial tree and permits use of a small brush to obtain cytologic specimens.

Mediastinoscopy is done to obtain tissue from the anterior mediastinal and hilar lymph nodes. An incision is made usually in the midline at the sternal notch, and blunt dissection is performed to the tracheal bifurcation in the pretracheal

space. If metastases are found in the nodes, a bronchogenic carcinoma is considered inoperable. Mediastinotomy is another surgical diagnostic procedure, in which a costal cartilage is removed, usually the third, the mediastinum is explored with a finger and biopsies taken. Both of these procedures may spare the patient an unnecessary thoracotomy.

PREOPERATIVE EVALUATION AND ANESTHESIA FOR THORACIC SURGERY

Most thoracic surgery is conducted under general anesthesia using endotracheal intubation and controlled respiration. In most cases pulmonary function can be estimated from the history, physical examination, and the patient's age. If any abnormality is suspected or there has been previous pulmonary or cardiac disease, pulmonary function tests should be performed. The most useful is to record the pulse and respiratory rate after climbing stairs. Specific tests can be done to measure the three main pulmonary functions: ventilation, perfusion, and diffusion. Ventilation is measured by determining the vital capacity (maximal volume expired following a maximal inspiration), timed vital capacity (volume expelled during one, two, and three seconds after a maximum inspiration), and maximum breathing capacity (maximum volume breathed in one minute). If these three tests fall below 50 percent of the predicted normal, a difficult postoperative course requiring respiratory support can be anticipated. Perfusion refers to the pulmonary capillary blood flow and is the result of the mean driving pressure in the right ventricle and the capillary resistance. When perfusion is inadequate, pulmonary arterial pressure is elevated and gas exchange is poor. Diffusion refers to the passage of gases across the alveolar capillary membrane. Blood gas studies estimate perfusion and diffusion. In the final analysis, however, no tests or values can replace good clinical judgment when contemplating pulmonary resection or cardiac procedures. Pulmonary function can be improved before operation by bronchodilators, expectorants, breathing exercises, antibiotics, and intermittent positive pressure breathing (IPPB).

During operation both lungs are ventilated through a firmly cuffed endotracheal tube, and secretions are repeatedly aspirated. This helps prevent postoperative atelectasis and pneumonitis. Spread of infectious material from one lung to the other is prevented by a double-lumen tube which occludes one major bronchus while permitting ventilation through the other. Selection of an anesthetic agent such as halothane allows a high concentration of oxygen to be administered throughout the procedure.

Finally the patient's position is important, more in pulmonary than in cardiac surgery. The lateral position is usually chosen for tumor removal. A semisupine position is best for patients with marginal pulmonary reserve. The semiprone position is chosen for patients with suppurative disease, since it allows better drainage and suction of secretion.

PULMONARY OPERATIONS

Thoracotomy is performed via an anterior, posterior, or lateral approach. The anterior approach least disturbs cardiorespiratory function but gives limited exposure. The posterior approach is best when dealing with suppurative diseases, since secretions are more readily evacuated and the bronchi are easily dissected and can be clamped early. The lateral approach gives the best technical exposure for hilar dissection but produces lung collapse and mediastinal shift. It is the most commonly used approach.

Pulmonary resections consist of pneumonectomy, lobectomy, segmental resection, or wedge resection. Pneumonectomy is performed for bronchogenic carcinoma when it is not possible to remove the entire lesion by lobectomy alone. Lobectomy is performed for bronchogenic carcinoma, tuberculosis, bronchiectasis, multiple lung abscess, giant bullae, and, occasionally, metastatic carcinoma. Segmental resection is performed for benign disease when it is important to conserve normal lung tissue. The main indication is for disease with segmental distribution, such as bronchiectasis. Other indications are lung abscess, cyst, metastatic carcinoma, and hamartoma. Wedge resections are not performed along anatomic planes and are done for well-circumscribed benign tumors, metastatic tumors, and localized inflammatory diseases.

THORACIC TRAUMA

Chest injuries can be either penetrating or nonpenetrating. Penetrating injuries arise from bullets or stabbings. Nonpenetrating injuries are the result of forceful contact with blunt objects as in automobile accidents, in falls, or from blasts. Chest injuries are often associated with injuries to the head, abdomen, spine, and extremities. The major alterations in cardiopulmonary physiology can be restored by quite simple procedures, and only a small percentage of patients require operation.

Clean penetrations, as with a knife, usually damage a single organ, lung, heart, or great vessel, and produce a hemothorax or pneumo-

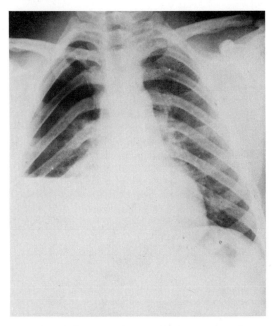

Figure 30–3. A stab wound of the chest has caused a hemothorax and pneumothorax. An air-fluid level is present, and there is partial collapse of the lung.

thorax (Figure 30–3). Penetrations below the fifth interspace may have transversed the diaphragm and injured the abdominal contents. Missile penetrations, as with bullets, produce more damage, both to the thoracic organs and to the chest wall, and may cause a tension pneumothorax. Blunt trauma always injures the chest wall and frequently the lung, heart, and great vessels. Blast injury frequently damages the lung and sometimes the heart, esophagus, and great vessels but infrequently affects the chest wall.

Initial Management

The history is important since visible injuries may be minimal. The patient is examined and vital functions are restored. If indicated, an endotracheal tube is inserted and intravenous fluids are administered. The type of chest wound is important. A missile penetration damages the chest wall, and there is a high likelihood of a valvelike sucking defect being present. Air enters the pleural space through the wound and the injured lung, producing a tension pneumothorax. The lung collapses and the mediastinum is shifted to the opposite side, compressing the venae cavae (Figure 30–4). The patient is cyanosed, the chest is tympanic, the trachea is deviated to the opposite side, and death occurs if the condition is not relieved.

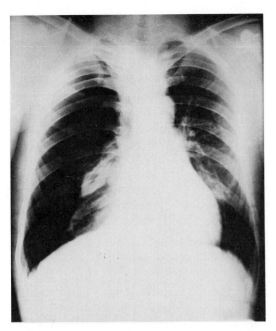

Figure 30–4. With a tension pneumothorax, the lung is totally collapsed and the mediastinum shifted under pressure to the opposite side.

The sucking wound is closed with whatever is available, preferably Vaseline gauze. A large-bore needle is inserted in the second interspace anteriorly. Air rushes out, with immediate improvement in cardiorespiratory dynamics. The occlusive dressing may be intermittently applied, removing it on expiration and re-positioning it on inspiration. A catheter is inserted at the needle site as soon as possible and attached to underwater seal drainage (Figure 30–5). The chest wound is debrided only after the general condition has been stabilized and the patient completely assessed.

Closed pneumothorax implies that air has entered the pleural space due to penetrating, blunt, or blast injury to the lung without defect in the chest wall. The condition is usually not urgent, and roentgenographic examination is generally possible. A catheter is inserted under sterile conditions in the second interspace anteriorly and attached to underwater seal drainage. Suction may be applied. If lung tissue or a major bronchus is not massively damaged, the lung usually expands and seals off the internal air leak. Subcutaneous emphysema may occur if air enters the mediastinum and the subcutaneous tissues of the chest, abdomen, and neck. The subcutaneous air does not cause any symptoms and becomes absorbed as the pneumothorax decreases.

A hemothorax may accompany any pene-trating or nonpenetrating chest injury with or without a pneumothorax. Blood in the pleural space may come from lung tissue, intercostal or internal mammary arteries, or the great vessels in the mediastinum. The patient may be short of breath, the chest is dull to percussion, and breath sounds are absent. The chest x-ray may initially show blunting of the costophrenic angle, and with further accumulation of blood, a line of density rises laterally up the chest wall. A fluid level means a hemopneumothorax. Blood must be removed from the pleural cavity and the continuing loss monitored. Pulmonary bleeding is low pressure and usually self-limiting, while bleeding from major pulmonary or systemic vessels is usually massive and continuous. Some authorities use repeated needle thoracentesis, but more effective drainage is obtained by inserting a catheter in the seventh interspace in the posterior axillary line. An anterior catheter should also be inserted if air is present. If continuous blood loss exceeds 300 ml per hour, thoracotomy is indicated.

When blunt trauma causes multiple rib, cartilage, or sternal fracture, an unstable chest wall results. Usually three or more ribs are involved. The flail chest results in paradoxical motion of the chest wall inward with each inspiration and outward with each expiration. The mediastinum tends to oscillate or "flutter" with each respiration. The diaphragm alone remains as the ventilating muscle. Air passes back and forth between the lungs (penduluft), adding to the hypoxia and hypercarbia. There is severe pain with each respiratory motion. Ventilation is severely affected and early hypoxic death can ensue. The chest wall can be initially stabilized by placing a sandbag over the

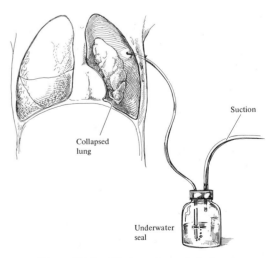

Collapsed lung

Suction

Underwater seal

Figure 30–5. Underwater seal drainage.

injured area. Definitive treatment formerly consisted of traction applied to the chest wall, using surgical towel clips and wires driven through the ribs (external splint). Recently endotracheal intubation or tracheostomy with the use of a volume respirator has replaced the older method (internal splint). The chest wall stabilizes usually within two or three weeks, and the patient can be gradually weaned off the respirator. Meticulous suctioning is necessary to avoid atelectasis or development of the "wet lung" syndrome. An associated pulmonary contusion is often present.

Tracheobronchial rupture is an infrequent occurrence following blunt upper chest or blast injury and is often associated with fracture of the clavicle and first rib. Hemoptysis and rapidly developing subcutaneous emphysema are prominent features. The airway may be obstructed, leading to rapid asphyxia. Chest x-ray shows mediastinal emphysema and possible atelectasis of a lobe or entire lung and a pneumothorax. Immediate bronchoscopy is indicated to confirm the diagnosis, followed by operative repair. Occasionally the injury is not recognized and mediastinitis develops with fever, pain, and shortness of breath. X-ray reveals widening of the mediastinum. A bronchogram confirms the diagnosis.

Hematomas of the lung, which may develop with any of the above-mentioned chest injuries, present on x-ray as a density in the lung field. They generally resolve without specific treatment, but occasionally a fluid-filled cavity develops, or even an abscess which requires surgical excision.

"Traumatic wet lung" describes a condition which sometimes follows a blunt or blast injury to the chest. This syndrome has several aspects. Ventilation is reduced because of pain from the injury to the chest wall and the upper abdominal contents. Visceral injury increases mucous secretion from the tracheobronchial tree, the mouth, and nasopharynx. Membrane damage may have caused local hemorrhage. Finally, local tissue injury and hypoxia may increase alveolar transudates. The situation is compounded if a head injury coexists. This ventilating inactivity is termed splinting. If unrelieved, secretions and transudates collect and atelectasis and pneumonia develop, resulting in hypoxia and death. The diagnosis can be made by hearing rales after the patient coughs or tries to cough. Audible gurgling sounds can be heard. The chest x-ray is nonspecific, but patchy infiltrates and pulmonary edema are usually present. Therapy is directed initially to increasing effective cough. Good nursing aid may help in splinting the patient as he coughs. Intercostal nerve blocks and small doses of narcotics can be used. Intermittent positive pressure breathing (IPPB) and, more recently, positive end expiratory pressure (PEEP) breathing with a mechanical respirator increase ventilation at the alveolar level and decrease alveolar fluid. Bronchodilators and steroids can reduce small airway obstruction.

DISEASES OF THE PLEURA

In health the pleural space is a potential space containing a few cubic centimeters of fluid which acts as a lubricant, permitting the moist surfaces of the visceral and parietal pleurae to slide freely with respiration. The presence of additional fluid is termed a pleural effusion. If infected, the effusion is an empyema. Noninflammatory causes of pleural effusions are cardiac failure, cirrhosis of the liver, nephrosis (transudates), primary or secondary pulmonary cancers, primary mesothelioma of the pleura, exudates, and traumatic hemothorax. Chylothorax is often present with lymphomas. Pleural effusions can also result from rupture of the esophagus with filling of the pleural space with gastric contents. A sterile inflammatory effusion may occur from an adjacent inflammatory disease such as pulmonary tuberculosis, subphrenic abscess, or pancreatitis. A number of viral infections can also cause polyserositis.

A pleural effusion results in shortness of breath, depending upon its size and speed of development. Pain on breathing may be present if the effusion contains blood or has occurred rapidly. It may be felt locally or, if the central diaphragm is irritated, can be referred to the shoulder. On inspection the affected hemithorax lags behind during inspiration. Palpation reveals a reduction of fremitus, flat percussion, and reduced breath sounds. The findings are most noticeable posteriorly and inferiorly. The trachea is moved to the opposite side with a massive effusion. On roentgenographic examination small collections of fluid blunt the costophrenic angle, while larger collections show the fluid rising laterally up the chest wall in the posteroanterior projection (Figure 30–6). Massive effusions obliterate the lung and shift the mediastinum to the opposite side. Longstanding effusions may be located in fibrous compartments or may be loculated, producing bizarre shadows.

Empyema may be acute or chronic. With an acute empyema infection reaches the pleural space from a penetrating wound, underlying lung infection such as pneumonia or lung abscess, a neglected subphrenic abscess, or following operation. The patient becomes toxic, febrile, and may be dyspneic. Roentgenograms

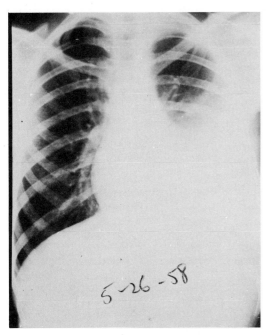

Figure 30–6. A pleural effusion may consist of pus, as in an empyema (exudate); clear or blood-stained fluid, due to primary or metastatic tumor (exudate); a transudate, associated with nephrosis, liver cirrhosis, or cardiac failure; or blood, as in trauma. This patient has tuberculosis.

initially show a pleural effusion, but within 10 to 15 days the pus becomes loculated and accurately localized. The exception is a streptococcal empyema which remains fluid and does not localize. Treatment is drainage using a chest tube or removal of a segment of overlying rib. In some cases thoractomy may be performed and the empyema excised with the involved pleura (decortication). A chronic empyema may give rise to a number of complications. An empyema necessitatis is spontaneous drainage of pus through the chest wall. A chronic sinus may occur associated with osteomyelitis of ribs. A neglected empyema may drain internally into a bronchus, forming a bronchopleural fistula. The patient coughs up large volumes of pus, and an air-fluid level is seen on roentgenograms. Systemic amyloidosis may occur from chronic sepsis.

A tuberculous empyema may occur with or without a demonstrable underlying pulmonary lesion as a complication of reinfection tuberculosis. The infection is often mixed, containing tubercle bacilli and pyogenic organisms. Treatment is initially medical, and surgical intervention is required for drainage or resection only if conservative measures fail.

Tumors of the pleura are either primary benign or malignant mesotheliomas or metastatic. Benign mesotheliomas are small, circumscribed, indolent lesions of little clinical consequence. They are removed when their true nature is in doubt on roentgenographic examination. Malignant mesotheliomas are initially localized but later become diffuse throughout the pleural space. There is a high correlation between industrial exposure to asbestos, chromium, and uranium and the development of mesothelioma. The tumors produce paraneoplastic syndromes of osteoarthropathy, hypercalcemia, and hyperglycemia as well as clubbing of the fingers. There is a rapidly developing bloody pleural effusion containing bizarre neoplastic cells. Thoracotomy may occasionally be necessary to establish the diagnosis. Resection may sometimes be curative but only for early localized lesions.

Metastatic tumors to the pleura are most frequently from the breast and lung, less commonly from the gastrointestinal tract. Lymphomas may also involve the pleura. Treatment consists of drainage of the effusion, radiotherapy, infusions of radioactive isotopes or chemotherapeutic agents, or systemic chemotherapy.

DISEASES OF THE TRACHEA

Diseases of the trachea are congenital, traumatic, inflammatory, or neoplastic. Symptoms are usually those of upper airway obstruction, an inspiratory wheeze or "asthma," although, pain, cough, or even hemoptysis may be present. The history is important. Congenital lesions produce symptoms from birth; post-traumatic lesions date from the time of injury; neoplasms are usually progressive. Special roentgenographic diagnostic studies are tomography, fluoroscopy, and contrast tracheography. Bronchoscopy and, when indicated, biopsy should be performed, and pulmonary function studies are desirable prior to operation.

Squamous cell carcinoma is the most common primary malignant tumor. Adenoid cystic carcinoma and carcinoid adenoma are less frequent. Benign lesions include papillomas, fibromas, and chondromas. Secondary neoplasms occur usually by direct extension from tumors of the thyroid, esophagus, larynx, or lung. Such extension almost always means a hopeless prognosis, and tracheal resection is rarely indicated. Primary malignancies, however, are amenable to surgical resection, as are benign lesions. Radiotherapy can be used as a preoperative adjunct.

Congenital lesions include tracheal stenosis, hypoplasia, and chondromalacia, a defect in

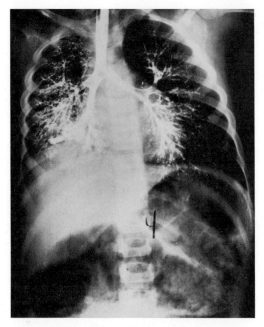

Figure 30–7. In bronchiectasis, a bronchogram is indispensable. All segments must be visualized and only those that are involved should be resected. In this patient the right middle and lower lobes are involved.

cartilage formation. Unless localized, these lesions are difficult to treat. Acquired tracheal stricture can occur as a complication of endotracheal tuberculosis. Other causes are direct external trauma, damage by a foreign body, or damage from intubation or a tracheostomy. A cuffed endotracheal tube can cause ischemic damage if not periodically deflated. Stenotic segments involving several cartilaginous rings can be successfully resected.

INFECTIOUS DISEASES OF THE LUNG

The indications for surgery for infectious diseases of the lung have decreased since antibiotics became available.

Bronchiectasis

Bronchiectasis means dilatation of the bronchi. It is invariably associated with infection of the bronchi and the surrounding lung. Although it is most often a complication of chronic bronchitis, it may also occur in tuberculosis or distal to an obstruction caused by an aspirated foreign body or an endobronchial neoplasm. There are large volumes of foul-smelling sputum and often hemoptysis, although a "dry" variety is recognized. Pulmonary fibrosis with respiratory

insufficiency can occur. The chest roentgenogram may be normal or show patchy pneumonia, especially in the basilar segments or the lingula. Bronchoscopy should be performed to determine the presence of a foreign body or tumor. A bronchogram delineates which segments are involved (Figure 30–7). Treatment consists of postural drainage, bronchodilators, and antibiotics. Operation is indicated for chronic, uncontrolled cases or for recurrent hemoptysis. The results are excellent after the affected segments are removed.

Lung Abscess

A lung abscess most often results from a gangrenous pneumonia. It also occurs after aspiration of a foreign body, such as a tooth during dental extraction, or gastric contents during anesthesia, or in the debilitated elderly patient. Most often a lung abscess occurs in the chronic alcoholic or drug addict following a period of respiratory depression when anaerobic streptococcal, staphylococcal, and fusospirochetal organisms drain into the superior segments of the lower lobes or the axillary subsegments of the upper lobes. Multiple lung abscesses may be hematogenous, following a staphylococcal septicemia. Pseudomonas abscesses can occur after trachcostomy. A local-

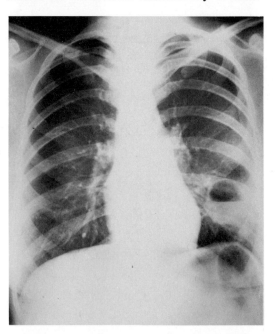

Figure 30–8. With a putrid lung abscess there is liquefaction necrosis. When an adjacent bronchus is eroded, the patient discharges the central contents and an air-fluid level can be seen on the chest roentgenogram.

ized pneumonia is quickly followed by a necrotizing liquefaction. The patient becomes acutely ill with chest pain and coughs up a large amount of putrid, rusty sputum when the material erodes through an adjacent bronchus. The chest roentgenogram initially shows a solid pneumonitic patch which, after evacuation of its liquid contents, has an air-fluid level (Figure 30–8). Treatment consists of anti-biotics, postural drainage, and bronchodilators. Bronchoscopy is indicated for drainage and, more important, to rule out the presence of an aspirated foreign body or endobronchial neo-plasm. Most lung abscesses resolve with conservative management, and only those that persist should be excised.

Pulmonary Tuberculosis

Pulmonary tuberculosis affects over 3.5 million people in the United States. Fifty thousand have clinically progressive disease or develop an exacerbation of quiescent disease, and 6000 may be expected to die. The majority are controlled by antituberculous drugs, and only 5 to 10 percent require surgical intervention. The general indication for operation is persistent cavitary or solid disease. Specific indications are listed in Table 30–2. The disease should be stable, and perioperative drug coverage is desirable (Figure 30–9). Pulmonary resection is the procedure of choice and can be carried out with a mortality of 1.5 percent for lobectomy or segmental excision and 10 percent for pneumonectomy. Thoracoplasty, removing ribs to collapse the lung, is rarely indicated. Lobec-tomy or segmentectomy successfully arrests the active disease in over 90 percent of patients and pneumonectomy, when indicated, in about 65 percent.

Fungal Infections

The three most important fungal infections in North America involving the lung are histo-

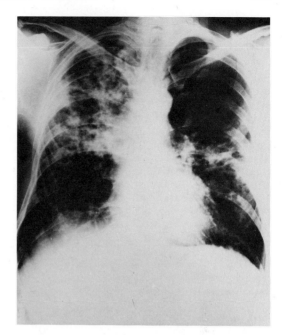

Figure 30–9. Pulmonary tuberculosis causes fibrosis and cavitations (honeycombing), most often in the upper lobes, and enlargement and calcification of the hilar lymph nodes.

plasmosis, coccidioidomycosis, and blastomy-cosis—all widespread and contracted by in-halation of the spores, although blastomycosis may enter through the skin. Histoplasmosis is endemic in the central United States in the Mississippi valley; coccidioidomycosis is seen in the San Joachim Valley of California and throughout the southwest; blastomycosis is found chiefly in the southeast and the northern central states. All three produce an acute fever with anorexia, cough, malaise, chest and muscle pain, and occasionally hemoptysis. Blastomycosis tends to spread to bones and produce local symptoms. Early chest roent-genograms show patchy infiltrates which later develop into nodular calcific lesions. Cavitary lesions are rare except in blastomycosis. The diseases are generally self-limiting and are often discovered incidentally on routine chest x-rays. Specific skin tests are usually not helpful due to the prevalence of the diseases and the presence of cross-reactivity. Complement-fixing serologic testing is helpful in blastomycosis where a high titer is of prognostic value. Diagnosis is made by culturing the organism from the sputum or tissues. The treatment is primarily medical, but surgery is indicated for progressive cavitary disease, destroyed lung tissue, or when a peripheral granuloma resembles a neoplasm (Table 30–2).

Table 30–2. INDICATIONS FOR SURGERY IN PULMONARY TUBERCULOSIS

Sputum persistently positive while on adequate medical treatment.
Bronchostenosis with distal collapse of lung tissue.
Tuberculous bronchiectasis.
Destroyed lobe or lung.
Massive hemoptysis.
Tuberculoma indistinguishable from a tumor.
Tuberculous empyema.
Lower lobe cavitation.
Upper lobe cavitation in certain patients (alcoholics, drug addicts, patients who cannot be relied on to take drugs).

CONGENITAL ABNORMALITIES OF THE LUNG: BULLOUS AND BLEB DISEASES

There are two types of chronic obstructive pulmonary disease (COPD), the result of bronchial tree obstruction. Type A (emphysematous or panlobular) obstructive pulmonary disease leads to dilatation of all elements of the respiratory tract and should be treated by operation when there are blebs and bullae. Type B (bronchitic, centrilobular) obstructive disease produces a diffuse air space disorder which should generally not be treated by operation. Blebs are small subpleural air spaces produced by air trapped in terminal respiratory divisions. Bullae probably have the same origin but larger collections of air. Both are multiple, progressive, and produce clinical pulmonary insufficiency. True lung cysts are rare and are lined by respiratory epithelium, cartilage, and smooth muscle. A pneumatocele is an air space resulting from inflammatory bronchial obstruction, especially complicating staphylococcal pneumonia in children.

Type A disease produces few symptoms other than dyspnea and distant breath sounds. The roentgenogram shows increased lung volume and sometimes bullae, and an increase in residual volume is prominent on pulmonary function testing. Type B disease is associated with severe coughing, copious sputum, wheezing, dyspnea, rales, recurrent infection, and cyanosis. The chest x-ray may show fibrosis or be entirely normal. Increased airway resistance with hypoxia and hypercapnia is noted on pulmonary function testing. Surgical therapy in type A disease is indicated when bullae produce shortness of breath or occupy more than 50 percent of the lung volume (vanishing lung). Removal of the bullae is technically simple, and results are gratifying and usually permanent. Surgical therapy in type B disease is unsatisfactory. Tracheal fenestration (a skin-lined tracheostomy) with repeated suctioning has been advocated, and thoracotomy with a plication procedure to expand lung volume has also been used.

Spontaneous pneumothorax occurs as a complication of bullous emphysema. There is sudden chest pain and dyspnea, and the collapsed lung is seen on roentgenography. The lung usually expands after insertion of a tube and establishment of closed underwater seal drainage. Surgery is indicated only if the leak persists or the pneumothorax is recurrent.

The congenital abnormalities of pulmonary agenesis or hypoplasia are of surgical interest only if they are associated with recurrent infections. Congenital pulmonary cysts may be single or multiple. Multiple cystic disease is rare and must be distinguished from pneumatoceles, as seen in staphylococcal pneumonia and mucoviscidosis. Single cysts should be removed when they expand to embarrass respiration and when they become infected. Congenital lobar emphysema occurs in the first six months of life. One or more lobes hyperinflate, probably due to cartilaginous bronchial defects, and compress adjacent lung tissue with respiratory distress. Prompt lobectomy is indicated.

In lobar sequestration bronchial connections of all or part of a lower lobe are absent, and the parenchyma is carnified and produces abnormal roentgenographic shadows. Removal is always required. A variety of vascular abnormalities exists, and these may produce murmurs, clubbing, cyanosis, and polycythemia. Angiography should be carried out, and when confirmed, the lesion should be removed.

TUMORS OF THE LUNG

Bronchial Adenoma

These neoplasms of low-grade malignant potential arise from the epithelium or the ducts and glands of the bronchi and are situated centrally in the trachea and major bronchi or in the periphery of the lung. The symptoms are usually long-standing. Central lesions produce cough, recurrent infection, and hemoptysis and sometimes wheezing, pain, and bronchiectasis. Peripheral lesions may be asymptomatic. The diagnosis is made by a combination of chest roentgenography, including oblique films, tomograms, and bronchograms, and by bronchoscopy. The tumors can be huge but are usually small. Opinions differ on the advisability of biopsy because of the possibility of severe bleeding. Histologically about 85 percent are carcinoids, and the remainder are adenoid cystic tumors. The carcinoid only rarely produces the carcinoid syndrome, and only about 10 percent metastasize to the regional nodes, while the adenoid cystic tumor is locally invasive, often recurs after removal, and metastasizes more frequently.

Treatment is lobectomy, segmentectomy, or a sleeve resection, depending on the site of the lesion. Bronchoscopic removal should be reserved for patients with a pedunculated lesion and those in whom thoracotomy is contraindicated. Radiotherapy is of little value for either lesion. The prognosis is excellent after removal of carcinoids but is poor for adenoid cystic tumors, with about two thirds of the patients ultimately dying.

Bronchogenic Carcinoma

The epidemic proportions of the largely preventable disease of lung carcinoma suggests a major failure on the part of health professionals to influence behavior patterns in the public. It would be difficult to imagine a parallel situation involving a preventable infectious or metabolic disease. About 90,000 new cases of lung cancer were seen in the United States in 1975 with 86,000 deaths. The incidence in the United States is exceeded in at least six major European countries and is twice as great in the United Kingdom. The sex ratio is about 6:1 for males over females, with a peak incidence in the sixth decade. It is the most common cancer in men and is responsible for 30 percent of all malignancies.

Sixty to 90 square meters of bronchial and respiratory epithelium are exposed to the air. This makes the lungs the largest surface target of the body to external carcinogens in the air (Table 30–3). The major factors are cigarette smoking and city living. Inflammatory changes in the lungs inhibit the discharge of particles by ciliary action and a decrease in macrophage activity increases exposure to the carinogens.

The incidence of tumors is 6:4 for right to left lungs, with most occurring in the upper lobes. About 50 percent are central, arising from the mainstem, lobar, or segmental bronchi, and 50 percent are peripheral, in the distal bronchi and bronchioles. The central tumors are firm and frequently obstruct, causing atelectasis, pneumonia, bronchiectasis, or abscess. Peripheral lesions are irregular, poorly demarcated from normal lung, tend to pucker the pleural surface, and do not obstruct. Microscopically the tumors are difficult to classify except for the well-differentiated ones. The World Health Organization classification is given in Table 30–4. Poorly differentiated tumors often show

Table 30–3. AIRBORNE CARCINOGENS ASSOCIATED WITH LUNG CANCER

AGENT	POPULATION
Cigarette smoke	Smokers
Hydrocarbons	Urban dwellers
	Coke oven operators
	Refinery workers
Asbestos	Construction workers
	Urban dwellers
Chromates, nickel, arsenic	Ore workers—chromium, nickel
Volatile fumes	Foundry workers, welders, steam fitters, cooks
Radioactive isotopes	Ore miners and smelter workers

Table 30–4. HISTOLOGIC CLASSIFICATION OF CARCINOMA OF THE LUNG*

Squamous cell carcinoma
Anaplastic small cell carcinoma
Adenocarcinoma
  Bronchoalveolar
  Giant cell
Large cell undifferentiated carcinoma
Mixed squamous cell and adenocarcinoma

* *Source:* World Health Organization.

multiple cell types. Surgical specimens have a high incidence of epidermoid carcinomas and a low incidence of small cell tumors, while the reverse occurs with autopsy material. This is due to the rapidly fatal outcome with small cell carcinomas.

Epidermoid carcinomas tend to have central location, have the most favorable prognosis, and metastasize primarily by the lymphatics. Adenocarcinomas and bronchoalveolar carcinomas are usually peripheral and metastasize late, either by the lymphatics or blood stream. The small cell or oat cell, anaplastic carcinoma, originally classified as a sarcoma or lymphoma because of its cellular nature, is central or peripheral, spreads early by the lymphatics and blood stream, and carries a hopeless prognosis. The large cell carcinoma is probably an anaplastic, clear cell variety of adenocarcinoma and has an intermediate prognosis.

There is usually a history of heavy cigarette smoking and urban living but this is not invariable. In 5 percent the disease is found in asymptomatic patients on a routine chest roentgenogram. Most, however, have symptoms for five to six months. These can be bronchopulmonary, intrathoracic, extrathoracic metastatic, or extrathoracic systemic. Bronchopulmonary symptoms are the result of irritation, ulceration, and obstruction within a bronchus. They are more frequent with central lesions and are therefore most often seen with epidermoid carcinoma. The percentage incidence of clinical features are cough (75), hemoptysis (57), chest pain (30), dyspnea (25), and fever (22). Intrathoracic spread affects the pleura, chest wall, and mediastinum. Fifteen percent of patients have one or more of the symptoms of hoarseness, superior caval obstruction, chest wall or arm pain, Horner's syndrome, dyspnea from a pleural effusion, or dysphagia.

Extrathoracic metastatic symptoms include malaise, weight loss, and fatigue. About 25 percent, especially with anaplastic tumors, present with evidence of such metastases, including bone pain, jaundice, ascites, ankle edema,

Table 30–5. CLINICAL MANIFESTATIONS OF CARCINOMA OF THE LUNG

Bronchopulmonary
- Cough
- Hemoptysis
- Chest pain
- Dyspnea (atelectasis)
- Fever
- Wheezing

Extrapulmonary Intrathoracic
- Hoarseness
- Superior caval syndrome
- Chest wall pain
- Arm pain
- Horner's syndrome
- Dysphagia
- Dyspnea (effusion)

Extrathoracic Metastatic
- Hemiplegia
- Epilepsy
- Personality changes
- Speech changes
- Bone pain or fracture
- Jaundice
- Ascites
- Masses (abdominal, nodes, subcutaneous)

Nonspecific
- Weight loss
- Malaise
- Weakness
- Anorexia

Table 30–6. PARANEOPLASTIC MANIFESTATIONS OF CARCINOMA OF THE LUNG

Metabolic
- Cushing's syndrome
- Antidiuretic hormone
- Carcinoid syndrome
- Hypercalcemia
- Gonadotropin
- Insulinlike activity

Neuromuscular
- Myopathy
- Peripheral neuropathies
- Subacute cerebellar degeneration
- Encephalomyelopathy

Skeletal
- Clubbing
- Pulmonary hypertrophic osteoarthropathy

Dermatologic
- Acanthosis nigricans
- Scleroderma

Vascular
- Migratory thrombophlebitis
- Nonbacterial verrucal endocarditis
- Arterial thrombosis

Hematologic
- Anemia
- Fibrinolytic purpura
- Nonspecific leukocytosis
- Polycythemia

convulsions, headache, nausea, diplopia, hemiplegia, and personality changes. Extrathoracic systemic manifestations occur in about 10 percent of patients and are the presenting symptoms in about 2 percent. Table 30–5 lists the main clinical manifestations of a bronchogenic carcinoma and Table 30–6 the paraneoplastic changes.

Roentgenographic Features. When detected roentgenographically, the tumor has probably already completed 75 percent of its natural history, from inception to death of the host. An important fact is that the x-ray abnormality frequently antedates clinical symptoms by over seven months. The abnormal findings on the chest x-ray are due to the tumor, obstructive lung changes, or local spread to other intrathoracic structures (Table 30–7). About 40 percent of patients have hilar changes from the primary tumor or its metastases, 40 percent have obstructive changes, 40 percent have peripheral masses, and 10 percent have extrapulmonary features. Squamous cell and small cell undifferentiated lesions tend to show central changes (Figure 30–10); adenocarcinomas, large cell undifferentiated, and bronchiolar carcinomas

tend to show peripheral changes. Special procedures include oblique views, tomography, bronchography, angiography, azygography, and isotope scans. Peripheral coin lesions may be particularly difficult to diagnose since they

Table 30–7. ROENTGENOLOGIC ABNORMALITIES ASSOCIATED WITH CARCINOMA OF THE LUNG

REGION INVOLVED	TYPE OF CHANGE
Hilus	Hilar prominence, no mass
	Hilar mass
	Perihilar mass
Parenchyma	Peripheral mass within lung
	Peripheral mass at chest wall
	Multiple masses
	Peripheral infiltrate
	Hyperlucency
	Peripheral collapse—segmental, lobar, total lung
Extrapulmonary	Mediastinal widening
	Erosions of rib or vertebrae
	Pleural effusion
	Elevation of diaphragm
	Obstruction on barium esophagram

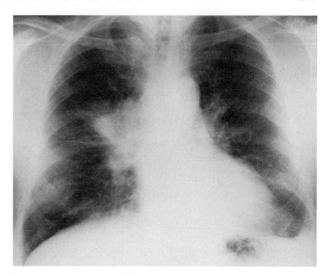

Figure 30–10. A centrally located bronchogenic carcinoma produces a hilar mass. Surrounding infiltrates cause a "sunburst" appearance. The tumor type is an epidermoid carcinoma.

may also be benign neoplasms, inflammatory lesions, or congenital abnormalities.

Diagnosis and Staging. The earliest diagnosis can be established by sputum cytology. If properly collected, early morning deep cough sputum is positive in about 85 percent of patients and sometimes antedates x-ray changes. In 25 to 50 percent of cases the lesion can be visualized via bronchoscopy with a rigid instrument. In addition, a direct biopsy can be taken and washings made for cytologic examination. Fiberoptic bronchoscopy permits more peripheral, although limited, visualization, and the brush technique can be used to obtain tumor cells. Biopsy of the scalene fat pad may reveal extrathoracic spread but should usually be performed only when nodes are palpable. Mediastinoscopy is done when roentgenograms indicate probable mediastinal node metastases. Operation is generally contraindicated when nodal metastases are present. A pleural effusion should always be aspirated and the fluid examined for cancer cells.

Proper staging at the time of diagnosis is essential to properly plan treatment (Table 30–8). The search for distant metastases includes bone survey, bone, liver, and brain isotope scans, marrow biopsy, and axial tomography of the brain. Patients with small cell carcinoma have 40 percent incidence of marrow invasion when first seen. Fifteen percent of patients examined transdiaphragmatically at thoracotomy have liver metastases.

Treatment. Operation is the only curative treatment for bronchogenic carcinoma. At the time of diagnosis about 50 percent of patients are found to have metastases. Contraindications to operation are extrathoracic metastases, certain local intrathoracic extrapulmonary extensions, and small cell carcinoma. Exceptions to operation for local spread are phrenic nerve paralysis and chest wall invasion in superior sulcus (Pancoast's tumor). A superior sulcus tumor should be treated by preoperative radiotherapy. Invasion of the atrium, vena cava, and pulmonary artery, and local invasion of ribs do not contraindicate an attempted curative operation. Medical contraindications are inadequate pulmonary reserve and cardiac disease. Age alone is generally not a contraindication to surgery.

Thoracotomy may be necessary to establish the diagnosis and to determine the extent of spread. One quarter to one half of those operated

Table 30–8. STAGING OF BRONCHOGENIC CARCINOMA (UTILIZING THE TNM SYSTEM)*

Stage I	T_1 N_0 M_0
	T_2 N_0 M_0
	T_1 N_1 M_0
Stage II	T_2 N_1 N_0
Stage III	T_2 N_2 M_0
	T_2 N_2 M_1
	T_2 N_0 M_1
	T_2 N_1 M_1
	T_3
	All small cell, oat cell lesions

* T_1: Lesion less than 3 cm, no proximal invasion
 T_2: Lesion greater than 3 cm, or proximal invasion or obstruction
 T_3: Any lesion with direct extension into adjacent structures
 N_0: No demonstrable node involvement
 N_1: Ipsilateral hilar involvement
 N_2: Mediastinal node involvement
 M_0: No distal involvement
 M_1: Contralateral node or extrathoracic metastases

on are found to have unresectable tumors. Extensive investigations, including mediastinoscopy, have in some centers eliminated many patients from thoracotomy and have reduced the number found unresectable at operation to about 5 percent. Total lobectomy or pneumonectomy are the surgical treatments of choice; segmental resection or wedge resection is rarely indicated. Lobectomy is generally preferred to pneumonectomy, since cure rates are the same for each and disability and mortality, especially in the aged, are less. The mediastinal lymph nodes are removed en bloc along with the lobe or lung. Some tumors cross fissures, making bilobectomy or pneumonectomy necessary. Palliative resection, however, leaving residual tumor is indicated only rarely, and then only to control pain, bleeding, or infection.

With the exception of the Pancoast tumor, preoperative radiotherapy has been found to be of no value, and it is possible that it even decreases survival. However, radiotherapy is indicated for small cell carcinoma, inoperable disease confined to one hemithorax, and for relief of bronchial obstruction associated with bleeding and infection. It also provides excellent palliation for bone pain from distant metastases and is of some value in treating cerebral or hepatic metastases. Cyclophosphamide may provide palliation for advanced disease, and recently combination chemotherapy has been found to be somewhat effective.

Results of Treatment. Five-year survival following attempted curative treatment of localized disease has improved from 9 to 25 percent between 1940 and 1964. The stage at treatment, localized, regional, or metastatic, however, has remained unchanged, while the percentage of patients undergoing treatment (surgery, radiotherapy, or chemotherapy) has increased from 36 to 74. Treatment and not earlier diagnosis is responsible for the improved results. The five-year survival following resection is about 20 percent, 30 percent with negative nodes, and 10 percent for positive nodes. Peripheral solitary alveolar cell carcinomas do best with a 50 percent five-year survival; epidermoid carcinomas are intermediate with 35 percent, and small cell carcinomas do poorest at 5 percent. Operation is not indicated for small cell carcinomas because the operative mortality is greater than the five-year survival. The best prognosis occurs when the tumor is small, peripherally located, and in an upper lobe.

The results of attempted curative surgery are superior to radiotherapy alone. After radiotherapy the five-year survival was about 7 to 8 percent compared with 30 percent after surgical resection. In those with small cell carcinomas, however, 5 percent survived five years after radiotherapy, while none survived this time after resection. Radiotherapy is indicated for those in whom resection is contraindicated because of poor pulmonary function or other diseases. It also provides useful palliation in those with distant metastases, local advanced disease, superior caval obstruction, and painful bony metastases. An obstructed bronchus, causing atelectasis and sepsis, can be opened in about 40 percent of cases. Multimodal therapy with surgery, radiotherapy, and immuno-chemotherapy in early cases may well produce the favorable results seen in other types of cancer.

Metastatic Tumors of the Lung

With few exceptions secondary tumors reach the lungs by the pulmonary arterial blood and may be multiple, bilateral, spherical, peripheral, or solid. Diffuse lymphatic permeation with or without pleural effusion may occur from tumors in the breast, stomach, prostate, pancreas, as well as primarily from lung. Direct pleural invasion from breast cancer is common but does not involve the lung parenchyma. About 10 percent of all metastatic pulmonary lesions are solitary, and in one half of these it is

Table 30-9. COMMON LESIONS OF THE LUNG*

NEOPLASMS	INFLAMMATORY LESIONS	PARASITIC LESIONS
Primary carcinoma	Tuberculoma and tuberculous	Hydatid cysts
Solitary metastases	lesions	*Ascaris lumbricoides*
Bronchial adenoma	Histoplasmosis	Mycetoma
Reticuloses	Coccidioidomycosis	*Malformations*
Neurogenic tumors	Cryptococcosis	Arteriovenous malformation
Mesothelioma	Nonspecific granuloma	Sequestrated segment
Leiomyoma	Chronic lung abscess	*Infarct*
Plasmacytoma	Lipoid pneumonia	
Endometriosis	Rheumatoid granuloma	

* A circumscribed, solitary, peripheral lung mass is termed a "coin lesion." It can be neoplastic, inflammatory, parasitic, congenital, or even an infarct.

the only known metastatic site. In patients with a known primary cancer it is often difficult to determine if the pulmonary lesion is a primary lung tumor or a metastasis. A list of the more common causes of coin lesions is given in Table 30–9. Solid metastatic lesions are asymptomatic which helps to exclude certain inflammatory conditions. Knowing the cell type of the original primary lesion may be helpful. If it were squamous, then a solitary lung lesion appearing later has a less than 50 percent chance of being metastatic. If it were adenocarcinoma, the chances are equal that the solitary lesion is either metastatic or a primary lung tumor. If the original primary was a sarcoma, the likelihood is high that a solitary lung lesion is metastatic.

The treatment of solitary lung lesions that appear after treatment of cancer elsewhere is surgical resection, but certain guidelines must be followed. First, the solitary nature of the lesion should be confirmed by tomography. Second, the primary disease must be controlled, and there should be no evidence of other metastatic spread. Finally, there should be a clear interval of three to six months since treatment of the primary tumor. Further waiting is not warranted since the lung lesion may be a new primary lung cancer and not a metastasis.

Resection of multiple metastatic lesions, segmental resection of recurrences, and even simultaneous bilateral thoracotomies have been employed. The results in patients with metastatic sarcomas are sometimes gratifying. Such extremes of therapy are justified when dealing with younger patients with an otherwise hopeless prognosis.

DISEASES OF THE MEDIASTINUM

The mediastinum must be considered separately because of the vital structures that it contains and its position within the bony framework of the thorax. The chief conditions of surgical importance are mediastinitis and tumors. In addition to posteroanterior and lateral roentgenograms of the chest, oblique views help to locate lesions anteriorly or posteriorly. Fluoroscopy determines if a mass pulsates, and a barium esophagram may locate a lesion by its deflection or intraluminal distortions. Tomography helps to locate masses accurately and can demonstrate calcification not seen on routine roentgenograms. Isotope studies include ^{131}I scans to demonstrate substernal thyroid extensions and ^{67}Ga scans to identify lymphomatous masses. Bronchoscopy permits visualization of primary endobronchial lesions and distortion of the tracheobronchial tree. Angiography may be indicated, especially if the mass is possibly an aneurysm or arteriovenous malformation. Biopsy material may be obtained at mediastinoscopy or at anterior mediastinotomy.

The mediastinum is divided into anterior, middle (visceral), and posterior (paravertebral) sections. Table 30–10 lists the chief space-occupying lesions of neoplastic, vascular, and congenital nature. Benign mediastinal tumors are usually asymptomatic and are discovered incidentally on x-rays but may cause cough, dysphagia, and feelings of pressure. The chief indication for their removal is the possibility that they may be malignant. Malignant mediastinal tumors can produce severe local symptoms due to pressure on the tracheobronchial tree, major vessels, and esophagus. Teratomas are usually malignant and occasionally present with endocrine abnormalities. Thymomas are often malignant, and about one half of adults with thymomas have myasthenia gravis. The disease does not respond well to thymectomy when a tumor is present.

Mediastinitis can be acute or chronic. Infections may reach the mediastinum from the neck (suppurative adenitis or tonsillar abscess), abdomen (subphrenic abscess), or mediastinal nodes (staphylococcal pneumonia), or from perforation of the trachea or esophagus. The

Table 30–10. COMMON LOCATION OF TUMORS AND CYSTS IN THE MEDIASTINUM*

ANTERIOR MEDIASTINUM	MIDDLE MEDIASTINUM	PARAVERTEBRAL SULCI
Thymoma	Enterogenous cyst	Neurilemoma
Teratoma	Lymphoma	Neurofibroma
Lymphoma	Pleuropericardial cyst	Ganglioneuroma
Thymic cyst	Mediastinal granuloma	Neuroblastoma
Substernal thyroid	Thoracic duct cyst	Fibrosarcoma
Ascending aortic aneurysm	Metastatic tumors	Lymphoma
	Lipoma	Paraganglioma
		Pheochromocytoma
		Duplication of the esophagus

* Space-occupying lesions of the mediastinum can be neoplastic, vascular, or congenital. Tumors can be cystic or solid. Most lesions are characteristically located in one of the three principal compartments.

most frequent causes are perforations of the esophagus occurring spontaneously after vomiting or after endoscopy. Acute mediastinitis has a rapid clinical course with high fever, pain in the chest, back or upper abdomen, dyspnea, and tachycardia and is frequently fatal. There may be fullness in the neck, and crepitus may be present if a perforated viscus has resulted in subcutaneous emphysema. Chest roentgenograms show widening of the mediastinum and loss of the cardiac borders. Subcutaneous emphysema will be seen if the trachea or esophagus has been perforated. A hydropneumothorax may also be present with perforation of the esophagus. Needle aspiration of the chest shows the presence of acid gastric content. An esophagram using water-soluble contrast medium is mandatory to locate the perforation.

A perforation is treated by immediate repair and wide drainage, using a neck approach if the cervical esophagus is involved or being done through the chest if the perforation is at a lower level. If an abscess has developed, it is drained either from above using a low collar incision or from below through the bed of a paravertebral segment of rib.

Chronic mediastinitis usually results from extension of a tuberculous or fungal infection from a mediastinal lymph node. A nonspecific fibrosing mediastinitis of unknown etiology has also been described. Symptoms are pain, fever, dysphagia, and cough, and superior vena caval obstruction may be present. There are usually no abnormal physical findings unless an abscess is causing local pain and redness in the neck or back. Roentgenograms in chronic mediastinitis show a contracted mediastinal silhouette and flecks of calcium. Specific drugs are given if tuberculous or fungal disease is present. Surgery is indicated only for drainage of abscesses. Fibrosing mediastinitis has been treated with steroids with little success, but operation is not indicated.

HEART

Embryology

The heart develops from a single, straight, pulsating tube within the pericardial sac of the 21-day embryo. It then elongates, forming an S-shaped curve. The caudal portion will become the sinus venosae and atria, and the cephalad portion the ventricles and bulbus cordis. Within seven days the ventricular septum and the atrial septum primum separate the right and left circulations. The sinus venosae and superior cardinal vein incorporate and drain into the right atrium, and a large pulmonary vein, from the differentiating lung, enters the left atrium. The bulbus cordis becomes the common aortic root, which leads distally into the truncus arteriosus. In the final separation endocardial cushions grow inward, dividing the atria from the ventricles by valves, and the truncus separates longitudinally, forming the aortic and pulmonary roots. These two divisions connect with the remnants of the briefly appearing aortic arches and incorporate the fourth and sixth arches respectively into definitive aortic arch and pulmonary arteries. The whole process is completed by the fortieth day, or within a brief span of 20 days.

Anatomy

The anatomy of the coronary arteries is most important, and surgery of the coronary arterial circulation now comprises about one half of all cardiac surgery. The right and left coronary arteries arise from the sinuses of Valsalva at the root of the aorta. The left coronary artery gives rise to the septal branch that supplies the region containing the conducting bundle, the anterior descending branch that supplies the anterior wall of the left ventricle, and the circumflex artery that is distributed in the posterior walls of the left and right ventricles. The right coronary artery, which is usually larger than the left, supplies the right ventricle and anastomoses through its posterior descending branch with the left system. It also has important communication with the circumflex artery.

Most of the venous return is through the coronary sinus to the right atrium. The anterior cardiac veins, however, drain directly into the right atrium, and a small portion of the ventricular wall drains directly into the right ventricle via the thebesian veins.

Special Diagnostic Procedures

Special studies are indicated following an adequate physical examination. Roentgenographic studies include posterior, anterior and lateral, right and left oblique views, and a barium swallow to determine displacement of the esophagus. Angiography is performed as part of the cardiac catheterization study. For right-sided studies the catheter is usually inserted into the femoral vein and advanced into the right ventricle. For left-sided studies the catheter is introduced into the brachial or femoral artery and then passes into the aortic root, coronary ostia, and left ventricle (Figure 30–11). Pressures can be recorded and blood samples obtained for gas analysis within the heart chambers, roots of the great vessels, and the peripheral lung (wedge position). Intra-

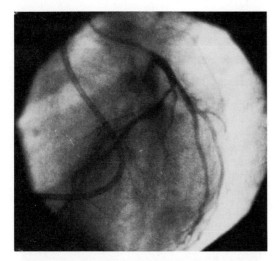

Figure 30–11. The coronary angiogram shows a high-grade obstruction in the left anterior descending coronary artery. A coronary bypass operation is indicated if intractable angina is present.

cardiac electrocardiography, phonocardiography, and cinematography are possible using special catheters.

Cardiopulmonary Bypass

Cannulation of the right atrium intercepts the venous inflow to the heart. The blood is drained either from the atrium directly or from the venae cavae, passed through an oxygenator, and then pumped under controlled conditions into the left-sided circulation: the aorta or a major artery such as the iliac. The aorta or pulmonary artery may then be occluded, establishing a total cardiopulmonary bypass. Only the partial bronchial venous return through the pulmonary veins and the venous return from the coronary circulation remain intact. These are drained from the left side by venting techniques. Intracardiac procedures are usually performed after stopping the heart beat by electrically induced fibrillation.

Congenital Lesions

Congenital lesions may be classified as those presenting with or without cyanosis. Cyanosis occurs when over 5 gm of reduced hemoglobin is present in 100 cm³ of blood. Minimal cyanosis is more readily recognized when there is capillary dilatation. The anatomic causes of desaturation of peripheral blood are a major venous-to-arterial or right-to-left shunt either in the heart or great vessels, or pulmonary factors reducing pulmonary blood flow or oxygenation in the pulmonary bed (Table 30–11). Congenital lesions

may also be classified according to the presence or absence of obstruction at the valves or in the major vessels. These are often associated with arterial-to-venous or left-to-right shunting of blood within the heart or the great vessels. A number of complex malformations have also been described.

In the tetralogy of Fallot there is a combination of a ventricular septal defect and obstruction to pulmonary outflow, producing a major right-to-left shunt with cyanosis. Other major malformations with cyanosis are transposition of the great vessels, tricuspid atresia, truncus arteriosus, and atresia or hypoplasia of the ascending aorta. Polycythemia with thrombosis and neurologic damage is a common sequel if these conditions are not treated.

Since left-sided pressures are higher at all levels, atrial, ventricular, or great vessel septal defects and aorticopulmonary communications result in left-to-right shunts. If untreated, serious overloading of the pulmonary vasculature produces irreversible pulmonary damage with cyanosis. The principal lesions are atrial (secundum and primum) and ventricular septal defects, atrioventricular canal, aorticopulmonary window, and patent ductus arteriosus. Total anomalous pulmonary drainage is clinically similar to atrial septal defects. The major obstructive lesions are stenosis of the pulmonary and aortic valves, coarctation of the aorta and muscular bands, or localized hypertrophy within the heart producing subpulmonic or subaortic

Table 30–11. THE MORE IMPORTANT CONGENITAL MALFORMATIONS OF THE HEART AND GREAT VESSELS

With Venous-Arterial Shunting	
Tetralogy of Fallot	Truncus arteriosus
Transposition of the great vessels	Atresia or hypoplasia of ascending aorta
Tricuspid atresia	

With Arterial-Venous Shunting	

Atrial septal defects
  Secundum defects
  Primum defects
	Aorticopulmonary window

	Patent ductus arteriosus
Ventricular septal defects	Anomalous pulmonary drainage
Atrioventricular canal	

With Obstruction	
Pulmonary stenosis	Coarctation of the aorta
Congenital aortic stenosis	Subpulmonic or subaortic stenosis

Complex Malformations	
Cor triatriatum	Anomalous origin left coronary vessel
Single ventricle	
Ebstein's anomaly	Congenital mitral stenosis
	Vascular rings

stenosis. The resulting cardiac hypertrophy can result in angina pectoris, cardiac failure, arrhythmias, and often sudden death.

Complex and rare malformations include cor triatriatum, single ventricle, Ebstein's anomaly, anomalous origin of the left coronary artery from the pulmonary artery, and congenital mitral stenosis. Defective development of the aortic arch can produce vascular rings which obstruct the trachea.

Acquired Heart Disease

The surgery of acquired heart disease (exclusive of trauma) is chiefly the correction of mechanical valvular defects and bypass of coronary artery stenosis. The latter accounts for about one half of all open cardiac procedures. Souttar performed the first intracardiac procedure in 1927. He unsuccessfully attempted to correct mitral stenosis by mechanical dilatation of the valve using a transventricular approach. In 1947 Bailey and Harken, working independently, corrected mitral stenosis by inserting a finger via the atrial appendix and fracturing the fused commissures. Initial results were encouraging, but stenosis often recurred and mitral insufficiency was sometimes produced. With the introduction of cardiopulmonary bypass more precise anatomic correction was accomplished by dividing the commissures and subvalvular fusions. In the early 1960s total valve replacement was performed using caged ball valves.

Mitral Stenosis. In mitral stenosis of rheumatic origin there are thickening and shortening of the leaflets of the valves and a fusion of the subvalvular chordae. The left atrial pressure increases and the chamber enlarges. The lungs become congested, leading to right heart strain and failure and often atrial fibrillation. Irreversible pulmonary vascular changes occur when pulmonary hypertension is of long standing. The first symptom is dyspnea, but later there are orthopnea, hemoptysis, and pulmonary edema. Peripheral embolism may occur as a result of dislodgment of clot from the fibrillating left atrium. The typical murmur is a diastolic rumble over the mitral valve. Chest roentgenograms and electrocardiograms are characteristic, and cardiac catheterization reveals a pressure gradient across the valve. Surgical correction produces good results only if preexisting cardiac and pulmonary damage is not severe.

Mitral Insufficiency. The most frequent cause of primary mitral insufficiency is rheumatic fever; less common are bacterial endocarditis, traumatic rupture of chordae, and myocardial infarction. Insufficiency may also occur from dilatation of the valvular annulus secondary to myocardiopathy. The combination of mitral stenosis and insufficiency on a rheumatic basis is common. The left ventricle ejects a portion of its output back into the left atrium. Both chambers enlarge, and pulmonary hypertension and left ventricular failure occur. The clinical features are fatigue, dyspnea, and palpitation, and with the onset of ventricular failure, there are paroxysmal nocturnal dyspnea and pulmonary edema. The murmur is systolic and apical. Roentgenography shows an enlarged left atrium and ventricle, and the electrocardiogram shows hypertrophy of both chambers. On cardiac catheterization a large regurgitant or pressure wave is seen in the left atrium, and cineangiography reveals free regurgitation of dye across the valve. Treatment in most patients is prosthetic replacement of the mitral valve. Annuloplastic repair can be carried out in a few younger patients.

Aortic Stenosis. Aortic stenosis is rheumatic in origin in about one half of patients. In the remainder it is the result of a congenital bicuspid valve or of atherosclerosis, usually also associated with extensive coronary atherosclerosis. The valve aperture is reduced by two thirds or more, producing ventricular systolic hypertension and a gradient across the valve. Concentric hypertrophy of the ventricle sustains cardiac output for a prolonged period. When failure occurs, ventricular end diastolic and left atrial pressures rise, with ensuing pulmonary edema. Symptoms may be mild or absent until late. Angina due to coronary insufficiency is present two to three years before frank decompensation. Syncope and sudden death from arrhythmia or rapid cardiac failure are the most frequent terminal events. Physical examination, x-rays, and electrocardiograms show massive left ventricular hypertrophy. A prominent precordial pulsation and an aortic thrill are felt. The pathognomonic murmur is a harsh systolic ejection sound heard over the aortic valve and transmitted into the neck. The peripheral pulse is weak and slowly rising (pulsus parvus and tardus). On cardiac catheterization extreme ventricular systolic hypertension is noted together with a gradient of 100 to 150 mm mercury across the valve. An elevated end diastolic pressure indicates a failing ventricle. Valve replacement is only for patients with high gradients or who have had symptoms of failure or coronary insufficiency, such as angina or syncope. Patients with mild gradients should be observed carefully and surgery should be deferred.

Aortic Insufficiency. The most common etiology is valvular damage due to rheumatic fever. Less common causes are congenital defects, bacterial endocarditis with leaflet perforation, dissecting aortic aneurysm, syphilis, and Marfan's syndrome. The changes produced in the valve by rheumatic fever are similar to those in the mitral valve. In endocarditis vegetations destroy part of the leaflets. A dissecting aneurysm deforms the annulus and prevents coaptation of the leaflets. Free regurgitation of blood places the left ventricle under great strain. This is compensated for by ventricular dilatation and hypertrophy, but eventually decompensation occurs, the ventricle dilates, end diastolic pressure rises, and pulmonary edema ensues. The patient develops palpitations, dyspnea, and angina and often excessive sweating. An enlarged heart with precordial heave is present on physical examination, together with a high-pitched diastolic decrescendo murmur along the left sternal border. The peripheral pulse is bounding (water hammer) due to the high systolic and low diastolic pressures. Capillary pulsation in the nail beds may be visible. Electrocardiograms and chest x-rays confirm the left ventricular strain. There may be no abnormality on cardiac catheterization if the disease is compensated, but left ventricular end diastolic pressures are elevated in decompensation. Cineangiography, however, shows regurgitation across the valve even in early cases. Valve replacement is indicated only when symptoms occur, and early operation is then necessary because of the rapid downhill course.

Tricuspid Disease. Tricuspid disease can be organic or functional. When it is organic, stenotic, or regurgitant, it is nearly always rheumatic in origin and is associated in 15 to 30 percent with mitral or aortic valvular disease. Functional tricuspid insufficiency in an anatomically undamaged valve is quite common as a result of right ventricular hypertension and dilatation. The increase in right atrial pressure results in hepatomegaly and ascites. In tricuspid regurgitation the liver pulsates, an hepatojugular reflex is present, as is a diastolic murmur at the lower end of the sternum. Tricuspid stenosis features a systolic murmur that is louder on inspiration. Right heart catheterization discloses an elevated right atrial pressure, a gradient across the valve when it is stenotic, and a prominent V wave when it is regurgitant. Cineangiography provides the best evidence of tricuspid insufficiency. Tricuspid stenosis should be treated surgically by commissurotomy or valve replacement during open heart operation for left-sided valvular disease. Treatment of tricuspid insufficiency, however, is controversial, most often annuloplasty being performed at the time of a major left heart valve operation.

Cardiac Trauma

Cardiac trauma results from penetrating injuries (knives, picks), perforating missiles (bullets, flying fragments), or direct contusing blows upon the anterior chest (steering wheels). Rarely do blast compressions or sudden decelerations of vehicles injure the heart, although the lungs and great vessels may be damaged. Since the heart is located anteriorly in the mediastinum, it is readily damaged by injuries to the sternum or precordial region. The thin-walled right ventricle lies deep to this region Sharp penetrations can be associated with survival because the pressure is low in this chamber. Perforations that extend deeply and into the high-pressure left ventricle rarely permit survival. A contusing and penetrating injury may damage not only the myocardial wall but also a coronary vessel, the septum, atria, intrapericardial portions of pulmonary arteries, or the conducting system.

The pathophysiology varies with the injury. In the most frequent event, penetration of the right ventricle or intrapericardial pulmonary artery, blood at a low pressure fills the pericardium. Tamponade occurs when 150 to 250 ml of blood has collected. Right atrial return is compromised, and shock develops within minutes to hours. Attenuation of heart tones, reduction in pulse pressure, dilated neck veins, and a rising central venous pressure are pathognomonic, though chest roentgenograms and electrocardiograms are often normal. The diagnosis is confirmed by pericardiocentesis. The needle is inserted immediately below the xiphoid process and the blood aspirated. Intravenous fluids are given rapidly to improve right heart filling. If the laceration is small, single or multiple aspirations may be adequate treatment since the low-pressure leak may seal spontaneously. If this measure fails, the patient should have immediate surgery. The atria are rarely penetrated since they lie posteriorly.

A massive hemothorax develops when the lacerating injury penetrates the pleural space. This produces the picture of hemorrhagic shock rather than tamponade. Blood pressure and central venous pressure are low, and the chest x-ray shows a massive effusion. Immediate blood replacement, chest tube drainage, and prompt operation are indicated.

Patients with penetrating wounds of the left ventricle rarely reach the hospital emergency room because of the high pressure of the escaping blood and the extensive myocardial disruption. Contusing injuries may also be fatal due to extensive damage to cardiac muscle. Progressive and intractable cardiac failure is present, and electrocardiograms show a pattern of massive infarction. Intra-aortic balloon pumping, a technique designed to relieve systolic load, has been applied with equivocal results.

Contusions or penetrations may injure a coronary vessel. The clinical presentation is that of an evolving myocardial infarction. Operation may be necessary to repair the myocardium, to repair a coronary artery, or to ligate the vessel and perform a coronary artery bypass graft. A delayed complication of a contusion injury is infarction of the intraventricular septum. Several days to weeks after the injury the patient may suddenly develop the picture of intraventricular septal defect requiring urgent repair. A ventricular aneurysm could also occur. A penetrating injury may rarely injure a cardiac valve.

Small foreign body missiles lodged in the heart need not be removed because they rarely erode or embolize. The chief indication for removal is the patient's anxiety.

Coronary Artery Disease

The most frequent acquired cardiac disease amenable to surgical treatment is segmental stenosis of the coronary arteries. Fully one half of all procedures requiring cardiopulmonary bypass are designed to relieve coronary obstructions. This is partially a response to a vast problem. Among Americans aged 18 to 79, there are 3.1 million with definite coronary artery disease and 2.4 million in whom coronary artery disease is suspected—that is, about 5 percent of all adults. Historically a large number of procedures such as internal mammary artery ligation, talc poudrage of the heart, and ligation of the coronary sinus have been performed and discredited. Vineberg in 1955 suggested tunneling the internal mammary artery through the ischemic ventricular muscle, and this procedure is still performed today. In 1966 Kahn and in 1967 Favoloro performed the first direct anastomoses between the ascending aorta and a patent coronary artery distal to an obstructive lesion using a segment of saphenous vein. This was made possible by Sones' development of coronary angiography. These advances produced an avalanche of surgery probably unequalled in the history of the art; nearly 30,000 bypass procedures were performed in 1974. They also produced one of the sharpest controversies to divide the profession. Basic questions are whether coronary bypass, although admittedly palliative for angina, could extend life and whether the surgery was worth the risk, morbidity, and cost. Advocates of medical therapy do not feel that it is. Most recent studies of groups of patients comparable in both age and extent of coronary disease indicate that at three

years' survival in surgical patients is 90 percent, while survival in medically treated patients is about 70 percent. Controlled and random prospective studies have not been performed. Long-term graft patency and the biologic fate of the grafts are still unknown. The recent procedure of directly anastomosing the internal mammary artery to the coronary arteries may answer these questions. The underlying disease of atherosclerosis is not affected by any procedure, however well conceived and executed.

The primary indication for coronary bypass surgery is stable and intractable angina without myocardial infarction. Crescendo angina, recent and increasingly severe, is also an urgent indication. Preinfarction angina, which refers to chest pain and electrocardiographic changes that do not abate with rest, oxygen, or vasodilators, is an emergency indication for surgery. Some feel that myocardial infarction should be treated by coronary bypass and infarctectomy. Myocardial failure without angina is sometimes due to "silent" coronary obstruction.

Coronary angiography is mandatory in all cases. The precise points of obstruction must be visualized and adequate vessels to accept the graft must be present distal to the obstruction. One, two, or three of the main vessels may be involved, such as the right, the left anterior descending, or the circumflex coronary artery (Figure 30–11). About 20 percent of patients with clinical angina do not have detectable coronary obstructions on angiography. Obstructive disease occurs in a single vessel in only about 20 percent of cases. Thus, 80 percent of patients receive from two to as many as five grafts. Patients with diffuse obliterative disease or with extensive myocardial fibrosis with failure are not good surgical candidates.

Previous myocardial infarction is not a contraindication to operation. A graft, however, should not be inserted into a vessel supplying an infarct scar, even though the vessel is open on angiography. The ejection fraction of the left ventricle (fraction of the diastolic volume ejected at full systole) is often improved by bypass surgery alone and may be considerably improved if an associated ventricular aneurysm is resected. Coronary bypass procedures are frequently performed in conjunction with valve surgery, especially aortic valve replacement. Some surgeons will also combine a bypass procedure with an internal mammary implant (Vineberg procedure) in selected cases.

Although the final evaluation of coronary bypass is not yet possible, certain facts are presently clear. It relieves angina dramatically in the majority of cases, unquestionably improves myocardial function by improving blood flow, and betters the length and quality of survival. The underlying disease process, however, is unaffected, making careful medical management a continuing requirement.

Pericarditis

Inflammation of the pericardial sac can be acute, chronic, adhesive, or constrictive. Acute inflammation can follow operation (postcardiotomy syndrome), be associated with metabolic disorders (uremia, myxedema), rheumatic fever, neoplasms, or with bacterial, viral, or tuberculous infection. Clinically there are persistent substernal pain, fever, malaise, leukocytosis, and a friction rub. The electrocardiogram will show S-T segment deviation and a deep S wave. Pyogenic or viral pericarditis tends to result in a large effusion and sometimes tamponade. In nonspecific pericarditis the treatment is rest, sedation, aspirin, and systemic steroids. Repeated pericardiocentesis is necessary if there is a large effusion, and, if indicated, antibiotics can be inserted through the same needle. Tuberculous pericarditis can be treated in the acute phase by antituberculous medication and early partial pericardiectomy. This prevents the development of chronic constrictive pericarditis and a more difficult surgical procedure at a later date. Drainage by pericardiotomy (window operation) may be indicated to control a life-threatening pyogenic or neoplastic effusion. A subdiaphragmatic approach is used to avoid contaminating the pleural space.

Tuberculosis causes constrictive pericarditis in only 20 percent of patients; in the remainder, the etiology is unknown. The peak incidence is in young adults. The parietal and visceral layers of the pericardial sac are thickened and generally fused, but pockets of fluid may be present. Patients are dyspneic, easily fatigable, and have hepatomegaly, ascites, dilated peripheral veins, and often a paradoxical pulse. The picture resembles congestive heart failure, but the heart is either normal or only slightly enlarged on chest x-rays. Stroke volume is decreased, diastolic filling impaired, the pressure in the right heart is increased, and the electrocardiogram shows low voltage with T-wave inversion. The presence of a calcific "eggshell" is pathognomonic. Only excision of the pericardium, usually through a median sternotomy, relieves the progressive symptoms. Partial cardiopulmonary bypass has recently reduced the risk of surgery and improved results.

Pacemakers

Complete heart block with AV dissociation and Adams-Stokes seizures is the main indication for permanent cardiac pacing. Life expectancy is less than three years. Fibrosis with damage to function of the conduction system is generally a disease of aging and may be associated with coronary artery disease. It may be congenital, occur in rheumatic carditis, or follow open cardiac surgery. When it develops in myocardial infarction, the need for pacing is not permanent. Indications for pacing have been expanded to include heart block that is not causing seizures but may cause heart failure or be responsible for fatigue, claudication, and even sexual impotency. Other indications are a bradycardia below 45 beats per minute, even without symptoms, and tachyrhythmias which may be dangerous. Over 125,000 pacemakers are now in use in North America. Transvenous pacing is the preferred technique except during cardiac surgery when electrodes are directly placed. Under local anesthesia and with fluoroscopic control, the wire catheter is inserted usually into the cephalic vein and advanced to the apex of the right ventricle. The electrocardiogram derived from the catheter tip ensures proper positioning. Threshold current measurements are taken to assure good electrical coupling to the endocardium. The pacemaker, or pulse generator, is then buried, under local anesthesia, in a skin pocket.

The two principal pacemakers are the fixed rate and the demand or standby types. With the latter the electrical impulse is not delivered unless the heart rate drops below a predetermined level, and this conserves battery power in patients with intermittent block. More important, however, it avoids delivering a pulse during the vulnerable period of the cardiac cycle when there is a slight risk of causing fibrillation. Some pacemakers sense the atrial P wave as a trigger for pulse delivery.

Pacemaker failure is a cause of constant concern. Battery life is usually 20 to 24 months but this cannot be relied upon. Recently developed isotope-powered units have much longer lives. The rate usually decreases as battery power is decreasing but with one type it increases. Other problems are case leakage, catheter breakage, and increasing electrical resistance at the catheter tip. Clearly, function must be monitored at predetermined intervals for replacement of the pulse generator or catheter. This can be done at hospital visits or, more conveniently, in the patient's home by using an electrocardiogram transmitter. Two self-attached wrist electrodes are inserted into the transmitter, which uses the telephone to communicate the signal to a central facility. The physician receives periodic reports and is alerted immediately in cases of rapid change in pacemaker function.

Temporary pacing is used largely in emergencies, such as heart block following myocardial infarction, cardiac surgery, or to resuscitate the patient with a Adams-Stokes attack. An immediate high-voltage external current can be delivered through the skin directly overlying the heart, but for only short periods because of the danger of burning the skin. A percutaneous wire electrode inserted into the mycocardium permits the use of a lower voltage. This technique is for short-term use only. If a complete or partial block is present following cardiac surgery, wire electrodes are sutured to the myocardium and led out through the skin. They can be cut flush and allowed to retract when no longer required.

When longer periods of pacing are required, a "floating" wire catheter is inserted into the antecubital or femoral vein and advanced into the right ventricle under electrocardiographic control. This equipment, including a battery-powered external pulse generator, is present on most emergency carts. The need for pacing may arise at any time in the operating room or coronary care unit. Temporary pacing is used prophylactically during coronary angiography and to protect patients with heart block and bradycardia who are undergoing elective major surgery. In most of these situations the demand mode is employed since the block is either temporary or anticipated. Because of prior indications patients coming to permanent pacemaker implantation usually already have temporary pacer wires in position. In fact temporary pacing is often used to evaluate the benefit of pacing before permanent pacemaker insertion.

Complications of temporary pacing that do not occur with permanent implantation are infection at the point of wire insertion, knotting of the thinner wire, loss of contact at the electrode tip, and arrhythmias. Perforation of the right ventricle by the electrode tip is not common but is also not serious. Tamponade does not occur unless the patient is anticoagulated. Intravenous lidocaine is used if dangerous tachycardias appear.

SUGGESTIONS FOR FURTHER READING

Comroe, Julius H.; Forster, Robert E. II; Dubois, Arthur R.; Briscoe, William A.; and Carlsen, Elizabeth: *The Lung*. Year Book Medical Publishers, Chicago, 1962.
This book has become a standard reference for students of pulmonary physiology. The theory and clinical applications of ventilation, circulation, and diffusion of gases are covered.

Gibbon, John H. (ed.): *Surgery of the Chest*. W. B. Saunders Co., Philadelphia, 1962.
The surgical management of chest diseases is treated by the most prominent authors. The text material and illustrations, exclusive of cardiac surgery, can be regarded as the best currently available.

Harken, D. E., and Clauss, R. H.: Valvular heart disease; tumors, pericardium and resuscitation. In: Blades, Brian (ed.): *Surgical Diseases of the Chest*. C. V. Mosby Co., St. Louis, p. 431, 1974.
A comprehensive review of these subjects including their management.

Hinshaw, H. Corwin, and Garland, L. Henry: *Diseases of the Chest*. W. B. Saunders Co., Philadelphia, 1963.
Many diseases of the chest are treated optionally by either medical or surgical intervention. The authors present a medical viewpoint.

Shields, Thomas W. (ed.): *General Thoracic Surgery*. Lea & Feibiger, Philadelphia, 1972.
A current and most comprehensive work covering all aspects of thoracic surgery, exclusive of cardiac surgery.

Taussig, Helen B.: *Congenital Malformations of the Heart*. Harvard University Press, Cambridge, 1960.
A classic and still the definitive treatise on the pathologic anatomy and pathophysiology of congenital heart disease.

Chapter 31

PERIPHERAL VASCULAR SURGERY

Worthington G. Schenk, Jr.

CHAPTER OUTLINE

Place of Surgery in the Management of
    Vascular Disease
Trauma
Arterial Embolism
Arteriosclerotic Occlusive Disease
    Lower Extremity
        Treatment
    Carotid Vertebral Occlusions
    Renal Occlusive Disease
    Arteriosclerotic Aneurysm of the
        Abdominal Aorta
    Visceral Mesenteric Atherosclerotic
        Disease

Lumbar Sympathectomy
Thoracic Sympathectomy
Thoracic Outlet Syndrome
Buerger's Disease
Arteritis
Veins
    Thrombophlebitis
    Varicose Veins
Amputations
Frostbite

PLACE OF SURGERY IN THE MANAGEMENT OF VASCULAR DISEASE

The proper management of blood vessels is the key to all successful surgery. This includes hemostasis without which surgery cannot be performed, the identification and ligation of those vessels required to successfully perform a surgical procedure, and the preservation of those vessels essential to the preservation of life and organ. The place that any treatment has in the management of a disease changes as knowledge increases. The present role of surgery in the management of arterial and venous disease is indicated in Table 31–1.

TRAUMA

As the number and speed of vehicles increase, vascular injuries will assume greater importance. The common lesions are the result of blunt trauma, penetrating injuries, such as stab or gunshot wounds, or complications of displaced fractures and dislocations. External or concealed hemorrhage may occur and may compromise or cause loss of an extremity or organ. The first-aid management of a bleeding, open vascular injury is to control hemorrhage. Most often this can be done by firm external pressure, either digitally or by using a compress. A tourniquet is rarely required to control arterial bleeding from an extremity. In the upper extremity the pressure must exceed 250 mm Hg pressure and in the lower extremity 350 mm Hg pressure. If applied as a narrow band, underlying structures are damaged. A broad band surgical tourniquet is rarely available at the site of first-aid treatment, and in a hospital or clinic it is usually possible to institute more definitive treatment. Perhaps the commonest error is to apply a tourniquet at a pressure less than arterial to control venous bleeding. The tourniquet permits arterial inflow but obstructs venous return and hence greatly increases the venous blood loss. Blood loss will decrease or stop when the tourniquet is removed. Venous bleeding from a leg or arm can often be controlled by elevating the wound above the level of the heart. Venous pressure is removed, the vessel collapses, and bleeding ceases. Blood loss from a defect in the aorta, left ventricle, or at any other site can generally be controlled by digital pressure over the defect. If external pressure does not control hemorrhage in a deep open wound, a hand should be inserted and control obtained by manual pressure. This will introduce contamination in the absence

Table 31–1. SURGERY IN THE MANAGEMENT OF VASCULAR DISEASE

DEFINITIVE	GENERALLY ACCEPTED BUT UNDER STUDY	EXPERIMENTAL
Arterial		
Trauma—lacerations	Sympathectomy for	Visceral occlusive
False aneurysms	extremity occlusive disease	disease
AV fistulas	Carotid-vertebral	Mesenteric
Embolectomy	reconstruction	Coronary
(extremity)	Renal occlusive disease	Embolectomy-
Lower extremity	especially with hypertension	pulmonary
occlusive disease		Congenital AV
		fistulas (cirsoid
		aneurysms)
Venous		
Trauma	Varicose veins	Caval interruption
	stripping	Compartmentation
		Filters (for emboli)
		Vein reconstructions
		Femoral valves
		Portosystemic shunts
		Venous thrombectomy

of aseptic technique but can prevent death from exsanguination.

A high incidence of suspicion regarding vascular injury should be based on the following six points:

1. The location of trauma, either open or closed, may suggest a vascular injury (Figure 31–1).

2. Evidence of major blood loss, either external or internal.

3. Absence of a pulse distal to a point of suspected vascular injury confirms a serious vascular injury. The presence of pulses offers no assurance that vascular injury has not occurred, as the injury may cause delayed thrombosis.

4. Reduced skin temperature or cyanosis of an extremity.

5. Hypesthesia or anesthesia of an extremity.

6. Marked swelling in the region of injury.

When a vascular injury is suspected, an angiogram may be obtained to confirm the diagnosis or the vessel may be explored surgically. The manner in which the most common vascular injuries occur is shown in Figure 31–2 and the types of injury in Figure 31–3.

Spasm of a vessel is perhaps the most treacherous of all diagnoses to make. It may cause the physician to adopt an unjustifiably optimistic attitude. The condition can occur but is exceedingly rare. Vascular contusion varies from a small swelling in the wall to complete occlusion. There is often an associated tear in the intima that acts as a valve and completely occludes the lumen. A vessel may be partially or completely disrupted. The anatomic defect of arteriovenous fistula usually is not seen immediately after a vascular injury but is identified weeks or months later. A side-by-side injury occurs in an artery and a vein; the arterial blood takes the path of least resistance and enters the vein, forming an arteriovenous fistula. High-output cardiac failure may result if the flow through the communication is large.

When a vascular injury is suspected or has been confirmed, operation should be performed promptly. A sufficient quantity of cross-matched blood should be available to replace losses that may occur during surgery.

At operation, *proximal and distal control* of the involved vessels should be obtained before the injured area is approached (Figure 31–4). A penetrating knife, stick, or other protruding missile which is still in place should be left undisturbed until definitive surgical treatment is undertaken. Massive and uncontrollable hemorrhage may occur on removing the foreign object that is acting as a tampon.

Once proximal and distal control has been achieved, the site of vascular injury is explored. In deciding how to manage the injury, expendable vessels must be considered (Figures 31–5). Most arteries can be ligated without risk to life, limb, or organ. A vascular reconstruction may be required later. There is an increased risk of sepsis and hemorrhage if a vascular repair is done in an open wound. For the vessels that cannot be sacrificed, some type of reconstruction must be carried out immediately (Figure 31–6). Generally puncture wounds and short lacerations can be repaired by direct suture. An end-to-end anastomosis can be done of a completely divided vessel. In low-velocity missile wounds the area of vascular damage can be excised and the vessel repaired by end-to-end anastomosis. In most vessels as much as 2 cm can be removed and an end-to-end anastomosis accomplished. An extensive intramural hematoma with intimal disruption and thrombosis is treated by excising the involved segment and reestablishing the circulation with autogenous tissue, most frequently the saphenous vein.

Prosthetic materials have proven unsuccessful in the management of open vascular injuries because of the high incidence of sepsis, thrombosis of the reconstructed vessel, or rupture of the suture line and exsanguination. For closed vascular injuries prosthetic materials may be used but are not as successful as autogenous tissue.

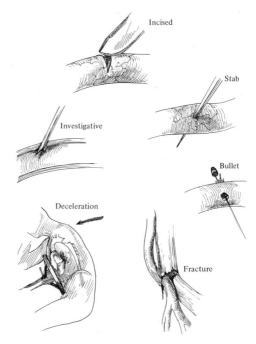

Figure 31-2. Vascular trauma may result from steering column of car, needle puncture, knife wound, impalement, bullet wound, or complicating fracture.

An arteriovenous fistula is usually repaired by dividing and ligating the involved vein. The defect in the artery is repaired by direct suture.

ARTERIAL EMBOLISM

Surgery plays an important role in the treatment of arterial embolism. Arterial emboli lodge at sites of bifurcations or at the origin of major branches (Figure 31-7). Examples are the bifurcation of the aorta, common iliac, and common femoral arteries and the trifurcation of the popliteal and brachial arteries. There is serious question as to whether carotid arterial emboli should be removed, because even under optimum conditions the embolus cannot be excised fast enough to prevent cerebral damage, often with some brain softening. If this has occurred, removal of the embolus with restoration of a full head of arterial pressure to damaged cerebral tissue can result in cerebral hemorrhage with much greater destruction of cerebral tissue. For the aorta and extremity emboli mentioned earlier, the diagnosis can be suspected from the history of sudden pain in the involved extremity followed by numbness and paralysis. On physical examination there will be obvious ischemia of the part with appropriate pulse losses, which in general will localize the

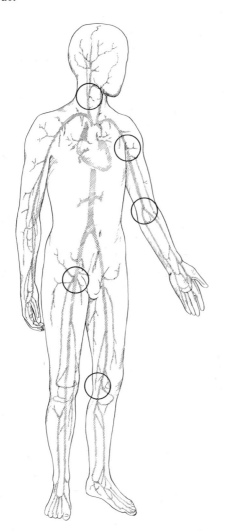

Figure 31-1. The common sites of vascular injury are the neck, axilla, front of elbow, groin, and posterior aspect of the knee.

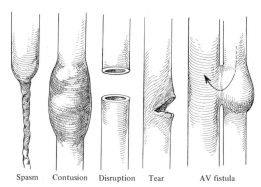

Figure 31–3. Anatomic defects that may result from arterial trauma: diffuse spasm, thrombosis, complete division, laceration with incomplete division, and arteriovenous fistula.

site of embolism so accurately that arteriographic study is superfluous and time wasting. The immediate management as soon as the diagnosis is made or suspected is systemic heparinization of the patient to prevent thrombosis in the small distal arterial channels. If this is not prevented, distal arterial thrombosis may militate against successful revascularization of the limb even though the major proximal embolus has been successfully removed. There is no firm deadline in hours beyond which embolectomy should not be done, but the sooner

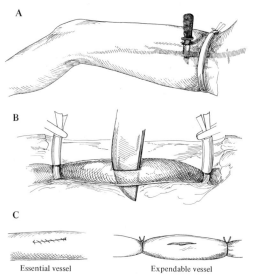

Figure 31–4. Control of hemorrhage from (*A*) penetrating knife wound, (*B*) proximal and distal control of vessel by tourniquets before withdrawal of the knife, and (*C*) direct suture repair of essential vessel or sacrifice of an expendable vessel.

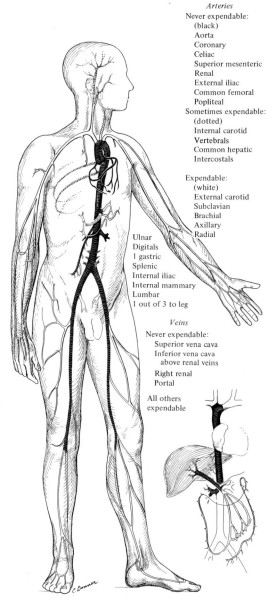

Figure 31–5. Arteries that cannot be ligated are shown as dark.

it can be performed, the more successful the outcome (Figure 31–8, *A*). Success rates over 85 percent in terms of saving life and limb can be expected if the embolus is successfully extracted within eight hours of its lodgement. After eight hours the embolectomy should probably be performed up to as long as 48 hours, but understandably the success rate in limb survival will be significantly reduced.

A major contribution to improvement of

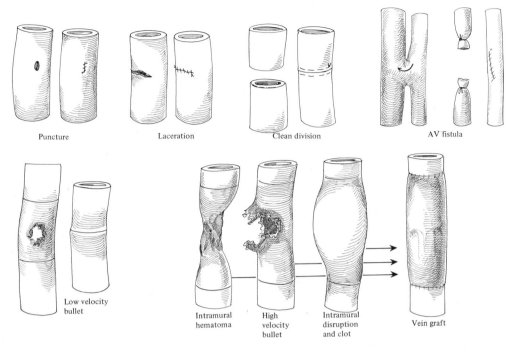

Puncture   Laceration   Clean division   AV fistula

Low velocity bullet   Intramural hematoma   High velocity bullet   Intramural disruption and clot   Vein graft

Figure 31–6. Vascular injuries and types of repair: puncture wound, direct suture; short laceration, direct suture; complete transection, end-to-end anastomosis; arteriovenous fistula, ligation and division of vein and arterial suture; low velocity missile, resection of up to 2 cm and end-to-end anastomosis; extensive intramural hematoma with intimal damage as well as large laceration and thrombosis, resection and insertion graft (most often saphenous vein).

morbidity and mortality in the management of arterial embolism was made by Fogarty (Figure 31–8, *B*). He developed a balloon-tipped catheter resembling a long ureteral catheter with an inflatable balloon at its distal end. The catheter can extract emboli lodged anywhere from the aortic bifurcation to the ankle. The common femoral artery is exposed under local anesthesia in the groin and proximal and distal control is obtained of the proposed site of arteriotomy. With the balloon deflated the catheter is inserted and the tip passed either around or through the clot as the catheter is inserted proximally or distally. The balloon is then filled with saline and the catheter extracted with the balloon distended, removing the embolus and any clot that may have propagated proximal and distal to it. Several passages are often required to remove all clots and to produce both good proximal arterial flow and good back bleeding from the distal arterial tree. Vessels in the upper extremity may be cleared of emboli and thrombi by introducing balloon catheters through the brachial artery exposed in the antecubital space under local anesthesia. Heparin may or may not be given after operation. Coumadin may be given indefinitely

when the source of the embolus was a fibrillating atrium.

ARTERIOSCLEROTIC OCCLUSIVE DISEASE

Lower Extremity

Perhaps the single most common clinical manifestation of atherosclerotic arterial disease is arterial insufficiency of the lower extremity. There is every reason to believe this a "diet-related" metabolic disease and hence preventable. However, once the atheroma have been deposited in the vessel wall with partial or complete arterial occusion, successful management is surgical.

The commonest site for atheromatous occlusion is the superficial femoral artery at the adductor hiatus in the lower third of the thigh. Another common location is the common iliac artery just distal to the aortic bifurcation. In addition, atheromatous occlusion may occur anywhere from the ankle to the renal arteries.

Patients present with claudication, that is with calf, thigh, or hip pain on exertion but no pain at rest, or with compromise of tissue, that is with pregangrenous changes usually in the toes,

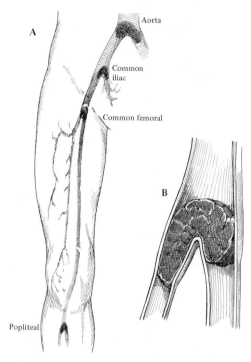

Figure 31–7. *A.* Common sites of embolism are bifurcations of the aorta, common iliac, common femoral, and popliteal arteries. *B.* Saddle thrombus at bifurcation of common femoral artery.

and accompanied by rest pain relieved only by dependency or exercise.

The characteristic finding on examination is that the distal part of the limb is cooler than the proximal part, that is, the toes are cooler than the heel and the heel is cooler than the knee. There is deep rubor of the foot on dependency and blanching on elevation. Frequently hair is absent from the extremity. Paradoxically the toenails become hypertrophic and thickened in the ischemic foot, while the skin becomes thin and atrophic. Pulses characteristically are absent in the distal portion of the extremity. It is often difficult to be sure whether or not a pulse is present at a given level. It is sometimes helpful to ask another examiner to palpate a pulse in the upper extremity. On counting, if 10 to 20 beats from the questionable distal pedal or popliteal pulse correspond with those in the upper extremity, then the pulse can be assumed to be present. The patient who presents with claudication may have pedal pulses. It is well to exercise the patient by jogging in place for several minutes and then repeat the examination, since exercise often results in loss of pedal pulses.

Auscultation in arterial occlusive disease may reveal the precise area of stenosis by the presence of a loud bruit. Sites to be regularly examined include the popliteal space, the superficial femoral artery at the adductor hiatus, and the common femoral artery at the inguinal ligament.

Clinical examination often gives a good lead as to the site of arterial stenosis or occlusion, but precise localization can only be obtained by arteriography, either by direct femoral puncture or aortography. For direct femoral puncture a #18 needle is inserted under local anesthesia, and 15 to 20 ml of contrast medium, usually 50 percent Hypaque, is injected. Since all the contrast media are painful on introduction into the arterial tree, the patient should be heavily sedated to prevent his sudden movement when the x-rays are taken. In occlusive disease two exposures at an internal of five to eight seconds are often necessary. This is because the dye reaches the distal patent arterial channel by collateral routes much more slowly than it would have reached it through the patent main arterial channel. It is this *distal patent channel* that is of crucial importance in an arterial reconstruction.

Aortography can be performed by direct needle puncture of the abdominal aorta through the left flank with the patient in the face-down position, or it can be done using the Seldinger technique by introducing a catheter either into

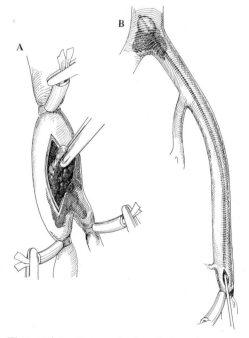

Figure 31–8. Removal of embolus at bifurcation of aorta. *A.* Embolectomy. *B.* Using Fogarty catheter.

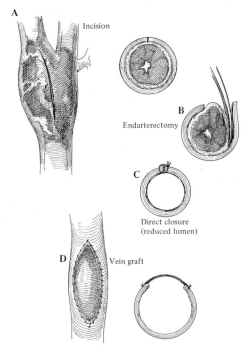

Figure 31–9. Technique of endarterectomy. Thrombosis of common carotid artery (*A*) treated by (*B*) endarterectomy, (*C*) without or (*D*) with application of a vein patch.

a femoral or brachial artery under local anesthesia and guiding the catheter into the aorta. The latter technique permits selective localization of the dye bolus within the aorta but occasionally results in arterial occlusion, perforation, or formation of a false aneurysm. Direct arteriographic study should be performed in almost every case of arterial insufficiency of the extremity.

Treatment. The three types of repair are endarterectomy, vein graft bypass, or prosthetic graft bypass.

In endarterectomy the atheroma along with the diseased intima and a portion of the media are removed from short segments of the artery (Figure 31–9). It has been particularly successful in obstruction of the common iliac artery and at the aortic bifurcation. Vein grafts, using most often the long saphenous vein but less commonly the cephalic vein, have been most successful in bypassing the obstructed superficial femoral artery (Figure 31–10). Prosthetic grafts have been most successful in bypassing the segment between the abdominal aorta and the common femoral artery when long segments have been occluded and endarterectomy does not appear feasible.

A salvage operation very helpful in poor-risk patients with unilateral iliac occlusive disease

has been the *crossover* graft. Under local anesthesia a graft, either saphenous vein or prosthesis, is placed between the common femoral on the side with a patent iliac system across the pubis subcutaneously to the common femoral on the occluded side. Axillofemoral grafts have also been used but not as successfully.

Recently arterial reconstruction has been performed using the implanted mandril technique and gas embolectomy. Sparks has developed a method whereby a very thin knitted dacron prosthesis, containing an inner silicone mandril, is inserted approximately where a bypass arterial reconstruction is planned. The most common sites are in preparation for femoropopliteal and axillofemoral bypasses. The prosthesis is left in position for six weeks during which it becomes infiltrated by ingrowth of host tissues. At a second operation the ends of the implanted prosthesis are dissected free, the central silicone mandril is removed, and the prosthesis is anastomosed, usually end-to-side, to the vessel above and below the segment to be bypassed. The advantages are the short time required for the second operation compared with that for dissection and insertion of a saphenous vein bypass and that the prosthesis in many ways resembles a normal artery. Disadvantages are the need for two operations and the six-week interval between them.

Sawyer has modified endarterectomy by introducing carbon dioxide gas into the vessel to separate the clot from the vessel wall. Its developers have had excellent results, but the procedure has not gained wide usage, suggesting that the technique is difficult to master.

Success rates for such reconstructions usually

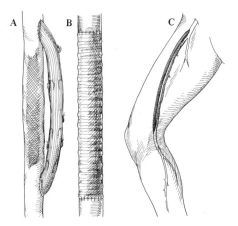

Figure 31–10. Thrombosis of superficial femoral artery (*A*) treated by (*B*) insertion of prosthetic graft or (*C*) autogenous long saphenous vein.

range around 80 percent for the initial procedure in restoring improved blood flow and approximately 50 percent patency after five years. This "failure" rate is undoubtedly in large part an expression of progression of the patient's atherosclerotic occlusive disease. Surgery does *not* cure atherosclerosis!

Carotid Vertebral Occlusions

The patient with carotid or vertebral occlusive disease may present with a complete stroke or a history of small strokes, that is, fainting, usually unilateral weakness, blindness, and aphasia clearing within minutes or hours. The carotid pulse is absent on the affected side, or an audible bruit on one or both sides indicates significant arterial narrowing. Only by arteriography can detailed knowledge of the distribution of the occlusive disease be obtained. Direct puncture of the common carotid arteries in the neck with injection of contrast medium excellently visualizes the common, internal, and external carotid vessels as well as the intracranial circulation. Aortic arch angiography, by introduction of a catheter with the Seldinger technique via a brachial or femoral artery, gives information about the subclavian arteries and the vertebrals as well as the origin of the carotids, but does not give the same degree of detail in the region of the carotid bifurcation. Operation is indicated when a significant unilateral stenosis is detected in the common carotid or at the origin of the internal carotid artery. Some consider that stenosis of a vertebral artery at its origin from the subclavian should be treated by operation; however, the results are not as good as with the carotid.

Operation can be under local or general anesthesia. The advantage with local anesthesia is that the patient can be asked to perform voluntary movements to be sure that cerebral blood flow is adequate during total carotid occlusion. Internal shunts, hypertensive drugs, and increased concentrations of carbon dioxide in the inhaled gas mixture have been used in an attempt to reduce postoperative complications when reconstruction is performed under general anesthesia. The surgical procedure usually consists of endarterectomy of the carotid bifurcation including the core, which usually extends a short distance up the internal carotid. The arteriotomy can usually be closed, but if this appears to produce stenosis, a vein patch graft can be used to close the arteriotomy (Figure 31–9).

Ninety-five percent of patients are improved by operation. However, it is difficult to evaluate patients with some neurologic deficit before operation because the natural course of the untreated disease involves improvement. However, in patients who had only transient phenomena preoperatively, their disappearance is evidence of the success of cerebral revascularization. The procedure has now been done a sufficient number of years for it to be established that the incidence of disabling strokes is less in patients who have had carotid stenosis treated by operation than in those treated conservatively.

Renal Occlusive Disease

The diagnosis of renovascular hypertension can only be made if patients with hypertension have renal arteriography. Physical examination is rarely helpful, and a bruit on auscultation over the renal area may be misleading. Split renal function studies have not been particularly helpful in detecting significant renal artery artery stenosis. The most useful chemical test is an increase in renin in the renal vein of the affected side.

A transabdominal approach is made to the stenotic renal vessel and an aortorenal bypass performed using an autogenous vein or prosthetic substitute. In about 20 percent reconstruction is not technically successful and nephrectomy must be performed. Hence it is important to be sure that the contralateral kidney is functioning adequately before attempting a unilateral reconstruction.

After reconstruction about one third become normotensive, another third have a reduced arterial pressure but are not normotensive, and roughly one third remain unchanged. Patients treated by nephrectomy have as good a chance of improvement as those with a successful reconstruction.

When hypertension is detected in a young female and coarctation has been excluded, the most likely renal arterial lesions responsible for the increase in pressure is fibromuscular hyperplasia. Unfortunately the condition is frequently bilateral so that complete surgical cure is not possible. However, if there is a significant difference between the two sides, unilateral reconstruction often results in improvement.

Bilateral nephrectomy and renal transplantation will play an increasing role in the management of hypertension. Particularly baffling, however, are the patients in whom hypertension persists *after* bilateral nephrectomy.

Arteriosclerotic Aneurysm of the Abdominal Aorta

Patients with an atherosclerotic aneurysm of the abdominal aorta may be asymptomatic or have flank, back, or abdominal pain. On physical examination the significant finding is a pulsatile abdominal mass. Only if both borders of the mass can be palpated is it definite that an aneurysm is present, since a tortuous abdominal aorta, particularly convex to the left, is occasionally misinterpreted as an abdominal aneurysm. Angiograms are rarely needed to confirm the presence and level of an abdominal aortic aneurysm since this can generally be outlined by palpation and defined by plain abdominal PA and lateral x-rays.

The indications for resection and prosthetic replacement are controversial. A symptomatic aneurysm should be resected regardless of the patient's age and complicating medical illnesses because the symptoms indicate progressive enlargement. The more difficult decision is in the patient who is found on routine examination to have a completely asymptomatic aneurysm. An aneurysm that is more than 6 cm at its widest point, on clinical examination, or on the PA x-ray is a greater hazard to the patient than a smaller aneurysm. The patient with significant cardiac or cerebral occlusive disease at the time an aneurysm is identified is more likely to die of his cardiac or cerebrovascular disease than from rupture of the aneurysm.

The most commonly employed procedure is excision of the infrarenal aortic aneurysm and reconstruction of the aorta with a prosthetic graft (Figure 31–11). Of growing interest is the use of an extravascular prosthetic graft. This should not be confused with the old and discredited technique of aneurysm wrapping with irritant substances, such as cellophane, which were hoped to provoke a fibrous reaction that would reinforce the aneurysm and prevent rupture. With external grafting the aneurysmal section of the vessel is freed from surrounding structures and is then completely encircled by a well-fitting prosthesis which is sewn in place over its external surface. This technique was

originally employed in poor-risk patients in whom interrupting circulation to the lower extremity, even temporarily, would carry high risk and in patients in whom the aneurysm extended above the renal vessels. The results have been so encouraging, however, that the indications for this procedure are increasing and now include the patient with the small aneurysm that is "too small to remove but too large to leave alone."

At least a 90 percent survival can be expected in patients having elective resection of abdominal aortic aneurysms. However, many do not survive the next five years because of atherosclerotic disease involving the coronary, cerebral, or renal vessels.

Frank rupture of an abdominal aortic aneurysm is a catastrophic illness in which survival can only be achieved by immediate surgical intervention. A number of patients present with rupture of a previously asymptomatic aneurysm. Resuscitation must be prompt with massive quantities of colloid and blood while prompt control of aortic inflow is being achieved by digital pressure until vascular clamps can be applied. Only about 20 percent of such patients reaching a hospital can be expected to survive.

Visceral Mesenteric Atherosclerotic Disease

Abdominal angina is postprandial abdominal pain resulting from superior mesenteric and celiac artery stenoses. Arterial stenosis has been demonstrated by angiographic techniques in a number of patients. The results of arterial reconstruction have been disappointing.

LUMBAR SYMPATHECTOMY

There is no uniformly successful clinical or laboratory test for selecting patients with arterial insufficiency of the lower extremity who will benefit from lumbar sympathectomy. A number of such patients, however, significantly improve after sympathectomy. Hence, in the patient who cannot have direct arterial reconstruction, sympathectomy should always be considered. The usual patient is one who has ischemia, often with ulceration or impending gangrene. The patient with claudication rarely benefits from sympathectomy because it is skin blood flow rather than muscle blood flow that is augmented by lumbar sympathectomy. The operation consists of unilateral or bilateral removal of the first to fourth or second to fourth lumbar ganglia. Ten percent phenol may be injected to produce temporary paralysis of the lumbar sympathetic nerves.

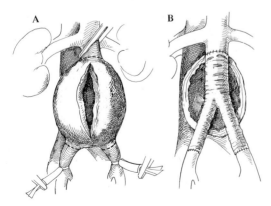

Figure 31–11. Resection of aortic aneurysm and insertion of a prosthetic graft.

THORACIC SYMPATHECTOMY

Raynaud's disease is the most common indication for thoracic sympathectomy. These patients have intermittent arterial spasm involving the small arteries of the fingers on exposure to cold. The debate as to whether the occlusive disease in the upper extremity is Raynaud's disease or Raynaud's phenomenon, possibly associated with scleroderma, is not important since thoracic sympathectomy may be helpful in both conditions. Another indication often seen in young women is hyperhydrosis, when large amounts of sweat drip from the hands almost continuously.

The approach to the thoracic sympathetic chain may be transthoracic, transaxillary, transcervical, or posterior extrapleural. Usually the second and third thoracic ganglia with the intervening chain are removed. The first or stellate ganglion may also be removed, but this produces a Horner's syndrome.

The results in Raynaud's disease and hyperhydrosis are excellent. In Raynaud's phenomena they are less certain.

THORACIC OUTLET SYNDROME

This is a clinical syndrome consisting of pain in the arm and/or hand accompanied by numbness and coldness of the hand. It is produced by compression of the neurovascular bundle supplying the arm and the hand as these structures leave the thorax. The compression takes place between a cervical rib and the first rib, between the scalenus anticus muscle and the first rib, or between the clavicle and the first rib. The symptoms are brought on by placing the arm in a certain position and may take the form of claudication. A typical example is the woman who experiences the symptoms only when hanging wash on the line with the arm extended over the head, thus accentuating the compression. The same may be true of a workman when required to work with the arms elevated over the head. The most useful clinical test is examining the radial pulse with the patient sitting relaxed with the arms at the side, and then while the patient braces his shoulders in the "military" position. The radial pulse may decrease or disappear. X-ray examination of the upper thorax discloses the presence or absence of a cervical rib.

Surgical management is excision of the cervical rib with or without division of the scalenus anticus muscle.

BUERGER'S DISEASE

The controversy continues as to whether thromboangiitis obliterans or Buerger's disease does or does not exist. The condition may be arterial atherosclerosis in a young adult which has resulted in ischemic ulceration with recurrent sepsis producing the so-called characteristic findings of inflammation along nerves and vessels. The entity may exist, but it is much rarer than once considered.

ARTERITIS

This group of poorly understood conditions includes arterial involvement in disseminated lupus erythematosus, scleroderma, dermatomyositis, and polyarteritis nodosa. They are probably collagen diseases of autoimmune origin. Their disseminated nature, atypical vessel involvement, and accompanying systemic disease should lead to the diagnosis. Biopsy of a superficial artery, such as the temporal artery, may be needed to establish the diagnosis. Treatment consists of giving systemic steroids.

VEINS

Thrombophlebitis

Thrombophlebitis means thrombosis and inflammation of a vein. The commonest site is the long saphenous system where the presenting symptoms are redness, tenderness, and swelling along the course of the vessel associated with a palpable thrombosed vein. The etiology of the condition is unknown; a bacterial or viral etiology has not been demonstrated. Treatment is bed rest until the acute symptoms have subsided and then gradual ambulation. Phenylbutazone may be of some value. Surgery is only indicated if the process extends, during observation, proximally toward the groin. Interruption of the saphenous vein at the saphenofemoral junction under local anesthesia should then be done and usually halts its progress.

Thrombophlebitis of the deep veins of the leg is a different and more serious problem. Obstruction to the major venous return from the extremity results in swelling of the foot and ankle and tenderness of the calf on palpation and on dorsiflexion of the foot (Homans' sign). Deep thrombophlebitis is particularly dangerous because it may lead to the formation of bland thromboemboli and pulmonary embolism and because the inflammatory process may destroy the venous valves causing chronic venous stasis disease. The management of deep venous thrombosis is bed rest with elevation of the extremity plus early and vigorous anticoagulation, first with heparin and then with Coumadin. There is no general agreement as to how long such anticoagulant therapy should be continued, but it probably should last for a minimum of several weeks and possibly for several months.

A common problem is recurrent thrombophlebitis involving either the superficial or deep venous system of the lower extremity. One course of management being investigated at present is administration of small daily doses of aspirin for its low-grade antiprothrombin activity effect.

Phlegmasia alba dolens or "milk leg" is an old name for deep thrombophlebitis in postpartum women. The term serves no useful purpose, however, since it merely describes the syndrome.

A more serious type of deep leg venous thrombophlebitis is phlegmasia cerulea dolens. While its pathogenesis is poorly understood, the condition is clearly a severe form of ileofemoral thrombophlebitis to be distinguished from the other milder forms of deep thrombophlebitis by two striking features:

1. The sequestration of fluid in the involved edematous extremity may be so gross as to produce life-endangering hypovolemic shock.

2. The circulation to the extremity may be so compromised by the venous obstruction, perhaps accompanied by arteriovasospasm, that part of the extremity may become gangrenous.

Management consists of bed rest with elevation of the extremity, prompt restoration of blood volume, and immediate and prolonged heparin therapy.

The clot has been removed successfully using a Fogarty catheter inserted under local anesthesia through a groin incision. A significant number of patients, however, with early successful thrombectomy, have on angiography been found to develop venous occlusion. This should not be interpreted as failure of the original procedure. Significant collaterals might have formed permitting the original site to rethrombose but without producing vascular insufficiency.

Phlegmasia cerulea dolens carries a high risk of pulmonary embolism. These patients are candidates for vena caval ligation, particularly if venous thrombectomy is performed.

Varicose Veins

Saphenous varicosities of the lower extremity may be asymptomatic or cause aching, heaviness, tiredness, and swelling. Many women consciously or subconsciously manufacture the symptoms when they object to the appearance of the prominent veins. Special tests, such as the Trendelenburg, can demonstrate certain hemodynamic features. The only test I have found clinically helpful in identifying the course

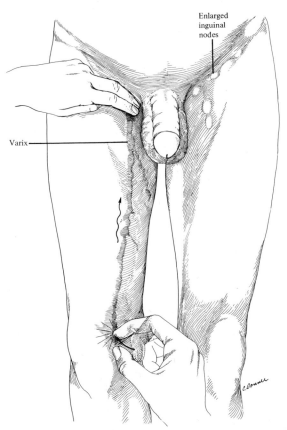

Figure 31–12. Percussion test for varicose veins. This is also useful to distinguish a saphenous varix from other groin swellings.

and severity of saphenous varicosities is, with the patient standing, to percuss a distended channel in the distal part of the limb and palpate the pressure impulse along the course of the distended vessel with its incompetent valves, which can be easily palpated at a higher level (Figure 31–12). The impulse depends upon the dilatation and degree of valvular incompetence. It is extremely important to examine for pedal pulses, because many patients have combined arterial and venous disease and attribute their arterial insufficiency symptoms to the prominent veins. Stasis changes such as discoloration, ulceration, and telangiectases about the ankle and leg are signs of long-standing deep venous insufficiency and not of the saphenous system. "Varicose ulcer" is therefore a misnomer since this rarely develops from a saphenous varicosity.

Stripping of the long and/or short saphenous veins from ankle to groin with ligation of the groin tributaries is a highly successful operation cosmetically and functionally (Figure 31–13).

It is impossible to predict if new varicosities

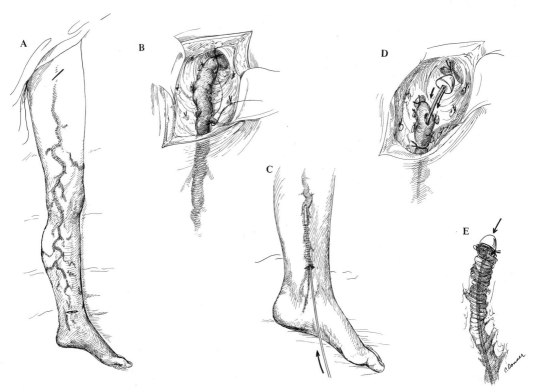

Figure 31–13.   Stripping of varicose veins. *A*. Incisions. *B*. Note ligature of long saphenous vein at saphenofemoral junction; groin tributaries are ligated and divided. *C*. Vein stripper is inserted at ankle. *D*. Long saphenous vein is divided at saphenofemoral junction, and stripper is in place; note ligature around distal vein snug on stripping shaft. *E*. Schematic view of stripping; tributaries are avulsed, and vein telescopes on stripper.

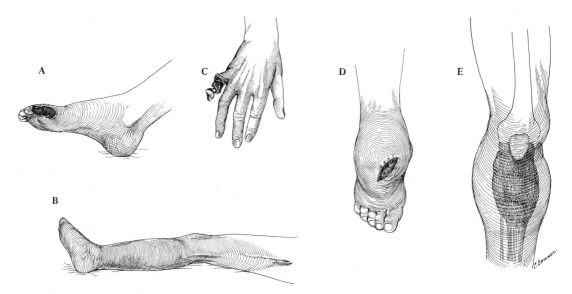

Figure 31–14.   Indications for amputation. *A*. Dry gangrene of toe from atherosclerotic occlusive vascular disease. *B*. Extensive moist gangrene following embolism of the superficial femoral artery. *C*. Traumatic amputation of finger. *D*. Gas gangrene of foot. *E*. Osteogenic sarcoma at upper end of tibia.

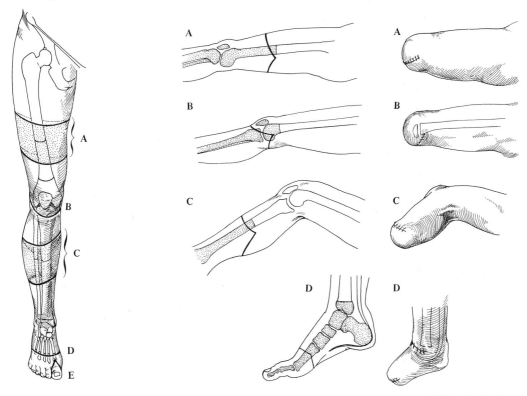

Figure 31–15. Sites for elective amputation in the lower limb. *A.* Lower to middle third of femur. *B.* Disarticulation of the knee. *C.* Mid tibia. *D.* Symes amputation at ankle.

will form because their etiology is still not known.

AMPUTATIONS

Amputation is indicated in limbs with dry and moist gangrene due to atherosclerotic occlusive vascular disease, in certain anaerobic infections, for major vascular trauma that cannot be repaired, and in treatment of certain malignant tumors such as osteogenic sarcoma (Figure 31–14). In the nonviable traumatized extremity a transverse or guillotine type of amputation without flaps and with no effort at stump reconstruction is indicated. The amputation is performed at the most distal site at which viability might be expected. This provides adequate open drainage of a contaminated wound. It is then possible at the definitive operation to provide the greatest length of stump.

Sepsis is rarely an indication for amputation except in gas gangrene (see page 139).

The site for elective amputation in the lower extremity has been found to be where ambulation using a prosthesis is most successful (Figure 31–15). In the upper extremity every effort

is made to preserve all viable tissues (see page 525).

In severe occlusive arterial disease it is often difficult for the physician and the patient to decide if an attempt should be made to save a "useless" extremity by a vascular reconstruction. In a bedridden patient is there reason to run the risks involved in attempted vascular reconstruction to save an extremity that will never be used for ambulation? In most instances amputation is safer.

FROSTBITE

Frostbite is thermal trauma to tissues resulting from exposure to a low temperature. The commonest parts involved are those usually exposed to the elements such as the external ear, tip of the nose, and the fingers and toes.

Cold injuries are classified in degrees similar to burns. In a first-degree cold injury edema develops within hours of the cold exposure and usually subsides in a few days with no residual defect. With a second-degree cold injury vesicles appear in 4 to 24 hours. After rupture of the vesicles or resorption of the fluid only the most superficial layers of skin are lost and there is no permanent cosmetic defect. Third-degree cold injury results in full-thickness destruction of skin, usually with cutaneous gangrene or eschar formation.

Fourth-degree cutaneous injury includes thermal trauma to structures deep to the skin such as nerve, tendon, or bone.

"Specific" treatment of frostbite remains controversial. Since blood vessels are particularly susceptible to cold injury, anticoagulants and sympathectomy should decrease sludging of blood with thrombosis. This has been confirmed in a number of animal studies. Military experience has not confirmed the regular benefit of anticoagulants, sympathetic block, or sympathectomy.

Although the advantage of fast rather than slow warming of the affected part as the initial management is still controversial, rapid warming appears to be desirable by applying warm packs or immersing the part at a temperature not exceeding body temperature. The affected parts are then protected similarly to burns, generally by applying an ointment to prevent adherence of dressings and covering this with a large protective bandage. Antibiotics and tetanus prophylaxis are indicated in third- and fourth-degree cold thermal injuries.

It is often difficult to differentiate between third- and fourth-degree cold thermal injuries. It may be felt that amputation is indicated when the skin becomes gangrenous and mummified. It is not unusual, however, that after weeks the skin slough separates and reveals viable deep tissues. Conservatism is therefore indicated in

treating cold thermal injuries. Only obviously nonviable tissues are debrided and only after waiting for at least partial spontaneous separation of the slough. Amputation may be required but should rarely be done less than several weeks after the thermal injury.

Repeated first-degree cold thermal injury may result in "trench foot," seen most often in soldiers exposed to chronic cold exposure and with the feet damp. The resulting late syndrome appears to be a causalgia-like state in which there is hypersensitivity of the affected part to touch and change in temperature, mild edema, and frequently some skin atrophy. A number of patients respond well to lumbar sympathectomy.

SUGGESTIONS FOR FURTHER READING

Beebe, H. G.: *Complications in Vascular Surgery.* J. B. Lippincott, Philadelphia, 1973.
A specialized presentation of the subject.
Eastcott, H. H. G.: *Arterial Surgery.* J. B. Lippincott Co., Philadelphia, 1969.
One of the authoritative texts on the subject.
Linton, Robert R.: *Atlas of Vascular Surgery.* W. B. Saunders, Philadelphia, 1973.
Well illustrated, concentrates on technique.
Wiley, F.: *Peripheral Arterial Disease.* W. B. Saunders, Philadelphia, 1966.
The subject is covered in depth.
"Atlas"-type volumes showing details of surgical techniques in vascular procedures with very brief related text.
Hershey, F. B., and Calman, C. H.: *Atlas of Vascular Surgery.* C. V. Mosby, St. Louis, 1963.
Julian, O. C.; Dye, W. S.; *et al.*: *Cardiovascular Surgery.* Year Book Publishers, Chicago, 1962.
Warren, Richard: *Procedures in Vascular Surgery.* Little, Brown & Co., Boston, 1960.

Chapter 32

UROLOGY

R. Roderick Shepherd

CHAPTER OUTLINE

Embryology
Renal Function
  Diuretics
  Urine Transport
Pain from the Urinary Tract
  Renal Pain
  Ureteral Pain
  Lower Tract Pain
Physical Examination
Investigations
  Urinalysis
  X-ray Studies
    Intravenous Pyelography
    Retrograde Pyelography
    Arteriography
    Venography
    Cystography
    Lymphangiography
  Endoscopic Examination
  Biopsy
  Exfoliative Cytology
  Ultrasound
  Radioisotopes
  Biochemical Tests
Urinary Calculi
  Diagnosis
  Treatment
    Renal Calculi
    Ureteral Calculi
  Surgical Management
  Subsequent Management
    Fluids
    Diet
    Urinary pH
    Drug Therapy
Trauma to the Urinary Tract
  Renal Trauma
    Penetrating
    Nonpenetrating
    Management
  Ureteral Injury
    Diagnosis
    Treatment
  Bladder Trauma

Urethral Injury
  Below the Urogenital Diaphragm
  Above the Urogenital Diaphragm
Genital Injuries
Acute Renal Failure
  Causes
    Prerenal
    Postrenal (Obstruction)
    Renal
  Diagnosis
  Management
Chronic Renal Failure
  Causes
  Management
Catheters
Urinary Tract Infections
Neurogenic Bladder
  Uninhibited Neurogenic Bladder
  Reflex Neurogenic Bladder
  Autonomous Neurogenic Bladder
  Motor Paralytic Bladder
  Sensory Paralytic Bladder
Scrotal Swellings
  Painful
  Nonpainful
Prostate
  Acute Prostatitis
    Symptoms
    Physical Examination
    Treatment
  Chronic Prostatitis
  Benign Prostatic Hypertrophy
    Treatment
Penis
  Hypospadias
  Epispadias
  Inflammatory Diseases
  Paraphimosis
Renal Transplantation
  Recipient Selection
  Donor Selection
  Surgical Technique
  Postoperative Care
  Results

Tumors of the Genitourinary Tract   Carcinoma of the Penis
    Wilms' Tumor (Nephroblastoma)   Urethra
    Renal Cell Carcinoma   Posterior Urethral Valves
    Carcinoma of the Renal Pelvis and Ureter   Urethral Stricture
    Carcinoma of the Urinary Bladder   Meatal Obstruction
    Carcinoma of the Prostate   Urethritis
        Treatment   Carcinoma of the Urethra
    Testicular Tumors
        Treatment

EMBRYOLOGY

The urinary tract is a frequent site of anomalies because of the complex nature of its development.

The nephrogenic cord, of mesodermal origin, gives rise to the rudimentary kidneys. The pronephros and mesonephros regress early in embryonic life, leaving only the mesonephric duct, which in the male becomes the vas deferens and epididymis. The distal part of the nephrogenic cord gives rise to the excretory part of the metanephros or definitive kidney. Differentiation of the nephrogenic cord occurs under the influence of the ureteric bud, an outgrowth of the mesonephric duct. Early generations of the ureteric bud form the collecting system of the kidney, and later generations stimulate the nephrogenic tissue to form the excretory units.

Abnormalities of position may be explained by failure of the nephrogenic cord to ascend from its pelvic origin to its normal lumbar position. Morphologic change may be from failure of rotation or from fusion of the anlagen of the two sides, producing horseshoe kidneys (Figure 32–1). Cystic kidneys may result from persistence of tubules which normally degenerate or from failure of the tubular components to join with their secretory counterparts.

The cloaca is subdivided by a mesodermal ingrowth, the urorectal septum, to produce the rectum dorsally and the urogenital sinus ventrally. The mesonephric ducts enter the urogenital sinus. The sinus has three subdivisions: (1) pars vesicourethralis, forming the bladder and urethra down to the prostatic utricle; (2) pars pelvina, forming the distal prostatic urethra and the membranous urethra in the male. In the female this forms most of the urethra and lower vagina. (3) Pars phallica, forming the bulbous and penile urethral and bulbourethral glands in the male, and the vestibule and bulbourethral glands in the female. The allantois regresses, leaving the urachus as a cord between the fundus of the bladder and the umbilicus. The mesonephric duct becomes incorporated at the level of the prostate, while the ureteric bud is carried cephalad and laterally. This produces a mesodermal component to the bladder, the trigone, in an otherwise entodermal structure.

Abnormality of the cloacal membrane produces ectopia vesicae. Urachal cyst or fistula may result from failure of obliteration of the allantois. The cloaca may persist if the urorectal septum fails to develop. Abnormal insertion of the mesonephric duct and ureteric bud into the urogenital sinus may produce a variety of ectopic ureteral orifices from the seminal vesicle to the vaginal introitus. The intermediate forms of ureteral ectopia are commonest.

Elevations of tissue in and lateral to the

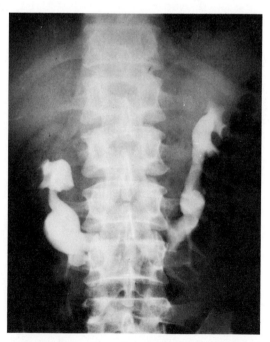

Figure 32–1. Horseshoe kidney. The polarity of the kidneys is changed with the lower poles closer than normal and the upper poles farther apart. The anterior and medial deviation of the calyces indicates the malrotation associated with this anomaly.

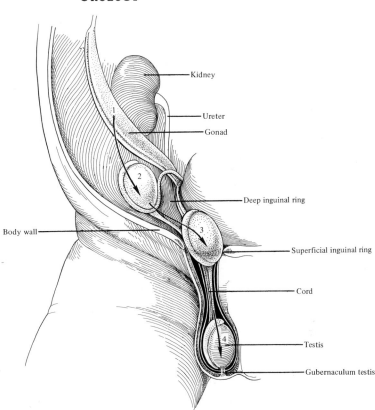

Figure 32–2. The testis descends from its origin beside the kidney through the inguinal canal to the scrotum.

cloacal membrane form the inner genital folds within which lies the genital fossa. Just cephalad the genital eminence appears as a precursor of the genital tubercle and phallus. Peripheral to the genital folds, genital swellings (labioscrotal folds) develop.

The posterior component of the cloacal membrane becomes incorporated into the anus and rectum. The anterior urogenital component of the cloacal membrane and the genital fossa become the pars phallica of the urogenital sinus, forming the bulbous and penile urethra in the male and bulbourethral glands, vestibule, and bulbovestibular glands in the female. Elongation of the genital tubercle forms the penis. The genital folds join to form the urethra, and the genital swellings enlarge posteriorly and fuse to form the scrotum. In the female the genital tubercle becomes the clitoris and the genital folds and swellings form the labia minora and majora.

The testicular anlage is close to that of the kidney. Proliferation of germ cells with invasion of mesenchyme results in the development of an embryonic testis which then joins with the mesonephric duct. Early descent to the level of the deep inguinal ring is probably due to embryonic growth (Figure 32–2). The factors

responsible for descent of the testis via the inguinal canal to the scrotum are not understood. The implication of the gubernaculum either as an anchor or tractor, although convenient to explain the descent, is difficult to support. The early position of the testis explains the lumbar origin of its blood, nerve, and lymphatic supplies.

RENAL FUNCTION

The kidneys play a major role in homeostasis (Tables 32–1 and 32–2). They excrete the products of metabolism and control the concentration of most constituents of the body fluids. The renal blood flow is about one fifth the cardiac output, and the volume of glomerular

Table 32–1. NORMAL VALUES IN THE SERUM

Blood urea nitrogen	10 to 20 mg/100 ml
Creatinine	0.7 to 1.2 mg/100 ml
Calcium	9 to 10.5 mg%
Phosphorus	2.5 to 4.5 mg%
Uric acid	2.5 to 7 mg%
Albumin	3.5 to 5 gm%
Globulin	2.5 to 3.5 gm%
Osmolality	285 to 295 mOsmol

Table 32–2. NORMAL VALUES OF CONSTITUENTS OF URINE

Chloride	170–250 mg/24 hr
Sodium	130–260 mg/24 hr
Potassium	25–100 mg/24 hr
24-hr protein	< 150 mg
Creatine clearance	80–120 ml/min
24-hr calcium	100–300 mg
24-hr uric acid	0.4–1.0 gm

filtrate is about one fifth the renal blood flow. Each kidney contains about 1,000,000 nephrons. The afferent arteriole carries blood to the capillaries in the glomerulus. The efferent arteriole divides to form a peritubular plexus around the tubules which drain into the renal veins. The tone in the efferent arteriole results in high pressure in the glomerulus and the production of a large volume of glomerular filtrate. The low pressure in the peritubular capillaries results in fluid readily being absorbed from the tubules. The long vessels that dip down into the medulla are called the vasa recta. A small amount of blood passes through arteriovenous shunts that bypass the glomerular and peritubular plexi. About 180 liters per 24 hours of glomerular filtrate enters Bowman's capsule in the glomerulus and is modified as it passes through the proximal tubule, the loop of Henle, and the distal tubules. Normally about 1500 ml of urine is formed every 24 hours. Glomerular filtrate has about the same constitution as plasma except for the almost complete absence of proteins. On its passage through the tubules the constituents are changed mainly as a result of absorption especially of water and glucose, but in addition tubular cells secrete substances such as potassium and hydrogen ions. In the proximal convoluted tubule active sodium reabsorption is followed by diffusion of water to reduce the volume of the filtrate by 80 percent. Also reabsorbed at this level are potassium, glucose, amino acids, and phosphate. Sodium and urea are recycled between the ascending and descending loops of Henle to produce a progressive increase in osmolality toward the area of the renal papillae. This is described as a countercurrent multiplier.

In the distal convoluted tubule antidiuretic hormone (ADH) activity permits inward passage of water and sodium to produce an isotonic urine, which may be concentrated further as the collecting ducts pass through the renal papillae.

Acid-base regulation in the kidney depends upon the bicarbonate buffer system and tubular secretion of H^+ in place of Na^+. The mechanism is aided by the enzyme carbonic anhydrase, and the newly formed bicarbonate is reabsorbed. Other mechanisms include transfer of hydro-

gen ion to convert buffer salts to acid salts. Ammonium excretion also helps reduce loss of Na^+. The free diffusion of NH_3 into the tubular lumen makes it readily available for combination with a variety of radicals (e.g., Cl^-, $SO_4^=$), after which it is held in the tubule for excretion (see page 100).

Diuretics

Abnormalities of body water distribution may require the use of diuretics. Certain of these agents are no longer clinically useful (e.g., alcohol, acidifying salts, xanthenes). Osmotic diuretics, such as mannitol, glycerol, and urea, induce water diuresis rather than natriuresis. They are of value in maintaining high urine flow rates and in states where a "dehydrating" action is desired, such as increased intracranial pressure. Thiazides, which are sulfonamide derivatives, are the most widely used. They inhibit reabsorption of sodium in the distal loop of Henle and in the proximal part of the distal tubule. Because they increase the amount of sodium delivered to the distal tubule, they increase the amount of sodium-potassium exchange at this site and may produce hypokalemia. Mercurial diuretics inhibit sodium reabsorption beyond the proximal tubule and at the same time inhibit potassium secretion, thereby reducing the problem of sodium loss noted with thiazides. The main disadvantage is that they require intramuscular injection.

Furosemide and ethacrynic acid inhibit sodium reabsorption in the loop of Henle.

Spironolactone inhibits the action of aldosterone, thereby sparing potassium and wasting sodium. It depends on the presence of filtered sodium at the distal reabsorption sites, and therefore is of little value when filtered sodium has been reabsorbed proximally. It also has the risk of causing hyperkalemia.

Triamterene acts directly on the distal tubular Na-K-exchange mechanism rather than by inhibiting aldosterone.

In all situations in which diuretic therapy is used, serum electrolytes, CO_2, and urea must be monitored in order to avoid electrolyte imbalance and related metabolic disturbances.

Urine Transport

The renal pelvic pressure is low and increases with filling of the pelvis. The ureteropelvic junction is open during the filling phase, but with the onset of a contraction wave, it closes and urine in the ureter is transported by contraction waves occurring at one to five times per minute. When flow rates are high, the ureter stays open and acts as a conduit. A rapid increase in ureteral pressure to above 20 mm Hg causes pain, but a slow increase to as much as 70 mm Hg may be asymptomatic.

The function of the bladder is storage and expulsion of urine. Patency of the urethra to allow voiding at an adequate flow rate is a prerequisite for normal micturition.

PAIN FROM THE URINARY TRACT

Renal Pain

Inflammation and increased intrarenal pressure are the main causes of renal pain. These may be aggravated by movement, percussion in the costovertebral angle, hydration, or traction on the renal pedicle, as in nephroptosis. Pain reflects more accurately the rate of onset of a disease rather than its gravity. Serious obstructive lesions may be silent.

Ureteral Pain

Ureteral obstruction by stone, clot, or tumor leads to ureteric colic. The pain is felt in the loin and lower abdomen in the distribution of the tenth thoracic dermatome and referred to the distribution of the genitofemoral nerve, in the testis, and upper-inner thigh (Figure 32–3). The accompanying distention of the renal pelvis can result in severe flank pain in the patient with a stone at the lower end of the ureter. Conversely a high obstruction may produce pain at a lower level.

Lower Tract Pain

Bladder infection leads to a dull, continuous suprapubic pain that may radiate along the urethra. Urine retention causes severe persistent

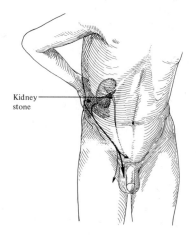

Kidney stone

Figure 32–3. The pain of renal colic is referred in the tenth thoracic dermatome from the costovertebral angle to the lower abdomen, scrotum, and inner thigh.

lower abdominal pain. Trigonal irritation produces pain that radiates to the tip of the penis.

Urethral pain from inflammation produces burning on micturition, strangury, and spasm at the end of micturition. Posterior urethral irritation leads to discomfort in the perineum and external meatus.

Prostatic disease may produce perineal pain and a feeling of rectal fullness. Testicular pain following an injury or infection is felt locally. A varicocele produces a feeling of heaviness in the testis. Pain may be referred to the testis along the spermatic cord, as for example with disease in the bladder, ureter, or kidney. This is the result of the testis and kidney having the same nerve supply, since both arise from the urogenital ridge.

PHYSICAL EXAMINATION

Systemic signs of renal failure are anemia, uremic odor, muscle irritability, stupor, and eventually coma. On inspection distention in a flank may indicate a large renal mass, while tenderness and immobility suggest perinephric suppuration. Bimanual palpation helps in the diagnosis of a renal swelling. The downward thrust of the diaphragm may aid in bringing the lesion from its protected position under the rib cage. A mobile kidney giving rise to pain may be felt on examining the standing patient. A distended ureter may be felt as a sausagelike mass and in the infant can readily be mistaken for a distended loop of bowel. Tenderness along the course of the ureter is often present with ureteral obstruction. The ectopic ureteral opening in the paraurethral region of the vagina may clarify the diagnosis in a patient presenting with fever, incontinence, or vaginal discharge.

When a lower abdominal mass is present, the old adage "pass a catheter before passing an opinion" is valid. The bladder may be further assessed by bimanual examination, best performed with the patient anesthetized. Under such circumstances areas of perivesical thickening, fixation, or induration of the bladder may be detected. This is of special value in patients with bladder tumors.

The foreskin is retracted to allow inspection of the glans and to exclude the presence of balanitis, carcinoma, or meatal stenosis. The penis is palpated for plaques of induration (Peyronie's disease), urethral induration, or diverticulum. The testis and epididymis are palpated to exclude neoplastic or inflammatory change. The vas deferens should be smooth and firm but not rigid. A varicocele, usually found on the left side, presents as a "bag of worms" and disappears in the recumbent position. Cord

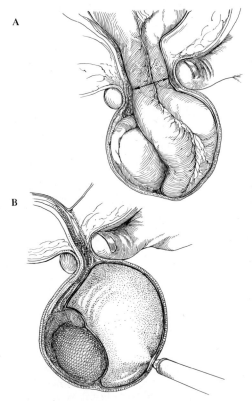

Figure 32–4. Differential diagnosis of scrotal mass. *A.* Inguinal hernia. Inability to define the upper limit of the mass suggests that it is of intra-abdominal origin. *B.* Hydrocele. The examiner is able to feel normal cord above the mass. Transillumination confirms the presence of fluid.

swellings may arise from within the scrotum or may originate within the abdomen. If the examiner is able to feel normal cord above the swelling, it is of scrotal origin. If the mass continues to the level of the external inguinal ring, then the diagnosis is most likely an inguinoscrotal hernia. Transillumination of scrotal masses is of great assistance in demonstrating fluid in a hydrocele (Figure 32–4). An increase in weight of a testis suggests testicular malignancy.

Rectal examination is performed using a well-lubricated index finger inserted gently so as to avoid anal spasm and pain. Noted are the perianal tissues, sphincter tone, rectal mucosal abnormalities, and the texture, size, symmetry, and presence of tenderness of the prostate. The prostate normally has a median sulcus and is firm and resilient but not hard in consistency. A specimen of prostatic fluid may be obtained for culture and microscopic examination by prostatic massage.

INVESTIGATIONS

Urinalysis

The three-glass test provides information about diseases at different levels in the renal tract. The initial specimen contains urethral debris and organisms, the second bladder urine, and the third specimen, obtained after prostatic massage, contains expressed prostatic secretions. Pus in the first glass suggests urethritis, in the second bladder infection or upper tract disease, and in the third prostatitis. In those with bladder infection all three specimens contain pus. Microscopic examination should be made for casts, crystals, bacteria, and red and white blood cells. Unspun urine is tested for sugar, protein, ketones, pH, and specific gravity. Twenty-four-hour collection may be required to assess creatinine clearance, protein loss, and the output of specific ions and amino acids.

X-ray Studies

The control film serves to identify normal landmarks and should be used to assess alteration in the skeleton, soft tissues, gas pattern, or calcification which may be of significance.

Intravenous Pyelography. The nephrogram and excretory phases of the intravenous pyelogram (IVP) are useful in assessing both form and function of the urinary tract. The contrast dose may be doubled to give better definition or may be given as a bolus or infused, and the degree of hydration of the patient may be varied. Tomography may help diagnose suspicious renal shadows, and a cine record is useful in assessing peristalsis and transit of urine. Fluoroscopy may help in dynamic studies. Views may be obtained in the erect, supine, prone, and oblique positions.

Retrograde Pyelography. The need for retrograde studies has decreased as a result of improvements in the intravenous pyelogram. When visualization of the upper tract is poor, a high-contrast medium injected directly into the ureter through a ureteric catheter provides better detail. Urine specimens may also be obtained for culture and cytologic studies.

Arteriography. Arteriography is performed to assess vascular integrity in trauma, to indicate vascular caliber in renovascular hypertension, and to clarify the nature of space-occupying lesions. Avascular cystic lesions are confirmed by a "claw" formed by the gradual thinning of normal parenchyma as it approaches the cyst margin. Small tortuous vessels which do not constrict on epinephrine injection are found in some renal tumors. These vessels tend to form a shunt through the kidney via venous sinusoids and produce early visualization of the renal vein. Arteriography may also detect arteriovenous malformations.

Venography. Venography is not commonly required in renal lesions. When venous invasion by renal tumor is suspected, an inferior vena cavagram may confirm involvement of that vessel. Venographic techniques can be used to sample renin output from each kidney. In patients with hypertension selective venography has been used to demonstrate adenomatous lesions associated with Conn's syndrome.

Cystography. The contour and ability of the bladder to empty can be assessed on views obtained in the course of the IVP. A marked dilution of contrast suggests a high volume of residual urine. Abnormalities of outline may be produced by diverticula or space-occupying lesions. The degree of emptying on the postvoid film gives a static appraisal of the state of bladder function. Cine studies of the contrast-filled bladder during micturition add information about the existence of vesicoureteral reflux, rate of emptying, and urethral caliber. When the urethral caliber is abnormal, a retrograde urethrogram, i.e., injection of dye into the urethral lumen from the meatus, is indicated. Urethral valves are only demonstrated on micturition.

Lymphangiography. This may be used to demonstrate the retroperitoneal lymph nodes and to detect their involvement by testicular and renal tumor.

Endoscopic Examination

The bladder can be visualized by cystoscopy. Changes in the bladder wall, ureteral orifices, trigone, bladder neck, prostatic fossa, and urethra may be diagnostic of certain diseases. A biopsy can be taken when necessary.

Biopsy

A renal biopsy may be taken using a needle inserted percutaneously or an open biopsy may be obtained. A needle biopsy of a palpable nodule in the prostate can be obtained by the transperineal or transrectal routes. Open biopsy can be performed by the perineal route but may cause impotence.

Exfoliative Cytology

Cancer cells can readily be identified in the urine. It is essential to obtain fresh urine, separate the sediment, and rapidly fix and stain the specimen.

Ultrasound

A fluid-solid interface can be identified with ultrasound and is useful to differentiate cystic from solid lesions.

Radioisotopes

Radioisotopes have diagnostic and therapeutic value in urology. The gamma radiation of diagnostic isotopes makes them readily detectable, while their short half-life makes them safe.

The isotope renogram, using ^{131}I hippurate or ^{203}Hg choromerodrin, provides a graphic representation of renal blood flow and tubular secretion with filling and drainage of the collecting system.

A renal scan provides information about the anatomy and function of the kidney. The blood supply to the kidney is recorded by a gamma camera after injection of the isotope ^{99M}Tc. Regions of altered vascularity are detected, and the size, shape, position, and function of the kidney can be determined. Resolution is less than that using radiologic techniques.

Biochemical Tests

The blood urea, blood urea nitrogen, and creatinine levels give basic information about kidney function. The acid phosphatase is increased in patients with metastases from carcinoma of the prostate. Blood and urine electrolyte and blood gas concentrations are frequently of value.

URINARY CALCULI

Calculi are a major cause of urinary tract disease. It is important that the patient who has had ureteric colic be fully investigated because there is a recurrence rate of 10 to 20 percent.

Calculi are the result of precipitates forming from the complex solution of cystalloids and colloids in urine. The basic problem is excess solute and insufficient solvent. The factors to be assessed include diet, dehydration, immobilization, urinary infection, obstruction, structural anomalies, and metabolic derangements, such as hyperuricuria, hyperparathyroidism, cystinuria, renal tubular acidosis, and hyperoxaluria.

The commonest stone components are calcium oxalate 50 percent, calcium phosphate 25 percent, and urate 10 percent. Less frequently encountered are cystine, xanthine, and ammonium magnesium phosphate. About 60 percent of stones in the kidney and ureter are calcium oxalate and calcium phosphate, while the commonest form of bladder calculus is magnesium ammonium phosphate.

The urinary pH is a critical factor in determining solubility. It may be altered by diet, medications, or by the presence of urea-splitting organisms, such as staphylococci, streptococci, or *Proteus mirabilis*. Infection may be the result of an obstruction producing urinary stasis. The solute load is important when there is an increased output in the urine or when there is dehydration with a normal output. Hypercalciuria occurs in those with hyperparathyroidism, vitamin D toxicity, bone metastases, multiple myeloma, thyrotoxicosis, milk-alkali syndrome, Addison's disease, infantile hypercalciuria, and osteoporosis. In many patients hypercalciuria is idiopathic.

The clinical presentation may be dramatic with ureteral colic or insidious with urinary infection or hematuria. Obstruction may occur at the infundibulum, the ureteropelvic junction, or anywhere along the ureter, but most commonly where the ureter crosses the iliac vessels and at the opening into the bladder. Calculous anuria occurs if both ureters are blocked, if the ureter of a solitary kidney is obstructed, or if impaction occurs at the bladder neck or the urethra.

Bladder calculi most often present with urinary symptoms from infection or mechanical trigonal irritation. An associated prostatism or neurogenic dysfunction may mask the symptoms.

Diagnosis

Urinary calculi are usually seen on abdominal x-ray. An intravenous pyelogram is essential to determine the state of the kidney on the affected side and also the function of the opposite kidney. When a stone is confirmed, the cause must always be considered.

Special attention should be paid to examination of the urine to determine the presence of infection, pH, and the rate of excretion of the chemicals constituting the stone. Increased blood values of urea and creatinine may indicate impairment of renal function. The blood calcium phosphate and uric acid are determined. It is also important to note the serum proteins to gain an estimate of the unbound calcium which is the active form.

Treatment

Urinary calculi may be treated conservatively hoping for spontaneous passage, or they may be removed.

Renal Calculi. Small renal calculi may be treated conservatively when there are mild symptoms and minimal obstruction. The calculi may disintegrate or pass spontaneously. The stone should be removed if it is increasing in size, causing obstruction, impairing kidney function, or associated with infection.

Surgical treatment consists of removing the stone, correcting any anatomic abnormality, and obtaining free drainage of urine. In younger patients an attempt is made to preserve renal parenchyma. In the elderly when operative risk is high, conservative management is indicated,

but if surgery is needed, nephrectomy is often the operation of choice.

Many procedures are available for removal of stones from the urinary tract. Pyelotomy offers least risk to renal parenchyma, while partial nephrectomy reduces the likelihood of recurrence by removing both the stone and diseased parenchyma. Nephrolithotomy can damage the renal tissue unless it is performed in the avascular plane between the anterior and posterior arterial divisions. Large branched calculi can be removed and the kidney preserved but nephrectomy may be necessary.

Ureteral Calculi. Expectant treatment is indicated in those with small calculi, less than 1 cm, which are likely to be passed spontaneously. The history, size of calculus, back pressure, and renal function must be considered. Additional factors are:

1. Economic status and occupation. Prompt intervention reduces loss of time from work.

2. Duration of symptoms. When short, the stone may rapidly be passed. When prolonged, renal damage may occur and removal is indicated.

3. Presence of infection. Urinary infection or fever demands prompt decompression of the obstructed kidney to prevent sepsis and impairment of renal function.

4. Persistence of impaction. A stone should be removed when it fails to move in four to six weeks.

Surgical Management

Small calculi, 5 mm or less, may be removed from the lower third of the ureter using a basket introduced into the ureter at cystoscopy, or the stone may be removed at operation by making an incision in the ureter (ureterolithotomy).

In the treatment of vesical calculi it is important to treat any associated outlet obstruction and urinary infection. The stone may be crushed using a lithotrite and fragments washed out. Open operation with an incision into the bladder (cystolithotomy) is required to remove large hard stones, foreign bodies, and to treat associated diverticula or outlet obstruction.

Subsequent Management

Treatment depends on the composition of the stone and the presence of urinary infection.

Fluids. A urinary output of about 2000 ml per 24 hours is essential. When a patient gets up to void at night, he should take more fluid to prevent the urinary concentration which normally occurs.

Diet. In those with calcium in the calculi the intake of milk and milk products should be restricted. This is often required in patients with idiopathic hypercalciuria. Oxalate excretion can be reduced by avoiding spinach, rhubarb, asparagus, chocolate, tea, and coffee.

Urinary pH. Urinary acidification is only necessary in those with triple phosphate stones associated with urinary infection. Acidification increases the incidence of other calculi. Alkalinization of the urine is essential in those with uric acid stones, and the urinary pH should be kept above 6.5. In cystinuria the pH should reach 8.0 with a urinary output of 3000 ml per day.

Drug Therapy. Allopurinol, a xanthine oxidase inhibitor, is given to patients with uric acid calculi. It acts by blocking the conversion of xanthine to uric acid.

D-Penicillamine combines with cystine to form a soluble complex and decreases urinary precipitation of cystine. This is useful in patients with cystinuria. The drug is expensive and toxic; therefore its use should be carefully supervised. A family history of the disease is generally present.

Hydrochlorothiazide, 50 mg twice daily, reduces stone formation in idiopathic hypercalciuria.

Neutral phosphate solution may reduce the recurrence of calcium oxalate or mixed calcium oxalate–calcium phosphate stones.

TRAUMA TO THE URINARY TRACT

Automobile accidents are the main cause of injuries to the urinary tract and generally result in blunt, nonpenetrating lesions. Penetrating injuries are usually from knife or gunshot wounds. The mechanism of injury and clinical presentation vary according to the site of the injury. There are, however, some features common to all. Bleeding may present as hematuria or a hematoma that may be complicated by sepsis or the late development of fibrosis and contracture. Urine in the tissues results in an inflammatory reaction which may be complicated by sepsis and tissue necrosis. Scar tissue may form as a result of tissue damage, organization of a hematoma, or loss of blood supply. The result may be renal ischemia with hypertension, renal failure, or obstruction to urinary flow. There are frequently associated injuries of the abdominal viscera, pelvis, spine, and major vessels.

In the patient with multiple injuries priority has to be given to the airway, control of bleeding, and treatment of oligemic shock. When the patient's general condition has been stabilized, the renal tract is considered. The patient is examined for bleeding from the urethra, tenderness and swelling in the loins, signs of peritoneal irritation, and extravasation of urine. Rectal and vaginal examinations are essential. The urine is examined for erythrocytes. An intravenous pyelogram is obtained, taking, if necessary, only one or two films. A urethrogram may be indicated if the patient is unable to pass urine. A cystogram is necessary if there is a possible bladder injury.

Renal Trauma

Penetrating. Penetrating wounds constitute only 10 percent of renal trauma but are associated with intraperitoneal injuries in 80 percent of cases. Physical examination should direct attention to the involved flank. Hematuria may be present, but its absence does not exclude renal injury. Abdominal x-rays and an intravenous pyelogram are essential to demonstrate the presence and extent of functional impairment and the state of the opposite kidney.

Nonpenetrating. The kidney is mobile but in the adult has considerable protection by bones. The child has greater risk of injury because the organ is more intraperitoneal, has less perirenal fat, and is relatively larger. Renal abnormalities such as hydronephrosis predispose to injury. The mechanisms include direct force when the kidney is crushed against the spine or perforated by a bony fragment, and indirect force the result of a fall on the buttock, or acute flexion or twisting.

Injuries include renal contusion, superficial cortical laceration, deep renal laceration, renal laceration involving the collecting system,

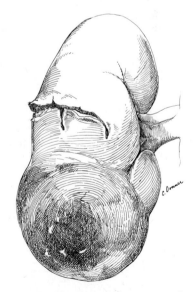

Figure 32–5. Nonpenetrating trauma has resulted in a hematoma in the lower pole of the kidney and a laceration at the center.

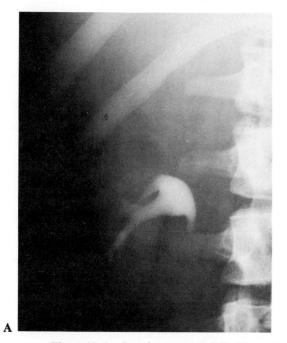
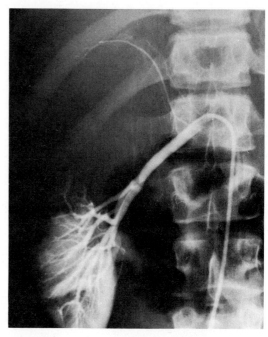

A   B

Figure 32–6. Renal trauma. *A.* IVP. The nephrogram and calyces representing the upper pole are not visualized. *B.* Arteriogram. The avulsed upper pole has no blood supply. A capsular vessel outlines the extent of the hematoma.

multiple renal lacerations, renal pelvic injury, and injury to the pedicle (Figure 32–5). Three degrees of severity are recognized: contusion, rupture, and severe rupture or injury to the pedicle.

Management. Following resuscitation, the decision is made to treat the renal lesion conservatively or by operation. The following observations and investigations should be considered:

1. Monitoring signs of oligemic shock.
2. Observing size of flank hematoma.
3. Repeatedly examining the urine for hematuria.
4. An intravenous pyelogram (Figure 32–6, *A*).
5. Retrograde pyelography is occasionally indicated.
6. Some recommend angiography in patients with all types of renal injury, while others reserve it for those with nonfunction of the kidney on pyelography. It is important to distinguish parenchymal damage from a pedicle lesion. If the injury to the pedicle is not repaired, ischemic necrosis of the kidney may occur. If the renal artery is not visualized, operation is indicated (Figure 32–6, *B*).
7. A renal scan may be performed to indicate integrity of blood supply and to delineate parenchymal tear. It also serves as a simple test if the indications for arteriography are not clear.

Operation should be performed if a hematoma in the loin is increasing in size, if transfusion is needed to maintain a stable state, or if there is massive hematuria. Penetrating injuries should be explored as a general rule.

If laparotomy is carried out for other reasons, a small retroperitoneal hematoma is best left alone. If the hematoma crosses the midline or extends into the pelvis, control of the renal pedicle should be obtained and the hematoma explored.

An injured kidney may be treated by local repair, partial or complete nephrectomy, or repair of the vessels or pelvis. Major segmental tears of the kidney can be repaired, preventing the complications associated with extravasation of urine and secondary hemorrhage. It should be noted, however, that extravasated urine can be reabsorbed without complication.

Patients treated conservatively are confined to bed until gross hematuria has cleared, and activity is limited as long as there is microscopic hematuria. Patients are given prophylactic antibiotics when there is a hematoma or urinary extravasation. A low-grade fever is common from reabsorption of a hematoma.

Follow-up includes pyelography to assess renal size and adequacy of drainage. Culture studies of the urine are needed to be certain that there is no urinary infection. Blood pressure is recorded for at least one year to detect hypertension which might occur on a renovascalur basis.

Ureteral Injury

Ureteral injuries may be penetrating, nonpenetrating, or iatrogenic. Surgical injuries to the ureter are most often associated with gynecologic, colonic, or urologic operations.

Diagnosis. Apart from direct visual recognition of the injury, diagnosis requires that ureteral injury be suspected and that its presence be proved, usually by radiographic techniques. Delayed recognition of ureteral injury may result in obstruction with loin ache, tenderness, low-grade fever, and leukocytosis. Anuria occurs if the injury is bilateral or to a solitary ureter. Urinary infection increases the rate of renal damage. Urinary extravasation may result in the presence of a mass, a fistula, or drainage of urine into the peritoneal cavity, resulting in malaise, ileus, or peritonitis. Infusion pyelography or retrograde studies confirm the diagnosis. When a fistula is present, injection of indigo carmine intravenously may confirm its origin in the urinary tract. This dye, placed in the bladder, is useful in differentiating a ureterovaginal from a vesicovaginal fistula; in the latter it will stain a vaginal tampon.

Treatment. Treatment entails repair or diversion when a ureter has been injured. Technique will depend on the time of recognition of the injury, the level of the ureter involved, the patient's condition, and whether or not the injury is bilateral.

When the injury is recognized at operation, ligatures are removed and ureteral viability observed. A ureteral splint may be left for 10 days when the ureter is injured by a clamp. A severed or resected ureter may be mobilized and reanastomosed or implanted into the bladder. When diagnosed late, renal function and drainage may be poor and systemic effects marked. When renal function is poor, drainage by nephrostomy is generally indicated. Reestablishment of urinary tract continuity may be by anastomosis, reimplantation, or nephrectomy if useful function cannot be regained.

Bladder Trauma

Bladder injuries are penetrating (internal or external) or nonpenetrating (intraperitoneal, extraperitoneal, or combined). A full bladder is especially liable to rupture in the dome or posterior wall following a nonpenetrating injury (Figure 32–7). Pelvic fractures are complicated by bladder rupture in 10 percent of patients. The injury results from perforation by bony fragments or from tears due to traction on the ligaments about the bladder base.

Diagnosis is suspected from the history of

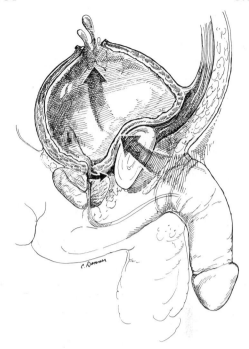

Figure 32–7. A nonpenetrating injury can cause intraperitoneal rupture of a distended bladder as well as a urethral tear.

trauma, pain on movement of the legs or on pelvic compression, and suprapubic discomfort. The patient may have an intense desire to void but be unable to do so. Catheterization may yield bloody urine. In the patient with intraperitoneal rupture signs of peritonitis occur. Extraperitoneal rupture may result in tracking of urine up the abdominal wall to the buttock, thigh, and inguinoscrotal regions. Signs of sepsis later become prominent.

A catheter is passed in patients with suspected bladder injury. A cystogram is obtained, taking anteroposterior and lateral views when the bladder is full and empty. The adult bladder should be distended with 300 ml of dye to identify a small leak. Treatment is by operative repair of the defect and drainage of the retropubic space. Catheter decompression is required postoperatively. Associated vascular and bony injuries may need treatment.

Urethral Injury

Injuries to the urethra may be penetrating or nonpenetrating and are situated above or below the urogenital diaphragm.

Below the Urogenital Diaphragm. Straddle injuries and urethral instrumentation are the common causes of injury to the urethra below the urogenital diaphragm. The injury may be simple contusion or complete or incomplete rupture. There are swelling, discoloration, and blood at the urethral orifice. Urethrography performed gently with an aqueous medium confirms the diagnosis.

Treatment is evacuation of hematoma, repair of the defect, and diversion of urine. Late repair of a neglected injury requires urethroplasty of the scarred segment.

Above the Urogenital Diaphragm. These lesions are among the most difficult and contentious of urologic problems. They are usually associated with pelvic fractures with marked displacement. The displacement may have been considerable, the bones returning to a near normal position. There is a perineal hematoma, blood at the external urethral orifice, and displacement of the prostate and bladder base recognized by rectal examination. X-ray of the pelvis, intravenous pyelography, and urethrography are usually needed. If urethrography fails to show loss of continuity, there is support for careful catheterization and drainage of the bladder until the hematoma disappears. In those with partial tear of the urethra traumatic catheterization may complete the injury. The bladder may be drained suprapubically, anticipating that the bladder base will return close to a normal location as the hematoma is absorbed. Alternatively primary debridement and repair may be performed. The bladder is drained suprapubically and an attempt made to reestablish urethral continuity by placing a catheter in the urethra and applying traction to return the bladder base and prostate to their normal positions. Impotence and incontinence may occur after severe urethral injuries.

Genital Injuries

Skin may be lost from the penis and scrotum by avulsion, when clothing is caught in machinery. The glans often escapes because the skin is more firmly adherent than in the shaft. A split-thickness skin graft is applied or the denuded penis covered by scrotal skin. When scrotal skin is lost, free grafts may be applied or the testes may be buried in the thigh or inguinal skin pouches.

Minor testicular injuries are treated by rest and ice packs. A testicular hematoma should be evacuated. Rupture of the tunica albuginea may result in complete loss of the seminiferous tubules. Leydig cells remain and maintain hormonal activity.

ACUTE RENAL FAILURE

Acute renal failure is diagnosed when urine output in an adult is less than 400 ml per 24 hours. A rising BUN and creatinine in the presence of a greater output also represents renal failure.

Causes

The causes of acute renal failure are:

Prerenal. These include fluid and electrolyte depletion, hemorrhage, septicemia, and myocardial infarction.

Postrenal (Obstruction). These include (1) bladder outlet—enlarged prostate, urethral obstruction; (2) ureteral obstruction—ligation, stone, retroperitoneal tumor, bladder tumor; and (3) renal tubular obstruction (see below).

Renal. These include (1) ischemic injury; (2) toxic injury—ethylene glycol, carbon tetrachloride, heavy metals; (3) hemolytic—e.g., transfusion mismatch; (4) crush, burn; (5) acute glomerulitis; (6) vascular occlusion—embolus, thrombus, aneurysm; (7) acute pyelonephritis, papillary necrosis; (8) hypercalcemia; and (9) precipitation—uric acid, myeloma, sulfonamide.

Diagnosis

The diagnosis is based on the history of onset and the degree of oliguria. Complete anuria suggests obstruction, necrosis, or vascular occlusion. Physical examination rapidly leads to the diagnosis when the cause is blood loss, sepsis, or fluid depletion. In acute tubular necrosis the urinary sediment contains casts consisting of renal tubular cells, coarse granular casts, and erythrocytes. In glomerulitis free erythrocytes are present. The urinary sodium concentration and serum and urine osmolality help establish the diagnosis. Renal failure due to prerenal causes results in a urine with a high specific gravity (> 1.020) and a high osmolality. The urinary osmolality is 50 to 100 mOsm per liter greater than the plasma osmolality. There is active renal tubular reabsorption of sodium, resulting in a urinary sodium of less than 25 mEq per liter. The urine-plasma creatinine ratio is greater than the normal ratio 20:1. Treatment is replacement of the blood volume deficit. The diuretic response in prerenal failure also confirms the functional integrity of the kidneys. Mannitol, 12.5 to 25 gm in 200 ml of fluid, given in 15 minutes produces a diuresis. Ethacrynic acid and furosemide may also be used to produce a diuresis without the risk of overloading with fluid. Anuria of obstructive origin is diagnosed by cystoscopy and retrograde pyelography. Acute tubular necrosis (ATN) generally results in oliguria but can be present with a urinary output of 1 liter in 24 hours. There is generally a history of hypotension or of administration of a nephrotoxic drug such as gentamicin or kanamycin.

The urine is isomotic with an osmolality within 50 mOsm per liter of that of the plasma and a urinary sodium concentration over 40 mEq per liter.

Management

Fluid intake should be limited to 400 ml per day plus measured loss. Daily body weight is the best indicator of fluid requirement. The patient in good balance should lose 200 to 300 gm per day. The potassium level in the plasma must be determined regularly and repeated electro-cardiograms obtained. Increasing levels may be controlled by Kayexalate (sodium polystyrene sulfonate) given by mouth or by enemas. An acute rise is treated by infusion of 10 percent calcium gluconate or 5 percent glucose and insulin. Peritoneal or hemodialysis may be needed to obtain an absolute reduction in body potassium.

Poisons, damaged tissues, and catabolic processes aggravate acidosis. Treatment is not required in most instances when the carbon dioxide content is above 18 mmole per liter. More profound acidosis is treated by intra-venous sodium bicarbonate solution, or by M/6 sodium lactate. An increase in urea and creatinine implies a build-up in other protein metabolic end products which give rise to uremia. The rate of rise may be slowed by debridement of devitalized tissues, drainage of collections of blood, and control of infection. Adequate carbohydrate intake, about 150 gm glucose daily, decreases protein catabolism and provides adequate caloric intake.

Urinary infection is treated by appropriate drugs, with dosage adjusted according to the degree of renal failure and the possibility of renal damage. Careful management is still needed during the diuretic phase after acute renal failure because marked fluid and electro-lyte losses may occur. Replacement must be adequate but not so great as to produce a forced diuresis. The volume of urine may not be adequate, and the BUN and creatinine levels may still rise even with a diuresis. As the BUN, creatinine, and electrolytes approach normal, the patient who can drink and who has access to fluid and salt will again be able to compensate for his own losses.

CHRONIC RENAL FAILURE

Chronic renal failure may be mild and evidenced only by laboratory measurements, or severe to the point of requiring fluid and dietary therapy, or dialysis. Nephron loss is associated with a decrease in flexibility of renal function until ultimately high flow rate through a reduced number of nephrons allows little opportunity for the tubule to modify the glomerular filtrate.

As nephron destruction progresses, the regulation of water, electrolytes, pH, and metabolic end products becomes impaired. The inability of the kidney to concentrate urine results in the production of urine of low specific gravity with consequent nocturia and polyuria.

Loss of tubular function results in reduced ability to recover bicarbonate and to form titratable acid. Ammonia formation is also impaired. This causes inability to handle hydrogen ion and the development of metabolic acidosis. Electrolytic disturbances include renal sodium loss with reduction in extracellular fluid volume and further impairment of renal per-fusion and function. Failure to exchange sodium for potassium results in hyperkalemia with its cardiac and neuromuscular complications. The decrease in calcium, increase in phosphate, and acidosis upset parathyroid function and in-crease neuromuscular excitability. Retention of metabolic end products results in nausea, vomit-ing, and neuropathies. There are anemia, a tendency to bleed because of impaired platelet function, abnormalities of prothrombin con-sumption, and poor capillary integrity.

Causes

The causes of chronic renal failure are:

1. Congenital: polycystic kidneys or obstruc-tion.

2. Infection: chronic pyelonephritis, specific inflammations such as tuberculosis.

3. Immunologic.

4. Obstruction: congenital obstruction with delayed presentation and outlet obstruction in the aged.

5. Hypertensive.

6. Other causes: infiltrations, gout, amyloid.

Management

When further loss of function can be pre-vented, anatomic abnormalities should be corrected. More often, treatment is conservative and is aimed at regulating body water, electro-lytes, acid-base balance, and preventing ac-cumulation of excessive metabolic end products. Fluid intake is limited to maintain body weight within 0.1 kg of the ideal weight each day. Sodium loss is treated by giving 5 to 15 gm sodium bicarbonate per day. This helps to correct the inability to excrete the high load of hydrogen ions. Hyperkalemia is avoided by eliminating foods high in potassium from the diet, such as chocolate and oranges. A total of 1500 to 2000 calories are given, with potassium limited to 40 mEq, sodium to 40 mEq, and protein to 40 gm. The patient adapts remarkably well to the low level of hemoglobin, often about 5 gm. Transfusion is only of temporary value. With increasing renal failure there are anorexia, neuropathy, hyperkalemia, and oliguria. Peritoneal dialysis may be used initially to correct the fluid and electrolyte abnormalities. In the chronic state hemodialysis is preferred with blood delivered through a variety of external arteriovenous shunts or internal arteriovenous fistulae.

CATHETERS

The urethral catheter provides the simplest form of urinary diversion, but improperly used it may result in sepsis and injury with stricture formation. The catheter is made of rubber, silicone, or metal with a straight or curved (coudé) end to glide over the bladder neck. The hole may be in the end or side. There may be an inflatable balloon to help retain the catheter in position. An additional channel may be incorporated to provide continuous irrigation. A two- or four-winged Malecot catheter or a circular de Pezzer catheter does not require a balloon to maintain it in position and is stretched over a stylet when it is introduced into the bladder. Calibration is in French units with one unit representing one third of a millimeter of diameter, for example 30 Fr = 1 cm.

The indications for catheterization are to relieve outlet obstruction, to decompress the bladder before operations especially in the pelvis, to measure residual urine volumes, to monitor urinary output in seriously ill patients, and to obtain urine under sterile conditions for bacteriologic examination.

Aseptic technique is essential when inserting the catheter. Topical anesthetic may be used but is no substitute for gentle technique. The catheter should readily find its way through the urethra and force should not be required. An indwelling catheter should be of adequate caliber but not of a size that will exert pressure on the urethra or impede the drainage of urethral secretions. A closed drainage system with strict asepsis is instituted if the catheter is left in position.

URINARY TRACT INFECTIONS

The presence of 10^5 organisms per milliliter of urine in two or more properly collected midstream specimens is diagnostic of urinary tract infection. Females are more prone than males, with a ratio of 3:1. During infancy the rate is particularly high in females, the result of fecal contamination of the perineum and the short urethra. Prostatic obstruction is responsible for a high incidence of infection in elderly males.

The organisms enter the urinary tract from the urethra, blood, or lymph. Predisposing causes are congenital abnormalities, outlet obstruction, the presence of calculi, and diabetes. If the rate of urine flow is low and the complete elimination of urine is not possible, the natural washing-out defense mechanism is impaired.

In the young fever and irritability are the main findings. Nausea, vomiting, and intestinal cramps may occur in those with pyelonephritis and may be accompanied by loin ache and tenderness. Frequency, urgency, and burning suggest a bladder infection. Urine may be obtained for bacteriologic examination by sampling a voided specimen, passing a catheter under sterile conditions, or by suprapubic aspiration. Further investigations include an intravenous pyelogram, voiding cystogram, and cystoscopy.

Fluids, antipyretics, and analgesics are given along with adequate dose of the correct antibiotics. A repeat culture should be obtained after three or four days to assess the efficacy of treatment. If a good response is obtained, treatment should be continued for at least 10 days for an acute infection, and for two or three weeks for a chronic infection. In a urinary tract with structural abnormality, infection may not be cleared until the appropriate surgery is performed. Urinary calculi should be removed. Vesicoureteral reflux, outlet obstruction, bladder diverticula, and strictures will require treatment.

NEUROGENIC BLADDER

The bladder and its sphincter mechanism must be regarded as a unit in the discussion of neurogenic disease. Normal bladder function implies a normal sensation of fullness, adequate control of the urge to void, easy initiation of the stream, free urinary flow, and complete emptying of the bladder. The mediation of such an act is complex and involves the nervous system from cortex to the sacral segments. Problems may develop at any level and may facilitate or inhibit bladder and sphincter activity. In every patient bladder activity is the composite effect of opposing forces:

$$\frac{\text{Expulsion}}{\text{Retention}} \approx \frac{\text{Detrusor} + \text{Intra-abdominal pressure}}{\text{Bladder neck} + \text{External sphincter} + \text{Urethra}}$$

Classification of neurogenic bladder may be confusing because of combining etiologic, neurogenic, and functional groups. If the nerve supply of the bladder is understood, one can construct a logical approach to treatment based on the site of the neurologic lesion.

Uninhibited Neurogenic Bladder

This bladder behaves as if there was lack of fine control of the time of voiding. This is seen in the newborn and in patients with cerebral atherosclerosis and after cerebrovascular accidents. It may also occur with brain tumor or trauma and in multiple sclerosis. The peripheral nervous circuits are intact. The bladder empties well but incontinence with urgency is present.

Reflex Neurogenic Bladder

The reflex arc mediated through the conus medullaris is intact, while influences above this level are lost. This is seen classically after a crushing injury to the spinal cord and in those with primary or secondary tumor involvement above the level of the conus, i.e., above the twelfth dorsal vertebra. Saddle anesthesia may be present and the bulbocavernosus reflex is hyperactive. The bladder empties incompletely and incontinence is common.

Autonomous Neurogenic Bladder

There is total isolation of the bladder from any neurogenic control as occurs with congenital disruption of function of the conus, e.g., spina bifida, myelomeningocele, or trauma to the conus medullaris, cauda equina, or pelvic nerves. There is marked motor and sensory impairment, and the bladder empties infrequently with poor flow. Overflow incontinence may be present.

Motor Paralytic Bladder

This may be seen after trauma or with neoplasm affecting the S_2, S_3, and S_4 parasympathetic nerve fibers, poliomyelitis, or herniated intervertebral disk. Sensation is intact but motor responses are lost. The bladder has no tone, and voiding must be assisted by manual compression or overflow will result.

Sensory Paralytic Bladder

This is a bladder incapable of transmitting sensory information to the central nervous system, as occurs in diabetes mellitus and tabes dorsalis. Awareness of bladder filling is lost and hypotonia results. The bladder empties seldom and incompletely, and overflow incontinence may occur.

Assessment of the bladder will allow its categorization into one of these groups, although incomplete lesions may complicate the picture. Testing of bladder innervation is aided by:

1. Bladder awareness of heat, cold, fullness.
2. Saddle sensation—sensory S_2, S_3, and S_4.
3. Bulbocavernosus reflex—intact sacral reflex arc.

4. Bladder tone—presence of normal higher controls.
5. Bladder capacity—presence of distention or of uncontrolled contractibility.
6. Residual urine—presence of coordinated efficient emptying.
7. Incontinence.

Cystourethrography helps in the assessment. Management is directed toward achieving continence with minimal residual urine. A history of strokes, injury, or acute disease suggests a neurogenic lesion. Other conditions such as diabetes or disseminated sclerosis may have a more insidious onset. Functional inquiry will delineate loss of urinary control, poor voiding, and frequency. There may also be constipation and impaired ambulation. Sexual function, erection, and ejaculation may be affected. Physical examination may reveal sacral anesthesia, decrease in anal tone, alteration in bulbocavernosus reflex, or cortico-regulatory upsets such as clonus, Babinski reflex, and hyperactive tendon reflexes. Investigations include urinalysis and culture, intravenous pyelography, and x-rays of the spine and pelvis. Observation of the patient voiding may aid diagnosis and may help predict the response to be found on cystometrography. Treatment includes maintenance of good urinary flow and a sterile urine. Altering the balance between expulsion and retention may require antispasmodics or parasympathomimetics as well as nerve blocks, mucosal blocks, or rhizotomies. Drainage may be improved by suprapubic or urethral catheters, by transurethral resection, or by ileal loop diversion. Instruction in compression voiding and the Credé expression of the bladder will aid hypotonic states. The high death rate of paraplegics in the past was the result of renal disease. Preservation of a healthy functioning upper urinary tract is essential.

SCROTAL SWELLINGS

Diagnosis of scrotal masses is possible in a high proportion of cases from the history and physical examination alone (Figure 32–8).

Painful

Painful scrotal lesions may be due to epididymo-orchitis, testicular torsion, orchitis due to viral infection (e.g., mumps), trauma, or from infection by pyogenic organisms disseminated by the blood stream.

Testicular torsion occurs mostly in the adolescent. An abnormal insertion of the cord into the testis leads to "bell clapper" deformity. Torsion is characterized by acute pain of sudden onset, usually preceded by a physical

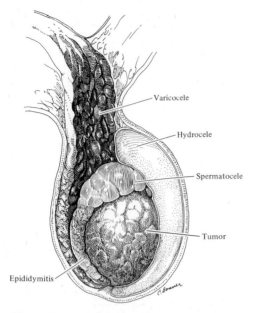

Figure 32–8. Conditions causing scrotal mass. Identification of each component of the scrotal contents allows accurate diagnosis of the mass.

movement which has allowed the twisting of the cord to occur with consequent venous occlusion. The history, the absence of inflammatory urinary symptoms, and marked testicular pain suggest the diagnosis. There are often considerable scrotal redness and swelling which may erroneously be thought to be the result of epididymo-orchitis. When the diagnosis is made early, a normal epididymis is palable. Treatment should be undertaken urgently. When the diagnosis is suspected, exploration with reduction of the torsion is carried out, and the testis is examined for viability. A nonviable testis is excised, but a viable testis is sutured to the scrotum to prevent recurrence. Prophylactic fixation of the uninvolved testis is also performed.

Epididymo-orchitis also results in a swollen, tender testis in which the pyogenic process involves the epididymis primarily and the testis secondarily. It occurs most often in young adults. Symptoms of lower urinary tract infection are often present, their onset being more gradual than with torsion. Treatment includes specific antibiotics, bed rest, scrotal elevation, and application of cold packs. Occasionally epididymo-orchiectomy is required. When doubt exists in the differentiation of torsion from epididymo-orchitis, exploration is indicated.

Orchitis may be the result of viral or bacterial infections or trauma. With mumps, symptoms occur four to six days after the parotitis. In

70 percent of cases the condition is unilateral, and in 50 percent there is some degree of atrophy of the testis. General measures usually suffice in treatment, but in addition estrogens, corticosteroids, or surgical decompression may be used.

Trauma to the testis may result in minor swelling, requiring only rest and analgesics. A more severe injury may produce a hematoma within the testis that ruptures through the tunica albuginea. Aspiration, evacuation of the hematoma, debridement of devitalized tissue, and repair of the tunica albuginea may be required. A minor injury may draw attention to a tumor.

Nonpainful

Hydrocele, a collection of fluid in the tunica vaginalis, may cause marked scrotal enlargement. In infants a communication with the peritoneal cavity may result in the fluid disappearing periodically. After two years the mass tends to be permanent and requires surgical treatment (Figure 32–9). Diagnostic features include a unilocular swelling which transilluminates and extends around the testis. Chronic epididymitis or orchitis or a testicular tumor may present as a hydrocele. It is therefore important to palpate the testis after aspiration of the fluid to be sure that underlying testicular abnormalities are not missed.

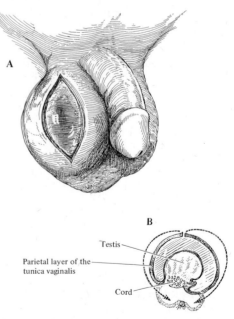

Figure 32–9. A hydrocele is repaired by making (*A*) an incision in the anterior wall of the sac and (*B*) suturing the edges behind the testis (Jaboulay repair).

A spermatocele is a postpubertal swelling which arises from the upper pole of the testis displacing the testis downward. The mass is round, often multilocular, and transilluminates. Aspiration yields opalescent fluid which may contain sperm. Surgical treatment is excision.

Varicocele presents as a "bag of worms" in the left hemiscrotum. It is the result of defective valves in the left testicular vein. The disappearance on recumbency is diagnostic. Failure of a varicocele to disappear on lying down or a rightsided varicocele suggests venous obstruction which may be on a malignant basis. Treatment entails ligation of the incompetent vessels at the level of the scrotum, inguinal canal, or retroperitoneum. In the subfertile male with a varicocele this procedure may result in improvement in the quality of the semen. Most require no treatment or use of a scrotal support.

A hematocele is a collection of blood in the tunica vaginalis that does not transilluminate. Treatment is bed rest, aspiration, or surgical drainage, depending on the severity of the lesion.

Gumma of the testis and tuberculous epididymitis are two painless lesions which are now quite uncommon. Diagnosis is made by the history, serology, and culture studies.

Testicular tumor is described on page 584. It is this diagnosis that must be kept uppermost on examination of the testes whether there be pain, fluid, or an accompanying hernia. Only by maintaining a high index of suspicion can this lesion be diagnosed early.

PROSTATE

Acute Prostatitis

The prostate may be the site of inflammation, benign hypertrophy, or malignant change. Prostatitis may be bacterial, fungal, viral, protozoal, or allergic in origin. Bacterial infection is most common; the others are rare and often difficult to prove. Infection may occur by direct extension from the urethra, by lymphatic spread from the rectum, or by the blood stream. Predisposing factors may be perineal trauma, fatigue, alcoholic excess, and sexual deprivation or overindulgence, but their importance is difficult to assess. Prostatitis is often a complication of benign prostatic hypertrophy and prostatic calculi.

The organisms involved are usually the pyogenic group, including staphylococci, streptococci, E. coli, and diphtheroids. The gonococcus may regain its former prominence.

The infection may be mild (catarrhal) and be associated with a posterior urethritis. It may spread to the prostatic ducts and acini to result in a follicular prostatitis. Further extension leads to parenchymatous inflammation and eventually to abscess formation with rupture into the urethra, ischiorectal fossa, or rectum. With spread of the inflammation the seminal vesicles become inflamed.

Symptoms. Prostatitis may present with chills, fever, myalgia, nausea, and vomiting. Local symptoms are perineal ache, low back pain, rectal discomfort, dysuria, frequency, urgency, and reduction in force of the urinary stream which may progress to complete urinary retention.

Physical Examination. A large, tense, tender, hot prostate may be felt on examination. Fluctuation with interspersed firm areas and extreme tenderness indicates abscess. Examination of urethral discharge and urinary sediment may give laboratory confirmation of the diagnosis.

Treatment. General treatment is rest, fluids, antipyretics, analgesics and antibiotics, according to the bacteriologic findings. Urinary retention is treated by insertion of a catheter. A transurethral or perineal approach is used to drain an abscess.

Chronic Prostatitis

Chronic prostatitis most often follows acute prostatitis and occurs most often in men over 50 years. Urethral discharge may be minimal and may present as a small, "morning drop" at the meatus. There may be frequency and urgency of micturition, sensation of bladder fullness, perineal and testicular discomfort, and lowback pain. The gland may feel boggy on rectal examination, and there may be profuse flow of prostatic fluid containing numerous white blood cells. The urine and prostatic fluid are examined microscopically and bacteriologically. Prolonged antibacterial therapy is indicated because antibiotics do not readily enter the prostatic acini. Prostatic massage may be worthwhile. It is essential to exclude urethral obstruction or any other predisposing cause. In selected cases transurethral resection may result in some improvement.

Benign Prostatic Hypertrophy

The etiology of benign prostatic hypertrophy is not known, but it is most likely the result of change with age in the hormonal status. The disease is rare in Chinese, Koreans, Japanese, Asiatic Indians, and Bantu. It occurs in the North American Negro about a decade earlier than in Caucasians. Prostatic atrophy can be produced by postpubertal castration and estrogen therapy. The target area of hormone imbalance is estrogen-sensitive connective tissue and smooth muscle in the periurethral tissue between the bladder neck and verumontanum. Hypertrophy in this region produces the condition known as prostatism.

The obstruction to flow results in frequency and nocturia. Other symptoms are hematuria, urgency, postvoid dribbling, and superimposed inflammation. Infection, once established, is difficult to eradicate because of the large volume of residual urine. Acute urine retention occurs when the obstruction is greater than the bladder's expulsive power. Acute retention is often precipitated by overdistention of the bladder, especially after operation. Bladder distention may be marked and may be undetected, especially when the onset of obstruction has been slow.

Rectal examination generally reveals prostatic enlargement. Investigations include examination of the urine, an intravenous pyelogram, and estimation of blood urea nitrogen and creatinine. Residual urine volume is assessed by passing a catheter after micturition, a postvoid film during intravenous pyelography, or at cystoscopy. In selected cases biopsy of the prostate, urethrography, and cystometrography may be helpful. Differential diagnosis includes prostatic carcinoma, prostatic abscess, neurogenic bladder, urinary tract infection, bladder neck dysfunction, urethral stricture, bladder calculi, and bladder tumors.

Treatment. The obstructing prostatic tissue should be removed surgically when the general condition and renal function are as good as possible and when any associated urinary infection has been controlled. The approach may be transurethral, retropubic, suprapubic, or perineal. The transurethral approach is used most commonly and requires a urethra of adequate caliber, and a gland which is not too large. The retropubic approach is used when the gland is large or the urethral lumen is small. The suprapubic approach is used when there is associated bladder pathology, such as a diverticulum or vesical calculus. The perineal route is only used when there is an area suggestive of carcinoma, and radical perineal surgery is contemplated.

PENIS

Hypospadias

The abnormal position of the urethra on the lower surface of the penis may be associated with a ventral band of fibrous tissue which causes a bending deformity of the penis referred to as chordee. This is accentuated by erection. The urethral orifice, which is often stenotic, may be coronal, penile, scrotal, or perineal in location. In those with severe deformity the child's sex may be in doubt and must be determined accurately before treatment is undertaken.

Correction of the chordee to produce a straight penile shaft results in a backward shift of the urethral meatus. A second procedure to create a new urethra is undertaken later. The foreskin provides valuable tissue for the reconstruction. Circumcision should therefore not be performed in children with hypospadias (Figure 33-9, page 592).

Epispadias

The urethral opening is on the dorsal aspect of the penis. The deformity is often associated with separation of the symphysis pubis and deficiency of the body wall below the umbilicus. There is often an imperfect bladder sphincter, so that urinary control is a chronic problem after correction of the defect.

Inflammatory Diseases

Phimosis (nonretractile foreskin) and balanitis (inflammation of the glans penis) are often associated. The tight foreskin leads to retention of organisms and cellular debris and predisposes to inflammation especially in diabetics. Phimosis is treated by circumcision. Balanitis responds to good hygiene following operation.

Paraphimosis

Paraphimosis occurs when the foreskin has been retracted proximal to the glans and cannot be replaced. Venous obstruction results in marked swelling. Treatment consists of gentle manual compression to reduce the edema so that the foreskin can be delivered over the glans. If the foreskin cannot be reduced, a dorsal slit under general anesthesia is required. Circumcision is necessary if the condition is recurrent.

RENAL TRANSPLANTATION

This procedure is now accepted therapy in selected cases of chronic renal failure and offers advantages over chronic dialysis, including freedom from dietary restriction, psychological and physical freedom from dependence on a mechanical device, return of normal hematopoiesis, spermatogenesis, and potency. The main problem in transplantation is graft rejection, which requires immunosuppression with its attendant risks.

Recipient Selection

Age limits are difficult to apply, and the upper limit of 50 years may often be exceeded in good-risk patients. In children transplantation offers hope for more normal growth and an escape from hemodialysis, which is technically difficult.

Creatinine clearance is usually less than 5 mg percent and serum creatinine greater than 10 mg percent when transplantation is undertaken. Potential recipients should be free from severe generalized arteriosclerosis, diabetes of juvenile onset, uncontrolled malignancy, uncontrolled infection, and systemic diseases with poor prognoses (e.g., scleroderma). They should have a normally functioning lower urinary tract. Urinary tract abnormalities requiring correction include outlet obstruction, vesicoureteral reflux, chronic pyelonephritis, and polycystic renal disease. Occasionally bilateral nephrectomy is performed in uncontrolled hypertension.

Donor Selection

Renal grafts may be obtained from living donors or from cadavers. The risk of rejection is reduced by selecting related donors and best of all identical twins. When numerous siblings are available, tissue matching allows selection of the best match. Major ethical considerations are to preserve the donor's health and to avoid pressure on an individual to donate a kidney. A living donor should be less than 55 years, free from significant disease, and must have adequate renal function to support life with a solitary kidney. Careful urinary tract investigations include urinalysis with culture, creatinine clearance, IVP, and aortography.

Cadaveric grafts are most often obtained from young victims of road accidents or subarachnoid hemorrhage in whom good renal perfusion has been maintained. Donors should be less than 65 years and free from malignancy, diffuse arteriosclerosis, and infections. Before kidneys are accepted, their function should have been assessed by urinalysis with careful examination of the sediment, BUN, creatinine, and two-hour creatinine clearance. Urine output must be maintained as an index of good renal perfusion.

Surgical Technique

Donor nephrectomy requires meticulous dissection of the renal arteries to avoid injury to polar vessels. Full vascular length should be maintained to facilitate anastomosis in the recipient. Hilar dissection is avoided to prevent devascularization of the ureter, and the ureter is removed without adventitial stripping.

The kidneys are cooled to reduce metabolic activity. Good results are now obtained in kidneys subjected to cold pulsatile perfusion for periods up to 24 hours prior to grafting.

Renal grafting is not technically complex, having been performed successfully in 1902. The iliac fossa is the common recipient site, and an extraperitoneal pouch is readily created. Vascular anastomoses are carried out followed by establishment of urinary continuity. Implantation of the donor ureter into the bladder is probably safest and simplest, although anastomosis of recipient ureter to donor renal pelvis has also been accomplished.

Postoperative Care

Protective isolation of the recipient is crucial, especially during the first week of immunosuppression. Catheter and drains are removed as soon as possible to prevent infection. Careful bacteriologic, hematologic, and biochemical surveillance is maintained. Early function of the graft may be poor, requiring hemodialysis. Problems may arise due to rejection, infection, drug toxicity, or urinary leakage. Chronic illness and immunosuppression constitute a risk to survival of both graft and patient and demand immediate correction.

Results

At all times patient survival must take precedence over graft survival. With the aid of HL-A matching, two-year graft survivals up to 70 percent may now be expected. Increasing incompatibility reduces chances of graft survival and carefully selected living related donors continue to show best overall results.

TUMORS OF THE GENITOURINARY TRACT

Tumors of the genitourinary tract are common. Many, unfortunately, remain silent until advanced. For this reason all urinary symptoms should be carefully evaluated.

Wilms' Tumor (Nephroblastoma)

This is an embryonal tumor presenting in 75 percent before five years, with equal sex incidence and bilateral in about 7 percent. The tumor is often large when diagnosed and may be detected by parents. Pain and hematuria occur in about one third of patients and hypertension in about 75 percent.

The diagnosis may be made on physical examination and confirmed by intravenous pyelography. Differentiation from neuroblastoma, renal cystic disease, and other retroperitoneal tumors can usually be made from the intravenous pyelogram. Treatment is by a combination of surgery, chemotherapy, and radiotherapy. Nephrectomy is performed through a transverse upper abdominal incision with ligation of the vessels prior to mobilizing

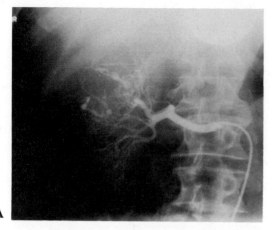
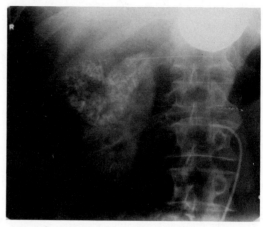

A   B

Figure 32–10. Renal cell carcinoma. *A.* Arterial phase shows irregular vessels with extension of the mass beyond the normal renal outline. *B.* Venous phase demonstrates sinusoids with "puddling" of dye in the tumor mass.

the tumor. Radiotherapy is given to the tumor bed after operation except in children below one year. Chemotherapy is often used, with dactinomycin and vincristine given especially to those with distant metastases.

Renal Cell Carcinoma

This is the commonest adult cancer of the kidney, with a peak incidence at about 60 years and twice as common in the male as the female. It arises from mature renal parenchyma and tends to reproduce the tubular architecture when well differentiated.

About 50 percent are asymptomatic when detected. Seventy percent of those with symptoms have hematuria. Pain consisting of a dull ache in the loin may be present, and about 50 percent have colic from passage of clots. A palpable mass is generally not present. Renal cell carcinoma may present as fever of unknown origin with polycythemia or with abnormal liver function tests without hepatic metastases.

The diagnosis should be suspected when there are hematuria and loin discomfort with or without a palpable mass. Intravenous pyelography may show a mass with caliceal distortion or with disruption of the normal renal outline. Nephrotomograms help to delineate the mass and differentiate solid from cystic lesions. Selective renal arteriography may demonstrate a classic tumor blush as well as early venous filling (Figure 32–10, *A* and *B*). When tumor neovasculature is less prominent, as when the center of the tumor is necrotic, careful examination of the periphery of the lesion will usually confirm its malignant nature.

Treatment is surgical with additional radiotherapy and chemotherapy in selected patients.

Radical nephrectomy is the operation of choice with early control of the renal pedicle and removal of the affected kidney contained within Gerota's fascia and the regional nodes. Postoperative radiotherapy is given if the tumor has extended beyond the renal capsule, or if there are metastases in the regional nodes or permeation of the renal veins.

Carcinoma of the Renal Pelvis and Ureter

These are urothelial lesions and are therefore usually transitional cell carcinomas. They present with bleeding or obstruction. Investigation includes cytologic examination of the urine and intravenous pyelography when a pelvic or ureteral filling defect is seen. The commonest reason for failure to make the diagnosis is acceptance of x-ray studies that fail to visualize the full length of the ureter. Retrograde pyelograms may be indicated to visualize the ureter more clearly. The tumors have a marked tendency to spread into the retroperitoneal tissues. Nephroureterectomy is the treatment of choice.

Carcinoma of the Urinary Bladder

This is the most important cancer of the genitourinary system. It occurs twice as often in males as in females, usually between 50 and 70 years, and can be produced by the chemical beta naphthylamine and by cigarette smoking. The tumors are usually transitional cell in type, although adenocarcinoma occurs in about 1 percent at the urachus and close to the bladder neck. Squamous cell carcinomas are present in about 5 percent and may be the result of chronic irritation by stone, infection, or parasites.

Gross hematuria is the presenting symptom

of most bladder tumors. Irritative symptoms such as frequency or urgency suggest invasion and more advanced disease. Diagnosis may be made while investigating microscopic hematuria. Before endoscopy intravenous pyelography is obtained to outline the upper tract. Cancer cells may be seen in the urine. Cystoscopy permits direct visualization of the tumor. The stage and grade of the lesion are determined by transurethral biopsy and bimanual examination while the patient is relaxed under anesthesia.

Increasingly aggressive treatment is required for increasing stage, grade, or multicentricity of the tumor. Prognosis is much worse when the tumor has penetrated deep muscle. Treatment requires assessing the tumor's stage and grade, the patient's age and general condition, and the previous treatments by operation or radiotherapy. The lesions may be classified as:

Phase I. Superficial growth (stage O, A, B) and low grade (I, II).
Phase II. Deep growth (stage B_2, C) and high grade (III, IV).
Phase III. Metastatic (stage D) and usually high grade.

Surgical treatments include transurethral resection, loop resection in the open bladder, partial cystectomy, and total cystectomy with urinary diversion. Radiotherapy may be given as teletherapy using a high-energy source, by implantation of radium needles or radon seeds, or by intracavitary balloon containing a radioactive isotope. Chemotherapy may be topical, applying thio-TEPA to multiple superficial lesions, or systemic, giving intravenous 5-FU to those with locally advanced disease or distant metastases.

Phase I tumors are usually controlled by transurethral resection and fulguration. Multiple lesions may be treated with intravesical thio-TEPA. If there is a rapid increase in the rate of recurrence or in the number of lesions, radiotherapy or operation should be considered.

Phase II tumors usually require total cystectomy with urinary diversion. Radiotherapy may be given prior to partial or total cystectomy or may be used as the only treatment. If the lesion is in the dome of the bladder, partial cystectomy may be adequate. In these patients accurate staging of the tumor is essential.

Phase III tumors. Local obstructive lesions may require endoscopy. Radiotherapy may help control pain and hematuria. Urinary diversion may relieve the exhausting frequency and discomfort from urine flowing through a bladder with ulcerated mucosa and reduced capacity.

Carcinoma of the Prostate

This disease is the second most frequent cause of death from cancer in the male. It is rare before 50 years and increases in incidence with age. Although changes in the hormonal environment have been implicated, the cause is not known. The tumor is an adenocarcinoma. Sarcomas occur rarely and most often in children. The disease is often asymptomatic and is discovered by careful rectal examination, looking for changes in the contour or consistency of the prostate. A hard, ill-defined region in the prostate suggests malignancy. It is essential, however, to establish the diagnosis microscopically either by needle biopsy or, if that is unsuccessful, by open perineal biopsy. About 50 percent of nodules are malignant. The commonest symptom of prostatic carcinoma is bladder neck obstruction.

Local spread of the tumor beyond the prostate to the seminal vesicles can be determined by rectal examination. The most frequent distant spread is to the pelvic and para-aortic lymph nodes, to bones, especially in the pelvis and lumbar vertebrae, and to liver, lungs, and supraclavicular nodes. The osteoblastic bony metastases may be diagnosed by skeletal survey, bone scan, and bone marrow cytology. The serum acid and alkaline phosphatase levels are increased.

Treatment. Treatment depends on the stage of the disease and the age and condition of the patient. Curative treatment is radical prostatovesiculectomy either by the perineal or retropubic route. It is possible in about 5 percent of patients who have early tumors and a life expectancy of at least 10 years (i.e., under age 70). "Cure" may also be obtained by radiotherapy.

It is important to appreciate that only about one patient in eight with prostatic cancer dies from that disease. Good palliation can be obtained by transurethral resection, estrogens, castration, ^{32}P, ^{198}Au, adrenalectomy, hypophysectomy, and radiotherapy. Transurethral resection may be used to correct obstruction and to control bleeding.

Estrogens provide the most important palliative treatment for advanced prostatic carcinoma. They relieve ureteral and bladder outlet obstruction, decrease bleeding, relieve bone pain from metastases, and increase survival.

Alteration of the tumor's hormonal milieu by castration may act in a way similar to oophorectomy for advanced carcinoma of the breast. Estrogens and castration may be used concurrently, but in some centers castration is performed only after estrogen therapy has failed.

Survival, however, is the same with both treatments. Adrenalectomy and hypophysectomy are only occasionally indicated in the patient in good general condition who has had a good initial response to castration and estrogens and has tumor, especially in bone and skin.

The primary tumor may be treated by teletherapy or local implantation of radon seeds or gold (^{198}Au). Metastases in bone tend to respond well to local radiotherapy, especially in patients with localized bone pain. Good palliation can often be obtained using radioactive phosphorus, ^{32}P, in those with widespread bony metastases causing pain or anemia.

Testicular Tumors

Tumors of the testis account for about 1 percent of male cancers but are of special importance because they occur most often in young men, aged 20 to 40. They tend to be asymptomatic and are often discovered by the patient or by a physician during a routine examination. A heavy mass in the testis is the most important finding. The incidence of testicular tumor in undescended testes is greater than that in scrotal testes. Tumors should be differentiated from other scrotal swellings such as hydrocele, spermatocele, epididymitis, orchitis, or connective tissue tumors. The presence of a hydrocele may be deceptive in that it may be produced by the tumor. Occasionally a testicular tumor may present with metastases in the lung or with pleural effusion, an abdominal mass from enlarged para-aortic nodes, liver metastases, and, rarely, endocrine changes such as gynecomastia. Preoperative investigations include an intravenous pyelogram, chest x-ray, and serum gonadotropins. Lymphangiography may be done to visualize the pelvic and para-aortic nodes but most commonly follows orchidectomy.

About 97 percent of testicular tumors are germinal, including seminoma, embryonal carcinoma, teratoma, teratocarcinoma, and choriocarcinoma. Mixed types are not uncommon. Solid tumors may originate from the interstitial cells or from the stromal elements of the testis.

Treatment. A diagnosis of testicular tumor calls for inguinal orchidectomy with removal of testis and spermatic cord to the level of the internal ring. Lymphangiography may then be done to attempt clinical staging. Further therapy depends on tumor type and stage. Tumors of the testis may be classified as stage A when the tumor is confined to the testis, stage B when subdiaphragmatic nodes contain metastases, and stage C when nodes above the diaphragm are involved or there are metastases in other organs. Patients with stages A and B

tumors which are not seminoma or choriocarcinoma should be managed by para-aortic lymph node dissection. Negative nodes at surgery preclude the need for further treatment. Positive nodes may indicate need for radiotherapy and chemotherapy.

Patients with seminomas have the best prognosis, with up to 90 percent five-year survival for those treated by orchidectomy and radiotherapy. The worst prognosis is in those with choriocarcinoma, where long-term survival is rare. Teratoma, teratocarcinoma, and embryonal carcinoma carry a five-year survival of about 80 percent when treatment is orchidectomy and node dissection. The importance of pathologic staging is shown in this group by the fact that survival is 87 percent when the nodes are negative and 66 percent when the nodes are positive but resectable.

Carcinoma of the Penis

This is a rare disease, occurring almost exclusively in those who have not been circumcised. The major factor in the association between the presence of the foreskin and carcinoma of the penis is probably hygiene. When cleanliness of the foreskin and glans is maintained, carcinoma is rare. A squamous cell carcinoma develops in the preputial cavity and presents with a foul discharge, bleeding, outlet obstruction, or metastases to the groin.

Treatment is local excision, usually with partial amputation of the penis. Clinically involved inguinal lymph nodes are removed by block dissection of the groin. Radiotherapy may be tried initially to the primary lesion provide it does not involve the urethra or the body of the penis. The prognosis in those with carcinoma of the penis is bad.

URETHRA

Posterior Urethral Valves

This abnormality, occurring in infant males, may present as abdominal distention, failure to thrive, urinary infection, or renal failure. The nature of the symptoms will be determined by the degree of renal damage and outlet obstruction. Diapers may mask the infant's failure to void freely.

Diagnostic radiologic findings of a dilated and elongated posterior urethra with a sharp cut-off of contrast at the level of the valves may be noted if a voiding study is obtained. Careful pyelographic and metabolic assessment is required. Metabolic deficits and obstruction must be corrected. Upper tract dilatation often requires supravesical diversion of the urine until relief from bladder wall obstruction is obtained. Destruction of the valves is carried out before urinary tract continuity is restored.

Urethral Stricture

Scarring of the urethra occurs as a result of external trauma, instrumental injury, either iatrogenic or self-inflicted, or as a late result of gonococcal urethritis. The fibrosis involves both mucosal and submucosal layers.

Symptoms relate primarily to slowing of the urinary stream. Secondary changes include urinary infection, upper tract dilatation and destruction, and formation of bladder calculi. Urethrography and urethroscopy will delineate the location and extent of the lesion.

Reestablishment of adequate urethral caliber may require dilatation with filiforms and followers or urethral sounds. Extensive strictures, or those that recur rapidly, may be relieved by urethroplasty, replacing the scarred segment with viable supple tissue. Surgery to correct urethral strictures from verumontanum to meatus is now possible.

Meatal Obstruction

A common finding in females complaining of frequency, urgency, and dysuria is a tight ring of tissue at the distal end of the urethra. Although the symptoms suggest infection, cultures often show no growth. This entity of "meatal stenosis" is frequently associated with spasm of the midurethral musculature. Dilation of the distal ring or meatotomy may cure the patient.

Meatal obstruction in the male may contribute to urethritis, enuresis, or frank outlet obstruction. Its cause is scarring subsequent to circumcision, meatitis, or transurethral surgery and catheter drainage. Dilatation or meatotomy will provide relief.

Urethritis

Acute urethral inflammation may be of bacterial, mycoplasmal, chemical, or protozoal origin. The infection may be a sequel to prostatic inflammation. Symptoms of itching, burning on urination, and urethral discharge are common. The investigation should include careful culture of urethral discharge. Gram stain of a foul discharge may reveal gonococci. Appropriate antibiotic therapy should be instituted.

Chronic urethritis may follow an acute attack or may arise primarily. Low-grade irritative symptoms and small volumes of clear, sticky discharge typify the ailment. Chronic prostatitis may be associated.

Following culture of urethral and prostatic secretion, antibiotic or antibacterial suppression should be instituted.

Carcinoma of the Urethra

This disease is uncommon and presents as urethral bleeding or with obstructive symptoms. Diagnosis may be suspected by the history and confirmed by inspection, endoscopy, and biopsy. Surgery and radiotherapy both contribute to therapy in varying degrees, depending on the site and stage of the lesion.

SUGGESTIONS FOR FURTHER READING

Campbell, M. E., and Harrison, J. H: *Urology*, 3rd. ed. W. B. Saunders Co., Philadelphia, 1970.
This standard reference is encyclopedic but some sections are out of date.
Emmett, J. L., and Witten D. M.: *Clinical Urography*, 3rd. ed. W. B. Saunders, Philadelphia, 1971.
This outstanding text has good correlation between clinical and radiologic findings.
Glenn, J. F., and Boyce, W. H.: *Urologic Surgery*. Harper & Row (Hoeber Medical Division), New York, 1969.
Comprehensive description of clinical urology and operative technique.
Netter, F. M.: *The Ciba Collection of Medical Illustrations*. Vol. 16. (Kidneys, Ureters and Urinary Bladder). Published by Ciba, 1973.
Classic illustrations with concise text.
Smith, D. R.: *General Urology*. 7th ed. Lange Medical Publications, Los Altos, 1972.
This is a concise, comprehensive, and up-to-date text.

Chapter 33

RECONSTRUCTIVE AND PLASTIC SURGERY

George P. Reading

CHAPTER OUTLINE

Principles of Plastic Surgery
  Definitions
  Techniques of Reconstruction
    Approximation
    Skin Grafts
    Uses of Skin Grafts
    "Take" of Skin Grafts
    Local Flaps
    Preincision or "Delay"
    Z-Plasty
    Distant Flaps
Congenital Anomalies
  Cleft Lip and Cleft Palate
    Treatment
  Ear Deformities
  Branchial Cyst
  Thyroglossal Cyst
  Hand Anomalies
    Supernumerary Digits
    Syndactyly
    Radial Club Hand
  Urogenital Anomalies
    Hypospadias
    Epispadias
Traumatic Defects and Deformities
  Facial Soft Tissue Injuries
    Initial Care

    Late Revision
  Facial Fractures
    Diagnosis
    Radiographs
    Treatment
  Eye Injuries
    Penetrating
    Conjunctival Foreign Body
    Abrasions and Lacerations
    Actinic Conjunctivitis
    Chemical Burns
  Hand Injuries
  Defects in the Lower Extremity
  Pressure Ulcers (Decubitus Ulcers)
Neoplastic Disease
  Cancer of the Skin
  Head and Neck Tumors
Aesthetic Surgery
  Aesthetic Rhinoplasty
  Skin-Tightening Procedures
    Rhytidectomy
    Blepharoplasty
    Chemosurgery
  Other Tightening Procedures
  Mammoplasty
    Reduction
    Augmentation

Plastic surgery is a specialized branch of surgery devoted to reconstruction of the skin, subcutaneous tissues, and deeper structures. As the name "plastic" suggests, it is largely concerned with changes in form or shape. The aim is to obtain primary wound healing with minimal scar formation in the skin, where disfigurement may be visible, or in deep tissues, where excessive scarring may impair function.

Frequently the plastic surgeon is called on to repair surface defects when simple methods will not suffice. He must also deal with defects in the deeper tissues such as the facial bones, tendons and nerves of the hand, and the nose, pharynx, and upper esophagus. The field of plastic surgery thus includes mostly the head, neck, hand, and less often the genitourinary system, trunk, and lower extremity. The underlying defects may be congenital, or follow trauma or resection of neoplasms. Aesthetic or cosmetic surgery is now an important aspect of plastic surgery.

PRINCIPLES OF PLASTIC SURGERY

Definitions

A *graft* is a tissue transplanted from one region to another without maintaining its blood supply. It must therefore live by imbibition of the fluids until a new blood supply is achieved from the recipient site. The most frequent grafts are skin, but free grafts of bone, tendon, cartilage, and fat are also used extensively. Vascular grafts are nourished by the blood within the lumen of the graft. Organ transplants may be called grafts but are connected by vascular anastomoses and are nourished through the vessels.

A *pedicle flap* contains several tissues that are moved from one position to another with some of the blood supply maintained. It usually consists of skin and subcutaneous tissues, but other tissues may additionally be transposed.

Grafts may also be described genetically. Those transplanted from one site to another in the same individual are called *autografts*; those between genetically identical individuals are *syngeneic*; those between individuals of the same species not genetically identical are *allografts*; and those between different species are *xenografts*.

Techniques of Reconstruction

Approximation. Simple defects may be closed by bringing one margin of the defect to the other. If the edges are undermined to avoid tension, the procedure is termed a local "sliding flap." If excessive tension cannot be avoided, some other method must be used. When revising scars, the careful approximation of tissues, layer by layer, is most important. The accurate approximation of the dermis, the strongest layer of the skin, is the most crucial element in the operation.

Skin Grafts. Defects may be closed by skin grafts when local approximation is not suitable. *Split-thickness skin grafts* consist of epidermis and the superficial portion of the dermis (Figure 33–1). The donor site heals by re-epithelialization from epithelial cells in the glands and hair follicles. In general, thin split-thickness grafts "take" better than thick split-thickness grafts, because there is less tissue to be nourished by the tissue fluids prior to ingrowth of blood vessels. However, a thick split-thickness graft functions better and has a better appearance. The thicker the split-thickness graft, the more difficulty in healing at the donor site. *Full-thickness skin grafts* include the epidermis and all the dermis. The donor site must be closed by approximation or grafting. Full-thickness grafts do not take as well as split-thickness grafts, but the functional and cosmetic results are better.

Uses of Skin Grafts. Skin grafts may be used anywhere a "take" is likely. Free skin grafts do not usually take on joints, tendons, bones, or cartilage. Defects over nerves and

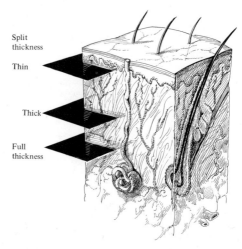

Figure 33–1. A free skin graft may be thin skin, thick skin, or full thickness depending upon the depth in the dermis at which the graft is cut.

large blood vessels can be covered by free grafts but are subjected to considerable trauma, and it is better to use a local or pedicle flap. Fascia, muscle, periosteum, and perichondrium are suitable recipient sites for free skin grafts. They also take on properly prepared granulation tissue, as for example a burn (see Chapter 15, page 267). Another common use is at the donor site following transfer of a flap.

Full-thickness grafts are used to cover small defects on the face, neck, and hands. The usual donor sites are the flexor creases in the groin and antecubital fossa for the hand and the retro-auricular skin and supraclavicular region for the face.

Split-thickness grafts taken from the "blush" region above the clavicles have a satisfactory color match with the surrounding skin when used on the face. Split-thickness grafts taken from below the blush region do not match.

"Take" of Skin Grafts. There are three phases in the establishment of a skin graft. First, the graft is nourished by plasma. Second, at about 24 to 48 hours, small vascular channels appear in the fibrin between the recipient site and the raw surface of the graft. These channels may supply the graft by direct anastomosis with the small vessels of the graft. Third, at about four days, new capillaries grow into the graft and lymphatics appear. The phases vary in duration. Sometimes it takes more than four days for vascularization to occur, whereas some grafts "pink up" in less than 24 hours.

The causes of failure to take are numerous. Anything that prevents the graft from intimate contact with the bed such as blood, serum, or pus results in failure. Insufficient tension allows wrinkling and failure of the graft to correspond to the minor irregularities of the bed. Excessive tension in the graft obliterates small blood vessels, and movement of the graft on its bed prevents vascularization. Movement is minimized by "tie-down" dressings. In addition, sutures are left long and tied over the dressing to hold it firmly in place and splints are used to keep limbs at rest. Limbs should be elevated to prevent edema.

A wound with an adequate blood supply is rapidly covered with granulation tissue and provides a satisfactory bed for skin graft. All necrotic or nonviable tissue must be excised. Alternatively wet or dry dressings may be applied three or more times per day to prepare the granulation tissue for grafting. If granulation tissue has been present for more than two weeks, it may be edematous and contain excessive fibrous tissue. It should then be excised before grafting.

The take of skin grafts in apparently clean wounds may be prevented by bacteria, such as the group A beta-hemolytic streptococcus which produces a potent epithelial toxin. The profuse exudate produced by *Pseudomonas aeruginosa* may float the graft off the recipient site. Any infections should be treated before grafting. Application of a nonviable skin graft, allograft, or freeze-dried skin to a granulating wound rapidly decreases the number of bacteria on the wound surface.

Local Flaps. Local flaps are frequently used to close defects and have the advantage over free grafts of producing a cover which includes vascularized subcutaneous tissue as well as skin. In addition, the skin adjacent to the defect is usually similar to the missing skin. Local flaps are often used to cover joints and bones in the hand and in the lower extremity. Local rotation flaps are particularly useful in the head and neck because of the rich blood supply. Defects produced by local rotation flaps may be closed by approximation but more often require a

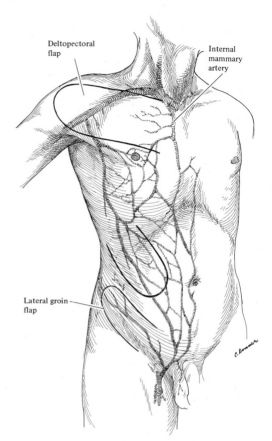

Figure 33–3. The deltopectoral, abdominal, and lateral groin flaps are shown based on their blood supply.

split-thickness skin graft, for example in management of decubitus ulcers.

Design. Local flaps must be large enough and have a good blood supply (Figure 33–2). It is important to note that the flap rotates from the corner of the pedicle rather than the center. Flaps in the head and neck may have long length-to-width ratios, but those in the extremities are best kept to a one-to-one ratio. Whenever possible the flap is made to include axial vessels in the pedicle (Figure 33–3).

Preincision or "Delay." If the survival of a flap is uncertain by virtue of its length-to-width ratio or anatomic position, its survival is enhanced by preincision or "delay." The margins of the flap are incised with or without undermining. There is then a compensatory increase in the blood supply carried by the planned pedicle. In general, a week or more should elapse between delay and transfer of the flap.

Z-Plasty. The Z-plasty is a special type of local flap (Figure 33–4). It involves changing the direction of a scar and lengthening it by making

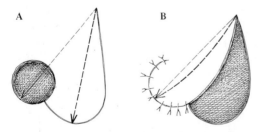

Figure 33–2. Skin flap. Note that the local flap rotates from the corner of the pedicle and not from the center.

two triangular local flaps, one at either end. The flaps are then switched so that each covers the other's donor site. The wound is now Z-shaped and at right angles to the scar. The scar is thus lengthened, and unscarred tissue is now present across the length of the original scar. Z-plasties are particularly useful at joints and in scars running in unfavorable directions, as for example across the wrinkle lines of the face.

Distant Flaps. Distant flaps require late division of the pedicle for the completion of reconstruction. Examples are the "cross-finger flap," the "cross-leg flap," those from the chest to the head and neck, or from the abdomen or thorax to the hand (Figure 33–5). The pedicle may be tubed or sutured to itself to close the raw surface. Alternatively a split skin graft may be used to close the raw surface of the pedicle. Skin grafting is usually needed to cover the donor sites. Distant flaps require about three weeks of attachment to the recipient site before the pedicle can be divided safely. It is often worthwhile to divide the pedicle in stages to avoid marginal necrosis of the flap.

Indirect flaps are distant flaps in which a tissue is transferred from one position on the body to another, using an extremity as a carrier. An example is a flap from the abdomen first attached to the wrist. After this attachment has matured, the opposite end of the flap is detached from the abdomen and then the wrist is carried to the recipient site, for example the leg. After a suitable time the pedicle to the wrist is divided and the reconstruction completed.

A recent development has been the use of free vascularized flaps or grafts consisting of subcutaneous tissue and skin based on discrete

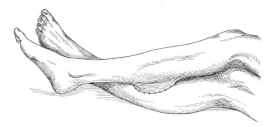

Figure 33–5. The cross leg flap is often used for the treatment of a compound fracture of the tibia.

arteries and veins and transferred by microvascular anastomosis of these vessels to vessels in the recipient area. The most commonly used donor area is the groin, supplied by the superficial circumflex iliac and superficial inferior hypogastric vessels.

CONGENITAL ANOMALIES

Cleft Lip and Cleft Palate

Cleft lip and cleft palate, occurring in about 1 out of 800 births, are among the most frequent congenital defects. The severity ranges from a small notch in the lip or a submucous cleft of the muscle and bone of the palate to a wide cleft involving both sides of the lips and the entire palate. The etiology is unknown. If a child is born with a cleft lip, the chance of a subsequent sibling having the same defect is about 5 percent. However, in those with a cleft palate alone the incidence of clefts in other siblings is small. Cleft lip with or without cleft palate seems to be genetically distinct from isolated cleft palate.

The lip is formed at about seven weeks after conception. Three masses of mesoderm penetrate the primordial lip composed of endoderm and ectoderm. If one of the lateral masses of mesoderm fails to penetrate, a cleft lip results on that side. Bilateral cleft lips occur when both lateral masses fail to penetrate. The rare median cleft is caused by failure of the central mass to develop.

The palate is formed by fusion of the lateral palatal shelves, first caudally and later over the tongue. The process starts at about seven weeks and is completed at about 12 weeks.

Treatment. Cleft lips are best repaired within three months of birth. If the clefts are approximated, edge to edge, the lip is too short from the nose to the vermillion border. Some sort of Z-plasty is usually employed to compensate for this shortening (Figure 33–6). The nose is always distorted. The results of operative treatment of cleft lip are excellent; those in balancing the nose are not as good.

The cleft palate is usually repaired at a later

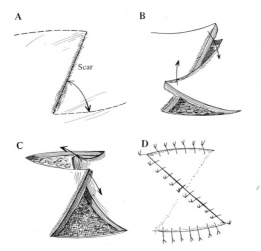

Figure 33–4. The Z-plasty is frequently used to change the direction of a scar.

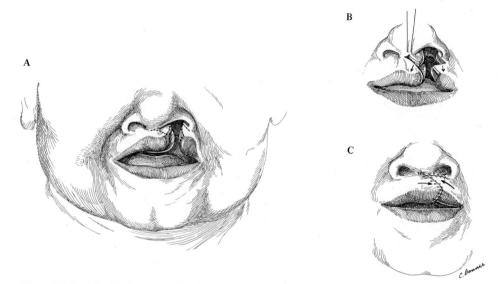

Figure 33–6. The Z-plasty is utilized in the repair of a cleft lip. In addition, nasal cartilage may be removed to correct the associated nasal deformity.

date because of the difficulty in maintaining the airway in the small infant, the importance of blood loss, and the small size of the structures. Some surgeons recommend that palatal repair should be done at five years or even later, because they believe that the trauma of operation may interfere with growth. However, speech is better if the palate is closed by 18 months when the first efforts at talking are usually made.

If a long mobile palate able to occlude the space between the nasopharynx and oropharynx is achieved, the patient usually speaks well. This result is obtained in about 75 percent of patients. Speech therapy, prostheses, and reconstructive operations are used in those with poor results.

The alveolar processes which carry the teeth are often deformed. Early or late bone grafting has been used to attempt to achieve a good bite. Otitis media is frequent in children with cleft palates. This is probably due to the proximity of the orifices of the eustachian tubes to the palatal muscles.

Ear Deformities

Protruding external ears are the most common deformity. The cause is failure of the ear cartilage to fold at the antihelix and increased depth of the concha. Repair should be done before the child starts school. A fold is produced in the cartilage, and/or the size of the concha is reduced by resection.

Microtia is a severe deformity from failure of the external ear to develop from the first and second branchial arches. Other structures

derived from these arches are often abnormal. The ears can be reconstructed by implantation of cartilage or prostheses beneath the skin to form a framework. The new ear is then elevated from the side of the head and a skin graft placed behind it. Results are generally disappointing. Sometimes reconstruction is not attempted, and a prosthetic ear is used.

Branchial Cyst

A branchial cyst is due to persistence of remnants of the second or third branchial clefts. The cyst is lined with stratified squamous epithelium. It may present as a mass in the neck along the anterior border of the sternocleidomastoid with or without episodes of infection, and there may be sinuses in the skin or internally in the pharynx.

Treatment is excision. The operation must be done carefully to avoid leaving remnants of the cyst and to avoid injuring adjacent structures, such as branches of the facial nerve.

Thyroglossal Cyst

A thyroglossal cyst arises from the embryonic thyroglossal duct, which lies between the median portion of the thyroid gland and the foramen cecum at the base of the tongue. Failure of the duct to close causes formation of a cyst or sinus. The cyst is a unilocular midline swelling which moves on protrusion of the tongue and on swallowing (Figure 33–7). It may be the site of recurrent infection. Treatment is excision of the entire cyst and/or fistula along with the central portion of the hyoid bone. Failure to remove a

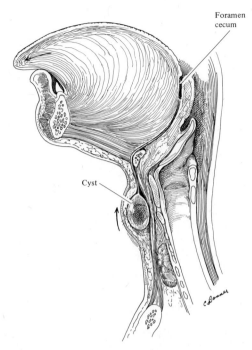

Figure 33–7. A thyroglossal cyst is attached to the base of the tongue by the remnant of the thyroglossal duct. The cyst therefore moves upward on swallowing and on protruding the tongue.

portion of the hyoid bone results in a high incidence of recurrence.

Hand Anomalies

When treating hand deformities, it is important to distinguish between cosmetic and functional problems. Severe deformities are compatible with excellent function. Care must be taken not to operate to improve appearance if there is a risk of impairing function.

Supernumerary Digits. Supernumerary digits are the most common anomaly in the hand and are familial. The extra digits may be at the ulnar or radial side of the hand and range from completely separate and normal digits to a small rudiment. The thumb may be double and have neither portion in the proper position or one may have the correct number of tendons and joints. There may be five fingers with no thumb.

Syndactyly. Syndactyly is fusion of two or more digits. The fingers may be intimately fused or connected only by a web of skin. The fingers should be separated and the adjacent sides covered with flaps or skin grafts (Figure 33–8). This is usually done after the child is 18 months old unless the fusion is producing deformity with growth of the hand.

Radial Club Hand. This deformity results from failure of the radius to develop. It produces radial deviation of the hand on the ulna and should therefore be corrected before contractures are established. A nonopposing thumb is often present.

Urogenital Anomalies

Hypospadias. Hypospadias, due to failure of the penile urethra to develop, is a common anomaly of the external genitalia. The urethra opens on the ventral surface of the shaft or in the perineum. There are congenital scarring and ventral contracture of the penis called chordee. The defect exists in varying degrees of severity. Treatment consists of straightening the penis by

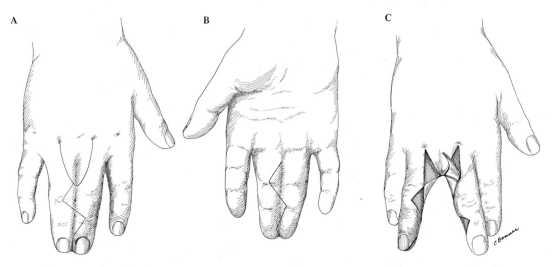

Figure 33–8. Syndactyly is treated by separation of the fingers and closing the defects with free skin grafts.

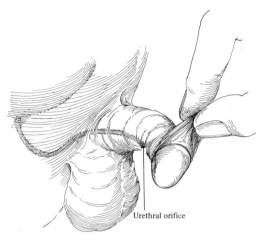

Figure 33–9. The first stage in the treatment of hypospadias is correction of the ventral curvature or chordee and covering the defect on the ventral surface with skin from the foreskin.

excising the ventral scar tissue and covering the ventral surface with skin (Figure 33–9). The external urethral orifice is displaced proximally. A skin tube is made using local flaps or skin grafts to reconstruct the urethra, either at the primary procedure or later (see page 580).

Epispadias. Epispadias is a defect of the dorsal surface of the penis and is often associated with extrophy of the bladder. Treatment is difficult. The pelvic bones are rotated into proper position before or at the time of reconstruction of the bladder and phallus.

TRAUMATIC DEFECTS AND DEFORMITIES

Facial Soft Tissue Injuries

Initial Care. Facial injuries are commonly caused by falls, assaults, and automobile accidents. Careful debridement is essential. Devitalized tissues are removed, the wound margins are carefully approximated, and hematoma and dead spaces avoided. Perfect anatomic alignment is essential for the margin of the lip, the alar margin of the nose, the eyebrows, and skin creases (Figure 33–10). The eyebrows should not be shaved. As little facial skin as possible should be excised. Apparently devitalized skin may survive due to the excellent blood supply of the face. The direction of the scar in relationship to the normal skin wrinkles is important in determining the final result. Scars that parallel wrinkles are most favorable.

Lacerations of the eyelids must be repaired with great care. Failure to carefully repair the margins may result in notching. Not recognizing a tear in the canaliculus will lead to epiphora, and excessive scarring in the lower eyelid will produce ectropion.

Late Revision. Unsatisfactory scars following primary repair of facial soft tissue injuries should be revised. It is important to wait for about one year until the scar has become soft and mobile and the initial hyperemia has gone. Initially unsightly scars may become acceptable when mature. Those that run across prominent wrinkle lines may be revised by changing the direction through W-plasties, in which a saw-toothed incision is made resulting in a zigzag scar, or by Z-plasties, in which the central limb of the Z is made parallel to the wrinkle lines. Other scars may be improved by simple excision and accurate approximation. In all cases the dermis must be accurately aligned and sutured.

Diffuse scars with sharp irregular margins similar to those caused by acne may be improved by dermabrasion, in which a sanding technique removes the outer layer of the skin. The regrowth of the epithelium results in a scar with more rounded margins which casts less visible shadows.

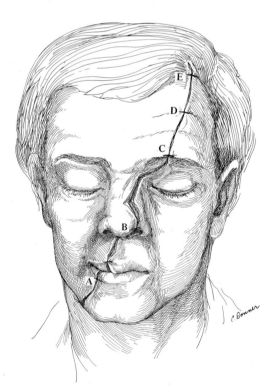

Figure 33–10. An extensive laceration of the face is repaired by accurately approximating anatomic landmarks.

Facial Fractures

Diagnosis. Physical examination can frequently diagnose facial fractures more easily than x-rays. The examination should be carried out as soon as possible after the injury, because swelling often obscures the findings. The nose is inspected and palpated for deformity. Examination with a speculum can demonstrate angulation of the septum or swelling indicating a septal hematoma. Palpation about the margins of the orbits demonstrates displaced fractures which are most commonly seen at the zygomaticofrontal suture lines and at the juncture of the zygoma and maxilla on the infraorbital rim. Extraocular movements should be tested and the patient asked about diplopia. If the floor of the orbit is fractured, the inferior orbital muscles may be caught in the fracture line and enter the antrum ("blowout fracture"). The patient cannot look upward and has diplopia. Fractures complicated by damage to the infraorbital nerve or the mental nerve produce anesthesia in their distribution on the face. Occlusion of the teeth must be evaluated by inspection. In those with bilateral subcondylar fractures of the mandible an open bite deformity may be present. The patient is asked to bite on a tongue depressor placed between the teeth. When the mandible or maxilla is fractured, there is twisting of the tongue depressor and pain at the fracture site. The mandible can be palpated externally and through the oral mucosa and deformities noted. The palate and upper jaw may be grasped in the hand and checked for abnormal mobility. The condyle of the mandible can be palpated through the external auditory meatus and its motion noted on moving the jaw. Cerebrospinal rhinorrhea should be suspected in patients with fractures involving the base of the skull and/or the cribriform plate.

Radiographs. Special x-rays are generally required. With a Water's view the infraorbital region is projected against the parietal occipital skull rather than against the mastoid air cells. Tangential x-rays of the zygoma reveal depressed fractures of the zygomatic arch. The anteroposterior skull x-ray with the mouth open reveals the ascending rami of the mandible. Intraoral dental films delineate fractures of the tooth-bearing portions of the maxilla and mandible.

Treatment. Facial fractures should be reduced early and, if unstable, held in position by direct wiring through small incisions in the skin. Normal occlusion between the upper and lower jaws must be maintained by wiring or fixing the jaws together until healing is achieved. Unstable fractures are fixed to the closest stable bone attached to the calvarium by using buried wire sutures.

Nasal Fractures. Simple deformities of the nasal bones and attached cartilages may be reduced early under topical and local anesthesia. The fragments are manipulated using an instrument in the nasal fossae and the fingers externally. If the reduction is unstable, splints and intranasal packing may be used but are often unnecessary. Septal hematomas and

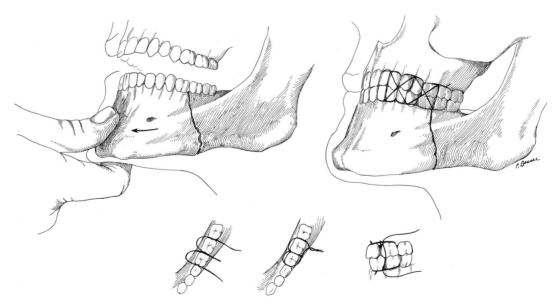

Figure 33–11. A fracture of the body of the mandible can be treated by interdental wiring.

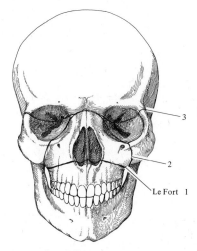

Figure 33–12. Fractures of the face are most likely to occur along Le Fort lines 1, 2, and 3.

deformities should be reduced. Complex nasal fractures may require open reduction.

Mandibular Fractures. Fractures of the tooth-bearing mandible are usually compound into the mouth, where they are exposed to saliva and have a high incidence of infection. If the maxilla is intact and adequate teeth are present, inter-dental fixation for four to six weeks may be sufficient (Figure 33–11). Liquid or semiliquid food is given during this period. Fractures through an edentulous mandible present special problems. A temporary prosthesis can be in-

serted to maintain proper alignment between the upper and lower jaws, while fixation between these structures is achieved by wire ligatures. Since the muscles attached to the inner and outer surfaces of the mandible tend to displace the fracture, open reduction and internal fixation are then required. Subcondylar fractures of the mandible can be successfully treated by inter-dental fixation even though accurate reduction has not been achieved.

Midface Fractures. Fractures of the maxilla are often associated with fractures of the zygomatic and nasal bones. The most severe midface fractures involve separation of the upper facial bones from the calvarium along the zygomaticofrontal and nasofrontal suture lines. The entire midface is supported only by soft tissue attachments (Le Fort 3) (Figure 33–12). A pyramidal fracture is through the nasal bones and between the zygoma and maxilla (Le Fort 2). A transverse fracture of the maxilla is the least severe (Le Fort 1). These fractures may involve disruption of the orbit. Careful reduction of the orbit is necessary to obtain normal function of the eyes (Figure 33–13). The floor of the orbit is reconstructed, using a small prosthetic implant or bone graft if a stable reduction cannot be achieved other-wise. In general, open reduction with interosseous wires is used in conjunction with stabilization of the maxilla to the mandible to treat midface fractures (Figure 33–14).

Timing of Treatment. Facial fractures are often associated with severe injury to other more vital structures. After assurance of an airway, which may require a tracheostomy, the treatment of facial fractures can be postponed for up to two weeks. After this period there is a fibrous

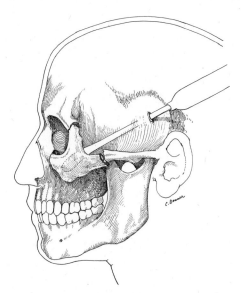

Figure 33–13. A depressed zygomaticomaxil-lary fracture is elevated to correct the facial deformity and diplopia.

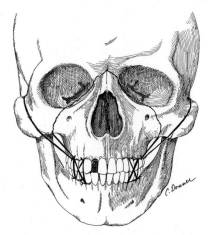

Figure 33–14. An extensive midface fracture is reduced and then stabilized by wiring the maxilla to the mandible.

union, often in malposition. The surgical treatment is then much more difficult.

Eye Injuries

Penetrating. Severe eye injuries, such as penetrating foreign body and intraocular hemorrhage, require the services of an ophthalmologist because of the serious potential for a permanent impairment of visual acuity and sympathetic ophthalmia. The simple application of a sterile dressing will suffice as a first-aid measure. Fortunately these severe injuries are rare, and the common minor injuries can be cared for effectively and safely by nonophthalmologists.

Conjunctival Foreign Body. The most commonly encountered problem, conjunctival foreign body, such as dust or cinder particle, can be removed under topical anesthesia with a moistened cottontip applicator. Embedded foreign bodies, however, will not adhere to the applicator tip and must be removed with a fine-pointed instrument by someone experienced in this procedure. Care should be taken to examine the conjunctival sacs completely by everting the lids to be sure all such material has been removed.

Abrasions and Lacerations. Corneal abrasions, which produce symptoms similar to those of conjunctival foreign bodies, can be demonstrated by fluorescein staining and heal 24 to 48 hours after the application of a sterile eyepatch. Most lacerations in the eyelids heal after suturing without residual disability, but those that transsect the lid margin or sever the duct apparatus require specialized repair techniques.

Actinic Conjunctivitis. Intense pain and photophobia develop several hours after exposure to the glare of a welder's torch. The patient usually attends the emergency room in the evening. Marked conjunctival reddening with a history as above will establish the diagnosis; the symptomatology can be completely alleviated by the application of a topical anesthetic. These agents should not be used more than once, pain control being provided thereafter by a systemic analgesic.

Chemical Burns. Immediate and copious irrigation should be used to remove and dilute the chemical agent. If available, sterile solutions are preferable, but time is of great importance and tap water or beverages may be used in emergencies.

Hand Injuries

Plastic surgeons have become involved in the treatment of hand injuries because of the importance of attaining proper skin coverage (see Chapter 28, pages 497–99). In general, patients do better when one surgeon cares for the entire hand with all of its defects.

Defects in the Lower Extremity

Injuries of the lower extremity resulting in open fractures are often associated with loss of skin. A common late problem is an open fracture of the tibia with failure to heal and/or with osteomyelitis and chronic draining sinuses. A crossleg flap is often needed. A flap is raised from one leg and applied to the defect in the opposite leg. The pedicle is left intact for three to four weeks, during which the two legs are fixed together in plaster. A skin graft is applied to the donor site and the raw surface of the pedicle. The pedicle is divided in stages, and the flap is placed in the defect. Another problem is loss of plantar weight-bearing skin.

Pressure Ulcers (Decubitus Ulcers)

An ulcer may form at the site of pressure over a bony prominence in patients with paraplegia, with anesthetic skin, and in the severely debilitated. Anesthetic skin is particularly subject to breakdown, probably because there is no pain to warn the patient of incipient damage but also because of impaired vasomotor responses. Common sites are the sacrum, great trochanter, and ischial tuberosity.

Conservative treatment consists of avoiding pressure to the region by frequent position changing, air mattresses, water beds, and occasionally placing the patient in a Stryker frame. The topical application of antibiotics and enzymes that digest necrotic tissue may be of value. Dry sterile dressings changed four times per day are most effective. Surgical treatment consists of debriding the ulcer and closing defects. The defects can usually be repaired by local rotation flaps after removing the bony prominence and excising the ulcer. Special care should be taken to prevent recurrence. Debilitated patients are not good candidates for extensive procedures because of difficulty in maintaining a healed wound even after adequate closure.

NEOPLASTIC DISEASE

Cancer of the Skin

Defects caused by resection or radiation of skin cancers often require repair of underlying defects of bone by bone grafts and skin coverage by local or distant flaps.

Head and Neck Tumors

Treatment of carcinomas in the mouth, pharynx, larynx, nasal sinuses, and nasal

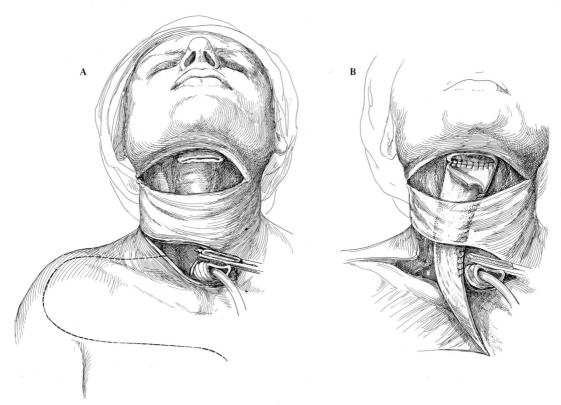

Figure 33–15. The deltopectoral or Bakamjian flap may be used to correct the defect following pharyngolaryngectomy for carcinoma.

cavities frequently results in major defects and deformities (see Chapter 16, page 275). In addition, a block dissection of the neck is often done. Reconstruction can be achieved by local flaps and skin grafts as well as by distant flaps from the forehead or neck. An example is the deltopectoral or Bakamjian flap (Figure 33–15). This is a medially based flap extending from the chest to the shoulder. Its axial vessels, which allow it to be used in a favorable length-to-width ratio, make it very versatile and able to cover many defects.

AESTHETIC SURGERY

Aesthetic or cosmetic surgery improves appearance beyond "normal" and toward an ideal of beauty held by the surgeon and the patient. Reconstructive surgery brings abnormal appearance or function toward "normal." The most common aesthetic operations include otoplasty for protruding ears, rhinoplasty, skin-tightening procedures, such as face lifts or rhytidectomies, and blepharoplasties, operations to elevate or to increase or decrease size of the breasts. The patient's

psychologic state must always be considered, and possible complications and expected results must be discused.

Aesthetic Rhinoplasty

This procedure is usually carried out through incisions within the lining of the nose. The skin and soft tissues are dissected away from the bony and cartilaginous framework. The framework is then rearranged by excisions, incisions, and fractures to achieve a straight, properly angulated nose with a narrow tip. The covering of skin and subcutaneous tissue is then allowed to settle back on the new framework. The results are usually excellent.

Skin-Tightening Procedures

Rhytidectomy.   Rhytidectomies (*rhytid*, wrinkle) or face lifts are done to improve the appearance of the sagging and wrinkled face (Figure 33–16). An incision is made within the hairline and in front of the ear. The skin and subcutaneous tissues are undermined anteriorly and inferiorly and then stretched superiorly and posteriorly. Excess skin is excised, and the skin

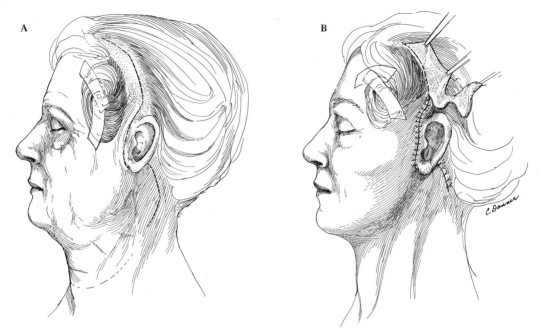

Figure 33–16. Rhytidectomy is performed to remove wrinkles and correct a sagging face.

is resutured in the new position. Care must be taken to avoid injuring the facial nerves. The results are good in selected patients.

Blepharoplasty.   Blepharoplasties are done to remove wrinkles and bagginess of the eyelids. The skin is excised along the lower margin of the lid and through a wrinkle line in the upper margin. There are often associated herniations of orbital fat through the orbital septum. This fat should be removed.

Chemosurgery.   Chemosurgery has been used to rejuvenate faces with "tissue paper" wrinkling. When skin is subjected to a second-degree or dermal burn, fine wrinkles are obliterated by the subsequent scarring. Caustic chemicals such as phenol and trichloracetic acid may be applied to the skin of the face. The inherent dangers of this procedure are obvious.

Other Tightening Procedures

Skin and fat have been excised in patients with redundancy of abdominal and thigh skin following weight loss.

Mammoplasty

Reduction.   Reduction mammoplasty may be done to decrease the size of the breasts. The indication may be entirely aesthetic or also functional if the patient has backache, ulcers where straps cross the shoulders, and maceration of opposing skin surfaces beneath the pen-

dulous breasts. A portion of the breast is excised and the skin refashioned to form a properly positioned skin brassiere. The nipple must be repositioned to the summit of the newly formed breast. In patients with a small degree of hypertrophy and sagging it is possible to preserve the innervation of the nipple, but in those with larger breasts it is safer to transplant the nipple as a free graft. Care must be taken to achieve symmetry of the breasts. The procedure can be used to correct asymmetric breasts.

Augmentation.   Augmentation mammoplasty has been used for many years to increase the breast size and improve the shape. Various fluids have been injected directly into the tissues. The character of these fluids ranges from paraffin in the early years of this century to liquid silicones more recently. The problems with injecting foreign materials include infection and reactions causing fibrosis and pseudotumors of the breast. It is impossible to remove injected materials without excising the breast. Injection of silicone fluids into the breast tissue is not legal in the United States at this time.

The usual technique for augmentation mammoplasty is to dissect a pocket behind the breast at the level of the fascia over or beneath the pectoral muscles and to insert a prosthesis. The prostheses have usually been made of a bag of silicone elastomer filled with physiologic solution or with a silicone gel. If the pocket and prosthesis are the proper size, the enlarged breast will feel and appear normal. Should infection ensue, the foreign body can be removed easily in one piece and perhaps later replaced.

In recent years, in patients with chronic nodular breast diseases or premalignant lesions requiring multiple biopsies or simple mastectomy, a subcutaneous mastectomy has been done and the breast contour filled out with a prosthesis. This replacement is carried out at the time of the excision or later, depending on local factors including bleeding and the previous scarring of the breast. This has been a most welcome alternative to simple mastectomy for some women with these problems.

SUGGESTIONS FOR FURTHER READING

Converse, John M.: *Reconstructive Plastic Surgery.* W. B. Saunders, Philadelphia, 1964.
    Five-volume, comprehensive text with chapters on basic principles as well as specific problems and procedures. The index is complete.
Grabb, W. C., and Smith, J. W.: *Plastic Surgery*, 2nd ed. Little, Brown and Co., Boston, 1973.
    A concise but complete, well-written and illustrated text.
Grabb, W. C., and Meyers, M. B.: *Skin Flaps.* Little, Brown and Co., Boston, 1975.
    These flaps, a major part of reconstructive surgery, are discussed clinically as well as experimentally by many authors.
Skoog, Tord: *Plastic Surgery.* W. B. Saunders, Philadelphia, 1974.
    The author presents a limited number of topics exquisitely with very fine illustrations.

Chapter 34

NEUROSURGERY

Donald H. Pearson and *John F. Mullan*

CHAPTER OUTLINE

Problems in Neurologic Surgery
Evaluation and Care of the Patient with
    Disturbed Consciousness
  Vital Signs
  General and Neurologic Examination
    Respiration
    Pupillary and Oculomotor Function
    Skeletal Muscle Responses
  Special Investigations
  Care of the Comatose Patient
Trauma to the Central Nervous System
  Anatomy of Head Injuries
  Clinical Syndromes of Head Injuries and
    Their Treatment
    Scalp Injuries
    Skull Fractures
    Brain Injuries
  Intracranial Hematomas
    Epidural Hematoma
    Subdural Hematoma
    Intracerebral Hematoma
  Summary of Management of the Acute
    Head Injury
  Trauma to the Spinal Column
    Types of Fractures
    Missile Injuries
    Syndromes of Incomplete Spinal Cord
      Injury
    Management of Spinal Injuries
    Management of Fractures
    Management of Neural Deficit
    Management of Paralyzed Patients
Brain Tumors and Increased Intracranial
    Pressure
  Increased Intracranial Pressure
    Cerebrospinal Fluid
    Cerebral Blood Flow
    Brain Volume
    Time Course of Intracranial Pressure
      Changes
    Treatment of Increased Intracranial Pres-
      sure
    Control of Brain Edema
  Clinical Syndromes of Brain Tumors
    Headache

    Vomiting
    Papilledema
    Brain Displacements
    Cerebral Irritation
    Cerebral Paralysis
  Classification of Brain Tumors
    Extracerebral Tumors
    Intracerebral Tumors
  Diagnosis of Brain Tumors
    Neurologic Signs
    Radiographic Studies
  Treatment of Brain Tumors
Subarachnoid Hemorrhage and Vascular
    Lesions
  Aneurysms
    Symptoms
    Nerve Compression
    Treatment
  Arteriovenous Malformations
  Arteriosclerotic Cerebrovascular Disease
    Hemorrhage
    Thrombosis
Spinal Column
  Anatomy
  Acquired Disorders of the Spine
    Cervical Disk Disease
    Thoracic Disk Disease
    Lumbar Disk Disease
  Tumors of the Spine
    Extradural Tumors
    Intradural Tumors
Infections of the Nervous System
  Infections of the Brain
    Infections of the Skull and Meninges
    Cerebral Abscess
  Spinal Epidural Abscess
Malformations of the Central Nervous System
    and Its Supporting Structures
  Embryology
    Primary Failure
    Failure of Separation
    Failure in the Development of Cere-
      brospinal Fluid Spaces
    Failure of Bone Development

PROBLEMS IN NEUROLOGIC SURGERY

The fundamental knowledge that every physician should have includes evaluation of coma, increased intracranial pressure, trauma to the central nervous system, spinal cord compression, brain tumors, vascular lesions of the central nervous system, brain infections, and developmental malformations of the central nervous system and its supporting structures.

EVALUATION AND CARE OF THE PATIENT WITH DISTURBED CONSCIOUSNESS

Every busy emergency room contains patients with altered states of consciousness ranging from lethargy through various degrees of obtundation to stupor and coma. Since the cause is often obscure, a checklist is useful to help evaluate and care for these patients rapidly. It is helpful to distinguish between consciousness as a state and the content of consciousness. Consciousness was formerly thought to be a mass action phenomenon of the brain. The degree of loss of consciousness was considered dependent on the quantity of nonfunctioning cerebral tissue present at any time. The anatomic substrate subserving consciousness is now known to be in the reticular core of the brain stem, a polysynaptic pathway running from the medulla to the thalamic reticulum which impinges upon most of the other neural systems. Integrity of this structure results in consciousness. The content of consciousness, on the other hand, depends upon the functional integrity of the cerebral cortex.

Consciousness is disturbed by cerebral or extracerebral causes. Most cerebral causes are anatomic in nature, while extracerebral causes are circulatory, respiratory, or metabolic. Since the degree of obtundation frequently heralds a life-threatening situation, every physician should know the priorities in care and evaluation.

Initial evaluation begins with a history; however, this may only be obtained from a friend or relative. A history of diabetes, intoxication, or epilepsy is important. While a history is being elicited, the vital signs are observed.

Vital Signs

Adequacy of respiration has first priority in the care of the obtunded patient. In coma there is often upper airway obstruction, particularly when the patient is supine. The tongue falls back against the posterior pharyngeal wall, the pharyngeal muscles are lax, and secretions are retained. The airway can be rapidly cleared by elevating the angles of the jaw and raising the base of the tongue forward. The pharynx is then inspected, and foreign material and secretions are removed manually or by suction. An oral airway may be inserted, and secretions are removed at frequent intervals. If ventilation is still not adequate, an endotracheal tube is inserted to establish controlled respiration. Tracheostomy is rarely required as an emergency procedure unless tracheal or laryngeal obstruction is present, as in severe injuries to the lower face or neck. Once adequate ventilation is established, the cardiovascular system receives attention.

Since the blood stream carries oxygen and nutrients to the brain, adequate circulation is essential. In oligemic shock two emergent problems coexist—cerebral damage and circulatory insufficiency. The two, however, are not always directly related. Generally a head injury does not cause shock. Conversely, consciousness is lost only in profound shock, since cerebral blood flow is maintained with a failing circulation at the expense of the systemic circulation. In the patient with multiple injuries without obvious external bleeding, hemorrhage into one of the body cavities must be suspected. Other causes of shock such as overwhelming sepsis or a failing myocardium should also be considered. A large-bore cannula inserted into a vein permits administration of fluids, medications, and volume expanders. A central venous pressure catheter is helpful in assessing cardiac efficiency and circulatory volume. Electrocardiographic evidence of myocardial damage or severe arrhythmia helps to diagnose cardiogenic shock.

General and Neurologic Examination

When the vital signs have been assessed and corrective measures undertaken, complete physical and neurologic examinations are performed. The patient is completely undressed, special care being taken if there is a possible spinal injury. In such a case the body is moved as a whole, preventing flexion or torsion of the cervical, thoracic, or lumbar spine. The patient is examined for wounds, fractures, contusions, hematomas, and petechiae. Palpation of the joints, the spine, and the abdomen and auscultation of the chest cavities help in planning appropriate x-rays.

Respiration. The pattern of respiration indicates the patient's metabolic status and also the level of a neurologic lesion. The "fruity" odor of the breath in ketosis or the urinary smell in uremia may indicate the diagnosis. Rapid deep hyperventilation is present in metabolic acidosis, as in uremia and diabetes, but also in the patient with midbrain compression secondary to increased intracranial pressure. Hypoventilation suggests drug overdosage or pulmonary disease with carbon dioxide narcosis. The respiratory pattern in the awake, conscious patient is rhythmic but is subject to changes induced by the cerebral cortex on the midbrain and medullary respiratory centers. As the cortical influences are removed in cerebral dysfunction, various forms of periodic breathing develop. Cheyne-Stokes respiration consists of regular oscillations between hyperpnea and apnea with a waxing and waning of respiratory effort in a regular periodic pattern. The central neurogenic hyperventilation of midbrain compression has been mentioned. Lesions at the level of the pons produce irregular breathing patterns such as gasping, inspiratory or expiratory pauses, ataxic or irregular breathing. Damage to the medullary respiratory centers usually results in respiratory failure preceded by irregular deep gasps culminating in apnea.

Pupillary and Oculomotor Function. The size and reactivity of the pupils are valuable indicators of intracranial pathology. An expanding intracranial lesion results in dilatation of the ipsilateral pupil. Paralysis of the parasympathetic fibers of the third cranial nerve that supply the pupillary constrictor muscle occurs when they are compressed against the tentorial edge by the herniated medial portion of the temporal lobe. An alternate cause is direct compression of the pupillomotor center in the ipsilateral hypothalamus. Figure 34–1 schematically demonstrates the distortion of the cerebral substance producing transtentorial herniation. A dilated pupil is a serious prognostic sign heralding

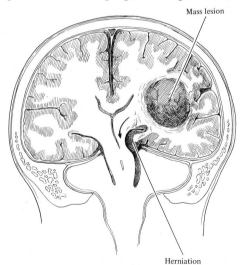

Mass lesion

Herniation

Figure 34–1. The mass lesion has caused transtentorial herniation of the medial portion of the temporal lobe against brain stem and hypothalamic structures. The patient had unilateral dilatation of the pupil.

transtentorial herniation. There is severe cerebral ischemia secondary to the increased pressure. The importance of unilateral dilatation of the pupil cannot therefore be overemphasized, since it usually signifies an expanding supratentorial hemispheric lesion.

Midbrain lesions produce midposition pupils that do not respond to light but may still respond by mydriasis to painful cutaneous stimuli, such as pinching the skin of the neck. Pontine lesions produce pinpoint unreactive pupils, while those in the medulla result in widely dilated and fixed pupils. Fixed dilated pupils signify severe brain stem damage and occur prior to death. However, the unresponsive patient with fixed dilated pupils due to oligemic shock can still recover if his circulatory volume is rapidly replaced. The brain stem of infants and young children is more resistant to injury and can recover in the presence of fixed and dilated pupils.

Overdosage of anticholinergic drugs can also cause fixed dilated pupils, while narcotic intoxication produces severely meiotic pupils which dilate on topical application of nalorphine.

Brain stem reflex integrity can be assessed by the oculomotor reflexes. The oculovestibular reflex is tested by placing ice water in the external auditory canal. A normal response is nystagmus or forced lateral deviation of the eyes. Its absence suggests severe brain stem disturbance. The oculocephalic reflex is tested by rapidly turning the head from side to side. Normally the eyes fix upon an object in the room. If the eyes passively follow the movement of the head, severe brain stem depression is present. These tests are more valuable in the long-term estimations of the level of consciousness than in the initial evaluation. Changes in their ease of elicitation or in the briskness of their response over a period of time help determine improvement or deterioration of brain stem function.

Skeletal Muscle Responses. The tone of skeletal muscles and the motor response to noxious stimuli are assessed in the arms and legs. The symmetry of responses is gauged by pinching the extremities to demonstrate hemiparesis. In early brain stem failure the muscles have increased tone. Described as paratonic rigidity, it is characterized by increased resistance to passive movement as though the patient were voluntarily resisting the movement. In advanced stages of brain stem compression the entire body becomes rigid so that passive motion is almost impossible.

In light coma the patient appears to evade or to brush away the source of irritation. As coma deepens more stereotyped movements occur, primitive extensor reflexes become prominent, and ultimately a decerebrate posture is assumed. Painful stimuli produce an opisthotonic position of the spine. There are adduction, extension, and hyperpronation of the arms, and extension and plantar flexion of the legs. With severe damage this position may be elicited by mild stimuli or may occur spontaneously. Decorticate posturing consists of flexion and internal rotation of the arms, and flexion of the wrist and fingers with the legs extended and internally rotated. Decerebrate or decorticate postures signify a severe cerebral injury with little chance of recovery. The prognosis is not as serious in infants and children as in adults.

Special Investigations

At the time of intravenous cannulation blood samples are taken for clinical chemical and hematologic studies. When the diagnosis is uncertain, 50 ml of 50 percent glucose may be given rapidly. This will help diagnose insulin coma and is not harmful when the coma has another etiology. Arterial samples are taken for blood gases and pH to assess the quality of ventilation and to determine the presence of acidosis or alkalosis. Changes in blood chemistries will suggest the metabolic causes of coma, from diseases of the liver, kidneys, or electrolyte imbalance. Samples are taken to determine the blood level of the common depressants such as barbiturates, alcohol, and, particularly in children, aspirin. In those with oligemic shock, blood is drawn for grouping and cross-matching. A urinary catheter is inserted to obtain a specimen for examination and for accurate recording of the urinary output.

X-rays of suspected injured regions are taken when the general condition is stable. Skull films are taken if there is evidence of head trauma. A single cross-table true lateral cervical spine film is essential as an initial evaluation for cervical spine injuries and can be performed as part of the skull examination. A chest x-ray is routinely obtained. A lateral decubitus view of the abdomen may demonstrate intraperitoneal air from a ruptured viscus. Spinal x-rays are indicated if there is tenderness, ecchymosis, or deformities, of the spine. Limb x-rays are taken when indicated.

An electrocardiogram is often necessary to evaluate the circulatory status. Electroencephalography is rarely needed as an emergency procedure, but an echoencephalogram may be useful.

Care of the Comatose Patient

Respiration is frequently a problem. Oral airways are only a temporary measure and should not be left in an unattended patient because they tend to become obstructed with secretions. Endotracheal intubation is often necessary. A tracheostomy is established if the patient remains comatose for more than two to three days. Secretions are frequently removed using a soft catheter.

Decubitus ulcers develop rapidly in patients who are unable to move freely. The position is changed at least every two hours and more often if any region is red or chafed. Alternating pressure mattresses, sheepskins, and gel floatation pads under pressure points are helpful. Temperature-regulated water beds are of great value, but they restrict access to the patient, making frequent inspection and physiotherapy more difficult.

Bowel care is best managed by the insertion of a mild laxative in suppository form at the same time each day.

Bladder infections are a major problem and should be prevented by sterile catheterization technique, prophylactic antibiotics, and maintenance of an adequate fluid output.

Adequate nutrition can be maintained in the comatose patient by frequent small feedings through a small nasogastric tube. The tube should be changed often and left out periodically to prevent damage to the esophageal mucosa. Care must be taken to prevent misplacement of the tube and pulmonary aspiration. Small dilute feedings are given initially and increased gradually to prevent vomiting and aspiration. The average adult will tolerate 2400 calories in 3000 ml of fluid given in six divided feedings per 24 hours.

Physiotherapy is mandatory to promote peripheral circulation and prevent joint contractions. It is useful if everyone who comes in contact with the patient spends a few seconds at gentle joint manipulation rather than relying on a once or twice daily visit by a physiotherapist.

TRAUMA TO THE CENTRAL NERVOUS SYSTEM

Trauma to the central nervous system is a major public health problem. The United States National Safety Council estimates that approximately one third, or 40,000, of the accidental deaths that occur each year are due to head injuries and that 11 percent of disabling injuries, or about 1,300,000, are to the head. Many head injuries are obvious on inspection, such as penetrating wounds, scalp lacerations, and severe contusions. It is the occult head injury with increasing intracranial pressure that needs to be recognized early so that lifesaving treatment is undertaken without delay.

The brain is enclosed within the cranium and tolerates increasing intracranial pressure poorly. The energy for the pressure build-up is derived from blood pressure. An expanding blood clot within the skull increases intracranial pressure until no further energy is available to drive blood into the brain. The intracranial pressure then equals the systemic blood pressure. Increasing intracranial pressure must be recognized and treated early if the patient is to be saved. The hallmark is a reduced level of consciousness, hence the stress laid on this as the most vital neurologic sign.

Anatomy of Head Injuries

The brain, enclosed in its bony carapace, floats in slowly circulating cerebrospinal fluid and is tethered at its base by the brain stem which exits through the foramen magnum. It is covered above by the smooth convexity of the skull interrupted longitudinally only by the sickle-shaped falx. Below it rests on the rough and irregular base of the skull. The most important sharp projections at the base are the sphenoid wings separating the temporal from the frontal fossae, and the triangular opening of the tentorium through which upper brain stem structures pass. The head is supported on the fulcrum of the atlanto-occipital joint.

The head is subject to two types of injuries, direct penetration and rapid acceleration or deceleration. Direct penetration presents no diagnostic problem. It is the acceleration-deceleration injuries, as when the head is propelled forward by a blow from a blunt object or rapidly decelerated in a vehicular accident, that produce the so-called occult head injury. In the acceleration-deceleration injury, the head pivots rapidly on the atlanto-occipital joint and the brain is ballotted about within the cranial cavity, striking the hard surfaces that confine it. Most damage occurs at the frontal, temporal, and occipital poles. In addition, since the base of the brain is tethered as it passes through the foramen magnum, traction and compression can occur within the brain stem and are probably responsible for the transient loss of consciousness interpreted as concussion.

Clinical Syndromes of Head Injuries and Their Treatment

Although they are frequently combined, it is convenient to separately discuss the clinical components of a head injury.

Scalp Injuries. The scalp is a specialized portion of the human integument, designed to fit closely over the smooth bony calvarium. It is richly supplied with blood vessels which anastomose freely between the dermis and galea. The vessels contract poorly when ruptured and can result in considerable blood loss. The blood vessels, while still bleeding freely, tend to retract between the two layers. Hemostasis can be obtained by placing a hemostat on the geleal layer and letting it flip back over the dermal layer, thus compressing the blood vessel and controlling the bleeding.

Scalp veins communicate with sinusoids in the diploic layer of the skull and with intracerebral veins. Infection may therefore pass from the scalp into the cerebral cavity, resulting in extradural abscess, meningitis, or brain abscess. Meticulous cleansing of all scalp wounds with adequate shaving, debridement, and accurate closure is therefore necessary. Hemostasis must be complete to prevent a subgaleal hematoma which provides an excellent nutrient medium for infection.

The galea is an aponeurosis for the insertion of the frontal and occipital muscles, and unless it is included in the sutures, separation and breakdown of the laceration may occur. The galea frequently retracts beneath the dermis and must be identified and included in every stitch when closing the laceration.

Skull Fractures. Skull fractures may be linear, comminuted, or compounded. Linear fractures usually radiate out from the point of maximum impact. They do not require treatment but are an index of the amount of trauma delivered to the head.

With depressed fractures the inner table is more extensively damaged than the outer table and overlaps adjacent bone. This produces the so-called double density sign on x-ray. In Figure 34–2 such a fracture may be seen on the calvarium. Depressed fractures that are not compounded do not need to be explored if their size suggests that at the moment of impact the dura was not torn and the brain lacerated. If there is any doubt, the fracture should be explored. All compound depressed fractures should be treated immediately by operation to provide adequate inspection and closure of the dura and, if necessary, debridement of the brain and removal of a hematoma or foreign material. Whether the bone fragments are elevated to their original position or discarded, leaving a hole in the cranial vault, depends upon the amount of wound contamination. A large vault defect can later be repaired by inserting a metal plate, autogenous bone usually from split ribs, or by using an acrylic plastic prosthesis.

Basilar fractures involve the base of the skull, the mastoid air cells, and the sinuses. They are frequently difficult, if not impossible, to visualize on x-ray but are indicated by air fluid levels in the sinus cavities and leakage of

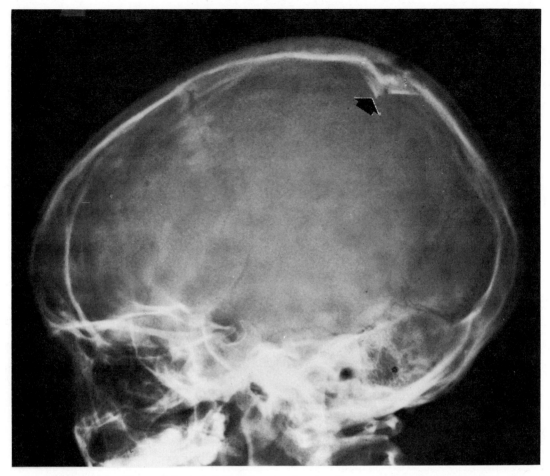

Figure 34–2. X-ray of depressed skull fracture showing the so-called double density sign.

cerebrospinal fluid through the ear or nose. Although most cerebrospinal fluid leaks close spontaneously within 7 to 10 days, those that persist require surgical repair.

Brain Injuries. Injuries to the cerebral substance may result in contusions, lacerations, and edema. Focal neurologic disturbances may or may not be present, and varying degrees of permanent neurologic deficits may result. Seizures are a common complication of interruption of cerebral tissue, occurring in about 30 percent of all cases; their onset may be months or years after the injury.

There is no treatment for damaged cerebral tissue, but the associated edema must be recognized and treated. The brain, like all tissues, responds to injury by swelling, but its tight confinement may further intensify the injury. Previously a large portion of the bony calvarium below the temporalis muscle was removed, and the dura was opened to permit expansion of the brain. Experience has shown that this does not lead to adequate decompression. Osmotic diuretics, such as urea, mannitol, and glycerol, are effective in reducing cerebral swelling. They are given intravenously or by nasogastric tube at a dose of 2 to 4 gm per kilogram every 24 hours. Changes in electrolyte and fluid balances must be looked for because large doses may produce cloudy swelling of the renal tubules and impair renal function. A catheter should always be in place in the comatose patient to monitor fluid output and prevent overdistention of the bladder.

In some centers a catheter is placed in a ventricle through a frontal or parietal burr hole to monitor the intracranial pressure by means of a strain-gauge manometer and to remove cerebrospinal fluid.

Intracranial Hematomas

Collections of blood within the skull produce clinical syndromes depending upon their location.

Epidural Hematoma. An epidural hematoma is probably the most acute neurosurgical emergency. The middle meningeal artery, the largest artery in the dura, enters the middle fossa through the foramen spinosum. It runs over the surface of the temporal lobe within the two leaves of the dura and is frequently torn when there is a fracture at the pterion above and in front of the external auditory canal. The artery may cause hemorrhage in the absence of a fracture. A hematoma rapidly forms in the potential space between the dura and calvarium. There is frequently an initial period of unconsciousness due to the concussive effect of the injury followed by an improvement. Compression and secondary loss of consciousness then succeed this so-called lucid interval. Hemiparesis is often present on the opposite side of the body. The uncus of the temporal lobe, ipsilateral to the injury, may herniate through the tentorial opening and compress the third nerve, producing pupillary mydriasis. By this time the disturbance of consciousness is usually profound. These signs may develop rapidly within minutes to several hours after the injury. An immediate temporal craniotomy, with removal of the epidural clot and clipping or coagulation of the bleeding artery, can be lifesaving.

Other small dural vessels produce epidural hematomas less frequently in the frontal and occipital areas. They are usually smaller and the progression of symptoms may be delayed over several days.

Subdural Hematoma. Subdural hematomas are frequent and are classified on a temporal basis as acute, subacute, or chronic.

The mortality of acute subdural hematomas is high, 80 to 90 percent, even if diagnosed and treated early. They are associated with a pulped, lacerated brain which cannot be repaired, even though the hematoma is recognized and evacuated rapidly. The signs are similar to those described for an epidural hematoma except that there is no "lucid interval."

A subacute subdural hematoma is a collection of blood on the surface of the brain associated with minor laceration of the cortex and hemorrhage from cortical vessels. Signs develop from several hours to several days after the injury and are similar to those of an epidural hematoma. There may or may not be a lucid interval. The diagnosis should be made and operation performed before signs of severe midbrain compression appear. Diagnosis can be determined by cerebral angiography. In Figure 34–3 a cerebral angiogram demonstrates the displacement of the cerebral vessels away from the inner table of the skull by a subdural hematoma.

A chronic subdural hematoma may occur at any age but is most prevalent in infants and elderly people. The interval between injury and the onset of signs may be weeks or months. In the infant the distensible skull can tolerate the initial solid hematoma without serious neurologic deficit. Similarly, in the elderly, the shrunken brain and widened subarachnoid space provide more room for the hematoma. There are a number of theories accounting for the delayed onset of symptoms. The most popular suggests that the hematoma gradually enlarges as the blood proteins break down, increasing the osmotic pressure and imbibing fluid. Another theory suggests that repeated bleeding occurs from the surface of the membrane formed around the hematoma. Signs develop slowly with increasing intracranial pressure. There is frequently a disturbance in the level of consciousness with few or no focal signs. Cerebral displacement in the elderly can result in coma with little increase in intracranial pressure. The possibility of a chronic subdural hematoma should always be considered in an elderly person who becomes confused and lethargic. Since these hematomas remain fluid, they may be diagnosed and treated by simple trephination. In the infant a generous craniotomy is occasionally required to remove the membrane and prevent constriction of the growing brain.

Intracerebral Hematoma. An intracerebral hematoma occurs alone or in combination with other syndromes of head injury. It is usually found in the frontal, temporal, or occipital lobes and may be associated with considerable brain maceration. An angiogram is indicated if an intracerebral hematoma is suspected. The clot is solid and cannot be removed by needling the cortex, but must be removed through a cerebrotomy in a region of the brain that will not result in serious neurologic deficit. The pulped tissue is often removed to provide internal decompression in case of cerebral swelling and also to remove nonfunctioning brain.

Summary of Management of the Acute Head Injury

The initial management of an acute head injury involves the total management of the critically injured patient. Attention must be paid to respiration and circulation. It must be stressed that low blood pressure is rarely a manifestation of cerebral injury, and if it is present, another cause must be sought. The early signs of increased intracranial pressure must be looked for before signs of midbrain compression begin. Deterioration in the level of consciousness is of paramount importance and must be frequently assessed. The clinical syndromes may present singly or in combination. If increased

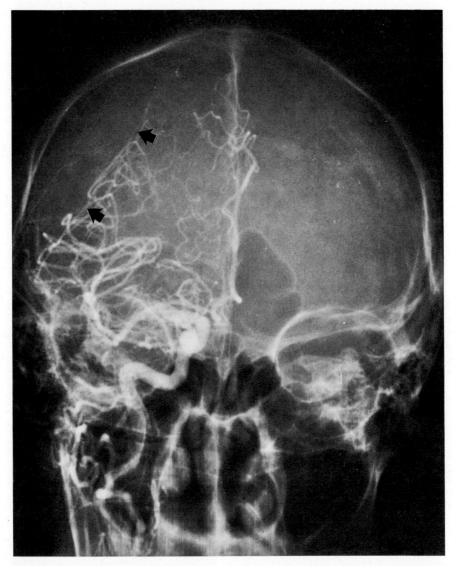

Figure 34–3. Carotid arteriogram demonstrates the presence of a subdural hematoma. Note that the cortical vessels are displaced from the inner table of the skull (arrows), and the shift of the normally midline anterior cerebral vessels.

intracranial pressure is suspected, 20 percent mannitol or urea in invert sugar should be rapidly administered to induce osmotic diuresis and shrink the cerebral substance. This also provides temporary relief from pressure in the patient with a hematoma during preoperative preparation.

In every severe head injury a cervical fracture must always be suspected. A single or stereo true lateral cervical spine should be obtained when taking a radiograph of the skull.

Lumbar puncture has no place in the evaluation of a head injury. Indeed, removing fluid from the spinal subarachnoid space in the presence of increased intracranial pressure may cause death.

TRAUMA TO THE SPINAL COLUMN

Trauma to the spinal column can result in bony injury, usually identified on x-ray, and neural damage, diagnosed by clinical examination. Occasionally severe neural loss can occur without evidence of bony damage, and in some regions severe bony damage can occur with little or no neural damage. As with a head injury

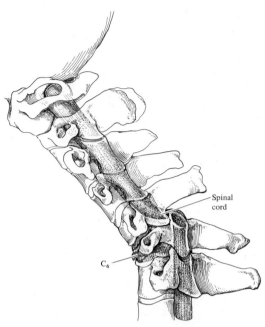

Figure 34–4. A typical crush fracture of the body of the sixth cervical vertebra associated with sharp forward flexion deformity. The spinal cord has been completely disrupted.

repeated neurologic assessment is essential for diagnosis and management of spinal column injuries.

Types of Fractures. Fractures occur predominantly in the mobile upper and lower ends of the spinal column, the cervical and lumbar regions. Thoracic fractures are less common but are particularly serious because of the severity of the spinal cord damage.

There may be simple crush fractures, comminuted fractures, or fracture dislocations. Occasionally there is also subluxation of one vertebra upon another with no visible fracture on x-ray. Fracture of a pedicle or facet can readily be missed.

In the neck a crush fracture generally involves a single vertebra, while in the thoracolumbar region several are generally involved, In Figure 34–4 a severe crush fracture of the body of C_6 is shown schematically. It is better to have several vertebrae crushed minimally than to have one completely collapsed, because the angulation of the cord is spread over a wider region. The cord is not damaged unless there has been subluxation or extrusion of disk material. Extruded disk material is most common in the cervical region.

Comminuted fractures are generally associated with a dislocated disk. In addition fragments of bone may be displaced posteriorly and compress the cord.

In a fracture dislocation the intra-articular joints have been subluxated, and the pedicles may be broken. Frequently displacement is more severe at the moment of impact and reduces spontaneously. An articular facet may slip in front of another, making reduction impossible. Many patients have irreversible spinal cord damage. Fracture and fracture dislocations are least serious in the region of the cauda equina which tolerates a greater degree of compression than the cord. Cord damage tends to be less in the neck because of a wide spinal canal. In the thoracic region there is virtually no free space in the spinal canal and minimal movement between the vertebrae; therefore neural damage is generally more severe.

Subluxation may be mild or severe. If mild, the bones may have slipped back to their normal position by the time of x-ray, but the unstable position may be demonstrated on repeat x-ray in slight forward flexion. Mild subluxations are not always associated with neurologic disturbance. Severe subluxations result in as much cord damage as fracture dislocations. In the cervical region subluxation of C_1 on C_2 is a common injury. Because of the wide spinal canal in this area, a surprising degree of dislocation can be tolerated without neural damage.

Spinal cord dysfunction varies from spinal shock through minimal compression to complete disruption. In spinal shock there is complete or incomplete loss of cord function below the level of injury for up to 24 hours. There may be some indication of return of function within a few hours, and complete recovery usually takes place. Minimal compression of the cord may be caused by an extruded fragment of a disk or by displacement of a vertebra. Severe compression or disruption of the cord results from fracture dislocation, severe subluxation, or a displaced disk or bone fragment. Damage caused by compression is only rarely reversible, while that caused by disruption is irreversible.

Missile Injuries. Missile injuries produce neural and bony disruption and should be treated like a compound fracture. This includes thorough debridement with primary closure of the wound unless the missile is small, the tract is long, and there is no indication for operation.

High-velocity missiles may cause damage by a disruptive force when they pass close to the cord. Complete paralysis can occur without evidence of mechanical compression.

Syndromes of Incomplete Spinal Cord Injury. There are two syndromes of partial cord injury in the cervical spine. The central cord syndrome occurs in hyperextension-flexion injuries of the cervical spine. There is greater weakness in the upper than in the lower extremities and non-specific or absent sensory changes. Hemorrhage occurs in the central substance of the cord. The medially placed fibers in the corticospinal tract to the hand and arm are damaged, while the more laterally placed fibers to the leg are spared. Sensory tracts may or may not be affected. The anterior spinal cord syndrome features acute anterior spinal cord compression by displaced bone fragments or portion of an intervertebral disk. The syndrome is characterized by complete paralysis below the level of the lesion with preservation of the posterior columns that transmit touch and proprioception. The affected region is supplied by the anterior spinal artery, while that portion which escapes damage is supplied by the posterior spinal arteries.

Management of Spinal Injuries. The patient may complain of severe pain in his neck or back, a penetrating wound may be present, or a neurologic deficit. The patient is often unconscious from a head injury, making diagnosis difficult. All severely injured patients must be transported in a neutral position without angulation of the spine.

High spinal injuries may produce severe hypotension. Neural shock from sympathetic paralysis and loss of vasomotor tone can be reversed by placing the patient in the Trendelenburg position. Rarely are fluids or sympathomimetic amines required. If the shock cannot be easily reversed, another cause must be sought, such as blood loss from a ruptured viscus.

Examination of the sensory dermatomes confirms the level of injury. In cervical fractures the level can also be determined by the motor power of the limb; C_5 supplies the shoulder, C_6 flexes the elbow and supinates the forearm, C_7 extends the elbow and wrist, C_8 flexes the wrist, and T_1 supplies the small muscles of the hand.

Severe fracture dislocations of C_3 to C_4 or at a higher level involve the phrenic outflow and are usually fatal. Dislocations at lower levels may also be fatal as edema ascends and compresses the respiratory center. Early mechanical respiration is necessary for survival.

Frequently a lumbar puncture with manometric studies helps assess damage. Compression of the veins in the neck raises the intracranial and intraspinal pressures. Normally the pressure in the lumbar manometer rapidly rises and falls when the jugular veins are occluded and then released. This may be accomplished by placing a blood pressure cuff around the neck, inflating it to diastolic pressure, and then releasing it. Absence of fluctuation signifies an obstruction to the free flow of cerebrospinal fluid between

needle and the neck. It may also be the result of an obstruction of the point of the needle, but this can be determined by gently pressing the abdomen and increasing pressure in the extradural spinal veins. This normally produces an increase in cerebrospinal fluid pressure, provided that the needle is not occluded. This test, though helpful, should not be relied upon since a partial spinal block may be present and give equivocal results.

In certain cases when an obstruction is suspected but cannot be confirmed by x-rays, contrast media may be injected through the lumbar needle and a careful myelogram performed. A disk fragment or an unsuspected bone fragment protruding into the spinal canal may be visualized.

Management of Fractures. In the cervical region crushed and comminuted fractures and subluxations are treated by skeletal traction until it is certain that there is no possibility of redislocation. Skull tongs are inserted through the outer table of the skull in the midlateral axis and traction applied for four to six weeks. Patients with subluxation generally wear a plaster or plastic cast for about the same time after skeletal traction is stopped. Operative fusion is usually required in subluxations at the C_1 to C_2 level because the bones rarely fuse spontaneously. The period of disability can be shortened by early fusion at other levels.

Fracture dislocations are reduced by applying up to 40 pounds of skeletal traction gradually over a few hours under x-ray control. Occasionally operative reduction is necessary for locked facets.

In the thoracic and lumbar regions crushed and comminuted fractures are treated by bed rest, usually for three to four weeks, until most of the pain has disappeared. The patient is then gradually ambulated while wearing a back support to reduce discomfort.

With a fracture dislocation of the thoracolumbar region an attempt is made to reduce the dislocation by applying traction in hyperextension. If this fails or if there are locked facets, operative reduction is necessary. The spine should be placed in the best position to prevent pain and decubitus ulcers at kyphotic protrusions of the spine.

Management of Neural Deficit. Operation is not indicated if there has been complete loss of function below the level of the injury. Operation is only indicated if pieces of bone or disk or foreign bodies, such as a bullet, continue to press on partially damaged but recoverable cord or if increasing paralysis is present.

The hemorrhagic cord lesion develops slowly after impact. It has recently been proposed that the cord be cooled at operation by local application of iced saline to decrease edema and prevent further neural damage. Osmotic diuretics, dexamethasone, dimethylsulfoxide, and hyperbaric oxygen have all been shown to improve recovery after experimental traumatic cord lesions, but their value in patients has not yet been established.

Management of Paralyzed Patients. Adequate ventilation must be established in the high cervical spine injury. A self-retaining catheter is inserted if bladder control is lost. The bladder must not be allowed to become overdistended, because if it is overstretched, a long time will be required to regain the original tone. Selected patients may be taught intermittent self-catheterization. The urine is routinely examined for microorganisms and appropriate antibiotics given when necessary.

The skin blanches if subjected to pressure and soon ulcerates if the pressure is sustained. Normally frequent movement prevents this, even during sleep. In paraplegia it is essential to change position frequently. Intermittent pressure mattresses and temperature-controlled water beds are useful. Alternatively the patient may be nursed on a Stryker frame in which he is sandwiched between canvas-covered frames and turned at least every two hours. The frame is particularly useful in the patient with an unstable spine.

Paralytic ileus is a common complication of spinal injury, necessitating continuous gastric suction and intravenous fluids. To prevent fecal impaction an enema is given usually daily. Paralyzed joints are regularly manipulated to prevent contractures. As paralyzed patients become depressed within a few days of their injury, psychotherapy and rehabilitation assist in their future self-care.

BRAIN TUMORS AND INCREASED INTRACRANIAL PRESSURE

Any expanding lesion within the skull produces a generalized increase in intracranial tension and displacement of brain substance from one compartment to another. The clinical picture depends on how rapidly the pressure changes occur.

Increased Intracranial Pressure

The three major intracranial components—cerebrospinal fluid, blood, and brain—all contribute to the maintenance of intracranial pressure relationships. If the skull was a closed cavity filled with an incompressible fluid, a small increase in volume would lead to a marked increase in pressure. When small volumes of saline are introduced into the skull of an experimental animal they are initially well tolerated with little increase in pressure. However, the "buffering" capacity quickly becomes exhausted, and further small increments of volume lead to an exponential increase in pressure.

Cerebrospinal Fluid. A decrease in the volume of cerebrospinal fluid is probably the first compensation for an increase in intracranial pressure. During intracranial surgery ventricular fluid is removed to lower intracranial pressure.

Cerebral Blood Flow. Cerebral blood flow remains constant although systemic arterial pressure varies widely. The intracranial arterial resistance declines to maintain circulation to the brain in the patient with increased intracranial pressure. The intracranial blood volume increases slightly as a result of dilation of the vessels. Cerebral blood flow thus remains constant as intracranial pressure increases until the pressure approaches the systemic diastolic pressure. At this stage the systemic blood pressure increases as the intracranial pressure rises (Cushing's reflex). Some of the highest systemic blood pressures recorded are seen in patients with intracranial hypertension. When the pressure head in the systemic circulation has been transmitted to the brain's capacitance vessels, no further blood can be accommodated. Intracranial pressure then approximates the systemic arterial pressure and blood flow to the brain ceases.

Precisely what controls the cerebral circulatory system is not known. The cerebral vessels are profusely innervated with sympathetic fibers from the cervical sympathetic chain. Their role in the regulation of the cerebral circulation is controversial. Recent evidence suggests that small cerebral vessels are directly innervated by adrenergic neurons within the cerebral substance. Some describe a myogenic reflex moderated by transmural pressure across arterioles. The cerebral vessels are uniquely sensitive to the level of intravascular P_{CO_2}. A high P_{CO_2} leads to marked dilation of the cerebral vessels and an increase in flow. What role these factors—myogenic, neurogenic and metabolic—play in cerebrovascular physiology remains to be defined.

Brain Volume. Brain tissue makes up the greatest bulk of the intracranial volume. The literature on brain edema is complex and many points of controversy exist. The brain's ability to swell enormously in response to noxious stimuli long thwarted surgical attacks on the central nervous system.

In an incompressible fluid pressure is transmitted equally throughout its entire volume.

The brain is not a fluid but has an elastic modulus; therefore it contains different states of tension. If a localized mass exists within the intracranial cavity, pressure is not distributed equally in all directions and displacement of brain can occur. This accounts for the many herniations of brain substance against and through apertures within the intracranial cavity. The most important are herniation of the midbrain downward through the tentorial opening, herniation of the middle portion of the temporal lobe across the tentorial edge against the brain stem, and herniation of the posterior fossa contents downward through the foramen magnum.

Time Course of Intracranial Pressure Changes. The time course of pressure changes within the cranial cavity is of great importance. Rapid changes are usually lethal, and only a small increase in intracranial volume can be tolerated acutely. However, a slowly growing brain tumor may be tolerated over a long period of time. A meningioma may occupy most of one frontal lobe without producing symptoms of increased pressure due to the slow wasting of cerebral substance and its substitution by the tumor mass. Similarly a rapidly growing glioblastoma can be accommodated for a time because it tends to destroy cerebral tissue.

The hallmark of increased intracranial pressure, papilledema, takes at least 24 hours to develop, usually much longer. Thus a rapid increase in intracranial pressure, as in a head injury, does not result in papilledema.

Treatment of Increased Intracranial Pressure

The ability to control or modify increased intracranial pressure has been responsible for many of the advances in neurologic surgery. Cerebrospinal fluid removal is the oldest method for treating pressure. However, the fluid should be removed from within the intracranial cavity, not extracranially; otherwise, incipient herniation can be converted to complete herniation with catastrophic results. Lumbar puncture is contraindicated in all cases of increased intracranial pressure when brain deformation is suspected. The release of pressure below the intracranial cavity will only complete the pressure shift, jamming the brain stem through the tentorial notch or the foramen magnum. The lateral ventricles are tapped through a fontanelle in infants or through a a burr hole in adults.

The risk of herniation is particularly high when a lesion is present in the posterior fossa, because vital brain stem structures are located there and the spinal fluid pathways may be obstructed at the aqueduct and in the fourth ventricle. It is common practice to reduce intracranial hypertension in posterior fossa tumors by a shunting procedure before operating on the mass. Fluid is removed by placing a small plastic tube in the lateral ventricle and implanting the other end in the jugular vein or peritoneal cavity, similarly to shunting procedures for hydrocephalus.

There are no means available of reducing the intracranial blood volume without aggravating the symptoms. Any respiratory obstruction with consequent CO_2 retention may cause cerebral vasodilatation and precipitate an uncontrolled rise in the intracranial pressure. The monitoring of respiration is therefore of paramount importance in intracranial hypertension.

The use of hypothermia to decrease cerebral metabolism and cerebral blood flow remains controversial.

Control of Brain Edema. The osmotic diuretics, hypertonic mannitol, glycerol, and urea withdraw fluids from all organs, including the brain. However, their relative failure to penetrate the blood-brain barrier increases their effectiveness in drawing water selectively from the brain. These agents are useful initially but can only rarely be used for long-term management of increased intracranial pressure. They act rapidly and can control intracranial pressure until more definitive treatment is performed, such as removal of a tumor or hematoma. Blood electrolytes must be watched because of the rapid shift in body fluids.

Dexamethasone, in divided doses to a total of 16 mg per 24 hours, decreases swelling around a tumor, probably through its action on the cellular membranes. Larger doses have occasionally been used. The drug is most effective in treating metastatic disease to the brain.

Clinical Syndromes of Brain Tumors

Brain tumors present clinically in four different ways: (1) they raise intracranial pressure; (2) they irritate the brain, giving rise to seizures; (3) they produce local loss of function by pressure or destruction; and (4) they herniate brain substance from one compartment to another. One or more of these mechanisms may predominate throughout the course of the illness. Supratentorial tumors increase intracranial pressure by their bulk or by obstructing the flow of cerebrospinal fluid. Posterior fossa tumors at an early stage produce obstruction by impinging upon the fourth ventricle. The classic signs of increased intracranial pressure are headache, vomiting, and papilledema.

Headache. Intracranial pain results from traction or distortion of the dura, of the bridging veins between the dura and the cerebrum, or of the large vessels of the cerebral hemispheres. A tumor may thus cause headache by local pressure and infiltrating the vessels in the dura or by blocking the flow of cerebrospinal fluid, distending the ventricles and stretching superficial blood vessels and brain coverings. The headache is usually of short total duration (months or, at most, one or two years), is a steady aching pain, becomes progressively severe in intensity, frequency, and duration, and eventually may be continuous. Characteristically it appears in the morning, sometimes upon arising, and disappears after a few hours. Any Valsalva maneuver, as on coughing or sneezing, increases venous pressure and precipitates the headache.

Vomiting.   Vomiting is prominent in tumors of the posterior fossa, especially those that impinge on the floor of the fourth ventricle. The patient, usually a child, has morning nausea which disappears in one or two hours. The vomiting is usually described as projectile in nature but need not be.

Papilledema.   Papilledema is the cardinal sign of increased intracranial pressure. First the retinal vessels do not pulsate, then the optic cup disappears, and soon the disk edges become blurred. As severe papilledema develops, the optic disk becomes elevated, the disk margins become obscured, and flame-shaped hemorrhages appear. With a rapid and severe increase in intracranial pressure the retinal hemorrhages escape from the plane of the retinal fibers and appear behind the vitreous body as small pools of subhyaloid hemorrhages.

Brain Displacements.   Experimentally it has been shown that high pressures upon the brain of up to 1000 mm of water can be tolerated for short periods and pressures of several hundred millimeters can be tolerated for longer periods with only the production of chronic papilledema. It is brain displacement that is responsible for the serious signs and symptoms. Tumor in the substance of the brain or on its surface gradually pushes the brain down into the tentorial opening and foramen magnum, resulting in tentorial or upper brain stem compression and foraminal or medullary compression.

Tentorial Compression.   Three factors are important: compression, stretch, and angulation. With descent of the brain a wider diameter of brain stem enters the tentorial ring and becomes compressed. The medial margins of the temporal lobes are squeezed through on one or both sides. The third and sixth nerves and the basal blood vessels are stretched. In Figure 34–5 the downward shift of the brain stem causes traction on the posterior cerebral artery

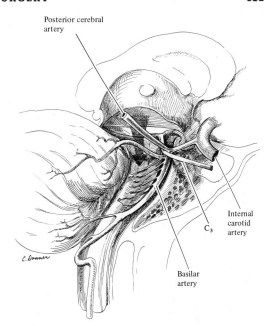

Figure 34–5.   Dislocation of the brain stem. As pressure increases above the tentorium, brain stem structures are displaced downward, creating traction on basilar structures, especially the third and sixth cranial nerves and the posterior cerebral artery.

and the third cranial nerve. Since the spinal cord is anchored by the first dentate ligament, the midbrain must angulate. Hemorrhages are frequently seen at autopsy in this region.

The sixth nerve runs a long course from the posterior fossa to the orbit and may be stretched and paralyzed at an early stage of tumor growth in both supratentorial and infratentorial lesions. Thus it is a poor locater of tumors. The function of the pyramidal tract of both sides, but especially the side of the tumor, is impaired. Asymmetric displacement may cause the contralateral pyramidal tract to be compressed against the tentorial edge and may give rise to false localizing lateral pyramidal signs. Compression and stretching of the third nerves result in dilatation of the pupils. Because the descent is usually asymmetric, pupillary changes are generally asymmetric, the side of the lesion usually leading. When there is full paralysis of both pupils in the adult, the condition is almost always irreversible. The child with fixed dilated pupils may recover if quickly decompressed.

Respiratory embarrassment is a prominent and serious component of the tentorial syndrome. The rate and depth of respiration increase and the respiratory pause is lost. With further damage there is forced respiration,

Table 34–1. CLASSIFICATION OF INTRACRANIAL TUMORS

INTRACEREBRAL	PERCENT*	EXTRACEREBRAL	PERCENT*
Neuroectodermal		Meningioma	28.0
Glial	(44)	Neurinoma	6.0
Astrocytoma (child)	6.0	Pituitary adenoma	(6.0)
Astrocytoma (adult)	12.0	Chromophobe	5.5
Astroblastoma	0.5	Eosinophilic	0.5
Spongioblastoma	0.5	Craniopharyngioma	2.0
Glioblastoma	22.0	Various	1.0
Oligodendroglioma	3.0	Dermoids and	
Ependymoma	4.0	epidermoids	
Medulloblastoma	2.0	Chordoma	
Colloid cyst	1.0	Melanoma	
Plexus papilloma	0.5		
Pineal	0.5		
Ganglioneuroma	0.5		
Mesodermal			
Hemangioendothelioma	3.5		
Various			
Dermoids and epidermoids			
Lipoma			
Aneurysm			
Percent	57		43
Approximately	60		40

* These figures are based upon the experience of the University of Chicago Clinics. The incidence of meningiomas is higher than average, which is about about 15 to 18 percent.

and eventually respiration becomes slow and irregular, culminating eventually in apnea.

Foraminal Compression. Tumors of the posterior fossa may embarrass the upper brain stem, but more characteristically they displace the tonsils of the cerebellum down into the foramen magnum. The resulting suboccipital pain is as a rule not severe, but the patient may hold his head stiff or to one side to obtain relief. Occasionally stretch paralysis of one or more of the cranial nerves may occur. Sudden herniation of the tonsils compresses the respiratory outflow and causes sudden death.

Cerebral Irritation. Epilepsy denotes irritation of brain substance. It is a common and often an early sign of extrinsic and intrinsic supratentorial tumors. Approximately 30 percent of patients who develop seizures for the first time after 20 years of age have a neoplasm. The seizure is frequently focal in nature and helps localize the tumor. If the tumor is situated near the central motor cortex, a jacksonian attack often ensues and culminates in a major generalized seizure.

Cerebral Paralysis. Localizing syndromes are produced by local pressure or invasion. The rapidly growing, malignant, intracerebral tumors quickly destroy wide areas of brain. Attention to the modalities of cortical function is helpful in localizing tumors. Benign tumors at the base of the brain compress the merging cranial nerves and produce neurologic dys-

function before there are signs of irritation, pressure, or displacement.

Classification of Brain Tumors

The incidence of central nervous system tumors is about the same as that of leukemia and is higher than that of carcinoma of the stomach. They may be classified into extracerebral and intracerebral groups (Table 34–1).

Extracerebral Tumors. Most extracerebral brain tumors are benign. The most frequent are meningiomas, neurinomas, pituitary adenomas, and craniopharyngiomas. Less frequent are dermoid and epidermoid tumors at the base of the skull.

Meningioma. About 15 percent of all brain tumors are meningiomas. They are solid encapsulated tumors, almost always attached to the meninges, probably arise from cells of the arachnoid granulations, and are generally related to the venous sinuses. They press against the brain and do not infiltrate it, but they may invade the dural sinuses and overlying bone. Infiltrated bone, particularly in the sphenoid wings, becomes thickened. The frequency is about the same along the sagittal sinus, over the convexity, attached to the sphenoid ridge, subfrontal or suprasellar, and in the posterior fossa and spinal canal. The tumors grow slowly, are rare in childhood, and are most frequent at 40 to 60 years. Treatment is surgical removal. Complete removal cures. If removal is incomplete, one or more subsequent removals may keep the patient relatively symptomfree over many years.

Neurinoma. A neurinoma is commonly found on the vestibular division of the eighth cranial nerve and less frequently on the fifth, ninth, and eleventh cranial nerves. In von Recklinghausen's disease the tumors may be multiple and are commonly found on the posterior roots of the spinal nerves. There are two theories on the origin of this tumor. It may arise from perineural fibrous tissue and be a perineural fibroblastoma, or it may arise from Schwann cells surrounding the nerve and be a schwannoma.

The acoustic neuroma may impair function of the lower cranial nerves and compress the cerebellum and brain stem. If sufficiently large it interferes with circulation of fluid in the posterior fossa and causes an increase in intracranial pressure.

Pituitary Adenomas. The chromophobe adenoma is the commonest pituitary tumor; the acidophilic and basophilic tumors are less frequent and rarely occur before the age of 20. The chromophobe adenoma is the largest and grows through the diaphragm of the sella to compress the overlying optic chiasm and hypothalamus. Eosinophilic tumors produce growth hormone and gigantism before the epiphyses are closed; later they cause acromegaly. True basophil tumors are rare. More frequent is hyperplasia of the basophilic cells associated with Cushing's syndrome. Most pituitary tumors are radiosensitive and long-term survival is common. If the tumor is large, endangering vision or compressing hypothalamic and other cerebral structures, surgical decompression may be necessary.

Craniopharyngioma. A craniopharyngioma is cystic in 80 percent and is derived from remnants of Rathke's pouch, the epithelial outgrowth of the nasopharynx which forms the anterior pituitary. It is usually situated above the sella turcica but may be intrasellar or both. The cyst contains oily fluid rich in cholesterol. Symptoms may arise in childhood, at puberty, or in the adult, usually by compression of the optic chiasm and by pituitary and hypothalamic dysfunction. This is the most common supratentorial tumor in childhood with the highest incidence at 12 years.

Treatment is by surgical removal or drainage supplemented by radiotherapy. If removal is incomplete, the tumor recurs and is fatal in a few years.

Intracerebral Tumors. Cells of the primitive neural tube give rise to the centrally placed ependymal cells, the ganglion cells or neurocytes in the cortex, and to the basal nuclei. They are supported by short branching cells of the astrocytic series and to a lesser extent by the oligodendroglia. Tumors can develop from the ependymal cells, the astrocytes, and the oligodendrocytes. Cells from the external granular layer of the cerebellum, which disappears in the first year of life, give rise to the medulloblastoma. More than half of all brain tumors belong to these four intrinsic types. In addition, tumors may arise within the brain from the choroid plexus, pineal gland, supportive connective tissue, or they may be metastatic from tumors elsewhere in the body.

Glioblastoma Multiforme. The glioblastoma is found most often in the central white matter and may grow across the corpus callosum. It is characterized by rapid growth and local invasion and destruction of tissue. There is often necrosis with formation of hemorrhagic cysts. The results of surgical removal are disappointing, but radiotherapy may give improvement for a few months. Recently chemotherapeutic agents have been tried in this most malignant of brain tumors with encouraging results. However, most patients die within a year of the onset of symptoms.

Cerebral Astrocytoma. The astrocytoma tends to infiltrate the hemisphere diffusely and develop cysts containing yellowish fluid. Common sites are the frontal, temporal, and parietal lobes. This tumor occurs in young adults and in the middle-aged. Symptoms usually precede diagnosis by about six months and survival is about six years. It is rarely possible to excise the whole tumor, but subtotal removal, which can sometimes be repeated, may prolong life.

Astrocytoma of the Cerebellar Hemisphere. Astrocytoma of the cerebellum is different from the supratentorial tumor in that it occurs mostly in children rather than adults, is almost invariably cystic, and contains a small nodule of tumor projecting into the cyst. Cure is frequent after surgical removal of the tumor nodule and drainage of the cyst into the cerebrospinal fluid pathway.

Astrocytomas of the Brain Stem and Spinal Cord. Like the diffuse astrocytoma of the cerebral hemisphere, these tumors grow diffusely and produce a general widening or "hypertrophy" of the nervous tissue rather than necrosis. Because of the respiratory importance of the brain stem and cervical cord, the prognosis of brain stem and upper spinal cord gliomas is poor. They cannot be treated surgically but radiotherapy may be of some benefit.

Oligodendroglioma. The oligodendroglioma occurs in adults and is situated most often in the cerebral hemispheres, especially toward the frontal and temporal lobes. It is usually a firm tumor with a deceptive appearance of encapsulation and is best treated by surgical excision and radiotherapy.

Ependymoma. The ependymoma arises from the ependymal lining of the ventricles, commonly the fourth, and may grow into the cerebral hemispheres with little or no attachment to the ventricles. It occurs most often in children and young adults. Treatment and prognosis vary according to the site. Patients with ependymoma of the fourth ventricles may receive temporary relief from removal of the obstructing mass if it is attached to the roof of the ventricle. Those in the cerebral substance are slowly progressive and moderately radiosensitive. Survival of many years may occur. Ependymomas sometimes seed to the ventricles and the subarachnoid pathways.

Medulloblastoma. The medulloblastoma occurs most often at five to nine years and is less common in children than astrocytoma of the cerebellum. It forms less than 20 percent of all brain tumors of childhood and adolescence. The tumor is situated in the vermis and roof of the fourth ventricle. Radiotherapy has produced some long-term survivals of 15 years and beyond. The tumor is infiltrative and cannot be totally removed, but operation may be needed to bypass the ventricle and establish diagnosis. Radiotherapy is given to the whole brain and spinal cord, because the tumor tends to spread by seeding throughout the cerebrospinal fluid pathway.

Choroid Plexus Papilloma. These tumors occur mainly in the first decade of life and are found in the fourth ventricles, the lateral ventricle, the third ventricles, and in the cerebellopontine angle. They may reach a large volume before blocking the cerebrospinal fluid pathways but can usually be completely excised.

Pinealoma. The more common pinealoma is benign and contains normal pineal tissue and epithelioid and lymphoid cells. The less common and rapidly malignant type consists of smaller, more homogenous cells. These tumors press upon the quadrigeminal plate and obstruct the aqueduct. In children they may cause precocious puberty.

Tumors from Supporting Connective Tissue. The hemangioendothelioma, a tumor of adults that occurs almost exclusively within the cerebellum, may be cured by total excision. It may be associated with angiomata of the retina and with polycystic kidney, pancreas, and liver. The malignant hemangiosarcoma and a few fibroblastic sarcomas may also be seen in the central nervous system.

Metastatic Tumors. Metastatic tumors are commonly from the lung, breast, kidney, thyroid, and malignant melanoma and occasionally from the bowel, uterus, ovary, and other sites. They are usually blood-borne but occasionally spread by contiguity from tumors in the nasopharynx and nasal sinuses. They are discrete masses within the cerebral substance, often multiple. In general there is no effective treatment, although deep x-rays may relieve headache and some thyroid metastases will respond to radioactive iodine. If the primary tumor responds to chemotherapy, so often will the cerebral metastasis. Hormonal therapy for metastatic breast carcinoma may also give relief. Occasionally surgical removal of a single metastasis from a slowly growing tumor is worthwhile.

Diagnosis of Brain Tumors

Tumors may be diagnosed by the neurologic signs they produce, by radiography, both plain and with contrast media, and by radioactive scanning agents.

Neurologic Signs. Brain tumors may be diagnosed by the focal neurologic findings they produce and by signs of increased intracranial pressure. The tumor may be large, as in the frontal and temporal lobes, before signs are present, while in other regions a small lesion may produce a focal neurologic deficit.

The visual system ramifies widely throughout the supratentorial space, lesions at various levels producing characteristic neurologic deficits from the optic nerve and chiasm to the occipital cortex. Figure 34–6 shows schematically how an examination of the visual fields can give important clues to the localization of lesions.

Lesions of the motor and sensory cortex at the lips of the central fissure and in the central and posterior portions of the internal capsule produce early signs of hemiparesis and sensory disturbances. Those in the speech areas at the lips of the sylvian fissure in the dominant hemisphere produce dysphasia, while those of the cerebellum cause nystagmus and disturbances of coordination, particularly if they involve the cerebellar nuclei. Brain stem lesions demonstrate their presence by abnormality of cranial nerve function.

Radiographic Studies. Plain x-rays of the skull should be taken in every case of suspected cerebral neoplasm. In selected cases tomography of the base of the skull may help delineate pathologic changes. Abnormalities in bony structures can be seen on plain radiographs, but to visualize nervous tissue and its supporting structures requires various methods of enhancing their contrast to x-rays.

Pneumography. Air may be introduced into

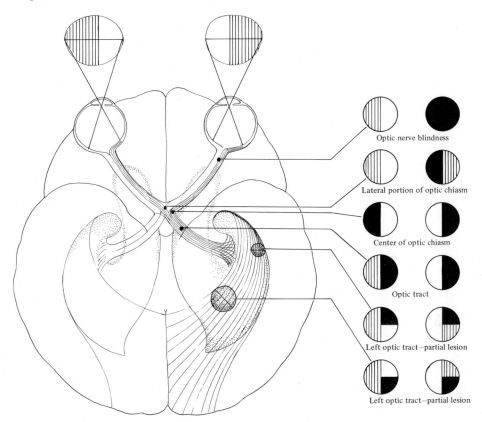

Figure 34–6. The visual pathways from the eye to the occipital cortex are shown. Lesions in the optic nerve, the optic chiasm, and the optic radiations produce characteristic localizing visual-field patterns.

the brain replacing cerebrospinal fluid from its normal pathways. It may be inserted by direct puncture of the ventricles in the adult, through burr holes in the calvarium. In the child needles are passed through the coronal suture next to the anterior fontanelle. This is the safest method when increased intracranial pressure is suspected since downward herniation through the foramen magnum can be prevented. Alternatively air can be introduced into the cerebral subarachnoid spaces and ventricles by the spinal route; 30 to 40 cc introduced into the lumbar subarachnoid space rises through the fourth ventricle into the lateral ventricular system. Radiographs are taken with the head in various positions to outline all portions of the ventricular system and the cisterns. The entire brain can be studied at one time, and lesions within the fluid-filled cavities may be directly visualized. Lesions remote from the ventricles or subarachnoid spaces cannot be directly seen, and their presence must be inferred by distortions of the ventricular system.

Angiography. The arterial system of the

brain is entered either by direct needle puncture of the carotid or vertebral arteries or indirectly through a catheter placed in a peripheral artery. Iodine-containing radiocontrast medium is injected under pressure as a bolus and rapid sequence x-rays are taken, visualizing the arterial and venous system. Displacement of normal vessels and the development of abnormal tumor vessels help diagnose and localize a tumor.

Brain Scans. Brain scans make use of the blood-brain barrier which excludes most forms of bloodborne substances from the cerebral tissues and retains them in the vascular space. Technetium 99-m (^{99M}Tc) injected intravenously is most often used. Tumors have a faultily formed or absent blood-brain barrier and retain the isotope. The advantage of this technique is that it is relatively noninvasive, i.e., no arterial puncture or invasion of the cerebrospinal fluid spaces is necessary. The disadvantage is that definition is poor and does not permit characterization of the lesion in all cases.

Computer-Assisted Axial Tomography. A narrowly collimated beam of x-rays is passed through the head and rotated circumferentially in a carefully chosen transverse plane. This plane is considered a "slice" through the head. The amount of radiation absorbed by the head at numerous points during the beam's 360° circumnavigation around the patient is recorded in the computer. The computer then reconstructs a picture of the slice two dimensionally, either on photographic film or on a cathode ray tube, using electronic image enhancement techniques. A good image of the cerebral tissue, the ventricles of the brain, and intracranial lesions is obtained.

Treatment of Brain Tumors

As with tumors elsewhere in the body, attempted curative treatment of brain tumors is largely surgical and aims at restoring normal intracranial pressure and removing the tumor.

Radiotherapy provides useful palliation of a number of cerebral tumors; for example,

medulloblastomas and pituitary tumors can occasionally be completely ablated by radiotherapy. Tumors of the astrocytic series and meningiomas can be temporarily controlled with radiation therapy, but few, if any, long-term "cures" result.

High-energy particles, such as protons, neutrons, and negative pi mesons, have recently been used and may provide better results than gamma rays, x-rays, or electrons.

Chemotherapeutic agents have been disappointing in the treatment of cerebral tumors. The nitrosourea group of compounds, BCNU (bischloroethylnitrosourea) and CCNU (chloroethylcyclohexylnitrosourea), are sometimes of value, especially for malignant astrocytomas.

SUBARACHNOID HEMORRHAGE AND VASCULAR LESIONS

There are few diseases of the central nervous system as dramatic as the onset of subarachnoid

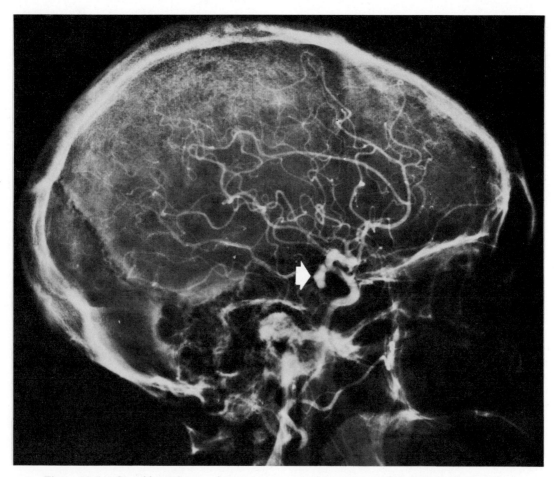

Figure 34–7. Carotid arteriogram demonstrates a saccular aneurysm of the intracerebral portion of the internal carotid artery at the junction of the posterior communicating artery.

hemorrhage, and its catastrophic consequences make it a not uncommon emergency room phenomenon. The so-called berry aneurysm on the circle of Willis is the most common source of the bleeding. The classic syndrome includes headache, stiff neck, and disturbance of consciousness. The astute physician recognizes the premonitory symptoms that frequently herald the disease.

It is the rapid onset of neurologic damage, at a time that can be easily fixed, which characterizes most diseases of the cerebrovascular system. Thus the layman's term "stroke" is descriptive, encompassing most syndromes described.

Aneurysms

Aneurysms are small outpouchings or swellings on the vessels at the base of the brain. Although rarely encountered in childhood, they are termed congenital. They occur at the bifurcation of vessels probably because of a congenital deficiency of muscle at these sites, and they enlarge under the force of intravascular pressure.

In Figure 34–7 an aneurysm of the posterior communicating artery is visualized during carotid arteriography.

Most aneurysms are 2 to 12 mm in diameter. The larger the aneurysm, the greater its tendency to rupture. Occasionally large aneurysms, 4 or 5 cm, may present as space-occupying lesions within the brain. About 35 percent of aneurysms are found on the internal carotid artery, most often at its junction with the posterior communicating artery, and the same percent on the anterior cerebral artery at its junction with the anterior communicating artery. Fifteen percent are found on each of the middle cerebral, the vertebrobasilar, and posterior cerebral arteries. Figure 34–8 shows a view of the base of the brain with its major arterial trunks and the circle of Willis where almost all aneurysms occur. Figures 34–9 and 34–10 show the blood supply of the brain and the anatomy of the cortex.

Symptoms. Most aneurysms are silent until they rupture. About one third of all patients die at or soon after their first hemorrhage. Survivors

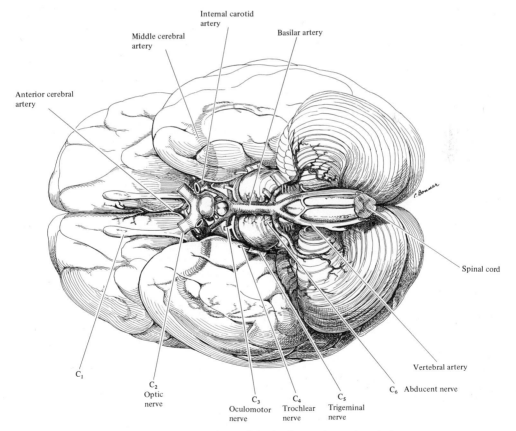

Figure 34–8. The major vessels at the base of the brain are shown in relation to nervous structures. Almost all aneurysms arise on these vessels.

A

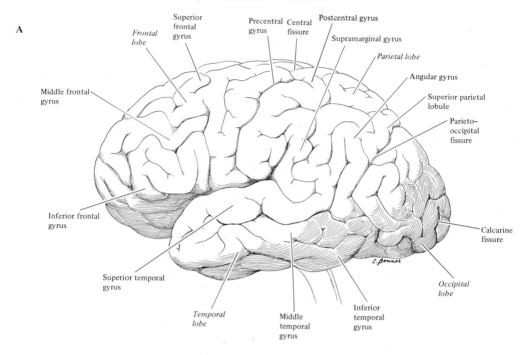

B

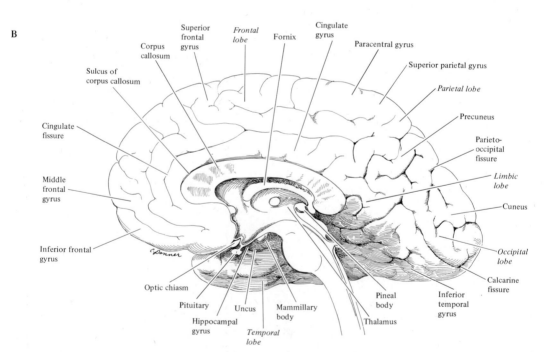

Figure 34–9. The surface anatomy of (*A*) the lateral and (*B*) the medial aspects of the cerebral hemisphere.

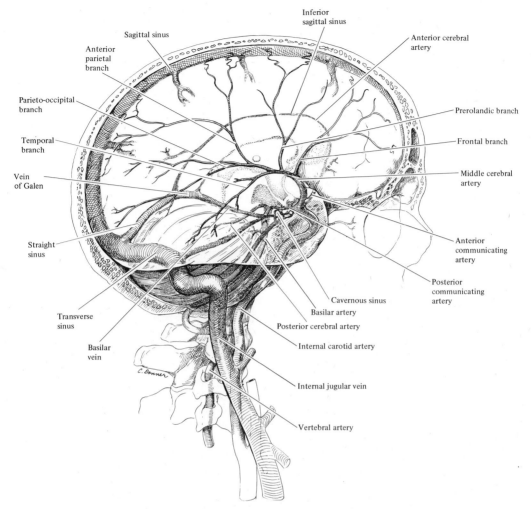

Figure 34–10. The arterial supply and venous drainage of the brain.

frequently give a history of one or more headaches subsiding spontaneously without subsequent neurologic deficit. These symptoms may be due to leaking of the aneurysm before its rupture. The headaches are sudden and extremely severe.

Hemorrhage from an aneurysm may occur into the subarachnoid space, the cerebral substance, or rarely the subdural space. Hematomas in the cerebral substance, fortunately uncommon, are treated as mass lesions and removed surgically if there are symptoms of transtentorial herniation. Subarachnoid hemorrhage causes a disturbance in consciousness which may be transient or prolonged, due to an increase in intracranial pressure or to spasm of blood vessels. Blood in the cerebrospinal fluid irritates the meninges and is responsible for the rapid onset of symptoms. Blood in the cerebrospinal fluid on lumbar puncture confirms the diagnosis.

Sometimes patients who have had only a small hemorrhage die or have permanent disability, such as prolonged coma, aphasia, or hemiplegia. Spasm of the cerebral vessels, which occurs protectively to limit the hemorrhage, becomes a pathologic problem that may persist for several weeks. The spasm, frequently seen on cerebral angiography, is usually close to the bleeding aneurysm but may be widespread throughout one or both hemispheres. There is no treatment for the vascular spasm.

Nerve Compression. The common aneurysm of the internal carotid at the origin of the posterior communicating artery may enlarge and press on the third and fifth cranial nerves. Oculomotor nerve paralysis produces a drooping eyelid, a dilated pupil, and weakness of the extraocular muscles. Fifth-nerve pressure usually results in headache in the distribution of the first division of the fifth nerve, in the frontal and retro-orbital regions. This is one of the few times when an aneurysm makes its presence known prior to rupture, and it demands immediate diagnosis and treatment.

Rarely an aneurysm near the junction of the ophthalmic and internal carotid artery presses upon the optic nerve causing partial monocular blindness, or a large anterior cerebral aneurysm may compress the optic chiasma mimicking a tumor. Aneurysms on the basilar artery may compress the cranial nerves that arise from the brain stem.

Treatment. Aneurysms so vary in their presentation and form that an abbreviated discussion of their treatment is difficult. The mortality for nonsurgically treated subarachnoid hemorrhage is 60 to 70 percent, with one half of patients dying within the first month from the initial or from subsequent bleeds. Surgical treatment should therefore be performed as early as possible after the initial rupture. Unfortunately it is at this time that the patient is often a poor operative risk because of the raised intracranial pressure, vascular spasm, and altered state of consciousness.

Surgical treatment aims at isolating the aneurysm from the cerebral circulation, strengthening the wall, or reducing the arterial pressure head presented to the fragile aneurysmal sac.

The preferred treatment is clipping or ligating the base of the aneurysm under direct vision, but this is only possible when the aneurysm is surgically accessible and when the sac has a narrow pedicle. Fortunately many aneurysms are of this type. In those that cannot be clipped the aneurysmal wall may be strengthened by encasing it with muscle, fascia, or plastic. An aneurysm may be thrombosed by injecting finely divided iron particles or inserting a thin, coiled copper wire.

Aneurysms of the carotid or middle cerebral arteries that are not amenable to direct attack are sometimes treated by ligation of the carotid artery in the neck. This lowers intraluminal pressure within the aneurysm and substantially reduces the chance of rupture. An adequate collateral circulation must be demonstrated before ligation to prevent ischemic infarction of the brain. Clamps may be placed which gradually occlude the carotid artery during hours or days to test for toleration of the treatment.

In patients in whom surgical treatment is not indicated, drugs may reduce the blood pressure, which is often elevated. An attempt may be made to promote healing of the aneurysm by preventing early dissolution of the clot. The potent antifibrinolytic agent, epsilon aminocaproic acid, given in large quantities, is the most effective drug. It may be given for the conservative treatment of an aneurysm and while waiting for the general condition to improve prior to operation.

Arteriovenous Malformations

A congenital arteriovenous malformation of the brain is a rarer cause of subarachnoid hemorrhage than an aneurysm. It probably results from an abnormal development of the primitive arteriovenous shunts between the arteries and veins of the central nervous system in fetal life. They may be so small that they are not recognized by standard angiographic techniques, while others may replace a lobe of the brain. They tend to enlarge slowly but do not present as mass lesions unless they rupture and form a hematoma.

They commonly present with focal or generalized seizures. Bleeding is less frequent than with an aneurysm and may occur in about 50 percent of patients. They may also produce increasing cerebral ischemia.

Operation is the treatment of choice when the lesion is well-circumscribed and located where surgical attack would not produce further neurologic deficit. Deep-seated lesions are best left alone.

Small pieces of muscle, fragments of autogenous clot, and inert plastic beads have been inserted into the feeding arteries to act as emboli through its parent vessel, usually the carotid. The feeding vessels may also be tied. Embolization and vessel ligation should be regarded as palliative procedures, since unless the entire arteriovenous shunt system has been obliterated, the malformation will persist and enlarge.

Arteriosclerotic Cerebrovascular Disease

Arteriosclerosis and hypertensive disease are the commonest cerebrovascular disorders. They may present suddenly as a "stroke" or as transient ischemic attacks produced by marginal cerebral perfusion or repeated embolization from a proximal arteriosclerotic plaque. They may present with hemorrhage or thrombosis.

Hemorrhage. Massive intracerebral hemorrhage is a frequent complication of hypertensive cerebral disease and also of arteriosclerosis. The vessels at greatest risk are the perforating vessels and the short central branches of the middle cerebral and anterior choroidal arteries. The hematoma presents as a deep mass lesion. The patient is frequently desperately ill. The surgical treatment of these hematomas is controversial, but if the patient is stable and the hematoma has been well localized by cerebral angiography, evacuation of the clot through a cerebrotomy can be lifesaving. Hematomas in the poles of the frontal, temporal, and occipital lobes are more readily dealt with surgically. A number of these may be caused by small "cryptic" arteriovenous malformations previously unrecognized. Signs of transtentorial herniation may occur rapidly. If the hematoma ruptures into the ventricular system, the patient appears more ill than with a subarachnoid hemorrhage from an aneurysm and generally dies.

Thrombosis. Cerebral thrombosis is the commonest cerebrovascular disease. The clinical picture depends upon the vessel involved, but the usual presentation is a sudden focal neurologic disturbance with little or no disturbance of consciousness. Since arteriosclerosis is a generalized disease, surgical treatment is only indicated if a well-circumscribed cervical or cerebral locus is the source of the symptoms.

The carotid arteries in the neck are frequently involved with localized atherosclerotic disease. Atheroma at the bifurcation of the common carotid may embolize distally, producing focal transient or permanent neurologic deficits. Occlusive disease without embolization may also produce transient or permanent neurologic deficits in the presence of distal disease in the small intracranial vessels. Transient ischemic attacks may occur from low perfusion of marginal areas of the cerebrovascular system. Atheromatous occlusion may also occur at the origin of the common carotid and vertebral arteries. All the vessels must be studied angiographically before surgical treatment is undertaken. Endarterectomy may be performed on one or more vessels to remove embolizing or occluding plaques and improve perfusion of the brain. With microneurosurgery embolectomy is now possible on small cerebral vessels, such as the middle cerebral artery. Small vessel perfusion can also be established by anastomosing the superficial temporal artery to the middle cerebral, thus increasing cerebral perfusion and bypassing more proximal intracranial disease. Operation cannot improve a fixed neurologic deficit.

SPINAL COLUMN

The spinal column provides support and form to the trunk and protects the spinal cord and nerves. To achieve flexibility the spinal column is arranged in segmental fashion with each vertebra jointed to its neighbor by a fibrocartilaginous semiliquid disk or shock absorber.

Anatomy

The segmental arrangement of the spinal column is important in diagnosis and treatment. The vertebral body is a large block of bone responsible for most of the strength of the column, while the neural arch, comprised of laminae and pedicles, is responsible for protecting nervous tissue. There are 7 cervical, 12 thoracic, and 5 lumbar segments. There are 8 cervical nerves, one more than the number of bony levels. Figure 34–11 shows the anatomic relationships between the exiting spinal nerves and the vertebral levels. The regions responsible for the most movement, the cervical and lumbar areas, have a larger neural arch, while the relatively rigid thoracic region has its nervous

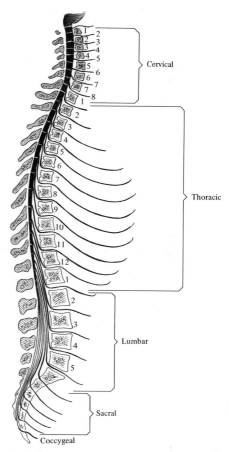

Figure 34–11. The figure demonstrates the segmental nature of the spinal column and the pattern of the emerging nerves. There are eight cervical nerves for seven vertebral levels. Below the cervical spine each nerve takes a progressively more downward course as it runs from the cord exit to the neural foramen. The cord ends at about the first lumbar vertebra.

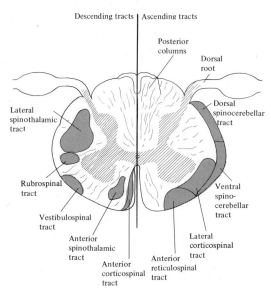

Figure 34–12. The major descending and ascending tracts of the spinal cord are shown. Of particular importance for purposes of the neurologic examination are the posterior columns, the lateral spinothalamic tract, and the corticospinal tract.

tissue closely encompassed by bone. Lesions causing compression in the cervical and lumbar areas can therefore be better tolerated than those in the thoracic area. The spinal cord ends at the level of the first lumbar vertebra. The nervous elements below that level are peripheral nerves.

The clinical problem is differentiating compression of nervous tissue from pathologic processes in neural tissue and distinguishing between spinal cord and peripheral nerve compression. Like acute brain compression, acute spinal cord compression is one of the most serious of all neurosurgical emergencies which must be recognized and treated immediately.

With movement the spinal column flexes and bends in its upper and lower portions, and the nervous tissue within the spinal canal moves during shortening and lengthening of the osseous canal. Immobilization and rest are therefore important in treating compressive disease of nervous tissue. Fibers conducting motor and sensory impulses are intermingled in the cauda equina and peripheral nerves. In the spinal cord they are collated in descending and ascending tracts (Figure 34–12).

Examination for disturbances of sensation in the spinal dermatomes gives information about the level of involvement, but it should be appreciated that the lesion may be cephalad to the signs. The dermatomes on the arm comprise C_4 to T_1 and those to the leg L_1 to S_1, and

neither is well represented upon the trunk (Figure 34–13).

Plain x-rays of the spine in at least two projections are essential in all suspected spinal column diseases. Note should be taken of the vertebral body, lamina, pedicles, articular processes, spines, intervertebral disks, and neural foramina.

Acquired Disorders of the Spine

The spine degenerates with age and continued use and occasionally in early life. The 23 intervertebral disks are most prone to degeneration They are soft and resilient in the center, firm and fibrous at the periphery, and contain a central nucleus pulposus enclosed in fibrocartilage. With use the nucleus pulposus loses its semifluid consistency, and the disk flattens and bulges at any weak spot in the periphery, most often on either side of the posterior longitudinal spinal ligament. The natural alignment of the vertebra at the intravertebral and interarticular joints is upset, and as a result spurs of bone are formed. This is osteoarthritis of the spine secondary to disk degeneration and is the commonest cause of chronic low back and neck pain. The osteoarthritic spurs may accumulate and press upon the neural elements within the spinal canal, particularly if the canal is congenitally small.

Prior to generalized chronic changes specific levels may become involved with degenerative disk disease. Force applied to a degenerating disk ruptures the annular ligament, and the nucleus pulposus extrudes posterolaterally on one or the other side of the posterior longitudinal ligament. The prolapsed disk presses upon the spinal nerve root and causes pain. Often the herniated disk repairs naturally. The soft protrusion becomes fibrosed and shrinks, and the nerve root accommodates as swelling produced by the initial injury subsides. Only those patients who remain symptomatic after conservative therapy should be considered for surgery.

Cervical Disk Disease. In cervical disk disease there are local tenderness and pain, most often radiating in the C_5–C_6 and C_6–C_7 distributions and less often the C_7–T_1 distribution. C_5–C_6 pain radiates to the radial fingers of the hand, C_6–C_7 to the middle fingers. Referred interscapular pain is common at both levels. C_5–C_6 herniation results in weakness of the biceps muscles, with absence or depression of its reflex, and C_6–C_7 prolapse includes weakness of the triceps muscle and decrease in its reflex contraction. Forceful compression of the cervical spine by pressure on the head may aggravate symptoms.

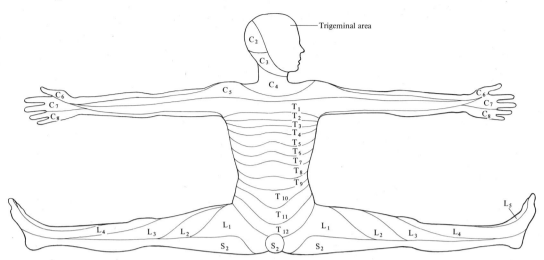

Figure 34–13. The cutaneous pattern of the spinal dermatomes. Note that C_5 to T_1 are on the upper extremity and L_1 to S_2 on the lower extremity.

The initial treatment of cervical disk disease without evidence of central protrusion is cervical traction using a head halter affixed to weights by a line over a pulley. The traction is adjusted until it is comfortable because painful traction is of no value. Subsequently it is often useful to immobilize the spine with a simple plastic collar to prevent the flexion and extension movement which aggravates the symptoms. Only those patients who have progressive weakness, who are not relieved by traction, or who have signs of spinal cord compression by a centrally protruding disk should be operated upon. An anterior approach may be used through the vertebral bodies and disk space, and this is combined with interbody fusion. Alternatively the posterior lamina and medial aspect of the pedicle may be removed, exposing the nerve and disk space.

Cervical spondylosis is advanced multilevel disk disease with hypertrophic osteoarthritis and pressure upon the cervical cord at several levels. Patients present with signs of slowly progressive upper and lower motor neuron paralysis. Immobilization and decompressive laminectomy have been performed, but the results are poor.

Thoracic Disk Disease. Thoracic disease is rare, but because of the narrow spinal canal, prolapsed disks constitute a serious and urgent problem. Frequently herniated thoracic disks are associated with major or minor trauma. Operation is indicated, but the results are often poor.

Lumbar Disk Disease. About 95 percent of lumbar disk herniations occur at the L_4–L_5 or L_5–S_1 levels; the remainder are mostly at L_3–L_4. The symptoms may arise acutely following a severe strain or sudden twist, or the onset may be gradual. There is pain in the back radiating to the buttock about the region of the sciatic notch and down the posterior surface of the thigh and outer aspect of the calf into the ankle. In the severe attack the patient may have difficulty standing or walking and feels relief only when he is lying down; coughing, straining, and sneezing give severe pain. There is frequently lumbar muscle spasm with scoliosis of the lower spine. The patellar reflex may be depressed in L_3–L_4 disk disease but is frequently intact at lower levels. The Achilles reflex may be depressed by either L_4 or L_5 root compression. Generally dorsiflexion of the great toe is weak in L_4 root compression, while plantarflexion is weak at L_5. At L_4–L_5 there may be hypalgesia over the dorsal and medial aspect of the foot. Protrusion at L_5–S_1 usually decreases sensation along the lateral and inferior aspect of the foot. Since there is considerable overlap in the distribution of these nerves, signs are not to be taken as absolute. Any maneuver that stretches the sciatic nerve, such as flexing the hip with the knee straight or bow stringing the nerve in the popliteal fossa, will reproduce or exacerbate the pain. Tenderness over the lower spine and the upper course of the sciatic nerve may be present.

Treatment of an acute sciatic attack is complete bed rest until the patient can lift his leg freely to 80° or 90°. This usually requires two to three weeks. The optimal position is "semi-Fowler," which has been shown to produce the lowest intradiscal pressure. Nonnarcotic analgesics and mild tranquilizers are useful initially. Steroids may also be given to decrease the inflammatory reaction. Once the patient is allowed out of bed, ambulation and return to work should occur gradually. The patient should not engage in strenuous physical labor for as long as three months.

Operation is indicated if there is muscle weakness and no improvement of pain despite bed rest. If a dropped foot is allowed to develop, operation may not restore full power. The economic consequences of prolonged bed rest or the occurrence of frequent attacks may be an indication for surgery.

If operation is contemplated, myelography is indicated, to confirm the diagnosis and to determine the level of one or more disk protrusions.

The operation consists of the simple removal of the extruded disk, with curetting of the disk space to extract any further material. It is usually necessary to remove a portion of the overlying lamina. Fusions for disk disease are no longer considered necessary.

Tumors of the Spine

Primary tumors of the spine are rare; most are metastases from disease elsewhere and may be extradural or intradural.

Extradural Tumors. The commonest extradural tumors are metastatic, usually from breast, lung, prostate, kidney, or thyroid. Less common are the lymphomas and multiple myeloma. They may compress the cord by extending into the extradural space or by destroying or collapsing the vertebra. They are treated by x-ray therapy before there is complete paralysis and if there is no myelographic block. Decompression by laminectomy is indicated when there is a block. The lymphomas tend to respond well to radiotherapy and chemotherapy, but decompressive laminectomy is sometimes required. Chemotherapy or hormonal manipulation may be useful, especially in carcinoma of the breast or prostate. Operative treatment does not prolong life but provides useful palliation, sparing the patient the misery of paraplegia, bed sores, and incontinence.

Primary tumors of the vertebral column are rare. Chordomas arise at either end of the spinal column in the sacrum or in the basisphenoid and are derived from remnants of the notocord. They are slowly growing tumors, relatively insensitive to x-ray but amenable to repeated surgical removal. They do not spread by metastasis. Chondrosarcoma and osteogenic sarcoma are rare and there is little effective treatment.

Intradural Tumors. These are extramedullary or outside the spinal cord and intramedullary or

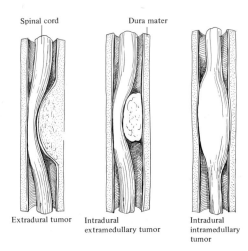

Figure 34–14. The three major types of spinal tumors are shown. They may generally be distinguished by myelography.

inside the spinal cord. The common extramedullary tumors are neurofibromas and meningiomas. The neurofibroma arises from the posterior roots or the peripheral nerves and may extend through the intervertebral foramen into the chest to form a "dumbbell" tumor. In von Recklinghausen's disease there may be multiple tumors within the spinal canal that can often be completely removed by surgical excision. The meningioma is an encapsulated tumor attached to the dura, commonly seen in women and with a predilection for the thoracic region. It can be removed completely, resulting in cure.

Intramedullary tumors are less common and are mainly astrocytomas and ependymomas of the cord. Astrocytomas produce a diffuse swelling with tumor cells intermingled with the normal cells in the fiber tracts. They grow slowly, are sometimes cystic and little can be done for them except decompressive laminectomy to minimize cord compression and to establish a diagnosis. Ependymomas are bulky tumors found commonly in the cauda equina. Complete surgical removal is rarely possible; however, subtotal removal may give useful palliation.

Intradural tumors are frequently insidious. They may present initially with local and radicular pain, or they may be painless but produce neurologic dysfunction, including sphincter disturbance. They frequently are misdiagnosed initially but should be recognized before the onset of irreversible cord symptoms.

Figure 34–14 shows the three major types of spinal tumors: extradural, intradural extramedullary, and intradural intramedullary.

INFECTIONS OF THE NERVOUS SYSTEM

Infections of the central nervous system produce systemic symptoms of toxemia, fever, and leukocytosis, and local destruction and compression of nervous tissue. Meningitis is rarely a surgical disease, although its complications may be treated surgically.

Infections of the Brain

These may be divided conveniently into local infections of the skull and meninges and cerebral abscesses.

Infections of the Skull and Meninges. An abscess may involve scalp, bone, epidural or subdural space, or all of these compartments. The infection may commence as a small scalp abscess or may extend from a middle ear, paranasal sinus, or mastoid infection. If restricted to the scalp, incision with drainage is all that is required. If bone is involved, necrosis and sequestration of the skull require wide removal of the infected region. Extradural and subdural abscesses are drained either through trephination, or when infected bone is removed. Subdural abscesses are particularly dangerous since the pus can spread widely within the intracranial cavity and cause meningitis, cerebritis, and cerebral edema. Cortical vein thrombosis may result in seizures. These desperately ill patients must have wide and effective debridement and decompression to survive. Intrathecal antibiotics may help in addition to systemic antibiotics.

Cerebral Abscess. Although cerebral abscess may occur by direct extension from an infected region in the head, it is more often the result of hematogenous spread, especially in those with lung abscess and congenital heart disease. Penetrating cerebral wounds are also a source.

Cerebral abscesses present as expanding intracranial lesions usually with considerable cerebral edema. Seizures frequently occur. The abscess begins in an area of diffuse cerebritis. As tissue liquefies the abscess enlarges, intracranial pressure rises, and death occurs from herniation of the brain. Alternatively death may occur from meningitis subsequent to rupture into a ventricle or the subarachnoid space.

Diagnosis is established by recognizing the signs of increasing intracranial pressure, with or without signs of focal neurologic deficits. The systemic signs of sepsis are often not present since the abscess is isolated in cerebral tissue. Brain scan or angiography confirms the diagnosis.

An abscess is treated by trephination over the site, puncture of the capsule, drainage of pus, and instillation of antibiotics. Frequently excision of the abscess and its capsule is necessary. The source of the abscess must be investigated and systemic therapy must be vigorous. Abscesses are not infrequently multiple.

An occasional complication of intracranial sepsis is obstructive hydrocephalus, secondary to arachnoid adhesions around the base of the brain, preventing proper absorption of cerebrospinal fluid. It is treated by shunting procedures.

Spinal Epidural Abscess

The most important infection of the spine is epidural abscess. It may arise hematogenously from foci of infection transmitted through the epidural veins or by direct extension from osteomyelitis of the spine. Occasionally it is seen following disk removal. The inflammation and edema produce intense pain. Even slight agitation of the bed is enough to produce severe pain. Compression of the spinal cord may be rapid. The diagnosis is made by the clinical signs and symptoms and by myelography. The condition must be recognized early and treated by immediate laminectomy and drainage of the epidural space before cord compression occurs. If the patient becomes paraplegic, he will remain so in spite of all subsequent therapy.

MALFORMATIONS OF THE CENTRAL NERVOUS SYSTEM AND ITS SUPPORTING STRUCTURES

Embryologic abnormalities of the central nervous system are numerous. Probably over half of all congenital malformations involve the brain, the spinal cord, or their supporting structures. The cause is usually obscure, but some can be traced to drugs or maternal infections in the first trimester of pregnancy.

Surgical treatment cannot correct the underlying condition; in most cases it makes the situation compatible with life or maximizes the potential for development of the nervous system.

Embryology

The central nervous system is formed by an invagination of the dorsal epithelium. The surrounding mesodermal somites form the skeleton and protective layers around the central nervous system. Normally the lips of the invaginated portion close and form a canal, the central canal of the nervous system, and the neural cord separates from the overlying skin. If these processes fail, there is an actual or potential communication between the central nervous system and the skin, and the mesodermal elements surrounding the cord may not

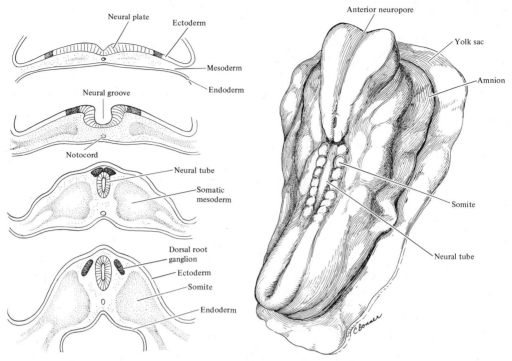

Figure 34–15. Various stages of the normal infolding of the neural canal are shown. Note that the center of the neural tube is completely closed early, while the cephalic and caudal ends close later.

develop normally. Figure 34-15 depicts the stages of the infolding of the neural tube.

Abnormalities may be described as:

1. Failure of the nervous tissue to develop.

2. Failure of the nervous tissue to separate adequately from the dorsal epithelium from which it is derived.

3. Failure of the cerebrospinal fluid spaces to develop.

4. Failure of the cranial sutures to remain open during the period of brain growth.

Primary Failure. This ranges from total failure of the brain development to lesser failures, such as agenesis of the corpus callosum which in its milder forms may be completely asymptomatic. There is no treatment for these anomalies.

Failure of Separation. The simplest failure of the neural cord to separate from the skin is spina bifida occulta. This occurs usually in the dorsal lamina of the lumbar and sacral region when the mesodermal structures fail to meet dorsally in the midline. It is usually an incidental radiologic finding of no significance. Occasionally, however, there is a cutaneous connection between the gap in the bone and a tiny pit in the skin, usually surrounded by abnormal skin containing hair. There may be a solid cord or epithelial tube connecting the pit to the central nervous system. A dermoid cyst or lipoma may form within this cord. Also infection may spread along the cord and cause meningitis. The pit with its cord or tube must be excised to prevent infection.

Occasionally a dermal cyst or lipoma may develop in the spinal canal with or without a dermal sinus and cause widening of the bony structures and gradual compression of nerve tissue. The cyst or lipoma tends to grow slowly and may not present until adult life. Cysts can usually be completely removed unless they have been complicated by infection. Lipomas may be embedded in the cord and can be only subtotally removed.

A cyst may develop in the neurenteric canal, a tract joining the lower end of the neural canal and the lower bowel. This is the result of persistence of a connection between the amniotic sac and the yolk sac which passes through the notocord. Neurenteric cysts are usually found anterior to the sacrum, and total removal is usually possible.

Failure in the Development of Cerebrospinal Fluid Spaces. Hydrocephalus is the most important of this group of anomalies and may be communicating or noncommunicating. In communicating hydrocephalus there is no obvious cause for obstruction in the ventricular or subarachnoid pathways. The absorptive mechanisms are deficient; for example, the arachnoid granulations in the sagittal sinus fail to develop. In noncommunicating hydrocephalus an obstruction is present, usually in the midline, in the third ventricle, aqueduct, or fourth ventricle. A common cause is failure of the aqueduct to form completely, known as aqueductal stenosis.

Frequently an early imbalance between the production and absorption of cerebrospinal fluid corrects itself, and the baby is normal. In a few the hydrocephalus is so severe that the fetus is not viable. Some infants with a delicate balance between secretion and absorption may have this balance upset by the trauma of birth. Hemorrhage into the cerebrospinal fluid may produce molecules too large for the inefficient absorbing mechanism to handle, and hydrocephalus results. Treatment is early shunting with careful follow-up and replacement of the shunts as necessary.

Shunting Procedures. If there is obstruction to the flow or inadequate absorption of cerebrospinal fluid, a shunt may be created to carry the fluid from the ventricular system to the blood stream. The most popular shunts are ventriculoatrial and ventriculoperitoneal. With a ventriculoatrial shunt a tube, containing a valve and pumping device, is placed in the lateral ventricle, brought out beneath the scalp and passed along the external jugular vein into the right atrium. The valve prevents regurgitation of blood into the tubing. The atrial end must be placed within the right atrium as thrombi may form on the tube if it is not in turbulent flow. As the child grows, the tube must be lengthened so that the distal end remains in the atrium. In the ventriculoperitoneal shunt the tube passes subcutaneously across the chest and abdomen and has the distal end implanted in the peritoneal cavity. Fluid is absorbed by the peritoneum and enters the vascular system. A pump is usually placed in the line to check that the shunt is functioning. A long loop is placed in the abdominal cavity to allow for growth. The ventriculoperitoneal shunt fails more frequently then the ventriculoatrial shunt because the distal end is often obstructed by omentum.

A ventriculosubarachnoid shunt is used mostly in older children and adults to bypass an obstruction in the ventricular system. Absorption of cerebrospinal fluid must be normal. The tube is passed below the cervical skin and inserted into the foramen magnum or the cervical subarachnoid space. A valve or pump is not needed and growth is not a problem, but the shunt does require a small craniectomy or laminectomy for insertion of the distal end.

Meningoceles. If there is an anomaly of fusion at a time when the intrauterine subarachnoid pressure is increased, the developing mesoderm might be weakened and allow the subarachnoid space to bulge and form a meningocele. In severe instances the central canal bulges and the sac contains nerve tissues. This is a myelomeningocele or in the cranium an encephalocele. Meningoceles and myelomeningoceles occur most often in the lumbar region and occasionally elsewhere, including into the nasal cavity. There may be associated anomalies, such as heart disease or hydrocephalus. The nervous system may be normal, or there may be partial or complete paralysis of the anal and urinary sphincters and the limbs. The meningocele or myelomeningocele may be completely or partly covered by skin. Operation does not improve any neurologic deficit but is aimed at skin closure to prevent meningitis. Many children develop hydrocephalus within a few months of operation. This is thought to be caused by a concomitant anomaly within the hindbrain known as the Arnold-Chiari malformation, that is, herniation of the cerebellar tonsils with elongation and kinking of the brain stem.

Failure of Bone Development. The posterior fontanelle closes by the sixth week and the anterior fontanelle by the tenth to the sixteenth month. Complete bony fusion of the cranium occurs later. When closure occurs during the period of growth of the brain a number of cranial deformities occur which are sometimes associated with mental and visual impairment. The four anatomic types are:

1. Premature closure of the sagittal suture, scaphocephaly. The skull becomes long and narrow as increased growth occurs in the coronal suture. This is the commonest anomaly.

2. Premature closure of the coronal sutures results in the skull becoming wide and short, brachycephaly.

3. Premature closure of the sagittal and coronal sutures produces a tower-shaped skull, turricephaly.

4. Crouzon's disease is premature closure of all the sutures associated with facial deformity.

Operation consists of reopening the sutures by a linear craniectomy through the suture or on both sides of it. Cosmetic results are best when the child is operated on prior to three months. To prevent recurrence a coat of inert plastic is placed between the bones to retard their growth.

SUGGESTIONS FOR FURTHER READING

GENERAL

Youmans, J. R. (ed): *Neurological Surgery*. 3 vols. W. B. Saunders Co., Philadelphia, 1973.
The most recent reference text on neurosurgery.

CNS TRAUMA

Evans, J. P.: *Acute Head Injury*, 2nd ed. Charles C Thomas, Springfield, Ill., 1963.
A description of the classical neurosurgical syndromes of head injury.

Plum, F., and Posner, J. B.: *The Diagnosis of Stupor and Coma*. F. A. Davis and Co., Philadelphia, 1966.
An excellent discussion of the pathophysiology of states of disturbed consciousness.

For trauma to the spinal column, see Youmans, above.

BRAIN TUMORS

Russell, D. S., and Rubinstein, L. J.: *Pathology of Tumors of the Nervous System*, 3rd ed. Edward Arnold, Ltd., London, 1971.
One of the standards in the field of neuropathology of tumors. Well illustrated.

SUBARACHNOID HEMORRHAGE

Fields, W. S., and Sahs, A. L. (eds.): *Intracranial Aneurysms and Subarachnoid Hemorrhage*. Charles C Thomas, Springfield, Ill., 1965.
Multiauthored symposium.

CONGENITAL MALFORMATIONS

Matson, D. D.: *Neurosurgery of Infancy and Childhood*, 2nd ed. Charles C Thomas, Springfield, Ill., 1969.
This definitive text includes excellent accounts of the surgical repair of childhood congenital anomalies.

Chapter 35

PEDIATRIC SURGERY

Stanley Mercer

CHAPTER OUTLINE

The Infant as a Surgical Patient
  Respiration
  Temperature Control
  Fluid and Electrolytes
    Body Water
    Electrolytes
  Blood Volume
  Renal Function
  Nutrition in the Surgical Neonate
Development of Intestines
  Atresia and Stenosis
  Duplications and Enterogenous Cysts
Abnormalities of Rotation
  Nonrotation
  Malrotation
Persistence of Vitello Intestinal Duct
  Fecal Fistula
  Cyst Formation
  Cord Persistence
  Meckel's Diverticulum
Mesentery of Ascending Colon
Omphalocele and Gastroschisis
Surgical Emergencies in the Newborn
  Cyanosis
    Pneumothorax
    Congenital Diaphragmatic Hernia
    Esophageal Atresia and Tracheoesoph-
      ageal Fistula
  Vomiting
  Abdominal Distention
  Failure to Pass Meconium

Pyloric Stenosis
Duodenal Obstruction
Jejunoileal Obstruction
Rectosigmoid Obstruction
Passage of Blood Rectally Within the First
  Year
  Acute Intussusception
  Differential Diagnosis
  Duplication of Bowel
  Meckel's Diverticulitis
  Other Conditions
Abdominal Masses in Childhood
  Genitourinary System
  Benign
  Malignant
  Other Systems
  Benign
  Malignant
  Clinical Examination
  Investigations
  Relationships Between Cancer and Con-
    genital Defects
Chronic Abdominal Pain in Childhood
Pigmented Lesions of the Skin
  Hemangioma
  Melanoma
Umbilical and Inguinal Swellings
  Umbilical Hernia
  Inguinal Hernia and Derivatives of the
    Processus Vaginalis

The development of pediatric surgery received its main incentive from the differences between the child and the adult. For example, the methods of maintaining homeostasis are much less well developed in the child, especially in the neonate, and disease processes, such as acute appendicitis, are often modified greatly. In fact some conditions, such as congenital anomalies and a number of cancers, are peculiar to childhood.

The care of the critically ill infant has markedly improved, largely because of the development of intensive care and better methods of maintaining nutrition and fluid and electrolyte balance. The team approach to patient care has meant greater sophistication in diagnosis and treatment. For example, the neonatologist working with the surgeon has led to marked reduction in mortality in surgical disease of the neonate. Although infants will respond well to proper surgical care, they will die rapidly if subjected to wrong management.

THE INFANT AS A SURGICAL PATIENT

The infant is not a miniature adult but should almost be regarded as belonging to a different species. The smaller and less mature the infant, the greater are the differences. The infant in the first 48 hours of life is a great deal sturdier than is commonly believed; nevertheless, he is less able to withstand undue stresses of surgery than an adult.

Respiration

An infant is less able than an adult to increase its oxygen intake by increasing the depth of respiration. Instead it increases the rate of respiration. This is less efficient and results in considerable loss of water and heat. The infant should therefore be nursed in a controlled environment. Restriction of chest movements by dressings must be minimized and the oxygen content of the air increased to reduce respiratory effort. Inhalation of greater than 30 percent oxygen for prolonged periods can produce retrolental fibroplasia. The temperature is kept at about 28°C for full-term babies and 30°C for premature infants, and the humidity of the incubator is maintained at 80 to 90 percent. Loss of fluid by respiration and insensible perspiration is then reduced by 50 percent.

Temperature Control

The temperature-control center in the neonate is poorly developed, and the surface area of skin is relatively larger than in the older child (Figure 35–1). The body weight of a 5-kg infant is about 10 percent of that of an adult. The surface area, however, is 20 percent of an adult's.[20] A six-year-old child weighing 16 kg has 25 percent of the weight and 50 percent of the surface area of an adult. The infant or child can therefore be cooled or heated more rapidly. This ease of cooling is of great value in treating convulsions due to hyperpyrexia. On the other hand, during surgical procedures in the newborn the body temperature can decrease rapidly. The first few degrees of cooling increase the oxygen needs, but further cooling decreases oxygen requirements. An infant's ability to initiate or sustain spontaneous respiration after an anesthetic is decreased until the body temperature rises to about 36°. The more premature the infant, the greater the problem.

Fluid and Electrolytes

The mechanisms for control of fluid, electrolyte, and acid-base balance are more poorly developed than in the adult. Four age groups behave somewhat differently: premature infants, i.e., less than 2.5 kg, full-term newborns, infants

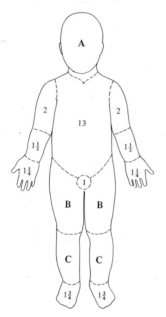

AREA	AGE 0	AGE 1	AGE 5	AGE 10	AGE 15	ADULT
A equals ½ head area	9½	8½	6½	5½	4½	3½
B " ½ thigh area	2¾	3¼	4	4¼	4½	4¾
C " ½ leg area	2½	2½	2¾	3	3¼	3½

Figure 35–1. The surface area of the neonate changes with age.

up to three years, and children over three years.

Body Water. The volume of body water is closely related to the age of the fetus in utero, the maturity at birth, and the age of the older child. Since fat is essentially water-free, the fatter the body, the smaller the percentage of water. The total body water is lower in females than in males, higher in children, especially newborns, and greatest in premature infants. The most rapid decline in total body water occurs in the first six months of life. Total body water in adult males is 60 percent of the weight in kilograms (72 percent "lean weight"), but in adult females it is only 40 to 50 percent. At birth the total body water is 80 percent of body weight.[21]

The relative daily intake and output of water are greater in the infant than in the adult. This is the result of the high basal heat production per kilogram, increased production of waste products and volume of urine, and loss of fluid by evaporation from the relatively large body surface. The water loss is about twice that of the adult and gradually decreases until 16 years. The daily turnover of water in an infant is one third of its extracellular water and is only about one seventh that in the adult. This is extremely important in the infant, because up to half of its extracellular water may be lost in 24 to 36 hours. Vomiting, hyperpyrexia, and sweating further increase the fluid loss. The infant can survive only three to four days without water, while the adult can survive 10 days or more.

Electrolytes. The water and salt needs in the first two to three days of life are minimal in the absence of marked fluid loss by vomiting or dehydration. The healthy, newborn, breast-fed infant normally receives little fluid or nutrition and loses weight. For basal requirements only about 30 percent of the stated amounts are given postoperatively in the first two to three days and 50 percent for the remainder of the first week (Figure 35–2).

Signs of dehydration—sunken fontanelle, dark dry skin, and dry mucous membranes—are not seen until about one sixth of total body water is lost. The best guides to dehydration and the adequacy of fluid intake are the volume and concentration of the urine. The volume of urine

is 25 ml per day during the second and third days and rises to 120 to 150 ml by the seventh day. Care must be taken to avoid overloading the circulation. Sclerema neonatorum can occur, especially in the premature infant and in the first few days of life, if the daily fluid replacement is less than 20 ml per kilogram.

Potassium loss is not important in the first week of life unless there is vomiting. Potassium should then be given intravenously but only if the urinary output is satisfactory and the potassium level in the blood is low. After the first week of life the newborn is able to conserve potassium more efficiently.

In the neonate requiring operation careful monitoring of serum calcium levels is essential, especially in the premature infant or child with a low birth weight. Hypocalcemia may develop very rapidly in those infants. Changes in magnesium usually accompany those of calcium.

Blood Volume

The normal blood volume in the normal newborn is 80 percent per kilogram of body weight and is slightly more in the premature infant. Blood loss must not be considered in terms of volume alone but must be related to the total blood volume and to the rate of loss. A loss of 50 ml of blood in a 3-kg infant represents a loss of about 20 percent of total blood volume (240 ml) and is equivalent to a loss of 1100 ml in a 70-kg adult with a blood volume of 5000 ml. Signs of advanced hypovolemic shock—loss of pulse and blood pressure and cyanosis—occur rapidly, often without the warning signs of a rising pulse and gradually falling blood pressure. The infant is much less able to restore its blood volume by mobilizing extracellular water than the adult. During operation in the neonate it is essential to weigh all sponges and accurately record blood loss.

Renal Function

Infants can excrete dilute urine almost as well as an adult but are unable to start excretion as quickly or excrete as rapidly as the adult. An overload of 50 ml is an addition of about 20 percent to the circulating blood and can cause heart failure. The volume of intravenous fluid must be calculated accurately, depending upon

Figure 35–2. Basal water and isotonic saline requirements.

Age	Water (ml/kg/24 hr)	Isotonic Saline
Premature infant	65	11
Full-term newborn	100	17
< 20 kg	135 to 200*	22
> 20 kg	100	11

*200 maximum in dehydrated child

body weight and maturity, and the physician should write an order for the exact rate per hour and the number of drops per minute. Infants concentrate urine poorly. To avoid administering excessive electrolytes, a solution of one third isotonic saline in 5 percent dextrose and water should be given rather than isotonic saline. The decreased ability of the infant's kidney to excrete concentrated urine and the increased metabolic rate present considerable difficulty in handling acid-base balance.

Nutrition in the Surgical Neonate

The normal infant on breast feeding receives little fluid or nourishment in the first few days of life. Consequently there is little need for caloric intake during that period following operation. Caloric needs, however, rise rapidly during the first month. During this time 100 to 125 calories per kilogram should be given to an infant before and after operation.

Intravenous hyperalimentation now plays an important role in maintaining nutrition in the seriously ill infant and especially in those that are premature (see Chapter 14). A baby can now be maintained in positive nitrogen balance and can grow and develop normally using only intravenous feedings.[4] Intravenous hyperalimentation may be used after correction of a small-bowel atresia. The baby may be unable to take oral feeds because of diarrhea due to a short-gut syndrome or because of disaccharide intolerance associated with a blind-loop syndrome. The short-gut syndrome results from resection of grossly distended bowel or from loss of absorptive surfaces of the small intestine because of multiple linked areas of atresia. The blind-loop syndrome is the result of incomplete bowel obstruction due to the great disparity between the dilated bowel above the original atresia and the much narrower unused bowel below. Intravenous hyperalimentation is often needed when the infant is treated by a number of staged procedures, for example repair of an omphalocele, when oral feeding is impossible or too dangerous. It is also indicated in the debilitated child in chronic or acute nitrogen imbalance during preparation for a major operation.

DEVELOPMENT OF INTESTINES

The development of the small and large intestine is described here in view of its importance in understanding congenital anomalies (Figure 35–3).

About the fourth week of development the midgut forms a solid tube and later becomes recanalized. Between the fourth and tenth weeks of development that portion of the midgut which is represented in the adult from the duodenojejunal junction to the transverse colon is herniated outside the abdominal cavity. It undergoes a rotation to the right through 90° and the prearterial segment increases in size more than the postarterial portion. The prearterial portion returns to the abdominal cavity first and the postarterial segment later, so that the latter portion comes to the ventral of the prearterial portion. At this stage that portion represented by the cecum lies to the left but later migrates to the right and eventually descends to the region of the right iliac fossa.

The prolongation of the midgut to the yolk sac normally becomes totally obliterated, and if it persists it forms a Meckel's diverticulum.

Atresia and Stenosis. If recanalization fails there may be a fibrous band connecting two parts of the intestines, while in other cases a diaphragm is present or simply an area of narrowing. The complete obstruction of the lumen presents within the first few days of life with vomiting, constipation, visible peristalsis, and increasing abdominal distention. Treatment consists of resecting the stenotic area with either a side-to-side anastomosis or preferably an end-to-end anastomosis. The latter may be very difficult because the lumen of the distal bowel is small. Atresia is most often due to intrauterine vascular accidents.

Duplications and Enterogenous Cysts. Abnormal recanalization probably accounts for these anomalies.[7] Double-barrelling may result in intestinal obstruction from enlargement of one portion. It may also present with melena because of venous congestion from pressure on the veins returning from the smaller portion or from ulcer due to ectopic gastric mucosa. Occasionally a large swelling results either from an enterogenous cyst or from occlusion at both ends of a double-barrelled portion of bowel. In treatment it is important to remember that the blood supply to either the cyst or bowel is the same so that a cyst cannot be removed without damaging the blood supply to the bowel. Similarly one portion of double-barrelled bowel cannot be removed. The condition, whether enterogenous cyst or double-barrelled bowel, is thus treated by resecting the affected portion of bowel.

Abnormalities of Rotation

Nonrotation. If the cecum does not pass across to the subhepatic region and subsequently descend to the right iliac fossa, then volvulus of the whole midgut is liable to occur. In these cases the bowel is simply attached posteriorly

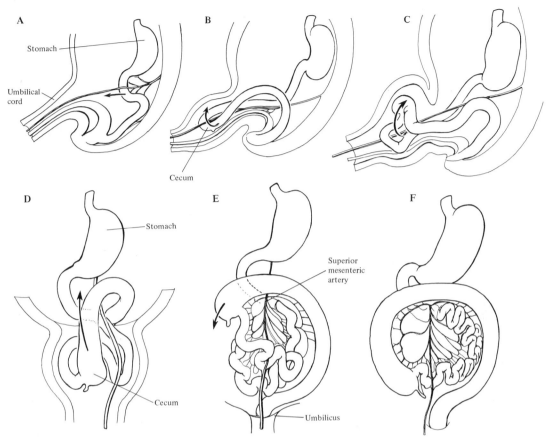

Figure 35–3. Development and rotation of small and large intestines. *A.* The loop of bowel forming the midgut enlarges. *B.* The loop then enters the umbilical cord. The distal portion thickens, forming the cecum. *C.* Rotation occurs as the loop commences to return to the abdominal cavity. *D.* The superior mesenteric vessels now lie ventral to the third part of the duodenum, and the cecum passes upward to the right subcostal region. *E.* The cecum commences its descent toward the right iliac fossa. *F.* The colon enlarges, taking on its adult appearance.

by a short mesentery which is usually called a duodenocolic mesentery. The obstruction may be either from obstruction at the duodeno-jejunal junction region simply resulting from the torsion or may be from pressure of the cecum on the third part of the duodenum. Clinically the child presents signs of acute high small bowel obstruction within the first few days of life. Immediate operation is essential. The volvulus is undone, and it is important always to free the cecum and allow it to stay in the left subcostal region. No attempt is made to place the large bowel in its normal position. In these cases it is as well at the conclusion of the operation to pass the stomach tube through the duodenum into the jejunum to make sure that all obstructions have been relieved.

Malrotation. The order of rotation may be reversed and the postarterial segment returned

to the abdomen first so that the transverse colon lines behind the small intestine. As with non-rotation this may be symptomless or cause intestinal obstruction.

Persistence of Vitello Intestinal Duct

Fecal Fistula. If this remains patent in its whole length, a fecal fistula results and, as already stated, it may be associated with lower intestinal atresia.

Cyst Formation. If a remnant persisted it may result in a raspberry adenoma at the umbilicus or in a cyst in a cord between the umbilicus and ileum, or sometimes in a cyst attached to the small bowel. These cysts may present simply as abdominal tumors.

Cord Persistence. Volvulus may result from persistence of the bowel between the ileum and the umbilicus, or a portion of the bowel may become twisted around a piece of intestine, leading to intestinal obstruction.

Meckel's Diverticulum. This is represented as a blind tube attached to the antimesenteric border of the ileum generally about 6 to 12 inches from the ileocecal orifice. There may or may not be a band passing from it to the umbilicus. There is frequently heterotopic gastric mucosa in the diverticulum which results occasionally in ulceration of the adjacent diverticulum or ileal mucosa. This ulcer may cause melena or may perforate, leading to peritonitis either local or generalized. Occasionally the diverticulum forms the apex of an intussusception (Figure 21-3, page 359).

Mesentery of Ascending Colon

There may be a mesentery to part or all of the ascending colon. If the cecum is abnormally mobile, it predisposes to volvulus of the cecum.

Omphalocele and Gastroschisis

An omphalocele is a defect in the umbilicus permitting escape of bowel into an amniotic-lined sac that is in continuity with parietal peritoneum. The sac may be intact or ruptured. Those with an intact sac may be treated with repeated application of antiseptic dressings, such as aqueous benzalkonium chloride, to promote covering of the sac with granulation tissue and later scar. Alternatively operation may be performed with primary closure if the amount of bowel that has entered the sac is small. In those with large omphaloceles skin coverage may be obtained by extensive undermining or applying a silon graft (silacylic-covered Dacron). Definitive repair is performed at a later age. Immediate operation is essential in those with a ruptured sac.

Gastroschisis is a defect in development of the abdominal wall lateral to the umbilicus, most often on the right side. No amnion covers the defect so that immediate operation is necessary.

SURGICAL EMERGENCIES IN THE NEWBORN

The size of the patient and lack of cooperation make diagnosis more difficult than in the adult. Some conditions can be diagnosed by observation, for example imperforate anus and omphalocele. Complicated investigations are rarely needed. A chest film and supine and cross-table lateral abdominal x-rays are often the main investigations. Air within the gut is an excellent contrast medium. Unless especially indicated. as in Hirschsprung's disease and occasionally esophageal atresia, contrast media are unnecessary and dangerous. Other diagnostic aids are the passage of a soft rubber catheter into the stomach and the insertion of a catheter into the rectum, combined with gentle colonic irrigation. It should be emphasized that many procedures in the newborn are potentially dangerous and should not be undertaken unless the examiner is entirely clear about their necessity and risk.

Cyanosis

Cyanosis may be transient and due to mucus, blood, or amniotic fluid in the mouth and nasopharynx. It may be secondary to congenital heart disease, a tension pneumothorax,[11,12] tracheoesophageal fistula, diaphragmatic hernia, or congenital lobar emphysema.

Pneumothorax. A spontaneous pneumothorax is suggested by early onset of cyanosis, diminished or absent breath sounds on one side of the chest, and deviation of the apex beat to the opposite side of the chest. An x-ray is essential to differentiate the condition from pneumomediastinum or diaphragmatic hernia. Chest x-ray is also essential because the lesion may be diagnosed clinically on the wrong side. Breath sounds are readily transmitted from one side of the chest to the other in the infant. Early diagnosis and treatment are imperative because the mediastinal shift can suddenly cause death. X-rays should therefore be done in the nursery, if possible without transferring the child to the radiology department. An infant laryngoscope, endotracheal tubes, and a 20-ml syringe for chest aspiration must be available upon suspicion of a pneumothorax. A tension pneumothorax may develop rapidly and cause death. If the pneumothorax is small and asymptomatic, the child should be kept under close observation. Air will absorb within two to three days, and complications are unlikely. A larger pneumothorax is initially treated by inserting a chest tube in the second intercostal space in the midclavicular line and establishing underwater seal drainage. Pneumothorax and pneumomediastinum may occur separately or together. The condition is often not diagnosed because it is not suspected. In a prospective study of the incidence of pneumothorax and mediastinum Steele[21] showed that pneumomediastinum was commoner than pneumothorax, and that the incidence of each was increased three to four times in infants who required intubation. About one third of infants with pneumothorax and one half of those with pneumomediastinum do not require treatment.

Congenital Diaphragmatic Hernia. This is one of the most rapidly life-threatening conditions in the neonate. If not corrected surgically, increasing amounts of bowel, stomach, liver,

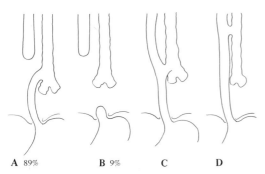

Figure 35–4.   Types of esophageal atresia.

and spleen are drawn up into the chest. The lung collapses on the affected side, and the mediastinum is shifted to the opposite side. The opposite lung then collapses, and venous return to the heart is impaired. If not operated on, the child is likely to die in the first few hours or days of life. If the defect is small and a sac is present, the patient may occasionally live for years without symptoms. The commonest type of diaphragmatic hernia is through the left posterolateral foramen of Bochdalek. Hernias through the foramen of Morgagni and the esophageal hiatus rarely require emergency treatment in the infant.

Esophageal Atresia and Tracheoesophageal Fistula. These occur together in about 90 percent of patients. The commonest type is atresia of the upper pouch with a fistula between the trachea, just above the bifurcation, and the lower pouch (Figure 35–4). The baby cannot swallow saliva and is often described as having "too much mucus." Saliva may flow out of the mouth or be aspirated causing cyanosis and choking. On feeding the infant swallows only a few milliliters before the blind pouch is filled and overflows. Effortless regurgitation of unchanged formula then occurs with cyanosis and choking. "Excess" salivation follows with regurgitation after only a few sucks and cyanosis after aspiration of saliva or formula. The diagnosis is confirmed by the inability to pass a soft rubber catheter into the stomach. A soft catheter may bend upon itself in the blind pouch and give the impression that it has passed into the stomach. If gas or fluid cannot be aspirated diagnosis may be confirmed by passing a radiopaque tube into the upper pouch. Air in the stomach means that a fistula is present. Closure of the fistula and reconstruction by suturing the proximal pouch to the distal esophagus should be undertaken. Note should be made of the passage of gas through the gut so that an associated duodenal or ileal atresia is not missed.

If there is no gas in the stomach, a fistula is not present. The lower segment of esophagus is then usually short or almost absent and primary reconstruction may not be possible. A gastrostomy is established for feeding. The upper pouch is continuously kept empty by suction to prevent aspiration. The two esophageal segments often grow together in weeks or months, and a primary anastomosis is then possible. Cervical cutaneous esophagostomy to drain mucus and saliva should not be established because it precludes any chance of primary reconstruction. The results of secondary reconstruction using stomach or bowel are generally unsatisfactory. Other congenital anomalies, especially imperforate anus, should be looked for in infants with esophageal atresia.

Vomiting

Vomiting should always be considered in relation to age at onset, force, and content.

A baby with esophageal atresia vomits after taking a few milliliters of the first feed. When obstruction is at the pylorus or lower, 30 to 40 ml can be taken before vomiting occurs. The neonate with an imperforate anus vomits and becomes distended after 12 to 18 hours. If the cardioesophageal sphincter mechanism is lax, as in chalasia,[15] the baby regurgitates during and after feeding, and pressure changes of gentle respiration cause reflux of feeds into the esophagus. If the baby cries or strains, the increased intra-abdominal pressure results in regurgitation. The reflux can be prevented by nursing the child almost erect in a chair. Gradually, over days or weeks, the sphincteric mechanism becomes normal.

The force of vomiting depends on the expulsive effort of muscle contraction. Food rolls out of the mouth when the lesion is in the esophagus. The powerful musculature in the stomach results in projectile vomiting when there is an obstruction at the pylorus or duodenum. It is important to exclude nonsurgical causes of vomiting such as cerebral hemorrhage, swallowed amniotic fluid, and infections. A baby who repeatedly vomits, especially if the vomitus is bile-stained, should be considered to have an obstruction until proven otherwise. Absence of bile may occur if the obstruction is above the entrance of the common bile duct into the second part of the duodenum.

Abdominal Distention

The lower the level of the obstruction, the greater the abdominal distention. The abdomen is not distended when the esophagus is obstructed unless there is a tracheoesophageal fistula that allows air to enter the stomach in large amounts but will not permit its escape. The baby with a gastroduodenal or high jejunal obstruction has localized epigastric distention and visible gastric peristalsis. When the obstruction is lower, there is generalized abdominal distention. The gas pattern on plain x-rays of the abdomen often establishes the diagnosis.

Failure to Pass Meconium

Meconium is passed in the first 12 hours by 70 percent of normal babies and in 12 to 24 hours by 95 percent.[19] Failure to pass meconium by 24 hours should be considered abnormal. Nonsurgical causes are prematurity and serious medical disorders. The insertion of a No. 10 rubber catheter into the anus stimulates passage of meconium and excludes imperforate anus and the rare condition of rectal atresia. It is not necessary to perform a routine digital rectal examination in the newborn and insertion of a thermometer is extremely dangerous. Instillation of 5 ml of isotonic saline into the rectum may initiate the passage of normal meconium or cause expulsion of a "meconium plug."[3] The meconium plug syndrome is not uncommon, occurring in about 0.5 percent of neonates, and causes obstruction and abdominal distention. The yellowish-gray head or caput meconium has a low water content and an increased surface tension and viscosity. It can therefore usually be washed out with isotonic saline. In meconium ileus there is inspissated tenacious meconium obstructing the terminal ileum, and the underlying disease is cystic fibrosis. Meconium plug may be confused with Hirschsprung's disease. The two conditions occasionally occur together.

In intestinal atresia absence of bile results in the meconium losing its normal greenish-black color and becoming grayish-yellow. Normal meconium may be passed in the baby with complete bowel obstruction. The probable explanation is that atresia with complete luminal obstruction may occur from failure of recanalization before bile was secreted, or from a vascular accident occurring after bile secretion had commenced.[1]

The level of the obstruction is usually established on plain x-ray of the abdomen. A barium enema may be useful in malrotation of the gut with duodenal compression and an incompletely descended cecum. Free gas in the peritoneal cavity denotes antenatal or postnatal rupture of gut.

Pyloric Stenosis

Pyloric stenosis is a progressive narrowing of the pyloric canal and the lower part of the pyloric antrum due to thickening of the muscle.

The condition is commoner in boys than girls, is sometimes familial, and the cause is not known. The obstruction to gastric emptying occurs gradually compared with the rapid and complete obstruction in duodenal atresia. At first the stomach can empty almost completely, vomiting is irregular and not projectile, and bile can regurgitate into the stomach and be present in the vomitus. Only later, when there is virtually complete obstruction, is bile absent from the vomitus. Vomiting becomes projectile when all the force of gastric peristalsis is directed upward rather than downward. The infant is constipated and rapidly becomes dehydrated and loses weight. Diagnosis is made by examining the child while feeding. The enlarged pylorus may be felt and gastric peristalsis may be seen. An upper gastrointestinal x-ray is rarely needed to establish the diagnosis. A nasogastric tube is inserted and intravenous fluids administered. Laparotomy is performed through a small upper abdominal incision. The hypertrophied muscle of the pylorus is incised longitudinally exposing the mucosa.

Duodenal Obstruction

A single bubble is present on x-ray in the baby with the rare condition of pyloric atresia. A distended stomach and duodenum, as in duodenal atresia, give a "double-bubble" appearance. Fluid levels are present unless the x-ray is taken very early or the baby has vomited. In duodenal atresia with complete obstruction air is not seen in the small intestine or colon. Minor traces of air indicate an incomplete obstruction, as in duodenal stenosis, annular pancreas, and malrotation of the intestine with obstruction of the third part of the duodenum. Atresia or stenosis is present in 20 percent with Down's syndrome. Duodenal atresia is treated by a posterior duodenojejunostomy if possible.

Jejunoileal Obstruction

Atresia, marked stenosis, and meconium ileus are the commonest causes of obstruction in the jejunum or ileum. Loops of gas-filled intestine and multiple fluid levels are seen unless the baby is x-rayed early. In meconium ileus the terminal ileum is obliterated by inspissated tenacious meconium. The diagnosis is made if there are specks of calcium in the right lower abdomen. These specks indicate prenatal perforation and calcified meconium peritonitis. A coarse granular appearance of the intestine suggesting bubbles of air within the meconium has been described.[14] Laboratory tests are of little value preoperatively in determining the underlying disease, cystic fibrosis.

Rectosigmoid Obstruction

Imperforate anus is diagnosed by observation and the rare rectal atresia by passage of a catheter. The distance separating the distal blind end of the bowel from the perineum is determined by taking x-rays with the baby inverted. The relation of the distal gas bubble to the perineum may, however, give a false idea of the actual gap. Unless the bowel is separated from the skin by a proctodael membrane ("covered anus"), it is best to establish a colostomy at birth and to perform a definitive pull-through operation at about one year when it is possible to accurately position the bowel within the puborectalis muscle sling.

Hirschsprung's disease and the meconium plug syndrome are indistinguishable on plain abdominal films. In each condition there are distended loops of bowel often with fluid levels. In addition, it is not possible in the neonate to distinguish with certainty small and large intestine, although the position of the distended loops may help differentiate small from large bowel obstruction. Loops of bowel of different diameters in the pelvis suggest distention of large and small bowel and the presence of a large bowel obstruction.

Hirschsprung's disease is generally symptomatic from birth.[23] The child may present with acute intestinal obstruction or with severe constipation dating from birth. The infant may have gross abdominal distention, anemia, and inanition. On rectal examination the rectum is not distended. In Hirshsprung's disease the bowel is aganglionic from the anus extending upward for a variable distance.[2] The zone may be only a few centimeters long, but most commonly it extends into the rectosigmoid and rarely involves all the colon. An area of normally innervated bowel separating aganglionic segments has been described on a few occasions.[8] Microscopically the ganglia are absent from the myenteric (Auerbach's) plexus and the submucosal (Meissner's) plexus, and the number of nerve trunks is increased. The abnormal bowel is contracted and does not contain meconium. Above this level the bowel contains meconium but does not become thickened and distended for two to five weeks.[5] On barium enema there is a narrow rectum and lower colon, and the contrast medium is slow to be evacuated. After six weeks the conelike junction of collapsed and distended bowel becomes more obvious.

A biopsy of rectal muscle confirms the diagnosis; that of mucosa and submucosa is less certain. If the diagnosis can be made with certainty or if dilated colon is found at operation without obvious cause for the obstruction, a colostomy should be performed in the dilated bowel. Several types of definitive procedure, to excise or otherwise deal with the aganglionic bowel, can be done later. The tradition has been to obtain a biopsy in all suspected cases of Hirschsprung's disease before making the colostomy in the newborn. Recently it has been suggested that this is not always necessary in the neonate.[10]

Passages of Blood Rectally Within the First Year

Strictly speaking melena is the passage of black tarry motions following the action of the intestinal enzymes on blood. When the source of the blood is the terminal ileum and right colon, the blood is red and evenly distributed through the feces. A source in the lower left colon and anorectum usually gives rise to red blood often on the surface of the motion. The rapidity of the blood loss influences the appearance of the blood. Rapid blood loss in a child with Meckel's diverticulitis may give rise to bleeding that may be thought to originate in the rectum. Also the age of the child is helpful. Bleeding at birth is often due to a congenital anomaly such as duplication of the bowel; at six months it is most likely due to intussusception, and in older children to Meckel's diverticulitis or a juvenile polypus.

Acute Intussusception. Acute intussusception occurs most often in well-nourished male children from six months to two years. The condition may be idiopathic when it is postulated that hypertrophied lymphoid tissue in the wall of the terminal ileum forms the apex of the intussusception. At the apex there may be an inverted Meckel's diverticulum, a polyp, or a benign tumor. The apex may be in the terminal ileum or may be the ileocecal valve.

The child suddenly cries and draws up his legs as if suffering from intestinal colic. He frequently vomits. The condition is intermittent, with the child often sleeping between attacks. As the apex of the intussusception advances, there is venous congestion with rupture of mucosal capillaries. In addition, mucous secretion is increased. This results in the passage of bloody, mucoid, "currant jelly" motions. If the condition is not corrected, gangrene generally occurs with peritonitis and death often within 24 to 48 hours.

The history should suggest the diagnosis. On examination the general condition depends upon the stage of the disease. The sausage-shaped intussusception is palpable in about 90 percent, generally lying in the distribution of the large bowel. The right iliac fossa characteristically feels empty. On rectal examination the intussusception may rarely be felt, and bloody mucus is present on the examining finger. The diagnosis can usually be made clinically. A barium enema is now generally performed to establish the diagnosis and to attempt a hydrostatic reduction.

A hydrostatic enema is performed if the child's general condition is good, the symptoms are of less than 24 hours' duration, and there are no signs of dilatation of the small intestine. A rectal tube is inserted, the bulb inflated, and the buttocks strapped together. It is most important that the hydrostatic pressure of the barium that is used does not exceed three and a half feet. Reduction of the bowel can be followed on fluoroscopy. It is essential that the barium be seen to flow into the terminal ileum, and that the child be closely observed for several days in the hospital following a successful hydrostatic reduction. If there is vomiting, intestinal colic, or anything to suggest recurrence of the intussusception, then laparotomy is indicated. At operation initial reduction is rapid, but there may be difficulty in completing the final reduction. Resection with end-to-end anastomosis is indicated if the reduction is unsuccessful or strangulation has occurred.

Differential Diagnosis

Duplication of Bowel. This may occur at any level from the mouth to the anus, although the terminal ileum is the most frequent site. The condition superficially resembles a mesenteric cyst. Pressure of the cyst on the normal bowel may result in intestinal obstruction or cause venous obstruction with bleeding.

Meckel's Diverticulitis

Heterotopic gastric mucosa in a Meckel's diverticulum may cause peptic ulceration in the diverticulum or less frequently in the adjacent ileum. There may be vague abdominal pain associated with the passage of blood.

Other Conditions. Other causes of passage of blood are a juvenile colorectal polypus, fissure in ano (see Chapter 22), gastroenteritis, parasites and blood dyscrasias, such as Henoch's purpura.

Necrotizing enterocolitis is an important neonatal disease associated with shock and/or sepsis. Decreased intestinal blood flow causes diffuse or patchy necrosis with diarrhea and bleeding. Perforation and local or generalized peritonitis may follow.

ABDOMINAL MASSES IN CHILDHOOD

Abdominal masses are not particularly common but are often serious and demand early diagnosis. About 50 percent of abdominal masses are due to constipation, hepatomegaly, and/or splenomegaly. The remainder are "sur-gical" and are usually asymptomatic. Over half are unilateral or bilateral swellings arising from the genitourinary system. Most are found in the first year, most often in the first month.[16]

Genitourinary System

Benign. These masses include (1) hydronephrosis, (2) multicystic kidney, (3) solitary cyst kidney, (4) ovarian cyst, (5) distended uterus and vagina due to vaginal atresia, and (6) urachal cysts.

Malignant. A malignant mass of the genitourinary system is Wilms' tumor.

Other Systems

Benign. These masses include (1) enteric cyst, (2) hepatomegaly—cysts, fat storage disease, and hemangioma, and (3) splenomegaly—blood dyscrasias.

Malignant. Other malignant masses include (1) neuroblastoma, (2) lymphoma of spleen and liver, and (3) retroperitoneal lymphoma and sarcoma.

Clinical Examination

It should first be determined if the mass is intraperitoneal or extraperitoneal. An intraperitoneal tumor is usually mobile, while a retroperitoneal tumor is fixed. Most bilateral masses arise from the kidneys and are usually benign.

Wilms' tumor is the commonest neoplasm of the kidney. It may be present at birth and may rarely be bilateral. The mass initially moves with respiration and then becomes fixed as the tumor increases in size and extends outside the capsule. The tumor is firmer than a kidney cyst or hydronephrosis and is smoother and less hard than a neuroblastoma. Abdominal neuroblastoma becomes fixed early to the posterior abdominal wall and is hard and irregular. Conjunctival or periorbital hematomas make the diagnosis of neuroblastoma almost certain (Figure 35–5). Prognosis is much worse for a neuroblastoma than a Wilms' tumor. These two tumors are among the commonest malignant masses in childhood.

Investigations

Plain x-ray of the abdomen may show displacement or enlargement of the renal outline and displacement of hollow abdominal organs. Calcification in the renal region suggests neuroblastoma. It is much less common in Wilms' tumor. Abnormalities of the vertebrae, especially in the cervical and upper thoracic regions, occur in about half the children with duplications of the bowel. Chest x-ray and a skeletal survey may reveal bony metastases.

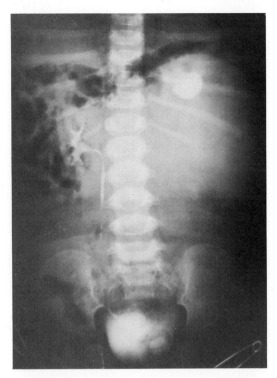

Figure 35–5. Wilms' tumor. A huge left-sided asymptomatic abdominal mass was present that moved with respiration and was smooth and firm but not hard. The intravenous pyelogram shows distortion and distention of the kidney and pelvis, displacement of intestinal gas shadows to the right, and a huge, opaque kidney mass.

Barium studies are of little help in diagnosis.

The findings on an intravenous pyelogram are often diagnostic when the mass is in the kidney. A retrograde pyelogram is rarely needed.

Angiography is often valuable in patients with retroperitoneal and especially renal masses.

Microscopic analysis of urine may show blood, bacteria, or tumor cells. Culture may reveal infection associated with renal disease.

Estimation of catecholamines may lead to a diagnosis of neuroblastoma.

Marrow studies are always indicated in patients with neuroblastoma.

Relationships Between Cancer and Congenital Defects

Many of the cancers in childhood may commence in utero.[13] A number are associated with congenital defects such as leukemia in Down's syndrome, glioma and medulloblastoma with certain phatomatoses and Wilms' tumor, primary liver tumors, and tumors of the adrenal cortex with congenital hemihypertrophy. Wilms' tumor

is also associated with genitourinary anomalies, hamartomas, aniridia[6] and other eye defects, mental retardation, and inner ear abnormalities. These relationships suggest that during embryologic growth specific developmental mechanisms are being shared. The possibility of an abdominal mass being malignant should always be considered in a patient with a congenital anomaly. Neuroblastoma does not seem to be associated with any congenital abnormality although it has a maximum incidence under five years. There is, however, some suggestion that opsoclonus and neuroblastoma are linked.

CHRONIC ABDOMINAL PAIN IN CHILDHOOD

Chronic or recurrent abdominal pain is a common and difficult problem, especially in children up to 12 years. In the past many children were treated by appendectomy; it is doubtful, however, if chronic appendicitis exists. Mesenteric adenitis, with nonspecific enlargement of the lymph nodes in the mesentery of the terminal ileum, probably rarely causes recurrent or chronic abdominal pain. There may be a psychogenic component to the pain. A history of functional intestinal disorder is often present in one or both parents. Constipation and "irritable colon" may be the diagnosis in some cases.[22] In those with the irritable bowel syndrome both parents have the syndrome in 50 percent, and both have migraine headaches in 10 percent. This suggests a psychic origin rather than "genetic or acquired familial disturbance." The fact that most patients are cured or are improved while in the hospital supports the psychic origin. Many improve with the onset of adolescence. A hiatal hernia, Meckel's diverticulitis, Crohn's disease, chronic pancreatitis, a duodenal ulcer, or an abnormal gallbladder are rare causes of abdominal pain. Kidney disease is usually easily eliminated. Abdominal epilepsy is not a convincing diagnosis, even in those with an abnormal EEG. It can be concluded that chronic abdominal pain is rarely surgical in nature, and appendectomy has no place in its treatment.

PIGMENTED LESIONS OF THE SKIN
Hemangioma

An intradermal hemangioma, or port-wine stain, persists for life and may be grossly disfiguring. However, no treatment may be necessary. Cosmetics may improve the appearance of facial hemangiomata, or occasionally skin grafting or a tattooing procedure may be indicated.

Capillary and cavernous hemangiomata grow rapidly in the first four to five months and then tend to self-cure in four to five years[17] (Figure 35–6). Parents are often concerned that the hemangioma is malignant. Bleeding is uncommon, and generally no treatment is indicated because of the likelihood of spontaneous regression. The lesion should not be irradiated because of the high incidence of radiation dermatitis and squamous cell carcinoma. Surgical excision or steroid therapy[24] should be reserved for the lesion that interferes with normal function or that occasionally fails to regress. Hemangioma of the parotid gland is the commonest tumor of that gland in childhood (Figure 35–7). It should be treated conservatively because of the risk of damaging the facial nerve at operation and the probability of self-cure. A bleeding diathesis may occasionally occur because of trapping of platelets and consumption of coagulation products.

Melanoma

Brown pigmented nevi are common in children (see Chapter 25). Grossly and microscopically the lesions may appear malignant, but malignancy rarely occurs before puberty.

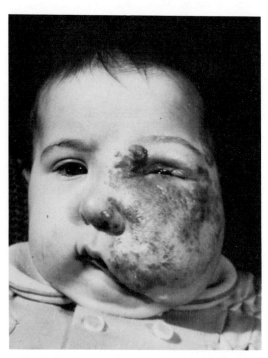

Figure 35–6. Hemangioma of face. Whitish areas of sclerosis suggest that spontaneous cure will occur. Total surgical excision is not practical in this area.

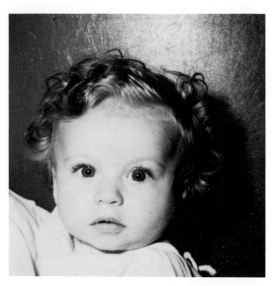

Figure 35–7. Hemangioma of parotid gland. The swelling is compressible, but there is often no skin manifestation of the hemangioma. Spontaneous solution occurred by four years of age.

UMBILICAL AND INGUINAL SWELLINGS

Umbilical Hernia

Umbilical hernia occurs where the umbilical cord passes through the linea alba. The opening normally closes by contraction of the surrounding fibrous tissue, and more than 95 percent have disappeared by two years. The hernia tends to persist when the opening in the linea alba is more than 1 cm in diameter and eccentric in relation to the umbilicus. Most of these lie in the upper margin of the umbilicus and are really supraumbilical hernias. Strapping is of no value. Operation is indicated if the hernia persists for three years. Strangulation is a rare complication.

Inguinal Hernia and Derivatives of the Processus Vaginalis

The processus vaginalis is a peritoneal pouch that passes through the inguinal canal and guides the testis from the abdomen to the scrotum. Normally the processus is obliterated before birth. If the testis fails to descend, the processus generally remains patent. All or part of the sac may persist (Figure 35–8).

Common abnormalities of the processus vaginalis are:

1. The entire processus may remain patent. The more premature the infant, the more likely is this to occur. The hernia is present at

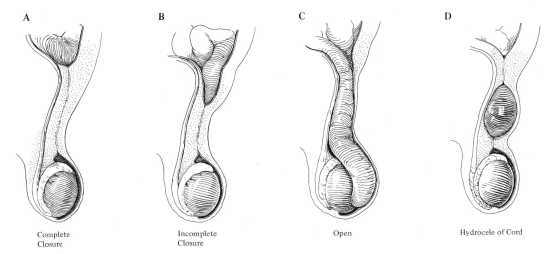

A — Complete Closure   B — Incomplete Closure   C — Open   D — Hydrocele of Cord

Figure 35–8. Anomalies arising from the processus vaginalis.

birth and tends to persist. The hernia should be repaired when the child is well and gaining weight, at about three months, because about 50 percent develop strangulation within six months.

2. The most common abnormality is persistence of the proximal part of the processus. The hernia tends to appear at some time after birth. Probably most of the inguinal hernias of early adult life are of this type and not acquired. All should be treated by operation since self-cure does not occur.

3. The distal part may persist and form a hydrocele. Most disappear in the first year. The size does not vary from day to day but gradually decreases.

4. Part of the processus may remain patent and form a hydrocele of the cord or of the canal of Nuck. This type usually disappears spontaneously.

5. There may be a patent processus connecting a hydrocele with a hernia. The hydrocele tends to vary from day to day in size because of the intraperitoneal connection. The hydrocele and hernia should be treated surgically because both will persist.

Views differ on how to manage the contralateral clinically normal side in a child with an inguinal hernia. Some advocate routine exploration of the normal side because of the high incidence of bilateral hernia. The incidence of unsuspected hernia has been reported to vary from 5 to 30 percent.[18]

CITED REFERENCES

1. Barnard, C. N.: The genesis of intestinal atresia. *Surg. Forum,* **7**:393, 1956, and *Lancet* **2**:1065–67, 1955.

2. Bodian, M., *et al.*: Hirschsprung's disease and idiopathic megacolon. *Lancet,* **1**:6–11, 1949.

3. Clatworthy, H. W., *et al.*: The meconium plug syndrome. *Surgery,* **39**:131–42, 1956.

4. Dudrick, S. J., *et al.*: Long-term total parenteral nutrition with growth, development and positive nitrogen balance. *Surgery,* **64**:134–42, 1968.

5. Ehrenpreis, F.: Megacolon in the newborn. *Acta Chir. Scand.,* Supp. **94**:112, 1946.

6. Haicken, B. N., and Miller, D. R.: Simultaneous occurrence of congenital aniridia, hamartoma and Wilms' tumour. *J. Pediatr.,* **78**:497–502, 1971.

7. Houston, H. E., and Lynn, H. B.: Duplications of small intestine in children. *Mayo Clin. Proc.,* **41**:246–56, 1966.

8. Keefer, G. P., and Mokrokistry, J. F.: Congenital megacolon (Hirschsprung's disease). *Radiology,* **63**:157–74, 1954.

9. Kieswatter, W. B., and Parenzan, L.: When should hernia in the infant be treated bilaterally? *JAMA,* **171**:287, **171**:287, 1959.

10. Leenders, E., *et al.*: Aganglionic megacolon in infancy. *Surg. Gynecol. Obstet.,* **131**:424–30, 1970. Hirschsprung's disease. *Surg. Clin. North Am.* **50**:907–17, 1970.

11. Leininger, B. J., *et al.*: Tension pneumoperitoneum and pneumothorax in the newborn. *Ann. Thorac. Surg.,* **9**:359–63, 1970.

12. Miller, R. D., and Hamilton, W. K.: Pneumothorax during infant resuscitation. *JAMA,* **210**:1090–91, 1969.

13. Miller, R. W.: Relationship between cancer and congenital defects: an epidemiological evaluation. *J. Natl. Cancer Inst.,* **40**:1079–85, 1968.

14. Neuhauser, E. B. D.: Roentgen changes associated with pancreatic insufficiency in early life. *Radiology,* **46**:319–28, 1946.

15. Neuhauser, E. B. D., and Berenberg, W.: Cardioesophageal relaxation as a cause of vomiting in infants. *Radiology,* **48**:480–83, 1947.

16. Raffensperger, J., and Abousleiman, A.: Abdominal masses in children under one year. *Surgery,* **63**:514–21, 1968.

17. Simpson, J. R., and Lond, M. B.: Natural history of cavernous hemangiomas. *Lancet,* **277**:1057, 1959.

18. Simpson, T. E., *et al.*: Further experience with bilateral operations for inguinal hernia in infants and children. *Ann. Surg.,* **169**:450–54, 1969.

19. Sherry, S. N., and Kramer, I.: The time of passage of the first stool and first urine by the newborn infant. *J. Pediatr.*, **46**:158–59, 1955.

20. Smith, C. A.: *The Physiology of the Newborn Infant.* Charles C Thomas, Springfield, Ill., 1959.

21. Steele, R. W., *et al.*: Incidence of pneumothorax and pneumoperitoneum. Spring 1970 meeting of the Pediatric Societies, Atlantic City. *Year Book of Pediatrics*, 1971.

22. Stone, R. T., and Barbero, G. J.: Recurrent abdominal pain in childhood. *Pediatrics*, **54**:732–38, 1970.

23. Swenson, O., *et al.*: New concepts of the etiology, diagnosis and treatment of congenital megacolon (Hirschsprung's disease). *Pediatrics*, **4**:201–209, 1949.

24. Zarem, H. A., and Edgerton, M. T.: Induced resolution of cavernous haemangiomas following prednisolone therapy. *Plast. Reconstr. Surg.*, **39**:76–83, 1967.

SUGGESTIONS FOR FURTHER READING

Ariel, I. M., and Pack, G. T.: *Cancer and Allied Diseases of Infancy and Childhood.* Little, Brown & Co., Boston, 1960.
A comprehensive review of malignant disease in pediatrics.

Gray, S. W., and Scandalakis, J. E. (eds.): *Embryology for Surgeons.* W. B. Saunders Co., Philadelphia, 1972.
The relation between embryology and clinical anomalies is fully discussed.

Mustard, W. T.; Ravitch, M. M.; Synder, W. H., Jr.; Welch, K. J.; and Benson, C. D. (eds.): *Pediatric Surgery.* 2 vols. 2nd ed. Year Book Medical Publishers, Chicago, 1969.
A standard complete reference book.

Rosenberg, H. S., and Bolande, R. P.: *Perspectives in Pediatric Pathology.* Vol. 2. Year Book Medical Publishers, Chicago, 1975.
Selected topics, such as Hirschsprung's disease, are presented in considerable detail from the viewpoint of the pathologist.

Rowe, M. I., and Marchildon, M. B.: Physiologic considerations in the newborn surgical patient. *Surg. Clin. North Am.*, **56**:245–61, 1976.
Selected topics of newborn physiology are discussed, such as birth weight gestational relationship, glucose metabolism, temperature regulation, calcium balance, infection, and fluid and electrolyte balance.

Smith, C. A.: *The Physiology of the Newborn Infant.* Charles C Thomas, Springfield, Ill., 1959.
An excellent review of the physiology of the neonate.

Touloukian, R. J.: Neonatal necrotizing enterocolitis: an update on etiology, diagnosis and treatment. *Surg. Clin. North Am.*, **56**:281–98, 1976.
A recent review of a condition that is of increasing interest.

Abdomen, clinical evaluation, 202, 203
  injuries, 176–78
  pain, 196, 200
Abetalipoproteinemia, 358
Abruptio placentae, disseminated intravascular coagulation, 212
Abscess, amebic, 332
  anorectal, 402–403, **403** *
  appendiceal, 392
  brain, 625
  breast, 446
  carbuncle, **135,** 136
  "collar button," **135,** 136, 502
  drainage, 129, 134, **134**
  epidural, 625
  furuncle, **135,** 136
  hand, 501–502
  liver, 332
  lung, 534–35
  pelvic, 252
  perirectal, 402, 403, **403, 404**
  peritonsillar, 273
  salivary gland, 274
  stress catabolic state, 34
  subphrenic, 252
Acanthosis nigricans, 437
Achalasia, 291–92, **292**
Achlorhydria, gastric cancer and, 309
Acid-base balance, 45–46. *See also* Acidosis; Alkalosis
  in shock, 45, 46
Acid citrate dextrose, 214
Acidosis, 99–100
  metabolic, 100
  respiratory, 101
Acinar cell adenocarcinoma, 349–50
Actinic conjunctivitis, 595
Actinomycin, 582
Actinomycosis, 128, 397
  "sulfur" granules, 128
Acupuncture, 192, 193
Adams-Stokes seizures, 547, 548
Addison's disease, 200, 201, 206, 207
  anesthesia, 232
  pigmentation, 437
  postoperative, 253
  skin pigmentation, 437
Adenitis, cervical, 273–74
  mesenteric, 390–91
Adenoids, hypertrophied, 273
Adenomatous polyp, 395
Adenosine triphosphate (ATP), 54
  in metabolic acidosis, 100
ADH. *See* Antidiuretic hormone
Adrenal, acute insufficiency, 488–89
  Addison's disease, 489

* Numbers in **boldface** type refer to pages on which illustrations appear.

adrenocortical tumors, 491, **491–92**
  adrenogenital syndrome and, 491
  aldosteronism, 490, 491
  anatomy, 487
  androgen-secreting tumors, 491, **492**
  anesthesia, 230, 231
  breast cancer and, 470
  catecholamines, 491–92
  Conn's syndrome, 490, 491
  cortex, 487–91
  Cushing's syndrome, 489–90. *See also* Cushing's syndrome
  estrogen-secreting tumors, 491, **491**
  function, 487–88
  hemorrhage, 488
  medulla, 491–93
  neuroblastoma, 493
  pheochromocytoma, 492, 493
Adrenalectomy, aldosteronism, 491
  carcinoma, breast, 470
    prostate, 584
  Cushing's syndrome, 490
  pheochromocytoma, 493
Adrenocortical steroids, in transplantation, 112
Adrenocorticotropic hormone (ACTH), 207, 488
Adrenogenital syndrome, 491
Adriamycin. *See* Doxorubicin
Adult respiratory distress syndrome (ARDS), 64, 65
Adynamic ileus. *See* Paralytic ileus
Agammaglobulinemia, Bruton type, 105, 114
  Swiss type, 105, 114
Albumin, 204
  ascites, 321
  ventilatory failure, 259
Alcohol, gastritis, 305
  hypomagnesemia, 98
  intravenous, 98
  sphincter of Oddi, 343
Alcoholism, cirrhosis, 336
  pancreatitis, 347
Aldosterone, 96, 206, 487, 488
  ascites, 321
  liver disease, 321
Aldosteronism, 490, 491
  anesthesia, 232
Alimentation (intravenous), 243, 244, 245
  burns, 264
  complications, 137, 244, 245
  fat deficiency, 98
  solutions, 244, 245
  stress catabolic states, 36
Alkaline phosphatase, 323, 461, 487
Alkalosis, hypokalemic, 97
  metabolic, 100–101

  respiratory, 101
Alkylating agents, 112, 153, 154
Allantois, 564
Allergic contact dermatitis, 132
Allergic reactions, 109, 110
Allografts, 110
Allopurinol, 571
Alpha-fetoprotein, 115, 323
Ambu bag, 170
Amebiasis, colon, 375
  rectum, 394, 397
Amebic abscess, liver, **327**
Ameloblastoma, 284
Amethocaine, 225
Amino acids, 98
  calorie-nitrogen ratio, 24, 25, 35
  hepatic protein synthesis, 9
Aminoglycosides, 132
Ammonia, encephalopathy, 322
  urine, 100
Amphotericin B, 128, 132
Ampicillin, 131
Ampulla of Vater, **348**
Amputation, hand, 499
  indications, **560**
  lower limb, **561**
  penis, 584
  rehabilitation, 525
Amylase, 307, 342, 345, 348
  pancreatic trauma, 346
Anaerobic clostridial myositis, 139
Anatomic snuffbox, 495
Androgens, 470
Anemia, 202
  blind-loop syndrome, 362
  burns, 263
  congenital hemolytic, 432
  gastrectomy, 304
Anesthesia, 222–32
  agents, local and regional, 225
  aldosteronism, 232
  antibiotics, 231
  antihypertensive medication, 231
  apparatus, 229, **229,** 230
  aspiration, 230, **230**
  cardiac arrest, 230
  complications, 230, 231
  cyclopropane, 227
  diazepam, 228
  diuretics, 231
  drug reactions, 230, 231
  endocrine disorders, 232
  endotracheal, 228, 229
  epidural, **224,** 225
  gallamine, 228
  general, 226–31
  halothane (Fluothane), 226
  hyperthyroidism, 232
  infiltration, **224,** 225
  Innovar, 227
  intravenous, **224,** 227, 228
  ketamine, 228

Anesthesia [*cont.*]
  malignant hyperthermia, 231, 232
  methoxyflurane (Penthrane), 227
  monoamine oxidase inhibitors,
    231
  neostigmine, 228
  nerve block, 224, **224,** 225, 277
  nerve compression, 235
  nitrous oxide, 226
  postoperative care, 242, 243
  pregnancy, 216
  premedication, 223
  propanidid, 228
  recovery room, 232
  regional, 223–26
  relaxants, 228
    tetanus, 138
  spinal, 225
  steroids, 230, 231
  thiopental (Pentothal), 227
  tranylcypromine sulfate
    (Parnate), 231
  tubocurarine chloride (curare),
    228
  types, 224
  vomiting, 230, **230**
Aneurysms, 556–57
  aortic, 556–57
  basilar, 620
  cerebral, **616,** 617, **617,** 620
    treatment, 620
  grafts, 557, **557**
  rupture, perforation, peptic ulcer
    vs., 308
  ventricular, 546
Angina, intestinal, 557
Angina pectoris, 546
Angiography, aorta, 554–55
  cerebral, 605, 615
  coronary, 546
  heart, 542
  hepatic, 325, **325**
  kidney, 572, **572, 582**
  pancreas, 346
Angle of His, 288
Ankylosing spondylitis, 518
Annular pancreas, 346
Annuloplasty, heart valves, 544, 545
Anoderm, 399
Anorectal prolapse, 405, 406, **407**
Antacids, 301
Antibiotics, 130–33
  agents. *See* individual agents
  anesthesia, 231
  burns, 265
  hypersensitivity, 132
  mechanism of action, 130
  prophylactic, 132, 133
  tetanus, 139
Antibodies. *See* Immunoglobulin
Anticoagulants, 211, 212. *See also*
    Coumadin; Heparin
  venous thrombosis, 248, 558, 559
Antidiuretic hormone (ADH), 96,
    566
  inappropriate secretion, 96
Antigens, carcinoembryonic (CEA),
    115
  histocompatibility, leukocyte-
    antigen (HLA), 111, 112
  tumor-specific, 115
Antihemophilic concentrates, 210
Antihistamines, 132

Antihypertensive drugs, 231
Antilymphocytic serum, 112
Antimetabolites, 254
Antiseptics, 133
Antithyroid drugs, 479
Antrectomy, 302
Anuria, 574
Anus, 398–408
  anatomy, 398, 399
  carcinoma, 406, 407
  cryptitis, 402
  fissure, 401, 402
  fistula, 403
  hematoma, 405, **406**
  hemorrhoids, 404, 405
  imperforate, 637
  incontinence, 404
  pain, 400, **400**
  perirectal abscess, 402, 403
  physiology, 399
  prolapse, 405, 406, **407**
  pruritus, 403
  stricture, 402
Aorta, aneurysm, 556, **557**
  embolectomy, 553, **554**
  rupture, 175, 176
Aortic valve, insufficiency, acquired,
    544–45
  stenosis, acquired, 544
    congenital, 543
Aortography, 554–55
Appendectomy, 392, **392**
Appendicitis, 389–93
  clinical manifestations, 389–92
  complications, 390
  differential diagnosis, 390–92
  in the elderly, 393
  in infants, 392
  pelvic inflammatory disease vs.,
    391
  in pregnancy, 216
  treatment, 392, **392**
Appendix, 389–93
  carcinoid, **393**
  mucocele, 393
Aprotinin, 349
Arnold-Chiari malformation, 627
Arrhythmias, 44, 56, 170
  postoperative, 254
Arterial disease, 551–59
  aneurysms, 556–57, **557**
  arteritis, 558
  atherosclerosis, 553–59
  Buerger's, 558
  carotid, 556
  embolism, 551–53, **554**
  endarterectomy, **555**
  grafts, **555**
  mesenteric, 557
  occlusive, of lower extremity,
    553–56
  Raynaud's disease, 558
  renal, 556
  vertebral, 556
Arteries, 549–59. *See also* specific
    arteries
  chemotherapeutic perfusion
    through, **156**
  diseases. *See* Arterial disease
  embolism, 551–53, **554**
  embryology, **527**
  grafts, 555, **555**
  superior mesenteric, 354

  trauma, 549–51, **551, 552, 553**
Arteriovenous malformations,
    cerebral, 620
  lung, 540
Arteritis, 558
Arthritis. *See also* Osteoarthritis
  degenerative, 518, 519
  pyogenic, 517
  rheumatoid, 202, 504, 517–18
Ascaris lumbricoides, 540
Ascites, cancer, 147
  cirrhosis, 321, 336
Ascorbic acid, 121
Aspiration, during anesthesia, 230
  in burns, 264
  head injury, 602
  in tracheoesophageal fistula, 635
Aspirin, 286, 305
Astrocytoma, 613, 624
Astrup technique, 102
Asynergy, 58
Atelectasis, 243, 246, **246,** 247
  postoperative, 258, 259
  regional hypoventilation, 81–82,
    81
Atherosclerosis, 122, 553–59
  cerebral, 620, 621
ATP. *See* Adenosine triphosphate
Atresia, intestine, 632
Atrial septal defects, 543
Atropine, 223
  sinus bradycardia, 254
  vagal blockage, 342
Australian antigen. *See* Hepatitis-
    associated antigen
Autoimmune disease, 109
Axillary nodes, 447–49
Azathioprine, 112, 121
Azide, 298

Bacillus Calmette-Guérin (BCG)
    vaccine, 115, 443
Bacitracin, 130
Bacteria. *See also* specific organisms
  culture, 128
Bacterial endocarditis, 133
Bacterial shock, gram-negative, 34,
    35, 126
Bacteroides, 128, 131, 358
Balanitis, 580
Barbiturates, 186, 194
Basal cell carcinoma, 439
Basal metabolic rate, 477
Basophilic adenoma, pituitary, 613
Bassini herniorrhaphy, **420**
Battered child syndrome, 513
BCG in immunotherapy, 115
Benzalkonium chloride, 634
Bernstein perfusion test, 286
Bicarbonate, 45–46
Biliary tract, 317
  anatomy, 317, 318, **318**
  atresia, 325, 329
  Courvoisier's law, 322
  roentgenography, 324–25
Bilirubin, 322
Billroth I and II gastrectomy, **302,
    303**
Biopsy, breast, 464
  cancer, 147–48
  excisional, 147, 148
  hepatic, 325
  incisional, 147, 148

kidney, 569
lip, 277
liver, 325
lung, 539
needle, 147, 148
rectal, 401
    Hirschsprung's disease, 637
tongue, 278
Birth injuries, 513
Bishydroxy urea, 443
Bites, human, 130
Bladder, urinary. *See* Urinary
    bladder
Blastomycosis, 535
Bleeding time, 209
Blepharoplasty, 597
Blind-loop syndrome, 362
Bloat syndrome, 290
Blocking factors, lymphocyte, 109,
    114
Blood, banked, 213–16
    coagulation, 207–13, **207–209.**
        See also Coagulation
    factors. *See* Coagulation
    peripheral flow, 56, 57
    transfusion. *See* Transfusion
    volume, 53, 55
Blood flow, regulation, 50, 51
Blood gases, 45. *See also* Carbon
        dioxide; Oxygen
Blood groups, 213, 214
Blood pressure. *See* Hypertension;
    Hypotension
Blood vessels. *See also* Arteries;
    Veins; specific vessels
    cancer spread, 145–47
    grafts, 122
    repair, 121, 122
Blood volume, in infancy, 631
Blowout fracture, 593
Body fluids. *See* Fluids and
    electrolytes
Body water, 94–97
    in infancy, 631, **631**
Bohr effect, 67
Boil, **135,** 136
Bone, chondroma, 523
    chondrosarcoma, 523
    congenital disorders, 509–11
    cyst, 523
    Ewing's tumor, 523, 524
    giant cell tumor, 523
    growth disorders, 511, 512
    healing, 122
    hyperparathyroidism, 521
    matrix, 508
    metabolic disorders, 520–22
    metabolism, 508, 509
    metaphyseal fibrous defect, 522
    metastases, 524
    multiple myeloma, 524
    osteoblastoma, 522
    osteocartilaginous exostosis, 523
    osteogenic sarcoma, 523
    osteoid osteoma, 522
    osteomalacia, 520–21
    osteoporosis, 521
    Paget's disease, 521
    parathyroid and, 486
    renal osteodystrophy, 521
    reticulum cell sarcoma, 524
    rickets, 520–21
    tumors, 522–24

Borrelia vincentii, 126
Boutonnière deformity, 500–501, **501**
Bowen's disease, 277, 406, 407
Bowman's capsule, 566
Boyle gas-oxygen apparatus, 229
Brachial plexus block, 224
Brachycephaly, 627
Brain, abscess, 625
    anatomy, **617, 618, 619**
    blood supply, **616, 617, 619**
    hematoma, epidural, 605
        intracerebral, 605
        subdural, 605
    infections, 625
    pneumography, 615
    subarachnoid hemorrhage, 616–20
    transtentorial herniation, **601**
    tumors, 609–16
        classification, 612–14
        clinical manifestations, 610–12
        diagnosis, 614–16
        increased intracranial pressure,
            609, 610
        intracerebral, 613–14
        metastases, 614
        tentorial compression, 611, 612
        treatment, 616
    visual pathways, 614, **615**
Brain stem dislocation, 611
    tractotomy, 191, **191**
Branchial cyst, 590
Breast, 445–73
    abscess, 446
    anatomy and development, 445,
        446
    anomalies, 446
    blood supply, 446
    cancer, 447–72
        biopsy, 464
        castration, 469, 470
        chemotherapy, 470–71
        comedo, 144, 450
        cytology, 455
        diagnosis, 454–61
        differential diagnosis, 461–64,
            462
        etiology, 447
        examination, **455, 456, 457**
        grading, 453
        hormones and, 469–70
        hypophysectomy, 469
        incidence, 447
        isotope scans, 460, 461
        male, 471, 472
        mammography, 458–60, **458,
            459, 460**
        medullary, 50
        microscopic classification, 450
        oophorectomy, 469
        operations, 464–67
        Paget's disease, 450
        papillary, 450
        prognosis, 453
        psychologic effect, 218
        radical mastectomy, 466–67
        radiotherapy, 467–69, **468**
        screening, 461
        spread, 447–49, **448, 449**
        staging, 450–53, **451, 452**
        thermography, 455, 458
        treatment, 464–71
    clinical examination, 454–55,
        456–57

cystosarcoma phylloides, 464
cysts, 463
    duct papilloma, 463
    embryology, 445
    fat necrosis, 464
    fibroadenoma, 463
    infections, 446–47
    lymphatic drainage, **448**
Broder's classification, 440
Bromsulphalein (BSP) test, 322
Bronchial adenoma, 536
Bronchiectasis, 534, **534**
Bronchoscopy, 528, 529
Bronchospasm, 243
Bronchus, carcinoid, 536
    carcinoma, 537–40
    ruptured, **176,** 532
Brooke formula, 265
Brown tumors, 521
Buccal mucosa, 275
    carcinoma, 280
Buerger's disease, 558
Buffers, 94, 100
Bupivacaine (Marcaine), 225, 226
Burkitt's lymphoma, 114, 153
    chronic malaria, 115
    spontaneous regression, 114
Burns, 261–68
    anemia, 263
    classification, 262, 263
    Curling's ulcer, 264
    depth of skin destruction, **262**
    edema, 54–55
    eye, 595
    heart failure, 263
    infection, 263, 264
    nitrogen loss, 264
    pathophysiology, 263, 264
    prevention, 268
    rule of nines, 263, **263**
    stress catabolic state, 34, 35
    treatment, 34–35, 264–68
        intravenous fluids, 265
        rehabilitation, 267, 268
        respiratory system, 264, 265
        skin grafting, 266, 267
        topical, 266
    types, 262
Bursa of Fabricius, 104
Bursal-dependent lymphocytes
    (B-cells), 104, 427
Bursitis, 519
Bypass procedures, blood vessels,
    122

"C" fiber system, 185
Cachexia, 201, 202, **202**
Calcaneal spur, 520
Calcitonin, 485
Calcium, bone metabolism, 484,
        485, 520, 521
    cardiac arrest, 256
    hyperparathyroidism, 485–87, 521
    pancreatitis, 345
Calculi, gallbladder. *See* Gallstones
    salivary glands, 274
    urinary, 569–71
Caloric requirements, 98
    infancy, 632
Calories, in catabolic state, 36
Canal of Guyon, 503
Canal of Nuck, 641
Cancer. *See also* specific sites

Cancer [*cont.*]
  biopsy, 147, 148
  cellular features, **142**
  immunotherapy, 115–16
  lymphangiosarcoma, 429
  lymphomas, 429, 430
  melanoma, 440–43
  metastases, 144–47
    bone, 524
    pleura, 533
    resection, 540, 541
  mononuclear cell infiltration, 114, 429, 450
  pain, 193–95
  paraneoplastic manifestations, 538
  sarcomas, 443–44
  skin, 438–43
  specific antibodies, 115
  specific antigens, 115
  spontaneous regression, 114
  spread, 141–47, **142, 143**
    esophagus, **293–94**
    hematogenous, 143, 144, 145
    larynx, **281**
    local, **142,** 143
    lymphatic, 143, **145**
    metastases, 144–47, **144, 145**
    theories, 146
    tongue, **276**
    transluminal, 144, **144,** 147
    transserous, 147
    vertebral venous system, **146**
  surgical treatment, 147–49
  treatment, 147–57
    chemotherapy, 153–57, **156**
    immunotherapy, 115–16
    palliative, 149, 153, 155
    radiation, **150–51**
  types of biopsy, 147–48, **147**
Candida albicans, 128, 264
Cannon's law, 291
Cantor tube, 415
Carbenicillin, 131
Carbenoxolone, 301
Carbon dioxide, endarterectomy, 555
  exchange, 67, 68
  respiratory acidosis, 242, 243
Carbon dioxide tension, acid-base balance, 93–94, 101, 102
  measurements, 66–67
Carbonic anhydrase, 68, 299
Carbuncle, **135,** 136
Carcinoembryonic antigen (CEA), 115
Carcinogenesis, esophagus, 292
  skin, 275
Carcinoid, appendix, 393, **393**
  lung, 536
  rectum, 396
  small intestine, 364–66
  trachea, 533
Carcinoid syndrome, 365, 366
  niacin deficiency, 365
Carcinoma. *See also* Cancer
  adrenocortical, 491–93
  ampulla of Vater, 344
  anus, 406, 407
  appendix, 393
  basal cell, 439
  biliary tract, 334
  bladder, 582, 583

bone metastases, 146, 323, 460, 461
brain, 609–16
breast, **452**
colon, 383–85, **383**
comedo, 144, 450
esophagus, 292–94, **293**
gallbladder, 330
kidney, 581–82, **582**
larynx, 281, **281**
lip, 276–77, **277**
liver, 334–35
lung, 537–40
mouth, 277–80, **279–80**
palate, 280
pancreas, 349–51, **352**
parathyroid, 486
parotid, **282**
penis, 584
prostate, 583–84
rectosigmoid, 396–98, **397–98, 401–402**
salivary glands, 281, 282
skin, 438–43
small intestine, 363–66
staging, 276, 450–53, 539
stomach, 309–12, **310**
testis, 584
thyroid, 482–84, **483**
tonsil, 280
trachea, 533
ureter, 582
urethra, 585
urinary tract, 581–84
Cardiac arrest, 243, 255, 256
  anesthesia, 230
  management, 170
  postoperative, 255, 256
Cardiac arrhythmias, 254
Cardiac output, 49, 50
Cardiac tamponade, 55, 56, 545
Cardiopulmonary bypass, 543
Cardiopulmonary surgery, 526–48
Cardiospasm. *See* Achalasia
Cardiovascular system. *See also* Arteries; Heart; Veins
  burns, 263
  history, 203, 204
  monitoring, 218, 219
  normal physiology, **50,** 51, **51**
Carotene, 357
Carotid arteries, injuries, 175
  occlusion, 556
Carpal tunnel syndrome, 503
Cascade systems, 207–209
Casilan, 345
Castration, breast cancer, 469–70
  carcinoma, prostate, 583
Catecholamines, 11, 12, 491, 492
  neuroblastoma, 639
Catgut, 236, 237
Catheter(s), urinary tract, 576
Catheterization, 576
Cation pump, 95
Causalgia, 196, 197
Cecum, volvulus, 387
Celestin tube, 294
Celiac disease, immunosuppression, 115
Cell, cancer, **142**
  electron microscopic features, **142, 143**
  generation cycle, **155**

Cellular immune response, 104, 105
Cellulitis, 133, 134, **134**
Central nervous system, 599–628
  anomalies, 625–27
  embryology, 625–26, **626**
  pain pathways, 182–85
  trauma, 602–609
Central venous pressure, 172
Cephalothin, 131
Cerebral arteries, **617, 619**
Cerebral palsy, 524
Cerebrovascular disease, 620–21
Cervical disk disease, 622, 623
Cervical fractures and dislocations, 606–609
Cervical lymph nodes, 428
Cervical rib syndrome, 558
Cervical spondylosis, 623
"C" fiber system, 185
Chagas' disease, 387
Chemotherapy, 153–57
  adjuvant to surgery, 155
  alkylating agents, **150,** 153, 154
  antimetabolites, 154
  breast, 470–71
  intraoperative, **156**
  melanoma, 443
  palliative, 155
  thio-TEPA, 467–69
  tumors, brain, 616
Chest, flail, **176,** 531, 532
  injuries, 170, 175, 176, **176,** 530–32
Cheyne-Stokes respiration, 601
Chi^2 test, 163
Children. *See* Pediatric surgery
Child's operation, 349
Chloramphenicol, 132
Chlordiazepoxide, 187
Chlorpromazine, 187
Chlorprothixene, 187
Cholangiocarcinoma, 334
Cholangiography, 323, **323,** 324, **324**
  operative, 324
  percutaneous transhepatic, 324
  transduodenal, 325
Cholangitis, acute suppurative, 330
Cholecystectomy, 330–32, **331**
Cholecystitis, **329,** 330–32
  pregnancy, 216
Cholecystography, 324
Cholecystokinin, 322, 356
Choledochal cyst, 329
Choledochoduodenostomy, 332
Cholelithiasis. *See* Gallstones
Cholesterol, biliary tract disease, 323, 324
  gallstones, 329
  intestinal bypass, 360–61
Cholestyramine, 344
  pruritus, 344
Chondroitin sulfate, 119
Chondrosarcoma, 523
Chordee, 592
Chordoma, 624
Christmas factor (IX), 210, 320
Chromophobe adenoma, 613
Chronic obstructive pulmonary disease (COPD), 536
Chylomicrons, 354, 427
Circle of Willis, 617
Cirrhosis, 338

esophagogastric varices, 336
Citrate, transfusions, 214, 215
Claudication, 553–54
Cleft lip and palate, 589, 590, **590**
Clindamycin, 131
Clinical trials, analysis of data,
  162–63
  chi² test, 163
  sequential analysis, 163
  student's *t*-test, 163
  controls, 159, 160, 161
  paired stratification, 161–62
  protocol, 161
  randomization, 161
  retrospective studies, 158, 159
Cloaca, 564
Clonal selection theory, 109
Clonorchis sinensis, 329
Clostridial infections, 126, 137, 138
Clostridial myonecrosis, 138, 139
Clostridium histolyticum, 139
Clostridium novyi, 139
Clostridium perfringens, 139
Clostridium septicum, 139
Clostridium sporogenes, 139
Clotting time, 210
Cloxacillin, 131
Clubfoot, 510
Coagulation, 207–13
  cascade system, 208–209, **208**
  clot formation, 207–209, **207**
  disseminated intravascular (DIC),
    212, 213
  evaluation, 209–11
  factors, 208–12, 320
  liver function, 320, 321
  tests, 209, 210
Coarctation of aorta, 543, 544
Cocaine, 225
Coccidioidomycosis, 535
Codeine, 187, 194
Colchicine, 154
Colectomy, 384
Colistin, 132
Colitis, Crohn's disease, 379, **379**
  ischemic, 385–87, **386,** 418
  pseudomembranous enterocolitis,
    375
  ulcerative, 375–79
    complications, 376–78, **376**
    diagnosis, **377,** 378
    pathology, 374–75, **375**
    toxic megacolon, 376–78
    treatment, 378
Collagen, 558
Collagen diseases, 369
Colles' fracture, 514
Collis repair, 290
Colloids, burns, 265
Colon, 371–88
  amebiasis, 375
  anatomy, 372
  arterial supply, 373
  carcinoid, 384
  carcinoma, 383–85
    chemotherapy, 155
    diagnosis, 384, 385
    etiology, 383–84
    operations, 384, 385, 397
    pathology, **383,** 384, **385**
    psychologic effect, 218
    radiotherapy, 152
    treatment, 384–85

ulcerative colitis, 379
  colostomy, 388
Crohn's disease, **379**
  diverticular disease, 380–83,
    380–81
  enterocolitis, 375
  function, **372**
  hematochezia, 388
  Hirschsprung's disease, 637
  megacolon, 387
  physiology, **372,** 373–74, **374**
  polyps. *See* Polyps, colorectal
  preparation for operation, 384–85
  radiation injury, 388
  trauma, 374–75
  tuberculosis, 375
  ulcerative colitis, 375–79, **375–77**
  volvulus, 387
Colon interposition, esophagectomy,
  290, 291
Colonoscopy, 400
Colostomy, care, 388
Colostrum, 446
Columns of Morgagni, 399
Coma, care of patient, 602
Common bile duct, anatomy, 317
  carcinoma, 335
  operations, 331, 332
Complement, 105–106
Compliance, 83
Complications (postoperative),
  241–60
  abdominal distention, 250, 251
  adrenal insufficiency, 253
  arrhythmias, 254
  atelectasis, 246, 247
  decubitus ulcer, 253
  dehiscence, 251, 252
  diabetes, 253
  evisceration, 251, 252
  fat embolism, 248, 249
  fever, 245, 246
  gout, 253
  hematoma, 252
  intraperitoneal abscess, 252
  organ failure, 253–59
  pancreatitis, 249, 250
  parotitis, 249
  psychiatric, 253
  pulmonary embolism, 247, 248
  stress ulcer, 250
  urinary, 252, 253
  ventilatory failure, 258–59
Computer-assisted axial tomography,
  616–16
Condylomata accuminata, 438
Congenital hemolytic anemia, 432
Conn's syndrome, 490, 491
Connell stitch, **415**
Consciousness, 600
Contractures, burns, 267, 268
  Dupuytren's, 503
  Volkmann's, 514
Coombs' test, 200, 210, 432
Cooper's ligaments, 446, 449
Coronary arteries, 542
Coronary artery disease, 546–47
  bypass operation, 546, 547
Corticosteroids, 200
Cortisol, 96, 488, 489
  Cushing's syndrome, 489, 490
Cortisone, Addison's disease, 207
  hyperparathyroidism, 487

immunosuppression, 112
  wound healing, 120
Cosmetic surgery, 596–98
Coumadin, 212, 248, 553
Courvoisier's law, 322, 344
Craniopharyngioma, 613
Creatine phosphokinase, myocardial
  infarction, 255
Creatinine clearance, 581
Credé bladder expression, 577
Crigler-Najar syndrome, 319
Critical point of Sudeck, 373
Critically ill, monitoring, **219**
Critically injured, 167–80, **168, 174.**
  See also individual organs
  abdominal injuries, 176, **176,** 177
  chest injuries, 170, 175, **175,** 176
  clinical evaluation, 173
  head and neck, 175, **175**
  incidence, 167
  initial resuscitation, 168
    airway, 170
  limb injuries, 178–79, **179**
  special procedures, 179
Crohn's disease, 366–69, **367, 368,**
  379
  colon, 379, **379**
  esophagus, 293
  obstruction, 417
Cronkhite syndrome, 395
Croup, 273
Crouzon's disease, 627
Cryotherapy, 276, 439
Crypts of Lieberkuhn, 355
Curare, 228
Curling's ulcer, 264
Cushing stitch, **415**
Cushing's disease, metabolic
  alkalosis, 101
Cushing's reflex, 609
Cushing's syndrome, 489–90, **489**
  basophilic adenoma, 613
Cyanosis, congenital anomalies, 543,
  544
  neonate, 634, 635
Cyclic AMP, 487
Cyclophosphamide, 154, 155, 312
Cyclopropane (trimethylene), 227
Cyst(s), bone, 523
  branchial, 590
  breast, 461, 463
  choledochal, 329
  congenital pulmonary, 536
  dermoid, 437
  enterogenous, 632
  epidermal, 437
  pancreatic, 346, 347
  pilonidal, 407
  presacral, 407, 408
  sebaceous, 437
  vitellointestinal duct, 633
Cystectomy, 583
Cystic fibrosis, meconium ileus, 636
Cystic hygroma, 444
Cystic mastitis, chronic, 461–63
Cystography, 569, 571, 573
Cystolithotomy, 570
Cystosarcoma phylloides, 464
Cystoscopy, 569
Cystourethrography, 577
Cytology, breast secretions, 455
  bronchial washings, 539
  esophagus, 286

Cytology [*cont.*]
 gastric juice, 311
 mouth, 275
 sputum, 539
 urine, 569

Da Nang lung, 64
Dactinomycin, 154, 155, 211, 582
Danlos' syndrome, 121
Darvon, 193
Decerebrate rigidity, 602
Decortication of lung, 533
Decubitus ulcer, 205, 602
Defecation, 373–74
Defibrillation, ventricular, 256
Degenerative disk disease. *See* Disk disease
Degenerative joint disease. *See* Osteoarthritis
Dehiscence, 251, 252
Delayed splenic hematoma, 431
Demerol, 223, 231
 pancreatic pain, 343
de Pezzer catheter, 576
DeQuervain's tenosynovitis, 504, 520
Dermabrasion, 592
Dermatitis, contact, 132
Dermatomes, **623**
Dermoid cyst, 437
Descending spinal trigeminal tract, 184, **184**
Dexamethasone, 610
 suppression test, 490
Dextran, 172, 265, 386
Diabetes mellitus, 205, 206, 253
 anesthesia, 232, 253
 carcinoma, pancreas, 350
 history, 205
 necrotizing cellulitis, 139
 postoperative, 253
 preoperative, 205–206
Diabetic necrotizing cellulitis, 139
Dialysis, 375
Diaphragm, hernia, acquired, 424
 congenital, 634, 635
 trauma, 176, 177, 178
Diarrhea, carcinoid syndrome, 365
 ulcerative colitis, 376
 vagotomy, 304
 Zollinger-Ellison syndrome, 353
Diazepam, 187, 223, 228
Dicumarol, 212
Diet, elemental, 205, 243, 244
 high-roughage, 382
Diethyl ether, 227
DiGeorge syndrome, 104–105, 114
Digitalis, 200
 arrhythmias, 254
 heart failure, 254, 255
 hypokalemia, 97
Dilantin, 195
2:4 Dinitrophenol, 298
Diphosphoglycerate, 46
Diplopia, facial fractures, 593
Disinfectants, 133
Disk disease, 519
 cervical, 622–23
 lumbar, 623–24
 thoracic, 623
Dislocations, acromioclavicular, 515
 ankle, 516
 fingers, 500
 hip, 515

congenital, 510
 shoulder, 514, 515
Disseminated intravascular coagulation (DIC), 212, 213
Diuretics, 566
 mercurial, 566
 ventilatory failure, 259
Diverticula, colonic, 380–83
 duodenal, 312
 epiphrenic, 291
 Meckel's, 359–60, **359,** 391, 634
 Zenker's, **290,** 291
Diverticulitis, appendix, 393
Diverticulosis coli, complications, 380, **380,** 381, **381,** 382
 diverticulitis, 380–83, **380**
 etiology, 380
 hemorrhage, 382
 obstruction, 417
 pathology, 380, 381
 treatment, 382–83
DNCB, 115
Donovan bodies, 402
Down's syndrome, duodenal atresia, 636
 leukemia, 639
Doxorubicin, 154, 155, 312, 471
Drainage, chest, 531, 533
 pelvic abscess, 252
 subphrenic abscess, 252
 underwater seal, **531**
 vagotomy, 297, 301
 wounds, 123, 238
Drugs. *See also* Antibiotics; Chemotherapy
 anesthetic. *See* Anesthesia
 immunosuppressive, **112**
Dubin-Johnson syndrome, 319
Ductus arteriosus, patent, 543
Dukes' classification, 385, 397
Dumping syndrome, 304
 operations, 361
Duodenum, 296–314, **312**
 atresia, congenital, 636
 diverticulum, 312
 mesenteric arterial obstruction, 312
 trauma, 309
 tumors, 312
Duplication, intestine, 632
Dupuytren's contracture, 503
Dyskeratosis, mouth, 275
Dysphagia, 285, 286
Dyspnea, 246, 248, 255

Ears, microtia, 590
 prominent, 590
 squamous cell carcinoma, 439
Ebstein's anomaly, 544
Echinococcus granulosus, 332
Ectopia vesicae, 564
Edema, cellular, 54–55
 cerebral, 610
 production, 53–54
Eggshell pericarditis, 547
Electrocardiography, Addison's disease, 207
 hyperkalemia, 97
 hypokalemia, 98
 myocardial infarction, 255
Electrolytes. *See* Fluids and electrolytes
Electromyography, 401

Elemental diets, 205, 243, 244
 gastrostomy, 205
 jejunostomy, 205
Embolectomy, **554,** 621
 cerebral vessels, 621
Embolism, aortic, 551, **554**
 carotid, 551
 fat, 248, 249, 513
 pulmonary. *See* Pulmonary embolism
Embryonal carcinoma, testis, 584
Emphysema, subcutaneous, 286
Empyema, 532, 533
Encephalopathy, 321, **321,** 322
Enchondroma, 523
Endarterectomy, 555, **555,** 621
Endarteritis obliterans, 128
Endocarditis, prophylactic antibiotics, 133
Endocrine glands. *See* individual glands
Endocrine system, history, 205
Endoscopy, colonoscopy, 400, 401
 esophagoscopy, 286
 gastroscopy, 305
 proctoscopy, 400, 401
Endotoxins, 126
Endotracheal intubation, 170, 205, 259
Enhancement, immune, 109
Entamoeba histolytica, 394
Enterogastrone, 356
Enterokinase, 342
Eosinophil(s), 119
Eosinophilic adenoma, pituitary, 613
Ependymoma, 614, 624
Epidermis. *See* Skin
Epididymitis, 577, 578
Epididymo-orchitis, 578
Epidural abscess, 625
Epidural anesthesia, 225
Epilepsy, abdominal, 639
Epinephrine, 15, 19, 491
 wound healing, 120
Epiphrenic diverticulum, 291
Epispadias, 580, 592
Epsilon aminocaproic acid, 209, 211
Epulis, 283, **283**
Erythrocytes, survival, 432
Erythromycin, 131
Escherichia coli, 128, 131, 132, 389
Esophageal varices, **334,** 336–37, **337**
Esophagitis, reflux, 287–91, 289, **289**
 fundoplication, 290, **290**
 operations, 289–91, **292**
Esophagoscopy, 286
Esophagostomy, cervical cutaneous, 635
Esophagus, 285–95
 achalasia, 291, 292
 Heller's operation, **292**
 carcinoma, 292–94, **293**
 palliative treatment, **294**
 treatment, 293, 294, **294**
 congenital atresia, 635, **635**
 corrosives, 287
 diverticula, **290,** 291
 esophagogastrectomy, **294**
 foreign bodies, 287
 hiatal hernia, 287–91
 paraesophageal, **288**
 sliding, **288**
 injuries, 287

investigations, 286, 287
Mallory-Weiss syndrome, 305, 308, 309
motility studies, 286
reflux, **289**
symptoms, 285, 286
varices. *See* Esophageal varices
Zenker's diverticulum, **290**
Estrogens, adrenal production, 488, 491
carcinoma, breast, 469
prostate, 583
Ethacrynic acid, 566, 574
Ether, diethyl, 227
Ethoheptazine (Zactirin), 193
Ethylenimine radical, 150, 153, 154
Evisceration, 251, 252
Ewing's sarcoma, 284, 523, 524
Exophthalmos, 475, 478
Extradural tumors, 624
Extraperitoneal injuries, **177**
Eye, trauma, 595
trigeminal neuralgia, 195

Face, fractures, 170
scars, 592
trauma, 592–95
Facial nerve, parotidectomy, 282, 283
Factors, blood. *See* Coagulation
Familial polyposis, 395
Fat(s), chylomicrons, 354
energy source, 9
metabolism, 8–9
synthesis, 14
Fat embolism, **249**
Fat necrosis, pancreatitis, 345, 348
Feces, carcinoma of ampulla of Vater, 344
impaction, 416
Felon, 501, **501**, 502
Felty's syndrome, 432
Feminizing tumors, 491, **491**
Femoral hernia, 421–23
Femur, amputation through, **560**
fractures, 515
Fetal antigens, 115, 311, 323
Fetor hepaticus, 321
Fibrinolysis, **207**
tests, 210
Fibroadenoma, breast, 463
Fibroma, 444
Fibromuscular hyperplasia, 556
Fibrosarcoma, 444
Fibrosing mediastinitis, 542
Fingers. *See also* Hand
amputations, 499
boutonnière deformity, **501**
fractures, 500, 513, 514
infections, 501, 502, **502**
nerve injuries, **497**
skin grafting, 499
tendon injury, 492, **498**, 500, 501
trigger finger, **503**
Fissure, anal, **400**, 401–402
Fistula, in ano, 403
arteriovenous, 551
intestinal, 361
vitellointestinal duct, 633
Flail chest, 79, 85–86, **176**
Flexor digitorum profundus, avulsion, 501
Flexor tendon injuries of hand, 130,

498, 501
Fluids and electrolytes, atomic structure, 92–93
buffers, 94
fluid compartments, 94–95
Henderson-Hasselbalch equation, 93
in infancy, 630–31
milliequivalent, 93
overhydration, 96–97
Ringer's lactate, 43, 55
underhydration, 96–97
5-Fluorouracil (5-FU), 154, 155, 312, 351, 385, 471, 583
Fogarty catheter, 553, 559
Foley catheter, 174
Foot, 520
club, 510
Köhler's disease, 512
Foramen, of Bochdalek, 424, 635
of Morgagni, 424, 635
of Winslow, 424
Foreign bodies, airway, 170
esophagus, 287
eye, 595
hand, 501
heart, 546
intestinal obstruction, 416
wound(s), 127
wound healing, 123
Fractures, 512–16
ankle, 516
arm, 514
birth injuries, 513
cervical spine, 170, **607**
clavicle, **176**
Colles', 514
complications, 513
compound, **179**
face, 170, 593–95, **592–94**
femur, 515
fingers, 500, 513
foot, 516
hand, 513, 514
hip, 515
humerus, 514
Le Fort lines, 594, **594**
leg, 515, 516, 595
mandibular, 593, **593**, 594, 595
maxillary, 175, **175**, 593–95
metacarpals, 513, 514
midface, **594**
milkman's, 521
nasal bones, 593–95
navicular (scaphoid), 514
nonunion, 513
nose, 593, 594
patella, 516
pelvis, **177**, 178, 515
phalanges, 500, 513, 514
rib, 176, **176**, 531, 532
skull, 175, 603–604, **604**
spine, 175, 178, 607, **607**
talus, 516
tibia, 516
zygomaticomaxillary, **594**
Freiberg's disease, 512
Frostbite, 561–62
Frozen shoulder, 519, 520
Fundoplication, **290**
Fungal infections, 535
Furosemide, 566, 574
Fusobacterium nucleatum, 126

Gallamine, 228
Gallbladder, carcinoma, 335
cholecystectomy, 330
diagnosis, 330
function, 317
stones. *See* Gallstones
Gallstones, formation, 329, 330
Ganglia, 502
Ganglioneuroma, 541
Gangrene, amputation, **560**
"dry," **137**
gas, 128, 138, 139
Meleney's postoperative, 126, **126**
"wet," **137**
Gardner's syndrome, 395
Gas gangrene, 128, 138, 139
Gastrectomy, Billroth I and II, **302, 303**
total, **311**
Gastric dilatation, burns, 264
Gastric secretion. *See also* Stomach, secretions
pregnancy, 216
Gastrin, 299, 342
Zollinger-Ellison syndrome, 352
Gastritis, atrophic, 305
cancer, 309
Gastrointestinal tract, changes in shock, 21
Gastroschisis, 634
Gastroscopy, 301, 305
Gastrostomy, 305, 306
elemental diets, 205
postoperative ileus, 250
"Gate" theory, 182, 192
Generation cycle, 154, 155, **155**
Genetic factors, carcinoma, breast, 447
polyposis coli, 395
Genitals, trauma, 574
Genitourinary tract, 563–85. *See also* Kidney; Urinary bladder; other structures
calculi, 569–71
embryology, 564–65
history, 204, 567
infections, 576
trauma, 571–74
Gentamicin, 128, 132, 574
Geriatric surgery, 217, 218
Gerota's fascia, 582
Giant cell tumor, bone, 523
Gilbert's disease, 318
Glanzmann's disease, 211
Glioblastoma multiforme, 613
Glomus tumor, 503
Glucagon, **12**, 345
for pancreatic pain, 343
in pancreatitis, 345
Glucocorticoids, 487, 488
Gluconeogenesis, 14, 15, 98
burns, 264
renal failure, 258
Glucose, 9–15
hypothalamic control, 9
Glucuronyl transferase, 319
Glycocalyx, 354, 355
Glycogen, 16–17
Goiter, clinical manifestations, 478
Golgi apparatus, 119
Gonorrhea, 579
urethritis, 585
Gout, 253, 521

Graft, mandible, 279, 283, 284
Graft-versus-host reaction, 109
Grafting. *See* Skin grafting;
    Transplantation
Gram-positive microorganisms,
    antibiotics, 131–32
Gram stain, 501
Graves' disease, 478–79
    treatment, 479
Grease injuries, 500
Griseofulvin, 132
Growth hormone, 15
Gubernaculum testis, 565
Gumma, 579
Gynecologic disorders, appendicitis
    vs., 391

Hallux valgus, 520
Halothane, 226, 227, 338
Halsted operation (radical
    mastectomy), 466
Halsted stitch, **415**
Hammer toes, 520
Hand, 494–504
    amputations, 499
    anatomy, 494–95, **495, 496**
    anomalies, 591
    burns, 267, 499
    cysts, 502, 503
    debridement, 498–99
    Dupuytren's contracture, 503
    felon, 501, **501,** 502
    ganglion, 502
    grease injuries, 500
    infections, 501, **501,** 502, **502**
    motor function tests, **497**
    nerve compression syndromes,
      503
    "no-man's land," 498
    palmar and thenar space
      infections, 502
    paronychia, 502, **502**
    rheumatoid arthritis, 504
    suppurative tenosynovitis, 502
    trauma, 595
    trigger finger, 503, **503,** 504
    tumors, 503
    wringer injury, 499
Hartmann's pouch, 330
Hashimoto's disease, 480, 481
Head, 273–84
    hematomas, 604, 605
      epidural, 605
      intracerebral, 605
      subdural, 605, **606**
    injuries, **175,** 602–606
      scalp, 603
    tumors, 275. *See also* specific
      areas
Headache, brain tumors, 610, 611
Healing (wound), blood vessels,
    121, **207**
    bone, 122
    collagen synthesis, 119–20, **120**
    epithelium, 121
    humoral factors, 120
    muscle, 121
    nerves, 121
    phases, 117–20, **118**
    tendon, 122
Heart. *See also* specific diseases
    acquired diseases, 544–47
    anatomy, 542

angiography, 542, **543**
aortic insufficiency, 61, 544, 545
aortic stenosis, 544
arrest. *See* Cardiac arrest
asynergy, 58
block, 547, 548
    pacemakers, 547–48
catheterization, 542–43
coarctation of aorta, 543
congenital diseases, 543, 544
coronary artery disease, 546–47
embryology, 542
failure, 43–44, 58–59, **58,** 62–63,
    62, 63
    acute, 58–59
    burns, 263
    intracardiac disorders, 60–61
    postoperative, 254, 255
investigations, 542, 543
massage, 256
mitral regurgitation, 61
murmurs, 544, 545
patent ductus arteriosus, 543
pericarditis, 547
septal defects, 543
tetralogy of Fallot, 543
trauma, 545–46
tricuspid disease, 545
venous return, 61, 62
Heartburn, 286
Heller myotomy, 292, **292**
Hemangioendothelioma, cerebellum,
    614
Hemangioma, 437, 639, 640
    hand, 503
    liver, 333
    parotid, 640
    sclerosing, 441, 442
    subcutaneous cavernous, 444
Hematocele, 579
Hematochezia, 388
Hematocrit, burns, 263
Hematoma, intracranial, 604, 605
    intramural, 551
    lung, 532
    neck, 170, 275
    retroperitoneal, 356, 515, 572
    subdural, 605
    subungual, 500
    wound healing, 119
Hemochromatosis, skin
    pigmentation, 437
Hemoconcentration, burns, 263
Hemodialysis, 575
Hemoglobin, buffer action, 94
    component therapy, 213
Hemophilia, 210, 213
    wound healing, 121
Hemophilus influenzae, 273
Hemorrhage, adrenal, 488
    cerebral, 620, 621
    classification, 170–73
    control, **237**
    diverticulosis coli, 382
    gastrointestinal, 304–309, **305, 306**
      operations, 306–308, **307, 308**
    hemophilia, 210, 213
    hiatal hernia, 289
    management, 172–73
    peptic ulcer, 304–307
    scalp, 603
    subarachnoid, 616–20
Hemorrhagic diatheses, **209**

Hemorrhoid(s), 404, 405, **405**
Hemorrhoidectomy, **406**
Hemostasis, 207–209
Hemothorax, 530–32
    treatment, 79–80
Hemovac, 238
Henderson-Hasselbalch equation,
    45, 93, 99–100
Henoch's purpura, 638
Heparin, 211, 248
Hepatectomy, 334, 335
Hepatic function, failure, **32**
    normal, 8–11
Hepatic vein thrombosis, 319
Hepatitis, halothane, 227, 338
    viral, 332, 333
Hepatitis-associated antigen (HAA),
    235, 236, 323
Heredity. *See* Genetic factors
Hernias, 419–24
    diaphragmatic, 424
    epigastric, 423
    external, **416**
    femoral, 421–23, **421, 422**
    hiatal, 287–91, **288, 290**
    incisional, 423, **423,** 424
    inguinal, **418,** 419–21, **419, 420,**
      421
    internal, 424
    paraesophageal, 287
    pregnancy, 216
    Richter's, 419
    scrotal, 420, 578
    sliding, **417,** 421
    spigelian, **416**
    strangulation, 414, 419
    umbilical, **422,** 423
Herniorrhaphy, Bassini, 420, **420,**
    421
Herpes zoster, perforated peptic
    ulcer vs., 308
Heterotopic tissue, pancreas, 346
Hexachlorophene (pHisoHex), 234
Hiatal hernia. *See* Hernias
Hip, degenerative arthritis, 518, 519
    dislocation, congenital, 510
Hirschsprung's disease, 637
Histamine, 118, 120, 127
Histiocytic sarcoma, 429
    bone, 524
Histocompatibility leukocyte
    antigen (HLA), kidney
    transplant, 108, 111, 113, 581
Histocompatibility tests, 111
Histoplasmosis, 535
Hodgkin's disease, 428–30
    chemotherapy, 154, 155
    immunosuppression, 115
    lymphangiography, 428
    mononuclear cell infiltration, 114
    stages, 429
    staging laparotomy, 430
    stomach, 311
Hollander test, 301
Homans' sign, 247, 558
Hormones. *See also* individual
    hormones
    adrenal, 487, 488
    thyroid, 476
Horner's syndrome, 558
Horseshoe kidney, **564**
Host defense, burns, 264
    immunotherapy, 115

tissue healing, **118,** 121, 126, 128
Hubbard tank, 266
Human immune globulin (Hypertet), 265
Human tetanus immune globulin (TIGH), 138
Humoral antibody, 105
Hürthle cell, 482
Hutchinson freckle, 441, 442
Hydatid cyst, liver, **325**
Hydatid disease, Casoni test, 110
liver, 332
Hydradenitis, 136, 147
Hydrocele, 568, 578, **578,** 641
Hydrocephalus, 625, 626–27
shunting procedures, 627
Hydrochlorothiazide, 571
Hydrocortisone, 231
Hydrogen ion concentration, 93
5-Hydroxyindole acetic acid, 366
Hydroxyproline, 120
17-Hydroxysteroids, 488
Hyperalimentation, infection, 137
intravenous, 244, 245
Hyperbaric oxygen, gas gangrene, 139
during radiotherapy, 151
Hypercalcemia, differential diagnosis, 485
hyperparathyroidism, 485–87
Hyperkalemia, 97
renal failure, 258
Hyperosmolar diuresis, intravenous alimentation, 245
Hyperparathyroidism, 485–87
pancreatitis, 345
Hypersensitivity, anaphylactic shock, 110
delayed reaction, 110
immune complex reaction, 110
iodine, 324, 325
Hypersplenism, 432
Hypertension, Conn's syndrome, 490
Cushing's syndrome, 489
fibromuscular hyperplasia, 556
MAO inhibitors, 187
due to pheochromocytoma, 492
portal. *See* Portal hypertension
postoperative, 243
renin, 556
Hyperthyroidism, 478, 479, **480**
anesthesia, 232
Hypnosis, 192
Hypocalcemia, 485
in infancy, 631
Hypokalemia, 97
digitalis, 97
diuretics, 254
paralytic ileus, 250
Hypokalemic alkalosis, 97
Hypoparathyroidism, 479
Hypophyseal portal system, **475**
Hypophysectomy, carcinoma, breast, 469
prostate, 584
Hypospadias, 580, 591, 592, **592**
Hypotension, postoperative, 243
Hypothalamus, metabolism, 10
temperature regulation, 128
Hypothermia, burns, 264
Hypothyroidism, 479–80
Hypoxia, 48, 49, 50, 67
causes, 44

postoperative, 243
stress ulcer, 304

Ileal conduit, 583
Ileostomy, 239, 378, 379, **379**
Ileum. *See* Intestine, small
Ileus, gallstone, 330, 332, 416
meconeum, 636
paralytic, 418, 419
postoperative, 250, **250,** 251
Imidazole carboxamide, 443
Immune competence, 104
Immune response, components, 106–108, **106**
primary and secondary, 108
theories, 109
Immunity, cancer, 113–16
Immunoglobulin, structure, **105**
types, 105
Immunologic tolerance, 108, 113
Immunosuppression, chemotherapy, 114, 115, 471
kidney transplants, 114, 115, 581
radiation, 152, 153, 468, 469
Immunotherapy, cancer, 115, 116
melanoma, 443
Imuran, 112
Incisions, **235, 236**
abdominal, 236, **236**
closure, **239**
Infarction, intestine, 362
Infections, 125–40. *See also* specific infections
abscess, **129, 134**
aerobic, 130–32
anaerobic, 126, **126,** 130–32
antibiotic therapy, 130–32
burns, 263, 264
diagnosis, 128, **129**
general factors, 128
lymphadenitis, 134, **134**
opportunistic, 126, 128
urinary tract, 576
Inflammatory response, 127
Inhalation anesthesia, 226–31
Innovar, 227
Instructional theory, 109
Insulin, **12, 16,** 342, 345
dumping syndrome, 304
Hollander test, 301
pancreatic function, 342
postoperative period, 253
resistance, 25–26
Intensive care unit, 243
Intermittent positive-pressure breathing (IPPB), 529, 532
Interstitial fluid, 53–54
Intestine, congenital anomalies, 632
large. *See* Anus; Cecum; Colon; Rectum
malrotation, 633
nonrotation, 632, 633
obstruction, **251,** 411–18, **412**
atresia, 636
Crohn's disease, 417
decompression, **413**
gallstone ileus, 332, 416
intussusception, 637–38
neonatal, 416
newborn, 635–38
pathophysiology, 412, 413
postoperative, **251**
strangulation, **413**

treatment, **230,** 414–16, **414, 415**
vitellointestinal duct, 633–34
small, 354–70. *See also* Duodenum
afferent (blind) loop syndrome, 362
anastomosis, **414**
anatomy, 354, 355, **355**
carcinoid, 364–66
Crohn's disease, 366–69, **367–68**
embryology, 632, **633**
infections, 369
investigations, 357, 358
Peutz-Jeghers syndrome, 363
physiology, 355–57, **357**
radiation enteritis, 369
short-bowel syndrome, 361, 362
transposition, 361
trauma, 362, 363, **363**
tumors, 363–66, **364, 365**
vascular insufficiency, 362
Intracranial hemorrhage. *See* Brain; Hematoma
Intracranial infections, 625
Intradural tumors, 624
Intralipid, 98
Intubation, endotracheal, 170, 205
intestinal obstruction, 415
Intussusception, 416, 637–38
Iodophors (Betadine), 234
Iopanoic acid (Telepaque), 324
IPPB. *See* Intermittent positive-pressure breathing
Isoproterenol, 57
atrioventricular block, 254
bronchospasm, 243
Isotopes. *See* Radioisotopes

Jaundice, causes, 318, 319, **319, 329**
hemolytic, 318, 432
obstructive, 319, 330
pancreatic disease, 343, 344
postoperative, 337, 338
Jejunoileal bypass, 360, 361
Jejunostomy, elemental diets, 205
Joints. *See also* specific joints
gout, 521
Juvenile polyp, 396

Kallikrein, 349
Kanamycin, 132, 574
Kaposi's sarcoma, 443
Keel operation, **423**
Keloid, 437
Keratoacanthoma, 438, **438**
Keratosis, actinic, 438
seborrheic, 438
Ketamine, 228
17-Ketosteroids, 207, 488
Kidney, acute tubular necrosis, 574, 575
arteriography, 568, 569
biopsy, 569
calculi, 569, 570, 571
carcinoma, 582, **582**
congenital conditions, 564
countercurrent multiplier, 566
cystic, 564
failure, acute, 44, 574, 575
chronic, 575–76
dialysis, 575
high-output, 258
postoperative, 256–58

Kidney [*cont.*]
function, 565–67
horseshoe, **564**
hyperparathyroidism, 486
infections, 576
radioisotopes, 569
trauma, 571–73 **571, 572**
Wilms' tumor, 581–82
Kienbock's disease, 512
Kirschner wires, 498, 514
Klinefelter's syndrome, 471
Knee, meniscus injuries, 516
Kocher maneuver, 514, 515
Kohler's disease, 512
Konyne, 210
Krause end bulbs, 436
Krebs cycle, 100
Kruckenburg tumor, 147
Kultschitzky cells, 364
Kupffer cells, 317
Kussmaul respiration, 100
Kveim test, 110
Kwashiorkor, 28–30

Lacerations, eye, 595
face, 592, **592**
scalp, 603
Lactic dehydrogenase (LDH),
myocardial infarction, 255
Laminar air flow, 264
Laryngectomy, 281
Laryngoscopy, 280, **280,** 281
Laryngospasm, 243
Larynx, carcinoma, 281, **281**
Lateral spinothalamic tract, 183
Lebske knife, 434
Lecithinase, 139
Left-to-right shunts, 543
Legg-Perthes disease, 511
Leiomyoma, 444
esophagus, 292
small bowel, 363
stomach, 305
Leiomyosarcoma, 305, 311
Leukocytes, acute appendicitis, 390
diagnosis of infection, 128
inflammatory response, 117, 118,
119, 127, 128, 134
Leukoplakia, 275, **275,** 276, **278**
Librium, 187
Lidocaine (Xylocaine), 225
arrhythmias, 254
cardiac arrest, 256
Ligaments, injuries, 516
Ligatures, 236–38
Lincomycin, 131
Lip, carcinoma, 276–77
cleft, 589, 590, **590**
operations, 277, 278, **278**
Lipase, 342
pancreatitis, 344
Lipids. *See* Fat(s)
Lipoma, 363, 443
Liposarcoma, 443
Liver, amebic abscess, **327**
anatomy, 315–18, **315, 316**
ascites, 321
biopsy, 325
bleeding factors, 320, 321
catabolic states, 30, 33
cholangiocarcinoma, 334
cirrhosis, **333,** 335, 336
encephalopathy, 321, 322

failure, 336, 337
function, normal, 8–11
halothane, 226, 227
hepatitis, 226, 227, 323, 332, 333
hepatitis-associated antigen
(HAA), 323, 332, 333
hepatocyte, **318, 319**
hepatoma, 334
hydatid disease, 332
investigation, 322–25
jaundice, 318, 319
lymphoreticular system, 317
metabolism, 30–33
metastases, 323, 325, 333, 334
obstruction, **332**
pain, 319, 320
protein, catabolic states, 7, 8
resection, 334, 335
segments, **315, 316**
shock, 30–33, **31**
transplantation, 338–39
trauma, **332,** 333
Lobar sequestration, 536
Lobectomy, 540
Lockjaw, 138
Long's measurements of glucose
turnover, 24
Loop of Henle, 566
Lucid interval, 605
Lumbar disk disease, 623–24
Lumbar puncture, 606, 610
Lumbar sympathectomy, 557
Lundh test, 345, 349
Lung, 68–72
abscess, 534, **534**
adult acute respiratory distress
syndrome, 64–65
anatomy, 527–28
biopsy, 529
blood supply, 68–72, **70**
bronchial adenoma, 536
bronchiectasis, 534
bullous disease, 536
carcinoma, 537–40, **538**
diagnosis, 537–39
etiology, 537
prognosis, 540
staging, 539
treatment, 539–40
compliance, **70,** 71
congenital anomalies, 536
embolism. *See* Pulmonary
embolism
embryology, 527, **527**
function, 68–72
function tests, 529, 530
great alveolar cells, 527
infections, 534–35
fungal, 535
intrapleural pressure, 72
lobar sequestration, 536
lobectomy, 540
mediastinoscopy, 529, 539
metastases, 540, 541
operations, 530
PEEP, **82**
pulmonary failure, **84**
radiography, 528
regional hypoventilation, 73–76,
74, 79–82, **79**
etiology, 80–81, **80**
stress catabolic state, 33, 34
tracheobronchial rupture, 532

tumors, 536–41
Lymph node, 425, 427
anatomy, 425, **427**
axillary, 447, 448
biopsy, 428, 429
breast, **448**
cervical, **276,** 428
excision, 429
function, 425, 427
Hodgkin's disease, 429, 430
metastases, 428
prophylactic excision for cancer,
149
Lymphadenitis, **134,** 428
Lymphangiography, 428
Lymphangiosarcoma, 429, 444
Lymphatic system, 425–29
cancer, **145**
development, 104, **104**
Lymphedema, 429
Lymphocytes, **106**
types, 427
Lymphogranuloma venereum, 402
Lymphomas, Burkitt's, 114
classification, 429
staging, 429, 430
Lymphoreticular system, 425–34, **426**
liver, 315
nodes, 104, 105, 425, 427
Peyer's patches, 104
shock, 28
thymus, 104, 433
Lymphosarcoma, 429
Lysolecithin, 347

Mafenide, 131, 266
Magnesium, **98**
deficiency in pancreatitis, 344
Malecot catheter, 576
Malignant hyperthermia, 231, 232
Mallet finger, 500
Mallory-Weiss syndrome, 305, 308,
309, **309**
Malrotation, intestine, 632, 633
Mammary dysplasia, 461–63
Mammary gland. *See* Breast
Mammography, 458–60, **458**
carcinogenesis, 458, 459
Mammoplasty, 597, 598
Mandible, Ewing's sarcoma, 284
fracture, 593, **593**
osteosarcoma, 283, 285
reconstruction, 279, 280
Mandril technique, 555
Mannitol, 566, 574
cerebral edema, 610
head injuries, 606
Marfan's syndrome, 511
Marjolin's ulcer, 440
Marlex mesh, 238
Marsupialization, pilonidal cyst, 407
Mast cells, 119
Mastectomy, **465**
psychologic aspects, 218
radical, 466
simple, 465–66
McVay repair, **420**
Meatotomy, 585
Mecholyl, 291
Meckel's cave, 184
Meckel's diverticulum, 359–60,
359, 360, 391, 634
heterotopic pancreatic tissue, 346

Meconium ileus, 636
Mediastinitis, 541–42
Mediastinoscopy, 529
Mediastinotomy, 529
Mediastinum, 541–42
Medulloblastoma, 614
Meissner's corpuscles, 436
Melanocyte-stimulating hormone
    (MSH), 440
Melanoma, 440–43, **440**
  BCG, 443
  childhood, 640
  clinical findings, 441
  differential diagnosis, 441
  prognosis, 442
  subungual, **440**
  treatment, 442–43
Meleney's gangrene, **126**
Meleney's ulcer, 136
Meningioma, 612, 613, 624
Meningocele, 627
  neurogenic bladder, 577
Meniscus injuries, 516
Mental retardation, 205
Mepivacaine (Carbocaine), 224, **225**
Meprobamate, 187
Meralgia paresthetica, 188
6-Mercaptopurine, 112
Mesenteric adenitis, 639
Mesenteric embolism, 362
Mesenteric stenosis, 557
Mesonephric duct, 564
Mesothelioma, 533
Metabolic acidosis, 100
  cardiac arrest, 170, 256
  oligemic shock, 172
  renal compensation, 100
Metabolic alkalosis, 100, 101
  pyloric stenosis, 308
  renal compensation, 101
Metabolism, bile, 318, 319
  bone, 508, 509
  burns, 264
  calcium, 484, 485
  catabolic state, 17–19, **18**
  depleted patient, 27–29
  glucagon, **12**
  hepatic role, 30–33
  hyperanabolic fed state, 16–17,
    16
  hypercatabolic state, 19–23, **20**
    gastrointestinal tract, 21
    muscle mass, 21
    shock, 19
  insulin, **12**
  nervous system, **10**
  normal, 10–11, **16**
  stress catabolic state, **22**, 23–27
  temperature, 26–27
Metacarpals, fractures, 513–14
Metaphyseal fibrous defect, 522
Metastases, bone, 146, **146**, 153,
    194, 460, 461
  establishment, 145, 146
  liver, 323, 325, 333, 334
  lung, 540, 541
  "skip," 144, **145**
  supraclavicular, 144, 145, **145**
Metatarsal fractures, 516
Metatarsalgia, 520
Metatarsus varus, 510
Methadone, 187
Methemalbumin, 348

Methotrexate, 154, 155, 312, 471
Methoxyflurane (Penthrane), 227
Methylprednisolone, 56
Metyrapone test, 489
Micelles, 356
Michelle clips, 238
Microsurgery, 499
Microtia, 590
Mikulicz's disease, 274, 282
Miller-Abbott tube, 415
Milliequivalent, 93
Milwaukee brace, 512
Mithramycin, 312
Mitral insufficiency, acquired, 544
  pathophysiology, 61
Mitral stenosis, acquired, 544
  congenital, 543
Mittelschmerz, 391
Mixed lymphocyte culture test, 111
Mok's chemosurgical technique, 439
Monitoring, 218, 219, **219**, 265
Monoamine oxidase inhibitors, 231
Monobloc technique, 149
Mononuclear cells, inflammatory
    response, 127
Morphine, 187, 223
  sphincter of Oddi, 343
Morton's toe, 520
Mousseau-Barbin tube, 294
Mouth. See Oral cavity
Mouth-to-mouth respiration, 170,
    256
Mucocele, appendix, 393
Mucopolysaccharides, 119, 120
Mucosa, colitis, ulcerative, **375**, 376
  gallbladder, 315
  small intestine, 354, 355, 356
  stomach, 296, 297
Mucous cysts, oral, 276
Multiple myeloma, 524
Mumps, pancreatitis, 347
Muscle, healing, 121
  metabolism, 9, 12–13
  tumors, 444
Muscle fibers, structure, 509
Musculoskeletal disorders. See
    Bone; Joints; Muscle
Musculoskeletal system, 507–25
  congenital anomalies, 509–11
  development and structure,
    508–509
  growth disorders, 511–12
  history, 205
Myasthenia gravis, 433
Mycobacterium tuberculosis, **132**
Mycosis fungoides, 443
Mycotic infections, 535
Mydriasis, 601, 605
Myelography, 624
Myeloma, multiple, 524
Myelomeningoceles, 627
Myocardium (infarction), 546
  heart failure, 58–59, **59**
  postoperative, 255
Myoglobin, 264, 265
Myonecrosis, 138, 139
Myxedema, 479, 480
  pericarditis, 547

Narcotics, anesthesia, 223
Nasogastric tube, abdominal
    injuries, 174
Nasogastric tube feeding, head

  injury, 602
Nasopharynx, carcinoma, 280, 281
Navicular, **495**
  fractures, 514
Neck, 273–84
  adenitis, 273, 274
  branchial cyst, 590
  cystic hygroma, 444
  penetrating wounds, 275
  radical dissection, 279, **279**
  thyroglossal duct anomalies,
    590–91, **591**
  torticollis, 510–11
Necrotizing enterocolitis, 638
Needle biopsy, 147–48, **147**
Neisseria, **130**
Neomycin, 132
Neoplasms. *See also* Tumors;
    specific names of tumors
  biopsy, 147–48, **147**
  immunobiology, 113–16
  spread, 141–47
Neostigmine (Prostigmine), 228
Nephrectomy, 572, 582
  transplantation, 580–81
Nephrocalcinosis, 486
Nephrogenic cord, 564
Nephrotomography, 582
Nerve(s), abducent, 611
  brachial plexus, 235
  facial, 196, 282, **282**, 283
  fibers, 183
  glossopharyngeal, 196
  hand, 496, **497**
  injuries, 121, 130, **497**, 498, 499
  Latarjet, 297
  lateral popliteal, 235
  median, **503**
  mental, 277
  oculomotor, 601, 611, 619, 620
  radial, **235**, **497**
  repair, 121, **498**
  spinal, **621**
  splanchnic nerves, 186
  trigeminal, **184**, 185, 195, 196, 620
  ulnar, **497**, 503
  urinary bladder, 577
  vagus, 196, 342
Nervous system, anesthetic
    complications, 235
  brain tumors, 609–16
  cerebrovascular disease, 620, 621
  embryology, **626**
  intracranial infections, 625
  malformations, 625, 626
  pain, **189–91**, 195, 196, 610, 611
  spinal cord injuries, 606–609
  trauma, 274, 275, 602–606
Nervus intermedius, 196
Neurenteric canal, 626
Neurilemmomas, 444
Neurinoma, cranial nerves, 613
Neuroblastoma, 638
  catecholamines, 639
Neurofibroma, 444, 613, 624
Neurofibrosarcoma, 444
Neurogenic bladder, 576, 577
Neuroleptic syndrome, 187
Neurologic examination, 600–602
Neurologic surgery. *See* Brain;
    Nerve(s), Nervous system;
    Spinal cord
Neurologic system, history, 205

Neuroma, 188–89, 444
Neurosurgery, **189–91,** 599–628
Neutral phosphate solution, 571
Nipples, abnormalities, 446
  Paget's disease, **455**
Nissen fundoplication, **290**
Nitrogen mustard, 112, 154, 155
Nitrous oxide, 226
Nodule at umbilicus (Sister Saint
    Joseph node), 310
"No-man's land," hand, 498
Norepinephrine, 15, 19, 491
Nose, aesthetic rhinoplasty, 596
  fractures, 593, 594
5'-Nucleotidase, 323
Nutrition, anabolic events, 10, 11,
    12, 13
  catabolic events, 15, 16
  elemental diets, 205, 243, 244
  neonate, 632
  parenteral, 205
  postoperative, 243–45
  starvation, 17–19. *See also*
      Starvation
Nystagmus, 614
Nystatin, 132

Obesity, short circuit, 360
Obstruction, intestinal. *See* Intestine,
    obstruction
Ochsner treatment, 392
Oculocephalic reflex, 601
Oculovestibular reflex, 601
Oldfield syndrome, 395
Oligodendroglioma, 613
Oliguria, 574, 575
  ADH release, 566
Omphalocele, 634
Omphalomesenteric duct,
    persistence, 633, 634
Oncology. *See* Cancer, Carcinoma;
    Tumors; specific tumors
Oophorectomy in breast cancer, 469
Operating room, 233–41
  air, 234
  aseptic procedures, 234
  incisions, 235, 236, **235–36**
  nerve compression, 235
  personnel, 234
  skin preparation, 234
Operation, control of bleeding, **237**
  drains, 238
  hazards, 235
  prostheses, 238
  sutures, 236, 237, 238
  topical irrigation, 238
Optic chiasm, **615**
Oral cavity, 275–80
  benign lesions, **274,** 275–76
  carcinoma, 275–80, **279–80**
  cysts, 274
  examination, 277, **277**
Orchidectomy, carcinoma, breast,
    471
  testis, 584
Organ failure, intravenous fluids,
    35–36
  stress catabolic state, 23–27
  treatment, 35
Orthopedic deformities, acquired,
    524–25
  congenital, 509–11
Orthopedic surgery, 507–12

congenital anomalies, 509–11
neuromuscular disorders, 524
osteochondroses, 511–12
Osgood-Schlatter's disease, 511
Osler-Weber-Rendu syndrome, 363
Ossification, 508
Osteitis deformans. *See* Paget's
    disease
Osteitis fibrosa cystica, 486, 521
  hyperparathyroidism, 486, 521
Osteoarthritis, 518, 519
  hip, 519
  knee, 519
Osteoblastoma, 522
Osteoblasts, 508
Osteocartilaginous exostosis, 511,
    523
Osteochondritis dissecans, 511
Osteochondroses, 511–12
Osteoclasts, 508
Osteogenesis imperfecta, 511
Osteogenic sarcoma, 523
  chemotherapy, 154
Osteoid osteoma, 522
Osteomalacia, 520, 521
  gastrectomy, 304
Osteomyelitis, 517
  terminal phalanx, 502
Osteopetrosis, 511
Osteoporosis, 521
  pancreatitis, 344
Ostium primum defect, 542, 543
Ovarian cyst, torsion, 391
Oxygen, arterial, **48**
  hyperbaric, gas gangrene, 139
    during radiotherapy, 151
  measurements, 46–50, **47, 48,**
    66–67
  mixed venous, 49
  postoperative, 243
  ventilatory failure, 259

Pacemakers, 547–48
  cardiac tamponade, 548
Paget's disease, bone, 521
  extramammary, 406, 407
  nipples, 450, 453, **455**
Pain, 181–98
  abdominal, 196, 200
  activation of pain inhibitory
      mechanisms, 192
  acupuncture, 192, 193
  amputation stump, 197
  anal, **400**
  anatomy and physiology, 182–86
  biliary, 186, 196, 319, 320, **320**
  cardiac, 185, 196
  causalgia, 196, 197
  cephalic neuralgias, 195, 196
  diverticulitis, 382
  drugs, 186–88
  esophagus, 286, 289, 293
  facial neuralgia, 196
  gastrointestinal, 185
  gynecologic, 186
  hepatic, 319, 320, **320**
  hypnosis, 192
  liver, 319, 320, **320**
  local anesthetics, **124,** 188
  monoamine oxidase inhibitors,
      187
  narcotic analgesics, 187
  pancreatic, 185, 186, **343–44**

paraphysiologic treatments, 192
pathways, 183–85, **184**
  "C" fiber system, 185
  lateral spinothalamic tract,
      183, 184
  quintothalamic tract, 184, 185
peptic ulcer, 301
placebo effect, 192
postherpetic neuralgia, 197
postoperative, 243
psychoaffective drugs, 187
psychologic, 197
referred, 185, 186, **200**
renal, 186, 196
renal colic, **567**
sciatica, 623–24
surgical relief, 188–92, **189, 191**
  brain stem tractotomy, 191, **191**
  cortical and subcortical
      sections, 192
  peripheral nerve section,
      188–89
  posterior rhizotomy, 189, **189**
  spinothalamic tractotomy, 190,
      190
  thalamotomy, 192
tabes dorsalis, 197
theories, 182
trigeminal neuralgia, **184,** 185,
    195, 196
urinary tract, 567
visceral, 185, 186
Palate, carcinoma, 280, **280**
  congenital cleft, 589, 590, **590**
Palmar space infections, 502
Pancoast tumor, 539
Pancreas, 340–53
  anatomy, 340, 341, 342
  carcinoma, 349–51, **352**
    periampullary, 349, 350, 351
  chronic pancreatitis, **350**
  congenital anomalies, 346
  endocrine-secreting tumors,
      351–53
  enzymes, **341,** 342
  islet-cell tumors, 351
  pain, 342, **342, 344**
  periampullary carcinoma, 349,
      350, 351
  physiology, 342
  pseudocyst, 347, **349**
  radiology, 345, 346
  scanning, 346
  tests of function, 345
  trauma, 346, 347, **347**
  tumors, 349–53, **352**
  weight loss, 344, 345
  Zollinger-Ellison syndrome, 351
Pancreatectomy, **352**
  chronic pancreatitis, 349
Pancreaticoduodenectomy, 351
Pancreatitis, 347–49, **348–50**
  acute, 347–49
    clinical manifestations, 348
    etiology, 347, 348
  biliary disease, 330, **348**
  chronic, 349, **350**
  complications, **349**
  hyperparathyroidism, 345
  mumps, 347
  postoperative, 249, 250
  pregnancy, 216
  skin pigmentation, 344

sphincteroplasty, 344
Pancreozymin, 342
Paneth cells, 355
Papillary carcinoma, breast, 450
    thyroid, 483
Papilledema, 611
Papilloma, choroid plexus, 614
    duct of breast, 463, 464
Paracentesis, abdominal trauma, 178
    peritoneal metastases, 157
Paraesophageal hernia, 287, **288**
Parafollicular cells, 485
Paralysis, median nerve, **496, 497**
    radial nerve, **496, 497**
    ulnar nerve, **496, 497**
    urinary bladder, 609
Paralytic ileus, 250, **250**, 418, 419
    hypercatabolic state, 21
    spinal injury, 609
Paraneoplastic syndrome, 533
Paraosteal osteogenic sarcoma, 523
Paraphimosis, 580
Paraplegia, 577, 609
    bladder dysfunction, 577
    epidural abscess, 625
Parasympathetic nervous system,
    9–11, **10**
Parathormone, 484, 485–87, **486**
    effect of hypomagnesemia, 344
Parathyroid, 484–87
    anatomy, **475,** 484
    crisis, 486
    function, 484, **486**
    hypercalcemia, 485–87
    hyperparathyroidism, bone
        changes, **486,** 521
    hypocalcemia, 485
    hypoparathyroidism, 487
    tests, 474
Parathyroid adenoma, 485–87
    calcitonin, 487
    calcium metabolism, 485–87, 521
    embryology, 484
    hyperparathyroidism, 485–87
    kidney transplants, 485
    peptic ulcer, 300, 486
Parathyroid hormone, 484, 485–87
Parathyroidectomy, 487
Parenteral alimentation, 243–44
Parenteral solutions, 98, 99, 205
Parietal cells, 297
Paronychia, 502, **502**
Parotid gland, acute infection, 274,
    274
    hemangioma, 640, **640**
    mixed tumor, **282**
Paratidectomy, 282
Parotitis, postoperative, 249
Paroxysmal tachycardia, 492
Partial prothrombin time, 210
Partial thromboplastin time, 248
Patella, fractures, 516
Patent ductus arteriosus, 543
Paterson-Plummer-Vinson
    syndrome, 277, 292, 309
P_{CO_2}. *See* Carbon dioxide tension
Peau d'orange, 449
Pediatric surgery, 629–42
    abdominal masses, 638
    anomalies of rotation, 632, 633,
        633
    appendicitis, 392
    chronic abdominal pain, 639

esophageal atresia, **635**
gastroschisis, 634
hemangioma, **640**
Hirschsprung's disease, 637
imperforate anus, 637
intestinal atresia, 632
intussusception, 416, 637–38
malrotation of intestine, 632, 633,
    633
Meckel's diverticulum, 359–60,
    359, 391, 634
meconium ileus, 636
neonatal emergencies, 634–38,
    635
omphalocele, 634
omphalomesenteric duct
    persistence, 633, 634
processus vaginalis, 640, 641, **641**
pyloric stenosis, 636
rectal bleeding, 637–38
rectal prolapse, 405
rectosigmoid obstruction, 637
tracheoesophageal fistula, 635
volvulus, midgut, 632–33
Wilms' tumor, 581–82, 638, **639**
Pedicle grafts, 589, **589, 596**
PEEP (positive end-expiratory
    pressure ventilation), **82, 84,**
    86, 87, **89**
    burns, 265
Pelvic abscesses, 252
Pelvic inflammatory disease, vs.
    appendicitis, 391
Pelvis. *See also* Hip
    fractures, 515
D-Penicillamine, 571
Penicillin, 131, 138
Penicillium notatum, 125
Penis, 580
    balanitis, 580
    carcinoma, 584
    epispadias, 580
    hypospadias, 580, **592**
    paraphimosis, 580
    phimosis, 580
Penrose drain, 238
Pentagastrin, 301
Peptic ulcer, 300–304, **300**
    bleeding, **300,** 304–307, **303, 305**
    dumping syndrome, 304
    duodenal, 301, **303, 305**
    endoscopy, 305
    gastric, 301
    hemorrhage, 304–307, **305, 307**
    hyperparathyroidism, 300, 486
    indications for surgery, 301
    pain, 301
    perforation, 307–308, **308**
    pregnancy, 216
    pyloric stenosis, 308
    rationale for operation, 301, 302
    steroid therapy, 301
    treatment, 301–304
        operations, **302, 303, 307**
        postoperative complications,
            302, 303, 304
        vagotomy, **298, 303**
    Zollinger-Ellison syndrome, 301,
        351, 352
Percussion test, 559
Periampullary carcinoma, 349, 350,
    351
Perianal hematoma, 405, **406**

Periarteritis nodosa, 362
Pericardiotomy, 547
Pericarditis, 547
Perineal prostatectomy, 583
Peripheral arterial disease. *See*
    Arterial disease
Peripheral neuropathies, 205
Peritoneal hemodialysis, 575, 576
Peritoneal lavage, 178, 179, 346, 347
Peritonitis, appendiceal rupture,
    390, 392
    ileus, 418, 419
    primary, 391
Permeation, lymphatics, 143, **143**
Peutz-Jeghers syndrome, 363, 395
Peyronie's disease, 567
Pezzer, de, catheter, 576
pH, alkalosis and acidosis, 99–102
    gastric juice, 298, 299
    urinary calculi, 571
Phagocytin, 119
Phalangeal amputations, 499
Phalangeal fractures, 500, 513
Phantom limb, 197
Phenol, 188
    nerve paralysis, 557
Phenothiazines, 186, 187, 200
Phenoxybenzamine, 57
Phentolamine (Regitine), 231
Phenylalanine mustard, 443, 471
Pheochromocytoma, 492, 493
    carcinoma, thyroid, 484
Phimosis, 580
Phlebitis, 558, 559
Phlegmasia alba dolens, 559
Phlegmasia cerulea dolens, 559
Phosphatase, alkaline. *See* Alkaline
    phosphatase
Phosphorus, bone metabolism, 487
Physiologic monitoring. *See*
    Monitoring
Pigment, bile, 318, 319, 322
Pigmented lesions of skin, 437
Pilonidal cyst, 407
Pinealoma, 614
Pitressin (vasopressin),
    gastrointestinal hemorrhage,
    337
Pituitary, adenomas, 613
    anatomy, **475**
    function, **475, 476**
    removal. *See* Hypophysectomy
Pituitary-thyroid axis, **476**
Plasma, burns, 265
    expanders, 172
Plasminogen, 211
Plastic surgery, 586–98
    aesthetic, 596–98, **597**
    cleft lip and palate, 589, 590, **590**
    decubitus ulcer, 205, 602
    deltopectoral flap, **596**
    dermabrasion, 592
    ear, 590
    face, 592, **592–94, 597**
    flaps, 588–89, **589, 596**
    mammoplasty, 597, 598
    mandible, 279, 280, **593**
    nose, 596
    skin grafting, 586–88, **587**
Platelet aggregation, 200
Platelets, **207**
    burns, 263
Pleura, effusion, 532, **533**

Pleura [*cont.*]
  empyema, 532, 533
  hemothorax, 531–32
  pneumothorax, 530–32
  tumors, 533
  underwater seal drainage, 531
Plummer-Vinson syndrome. *See*
    Paterson-Plummer-Vinson
    syndrome
Pneumonectomy, 540
Pneumonia, aspiration, 230, 635
Pneumothorax, **176,** 530–32, **531**
  bullous emphysema, 536
  intravenous hyperalimentation,
    244
  neonate, 634
  treatment, 79–80, 170
Poliomyelitis, 524
Polycythemia, 542, 582
Polydactyly, 510
Polyglycolic acid, 237
Polymorphonuclear leukocytes, 127
Polymyxins, 132
Polyp(s), colorectal, 394–96, **395**
  gastric, **305,** 309, 311
  Peutz-Jeghers, 363
Polyvinylpyrrolidone (PVP) test, 358
Portal hypertension, 335–37
  classification, **332,** 335, 336
  complications, 336
  operations, 337
  treatment, 337, **338**
Portal triad, **317**
Portography, **335,** 336, **336**
Positive end-expiratory pressure
    ventilation (PEEP), 65, 532
Postherpetic neuralgia, 197
Postoperative complications. *See*
    Complications (postoperative)
Postprandial alkaline tide, 299
Potassium, aldosteronism, 490
  cardiac arrest, 255
  electrocardiographic changes, 97
  hyperkalemia, 97
  hypokalemia, 97
  hypokalemic alkalosis, 97, 98
  infancy, 631
  renal failure, 575
Pouch of Douglas, 252
Prausnitz-Kustner (PK) test, 110
Precipitated tetanus toxoid (PPTD),
    138
Prednisone. *See* Cortisone
Pregnancy, breasts, 445
  coagulation, 212
  ectopic, 391
  surgery, 216, 217, **217**
Preoperative assessment and care,
    199–221, 242
Primary idiopathic
    thrombocytopenia, 432
Proaccelerin, 320
Procaine (Novocaine), 225
Processus vaginalis, 420, 640, 641,
    641
Proctitis, amebic, 394
  ulcerative, 394
Proctoscopy, **401, 402**
Propanidid, 228
Propantheline, 343
Propoxyphene, 193
Propylthiouracil, 479
Prostate, 579, 580

benign hypertrophy, 579, 580
  carcinoma, 583–84
  examination, 568
  infections, 579
  operations, 580, 583
Prostatectomy, 580, 583
Prostatitis, 579
Prostatovesiculectomy, 583
Prostheses, 238
  arteries, 551
  blood vessels, 555
  breast, 597, 598
  hip, 519
  infection, 123
  prophylactic antibiotics, 132, 133
  Teflon, 127
Protamine sulfate, 212
Protein, burns, 263, 265
  catabolic states, 78
  deficiencies, 204
  synthesis, 13
Proteus mirabilis, 375, **569**
Prothrombin time, 210
Pruritus, jaundice, 322, 344
Pruritus ani, 403
Pseudomembranous enterocolitis,
    375
Pseudomonas aeruginosa, 128, 131,
    264, 534–35, 588
Psychiatric complications,
    postoperative, 253
  preoperative, 218
Psychologic preparation,
    preoperative, 218
Pulmonary artery, embolectomy,
    248
  stenosis, 543
Pulmonary edema, Swan Ganz
    catheter, **62**
Pulmonary embolism, 247, **247,** 248,
    248
  fat, 249
Pulmonary failure, 44, 73–79, **74,**
    75, 77, 78
  etiology, 65
  physiology, 72–76
  positive end expiratory pressure,
    65
  sepsis, 84–85
  stress catabolic state, 34
  trauma, **86**
  treatment, 34
Pulmonary function, normal, 66–67
  tests, 204, 529
Pulmonary insufficiency, 258, 259,
    532
Pulmonary thromboembolism, heart
    failure, 58
Puncture wounds, neck, 275
  tetanus, 137, 138
Pupils, head injury, 601, **601**
Purpura, Henoch's, 638
  idiopathic thrombocytopenic, 210
Pyelography, 568, **572**
Pyloric obstruction, carcinoma,
    stomach, 310
  peptic ulcer, 308
Pyloric stenosis, congenital, 636
Pyloroplasty, 301, 302, 307, 308
Pyridoxilidine glutamate, 325
Pyrogen, 128

Quintothalamic tract, 184, 185

Radial club hand, 509, 591
Radial nerve palsy, 497
Radial ulnar synostosis, 509
Radical mastectomy, **465,** 466
Radical neck dissection, **279**
Radiocarpal joint, ganglion, 502
Radioisotopes, bones, 460, 461
  brain, 615
  kidney, 569
  liver, 461
  Paget's disease of bone, 461
  parathyroid adenoma, 487
  scanning. *See* Scanning
  spleen, 430
  thyroid, 477
Radiology, pregnancy, 216
Radiotherapy, bladder, 583
  brain, 616
  breast, 467–69
  carcinogenesis, skin, 150, 440
    thyroid, 482
  with chemotherapy, 152
  colorectum, 385, 397, 398
  curative, 152
  effect on DNA, **150**
  endotherapy, 150
  enteritis, 369, 388
  esophagus, 293, 294
  fractionation, 152
  immunosuppression by, 152, 153,
    468, 469
  lip, 277
  mechanism of action, 151, 152
  melanoma, 443
  with operation, 152, 153
  oxidizing radicals, 150, 151
  oxygen effect, 150, **150,** 151, **151**
  palliative, 153
  postoperative, 152, 153, 467–69
  preoperative, 152, 467
    bronchogenic carcinoma, 152
    colon, 152
  principles of treatment, 149–53
  proctitis, 394
  radiation injury, 388, 394
  seminoma testis, 584
  teletherapy, 149–50
  thyroid, 484
  tissue transplantation, 112
Radius, absence, 509, 591
Ranula, 274, **274**
Rathke's pouch, 613
Rauwolfia derivatives, 200
Reconstructive surgery. *See* Plastic
    surgery
Recovery room, 232, 242
Rectal shelf, 147, 455
Rectocele. *See* Anorectal prolapse
Rectum, 394–98
  abdominoperineal resection, 378,
    379, 397, 398
  abscess, 402, 403
  anatomy, 394
  carcinoid, 396
  carcinoma, 396–98, **397, 398**
    chemotherapy, 398
  digital examination, **401**
  examination, 568, 580
  polyps. *See* Polyp(s), colorectal
  proctoscopy, 400, 401
  prolapse, 405–406, **407–408**
  trauma, **177,** 374–75
Red cells, 432

Red degeneration of fibroid, 216
Reed-Sternberg cells, 429
Reflux esophagitis, 288–91
  operations, 289, 290, 291
  stricture, 290, 291
Regitine, 57
Rehabilitation, amputation, 525
  hand trauma, 499
Reidel's thyroiditis, 481
Relaxants, 228
Renal disease. *See* Kidney
Renal failure, 44
Renal function, infancy, 631–32
Renin, hypertension, 556
Renography, 569
Respiration, acid-base disturbances,
    101, 102, 243
  head injury, 600, 601
  infancy, 630
  monitoring, 218, 219, 265
  weaning from ventilator, 259
Respiratory acidosis, 243
Respiratory alkalosis, 101, 102
Respiratory complications, 246, 258,
    259
Respiratory system, history, 204
Reticulum cell sarcoma. *See*
    Histiocytic sarcoma
Retrograde pancreatography, 346
Reverse transcriptase, 115
Rheumatoid arthritis, 517, 518
  hand, 504
Rhinoplasty, 596
Rhizotomy, posterior, 189
Rhytidectomy, 596–97, **597**
Rib(s), cervical, 558
  fractures, 176, 531, 532
Ribonuclease, 342
Richter's hernia, 418, 421
Rickets, 485, 520, 521
  renal osteodystrophy, 521
Right-to-left shunts, 543
Ringer's lactate solution, 172
  burns, 265
Risus sardonicus, 138
Roentgenography. *See also*
    individual sites and diseases
  abdominal trauma, 176. *See also*
    individual organs
  aneurysm, 557
  biliary tract, 324–25
  bone disorders. *See* individual
    disorders
  brain, 615
  breast, 458–60
  colon. *See* individual diseases
  esophagus, 286
  fractures. *See* Fractures
  heart disease, 542, 543
    coronary arteriography, 546
  hemorrhage, gastrointestinal, 306,
    388
  Hirschsprung's disease, 636
  hyperparathyroidism, 486
  intestinal obstruction, 414
  lung, 528
  mediastinum, 541
  pancreas, 345, 346
  paralytic ileus, 250, 251
  peptic ulcer, 301
  salivary glands, 274
  subphrenic abscess, 252
  tracheoesophageal fistula, 635

Roux-en-Y anastomosis,
    esophagojejunostomy, 311
  pancreatic disease, 349, 351
Ruffini endings, 436

Saint's triad, 380
Salicylates, 188
Salivary glands, 274, 281–83
  calculi, 274
  carcinoma, 281, 282
  Mikulicz's disease, 274
  mixed tumor, 281–83, **282**
  papillary cystadenoma
    lymphomatosum, 282
  tumors, 281–83
Salpingitis, 391
Saphenous varix, **559**
Saphenous vein(s), bypass
    operations, 546, **555**
  operation, 559–60
  percussion test, 559
Sarcoidosis, Kveim test, 110
Sarcoma. *See also* individual tissue
    and organs
  antibodies, 115
  Ewing's, 284, 523, 524
  lymphangiosarcoma, 429
  osteogenic, 523
  soft tissues, 443, 444
Scalenus anticus syndrome, 558
Scalp hemorrhage, 603
Scanning. *See also* Radioisotopes
  liver, **326, 327**
    amebic abscess, **327**
    cirrhosis, **328**
Scaphocephaly, 627
Scheuermann's disease, 512
Schilling test, 358
Schwannoma, 613
Sciatica. *See* Disk disease, lumbar
Sclerosing adenosis of breast, 461
Sclerosing hemangioma, 441, 442
Scoliosis, congenital, 510
  idiopathic, 512
Scopolamine (hyoscine), 223
Scrotum, differential diagnosis, 577,
    578, **578**, 579
  examination, 568, **568**
  hematocele, 579
  hydrocele, 578, **578**
  spermatocele, 579
  varicocele, **578**, 579
Sebaceous cyst, 437
Secretin, 342
Secretin-pancreozymin stimulation
    test, 345
Seldinger technique, 556
Seminoma, 584
Sengstaken-Blakemore tube, 305,
    337, **337**
Sepsis, stress catabolic state, 34
Septic arthritis, 517
Septic shock, 34
Septicemia, 137
Sequential analysis, 163
Serotonin antagonists, dumping
    syndrome, 304
Serum glutamine oxaloacetic
    transaminase (SGOT), 322
  myocardial infarction, 255
Serum hepatitis, blood transfusion,
    215
Seton for fistula in ano, 403

Shiner capsule, 358
Shock, acid-base balance, 45–46,
    99–100
  catabolic state, treatment, 33–37
  definitions, 50, 55, 56
  endotoxin, 126
  heart failure, 58–59, **59**
  hypercatabolic state, 19–23
  low cardiac output, **55**, 57–61
  lymphoreticular system, 28
  mechanisms, 55–56, **55**
  oligemic, 28, 43, 170–73
  septic, 28, 34, 126
    definition, 42
  stress catabolic state, 23–27
  venous return to heart, 52, 53
Sialadenitis, 274
Sialography, 274
Sigmoidoscopy, **401, 402**
Silon graft, 634
Silver nitrate, 266
Silver sulfadiazine (Silvadene), 266
Simple mastectomy, 465, 466
Sister Saint Joseph node, 310
Skeletal muscle, reflexes, 60, 602
Skeleton, development, 508, 509
Skin, 435–43
  anatomy, 261
  basal cell carcinoma, 439, **439**
  benign diseases, 437–38
  cancer, 438–43
  functions, 261, 262, 436
  grafts, **267, 587–89**
  keloid, 437
  pigmentation in pancreatitis, 344
  pigmented lesions, 437, 438,
    440–43
  squamous cell carcinoma, 439,
    439, 440
  structure, 435–36
  systemic diseases, 437
  warts, 438
Skin grafting, Bakamjian flap, 596,
    596
  burns, **262**, 266, 267, **267**
  distant flaps, 589, **589**
  full-thickness, 587, **587**
  genetic description, 587
  hand, 499
  local flaps, 588–89, **588, 589**
  pedicle, 280, 589
  split-thickness, 587
  take, 587–88
  Z-plasty, 588, 589, **589**, 592
Skin tumors. *See* individual tumors
Skull, fractures, 603–604
Sliding hernia, **417**, 421
Slipped femoral epiphysis, 512
Small intestine. *See* Intestine, small
Sodium, cation pump, 95
  hypernatremia, 97
  hyponatremia, 97
  parenteral administration, 98, 99
Sodium polystyrene sulfonate, 575
Space of Disse, 13
Spermatocele, 579
Spherocytosis, hereditary, 432
Spigelian hernia, **416**
Spina bifida, 510
Spinal anesthesia, 225
Spinal column, 621–25
  anatomy, 621, 622
  disk disease, 622–24

Spinal column [*cont.*]
  tumors, 624, **624**
  trauma, **175,** 606–609, **607**
Spinal cord, **621**
  anatomy, **622, 623**
  cordotomy, **189–91**
  injuries. *See* Trauma, spinal
    column
  tumors, **624**
Spinothalamic tractotomy, 190, 191,
  191
Spironolactone, 566
Spleen, 430–33
  anatomy, 430–31, **431**
  congenital hemolytic anemia, 432
  cysts and tumors, 432, 433
  effect of epinephrine, 431
  function, 431
  Hodgkin's disease, 430
  hypersplenism, 432
  organ transplantation, 112
  primary idiopathic
    thrombocytopenia, 432
  radioisotope scanning, 430
  secondary hypersplenism, 432
  trauma, 431, 432
Splenectomy, 433
  Hodgkin's disease, 430
Splenomegaly, portal hypertension,
  322
Splenorenal shunt, 337
Spondylosis, 235
Sprengel's shoulder, 509
Stab wounds, abdomen, 176–77,
  176, 362
  chest, 176, **176,** 530, 531
  neck, 175
Staging of tumors, bladder, 583
  breast, 450–53, **451**
  head and neck, 276
  lung, 539
Staphylococcal enterocolitis, 375
Staphylococcus aureus, **131, 136,
  234, 249**
  pyogenic arthritis, **517**
Starling's law, 53, 95
Starvation, 17–19, **18**
Steatorrhea, gastrectomy, 302, 303
  pancreatitis, 344, 345
Stercobilinogen, 319
Stomach, 296–314
  acute dilatation, 250
  anatomy, 296–98
  aspiration, 230, 635
  carcinoma, 309–12
    investigation, 310, 311
    pathology, 309, 310, **310**
    treatment, 311,**311,** 312
  injuries, 309
  leiomyosarcoma, 311
  lymphoma, 311
  Mallory-Weiss syndrome, 305,
    308–309, **309**
  peptic ulcer, 300–302, **306**
  physiology, 298–300, **299**
  pyloric stenosis, acquired, 308
    congenital, 636
  secretions, 298, 299, **299**
    magnesium, 98
Stomatitis, ulceromembranous, 126
Strangulation, hernias, 419, 423
  intestinal obstruction, 414, 415
  volvulus, 387

Streptococcal myositis, 139
Streptococcus faecalis, 389
Streptococcus hemolyticus, 126, 134
Streptomycin, 132
Stress ulcer, 264, 304
Stroke patients, rehabilitation, 524
Stryker frame, 595, 609
Stuart factor, 320
Student's *t*-test, 163
Subarachnoid hemorrhage, 616–20
Subcutaneous emphysema, 286
Subdural hematoma, 605
Subphrenic abscess, 252
Succinylcholine (Anectine), 228
Sulfasuxidine, 131, 402
Sulfisoxazole, 131
Sulfoglycoprotein, 115, 311
Sulfonamides, 131
Sulfur granules, 128
Supernumerary digits, 591
Suppuration, 128
Supraventricular arrhythmias, 254.
  See also Arrhythmias
Surface area, infancy, **630**
Surfactant, 527
Surveillance, immune, 108–109
Sutures, 236–38
Swan Ganz catheter, **62**
Sympathectomy, **189**
  lumbar, 557
  thoracic, 558
Sympathetic nervous system, 9–11,
  10
  metabolism, 6–7
Syndactyly, 510, 591, **591**
Syphilis, proctitis, 394
  testis, 579

Tabes dorsalis, 197
Tail of Spence, 446
Tamponade, cardiac, 545
  pacemakers, 548
  esophagogastric varices, 337
  etiology, 59–60, **60**
Taractan, 187
Temperature, infancy, 630
  regulation, 26
  stress catabolic state, 26, 27
  thermoneutral zone, 26
  wound infection, **129**
Tendon(s), hand, 494, 495
  repair, **498**
Tendonitis, 519, 520
Tennis elbow, 520
Tentorial compression, 611, 612
Teratocarcinoma, testis, 584
Teratoma, mediastinum, 541
  sacrococcygeal, 408
  testis, 584
Testes, carcinoma, 584
  embryology, **565**
  orchitis, 578
  torsion, 577, 578
  trauma, 578
  undescended, 565
Testosterone, 344, 488
  breast cancer, 469
  pruritus, 344
Tetanus, 137, 138
  immunization, 138
  prophylaxis, 130
  treatment, 139
Tetanus neonatorum, 138

Tetracyclines, 131
Tetralogy of Fallot, 543
Tevdek, 237
Thal repair, 290
Thermography, breast, 455, 458
Thiazides, 566
Thiopental (Pentothal), 227
Thio-TEPA, 153, 154, 471, 583
Thoracic duct, cancer spread by,
  143, 144, 145
Thoracic outlet syndrome, 558
Thoracotomy, 530
Thrombin time, 210
Thromboangiitis obliterans, 558
Thrombocytopenia, causes, 211
Thrombophlebitis, 558, 559
Thrombosis, 247, 248
  anticoagulation, 200, 248
  carotid arteries, 621
  cerebral, 621
  mesenteric, 362
  portal vein, 344
  veins, 247
  vertebral arteries, 621
Thymectomy, 434
Thymic-dependent lymphocytes
  (T-cells), 104, 427
Thymus, 433, 434
  anatomy, 433
  function, 433
  immunity, 104, 105
  myasthenia gravis, 433
  organ transplantation, 110
  tumors, 433
Thyrocalcitonin, 485
Thyroglossal cyst, 590–91, **591**
Thyroid, 474–84
  adenoma, 482
  anatomy, 475, **475**
  carcinoma, 482–84, **483**
  examination, **478, 480**
  exophthalmos, 475, 478
  function, 474, **476**
    tests, 476–77
  Graves' disease, 478, 479
  Hurthle cell tumor, 484
  hyperthyroidism, 478–79, **480**
  hypothyroidism, 479, 480
  nontoxic goiter, **480,** 481
  radioactive iodine, 484
  radiotherapy, 484
  scanning, 477
  solitary nodule, 481, 482
  T-4 and T-3, 476
Thyroid-stimulating hormone (TSH),
  476
Thyroidectomy, 475, 479, 481, **482,**
  483, 484
Thyroiditis, 480, 481
Thyrotoxicosis, 478, 479
Thyrotropin-releasing hormone
  (TRH), 476
Thyroxine, 476
L-Thyroxine (T-4), **476**
Tibia, fractures, 516
Tic douloureux. *See* Pain, trigeminal
  neuralgia
Tolbutamide, 351
Tongue, biopsy, 278, **278**
  carcinoma, **276,** 277, 278
  leukoplakia, **275**
Tonsil(s), 273, 280
Tonsillitis, 273

Topical anesthesia, 223
Torticollis, 510–11
Tourniquet, 499, 549
Toxic megacolon, 376–78
Trace elements, wound healing, 120, 121
Trachea, 533–34
  opening in. *See* Tracheostomy
  stricture, 533–34
Tracheoesophageal fistula, 635
Tracheostomy, 170, 247, 259
  burns, 265
  care, 87
  neck trauma, 275
  technique, 43, **169**
  tetanus, 138
Tract of Lissauer, 183
Tranquilizers, 200, 223
  peptic ulcer, 301
Transfusion, banked blood, 213–16
  citrate toxicity, 215
  complications, 214, 215
  frozen red cells, 215
  massive, 215, 216
  oligemic shock, 170–73
  typing and cross matching, 213, 214
Transplantation, bone, 113
  histocompatibility tests, 111
  kidney, 113, 580, 581
    donor selection, 581
    glomerulonephritis, 113
    technique, 581
  liver, 113, 338, 339
  mixed lymphocyte culture test, 111
  rejection, 112
  skin, 113
  terminology, 110–11
  thymectomy, 433, 434
Transurethral resection, 583
Tranylcypromine sulfate (Parnate), 231
Trauma, **169, 174**
  abdomen, 175, **176.** *See also*
    individual organs
  arterial, 549–51, **551–52**
  biliary tract, extrahepatic, 333
  bladder, 573
  central nervous system, 602–609
  chest, **176,** 530–32, **530, 531**
  colorectum, 374, 375
  diaphragm, 176, 178
  duodenum, 309
  eye, 175, 595
  face, 592–95, **592**
  genitals, 574
  hand, 496–501, 595
    anesthesia, 498
    rehabilitation, 499
  head, **175,** 274, 275, 602–606
  heart, 545–46
  kidney, 571–73
  liver, 333
  lung, 530–32
  mouth, 175
  neck, **175,** 274, 275
  pancreas, 346, 347
  pelvis, **177**
  small intestine, 362, 363
  spinal column, **175,** 606–609, **607**
    management, 608, 609
  spleen, 431, 432

stomach, 309
testes, 578
ureter, 573
urethra, 573, 574
urinary tract, 571–74
Traumatic wet lung, 532
Trench foot, 562
Trendelenburg position, 81, 235, **401**
Trendelenburg test, 559
Treponema pallidum, 402
Triage, 168
Trianterene, 566
Trichloroethylene (Trilene), 227
Tricuspid stenosis and insufficiency, 545
Tricuspid valve, 545
Trigeminal nerve, 184, **184,** 185
Trigeminal neuralgia, 185, 195
Trigger finger, 503, **503,** 520
Triiodothyronine (T-3), 476, **476**
Tubercle bacillus, 402
Tuberculosis, bone and joint, 517
  cervical, 428
  colon, 375
  constrictive pericarditis, 547
  empyema, 533
  epididymis, 579
  lung, 535, **535**
  Mantoux test, 110
Tumors. *See also* Cancer;
    Carcinoma; specific tumors
  antibodies, 195
  antigens, 115
  biopsy, 147–48
  larynx, **280, 281**
  lip, 277
  oral cavity, **279, 280**
  nodes metastases system (TNM), 276, 450–53, 539
Turcot syndrome, 395
Turricephaly, 627
Tylosis, 292

Ulcer(s), decubitus, 205, 253, 595
  Marjolin's, 440
  peptic. *See* Peptic ulcer
  stress, 264, 304
    hypercatabolic state, 21
  varicose ulcer, 559
  venous stasis, **136**
Ulcerative colitis. *See* Colitis, ulcerative
Ulcerogenic tumors of islets, 301, 351–52
Ulnar nerve, 495
Ultrasound, 569
  pancreatic cyst, 346
  thyroid, 482
Ultraviolet, air sterilization, 234
  carcinogenesis, 439, 440
Umbilical hernia, 640
Umbilicus, omphalocele and gastroschisis, 634
  omphalomesenteric duct persistence, 633, 634
Underwater seal drainage, **531**
Urachal cyst, 564
Urachus, 564
Uremia, 574–76
  pericarditis, 547
Ureter, calculi, 570
  carcinoma, 582

ectopic, 564
trauma, 573
Ureteroileostomy, cutaneous, 583
Urethra, 584–85
  carcinoma, 585
  meatal stenosis, 585
  stricture, 585
  trauma, **177,** 573, **573,** 574
  valves, 584–85
Urethrography, 574, 585
Urethroplasty, 585
Urethroscopy, 585
Uric acid, gout, 253, 521
Urinalysis, 568
Urinary bladder, calculi, 570
  carcinoma, 582–83
  diverticulum, 576
  exstrophy, 564
  infection, 252, 253
  neck obstruction, 574, 584
  neurogenic, 576, 577
  retention, 252
  trauma, 573, **573**
  tumors, 582, 583
Urinary retention, postoperative, 252
Urinary tract. *See also*
    Genitourinary tract; Kidney;
    Urinary bladder
  anomalies, 591–92
  calculi, 569–71
  catheters, 576
  diagnosis, 567–69
  embryology, 564–65
  infections, 576
    postoperative, 252–53
  pain, 567
  tumors, 581–84
  urinalysis, 568
Urine, acute retention, 580
  diversion, 583
  hyperparathyroidism, 486, 487
  osmolality, 574
  pH, 100
  renal failure, 574
Urobilinogen, 319
Urology, 563–85

Vagotomy, peptic ulcer, 297, 298, **298,** 301, 302, **303**
  reflux esophagitis, 290
Vagus nerve, 297, 298
  gastric secretion, 298, 299, **299**
Valium. *See* Diazepam
Valve replacement, 544, 545
Valves, heart. *See* individual valves
Valvulae conniventes, 354
Vancomycin, 131
Varices, esophageal. *See*
    Esophageal varices
Varicocele, 579
Varicose ulcer, 559
Varicose veins, 559, **559,** 560
  operation, **560**
Vascular disease. *See* Arteries;
    Cardiovascular system;
    Heart; Nervous system;
    Veins
Vasodilators. *See* individual agents
Veins, 558–61
  grafts, 546, 547
  ligation or division for pulmonary emboli, 248

Veins [*cont.*]
  percussion test, 559
  portal, **316**
  thrombophlebitis, 558, 559
  thrombosis, 265
  varicose, 559, **559,** 560
  varicose ulcer, 559
Vena cava, inferior, ligation, for
    pulmonary embolism, 248,
    248
Venous insufficiency, 248, 558, 559
Venous pressure, **51,** 52
  central, 61–64
Ventilators, 87–88
  weaning, 88–89, **89**
Ventilatory failure, 170
Ventricles of heart, aneurysms, 546
  arrhythmias, 44, 56, 254
  defibrillation, 256
  failure, **58, 62**
  outflow obstruction, 57–59, **57,
    63**
Ventricular septal defects, 543
Verruca plantaris, 438
Verruca vulgaris, 438
Vertebral venous system, 146
Villous adenoma, 395, **396**
Vincent's angina, 126
Vincristine, 154, 443, 582
Vineberg procedure, 546
VIP pneumonic, 43–44
Visceral pain, 185, 186
Visual pathways, **615**
Vitamin(s), deficiency in
    pancreatitis, 344
  intravenous requirements, 98

Vitamin A, wound healing, 120
Vitamin B$_{12}$, 358
Vitamin C, 99, 121
Vitamin D, 484
Vitamin K, 211, 212, 213, 323
Vitellointestinal duct, 633–34
Volkmann's contracture, 499
Volvulus, 416, 417
  cecal, 634
  colon, 387
  midgut, 632–33
  sigmoid colon, **412**
Vomiting, anesthesia, 230, **230**
  brain tumors, 611
  intestinal obstruction, 413
  Mallory-Weiss syndrome, 305,
    308, 309
  newborn, 635
  pyloric stenosis, 308, 310
von Gierke's disease, 320
von Recklinghausen's disease, bone,
    486, 521
  multiple neurofibromas, 444, 613,
    624
von Willebrand's disease, 210, 213

Waldeyer's ring, 273
Warren distal splenorenal shunt, 337
Warthin's tumor, 282
Water. *See also* Fluids and
    electrolytes
  ADH release, 96, 566
Water hammer pulse, 545
Water retention, burns, 263
Water's view, 593
Watery diarrhea, hypokalemia, and

    achlorhydria (WDHA)
      syndrome, 353
Weaning from ventilator, 259
Web-space infection, 502
Weed system, 203
Wegener's granulomatosis, 369
Weight, body, fluids, 95, 96, 97
Weil's pneumonic, 43–44
Whipple resection, 309
Whipple's triad, 351
Wilms' tumor, 581–82, 638, **639**
  chemotherapy, 154
Wounds. *See also* Trauma
  care, 122–23
  chest, 175, 176, 530, 532
  classification, 239
  closure, 238, 239
  collagen, 120
  debridement, 129–30, **129, 130**
  dehiscence, 251, 252
  drainage, 123, 238
  healing, 117–21, **118**
  skin grafts, 587–89
Wringer injury, 499
Wryneck, congenital, 510

Xenograft, 110
Xeroradiography, 460
X-rays. *See* Roentgenography
Xylocaine, 225
D-Xylose excretion test, 358

Zenker's diverticulum, 286, 290
Zollinger-Ellison syndrome, 30, 307,
    312, 351–52
Z-plasty, 588, 589, **589**